CUTANEOUS
PATHOLOGY

John C. Maize, M.D.
Professor and Chairman
Department of Dermatology
Professor
Department of Pathology and Laboratory Medicine
Medical University of South Carolina
Charleston, South Carolina

Walter H. C. Burgdorf, M.D.
Clinical Lecturer
Department of Dermatology
Ludwig Maximilian University
Munich, Germany

Mark A. Hurt, M.D.
Private Practice
Cutaneous Pathology
St. Louis, Missouri

Philip E. LeBoit, M.D.
Associate Professor
Departments of Clinical Pathology and Dermatology
University of California, San Francisco
School of Medicine
San Francisco, California

John S. Metcalf, M.D.
Professor
Department of Pathology and Laboratory Medicine
Director of Surgical Pathology
Medical University of South Carolina
Charleston, South Carolina

Tim Smith, M.D.
Professor
Department of Pathology and Laboratory Medicine
Director of Anatomical Pathology
Medical University of South Carolina
Charleston, South Carolina

Alvin R. Solomon, M.D.
Professor
Department of Dermatology
Director of Dermatopathology
Emory University School of Medicine
Atlanta, Georgia

CUTANEOUS
PATHOLOGY

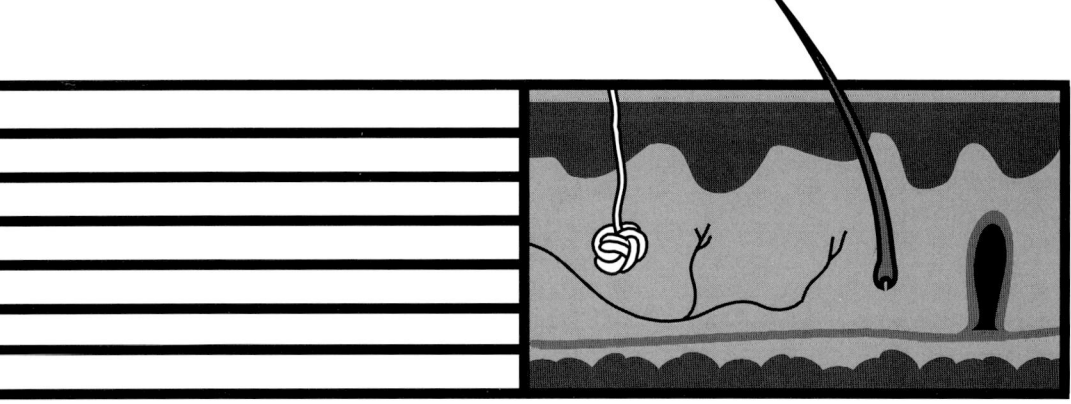

Churchill Livingstone

A Division of Harcourt Brace & Company

Philadelphia   London   Toronto   Montreal   Sydney   Tokyo

CHURCHILL LIVINGSTONE
A Division of Harcourt Brace & Company

The Curtis Center
Independence Square West
Philadelphia, Pennsylvania 19106

Library of Congress Cataloging-in-Publication Data

Cutaneous pathology / John C. Maize ... [et al.].

p.   cm.

Includes index.

ISBN 0–443–08717–2

1. Skin—Diseases.   2. Skin—Histopathology.   I. Maize, John C.
  [DNLM: 1. Skin Diseases.   WR 140 C9888 1998]

RL71.C945   1998   616.5—dc21
DNLM/DLC   98-16468

CUTANEOUS PATHOLOGY   ISBN 0–443–08717–2

Last digit is the print number: 9   8   7   6   5   4   3   2   1

PREFACE

The objective of this book is to provide students, residents, and practitioners of dermatology and pathology with a concise guide to the histopathologic differential diagnosis and definitive diagnosis of diseases of the skin. It is meant to be easy to use and pragmatic. We have aimed to provide the reader with a systematic method of approaching the histopathologic differential diagnosis of skin diseases by presenting either an algorithm or guidelines for differential diagnosis in each chapter. Because pathology is a visual specialty, considerable care has been given to including illustrations of the highest quality and teaching value. We owe a debt of gratitude to A. Bernard Ackerman for the concepts and techniques that he has pioneered in his many publications that have advanced the teaching of dermatopathology. These include the use of pattern recognition, decision trees, criterion-based diagnosis, and leader lines pointing out the important features of photomicrography. We have used these tools to enhance the usefulness of this text.

We have not had as a primary goal the development of an exhaustive reference work. In regard to the scope of the contents, we have drawn on our own experiences to present a broad spectrum of dermatopathology that includes the inflammatory and neoplastic diseases that make up the vast majority of day to day practice. We have provided what we think are readily available, useful, and relevant references. Encyclopedic textbooks of dermatopathology and abundant monographs are available to those who are interested in further study of specific subject areas.

The authors are indebted to several colleagues: Richard L. Dobson, M.D., for editing the manuscript; James Nicholson for the preparation of the photomicrographic images; Mark Wick, M.D., for contributing to the preparation of some of the manuscripts; and W. Ray Gammon, M.D., John R. Stanley, M.D., and Kim B. Yancey, M.D., for their review of Chapter 11. The authors are also indebted to the many colleagues who have submitted specimens to their laboratories in the last several years.

NOTICE

Dermatology is an ever-changing field. Standard safety precautions must be followed, but as new research and clinical experience broaden our knowledge, changes in treatment and drug therapy become necessary or appropriate. Readers are advised to check the product information currently provided by the manufacturer of each drug to be administered to verify the recommended dose, the method and duration of administration, and contraindications. It is the responsibility of the treating physician relying on experience and knowledge of the patient to determine dosages and the best treatment for the patient. Neither the Publisher nor the editor assumes any responsibility for any injury and/or damage to persons or property.

THE PUBLISHER

CONTENTS

1

THE NORMAL SKIN

The fact that, in most dermatological text-books, the microscopic anatomy is merely a sort of ornamental addition, is but too well justified; for when two skin diseases, clinically distinct, give, microscopically, the same appearances, or where the microscope shows differences where clinically none exist, it is clear that something wants elucidation.

Paul Gerson Unna[1]

THE DERMATOPATHOLOGIST'S APPROACH TO NORMAL SKIN

The accumulated data on the anatomy and physiology of the skin are enormous. Therefore, in a textbook of cutaneous pathology, it is practical and desirable to focus on cutaneous anatomy and physiology in relation to the context in which diseases of the skin are diagnosed histopathologically: light microscopy.

NORMAL SKIN

The skin is 1.8 m^2 and weighs approximately 4 to 5 kg in an average 70 kg man. The surface area of the skin is actually greater than the calculations of the gross dimensions because of two factors: the complex contours of its surface and the surface area of the adnexal epithelia (eccrine, apocrine, and folliculosebaceous) in direct continuum with the surface. Additional variables, such as percent surface area, whole skin thickness, volume, specific gravity, and weight, may be of value in certain contexts[2] (Table 1-1).

The principal vital functions of the skin include barrier protection (physical, chemical, and solar) thermoregulation, immunoregulation, and perception (touch, pressure, and pain) (Table 1-2).

Surface Anatomy

The topographic or surface anatomy of the skin varies considerably from body site to body site and in relation to patient age. On close inspection, the skin is a complex terrain of peaks and valleys. Detailed discussions of the surface anatomy are addressed in greater detail in research papers and textbooks of clinical dermatology.

Histologic Anatomy

The typical hematoxylin and eosin (H&E)-stained section after formalin fixation is oriented at a plane perpendicular to the skin surface. From this perspective, from external to internal, there are three principal divisions of the skin: the epithelial portion (including the epidermis, the folliculo-sebaceous-apocrine units, and the eccrine glands), the dermis, and the subcutis (Fig. 1-1). The epidermis (including the adnexa) and dermis are separated by a basement membrane. As a rule, there is a reduction, thinning, or loss of virtually all cutaneous elements with aging.[3] Regional variations are depicted graphically in Figure 1-2.

Cutaneous Epithelium

The epithelial portions of the skin include the *epidermis* and the *adnexal epithelium*, both of which are connected in an uninterrupted continuum. The adnexal epithelium includes the folliculo-sebaceous-apocrine units and the eccrine (sweat) glands.

Epidermis

The epidermis is the superficial layer of stratified cells covered by a thin layer of devitalized cells, the *stratum corneum*. The epidermis is thin at birth and increases to its maximal thickness at puberty. This is maintained until the fifth to sixth decades of life, when thinning begins.[4] The thickness range is between 0.027 and 1.4 mm, depending on site and age.[4]

By light microscopy, the epidermis is characterized by an undulating pattern of epithelial extensions into the papillary dermis (rete ridges) with corresponding epidermal thinning into which the papillary dermis extends, the *dermal papillae*[5] (Fig. 1-3). Although there is a wide variation in patterns from site to site, the "sine-wave" periodicity usually remains. Typical periodicity is

Table 1-1. Summary of Data on the Physical Dimensions of the Skin

Item	Quality	Remarks
Surface area		
Total	1.8 m^2 (20 ft^2)	Average adult of 170 cm and 70 kg
Regions	Head and neck, 9%	
	Each upper limb, 9%	
	Each lower limb, 18%	
	Anterior trunk, 18%	
	Posterior trunk, 18%	
	Perineum and genitals, 1%	
Thickness		
Whole skin	2 mm	Averages for most of the skin
Epidermis	0.12 mm	
Dermis	1.8 mm	
Subcutis	0.08 mm*	
Volume	3,600 mL (3.6 L or 3.7 qt)	Average adult
Specific gravity		
Glabrous skin	1.10	Probably not influenced by age, sex, or race
Nail	1.30	
Hair	1.31	
Weight		For an average adult, exclusive of the total weight of the extruded hair shafts, which would be a variable quantity
Entire skin	4 kg or 8.8 lb	
Epidermis	225 g or 0.5 lb	

(Adapted from Leider and Buncke,[2] with permission.)
* The zone where dermis and subcutaneous fat intermingle.

Table 1-2. Vital Skin Functions and Histologic Correlates

Function	Structure(s)
Barrier protection	Skin as a whole
Ultraviolet protection	Melanocytes
Infections	Keratinocytes
Fluid homeostasis	Keratinocytes
Protection from trauma	Epidermis and dermis
Thermoregulation	Blood vessels in superficial and deep dermal plexus
Immunoregulation	Langerhans cells
	Inflammatory cells of all types in reserve
Sense perception	Peripheral nerve trunks (pain, touch, temperature)
	Pacini-Vater corpuscles (pressure)
	Meissner's corpuscles (discriminant touch)
	Merkel cells(?)

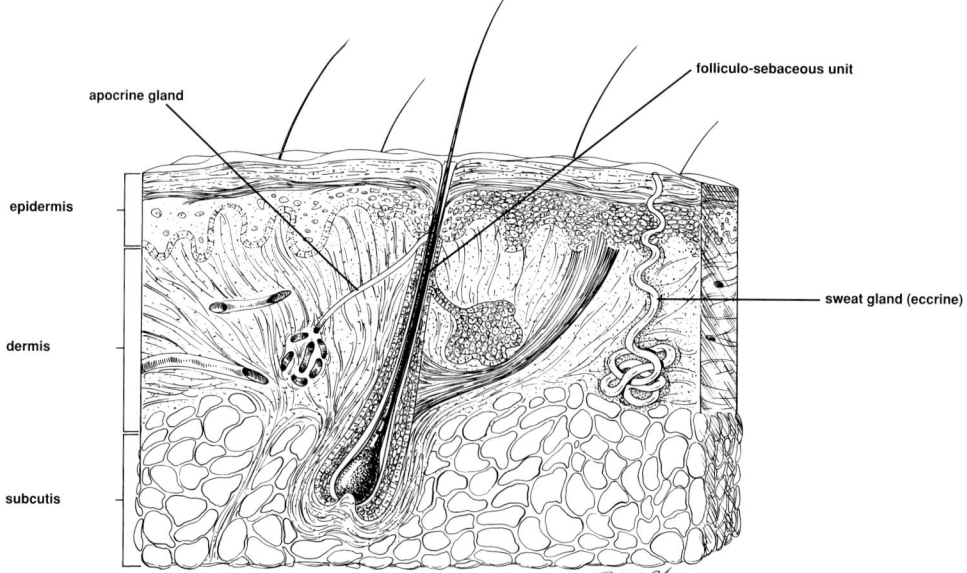

Figure 1-1. The three principle divisions of the skin are, from superficial to deep, the epidermis, dermis, and subcutis.

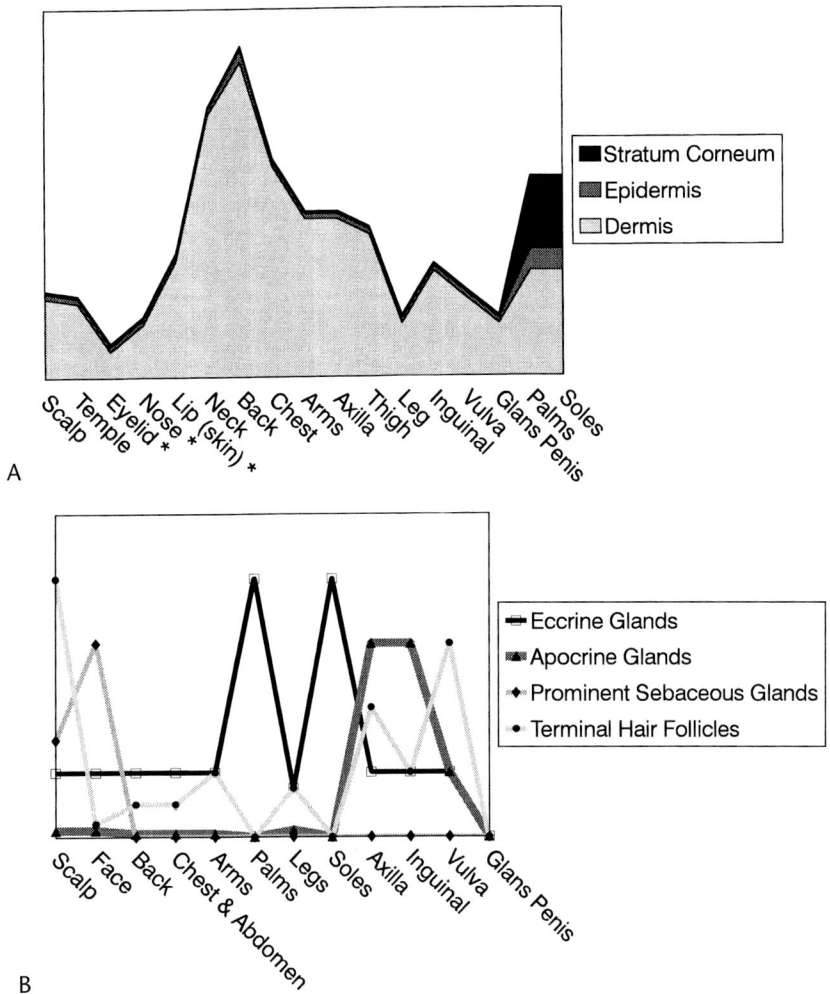

A

B

Figure 1-2. Regional histologic variation by (**A**) relative thickness and (**B**) distribution of the adnexa. *Not counting underlying skeletal muscle.

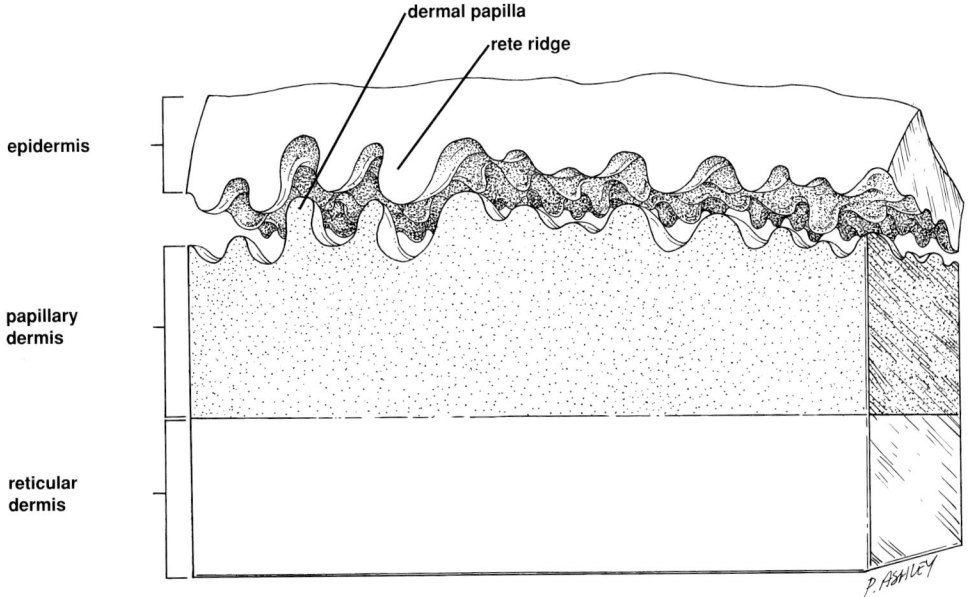

Figure 1-3. Relationship of the rete ridges to the dermal papillae. The epidermal rete ridges and dermal papillae have an inverse relationship. (Adapted from Ragaz and Ackerman,[5] with permission.)

Figure 1-4. (**A**) Diagram illustrating the three zones of vital epidermis plus the stratum corneum. (Adapted from Ackerman,[62] with permission). (**B**) Section of skin from a nonacral site containing three to eight layers of cells, a thin granular zone, and a prominent "basket weave" orthokeratotic pattern in the stratum corneum. (**C**) Section of acral skin illustrating the three zones of vital epidermis plus the stratum corneum. The stratum lucidum, seen here just above the granular layer, is not present in nonacral sites. Note also that the stratum corneum is at least three times as thick as the nonacral skin shown in B.

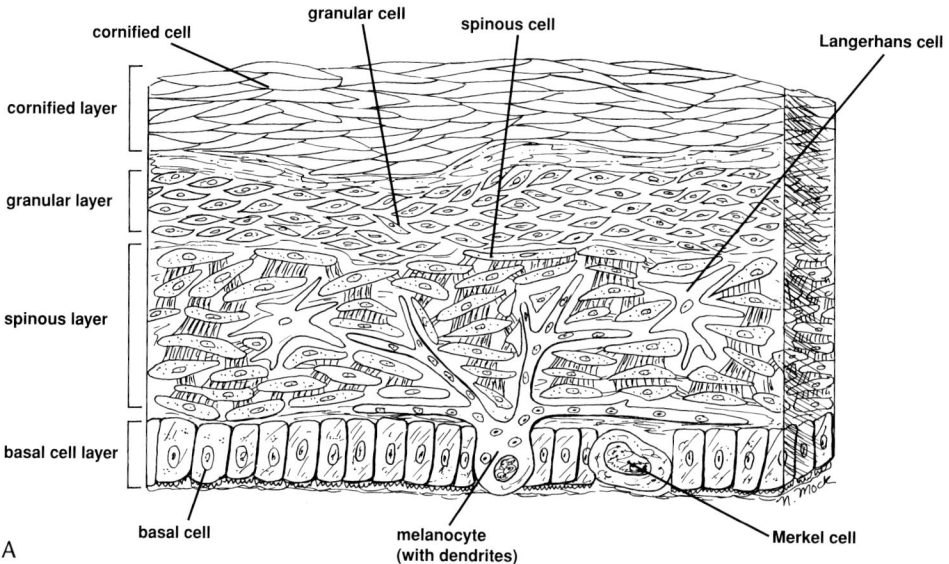

A

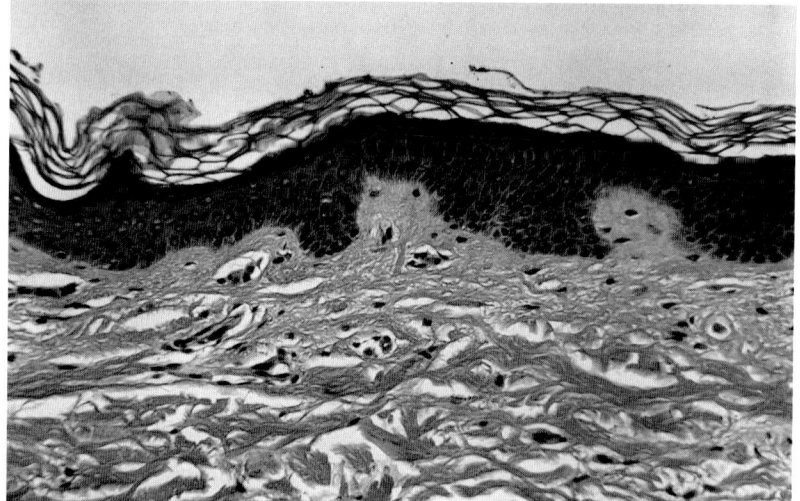

B

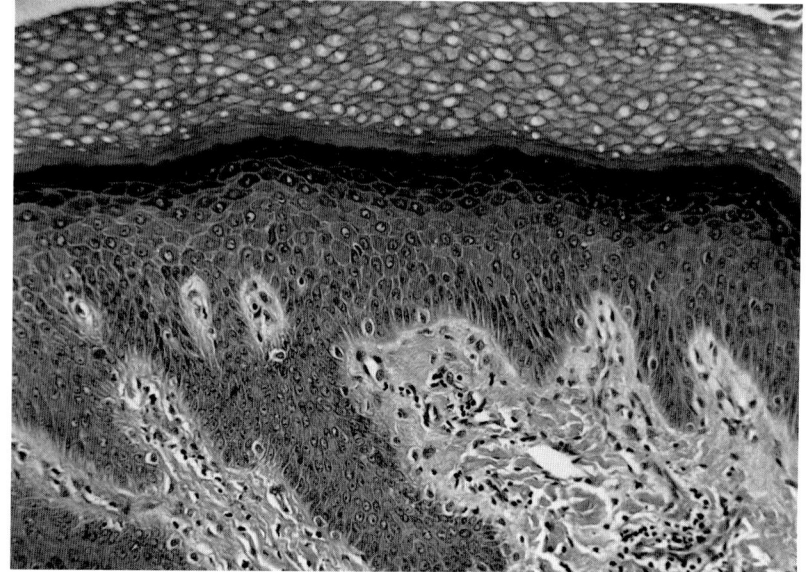

C

approximately 0.1 mm from rete ridge to rete ridge. The rete ridges are more pronounced on acral areas than proximal areas. In addition, they are more pronounced on dorsal skin than ventral skin. In facial regions, the rete ridges are diminished or absent.

There usually are three distinct zones in the vital portion of the epidermis, from superficial to deep: the granular layer, spinous (malpighian) layer, and basal layer (Fig. 1-4). These layers are composed primarily of *keratinocytes* in varying stages of maturation. Additionally, in the basal layer there exists a smaller population of cells with variable amounts of pigment and relative clearing of the cytoplasm—the *melanocytes*. Finally, classes of cells are present that are not readily identified by H&E stains. These are *Langerhans cells, Merkel cells, indeterminate cells*, and the *clear cells of Toker*.

Ultrastructurally, keratinocytes are interconnected by various types of junctions, principally desmosomes, but also macula adherens. The basal keratinocytes are anchored to the basement

Figure 1-5. Keratinocyte maturation proceeds from basal cell to granular cell and, ultimately, to a cornified cell. (From Freeman,[7] with permission.)

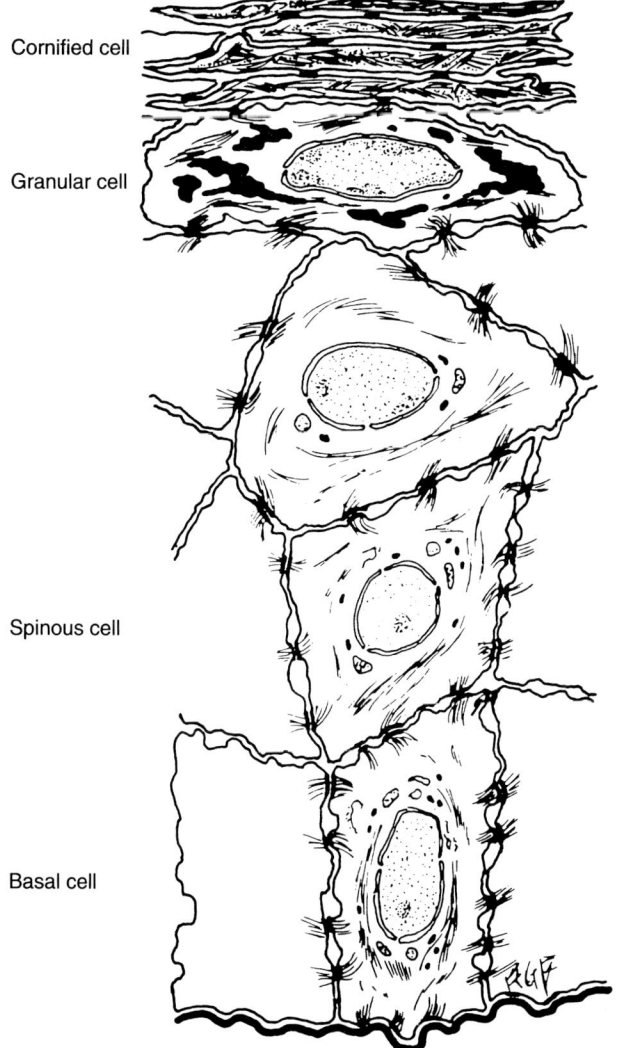

Cornified cell

Granular cell

Spinous cell

Basal cell

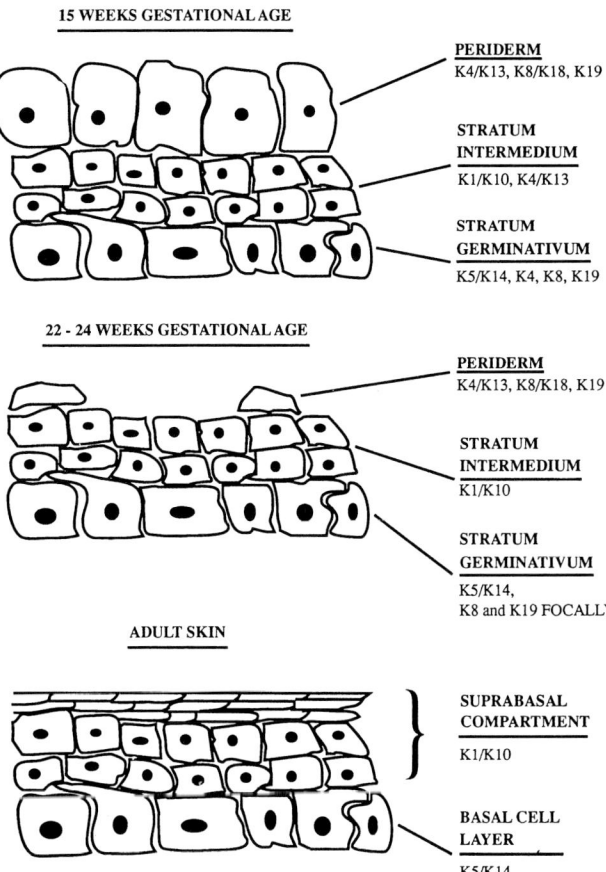

15 WEEKS GESTATIONAL AGE

PERIDERM
K4/K13, K8/K18, K19

STRATUM INTERMEDIUM
K1/K10, K4/K13

STRATUM GERMINATIVUM
K5/K14, K4, K8, K19

22 - 24 WEEKS GESTATIONAL AGE

PERIDERM
K4/K13, K8/K18, K19

STRATUM INTERMEDIUM
K1/K10

STRATUM GERMINATIVUM
K5/K14,
K8 and K19 FOCALLY

ADULT SKIN

SUPRABASAL COMPARTMENT
K1/K10

BASAL CELL LAYER
K5/K14

Figure 1-6. Keratin expression in fetal and adult skin. (From Smack et al,[8] with permission.)

membrane by hemidesmosomes. The keratinocytes, melanocytes, and Merkel cells are also connected by sparse numbers of junctions, principally of the macula adherens type. Langerhans cells contain no junctional components.

The epidermal keratinocytes move from basal cell layer to superficial layer in an organized fashion[6,7] (Fig. 1-5). The turnover of the viable epidermis, from basal cell to desquamation, requires approximately 1 month. The keratinocytes gradually differentiate as they ascend within the epidermis, producing a family of keratin proteins[8] as well as many organelles and cytokines (Fig. 1-6). As keratinocytes approach the surface, they accumulate numerous intracytoplasmic basophilic granules. In the stratum corneum, the anucleate squames are gradually shed.

Keratinocytes.   Most of the cells of the epidermis are keratinocytes. The basal or germinal cell is partially in contact with the basement membrane. This cell is the smallest of the keratinocytes and has the highest nuclear/cytoplasmic ratio. It is more basophilic than superficial squames and contains numerous cytoplasmic ribosomes, bundles of tonofilaments, and fewer cytoplasmic filaments.

The midlevel keratinocyte is characterized by numerous peripheral spiny processes (desmosomes) that join the keratinocytes to each other. The cytoplasm is amphophilic to eosinophilic, with a "glassy," hyalinized quality.

Ultrastructurally, the cytoplasm contains numerous intermediate filament proteins in addition to features typical of all cells undergoing synthetic functions. The periphery contains numerous desmosomes, some of which may occasionally be found within the cell cytoplasm. The nucleus is oval to round, usually with a prominent nucleolus. There may be one or more nucleoli; usually there is a diffuse chromatin pattern.

The granular keratinocyte[9] contains numerous cytoplasmic keratohyal in granules, ranging from less than 1 to approximately 2 μm in greatest dimension, that are histidine-rich precursors to filagrin, a protein that promotes keratin filament aggregation in the stratum corneum.[10] The nuclei are similar to the midlevel keratinocytes.

The stratum corneum is composed of stratified, anucleate squames. These typically have a periodic pattern by light microscopy, usually termed *basket weave orthokeratosis*. A variation that may be considered within the normal spectrum is *compact orthokeratosis*, characterized by a confluent layer of orthokeratotic squamous cells. By contrast, the term *parakeratosis* is applied to patterns of keratinization in which the keratinocytes of the stratum corneum retain their nuclei; this finding should be considered outside of the normal range. In palmar and plantar skin, a thin band of stratum corneum that stains poorly with H&E is termed the *stratum lucidum*.

Melanocytes. Melanocytes reside in the basal layer of the epidermis and are distributed regularly. With H&E stain, melanocytes are round to oval cells with a slightly higher nuclear/cytoplasmic ratio than the surrounding keratinocytes. As a rule, their cytoplasm is clear and contains finely granular melanin pigment. The nuclei are relatively uniform and contain one or two small nucleoli; occasionally, cytoplasmic "pockets" may be observed within the nuclei. These are termed *nuclear pseudoinclusions*.

Histochemically, there is a strongly positive reaction for argyrophil and argentaffin stains. These reveal numerous dendritic processes attracting the melanocytes to the adjacent keratinocytes to produce a melanocyte-keratinocyte unit[11] (Fig 1-7).

Immunohistochemically, some of the more useful markers for melanocytes are S-100 protein and HMB-45. The former is nonspecific but highly sensitive for melanocytes, while the latter is usually absent in normal melanocytes but is useful to detect hyperplasias and malignancies of melanocytes.

Ultrastructurally, melanocytes have abundant cytoplasm with sparse organelles, including melanosomes. The nuclei have relatively evenly dispersed chromatin and occasional nucleoli. Although melanocytes lack cell-to-cell connections to surrounding keratinocytes, they are attached to the basal lamina by anchoring filaments and structures similar to hemidesmosomes.[12]

Melanocytes produce two types of melanin, pheomelanin (red) and eumelanin (yellow, brown, or black), that serve an important ultraviolet light barrier function. The biochemical pathways of melanin production and transfer via dendritic processes to keratinocytes are complex. Detailed descriptions of melanin biosynthesis are available elsewhere.[11] The essential pathways are illustrated in Figure 1-7.

Skin color is also caused primarily by melanin. The differences in clinical hue are related not to the total number of melanocytes per unit area, which is relatively constant from race to race, but to the number and physical characteristics of the melanosomes within the keratinocytes.[13,14] As a rule, clinically dark skin is characterized by melanosomes that are more numerous and clumped centrally within the keratinocyte, especially the basal cells. By contrast, both the number and central clumping of melanosomes are less in lighter skin.

Figure 1-7. Epidermal-melanin unit and melanin synthesis. (From Jimbow et al,[11] with permission.)

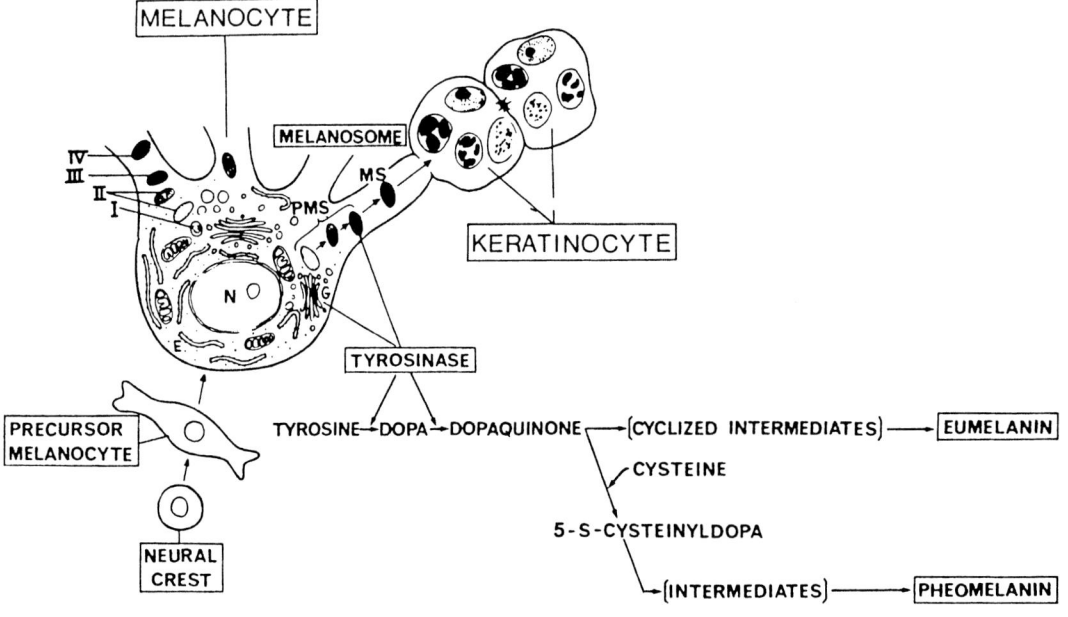

Langerhans Cells. Langerhans cells are dendritic, antigen-processing cells that originate from cells in the bone marrow.[15] They are not readily apparent in the spinous layer of the epidermis in H&E-stained sections. They account for less than 10% of the total cell population. S-100 protein staining highlights their complex dendritic processes and makes them easily observable.

Ultrastructurally, Langerhans cells contain organelles and phagolysosomes, similar to other types of macrophagic cells. The cytoplasm is abundant and contains small vesicles, multivesicular bodies, lysosomes. They lack filaments or cell-to-cell connections, such as desmosomes, but contain a diagnostic organelle, the Birbeck or Langerhans cell granule. This "granule" is a trilaminate rod-like structure terminating in a semicircular fashion likened to a tennis racket. It measures approximately 4 nm in width and 15 to 50 nm in length. The rod-like portion has been shown to be in contiguity with the cell membrane.[16] The nuclei are often multilobulated and may contain nucleoli.

Langerhans cells are thought to function in antigen presentation to T cells, immunosurveillance, allograft rejection, and delayed hypersensitivity.[17,18] They are the only cells in the epidermis known to contain receptors for Fc, IgG, and C3.[19] In addition, Langerhans cells also express T6 and Ia antigens.[20] A class of cells with all the structural properties of Langerhans cells except for Birbeck granules is termed *indeterminate*.

Merkel Cells. Merkel cells are nondendritic, neuroendocrine type I mechanoreceptors located in the basal zone of the epidermis. They are relatively sparse except in the face, particularly around the nose and mouth, digits, follicular outer root sheath,[21] and eccrine ducts.[22] These cells are relatively inapparent in H&E-stained sections and are not identified routinely.

Ultrastructurally, Merkel cells are characterized by abundant paranuclear cytoplasmic keratin filaments[23] and peripheral cytoplasmic collections of dense-cored granules ranging from 80 to 200 nm in diameter.[24] Desmosomes and desmosome-like junctions join them to keratinocytes.

Clear Cells (of Toker). The clear cells of the epidermis were first described in the nipple.[25] The function of these cells is, for the most part, unknown.

Adnexa

The cutaneous adnexa consists of epithelial structures in contiguity with the surface epithelium but, in addition, is characterized by specialized structures with specific functions not found in the surface epithelium. These include the *folliculo-sebaceous units* and *gland units* of apocrine and eccrine (sweat) secretion.

Folliculo-Sebaceous-Apocrine Unit. The folliculo-sebaceous unit consists of the hair follicle, the sebaceous gland, and their respective synthetic products: hair and sebum. The folliculo-sebaceous units are located throughout the body, with the exception of the glabrous skin of the palms, soles, glans penis, and portions of the vulva. It has been estimated that approximately 5 million units are present in adults, approximately 2% (100,000) of which are terminal hairs of the scalp.[26,27] In some cases, apocrine ducts join the infundibular portions of the folliculo-sebaceous unit, resulting in a *folliculo-sebaceous-apocrine unit*.

Hair Follicle. There are two morphologically recognizable types of human folliculo-sebaceous units: *vellus* and *terminal*. They are similar in structure but differ in size and function. In vellus folliculo-sebaceous units, the hair follicle and hair shaft is small, often extending no deeper than the level of the sebaceous gland. By contrast, terminal hair units typically extend into the subcutis while their corresponding sebaceous glands reside in the mid-dermis (Fig. 1-8).

The classic concept of the microanatomic structure of the hair follicle is as follows, from superficial to deep: the *infundibular* portion (connecting to the epidermis), the *isthmus* or middle segment (connecting to the sebaceous gland duct and acinus), and the *inferior* segment (including the hair stem with its specialized coverings, bulb, and follicular papilla). In a slightly different, *anatomic-physiologic* conceptualization of the hair follicle, it is divided into an upper and lower segment only. In this model, the infundibulum and isthmus are attributes of the upper segment (permanent), while the stem and bulb are attributes of the lower segment (transient)[28,29] (Fig. 1-9). The boundaries of the divisions of the hair follicle are listed in Table 1-3.[28,29]

The infundibular portion of the hair follicle joins the epidermis and is not appreciably different from the surface epithelium.

At the isthmus, the follicle narrows and joins with the openings to the sebaceous glands via the sebaceous ducts. The keratinization pattern in this zone, *tricholemmal* or *isthmus-catagen* keratinization,[30] is different from that of the surface and is especially noticeable in this region during the catagen phase of the follicular cycle, described below. The most striking difference in keratinization is that it is abrupt and compact, with the follicular keratinocytes lacking a granular zone. At the boundary of the isthmus and the stem is the *bulge* (der Wulst), which is actually a number of exophytic emissions that serve as the insertion point(s) of the arrector pili muscle (Fig. 1-10).

The inferior (transient) segment is composed of the hair follicle stem and bulb (Fig. 1-11). From inferior to superior, the *bulb* contains the follicular papilla, matrix, keratatogenous zone of the hair, and the follicular sheaths to the level of the A-fringe. The follicle continues as the *stem* to the level of the isthmus and consists of the follicular sheaths and the hair shaft.

The follicular papilla, or papillary mesenchymal body,[31] which is the mesenchymal contribution to the hair follicle, is composed of numerous semiparallel, fusiform cells that protrude into the sac of epithelial cells constituting the base of the hair bulb (Fig. 1-12).

The hair *matrix* is epithelial and is the source of the hair. It consists of basaloid cells that contact the dermal papilla and coalesce into an apex, ultimately differentiating through a keratogenous zone into the hair proper. The matrical cells have a characteristic growth pattern with three distinct zones. The zone adjacent to the follicular papilla below the critical line is composed of palisaded basaloid cells oriented perpendicular to the papillary-matrical junction. Variable numbers of melanocytes may be observed in this region, depending on race or if the hair has become depigmented with age (Fig. 1-12). Within a few cell layers there are numerous matrical cells in mitosis; they are relatively uniform, crowded, and overlapped and have a prominent vesicular nucleus with conspicuous nucleoli. This morphologic pattern of cells dominates as the supramatrical zone to approximately half its extent, terminating at the B-fringe, at which point the cell nuclei become fusiform and eventually slit-like in the

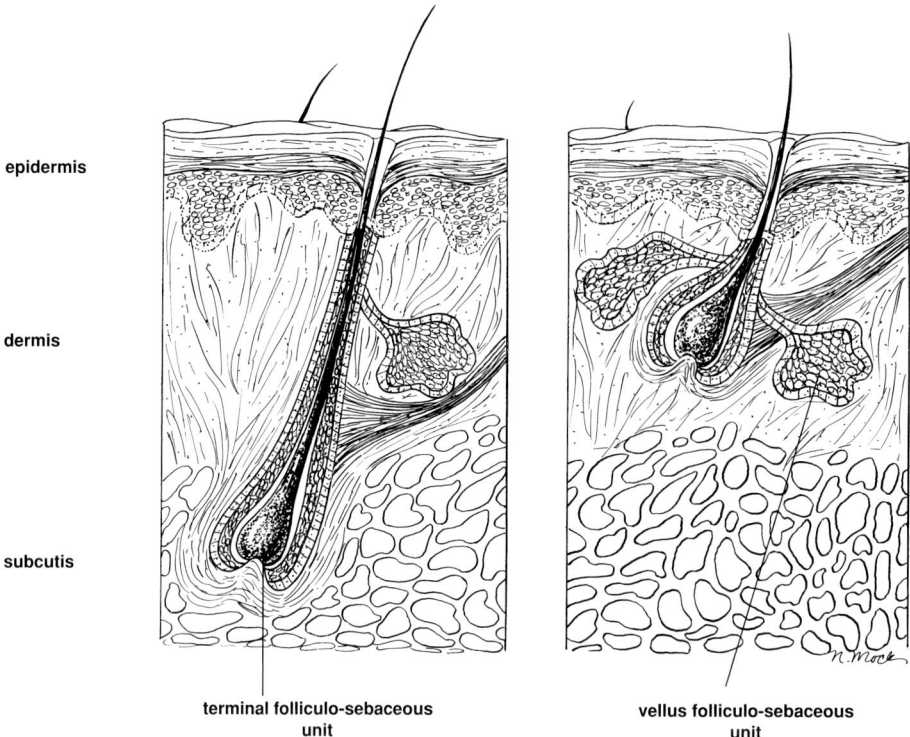

epidermis

dermis

subcutis

terminal folliculo-sebaceous
unit

vellus folliculo-sebaceous
unit

Figure 1-8. (**A & B**) Comparison of vellus and terminal folliculo-sebaceous units. Note that the vellus unit extends into the dermis only, while the terminal unit frequently extends its bulb into the subcutis.

Figure 1-9. Divisions of folliculo-sebaceous unit. (**A**) Classic (anatomic) division of the folliculo-sebaceous unit. (From Ackerman et al,[29] with permission.) (**B**) Anatomic-physiologic division of the folliculo-sebaceous unit. (Adapted from Jakubovic and Ackerman,[28] with permission.)

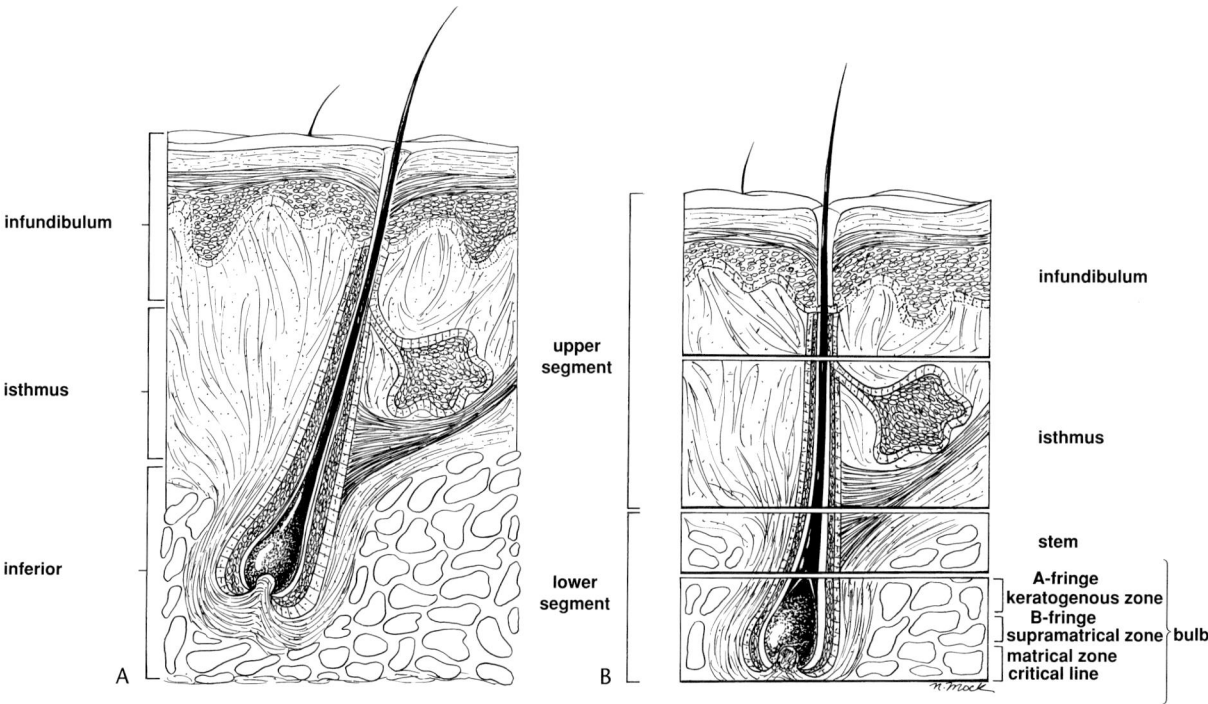

infundibulum

isthmus

inferior

upper
segment

lower
segment

infundibulum

isthmus

stem

A-fringe
keratogenous zone
B-fringe
supramatrical zone ⎫ bulb
matrical zone
critical line

Table 1-3. Hair Follicle Boundaries and Components

Segment	Division	Zone	Boundary	
Upper (permanent)	Infundibulum		Sebaceous duct	Ostium at surface
	Isthmus		Bulge	Sebaceous duct
Lower (transient)	Stem		A-fringe	Bulge
	Bulb		B-fringe	A-fringe
		Keratogenous	Critical line	B-fringe
		Supramatrical	Base	Critical line
		Matrical		

	Definitions of selected areas of the hair follicle
Critical line	The site where the diameter of the bulb and papilla are the greatest
B-fringe	Below Adamson's fringe: the upper part of the supramatrical zone at which trichohyalin granules from Henle's layer are lost
A-fringe	Adamson's fringe: the upper part of the keratogenous zone at which trichohyalin granules from Huxley's layer are lost

(Data from Jakubovic and Ackerman[28] and Ackerman et al.[29])

Figure 1-10. Follicular (arrector) muscle insertion into the follicular bulge, the boundary separating the isthmus (superficial) and stem (deep).

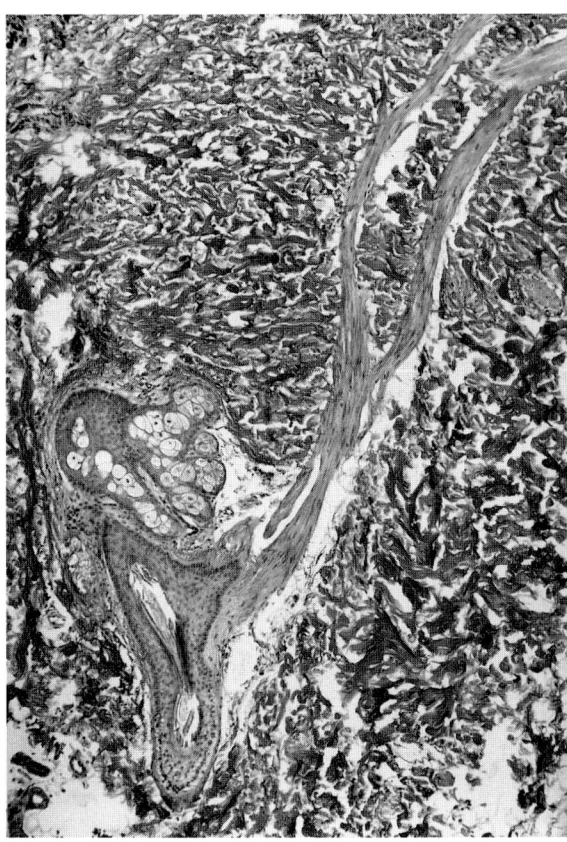

Figure 1-11. Lower (transient) segment, consisting of the stem (superficial) and bulb (deep) of an anagen hair follicle. The bulb and stem are bounded by the A-fringe, the point at which Huxley's layer loses its trichohyalin granules.

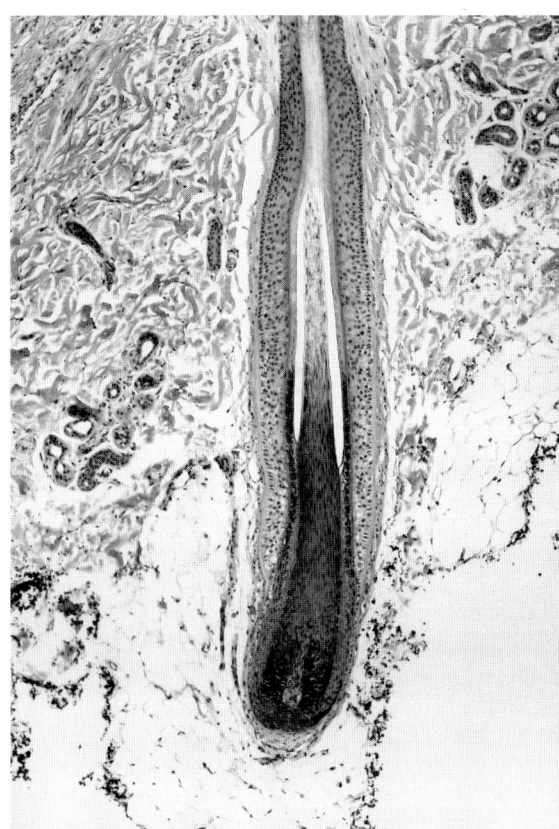

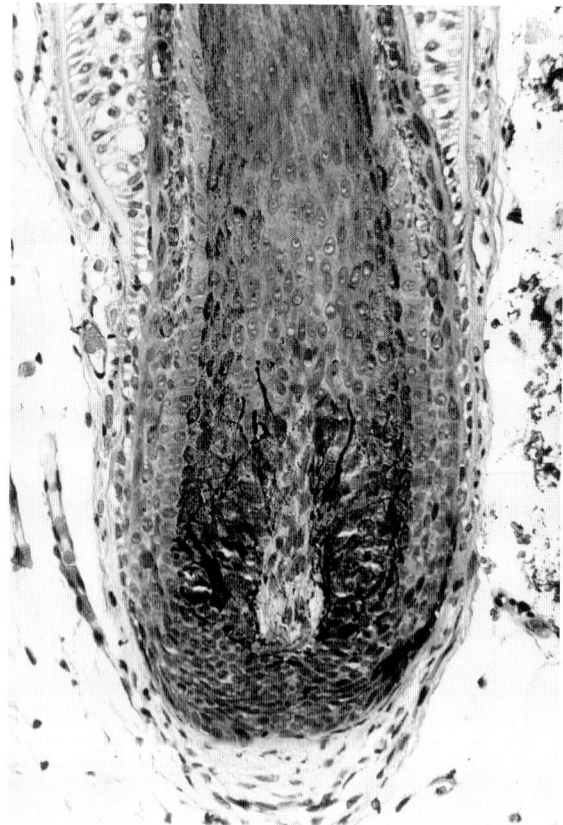

Figure 1-12. Bulb of an anagen hair follicle. At the base and in the center of the bulb is the follicular papilla, which is responsible for inducing the hair. At the base, surrounding the papilla, is the matrix. Note the prominent dendritic melanocytes located at the papillary-matrical interface. Above the critical line, the matrical cells differentiate into those that will become the cornified hair shaft.

keratogenous zone. Ultimately, the nuclei disappear as keratinization is completed, resulting in the hair proper. In the center of the matrix, a medulla is present that becomes the medulla of the hair proper.

In the bulb/stem of the lower segment, there are several specialized layers and membranes not observed elsewhere in the follicle or on the surface that culminate in the formation or housing of the hair proper. From outer to inner, these are as follows[29] (Fig. 1-13A):

1. The *perifollicular fibrous sheath* consists of a thin layer of fibrous tissue that surrounds the follicle at all layers and is analogous to the papillary dermis of the epidermis.

2. The *glassy* or *vitreous* layer corresponds to the basement membrane of the surface epidermis, with which it is contiguous.

3. The *outer root sheath* consists of one or more layers of glycogenated clear cells that begin as a single layer in the bulb, develops several layers near the B-fringe (below) of the follicle and terminates at the infundibulum.

4. The *inner root sheath* consists of three distinct layers, each of which emerges from the hair matrix, terminates in the isthmus, and keratinizes via keratohyalin granules. These layers are *Henle's layer*, *Huxley's layer*, and the *cuticle*.

   A. Henle's layer is the outermost layer, composed of one layer of cells that keratinize closest to the matrix. The point at which its keratinization ends has been termed the *B-fringe*[29] (Fig. 1-13B). The remainder of Henle's layer is an acellular membrane extending to the isthmus.

   B. Huxley's layer is the middle layer, composed of two rows of cells that begin to develop trichohyalin just below the B-fringe. The cells contain numerous large trichohyalin granules that extend well above the B-fringe. Keratinization is abrupt at the point at which the hair proper separates from the cuticle, also called the *A-fringe*[29,32] (Fig. 1-13C). The remainder of Huxley's layer is an acellular membrane extending to the isthmus.

   C. The *inner root sheath cuticle* is the innermost layer, adjacent to the cuticle of the hair proper, and consists of a single row of vertically oriented, flattened, clear cells. It is observed best at the periphery of the matrix in the hair bulb as Huxley's layer begins. Few keratohyalin granules are noted, observed best between the A- and B-fringes. Above the A-fringe, the cells are difficult to distinguish from Huxley's and Henle's layers as they terminate in the isthmus.

5. The *hair proper* consists of the terminal differentiation of the central portion of the matrix in the hair bulb. It is composed, from external to internal, of a *cuticle*, a *cortex*, and a *medulla*.

   A. The cuticle consists of a thin layer of cells that begins in the bulb and grows in a tapered fashion at the periphery of the cortex throughout the length of the hair. These interdigitate with the inner root sheath cortex until they separate at or around the A-fringe region (Fig. 1-13D).

   B. The cortex consists of most of the hair proper and of that portion of the hair that emerges from the matrix of the

Figure 1-13. (A) Layers of the follicular bulb and lower stem. (Adapted from Ackerman,[62] with permission.) (B) B-fringe region of the hair follicle is the point at which Henle's layer of the inner root sheath cornifies. (C) A-fringe region of the hair follicle is the point at which Huxley's layer of the inner root sheath cornifies and marks the boundary between the stem and bulb of the hair follicle. (D) Hair proper viewed at the level of the A-fringe (mid-photograph). The bulb region is inferior, and the stem region is superior. Note that most of the hair proper, at this level, is in transition from the keratogenous zone in the bulb to the cornified state in the stem and higher. Note also that the cuticle of the hair separates from the cuticle of the inner root sheath just below the A-fringe. The medulla cannot be seen in this figure.

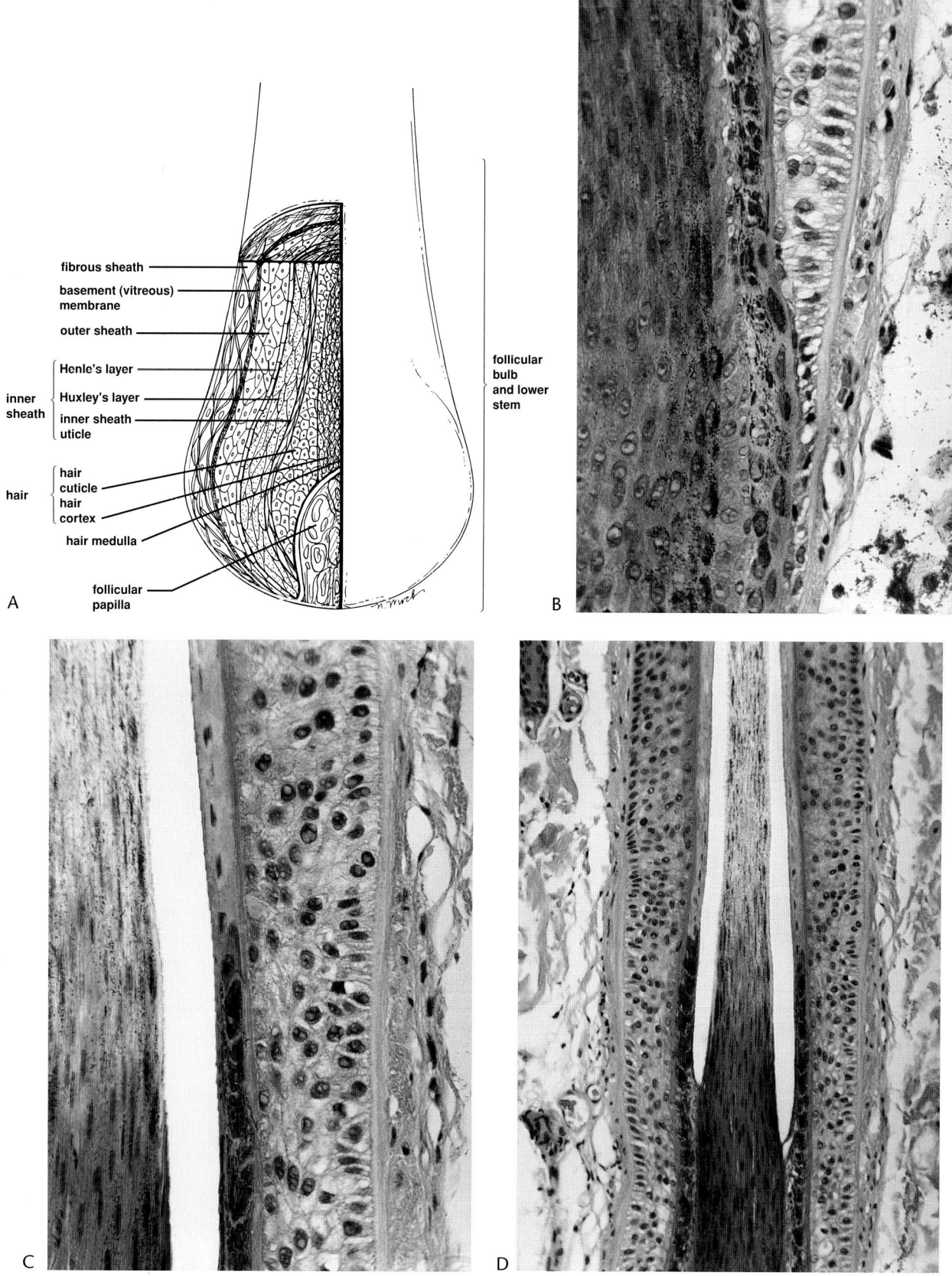

A

fibrous sheath

basement (vitreous) membrane

outer sheath

inner sheath {

Henle's layer

Huxley's layer

inner sheath uticle

hair {

hair cuticle

hair cortex

hair medulla

follicular papilla

follicular bulb and lower stem

B

C

D

hair bulb. At the A-fringe, the hair cornifies into an anucleate, keratinous shaft that eventually emerges from the follicular ostium.

C. The medulla consists of a central row or rows of cylindrical cells parallel to the long axis of the hair located in the central portion of the hair. It may be present in some terminal hairs, but is absent in vellus hairs.

Hair Follicle Cycle. Hairs cycle continuously in humans, in contrast to many other animal species. There is continuous shedding and continuous regeneration, resulting in the appearance of a stable hair population.[33] There are three phases that one may identify in the hair cycle: *anagen, catagen,* and *telogen*[34] (Fig. 1-14).

The anagen phase is the longest, consisting of the growth phase of the hair follicle. It lasts approximately 3 years or longer, and 90% of the hair follicle population at any given point in time is in this phase. The morphology of the anagen hair follicle is that of the typical, normal hair described above.

At the end of the anagen phase, the hair begins a process of involution, the catagen phase. This phase is the shortest, usually lasting only a few weeks. The earliest sign of catagen is apoptosis of the follicular keratinocytes. The matrix ceases proliferation, loses contact with the follicular papilla, and gradually recedes to the level of the bulge. The result is a "club" hair composed of the remaining papilla and fibrous track or root sheath as the epithelial stem of hair sheath involutes (Fig. 1-15). There is an abrupt transition from the epithelium to the hair, a pattern known as *isthmus-catagen keratinization* or *tricholemmal keratinization.*

Telogen, or the resting phase, lasts approximately 2 to 6 months. Morphologically, it is characterized by a follicle that terminates at the level of the bulge; it consists of a sac of outer root sheath epithelium surrounding the hair proper. The transition from the epithelium to the hair is that of a tricholemmal keratinization pattern. The fibrous root sheath extends deeply from the base of the follicle. The residual follicular papilla is inconspicuous.

As the new anagen phase begins, the root of the telogen hair develops a new germ that gradually grows along the fibrous root sheath, ultimately re-establishing itself for a new growth cycle. The old hair is usually shed during this process.

Figure 1-14. Follicular cycle. (**A**) Anagen. (**B**) Catagen. (**C**) Telogen. (**D**) Early anagen. (Adapted from Mehregan and Hashimoto,[34] with permission.)

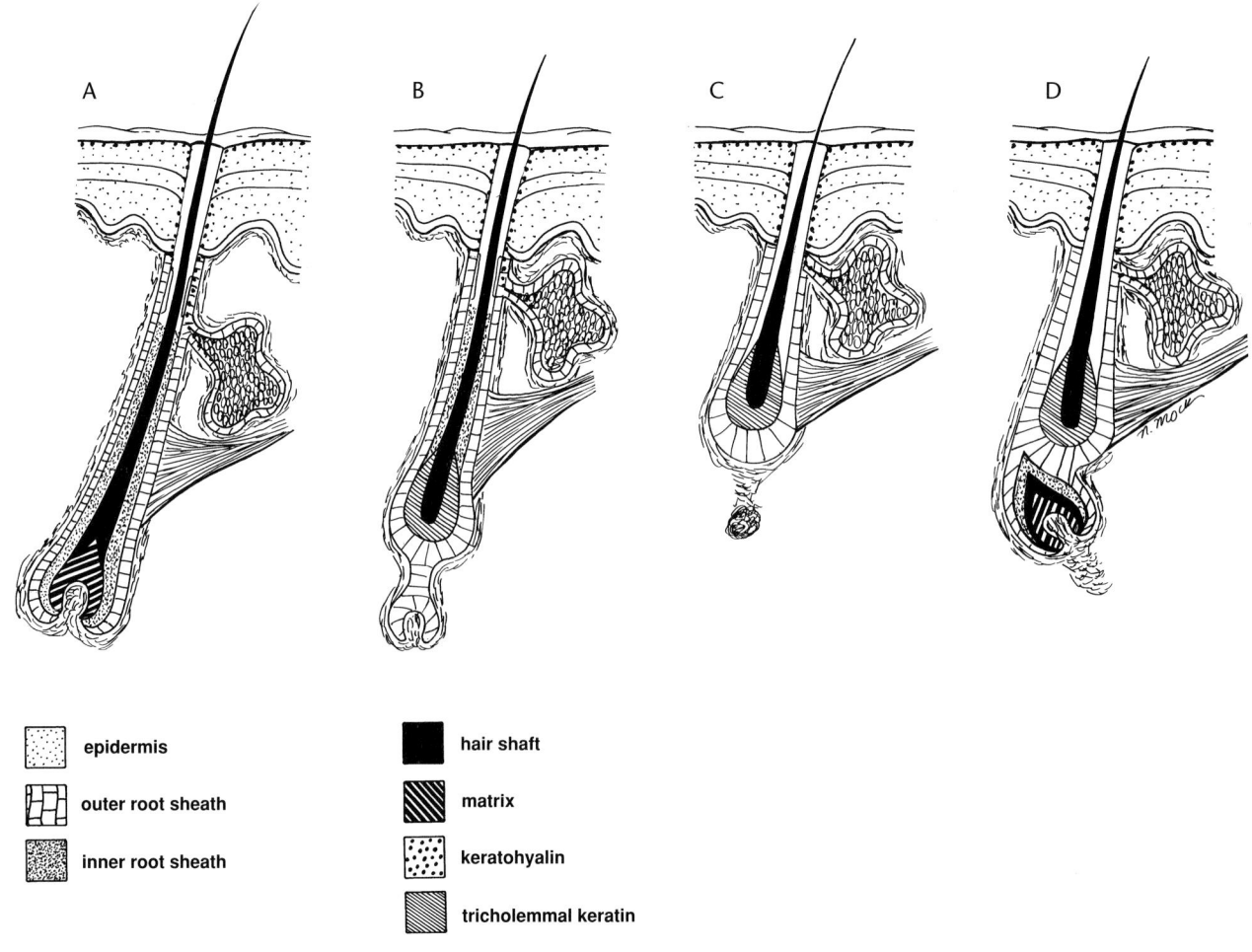

epidermis

outer root sheath

inner root sheath

hair shaft

matrix

keratohyalin

tricholemmal keratin

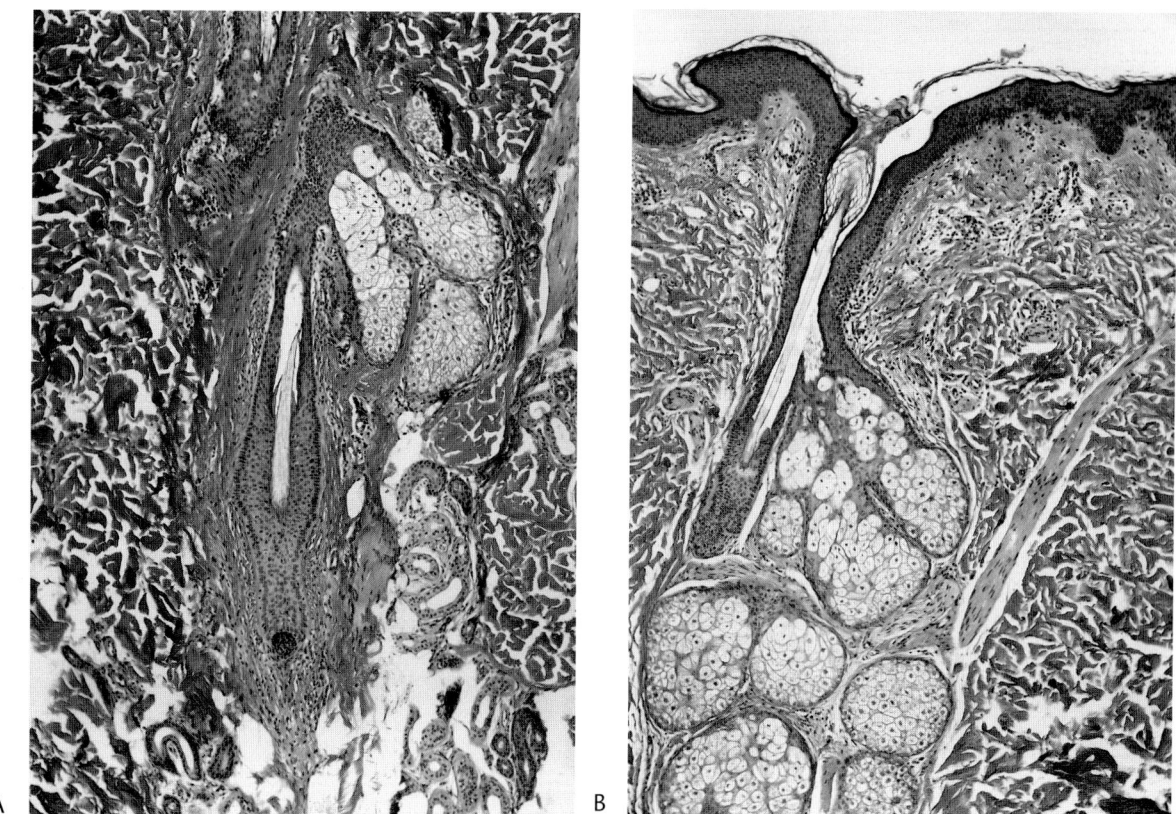

A   B

Figure 1-15. (**A**) Mid-catagen hair follicle with club hair. Note that the follicular papilla is small, no longer contained within the bulb claw, and is juxtaposed to the residual lower segment. The fibrous sheath is now a track that extends from the papilla and deep to the follicle. (**B**) Late catagen hair follicle with prominent sebaceous gland and arrector muscle. In late catagen, the follicular papilla is minuscule but still present. Note the club hair.

Figure 1-16. Diagram of a sebaceous gland attached to hair follicle compared with a free sebaceous unit opening to the surface.

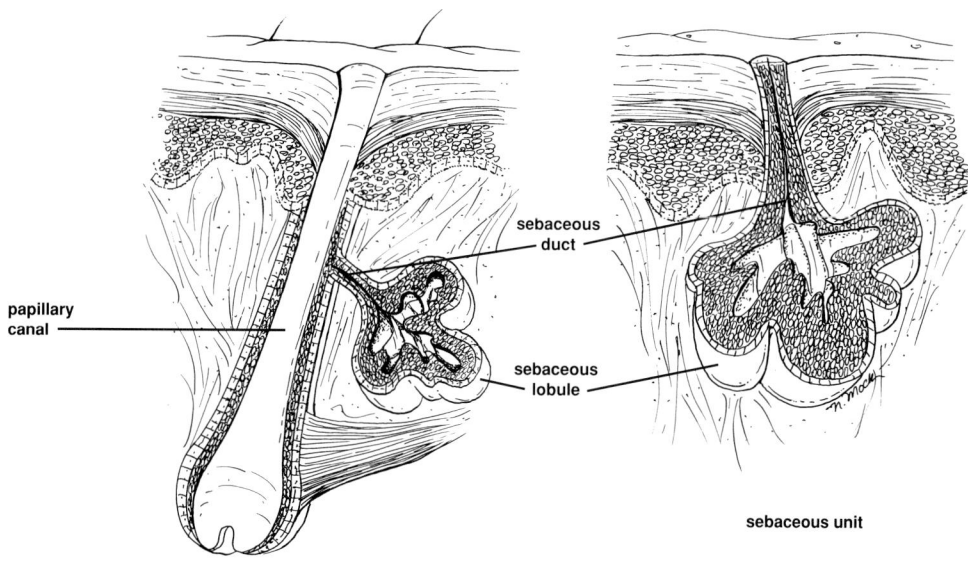

papillary
canal

sebaceous
duct

sebaceous
lobule

folliculo-sebaceous unit

sebaceous unit

The follicular papilla is thought to be necessary for the development of new hair. This theory has been challenged[35–37] by the hypothesis, from studies on mice, that the bulge is the cause of the hair cycle (the "bulge-activation hypothesis"). However, based on a comparison of the anatomy and physiology of the human hair with that of other species, the "germ as necessary for the follicular cycle" theory appears to be the true one, at least in humans, and perhaps in other mammals.[38–41]

Cutaneous Glands   *Sebaceous Glands.*   The sebaceous glands are holocrine glands that produce an oily substance, *sebum*. They are usually part of the hair follicle unit, the *folliculo-sebaceous unit*, but they can be self-contained units, especially in some locations, such as the lips. Their ducts arise at the level of the follicular isthmus, where they communicate directly with the pilary canal (Fig. 1-16).

Sebaceous glands are located throughout the body except on

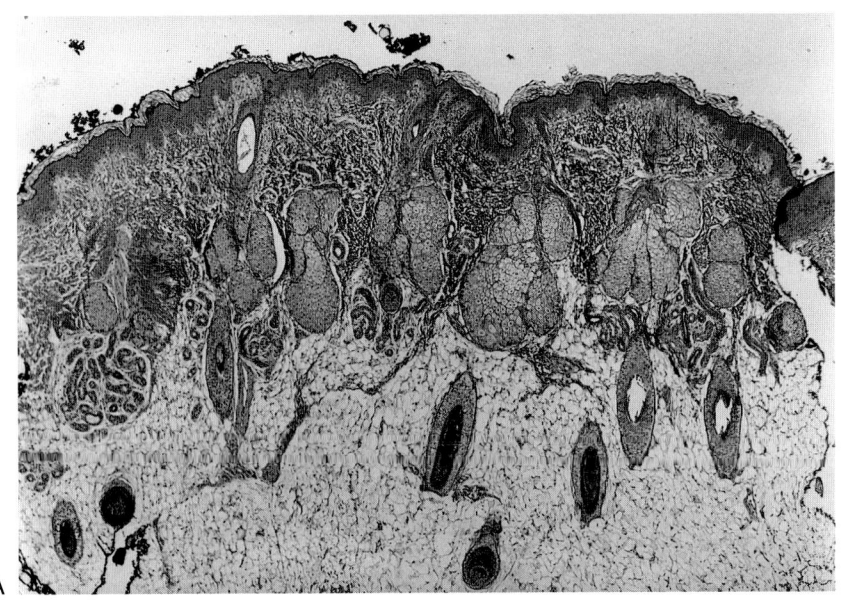

A

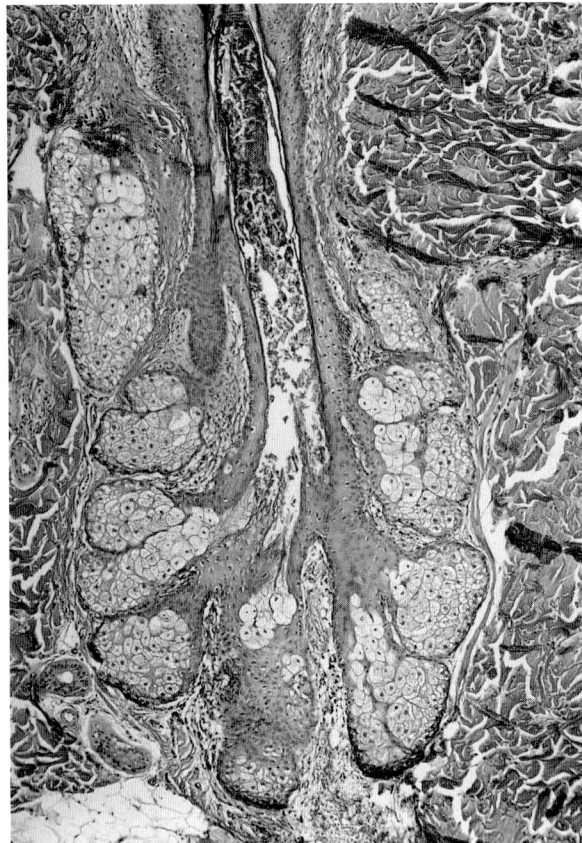

B

Figure 1-17.   (**A**) Sebaceous glands from the scalp of a newborn. Most of these glands are associated with anagen hair follicles. There are two to five lobules per gland seen in this two-dimensional plane. (**B**) Sebaceous gland of an adult. This gland has five lobules that all connect to the sebaceous duct where the sebum is eliminated.

the palms, soles, digits, dorsal feet, and portions of the genitalia. They are concentrated most heavily on the face and neck, where the sebaceous lobules are large and often associated with vellus hair follicles. These are often referred to as *sebaceous follicles*. In addition, sebaceous glands free of hair follicles are observed often on the oral mucosa (Fordyce spots), the nipple (Montgomery's tubercles)[42,43], the labia minora, the penis (glands of Tyson),[44] and the tarsal plate of the eyelids (meibomian glands).

The sebaceous gland secretory portion consists mainly of multiple lobules, or acini, that contain sebocytes in various stages of development. These are most notable on the face and least on areas such as the back. There may be one to many lobules in a sebaceous gland unit (Fig. 1-17), but most have only a few.[45] The acini connect via separate ductal systems to the pilary canal at the follicular isthmus. Free sebaceous glands connect directly to the surface via a similar ductal system (Fig. 1-18).

The *mantle* emerges as an appendage from the lower portion of the follicular infundibulum and surrounds it like a cloak or skirt.[46–48] It is especially noticeable in vellus hairs of the face (Fig. 1-19). The mantle cells also contain foci of sebaceous differentiation. It probably represents an involutional phase or resting phase of the sebaceous lobule.

In the mature sebaceous gland acinus (Fig. 1-20), the germinative layer, within one to two cells, begins to acquire visible lipid droplets. Toward the ductal portion of the lobule, the sebocytes are filled with small circular (spherical) lipid droplets and contain a central nucleus with one or more conspicuous nucleoli. The nucleus is characteristically indented over its entire surface by small convexities of lipid droplets, a feature that is often helpful in identifying sebaceous differentiation in tumors that are composed of mostly basaloid cells.

The sebocytes contain cytoplasmic periodic acid-Schiff (PAS)-positive glycogen granules in the germinative layers. The granules diminish as the cells mature. A rich, anastomotic network of nerve fibers, venules, and capillaries surrounds the sebaceous units.

Apocrine Glands, Eccrine (Sweat) Glands, and Other Glands. The apocrine and eccrine glands, other than sebaceous glands, are the classic glands of the skin and are characterized by tubular secretory units located in the dermis and/or subcutis. They eliminate their product via a duct that terminates in the stratum corneum (eccrine or apocrine) or follicular infundibulum (apocrine) (Fig. 1-21).

Morphologically, with the exception of growth pattern, there are no significant differences between the ducts of eccrine and apocrine glands. The principal differences are identified in the secretory portions.

The apocrine gland produces its product by an exudative process of "pinching off" portions of its acinar cells into the tubular lumen, often termed *decapitation secretion*. The eccrine gland produces its product principally by merocrine or transudative secretion. A third type of gland, which is composed of a mixture of the two other types, is termed *apoeccrine*.[49] Recently, a fourth type of gland, termed the *anogenital gland*,[50] was described. It shares features with mammary glands. A summary[50] of these glands is presented in Table 1-4. Mammary glands, although apocrine in their secretory pattern, are not discussed here.

Eccrine glands are located in highest density in the palms and soles; however, they are virtually ubiquitous, with the noted exception of the nail beds, lips, labia minora, glans penis, and inner prepuce. They total approximately 2 to 4 million units.[51,52] Apocrine glands are observed in greater numbers in the axillae, anogenital areas, eyelids, external ear, and (occasionally) the areola. The apoeccrine glands are concentrated in adult axillary areas.[49]

In the dermis, the eccrine secretory unit, the *coil*, is located in the deep reticular dermis and is invested within a small lobule of adipose tissue, the *adnexal fat pad*, which in most cases is contiguous with the subcutis (Fig. 1-22). The sweat gland (eccrine) coil is characterized by closely apposed tubular acini composed of *light* (clear) and *dark* cells. These are associated with a myoepithelial cell layer that abuts the basement membrane. The apocrine coil is arranged similarly, but the cells are uniform and lack features of light and dark cells. In addition, the apocrine coils are located within the superficial subcutis. The apoeccrine coils have mixtures of both types—apocrine and eccrine.

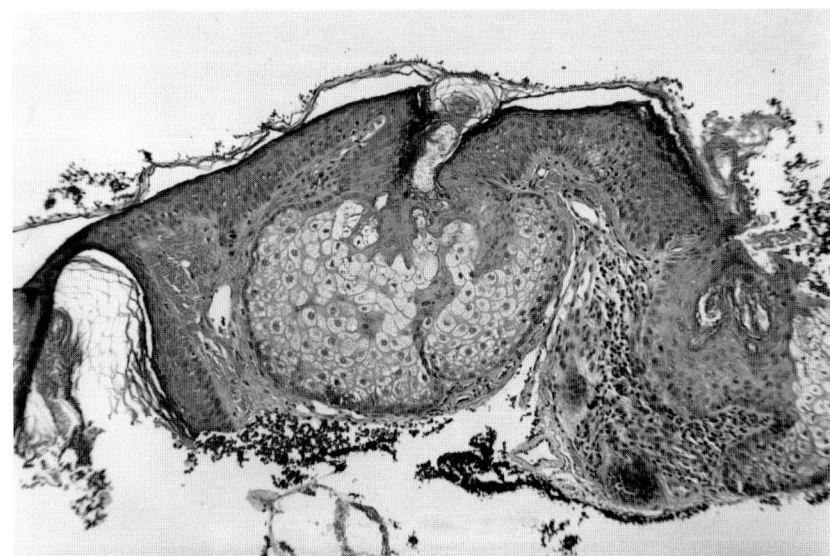

Figure 1-18. Free sebaceous lobule. Note that the lobule opens directly to the surface; it is not connected to a hair follicle.

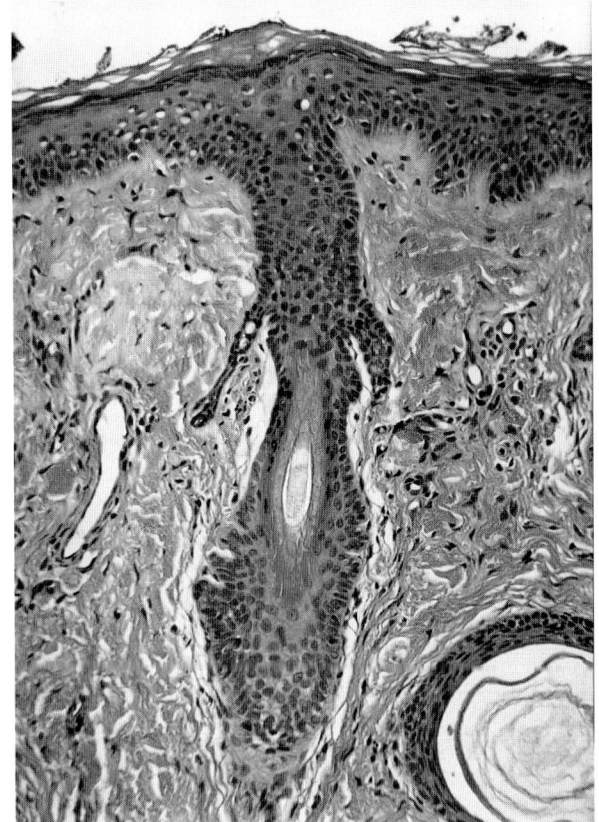

A

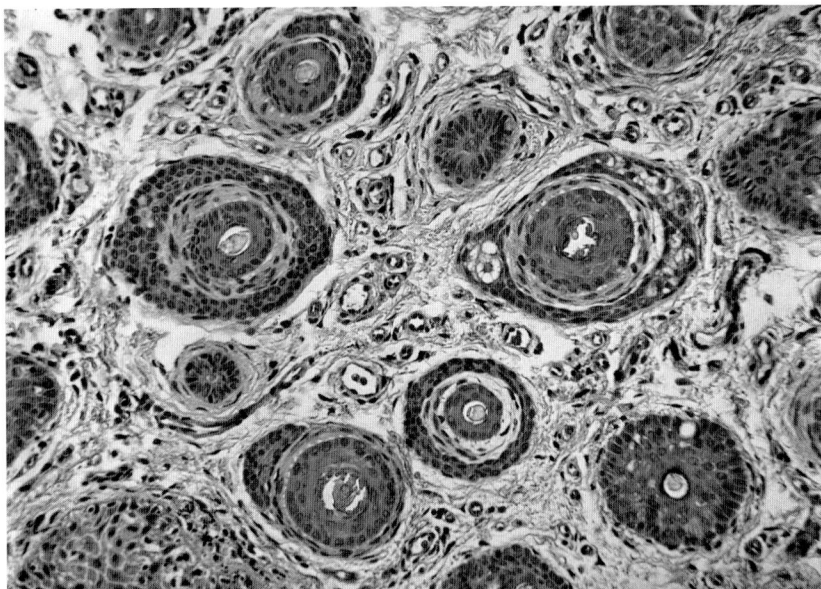

B

Figure 1-19. (**A**) Vellus hair follicle, longitudinal section. Note that the mantle extends diagonally toward the reticular dermis on either side of the hair follicle. Sebocytes are observed frequently within the mantle. (**B**) Vellus hair follicles, horizontal section at level of the isthmus. There are three mantles that form a circle (cloak) around these hair follicles. Note the obvious sebocytes in one of the mantles.

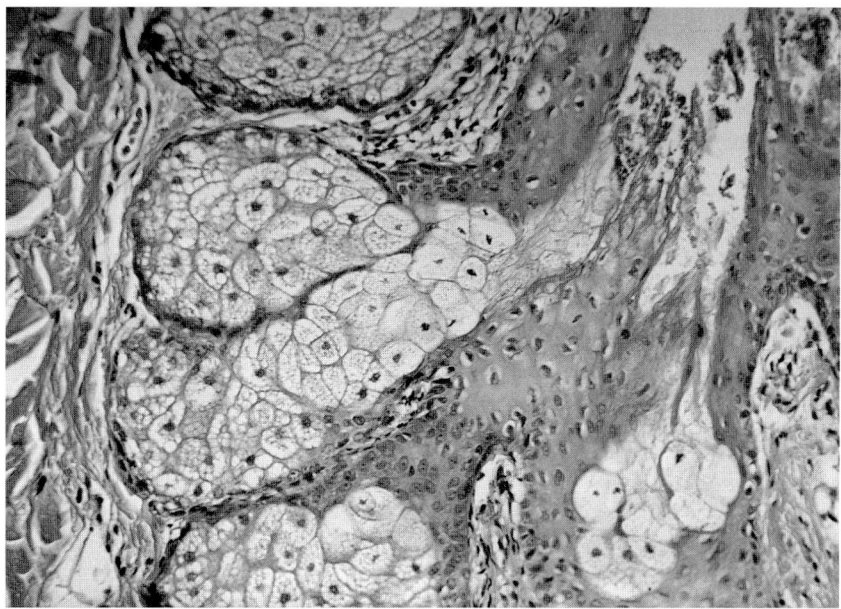

Figure 1-20. Magnification of a sebaceous lobule revealing that lipidization of the sebocytes occurs quickly in the maturation sequence. Note also that the sebocyte nuclei are centrally located and surrounded by spherules of lipid that indent the nuclei. As the entire cells eliminate into the duct (i.e., holocrine elimination), the outlines of the effete sebocytes are conspicuous.

Figure 1-21. Cutaneous gland structure in general, apocrine and eccrine. The eccrine units connect to the surface directly, while the apocrine units may connect to the surface or to the follicular infundibulum.

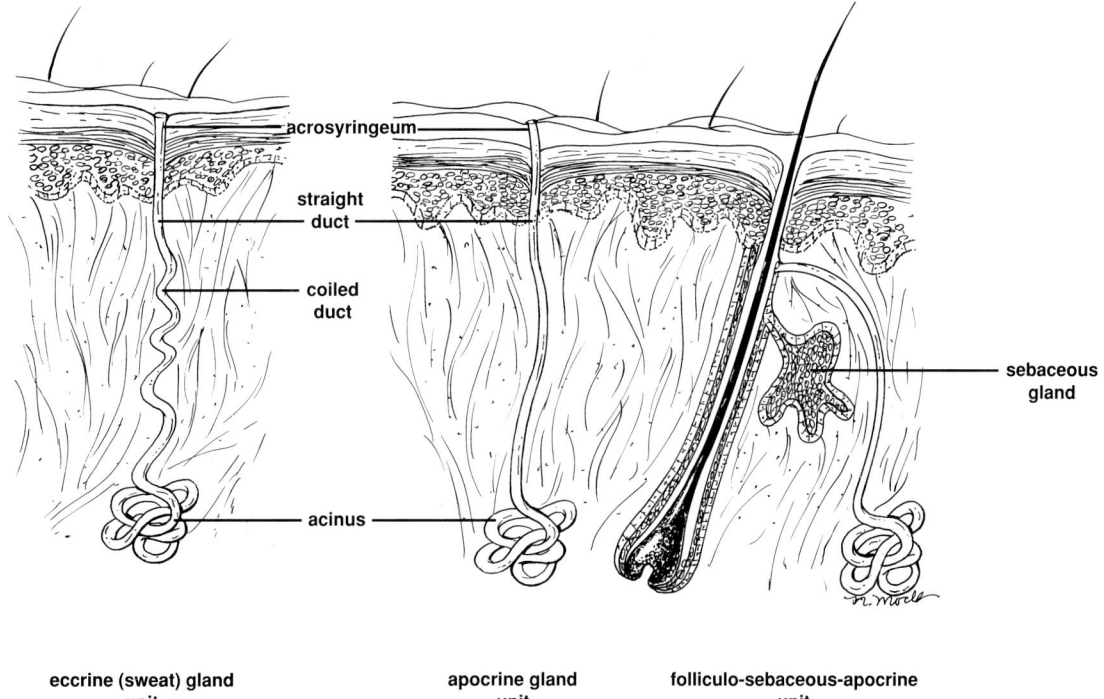

acrosyringeum

straight duct

coiled duct

sebaceous gland

acinus

eccrine (sweat) gland unit

apocrine gland unit

folliculo-sebaceous-apocrine unit

Table 1-4. Main Histologic Features of Glands (Nonsebaceous) in the Skin with Mammary Gland for Comparison

	Eccrine	Apocrine	Apoeccrine	Anogenital	Mammary
Glandular size	Small	Large	Intermediate and variable	Large and variable	Very large
Glandular form	Simple coiled narrow duct	Wide coiled duct with occasional diverticula	Simple coiled duct with wide and narrow segments	Wide coiled duct with irregular acini, diverticula, short branches, and occasionally lobuli	Very wide duct with irregular diverticula and branches; many lobuli in female
Ductal opening	Surface	Hair follicle	Surface	Surface	Surface nipple
Excretory duct size	Long and narrow	Short and wide	Long and narrow	Long and wide	Very long and wide
Lining					
Upper portion	Multilayered squamous	Multilayered squamous	Not described	Multilayered squamous	Multilayered squamous
Intermediate portion	Multilayered squamous, with cuticular-like surface	Simple columnar with snouts; myoepithelium	Not described	Simple columnar with snouts; myoepithelium	Simple columnar, occasionally with snouts; myoepithelium
Lower portion	Basal clear cells and luminal dark cells; canaliculi; myoepithelium	Simple columnar to cuboidal, occasionally snouts rich in cytoplasm; myoepithelium	Eccrine-like and apocrine-like segments	Simple columnar with snouts; cuboidal in acini and diverticula; myoepithelium	Simple columnar with snouts; columnar to cuboidal in acini; myoepithelium
Basement membrane	Thick	Thin	Not described	Thin to thick	Thin to thick
Stroma	Little and loose	Little and loose	Not described	Abundant and loose to dense	Abundant and loose to dense

(From van der Putte,[50] with permission.)

Figure 1-22. Adnexal fat pad with sebaceous lobules and sweat gland lobules in adult neck skin. This scanning magnification illustrates the relationship between adipose tissue, adnexa, and dermis. Note the diagonal extensions of adipose tissue into the reticular dermis, ending with sebaceous glands. Just deep to the sebaceous glands are sweat gland lobules, which are not visualized well at this low magnification.

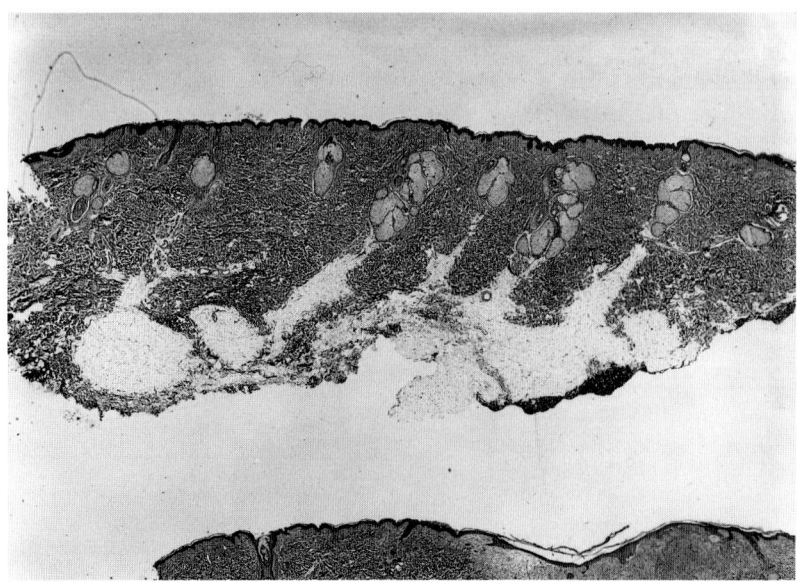

Regardless of coil type, the excretory ducts are similar. A portion of the eccrine duct may be within the coil, while the apocrine duct does not have a significant portion in the coil. The ducts are composed of two cell layers: *luminal* (or apical) and *basal*.

The coiled portion of the eccrine duct is convoluted, but distinct from the tubular acini. As the coiled portion of the duct enters the dermis, it becomes relatively straight and perpendicular to the skin surface, thus its designation as the *straight* duct. At the point where the straight duct enters the epidermis, it is termed the *acrosyringium*. The acrosyringial portion of the eccrine duct spirals through its course in the epidermis and stratum corneum (Fig. 1-23). The apocrine duct, which may eliminate through either the follicular infundibulum or the epidermis, is straight throughout its course in the epidermis and stratum corneum.

Gland Coil and Duct Apocrine Acinar Cells The cells of the apocrine coil are arranged in a single layer of columnar cells that rests on a layer of myoepithelial cells and, in turn, on a basement membrane. The apocrine cells contain an eosinophilic cytoplasm and small vesicular nucleus. Characteristic of these cells are small apical extrusions of cytoplasm, so-called decap-

Figure 1-23. Acrosyringium in the palm of an adult. This acrosyringium is sectioned such that only three portions of the spiraled intraepidermal duct are present. Several lumina of the intracorneal portion of the acrosyringium are also present.

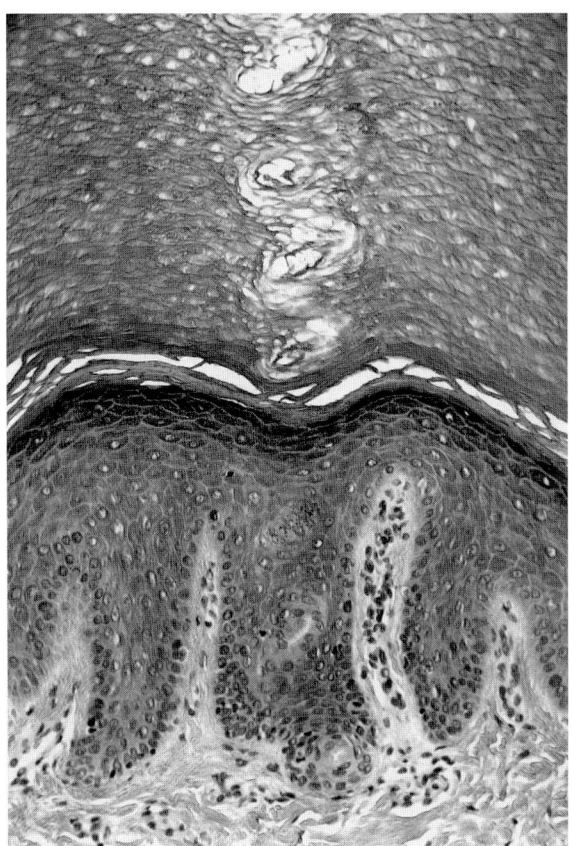

itation secretion[53] (Fig. 1-24). In the cell cytoplasm, there are large PAS-positive, diastase-resistant sialomucinous granules; often, iron is observed. Occasionally, mucinous metaplasia is observed in these cells.[54]

Ultrastructurally, the large granules correspond to "dark" granules and are lysosomes, evidenced by the presence of acid phosphatase and β-glucuronidase. They are dense, approximately 5 μm in diameter, and contain lipid particles, ferritin, and myelin figures. In addition, a "light" granule, with features of mitochondria, is also present.

Eccrine Acinar Cells. There are two types of secretory cells in the eccrine gland acinus: the *light* or clear cell and the *dark* cell. With H&E stain, the clear cells are more prominent at the basement membrane (Fig. 1-25). PAS stain accentuates the glycogen within the cell cytoplasm. The dark cells, which are mucin rich, are more prominent at the acinar apex and contain acid mucins (Alcian blue, pH 2.5).

Ultrastructurally, the clear cells have a highly complex basolateral cell membrane rich in paranitrolphenyl phosphatase, indicating Na-K-ATPase activity and suggesting that this is the site of active transport of ions in sweat secretion.[55] In addition, the clear cells contain numerous mitochondria, in contrast to most of the dark cells.

Functionally, the product of the clear cell is a serious isosmotic fluid that is gradually diluted as it nears the acrosyringium (except in certain diseases such as cystic fibrosis). The final product is a hypotonic, watery solution termed *sweat*.

The myoepithelial cells contain numerous myofilaments and contract in response to cholinergic, but not adrenergic, stimuli.[56]

Nail The nail[57] is an adnexal structure of the skin, located at the distal dorsal surfaces of the fingers and toes, that functions as a protective barrier for the digits. Nails grow more quickly in summer than in winter. In addition, some altered physiologic states, such as pregnancy, result in a more rapid rate of nail growth. Further information on nail kinetics is available elsewhere.[57,58]

Grossly,[57] from proximal to distal (Fig. 1-26), the nail unit consists of a *proximal nail fold*, the distal portion of which is termed the *cuticle*. The *lateral nail folds* are continuous with the proximal fold and are found at the periphery. Beneath the proximal nail fold and hidden from view is the germinal portion of the nail, the *matrix*. The exposed surface of the nail is termed the *nail plate*. The *lunula* (half moon) is a white crescentic zone located proximal to the nail plate, its convex surface pointed distally. The lunula is best observed on the thumb, but may be visible in the nails of the other digits.

Histologically,[59] the matrix (Fig. 1-27) begins at the angle of the inferior, clinically hidden portion of the proximal nail fold. It is continuous with the *keratogenous zone*, which corresponds to the lunula and consists of the distal matrix that gradually merges deep in an angular fashion with the *nail bed* and superficially with the *nail plate*. The nail bed epithelium terminates at the point where it develops characteristics of volar skin, termed the *hyponychium*, which is the portal of entry for microorganisms in nail infections. The hyponychium terminates at the *distal grove*, where the exposed surface of the skin begins.

The matrical zone[59] is characterized (Fig. 1-28) by a sharply accentuated, longitudinally parallel, villous rete ridge pattern.

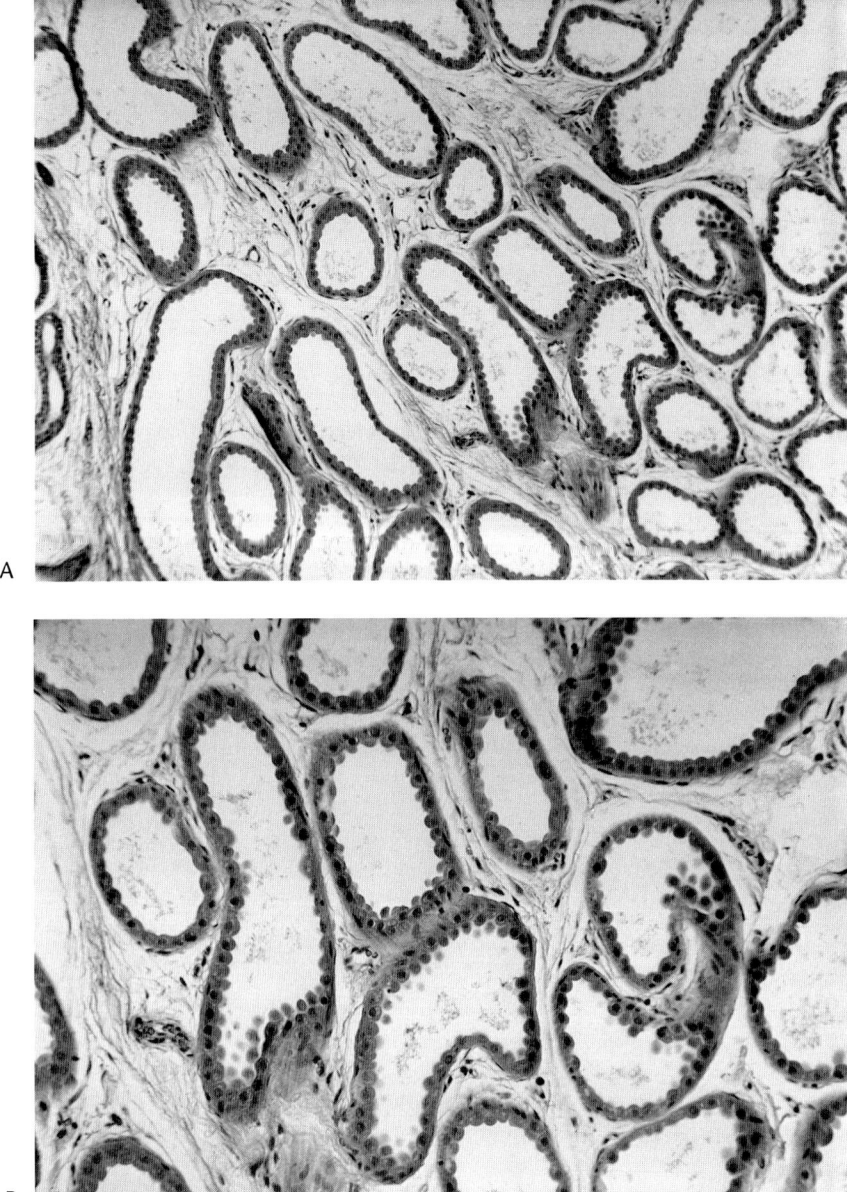

Figure 1-24.   Apocrine coil, medium- and high-power views. **(A)** The coil contains numerous secretory tubules separated by delicate stroma. **(B)** Note the apical apocrine cells. This hallmark feature, the "pinching off" or "decapitation secretion," is the fundamental feature of apocrine secretion.

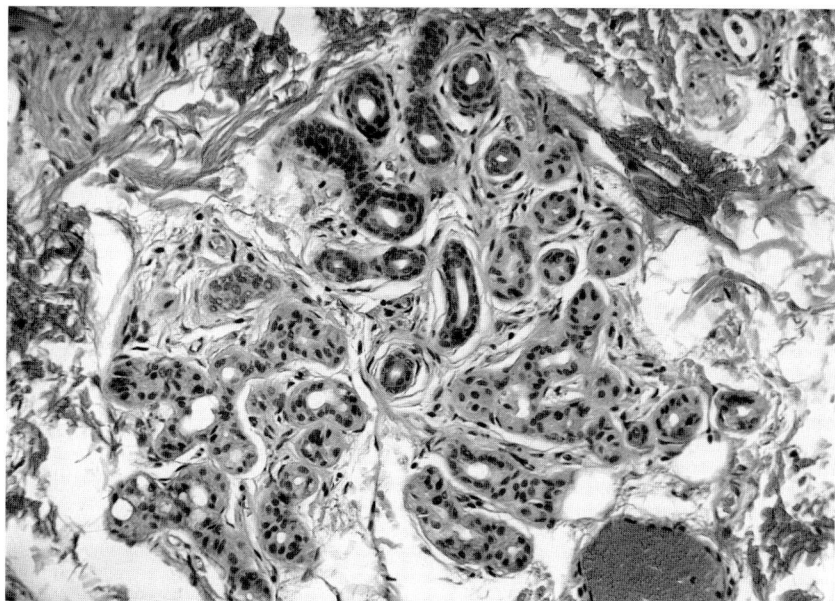

Figure 1-25. Eccrine coil. The acinus consists of small tubular glands that are closely apposed. Several sections through the coiled portion of the duct (superficial) are also present.

The maturation process is similar to that of hair matrix, beginning with the basal epithelium that matures in an angle oriented toward the distal portion of the nail. As the matrical cells differentiate and progress to the superficial layers, their nuclei flatten and the cytoplasm becomes eosinophilic and devoid of intracytoplasmic granules, in contrast with epidermal maturation. The distal area of the matrix, the keratogenous zone, sharply but gradually merges with the nail bed and nail plate. Melanocytes are observed easily in the matrical zones of dark-skinned persons and with difficulty in lighter skinned persons.

The nail bed begins at the lunula or the distal portion of the keratogenous zone. This is the dominant structure of the nail as it covers virtually the entire nail surface. In sections from this area, a ridged pattern may or may not be observed (depending on the plane of section) at the deep portion because of its longitudinal grooved structure. Small blood vessels contained within the ridges give rise to "splinter hemorrhages" from trauma and in certain disease states. The nail bed epithelium is composed of a relatively uniform population of keratinocytes lacking mitoses. In addition, there is no superficial granular layer.

Figure 1-26. Surface anatomy of a nail. This diagram illustrates the four epithelial components: I, matrix; II, nail bed; III, hyponychium; and IV, proximal nail fold. (From Zaias,[57] with permission.)

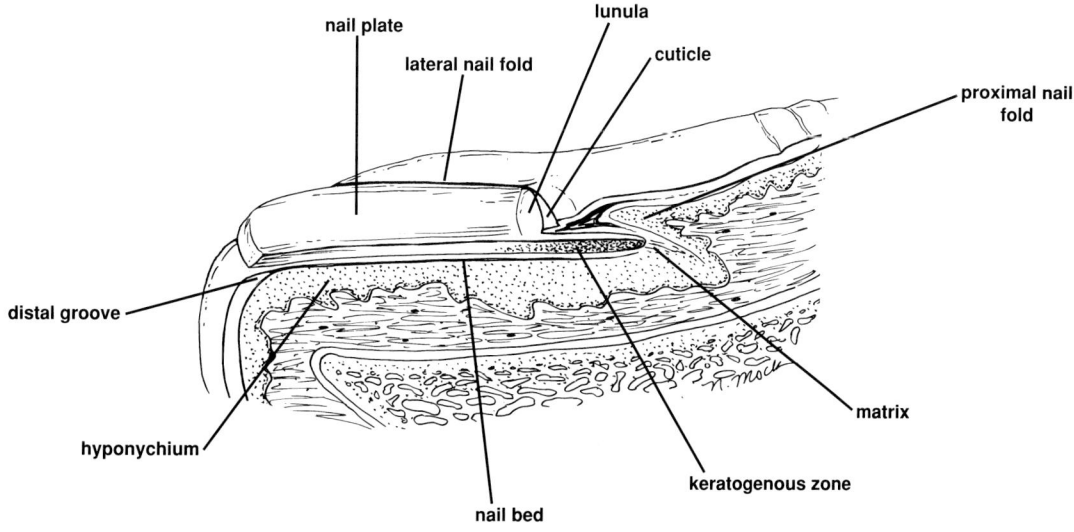

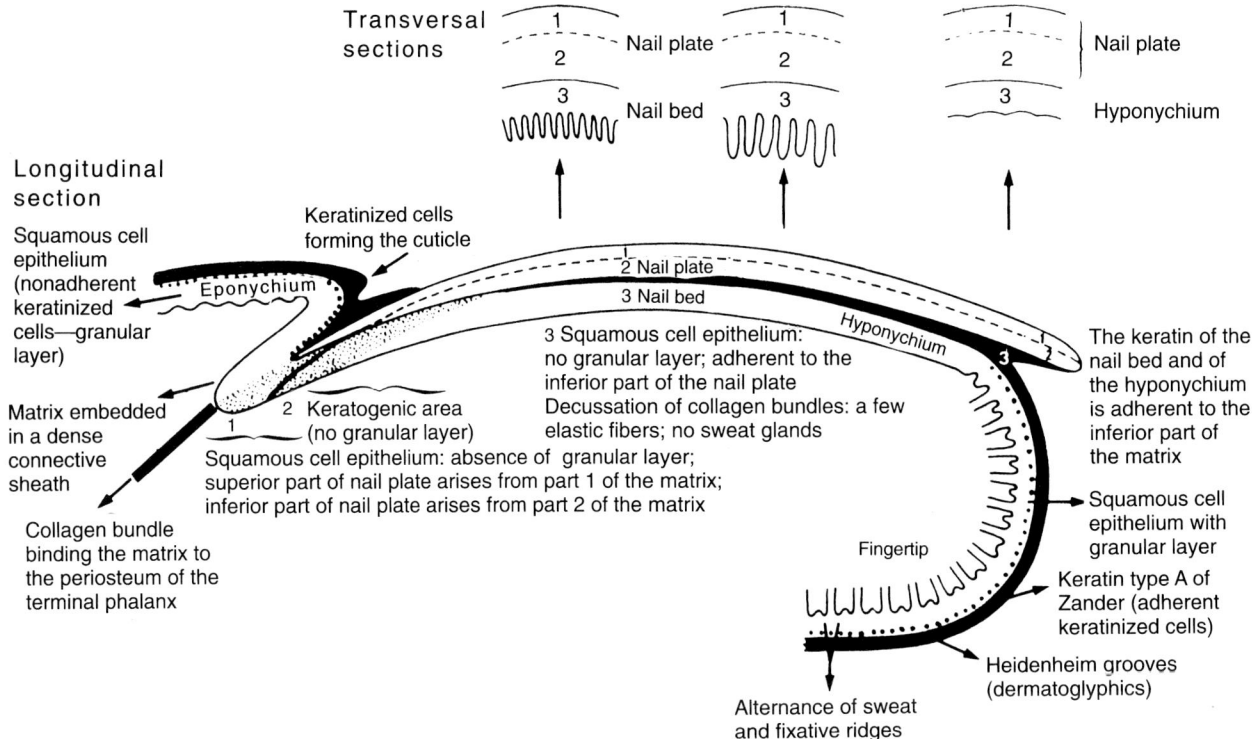

Figure 1-27.   Diagram of the histologic anatomy of a nail. (From Achten et al,[59] with permission.)

Basement Membrane

The cutaneous basement membrane separates the epidermis and adnexa from the dermis and functions as the mediator of epithelial-dermal integrity. It is a physiologically dynamic, continuous, acellular structure composed of substances, principally proteoglycans, synthesized by the surface and adnexal epithelium as well as cells within the dermis.

By light microscopy, the basement membrane is relatively inconspicuous. It is closely apposed to the basal layer of the epidermis and can be accentuated by the PAS stain that highlights

the hydroxyl groups of proteoglycans. The average thickness is approximately 0.5 to 1 μm.

Ultrastructurally, there is a more complex structure to the basement membrane. There are two distinct zones (Fig. 1-29): the superficial *lamina lucida* and the deeper *lamina densa*.[60,61] The lamina lucida is approximately 8 nm thick and directly contacts the basal cell membrane. It is composed of laminin, fibronectin, and bullous pemphigoid antigen. Anchoring filaments from the subbasal cell dense plate of hemidesmosomes traverse the lamina lucida and insert into the lamina densa.

The second portion, the lamina densa, is electron dense, mea-

Figure 1-28.   Longitudinal and cross-sections of the nail with eponychium, matrix, nail bed, and hyponychium. 1, the proximal part of the matrix gives rise to the upper nail plate; 2, the distal part of the matrix gives rise to the lower nail plate; and 3, the nail bed gives rise to the subungual keratin. (From Achten et al,[59] with permission.)

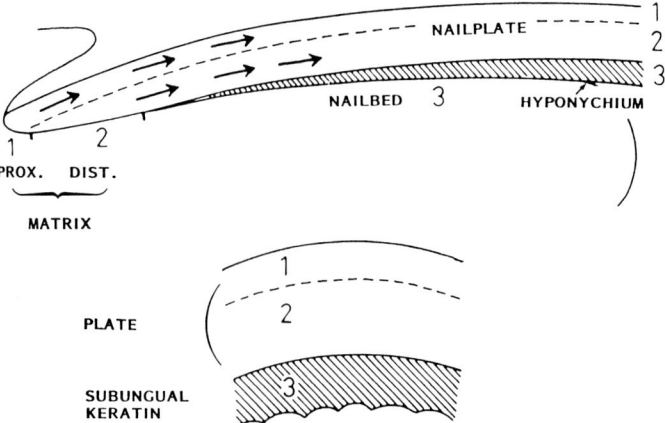

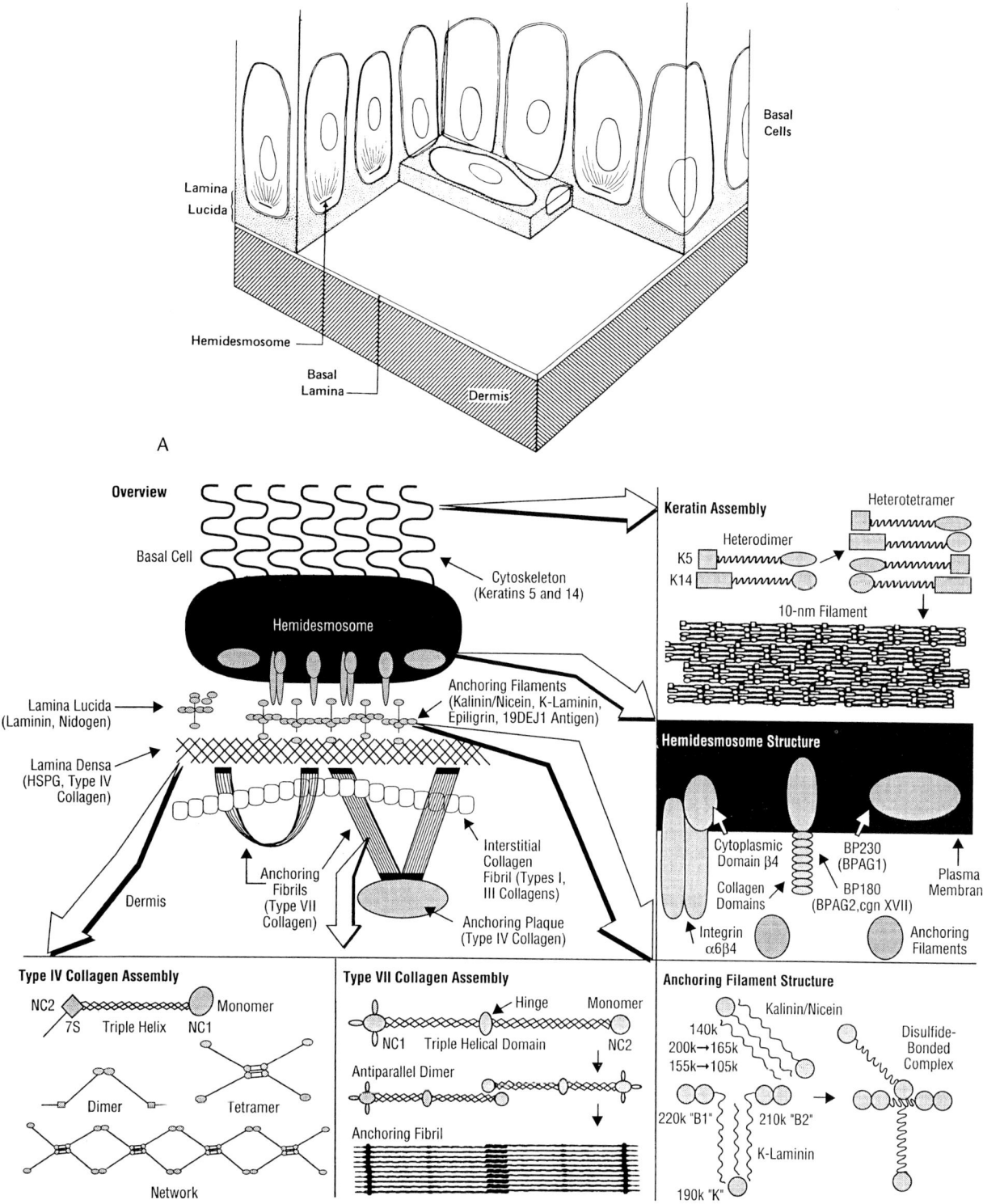

Figure 1-29. **(A)** Schematic of the basement membrane. (From Diaz,[60] with permission.) **(B)** Top left, molecular organization of the dermal-epidermal basement membrane. Top right, basal cell keratin filament assembly. Center right, structure of hemidesmosomal components. Bottom left, assembly of type IV collagen network. Bottom center, assembly of type VII collagen into anchoring fibrils. Bottom right, structure of anchoring filament components kalinin/nicein and K-laminin. HSP6, heparan sulfate proteoglycan. (From Marinkovich,[61] with permission.)

Figure 1-33. Vascular supply of the skin. (Adapted from Bacon and Niles,[69] with permission.)

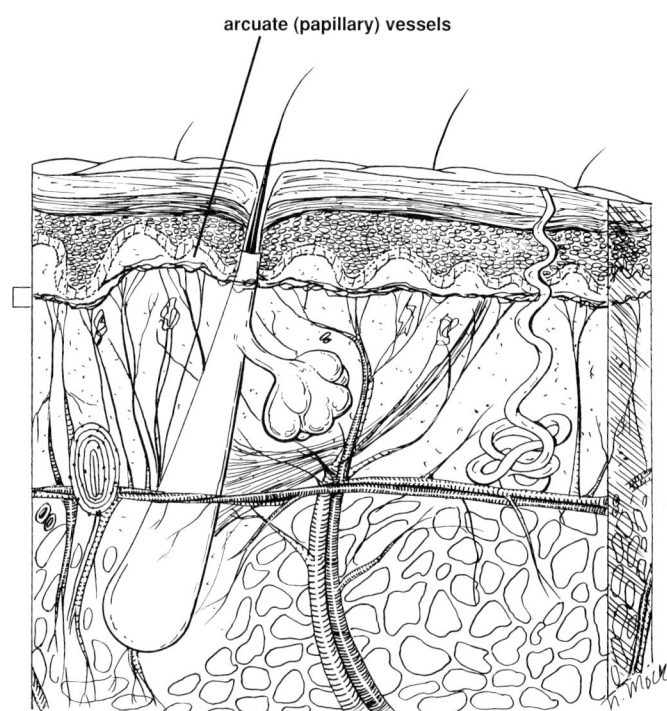

arcuate (papillary) vessels

superficial plexus

deep plexus

ily within the fibrous septa. Small feeder vessels coalesce in the deep dermis to form the *deep dermal plexus*. Communicating vessels ascend and descend perpendicular to the surface skin in the superficial dermis, coalescing once more to form the *superficial vascular plexus*, composed largely of venules and capillaries. Small arcuate capillaries (Fig. 1-33) emerge from the superficial plexus and supply the dermal papillae.[69] The capillary loops decrease in density with age. Not only is there a striking loss of their regular arrangement, but also there is an increase in the tortuosity of the horizontal vessels of the superficial vascular plexus. This change does not appear to affect the heterogeneity of tissue perfusion in older persons.[70]

The cutaneous adnexa receive branches from the ascending and descending vessels perforating the dermis midway between the superficial and deep plexuses. Capillaries converge in the follicular papilla as well as around and within all gland lobules.

Arteriovenous anastomoses, glomus bodies, are present within the reticular dermis and are especially prominent at acral sites, such as fingers and toes.[71] These anastomoses are composed of one to several thick-walled vascular channels, the Sucquet-Hoyer canals, that branch from the arteriole and communicate directly with a venule (Fig. 1-34). The glomus bodies serve a thermoregulatory function in the skin, diverting blood flow away from the skin as external temperature decreases.

Cutaneous lymphatics[72] are abundant but difficult to identify in routinely prepared sections. Architecturally, the lymphatics generally parallel the venous system. Lymphatic capillaries are simple tubes devoid of a basement membrane and lined by a single layer of endothelial cells, but are cuffed by elastic fibers. All lymphatics, even in the superficial dermis, contain valves (in contrast to superficial veins) (Fig. 1-35). Postcapillary lymphatics are located deep in the dermis and contain valves as well as smooth muscle. The deep lymphatics exist at the border of the dermis and subcutis. These are similar to veins.

Figure 1-34. Glomus body. There are two thick-walled vessels with several smaller caliber vessels in between. The smaller vessels contain multilayers of myoid cells that respond to temperature and act as vascular shunts.

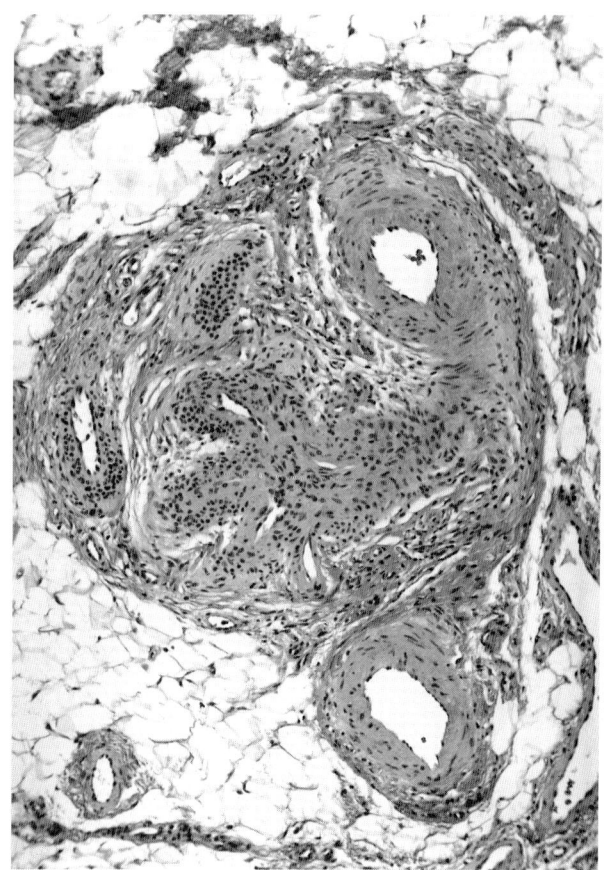

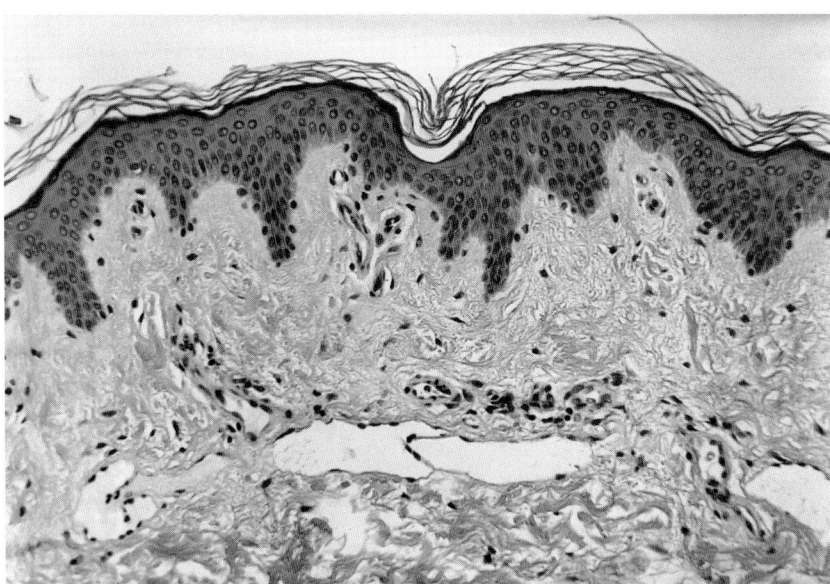

Figure 1-35. Cutaneous lymphatic with valve.

Cutaneous Nerves and Specialized Sensory Structures

The skin contains a rich network of nerves that innervate all aspects, from the epidermis to the dermis, the adnexa, and the blood vessels. Nerves are responsible for sensory and autonomic functions, the latter of which are responsible for the functional aspects of the glands and the arrector pili muscle. In addition, vascular shunts are regulated by nerves in an intricate autonomic nerve plexus.

The intraepidermal nerves are both myelinated and unmyelinated. They pierce the papillary dermis vertically and insert into the epidermis throughout its extent. In the most superficial aspects of the papillary dermis, sensory end-organs are commonly present[73] (Table 1-5). In the genital region, these are termed *genital corpuscles*. Similar end-organs are also identified in mucocutaneous junctions, such as the lip. Larger end-organs, termed *Meissner's corpuscles* (Fig. 1-36), are prominent especially in the hands and feet and are identified at the superficial tips of the papillary dermis. *Vater-Pacini corpuscles*, by contrast, are located in the deep aspects of the skin and are responsible for the registration of vibration and pressure. These are characterized by a central neural core surrounded by peripheral lamellar wrappings, giving rise to an "onion skin" appearance (Fig. 1-37).

Table 1-5. Morphologic and Physiologic Features of Cutaneous Sensory End-Organ Units

Morphologic Type	Nerve Type	Physiologic Type	How Stimulated	What Registered	Clinical Sensation
Hair disc	A	Type I	Low threshold	Displacement	?
Merkel cell complex	A	SAI	Mechanoreceptor	Displacement	Pressure
Ruffini ending (?)	A	Type II; SA II	Mechanoreceptor	Displacement	?
Hair palisade	A	GI hair	Mechanoreceptor	Displacement velocity	Hair movement
Meissner's corpuscle	A	RA field receptor	Mechanoreceptor	Displacement velocity	Tapping
Hair follicle	A	D hair	Mechanoreceptor	Displacement velocity	?
Nerve network (?)	C	C-mechanoreceptor	Mechanoreceptor	Displacement velocity	?
Pacinian corpuscle	A	Pacinian corpuscle	Mechanoreceptor	Vibrations	Buzzing
Nerve network	C, A delta	Cold receptor	Thermoreceptor	Cooling	Cold
Nerve network	C	Warm receptor	Thermoreceptor	Warming	Warm
Nerve network	A delta	Myelinated	Nocireceptors	Noxious deformation	Sharp pain
Nerve network	C	Unmyelinated	Nocireceptors	Noxious heat, chemicals	Dull pain, sharp pain, aching

(Adapted from Winkelmann,[73] with permission.)

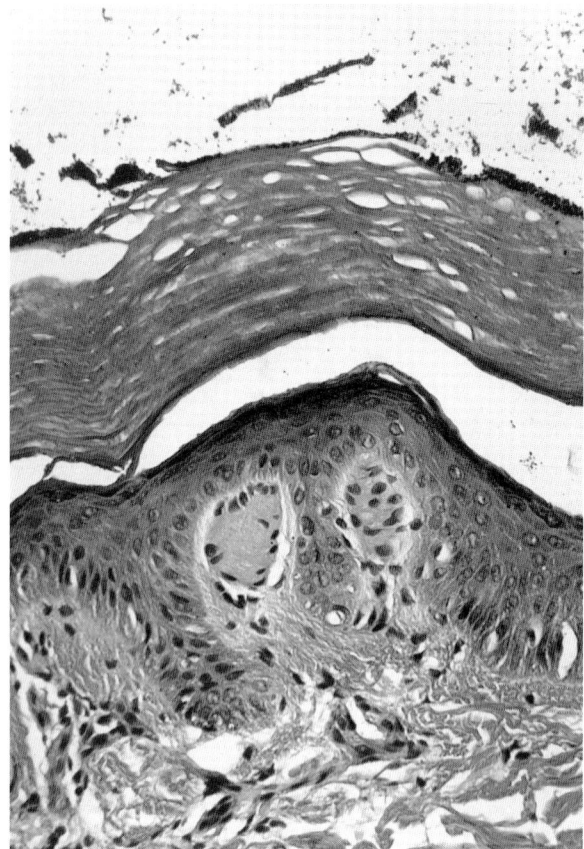

Figure 1-36. Meissner's corpuscles. These are sensory end-organs composed of unmyelinated nerve fibers in layers that are supported by Schwann cells, as well as fibrous and elastic tissue.

The adnexa are innervated throughout, the most stereotyped of which are the vellus hair follicles. A rich network of myelinated and nonmyelinated fibers encase the follicular fibrous sheath inferior to the sebaceous gland and form a palisaded end-organ, sometimes referred to as the nerve "stockade," which registers hair movement[74] (Fig. 1-38).

The innervation of the glands is a rich network of fibers that infiltrate and encase the entire acinus.

Cutaneous Muscle

Smooth and skeletal muscle are found in the skin. Smooth muscle is an integral part of the folliculo-sebaceous unit. The follicular muscle, muscle of hair erection,[75] or *arrector pili* muscle, originates at or around the bulge of the follicle and inserts on the undersurface of the epidermis (Fig. 1-39). Smooth muscle is also found as fascicles present at various levels in specialized areas of the dermal skin such as the nipple (areolar muscle) and scrotum (dartos muscle). The muscle fibers are characteristic in that they contain central, ovoid nuclei in contrast to skeletal muscle.

Skeletal muscle is present in the dermis of two body regions, the neck and face. In the neck, the skeletal muscle is referred to as the *platysma*. In the face, it consists of the muscles of facial expression. It is usually located in the deeper portions of the dermis. The skeletal muscle is striking for its cross striations and peripherally located, round nuclei.

CUTANEOUS EMBRYOLOGY AND FETAL MORPHOGENESIS

The skin is derived principally from ectodermal and mesodermal components. The epithelium/adnexa are derived from neuroectoderm, as are the melanocytes (neural crest), presumably the Merkel cells, and the cutaneous nerves. The dermis and subcutis are derived from the mesoderm, as is the vasculature. Table 1-6 summarizes some of the major events in cutaneous development.[66] As a point of reference, this text uses the term *embryo* to refer to the conceptus from approximately days 20 to 60 after which it is referred to as the *fetus*.

Epidermis

The earliest light microscopic evidence of a layer of cells separate from the neuroectoderm is observed usually during embryonic de-

Figure 1-37. Vater-Pacini corpuscle. This is a large sensory end-organ composed of an "onion skin" layering of Schwann cells and fibrous and elastic tissue around a central axon.

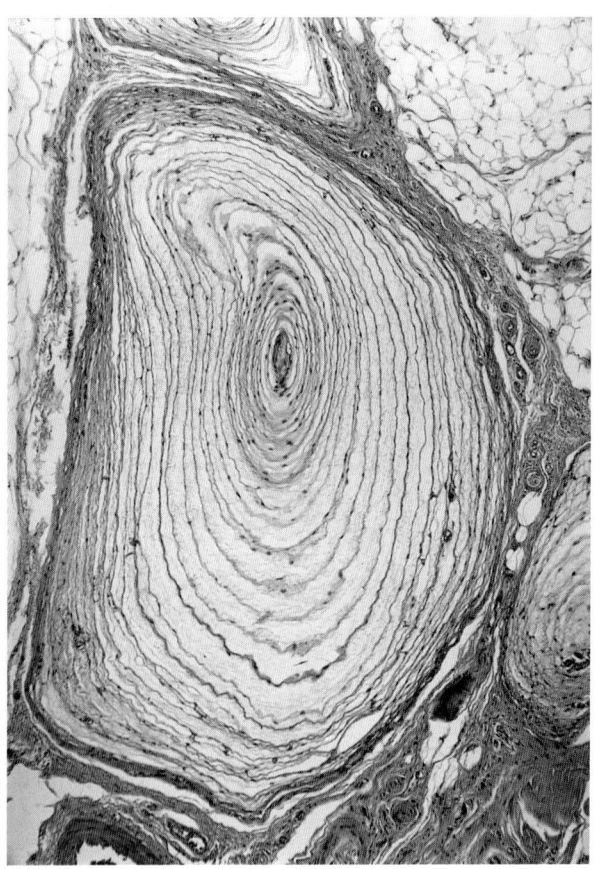

ferentiate into follicular and sebaceous sections of the unit.[48,80] Fetal folliculo-sebaceous units, *lanugo*, form at approximately 3 to 4 months, or approximately 1 to 2 months before the epidermis. Sebaceous glands also begin their holocrine elimination during this time, mixing with cells from the surface to form the vernix caseosa.

The eccrine glands are first observed at 3 months gestation on the palms and soles and at 5 months elsewhere.[51,52,81,82] They begin as buds that develop into cords of cells connecting with the epidermal ridge. Secretion begins by the seventh month in some zones of the body.

The nails begin forming from basal cells of the digits around the time that the palmar sweat glands develop.

Basement Membrane

In the embryonic phase, the interface between the dermis and epidermis is a simple structure, initially containing only type IV collagen and laminin. By approximately 3 months' gestation, virtually all phenotypic markers of the adult basement membrane are present.

Dermis

The embryonic dermis consists of a cellular mesenchyme and a matrix rich in hyaluronic acid. Several types of collagen are pre-

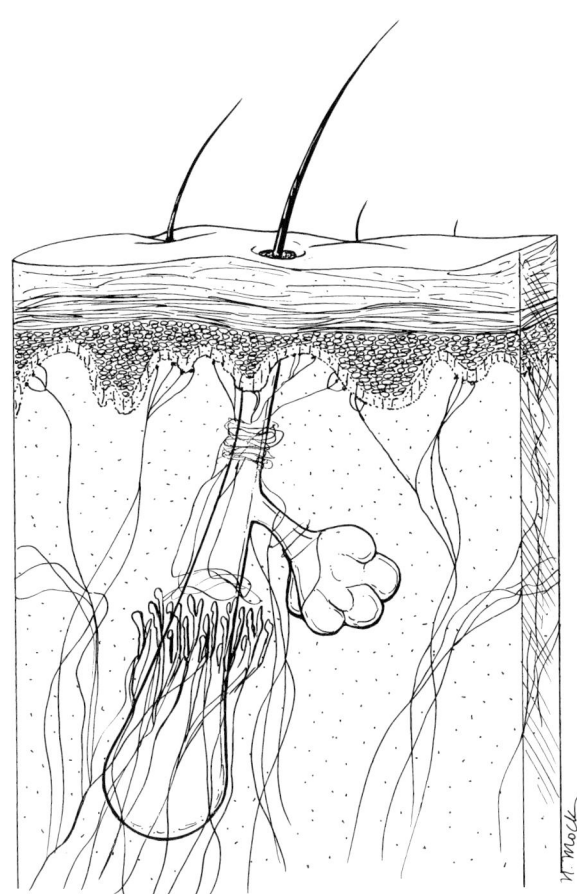

Figure 1-38. Nerve "stockade," a sensory organ that registers motion of the hair follicle. (Adapted from Montagna et al,[74] with permission.)

velopment. The earliest epithelial surface layer is termed the *periderm* and consists of a single layer of cells superficial to a basal layer. The periderm is unique to developing skin,[76] as it lacks mature keratins and filaggrin, which are observed in mature skin. During the third month, the epidermis develops a stratified layer of cells interposed between the periderm and basal cell layer (Fig. 1-40). These cells synthesize keratin filaments and desmosomes. By the sixth month, the keratinocytes produce keratin and keratohyalin granules sufficient for light microscopic identification. In this period the stratum corneum forms and the periderm desquamates into the amniotic fluid.[77] In the third trimester, the fetal epidermis continues to mature and is morphologically similar to adult epidermis.

Other cells of the epidermis, such as Langerhans cells and melanocytes, can be identified as soon as the second month.[78,79]

Adnexa

The adnexa develop between the third and sixth months of gestation and are first perceived as periodic invaginated buds of basaloid epithelium within the dermal mesenchyme.

The folliculo-sebaceous units begin as several bulges from the surface that gradually extend into the dermis and eventually dif-

Figure 1-39. Follicular muscle. The smooth muscle extends diagonally from the bulge of the hair follicle at the lower portion of the isthmus and inserts into the undersurface of the epidermis.

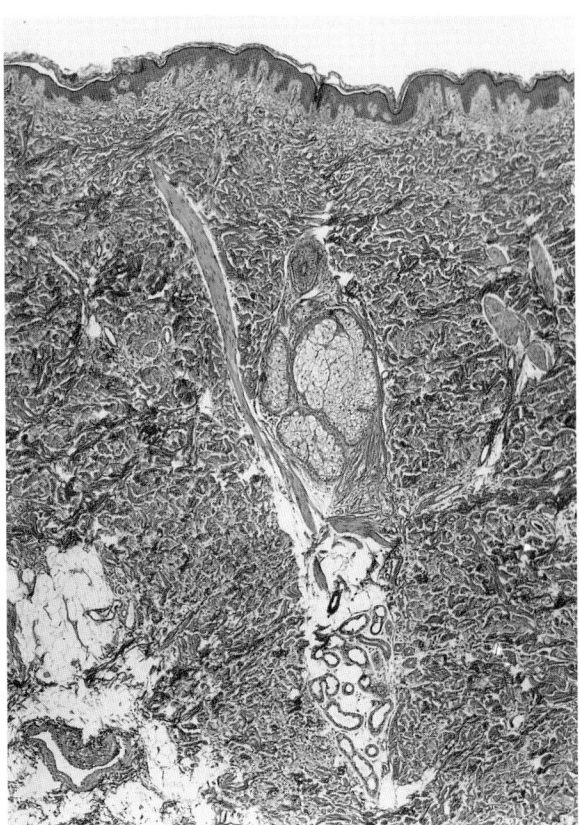

Table 1-6. Chronology of Major Events in Cutaneous Embryogenesis

Structure	Month 1	Month 2	Month 3	Month 4	Month 5	Month 6	Month 7
Epidermis							
Basal layer	X						
Periderm	X						
Spinous layer		X					
Granular layer						X	
Stratum corneum						X	
Immigrant Cells							
Melanocytes with premelanosomes		X					
Melanocytes that synthesize melanin				X			
Melanosome transfer to melanocyte						X	
Langerhans cells			X				
Merkel cells				X			
Adnexa							
Hair follicle development begins			X				
Sebaceous gland primordium				X			
Sebaceous gland function					X		
Apocrine gland primordium						X	
Apocrine gland function							X
Eccrine duct and gland functional						X	
Nail fold matrix and primordium forms			X				
Nail plate forms				X			
Dermis							
Papillary and reticular dermis formed				X			
Dermal papillae formed					X		
Dermis/subcutis boundary formed		X					
Panniculus adiposus established				X			

(Adapted from Holbrook and Wolff,[66] with permission.)

sent in the mesenchyme, which is the matter from which the vasculature and pilar muscles develop.

By the end of the first trimester, the fetal dermis is differentiated into an adventitial and a reticular dermis. In addition, the vascular plexuses are evident.[83] Associated mononuclear cells, such as macrophages and mast cells, are also present.

At the end of the second trimester, the dermis is easily identified as papillary and reticular. Elastic tissue is synthesized during this period,[84] but does not reach full development until after birth and into the first several years of life.

Subcutaneous Tissues

Lobules of highly cellular adipose tissue are first identified in the fourth month of gestation. After this, a highly variable accumulation of adipose tissue is acquired in the subcutaneous region.[85]

Figure 1-40. Fetal skin at 17 weeks' gestation. Note that the epidermis has developed several layers between the basal layer and the periderm. Also note the bud protruding from the surface; this is a primitive adnexus. The dermis is a loose, mesenchymal meshwork that contains one developing hair follicle.

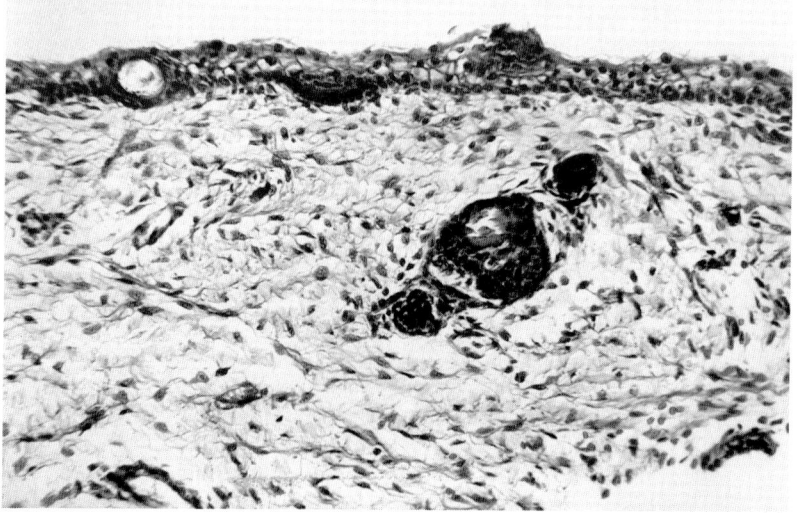

REFERENCES

1. Unna PG: Author's preface. p. vi. In: Histopathology of the Skin. Macmillan, New York, 1896
2. Leider M, Buncke CM: Physical dimensions of the skin. Determination of the specific gravity of skin, hair, and nail. AMA Arch Dermatol Syph 69:563, 1954
3. Montagna W, Carlisle K: Structural changes in aging skin. Br J Dermatol 122:61, 1990
4. Southwood WFW: The thickness of the skin. Plast Reconstr Surg 15:423, 1955
5. Ragaz A, Ackerman AB: Subtle clues to diagnosis by gross pathology. Superficial atrophy: loss of papillary dermis and epidermis. Am J Dermatopathol 2:337, 1980
6. Halprin KM: Cyclic nucleotides and epidermal cell proliferation. J Invest Dermatol 66:339, 1976
7. Freeman RG: The keratin. A biological unit of the epidermis. Am J Dermatopathol 1:35, 1979
8. Smack DP, Korge BP, James WD: Keratin and keratinization. J Am Acad Dermatol 30:85, 1994
9. Holbrook KA: Biologic structure and function. Perspectives on morphological approaches to the study of the granular layer keratinocyte. J Invest Dermatol 92:84S, 1989
10. Bernard BA, Robinson SM, Vandaele S et al: Abnormal maturation pathway of keratinocytes in psoriatic skin. Br J Dermatol 112:647, 1985
11. Jimbow K, Quevedo WC Jr, Fitzpatrick TB, Szabó G: Biology of melanocytes. p. 261. In Fitzpatrick TB, Eisen AZ, Wolff K et al (eds): Dermatology in Clinical Medicine. 4th Ed. Vol. 1. McGraw-Hill, New York, 1993
12. Tarnowski WM: Ultrastructure of the epidermal melanocyte dense plate. J Invest Dermatol 55:265, 1970
13. Szabó G, Gerald AB, Pathak MA, Fitzpatrick TB: Racial differences in the fate of melanosomes in human epidermis. Nature 222:1081, 1969
14. Goldschmidt H, Raymond JZ: Quantitative analysis of skin colour from melanin content of superficial skin cells. J Forensic Sci 17:124, 1972
15. Katz SI, Tamaki K, Sachs DH: Epidermal Langerhans cells are derived from cells originating in bone marrow. Nature 282:324, 1979
16. Hashimoto K: Lanthanum staining of Langerhans' cell. Communication of Langerhans' cell granules with extracellular space. Arch Dermatol 102:280, 1970
17. Shelley WB, Juhlin L: Langerhans cells form a reticuloepithelial trap for external contact antigens. Nature 261:46, 1976
18. Hunter JAA: The Langerhans cells: from gold to glitter. Clin Exp Dermatol 18:569, 1983
19. Stingl G, Wolff-Schreiner EC, Pichler WJ et al: Epidermal Langerhans cells bear F_c and C_3 receptors. Nature 268:245, 1977
20. Klareskog L, Malmnäs Tjernlund U, Forsum U, Peterson PA: Epidermal Langerhans cells express Ia antigens. Nature 268:248, 1977
21. Santa Cruz DJ, Bauer EA: Merkel cells in the outer follicular sheath. Ultrastruct Pathol 3:59, 1982
22. Narisawa Y, Hashimoto K, Kohda H: Merkel cells in human fetal eccrine glands. Br J Dermatol 129:541, 1993
23. Moll R, Moll I, Franke WW: Identification of Merkel cells in human skin by specific cytokeratin antibodies: changes of cell density and distribution in fetal and adult plantar epidermis. Differentiation 28:136, 1984
24. Mérot Y: Immunohistochemistry of the Merkel cell. Semin Dermatol 7:269, 1988
25. Toker C: Clear cells of the nipple epidermis. Cancer 25:601, 1970
26. Szabó G: The regional anatomy of the human integument with special reference to the distribution of hair follicles, sweat glands, and melanocytes. Philos Trans R Soc Lond Ser B 252:447, 1967
27. Price ML, Griffiths WAD: Normal body hair—a review. Clin Exp Dermatol 10:87, 1985
28. Jakubovic HA, Ackerman AB: Structure and function of skin: development, morphology, and physiology. p. 3. In Moschella SL, Hurley HJ (eds): Dermatology. 3rd Ed. WB Saunders, Philadelphia, 1992
29. Ackerman AB, de Viragh PA, Chongchitnant N et al: Anatomic, histologic, and biologic aspects of hair follicles and hair. p. 35. In Ackerman AB (ed): Neoplasms with Follicular Differentiation. 1st Ed. Ackerman's Histologic Diagnosis of Neoplastic Skin Diseases: A Method by Pattern Analysis. Lea & Febiger, Philadelphia, 1993
30. Pinkus H: "Sebaceous cysts" are trichilemmal cysts. Arch Dermatol 99:544, 1969
31. Brooke JD, Fitzpatrick JE, Golitz LE: Papillary mesenchymal bodies: a histologic finding useful in differentiating trichoepitheliomas from basal cell carcinomas. J Am Acad Dermatol 21:523, 1989
32. Adamson HG: Observations on the parasites of ringworm. Br J Dermatol 7:201, 1895
33. Chase HB: Growth of the hair. Physiol Rev 34:113, 1954
34. Mehregan AH, Hashimoto K: Normal structure of skin. p. 5. In Pinkus' Guide to Dermatohistopathology. 5th Ed. Appleton & Lange, E. Norwalk, CT, 1991
35. Cotsarelis G, Sun TT, Lavker RM: Label-retaining cells reside in the bulge area of the pilosebaceous unit: implications for follicular stem cells, hair cycle, and skin carcinogenesis. Cell 61:1329, 1990
36. Sun TT, Cotsarelis G, Lavker RM: Hair follicle stem cells: the bulge-activation hypothesis. J Invest Dermatol 96:77S, 1991
37. Holecek B-U, Ackerman AB: Bulge-activation hypothesis: is it valid? Am J Dermatopathol 15:235, 1993
38. Ackerman AB: Bulge-activation hypothesis. Part 1—a hair is not a follicle. Dermatopathol Pract Concept 1:53, 1995
39. Radonich M, Misciali C, Ackerman AB: Bulge-activation hypothesis. Part II—the bulge is not a bulge. Dermatopathol Pract Concept 1:77, 1995
40. Ackerman AB, Misciali C, Radonich M: Bulge-activation hypothesis. Part III—a mouse is not a man. Dermatopathol Pract Concept 1:146, 1995
41. Dunstan RW, Linder KA: Mammals, other than man, do not have follicular bulges: implications for the bulge-activation hypothesis. Dermatopathol Pract Concept 1:154, 1995
42. Montagna W, Yun JS: The glands of Montgomery. Br J Dermatol 86:126, 1972
43. Smith DM, Peters TG, Donegan WL: Montgomery's areolar tubercle. Arch Pathol Lab Med 106:60, 1982

44. Hyman AB, Brownstein MH: Tyson's glands. Ectopic sebaceous glands and papillomatosis penis. Arch Dermatol 99:31, 1969

45. Montagna W, Kligman AM, Carlisle KS: Glands. p. 225. In Atlas of Normal Human Skin. Springer-Verlag, New York, 1992

46. Zimmerman KW: Über einige formverhältniβe der haarfollikel des menschen. Z Mikrosk Anat Forsch 38:503, 1935

47. Steffen C: Mantleoma. A benign neoplasm with mantle differentiation. Am J Dermatopathol 15:306, 1993

48. Steffen C, Ackerman AB: Embryologic, anatomic and histologic aspects. p. 27. In Neoplasms with Sebaceous Differentiation. 1st Ed. Ackerman's Histologic Diagnosis of Neoplastic Skin Diseases: A Method by Pattern Analysis. Lea & Febiger, Philadelphia, 1994

49. Sato K, Leidal R, Sato F: Morphology and development of an apoeccrine sweat gland in the human axillae. Am J Physiol 252:R166, 1987

50. van der Putte SCJ: Anogenital "sweat" glands. Histology and pathology of a gland that may mimic mammary glands. Am J Dermatopathol 13:557, 1991

51. Kuno Y: Human Perspiration. Charles C Thomas, Springfield, IL, 1956

52. Montagna W, Parakkal PF: The Structure and Function of Skin. 3rd Ed. Academic Press, San Diego, 1974

53. Schaumberg-Lever G, Lever WF: Secretion from human apocrine glands. J Invest Dermatol 64:38, 1975

54. Winkelmann RK, Hultin JV: Mucinous metaplasia in normal apocrine glands. Arch Dermatol 78:309, 1958

55. Sato K, Kang WH, Saga K, Sato KT: Biology of sweat glands and their disorders. I. Normal sweat gland function. J Am Acad Dermatol 20:537, 1989

56. Sato K, Nishiyama A, Kobayashi M: Mechanical properties and functions of the myoepithelium in the eccrine sweat gland. Am J Physiol 237:C177, 1986

57. Zaias N: Anatomy and physiology. p. 3. In The Nail in Health and Disease. 2nd Ed. Appleton & Lange, E. Norwalk, CT, 1990

58. Zaias N: Kinetics. p. 33. In The Nail in Health and Disease. 2nd Ed. Appleton & Lange, E. Norwalk, CT, 1990

59. Achten G, André J, Laporte M: Nails in light and electron microscopy. Semin Dermatol 10:54, 1991

60. Diaz LA: Molecular dissection of the dermal-epidermal junction. Am J Dermatopathol 2:79, 1980

61. Marinkovich MP: The molecular genetics of basement membrane diseases. Arch Dermatol 129:1557, 1993

62. Ackerman AB: Skin: structure and function. p. 3. In Histologic Diagnosis of Inflammatory Skin Diseases. A Method by Pattern Analysis. 1st Ed. Lea & Febiger, Philadelphia, 1978

63. Headington JT: The dermal dendrocyte. Adv Dermatol 1:159, 1986

64. Cerio R, Griffiths CEM, Cooper KD et al: Characterization of factor XIIIa positive dermal dendritic cells in normal and inflamed skin. Br J Dermatol 121:421, 1989

65. Nestle FO, Nickoloff BJ: A fresh morphological and functional look at dermal dendritic cells. J Cutan Pathol 22:385, 1995

66. Holbrook KA, Wolff K: The structure and development of skin. p. 97. In Fitzpatrick TB, Eisen AZ, Wolff K et al (eds): Dermatology in Clinical Medicine. 4th Ed. Vol. 1. McGraw-Hill, New York, 1993

67. Lasser A: The mononuclear phagocytic system: a review. Hum Pathol 14:108, 1983

68. Tucker SM, Linberg JV: Vascular anatomy of the eyelids. Ophthalmology 101:1118, 1994

69. Bacon RL, Niles NR: Integument. p. 213. In Medical Histology. A Text-Atlas with Introductory Pathology. 1st Ed. Springer-Verlag, New York, 1983

70. Kelly RI, Pearse R, Bull RH et al: The effects of aging on the cutaneous microvasculature. J Am Acad Dermatol 33:749, 1995

71. Mescon H, Hurley HJ, Moretti G: The anatomy and histochemistry of the arteriovenous anastomosis in human digital skin. J Invest Dermatol 27:133, 1956

72. Ryan TJ, Mortimer PS, Jones RL: Lymphatics of the skin. Int J Dermatol 25:411, 1986

73. Winkelmann RK: Cutaneous sensory nerves. Semin Dermatol 7:236, 1988

74. Montagna W, Kligman AM, Carlisle KS: Skin sensory mechanisms. p. 191. In Atlas of Normal Human Skin. Springer-Verlag, New York, 1992

75. Radonich MA, Paredes B, Ackerman AB: Sites of attachment of the muscle of hair erection. Dermatopathol Pract Concept 1:229, 1995

76. Holbrook KA, Odland GF: The fine structure of developing human epidermis: light, scanning, and transmission electron microscopy of the periderm. J Invest Dermatol 65:16, 1975

77. Holbrook KA, Odland GF: Regional development of the human epidermis in the first trimester embryo and the second trimester fetus (ages related to the timing of amniocentesis and fetal biopsy). J Invest Dermatol 80:161, 1980

78. Foster CA, Holbrook KA: Ontogeny of Langerhans cells in human embryonic and fetal skin: cell densities and phenotypic expression relative to epidermal growth. Am J Anat 184:157, 1989

79. Holbrook KA, Underwood RA, Vogel AM et al: The appearance, density and distribution of melanocytes in human embryonic and fetal skin revealed by the anti-melanoma antibody HMB-45. Anat Embryol 180:443, 1989

80. Ackerman AB, de Viragh PA, Chongchitnant N et al: Embryologic aspects. p. 21. In Neoplasms with Follicular Differentiation. 1st Ed. Ackerman AB (ed): Ackerman's Histologic Diagnosis of Neoplastic Skin Diseases: A Method by Pattern Analysis. Lea & Febiger, Philadelphia, 1993

81. Hashimoto K, Gross BG, Lever WF: The ultrastructure of the skin of human embryos. I. Intraepidermal eccrine sweat duct. J Invest Dermatol 45:139, 1965

82. Ellis R: Eccrine sweat glands: electron microscopy, cytochemistry, and anatomy. p. 223. In Normale und pathologische anatomie der haut. Jadassohn J (ed): Handbuch der haut- und geshlechtskrankheiten. Vol. 1. Springer-Verlag, Berlin, 1967

83. Johnson CL, Holbrook KA: The development of human embryonic and fetal dermal vasculature. J Invest Dermatol 93:10S, 1989

84. Deutsch TA, Esterly NB: Elastic fibers in fetal dermis. J Invest Dermatol 65:320, 1975

85. Ryan TJ, Curri SB: The development of the adipose tissue and its relationship to the vascular system. Clin Dermatol 7:1, 1989

2

PROCUREMENT, PROCESSING, AND STAINING TECHNIQUES FOR DERMATOPATHOLOGIC SPECIMENS

BIOPSY TECHNIQUES IN DERMATOLOGY

The specific procedures used to perform biopsies of cutaneous lesions are usually left to the discretion of the attending clinician. This is not a problem if the operator is aware of the specific advantages and disadvantages of various techniques, as applied to specific classes of skin lesions. However, it may prove to be a disaster if the dermatologic surgeon is inexperienced in such matters. Enzyme histochemistry, immunohistology, or electron microscopy—both of which are greatly affected by nuances in tissue preservation—may be necessary in some instances to obtain a firm diagnosis. Because the clinician may not be able to anticipate these possibilities before obtaining the tissue sample, a predetermined routine should be followed in doing so.[1]

There are basically four generic categories of procedures that may be used in any given case. These include punch biopsies; shave or excisional biopsies done with a scalpel; electrosurgical excisions; and laser-mediated biopsies. In choosing one of these options, the operator should be cognizant of the two opposing "forces" that affect the final decision on this matter. On the one hand, the patient is often preoccupied with the cosmetic effects of a biopsy, and this typically induces the surgeon to limit the size of the sample as much as possible. On the other hand, the degree of difficulty with which the microscopic diagnosis is made by the pathologist—a factor that is often predictable by the amount of material that will be required to study the disease process adequately—must also be considered.

The cardinal rule is that a properly done biopsy is virtually never cosmetically deforming if it can be accomplished in an outpatient setting by a competent operator. By contrast, specimen inadequacy and marked artifactual changes in tissue are problems relating to faulty procedure that account for the great majority of diagnostic obstacles that dermatopathologists encounter. There is nothing quite so aggravating for the clinician (and the patient) as to be informed that a second biopsy will be necessary because of these deficiencies, adding additional expense, time, and anxiety to the situation.

As an example, it is well known that malignant hematolymphoid proliferations and certain metastatic carcinomas are composed of extremely fragile cells that are exquisitely susceptible to the compressive or shearing effects of some biopsies.[2] Moreover, it is probable that several cubic millimeters of tissue will be necessary for the complete pathologic characterization of such lesions. Hence, a small shave or punch biopsy specimen would be predictably unsuitable in these circumstances. When in doubt, the clinician should contact the pathologist *before* that procedure is done and inquire about recommended handling of the tissue sample and its minimally acceptable size based on the likely diagnostic possibilities.

Other procedures causing reproducibly detrimental physical effects on cutaneous specimens are electrocautery and laser excision. These methods are used widely because of their ease of performance and the limitation of *surrounding* tissue damage. Nonetheless, *lesional* cells in the specimen are often rendered unrecognizable because of widespread thermal coagulation, precluding histologic interpretation altogether. It should therefore be obvious that extensive cauterizing techniques must be avoided for diagnostic purposes.

Several adjunctive pathologic studies (see below) require specimens that have been handled in a special manner (Table 2-1). Again, they can be obtained prospectively following preprocedural consultation with laboratory personnel.

Table 2-1. Specimen Processing in Dermatopathology

Pathologic Technique	Recommended Fixative	Processing Time	Comments
Conventional histology	NBF or FA[a]	1 day	Tissue should be sectioned at 2–3 mm for good fixation
Immunohistology	NBF or FA[b]	2–3 days	Technique can be applied to frozen or fixed sections
Electron microscopy	2% Phosphate-buffered glutaraldehyde	3–4 days	Tissue must be minced into 1- or 2-mm cubes
Immunofluorescence	None, if tissue is flash frozen; 95% ethanol or acetone for touch-preparations; Michel's medium for transportation	1–2 days	Tissue can be held in Michel's medium for up to 48 Koans; frozen tissue must be kept at −70°C until use
In situ hybridization	NBF or FA for DNA studies; frozen tissue preferred for RNA studies	1 week	DNA studies can be done on frozen or fixed tissue

Abbreviations: NBF, neutral buffered 10% formalin; FA, NBF-ethanol (50:50).
[a] Tissue for routine histology can be fixed in B5 or Bouin's solutions to improve nuclear morphology, but these preservatives require special processing and compromise immunohistology.
[b] Certain tissue antigens (e.g., light chain immunoglobulins) are detectable only by frozen section immunohistochemistry.

IDENTIFICATION AND ORIENTATION OF THE BIOPSY SPECIMEN

There is nothing quite so exasperating for the pathologist as to receive a specimen that is unoriented and for which no anatomic location is given on the request form for pathologic examination. A lack of meaningful clinical history or a failure to list potential clinical diagnoses often compounds such omissions. These problems usually cannot be solved by the dermatopathologist; they typically require a laboratory visit by, or a telephone conversation with, the responsible physician. In many instances, it would be medicolegally dangerous to attempt a morphologic interpretation in the absence of such information, and this practice is inadvisable. On occasion, a specimen may be received that is so poorly labeled that the identity of the patient is in question. Such a submission should never be accepted by the laboratory unless the clinician is willing to provide written documentation verifying its origin and to accepting exclusive medicolegal responsibility for its interpretation.

If a skin lesion is a suspected malignancy for which a diagnostic biopsy is also intended to be a complete excision, the clinician should provide some means of identifying the superior, inferior, medial, and lateral borders of the tissue sample. This can be accomplished by attaching sutures of differing lengths or types to the specimen and sending a corresponding "map" of the tissue to the laboratory along with the dermatopathology request form.[3] Alternatively, indelible (e.g., tattoo) ink of various colors can be affixed to the borders of the specimen and identified accordingly. As a minimal requirement—for example, in very small excisional biopsies—at least one pole of an elliptical or circular tissue fragment should be labeled by such means. Punch biopsies and shaves are seldom oriented.

The clinician should be discouraged from attempting to prospect the specimen further before it is examined by the pathologist, except in very well-defined settings. When they are improperly performed, transections of ellipses and bisections of punch biopsy samples often confound subsequent orientation steps and may mechanically damage the lesion that is intended for study. The only acceptable reason for undertaking further clinical manipulation of the tissue sample is that of preparing cellular "touch" preparations in examples of suspected hematolymphoid disease. The latter can be obtained if the operator bisects a lesion at its bulkiest point and touches the cut surface of the tissue gently to glass slides in a serial fashion[2] (Fig. 2-1). When this is done, special care should be taken subsequently to orient both halves of the resulting two-part specimen for the pathologist. Moreover, all air-dried or fixed touch preparations must be labeled with the patient's name, date of birth, and the date on which the procedure was performed.

PREPARATION OF FROZEN SECTIONS

The widespread use of the Mohs chemosurgical technique in dermatology has made the interpretation of frozen tissue sections an important facet of this specialty.[4] Most Mohs surgeons are well trained in the procedural aspects of the frozen section (FS) method. However, these are reviewed briefly in this section for the benefit of other practitioners.

The purpose of obtaining FS examination is twofold; it may be used either to secure a rapid diagnosis for a lesion with unknown histologic attributes or to confirm that margins of excision are uninvolved by the pathologic process in question. Because of the potential distortion of morphologic detail that this procedure may induce, the first of the cited applications is not one that should be used frequently. With respect to the analysis of excisional margins, the operator must be certain to supervise the orientation and labeling of all specimens, as outlined above. This makes the availability of indelible ink an absolute requirement in the Mohs laboratory.[5]

Following such steps, one must be certain that the tissue sample is small enough to ensure rapid and uniform freezing and ease of sectioning with the cryomicrotome ("cryostat"). The specimen is usually placed in a small pool of gelatinous, water-soluble mounting medium (e.g., Cryogel) that has been applied to a precooled Teflon or metal "chuck." After making sure that the tissue is properly oriented on the flat surface of the chuck, it is then totally covered with additional mounting medium, fashioned into a circular pledget. Next the chuck is placed on the freezing plate in the cryostat. It must be recognized that the metal cooling "plates," which are incorporated into many cryostats, produce a slow freeze and therefore significant ice crystal distortion. Some degree of freeze artifact is present in all frozen sections, and we learn to interpret through the artifact. Little artifact is produced if the chuck is immersed in a bath of isopentane suspended in an outer container of liquid nitrogen. These devices are available commercially, and they allow for virtually instantaneous freezing of the mounting medium with minimization of ice crystal formation. The latter eventuality is undesirable, because entrapment of ice in the specimen (caused by slowly decreasing temperature) will cause significant microanatomic distortion (Fig. 2-1) and may interfere with microscopic interpretation.

The microtome in any cryostat must be affixed in such a manner that uniform sections of reproducible thickness (approximately 10 μm) can be prepared. Regular maintenance regarding the sharpness and integrity of microtomy blades is essential to this process. After "facing" the frozen block with the blade to obtain a smooth, flat tissue surface the operator cuts a section that can be kept flat by manipulation with a camel-hair brush. These are then apposed to an acid-cleaned glass slide that has been kept at ambient temperature, causing the tissue to adhere quickly. To eliminate concerns about the subsequent loosening of this bond, slides that have been pre-coated with albumin, poly-L-lysine, or a chrome-alum gel may be utilized.[6]

Most FS laboratories employ a brief (30 to 60 second) fixation step immediately after mounted sections are prepared, in Copland jars containing 95% ethanol. The slides may then be stained with hematoxylin and eosin (H&E), a "polychromatic" or metachromatic reagent such as methylene blue, or other reagents. Following dehydration in graded alcohols and xylene, a mounting medium (e.g., Permount) is placed over the tissue, and a glass coverslip is applied. The addition of a few drops of xylene to the mounting medium will slightly lessen its viscosity and help to prevent the entrapment of air bubbles under the coverslip.

If the surgeon wishes to keep some unstained frozen sections for future studies, such as those involving immunohistochemistry, one may remove slides from the alcohol fixative and place them promptly in a –20° or –70°C freezer. They can be kept in such devices indefinitely for further analysis.

Specific problems connected with poor microtomy technique are considered subsequently in this discussion. However, the most common difficulty seen in the FS area can be ascribed to improper calibration of the cutting interval between successive sections. Overly thick sections may result in consumption of the tissue before a suitable slide is obtained for microscopic examination; by contrast, it is extremely hard to obtain very thin sections without causing them to fold on themselves or shred. Thus, it is imperative that the cryostat be checked frequently to make certain that it is set up properly from a technical viewpoint. There is no substitute for practice and experience on the part of the operator with regard to procurement of optimal FS preparations. Tissue sectioning is as much art as science. The labeling of specimens subjected to FS examination should be no different than that of other tissue samples. The remnant tissue should

Figure 2-1. Severity of damage that can be produced by freezing. This freeze artifact is seen in skeletal muscle as small holes representing the formation of ice crystals. Similar damage is produced by freezing in smooth muscle, epidermis, and tumor cells. (H&E, × 100.)

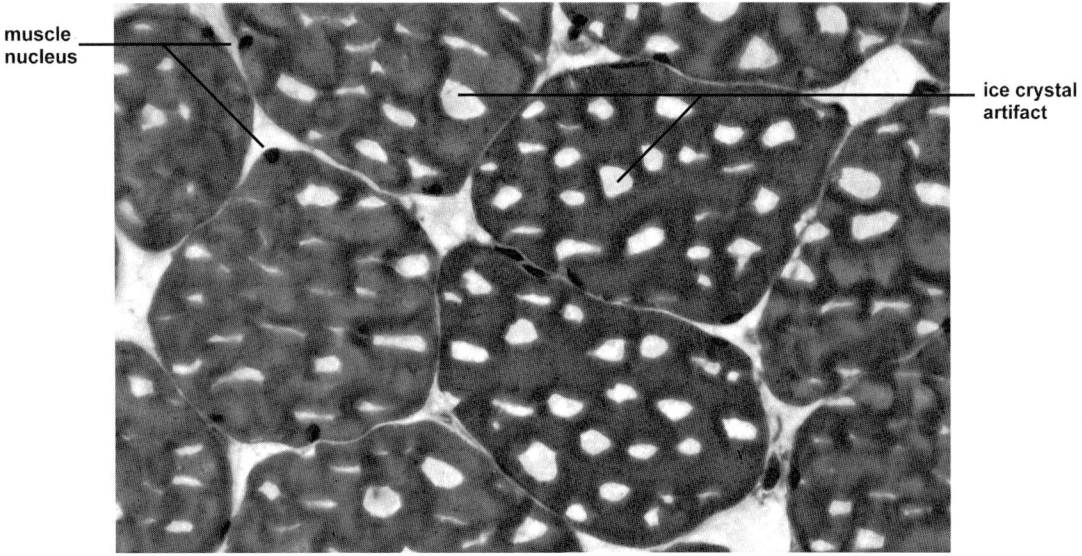

be placed in a plastic cassette that is suitably labeled with the accession number of the case and/or patient name and kept together with corresponding paperwork for transmittal to the histology laboratory. Under no circumstances should unlabeled frozen tissue be allowed to accrue in the FS laboratory, lest disastrous errors in identification occur.

FIXATION OF BIOPSY SPECIMENS

Questions often asked of the pathologist concern the choice of one fixative solution over another for the preservation of various cutaneous specimens. There is no "universal" fixative in dermatopathology, because skin samples may be used for an ever growing number of investigative analyses, many of which demand that special processing measures be applied in order to procure optimal results. Selected immunohistologic studies, electron microscopy, and genotypic assessment represent three advanced modalities of pathologic evaluation that are associated with specific fixation requirements. Laboratory specialists are continuing to develop procedural modifications to lessen the need for such provisions, but they do still exist.

In the ideal situation, it would be best to submit all skin biopsies in their fresh state in physiologic saline solution and for the pathologist to subdivide these specimens into several parts for diagnostic eventualities. Nevertheless, this is seldom practical for two main reasons. First, outpatient specimens are commonly submitted over long distances from the dermatopathology laboratory, increasing the likelihood that unfixed tissue will undergo autolysis before received. Second, cutaneous biopsies are rarely generous in size, making judiciousness in the selection of special studies an important point. The latter issue again emphasizes the wisdom of preprocedural consultation with the pathologist if unconventional evaluations are desired.

In the great majority of cases, the clinician requesting histologic examination of a skin biopsy is interested in a "traditional" interpretation based on microscopic findings as seen with the H&E stains. With this stipulation in mind, most laboratories have advocated the use of formalin as the fixative of choice. Nonetheless, the following sections briefly review the chemical characteristics of preservative solutions in a broader sense so that exceptions to the above-cited situation may be addressed.

General Considerations

The preservative effects of certain chemicals have been recognized for thousands of years, dating back to the ancient Egyptians. On an empiric basis, therefore, various fixatives have been employed to preclude bacterially mediated putrefaction of human tissues since the inception of pathology as a discipline.

In the past century, detailed studies of these agents have elucidated the probable mechanisms responsible for these beneficial effects.[7–10] In addition to antibacterial effects, fixatives also enhance the differences in refractive indices between dissimilar tissue constituents, allowing for greater resolution with light microscopy. Moreover, they augment the affinity that chemical dyes have for particular cellular elements. It is now known that chemical fixatives can be divided into two broad categories—coagulating and noncoagulating—with respect to their effects on proteins, which form the framework of virtually all cells.

Further subdivision into aqueous and nonaqueous agents, as well as additive or nonadditive preservatives, is also possible.[11]

Specific Fixatives

Formalin

Formalin represents a 37% to 40% aqueous solution of formaldehyde, the latter of which is marketed commercially in the United States. Because the former reagent is characteristically used at a 10% dilution, the final formaldehyde concentration is 3.7% to 4%. Various other chemicals have been added to formalin to alter its stability and preservative capabilities, including calcium chloride, calcium carbonate, ammonium bromide, sodium chloride, sodium phosphate, sodium hydroxide, and absolute ethyl alcohol. Among these mixtures, that consist of formalin, distilled water, and monobasic/dibasic sodium phosphate is the most widely employed and is known as *10% neutral buffered formalin* (NBF). *Paraformaldehyde* is a polymerized form of formaldehyde admixed with methanol; it is generally employed as a fixative for specialized immunohistologic procedures, particularly when combined with periodate and lysine (the "PLP" solution).[12]

Although it is a general-purpose fixative and yields good morphologic detail when prepared properly, NBF does have some disadvantages in tissue pathology. First, any solution containing formaldehyde is potentially carcinogenic, and levels of formalin vapor in the ambient air of the laboratory must be measured regularly by governmental regulation. The maximum permissible exposure limit for any individual employee is 1 part per million over an 8-hour period, as established by the Occupational Safety and Health Administration.[13] Second, poorly prepared NBF, which has been buffered erroneously and has a pH outside of the physiologic range, may cause unwanted precipitates of "black acid hematin pigment" in tissue sections. The latter has a dark particulate appearance and may simulate microorganisms on a histologic slide. These two possibilities can be distinguished through the use of polarization microscopy, because hematin pigment is birefringent whereas microorganisms are not.[11] Third, NBF that is exposed to ambient air for prolonged periods (as with large "batches" that are diluted for use in the gross laboratory) will develop high levels of formic acid. The latter is detrimental to protein substructure and may accentuate the formation of methylol bonds between polypeptides. This effect can "mask" proteinaceous epitomes that correspond to the targets of immunohistologic antibody reagents.[14] Finally formalin has a limited capacity for tissue penetration, 1 mm/h, and specimens fixed in it must not be too thick or autolysis will outpace fixation. Despite these drawbacks, formalin is inexpensive and widely available, and it is therefore ubiquitously employed as the fixative of choice for clinical specimens. Some laboratories prefer to use NBF-ethanol (mixed in equal volumes), because it affords a greater degree of tissue penetration than formalin alone.

B5, Zenker's and Helly's Solutions

B5, Zenker's, and Helly's solutions were introduced because of their superiority over NBF in the preservation of nuclear detail.[7,8] They are fixatives based on the inclusion of mercuric chloride, with or without sodium acetate, potassium dichromate, sodium sulfate, acetic acid, and formaldehyde as additional constituents. Because of the excellent morphologic detail that is achievable with these solutions, many laboratories prefer them for the routine preparation of H&E-stained sections. Nevertheless, there are three distinct disadvantages of B5, Zenker's, or Helly's reagents compared with NBF. Tissue sections must be removed from the former three fixatives after no more than 8 hours and placed into 70% ethanol; if this is not done, specimens will become extremely brittle and virtually impossible to section.[11] Also, the presence of mercuric chloride will cause deposition of pigment in microscopic preparations, which must be removed with iodine before final staining procedures are done. Finally mercury-based solutions are powerful coagulating agents and therefore damage many cytoplasmic proteins. This effect commonly renders tissue sections unsuitable for a variety of immunohistochemical studies.[15]

Bouin's Solution

Bouin's fixative is also based on formaldehyde as a major component, together with picric and acetic acids in aqueous solution. Like B5, this reagent affords excellent preservation of nuclear morphology, but suffers from the same failings pertaining to brittleness of tissue, pigment deposition, and adverse effects on cytoplasmic polypeptides. In addition, Bouin's-fixed specimens acquire a yellow color (because of the effects of picric acid) that must be removed by post fixation washing in alcohol and lithium carbonate. Bouin's fixative is preferred for visualization of delicate mesenchymal tissues because of its superior differentiating abilities in regard to these elements.[11] Accordingly, some "stromal" special stains (such as the Masson trichrome method [see below]) are best performed on specimens preserved in this solution.

Acetone and Alcohols

Acetone and alcohols are rapidly acting fixatives with good penetration of tissue. They also afford better preservation of some cytoplasmic enzymes than formaldehyde-based solutions do in paraffin sections. However, two major disadvantages attend the use of these organic reagents. They cause striking shrinkage of tissue because of their dehydrating effects, thereby altering morphologic details appreciably. Also, acetone and methyl or ethyl alcohols are relatively expensive, and they require special storage and inventory procedures because of possible abuse by laboratory workers as inebriants. In current practice, these agents are usually applied only in the fixation of touch preparations and are not commonly used in the processing of biopsy specimens. Similar comments apply to Carnoy's solution, which consists of ethyl alcohol, chloroform, and acetic acid.

Decalcifying Solutions

Decalcification of tissue specimens may be required in dermatopathology because of obvious foci of calcium salts, as suggested by clinical findings or difficulty in performing the biopsy procedure. In these circumstances, two main methods exist for the removal of such minerals from the specimen before sectioning can occur. One employs simple acids (hydrochloric or nitric) to solubilize calcium deposits, while the other uses chelating agents (ethylenediaminetetraacetic acid [EDTA]) to accomplish this task. The second of these methods is much "gentler" and does not cause the loss of microscopic detail that acid decalcification may incur. Fixation is allowed to progress in concert with decalcification with both acidic or EDTA reagents, because they are commercially marketed as mixed solutions containing formaldehyde.

Glutaraldehyde

Glutaraldehyde is similar in chemical activity to formaldehyde; both cause cross-linkage of proteins in tissue.[7] However, glutaraldehyde penetrates specimens very slowly, making the size of the tissue sample a critical determinant of fixation with this reagent. Moreover, 2% to 4% glutaraldehyde (representing the usual working concentration) has a propensity to cause brittleness of specimens that are immersed in it for more than 2 to 3 hours; transfer to a buffer solution is absolutely necessary after this point. For these reasons, among others, glutaraldehyde is not used often for the preservation of biopsy samples that are intended for light microscopy. However, it is the preferred fixative for electron microscopy, wherein specimens are very small and limited "hardening" of tissue may actually be morphologically advantageous.

Other Factors Influencing Fixation

There are several considerations in the fixation of tissue, including temperature, size of the sample, the volume ratio of tissue to fixative solution, the duration of fixation, and the pH of the solution. Recently, the rapid but controlled elevation of temperature with microwave ovens has been used as an independent means of fixation by coagulation of tissue proteins. Surprisingly, this process appears to have little adverse effect on staining characteristics, even with immunohistologic methods. However, it must be emphasized that careful control is the key to thermal fixation; overheating may completely destroy the specimen if it is allowed to reach an extreme level (e.g., over 65°C). In a more conventional context, there are really no compelling reasons to employ fixative solutions at one temperature versus another.

Specimen size is, by contrast, a potentially crucial factor affecting quality of fixation, and this determinant goes hand in hand with the volumetric relationship between a tissue sample and the solution in which it is immersed. Large, extremely thick specimens will be inadequately penetrated by most fixatives, allowing autolysis to proceed unchecked in their central areas. This results in eventual loss of the unfixed foci during microtomy, yielding microscopic sections that resemble doughnuts (Fig. 2-2). Because penetration is facilitated by minor thermal or mechanical currents in the fixative solution, large specimens that are covered with an inadequate volume of preservative will predictably be underfixed. An experienced histotechnologist typically detects this problem on attempting microtomy of the tissue and will "run the specimen back" for more prolonged fix-

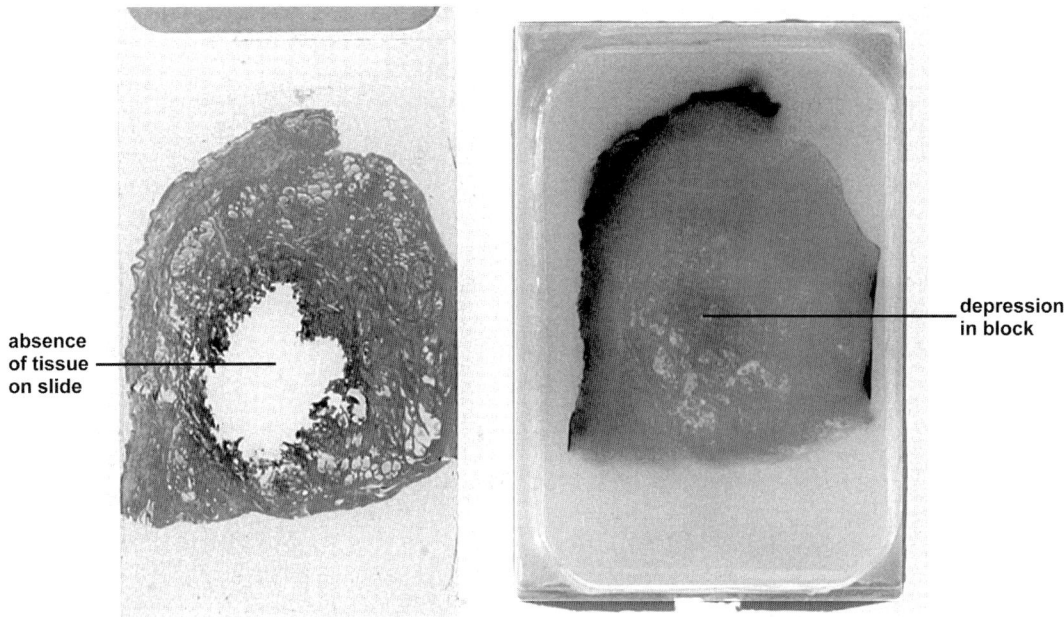

absence
of tissue
on slide

depression
in block

Figure 2-2. A block and the resulting slide from tissue that was too thick for processing. Slices of tissue that are greater than 2 to 3 mm will result in paraffin tissue blocks that are collapsed in the middle. This occurs because the time cycle was not adequate for the solutions to infiltrate into the thick tissue. The resulting slide also has a hole in the middle where the tissue was improperly processed. The tissue illustrated is a portion of prostate gland, but the same artifact commonly occurs with subcutaneous adipose tissue.

ation and reprocessing. However, this consumes additional time and should be unnecessary. There is a maximum recommended period of fixation with several preservatives over which unwanted changes reproducibly occur in tissue biochemistry. Specimens that are immersed in the most commonly used preservative NBF, should ideally be processed for immunohistochemistry within 8 to 12 hours.[15]

The pH of fixatives is not critical for light microscopy, except that certain unwanted pigmentary deposits may be seen with unduly acidic preservatives. Nonetheless, hyperacidity is extremely detrimental to cellular ultrastructure, and also to the maintenance of tissue antigenicity.[11–15] For these reasons, it would be wise to control pH within the physiologic range during fixation in the event that electron microscopy or immunohistology is necessary diagnostically.

Tissue Processing and Preparation of Microscopic Sections

Because most commonly employed fixatives are aqueous in nature, the next step in tissue processing is usually that of dehydration and "clearing" (removal of all water from the specimen). Graded solutions of ethanol are used for this purpose, and these must be changed frequently to maintain their desiccating properties. A variety of clearing agents are available, but the most common are xylene and limonene derivatives. In likeness to the alcohols, such reagents may be contaminated by water with repeated use and should be monitored closely for this problem.

Xylene is inexpensive and does not leave a residue on glassware or other instrument parts in the histology laboratory. In light of these virtues, it is the most popular clearing agent. Xylene fumes are potentially toxic to technologists, making careful storage, controlled disposal, and environmental monitoring mandatory. In addition, xylene may damage the protein substructure of certain fragile tissue antigens.[15] Limonene-type clearing agents are derived from plants and are biodegradable. They have a strong odor—like that of lemons or oranges—that is alternatively perceived as pleasant or noxious by various technologists. Other disadvantages of limonenes are that they leave a residue on mechanical tissue processors and may sometimes interfere with the adherence of tissue sections to glass slides. Moreover, the microtomy of specimens that have been cleared in limonenes is said to be much easier than that encountered with xylene.[11]

In the relatively early days of histotechnology, all dehydration and clearing steps were done by hand. Over the past 35 years, however, a variety of automatic tissue processors have been engineered and marketed. These are used widely at present and may be divided into two main groups, "open" and "closed." Open processors mechanically transfer baskets containing tissue cassettes from one "station" (chemical bath) to another on a computer-driven schedule. The latter may be altered by the operator to change the time of dehydration, clearing, or other steps. Closed instruments vary the solutions to which each specimen basket is exposed by pumping chemicals in and out of fixed chambers, again according to a programmed schedule. In other words, open processors move specimens, whereas closed processors move chemical solutions.

Each of these two types of instruments has advantages and disadvantages. Open processors show a low incidence of reagent contamination from one station to another, but they are subject to the mechanical "hangup" of specimen baskets in transit. Closed processors do not suffer from the latter drawback, but they are subject to chemical carryover from one reagent pumping step to another. This potentially compromises the dehydration-clearing sequence. On balance, individual experience on the part of technologists and pathologists ultimately determines which type of processor will be chosen.

EMBEDDING AND SECTIONING OF BIOPSY SPECIMENS

The final stations in any tissue processor infiltrate all specimens with paraffin or another wax-based embedding medium. Thereafter, the technologist removes each biopsy (one at a time) from its metal or plastic cassette and proceeds to embed it in a rectangle of additional liquid wax, with attention to the proper orientation of the tissue sample. The pathologist may direct this process by notching or inking one or several surfaces of the specimen or providing a "map" in accompanying paperwork that indicates whether these should be placed face-down or face-up. Such provisions are usually necessary only with large pieces of tissue. In other cases, technologists accustomed to handling skin biopsies will, as a matter of routine, orient the epidermis perpendicularly to the bottom of the cassette mold and facing one of its long sides (Fig. 2-3).

The embedding step is a potential source of great irritation to the pathologist if it is done improperly. With few exceptions, cutaneous specimens that are oriented improperly (e.g., with the skin surface facing the bottom of the cassette) cannot be interpreted microscopically, necessitating that the block be remelted and re-embedded. This takes time and, in the process of facing the poorly oriented specimen for preparation of initial sections, valuable tissue may be lost. Another advisable tenet concerns the orientation of the epidermis within any given block at the embedding step. All fragments of each specimen should be placed in wax in such a way that the microtome blade will first meet the *dermis* when the paraffin block is cut and, as far as possible, so that the skin surface is parallel to the edge of the blade. These provisions go a long way toward avoiding microtomy artifacts.[16]

To circumvent embedding difficulties, some pathologists have taken to *pre*-embedding small skin biopsies in agar before they are put in cassettes for fixation. This does ensure proper orientation, but agar will not "fix" in the same manner that tissue does, nor will it respond similarly to dehydration, clearing, and infiltration by wax. All of these factors may cause the tissue to "pop" free of the surrounding agar after embedding and during tissue sectioning, defeating the purpose of the agar impregnation step altogether.

Paraffin is still the most widely used embedding medium, but some laboratories have opted to employ Carbowax as a substitute. The latter compound is a water-soluble wax, making dehydration and clearing of the tissue unnecessary and allowing for direct infiltration of formalin-fixed tissue with embedding medium in the tissue processor.[11] This element of simplicity is attractive, but Carbowax has drawbacks. One concerns the dissolution of the embedding medium when microtomized tissue "ribbons" are placed in a water bath prior to mounting them on glass slides. This unwanted eventuality makes it difficult for the technologist to keep the tissue section flat, resulting in undesirable folds in the final stained slide. Furthermore, there are irregularities in antigen preservation when Carbowax-embedded tissues are studied immunohistologically. The temperature of paraffin or Carbowax stations in the tissue processor, and at the embedding center, must be monitored closely. Overheating the wax will cause unwanted thermal artifacts in the tissue and compromise its cellular detail. Excessively cool wax fails to infiltrate the specimens adequately.

Another class of embedding compounds that is presently in

Figure 2-3. Note that the epidermis is oriented perpendicular to the long axis of the tissue block. This is the proper orientation for cutting skin and results in much better sections than if oriented otherwise.

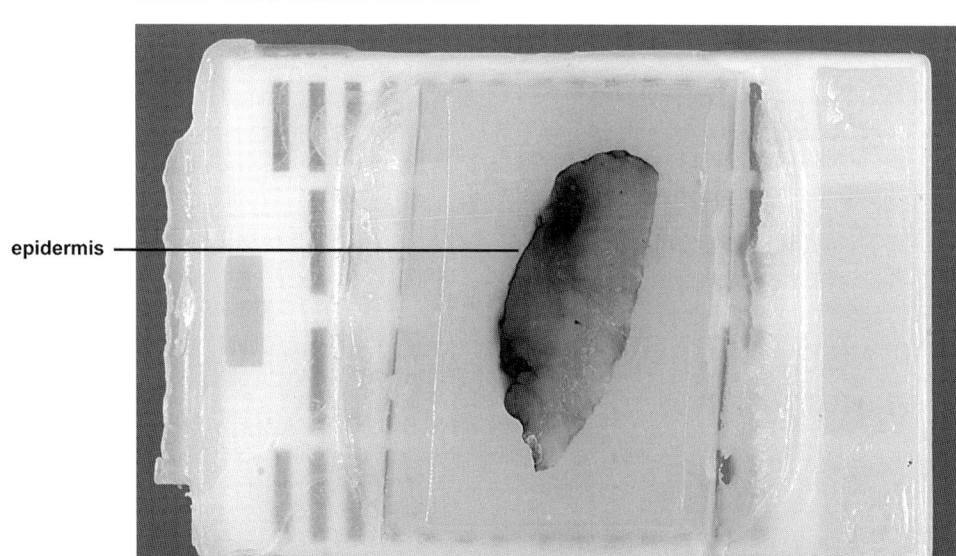

vogue in some centers is represented by polymeric plastic resins such as glycol methacrylate or epoxy. Disadvantages of these compounds include the necessity of cutting corresponding tissue sections with a glass or diamond knife microtome and the requirement for a "transitional fluid," such as propylene oxide, to embed the tissue after dehydration and clearing.[11] Moreover, plastic sections are difficult to stain with the same intensity as that seen in paraffin-embedded preparations. The main advantage of plastic media is that extremely thin, flat sections may be prepared by experienced microtomists, providing exquisite cellular detail. In addition, some enzyme-histochemical staining methods that otherwise require the use of frozen sections are possible with specimens embedded in epoxy or glycol methacrylate.

Histomicrotomy is a seemingly straightforward process, representing the cutting of serial paraffin-embedded sections with a tissue microtome. Nevertheless, this technique has many hidden traps that relate to the proper maintenance, calibration, and orientation of cutting blades; preparation of paraffin blocks; and dexterity of the technologist. Microtome blades that are dull or nicked will produce "chatter" or "venetian blind" artifacts in tissue sections. In addition, the "clearance angle" (between the tissue block and the microtome knife) is crucial to good technique. It should approximate 3 to 8 degrees. If the angle is too narrow, alternately thick and thin sections are cut, or they are folded on themselves.[17–19] An excessive clearance angle causes chattered or otherwise hideous sections and may preclude the ability of the technologist to obtain a tissue ribbon. Even worse are the effects of loose microtome blades or tissue blocks in the microtome chuck. These deficiencies may shatter the paraffin block entirely or deeply groove the tissue specimen. A block that is mounted crookedly in the microtome chuck will produce irregular ribbons or cause individual sections in the ribbon to break free from one another.

Regardless of whether one uses paraffin or carbowax as an embedding medium, there is still a need to refrigerate tissue blocks before microtomy is attempted. This step hardens the wax slightly and allows for crisp sections to be cut. Warm blocks will yield wrinkled ribbons or cause successive sections to anneal to one another. In addition, failure to moisten the surface of blocked tissue suitably before cutting it yields an excessive number of knife marks or fragmented sections. The technologist can simply rub a wet finger over the block several times prior to microtomy, if the specimen is small. If it is large, and particularly if the tissue is heavily cornified, a wet piece of cloth or cotton soaked in 5% ammonium hydroxide may be applied for 2 or 3 minutes to rehydrate the tissue face.[17]

Another problem that is sometimes seen at this step is the tendency for ribbons to "fly" onto the knife blade. This is the result of static electricity between the wax or tissue and the metal blade and also may be avoided by slightly moistening the knife and the block surface before each ribbon is prepared.

MOUNTING OF TISSUE SECTIONS

The wax ribbon of serial tissue sections can be removed from the microtome knife as it is cut by using a wooden tongue-depressor blade. In this process, the operator exerts slight traction on the end of the ribbon, stretching it gradually over the wooden blade, and subsequently depositing it on the surface of a warm water bath at the cutting station. The temperature of such flotation devices should be kept at 5° to 10°C below the melting point of the embedding wax. If it is too hot, desiccated-looking sections will result; by contrast, cool flotation baths produce excessive wrinkling of the tissue.

To facilitate the process of obtaining a smooth, unwrinkled, paraffinized ribbon of tissue, it can be stretched by slight traction on its ends while floating in the warm water bath. Also, adding a few milliliters of ethyl alcohol to the water is beneficial in this regard. The ribbon must not be left in the bath for more than 1 or 2 minutes, or spurious overhydration of the tissue will be produced. This effect simulates the appearance of edema fluid microscopically.[16] Because tissue sections do not adhere well to untreated glass slides, a bonding agent also must be a component of the water bath. Elmer's glue, albumin, and poly-L-lysine are all suitable additives of this type.

One of the most dangerous of all mistakes in the histology laboratory can take place when mounting sections from flotation baths. Friable tissue may "shed" small fragments that float free on the surface of the water, and these may be inadvertently picked up when mounting slides from subsequently processed, unrelated cases. Derisively known as "floaters," these stray pieces of tissue commonly cause agonizing interpretative problems for the pathologist. For example, it is not difficult to envision a small piece of a malignant melanoma that may find its way onto slides of a melanocytic nevus, a ribbon of which is mounted subsequently in the same water bath. Technologists must be impressed with the tremendous medicolegal liabilities that such a mistake incurs, and they must routinely skim, or otherwise clear, the surface of the water bath between cases. An alternative source of floater-type artifacts is the "tongue blade metastasis," wherein tissue adheres to a wooden applicator stick that is used to float successively prepared ribbons from two different cases.[11]

With respect to optimizing the cost of slide preparation, we recommend that as many individual sections as possible from the same ribbon be mounted on one slide. It is not difficult for adept technologists to include 10 to 15 cuts of a specimen on each slide, arranged in a serial fashion. Also, in light of the limited size of most cutaneous biopsies, it is advisable to save any unmounted paraffin ribbons (with appropriate identification) from dermatopathology cases for 1 week after they are accessioned. Re-mounts can be prepared from these directly, without the need for further microtomy of the tissue block.

Finally, the identification of tissue sections must be scrupulously maintained throughout the remainder of their sojourn in the histology laboratory. Such a necessity is ensured by having the technologist scratch the case and block numbers onto one end of all mounted glass slides with a diamond knife.

GENERAL STAINING AND COVERSLIPPING PROCEDURES

Once the tissue has been affixed to glass slides, paraffin is removed prior to the staining procedure. This is accomplished by placing the sections in a carrier, heating them to 56°C for at least 1 hour (to evaporate water from the glass slides), and immersing them for 3 to 5 minutes in each of three or four successive containers of a clearing agent (xylene or a limonene derivate [see above]). Most histologic dyes penetrate tissue best if it has been rehydrated; thus, passage of the slides through containers of graded ethanol solutions (absolute, 95%, 70%) and distilled water is necessary before staining can be undertaken. The importance of proper paraffin clearance with regard to final results cannot be overemphasized. If a sizable quantity of wax remains in the sections, dyes will not be able to penetrate them and impregnate constituent tissues.

The majority of diagnostic dermatopathology laboratories employ H&E as the stain of choice for microscopic interpretation. There are two principal procedures for applying these dyes—the progressive method and the regressive technique. The former is usually preferred, and it is characterized by sequential staining with hematoxylin (for roughly 15 minutes) and eosin (for 1 to 3 minutes). These steps are separated by application of ammonia water or lithium carbonate as "bluing" agents for hematoxylin, which is actually a chemical "lake" of hematein and a mordant such as ammonium aluminum sulfate.[20] In addition, copious rinses with water must be ensured after exposure of the tissue to hematoxylin and ammonia or lithium. The progressive H&E method is so named because the technologist can monitor the depth of staining as it develops and terminate each step appropriately. This procedure is desirable because it can compensate for the effects of various fixatives that enhance the uptake of either hematoxylin (formaldehyde, osmium, heavy metals) or eosin (picric acid). Retrogressive H&E staining is a technique wherein tissue is purposefully overimpregnated with hematoxylin and then modified to suit the operator by decolorization with dilute hydrochloric acid. Final results are much more difficult to control in this procedure, and it requires a highly experienced technologist to achieve good nuclear detail in the ultimate product.

With regard to eosin as a "counterstain" for hematoxylin, two points merit further mention. One is that eosin is a "differentiating" stain that dissimilarly impregnates tissues of varying chemical structure and molecular density. As such, it requires the same amount of technical attention as hematoxylin in a progressive H&E method. Different connective tissues should be stained to variable degrees in a properly performed procedure of this type; however, overly rapid passage of sections through ethanol solutions, *after* exposure to eosin, interferes with this effect and should be discouraged. Also some workers prefer to use a *combined* eosin reagent (incorporating such dyes as phloxine or safran) to enhance its differentiating properties.[11]

In addition to the H&E technique, there are many other specialized staining methods that are pertinent to pathologic diagnosis. These are discussed specifically later in this chapter.

Inasmuch as most laboratories use Harris hematoxylin which is insoluble in alcohol the final preparation of H&E-stained microscopic sections involves dehydration in graded alcohols and several changes of a clearing agent. Subsequently, a drop of synthetic mounting medium (such as Permount) is placed over the tissue after blotting away excess clearing solution, and a glass coverslip is affixed. The latter steps sound simple enough, but they actually require some technical finesse. Experienced technologists often dilute the mounting medium slightly with a few drops of clearing agent, and also leave a very small amount of clearing solution on the glass surface surrounding the tissue. These provisions ensure that the mounting medium will dis-

perse evenly under the glass coverslip to the exclusion of entrapped air bubbles. Excess mounting medium must be carefully blotted from the area around the attached coverslip, because it may otherwise diffuse over the surface of the slide. This unwanted phenomenon results in "blobs" of Permount on the coverslips (interfering with microscopy) or on the sides of the glass slides (causing them to stick to other surfaces or to one another). Under no circumstances should newly mounted sections ever be stacked on top of one another or immediately placed in vertical slide boxes or small plastic carriers. These maneuvers make it virtually certain that sections will stick to one another, to plastic surfaces, or to struts in slide boxes, as the mounting medium hardens. The latter process can be accelerated by brief and gentle warming in a drying oven into which forced air is pumped.

With regard to labeling, some laboratories attach gumbacked labels to coverslipped sections on which corresponding case and block numbers are then written or typed. Others prefer to use slides with a frosted area on one end, where these numbers can be written in indelible ink. Whichever procedure is followed, laboratory workers must be certain to check all labels against block designations and diamond knife-etchings on the slides. The crucial nature of this step cannot be overstated in reference to the dermatopathology laboratory, where gross characteristics of differing specimens are of little help in distinguishing one from the other. In other words, nearly all shave samples and 3- or 5-mm punch biopsies look alike when they are stained and mounted. If a mistake occurs that compromises the identity of any given case, the pathologist and responsible clinician should be informed immediately. Such errors commonly result in the need to rebiopsy the patients concerned to avoid potential diagnostic disasters.

SPECIFIC "SPECIAL" HISTOCHEMICAL STAINS

For purposes of differential diagnosis, it is often desirable to evaluate biopsy specimens for their content of such tissue constituents as glycogen, vicinal glycol, glycoproteins, mucosubstances, iron, melanin, calcium, lipofuscin, elastin, collagen, amyloid, muscular proteins, fat, nucleic acids, nucleoproteins, neural elements, specific enzymes, and microorganisms. These moieties comprise the targets of predefined "special" histochemical stains in which the chemical affinities of various biological components for several dyes have been exploited. A comprehensive discussion of the specific reactions involved, the detailed methods behind such stains, and all the circumstances in which they might be applied is clearly beyond the scope of our consideration. However, these topics have been well covered in previous textbooks and review articles to which the interested reader is directed.[11,20–26] General principles and pertinent brief summaries of selected histochemical methods are provided in the following sections.

Glycogen, Glycoproteins, and Mucosubstances

The periodic acid-schiff (PAS) procedure is used to visualize deposits of glycogen in tissue, as well as to label glycoproteins or mucinous cell products that contain vicinal glycol residues.[27] To distinguish between simple glycogen and the latter chemical substances, one usually exposes two serial tissue sections to the

PAS reaction. One of them is, however, modified by prior incubation with diastase or amylase; this step dissolves glycogen but does not interfere with the ability of sugars in glycoproteins or vicinal glycols in mucin to combine with Schiff's reagent and yield a bright red reaction product. Thus, pathologists commonly request that PAS stains be done "with and without" diastase or amylase.

Glycogen is seen in normal skin in the acrosyringia of sweat ducts and in pilar epithelium.[22] The detection of this polysaccharide may be important in the recognition of various cutaneous adnexal tumors, metastatic carcinomas of the skin, and clear cell acanthomas. It also plays a role in the distinction between poorly differentiated epithelial neoplasms (which are potentially PAS positive) and malignant hematopoietic tumors (usually PAS negative) with which they may be confused.

The glycoproteins of greatest interest in the skin are those that are components of basement membranes, together with collagen type IV and laminin. They are well seen with the PAS technique after prior diastase digestion of tissue sections (PAS-D), and thickening of the epidermal basement membrane—as seen in lupus erythematosus and other chronic interface dermatitides—is often spectacularly visualized with this procedure. Characteristic alterations in the basement membranes of papillary dermal blood vessels in porphyria cutanea tarda also are demonstrable by using PAS-D stains.

Mucosubstances that react with PAS-D are commonly called *epithelial mucins* (more appropriately, *glandular* mucins), and they tend to contain sialic acid residues.[28] As one would expect, connective tissue mucins are PAS-D-nonreactive. Hence, this method can be employed to identify selected constituents of the normal skin; apocrine glands are the only structures that produce glandular mucin, whereas dermal ground substance, blood vessels, papillae of anagen hairs, nerves, and intercellular intraepidermal spaces contain stromal mucosubstances. Stains in this category may distinguish cellular proliferations that produce glandular mucin (e.g., adenocarcinomas, Paget's disease) from those that synthesize "stromal" (mucopolysaccharide- or sulfated acid-rich) mucin (e.g., pseudoglandular squamous cell and basal cell carcinomas).[29] One more procedure that is sometimes used to recognize epithelial mucin the *mucicarmine* technique is not as well characterized as PAS-D with regard to its biochemical modus operandi. Nevertheless, staining results with these two methods are largely equivalent (including the color of the reaction product), with the possible exception that mucicarmine is less sensitive.

If a distinction between the nonglandular mucins is desirable, the aldehyde-fuchsin stain (AFS) can be performed along with the PAS-D, colloidal iron, Alcian blue, azure-A, and toluidine blue procedures. If it is done at a pH below 1.0, the AFS yields green-blue positivity in tissues that contain primarily sulfated acid mucosubstances.[11] By contrast, acid mucopolysaccharides such as hyaluronic acid, heparin, and chondroitin/dermatan/keratin sulfates constitute the major components of other stromal mucins.[23] All of these moieties are potentially visualized with colloidal iron or Alcian blue, both of which yield light-blue positivity; azure-A, showing red reactivity; and toluidine blue, producing lavender or purple positivity. A side benefit of toluidine blue is that it can be used to label mast cells in tissue, owing to the presence of heparan sulfate in mastocytic granules.

By manipulating either the tissue or the reaction conditions, further information may be obtained. Prior digestion of sections with hyaluronidase greatly decreases staining of ground substances with both the Alcian blue or colloidal iron procedures. Pretreatment with neuraminidase will abrogate the labeling of sialomucins, but they are intensely stained with the Alcian blue method when it is done in a milieu containing high concentrations of magnesium chloride at pH 2.5.[24] Similarly, decreasing the pH to less than 1 results in preferential Alcian blue staining of sulfated glycosaminoglycans such as heparin or dermatan sulfate, but the same step abolishes the recognition of acid mucopolysaccharides by toluidine blue.[23]

The stromal mucins are important to the diagnosis of several dermatologic diseases. Follicular and focal mucinoses feature the deposition of colloidal iron/Alcian blue-positive mucosubstance in the hair follicles or dermis, respectively. Myxedema, myxoid cysts, and lichen myxedematosus show regional or diffuse increases in the stromal mucin content of the corium. Necrobiotic processes may be separated from one another with the methods presented in this section; the central areas of granulomas in granuloma annulare contain much more hyaluronic acid than do those of necrobiosis lipoidica or rheumatoid nodule.[30] Finally, cutaneous lupus erythematosus, dermatomyositis, and malignant papulosis all may demonstrate the augmentation of dermal stromal mucin.[31]

Another exciting category of histochemical reagents is represented by the lectins; these proteinaceous products of various plants show preferential and differential affinity for particular carbohydrate residues.[32] It is now known that some—such as peanut, soybean, and wheatgerm agglutinins—bind to sulfated or sialated mucins, whereas others (concanavalin A and Lens culinaris agglutinin) do not.[33] In addition, *Ulex europaeus* I agglutinin recognizes poly-L-fucose residues that appear to be integral components of a panendothelial determinant, and they also are seen in adnexal epithelium in patients with blood group O.[34] Very few reports on cutaneous diseases have incorporated lectin histochemistry into the assessment of these processes,[35] but it is anticipated that this situation will change rapidly in the near future.

Amyloid

Amyloid is a peculiar tissue substance that is unique to pathologic conditions. It is principally a fibrillar protein that forms rods of variable length and 7.5 to 10 nm in diameter and that tend to aggregate extracellularly in a "tangled" configuration. A secondary, minor component of amyloid is sulfated proteoglycan, accounting for approximately 10% by weight.[36] It accounts for the fact that amyloid has some chemical similarities to polysaccharides and certain mucosubstances, such as an affinity for iodine and metachromatic labeling with toluidine blue.[11]

Detailed studies on linear amyloid fibrils have shown that they aggregate in "β-pleated sheets" as seen by x-ray crystallography.[36] This property has been exploited histopathologically, together with dyes that preferentially impregnate amyloid protein and proteoglycan. The latter stains, such as Congo red, Sirius red, Lieb's crystal violet, and thioflavine-T, are used to impart a red, magenta, or fluorescent yellow-green color to amyloid deposits, respectively. Polarization microscopy of sections labeled with Congo red shows a characteristic "apple green" dichroism in amyloid deposits because of its physicochemical attributes.

There are advantages and disadvantages to some of the above-cited methods. Sections stained with Congo red must be meticulously prepared at a thickness of 8 to 10 μm; if they are too thin or thick, the amyloid deposits will be a faint red or yellow on polarization rather than apple-green. We have also noticed that the use of unmatched polarizing microscopic lenses may cause similar problems. Lieb's stain is soluble in organic compounds, necessitating that sections cannot be coverslipped in a conventional fashion. Glycerol has been employed as a mounting medium, but it allows for the diffusion of crystal violet from the amyloid with the passage of time. Modified Apathy's medium (a mixture of acacia, cane sugar, water, sodium chloride, and thymol) is a suitable alternative, as are polymeric compounds such as Crystal Mount (BioMeda Laboratories).[11] As stated above, the thioflavine-T procedure must be interpreted by fluorescence microscopy and is therefore not widely used. Regardless of which specific type of amyloid one encounters in an individual case, all of them show nearly identical staining properties.[36]

Minerals and Pigments

There are a number of minerals and pigments in tissue that have dermatopathologic relevance. These can be localized and identified with histochemical methods.

Iron is detected with Perl's reaction, also known as the Prussian blue procedure. When loosely complexed with protein, ferric ions will combine with acidified potassium ferrocyanide to yield a deep-blue product that is insoluble.[20] Because of potential confusion with structures that hematoxylin may impregnate, Prussian blue tissue sections are counterstained with nuclear fast red.

Melanin is derived from tyrosine-containing compounds, and it is typically bound to protein in tissue. This pigment is capable of reducing silver nitrate solutions to metallic silver, which is deposited in tissue sections as a black precipitate in the Fontana-Masson technique.[24] Alternatively, solutions containing ferrous ions can be used to form complexes with melanin, and these are subsequently detectable as a blue product with the Turnbull reaction.[11] In the assessment of heavily melaninized cutaneous lesions, it is sometimes necessary to bleach the pigment to allow for evaluation of cellular detail. This can be accomplished by treating tissue sections with 10% hydrogen peroxide for 1 to 2 days or with 0.25% potassium permanganate for 1 to 4 hours, followed by 1% oxalic acid.[24] Lastly, one can capitalize on knowledge of the biochemical pathway whereby melanin is formed by melanocytes in order to visualize nonpigmented cells of this type. The DOPA reaction involves the exposure of tissue sections to a dilute solution of 3,4-dihydroxyphenylalanine. Melanocytes that contain DOPA oxidase will convert this compound to melanin, which may then be detected by one of the above-cited methods. Unfortunately, the DOPA reaction mandates the use of frozen sections, inasmuch as melanocytic enzymes are largely inactivated by routine tissue processing.[37]

Calcium typically is hematoxylinophilic on H&E stains. To confirm its presence definitively in such conditions as calcinosis cutis and pseudoxanthoma elasticum, one of two procedures should be used—either the von Kossa technique or the alizarin red method.[21] The first of these employs a solution of silver nitrate; calcium carbonate will combine with the latter compound to form silver carbonate, which, on exposure to ultraviolet light or sunlight, is reduced to elemental silver in a black precipitate. Unfortunately, formalin pigment will produce an identical result. This problem makes the alizarin red technique, wherein the dye chelates directly with calcium ions to form an orange-red complex, preferred. Alizarin red-stained sections are not counterstained, and the resulting calcium complexes show birefringence on polarization microscopy.[11]

Uric acid deposits are seen in the skin in gouty tophi. These are difficult to visualize in sections that are fixed with aqueous solutions, because urates are dissolved in the course of routine processing. Alcohol-fixed tissues are therefore best used in this context. Uric acid reduces the silver ions in a 5% silver nitrate solution to their metallic form, giving a black precipitate over the gouty deposits.[26] When employed as a part of the Gomori methenamine silver procedure, this reaction is useful diagnostically. Sections are counterstained with Light Green solution.

Lipids

Lipids in the skin and its adnexae may be of diagnostic importance in several settings. For example, it may be desirable to confirm the biochemical nature of apparent xanthomas, and the granulomas of necrobiosis lipoidica characteristically contain a central area of lipid deposition.[30] Cholesterol emboli may affect the skin by causing microinfarction of it, and sebaceous tumors are definitively identified by the demonstration of cytoplasmic fat in the neoplastic cells.

An inviolate requirement for visualization of lipids in clinical specimens is that frozen tissue, or, at the very least, unembedded formalin-fixed tissue must be available for study.[29] This is because the alcoholic and clearing agent steps in tissue processors otherwise dissolve all fat before sections are prepared for microscopic analysis.

Three major staining techniques are applicable to this problem. The oil red O and Sudan black B methods utilize dyes that are miscible in fat and therefore impregnate it.[24] These yield red and black products, respectively, as their names suggest. The third procedure is probably the best from a technical perspective, because it provides microscopic preparations of higher quality. This is the osmium tetroxide stain with periodic acid as a differentiating agent, wherein osmium fixes lipids and stains them black. Because this chemical is insoluble in organic compounds, frozen tissues labeled with 1% osmium can be post fixed in formalin and processed routinely.[11] The result is a histologic section with good cytologic detail as opposed to the suboptimal architecture that one sees in frozen sections. Nevertheless, procedures employing osmium tetroxide do have a significant disadvantage. It is a very caustic and potentially toxic compound, and technologists must work in a fume hood to avoid such dangers. Disposal of the reagent is accordingly difficult as well.

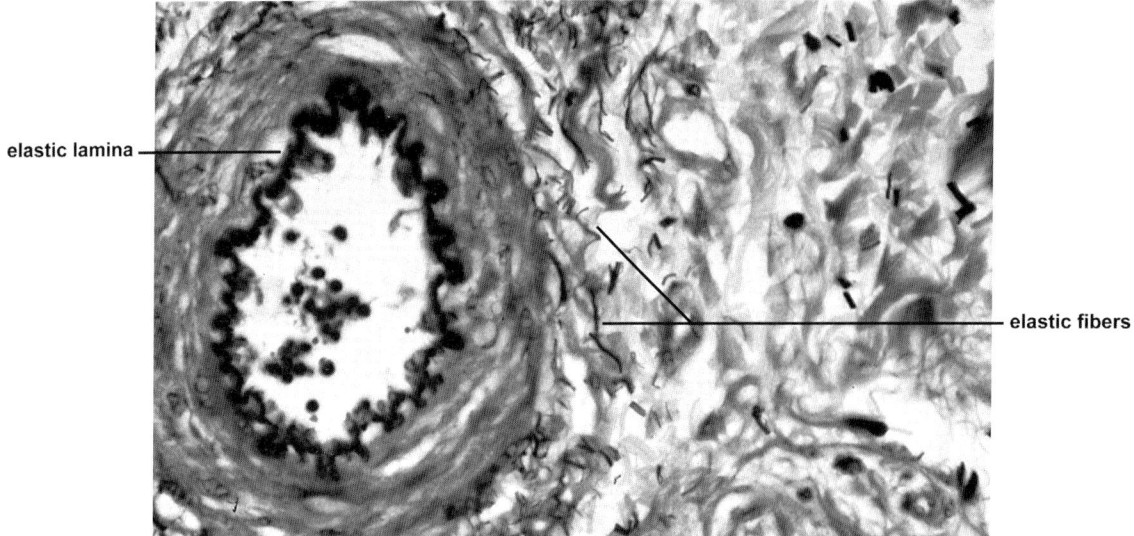

elastic lamina ———

——— elastic fibers

Figure 2-4. A high-power photograph of an elastic stain, the Veerhoff-van Gieson stain. Elastic fibers are black in the internal elastic lamina of an artery as well as in the connective tissue of the subcutis. (Veerhoff-van Gieson, ×150.)

Nucleic Acids and Nucleoproteins

Before the advent of flow cytometry and in situ hybridization, histochemical methods were developed to aid in assessing the amount of nucleic acid that malignant cells contain. The latter procedures are still useful in selected instances, particularly when coupled with morphometric (densitometric) techniques. There are two stains that are appropriately categorized as semi-specific for nucleic acids: the Feulgen method and the methyl green-pyronine MGP procedure.

The chemical basis for the Feulgen stain is predicated on the fact that controlled acid hydrolysis can be used to digest purine bases in deoxyribonucleic acid (DNA), producing aldehyde groups that are capable of combining with the Schiff reagent.[11] Therefore, the method is an indirect one requiring modification of the target compound. The reader will recall that Schiff conjugates yield a red color, representing the desired end product of the Feulgen stain. The hydrolytic step in this procedure is fixative dependent; formalin yields the most consistent results and requires only short exposure of tissue sections to acid, whereas specimens preserved in heavy metal fixatives must be digested for a longer period. Bouin's solution is itself hydrolytic and therefore renders tissue unsuitable for studies with the Feulgen reaction. Ribonucleic acid (RNA) is not sensitive to hydrochloric acid, and is not labeled in this procedure.

By contrast, the MGP technique depends on differential affinities of DNA and RNA for the two dyes used in this reagent. These affinities are presumably based on the tendency for methyl green to associate with large polymers (DNA), whereas pyronine intercalates with smaller polymeric compounds (RNA). As one would expect, nuclei are stained green with MGP, and the cytoplasm (where the majority of intracellular RNA resides), is red.[38] It should be remembered that pyronine is not specific for RNA; this dye also labels keratin and the granules of mast cells or eosinophils. Therefore, neoplasms

showing mastocytic, granulocytic, or keratinocytic differentiation are not reliably assessable with MGP. It is most often used in helping to confirm a plasmacytic or immunoblastic lymphoid phenotype in malignant lymphomas, where high levels of both DNA and RNA are expected.

Exclusive of immunohistochemical evaluation for cell phase-dependent nuclear antigens, or flow cytometric measurement of S-phase populations, there is only one method for the estimation of actively dividing cells. It is an indirect one, and is known as the *Ag-NOR* procedure. This acronym stands for silver (Ag)-stained *n*uclear *o*rganizer *r*egions, which are complexes of nuclear proteins and ribosomal RNA genes. They have been localized to five chromosomes in humans and tend to increase in number, size, and density in proliferative cell populations.[39] Preliminary studies have suggested, for example, that cells in benign melanocytic lesions have few, compact Ag-NORs, whereas those in malignant melanomas tend to show multiple coarse intranuclear bodies of this type.[40]

The Ag-NOR reagent is somewhat complicated to prepare and utilize. It consists of freshly dissolved gelatin and formic acid, which are mixed with silver nitrate solution prepared with deionized distilled water. The final product is a colloidal suspension; it is applied to deparaffinized-rehydrated or frozen sections of tissue and incubated in the dark for 30 minutes. Ag-NORs are visible in the sections as distinct, dark, intranuclear bodies when the procedure is performed properly.[41] However, slight variations in incubation time or reagent preparation can result in abundantly but nonspecifically deposited silver, producing "dirty" slides that are difficult to interpret.

Mesenchymal Structures

The skin contains several "connective" tissues and derivatives of embryonal mesenchyme, which figure into the assessment of selected inflammatory, degenerative, and neoplastic diseases.

These include collagen types, elastic tissue, muscle, and nerve, as well as fat and ground substances, discussed earlier.

One of the most widely used histochemical methods for the evaluation of these tissue components is the Masson trichrome technique. It is a mixture of three dyes—Biebrich's scarlet hematoxylin, and aniline blue—as well as phosphotungstic or phosphomolybdic acid. The latter compounds alter the affinity of various mesenchymal tissues for the dyes, causing differential staining.[11] Collagen and elastin are stained blue and muscle is red with the trichrome procedure, whereas nuclei are black and nonmuscular cytoplasm is also red. Attention to fibrillation of the cytoplasm is necessary on high-power microscopy to distinguish myogenous from nonmuscular cells.

Elastic tissue is best seen with Verhoeff's method (and a modification known as the Verhoeff-van Gieson method) or the aldehyde fuchsin elastic stain. In the first of these, a chemical "lake" of hematoxylin and ferric chloride is the principal staining reagent. Elastic tissue has a strong affinity for the latter complex and therefore resists decolorization better than other tissue components in this regressive staining technique. Elastic fibers are blue-black (Fig. 2-4), collagen is red, nuclei are blue, and other tissues are yellow in the version of Verhoeff's method where van Gieson's reagent is used as a counterstain.[24] This procedure is an excellent one for the demonstration of elastic tissue abnormalities, such as those seen in elastofibroma dorsi, pseudoxanthoma elasticum, and solar elastosis.

In the aldehyde fuchsin elastic stain,[42] basic fuchsin is combined with hydrochloric acid and paraldehyde to yield aldehyde fuchsin. This reagent has the ability to form Schiff bases and shows a strong affinity for elastic fibers. The latter acquire a dark-blue or purple color, and Light Green is usually used as a counterstain.

Nerve fibers may be visualized through staining either their neuronal processes or the myelin surrounding them. Silver methods such as the Bodian stain are used to accomplish the for-

mer task, whereas the Luxol fast blue technique is employed to delineate myelin in tissue. The Bodian method is a complicated procedure using silver proteinate, gold chloride, hydroquinone, sodium thisulfate, hydrochloric acid, and aniline blue. It was designed as a regressive staining technique to selectively impregnate neuronal processes with elemental silver, yielding a black precipitate on these elements[43] (Fig. 2-5). Nuclei are black, and surrounding tissues are blue. In the Luxol fast blue procedure, sulfonated copper phthalocyanine is used in an acid-base reaction to replace the bases of lipoproteins in myelin. As its name suggests, this dye has a blue color in the final staining product.[26]

Another cellular grouping of interest in dermatopathology is that called the "diffuse neuroendocrine system." It includes Merkel cells of normal skin and "Merkel cell carcinomas." Silver impregnation techniques also are employed to delineate neurosecretory granules in neuroendocrine cells. The Grimelius and Churukian-Schenk procedures are useful in this context.[44,45] Both of them are predicated on the knowledge that neurosecretory granules have the ability to bind silver ions (i.e., they are argyrophilic); a reducing substance is then applied to tissue sections to yield a precipitate of black elemental silver. Argyrophilic techniques are influenced by fixation. Formaldehyde-based solutions produce inconsistent positivity, whereas this is one situation where Bouin's fixative gives superior results. Also, melanosomes are reactive with the Grimelius and Churukian-Schenk methods, necessitating concomitant performance of the Fontana-Masson stain before interpreting an argyrophilic cellular proliferation as neuroendocrine in nature.

Microorganisms

The range of infectious agents that are evaluated in cutaneous diseases is broad. It includes conventional bacteria, spirochetes, mycobacteria, fungi, protozoan organisms, and nematodes.[11] A complete discussion of the histochemical methods used to iden-

Figure 2-5. Bielchowsky silver stain of peripheral nerve. The nerve fibers (axons) appear as linear black lines. This effect is produced by precipitation of silver salts onto the axon. (Bielchowsky, × 200.)

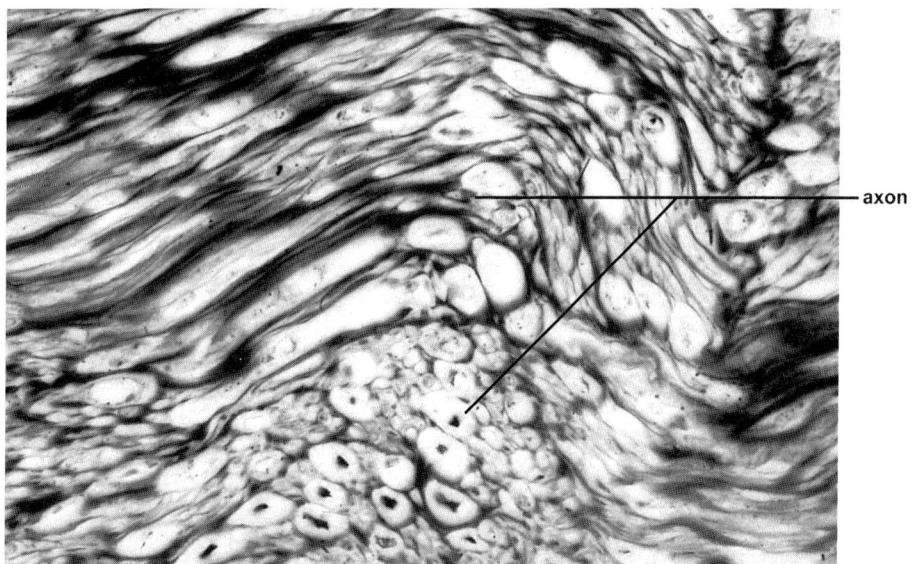

axon

Table 2-2. Histochemical Methods for Identification of Microbes

Class of Organism	Stains	Biochemical "Targets"	Comments
"Conventional" bacteria	Brown-Hopps modification of Gram stain	Peptidoglycans and lipopolysaccharide in bacterial walls	Superior to Brown-Brenn method
Fungi	Hotchkiss-McManus version of PAS technique	Polysaccharides in fungal walls	Diastase digestion suggested
	Grocott's methenamine silver nitrate procedure	Polysaccharides in fungal walls	Also will stain *Nocardia* and *Actinomyces*
	Mucicarmine method	Mucinous material in capsules of *Cryptococci*	Only used for *Cryptococcus neoformans*
	Biotinylated lectins (soybean and succinylated wheatgerm)	Polysaccharides in fungal walls	Requires detection by ABC technique
Mycobacteria	Kinyoun's method	Complex lipids in bacterial walls	Does not label "atypical" organisms; will also stain *Nocardia*
	Fite's technique	Complex lipids in bacterial walls	Preferred method for *Mycobacterium leprae* and other "atypical" organisms
	Auramine-rhodamine procedure	Unknown	Requires fluorescent microscopy
Spirochetes	Warthin-Starry technique	Argyrophilic proteins in bacterial walls	
	Dieterle method	Argyrophilic proteins in bacterial walls	
Nematodes	Grocott's methenamine-silver-nitrate technique	Polysaccharides in chitinous coat of organisms	Organisms usually seen well with H&E
	PAS-D method	Glycoproteins in chitinous coat or organisms	Organisms usually seen well with H&E
Rickettsiae	Giemsa or methylene blue technique	Unknown	Specific identification requires immunohistology
Leishmania	Giemsa or methylene blue techniques	Unknown	Specific identification requires immunohistology
Viruses (herpes simplex virus; cytomegalovirus; Orf; varicella-zoster virus)	Methyl green-pyronine Y method	Viral DNA or RNA	Used for confirming generic nature of viral inclusions; specific identification requires immunohistology

Abbreviations: PAS, periodic acid-Schiff method; PAS-D, PAS with diastase; H&E, hematoxylin and eosin; DNA, deoxyribonucleic acid; RNA, ribonucleic acid.

tify these microbes is not within the scope of this chapter. However, a summary of such techniques is given in Table 2-2.

Cytoplasmic Enzymes

Similarly, a large number of cytoplasmic enzymes has been assessed in cutaneous lesions using histochemical procedures. In particular, phosphorylase, succinic dehydrogenase, leucine aminopeptidase, indoxyl esterase, and cytochrome oxidase are thought to be helpful markers of eccrine differentiation in adnexal neoplasia. By contrast, acid and alkaline phosphatases, adenosine triphosphatase (ATPase), β-glucuronidase, acetate esterase, and monoamine oxidase are used as evidence for apocrine differentiation.[46] The methodology for each of these techniques has been outlined in other sources[37,46] and is merely ref-

erenced here. Most of them are based on the ability of any given enzyme to hydrolyze or oxidize a colorless insoluble compound to yield a colored precipitate. Appropriate counterstains are then applied to yield the final histologic product.

The procedures just mentioned are not used much currently because immunohistochemistry has largely superceded the application of enzyme histochemistry in dermatopathology. However, one that has not been cited is the naphthol AS-D chloroacetate method, also known as the *von Leder stain*. It is very useful in identifying immature granulocytes in suspected leukemia cutis cases or, perhaps more importantly, in recognizing tissue mast cells. The red product in this stain derives from the inclusion of Fast Garnet as the active dye.[47] Contrary to metachromatic techniques such as the toluidine blue stain, which is also employed for the labeling of mast cells, the von Leder procedure is not dependent on the integrity of mastocytic granules to produce a positive result.

IMMUNOHISTOCHEMICAL TECHNIQUES

Immunohistochemistry is still regarded by some pathologists as a "new" technology. This is really not an accurate perspective, because immunofluorescence, the prototype of immunohistologic procedures, was introduced over 50 years ago.[48] It is true that immunologic analysis of routine pathologic specimens did not gain wide acceptance until the 1970s,[49] but this discipline has literally exploded in scope since then. The following sections present a summary of various immunohistochemical procedures applicable to dermatopathology.

Immunofluorescence Techniques

Coons et al[48] were the first to describe the attachment of fluorescent chemical ligands to antibodies as diagnostic reagents.[48] The most widely used of these moieties is fluorescein isothiocyanate (FITC), which produces yellow-green emission when excited by ultraviolet light. Immunofluorescence is best performed on frozen sections prepared from specimens kept in saline for short periods after procurement, samples that are flash-frozen immediately after biopsy, or tissue that has been transported in Michel's medium. The latter solution allows for preservation of tissue-bound immunoglobulins for 1 or 2 days, owing to its content of N-ethylmaleimide and ammonium sulfate.[50] These chemicals must be removed from the specimen by thorough washing in buffer prior to immunolabeling, or poor results will be obtained. Similarly, unbound serum proteins must be rinsed out of all skin biopsies with saline before immunofluorescent ligands are attached to preclude the presence of high "background" staining in final microscopic preparations.

For "direct" immunofluorescent microscopy, cryostat sections are cut at 2 to 4 μm and mounted on adhesive-coated glass slides. They are then incubated at room temperature for 30 minutes with specific, FITC-labeled antisera (to immunoglobulins A, E, G, and M; fibrinogen; and complement fractions [such as C3]), rinsed, mounted in glycerol, and coverslipped. If the targets of the antibodies were affixed to the tissue in vivo, they will be visualized as fluorescent green deposits in the epidermis, the dermis, or both by ultraviolet microscopy. Permutations and patterns of stains for immunoglobulins or other reactants are provided in other chapters of this text and can be used to classify the immunologically mediated diseases of the skin.[6]

Direct immunofluorescence has the major limitation that morphologic detail is poor, and it may be necessary to switch back and forth between phase microscopy and ultraviolet illumination to determine the cellular locale for the reactants. In addition, collagen in the tissue may autofluoresce and complicate the interpretation. Moreover, immunofluorescence preparations fade after several days, and photomicrography is necessary for long-term documentation of results. Paraffin sections are suboptimal substrates for this procedure, but they may occasionally be rendered suitable by pretreatment with proteolytic enzymes and 0.1% ammonium hydroxide.[15]

"Indirect" immunofluorescence does not employ patient tissues as analytes, but rather uses serum taken from patients who are presumed to have circulating antibodies to cutaneous components. Normal substrate skin can be obtained from volunteers (or from previous diagnostic cases showing no immunologic abnormalities), or cross-reactive tissues such as animal esophagus can be procured from commercial vendors. These are exposed to patient serum for 30 to 60 minutes at room temperature, rinsed, and incubated with FITC-labeled antisera as cited above. Positive results may *indirectly* confirm the presence of circulating antibodies to keratinocyte attachment plaques (in pemphigus), bullous pemphigoid antigen (BPA), epidermolysis bullosa acquisita antigen (EBAA), and other tissue complexes.

To definitively distinguish anti-BPA from anti-EBAA, the "saline split skin" procedure must be used in indirect immunofluorescence. Normal skin is soaked in 1 M saline according to a predetermined protocol, causing the epidermal basement membrane to split between its laminae densa and lucida. Because BPA and EBAA are dissimilarly located in one or the other of these layers, immunofluorescent labeling for BPA is seen in the base of the artificial "blister," and EBAA is localized to its "roof."[51,52]

Indirect Antibody Procedures

Because of the morphologically suboptimal nature of immunofluorescence, pathologists were driven to develop alternative immunohistologic procedures that could be applied to conventional (fixed, paraffin-embedded) specimens. Antigens are localized in such samples indirectly, but they can be seen with a high level of resolution and clarity. Several indirect techniques are available, as outlined below.

The Peroxidase-Antiperoxidase Method

Sternberger and colleagues[53] can be credited with devising the first practical immunohistologic technique, the peroxidase-antiperoxidase (PAP) procedure. It is based on the ability to complex two immunoglobulin (Ig) G molecules to several horseradish peroxidase molecules in vitro via the Fab fragments of the antibodies. Rabbit immunoglobulins are most often used for this purpose. A specific rabbit antiserum against an antigen of interest is first incubated with test tissues, followed sequentially by application of a generic antirabbit immunoglobulin and the immunoglobulin-peroxidase complex. Peroxidase is capable of oxidizing 3,3′-diaminobenzidine hydrochloride (DAB) or 3-amino-9-ethylcarbazole (AEC) to their insoluble forms in the presence of hydrogen peroxide. This step produces brown-black and red precipitates, respectively, allowing for localization of bound rabbit immunoglobulin/anti-rabbit immunoglobulin/rabbit immunoglobulin-peroxidase complexes in tissue.

We prefer DAB over AEC, because the former compound gives a denser product and is insoluble in organics. By contrast, AEC dissolves in clearing agents and Permount, and sections must be mounted with an aqueous medium or polymeric resin. Glycerol medium is suitable for short-term study of AEC-labeled sections, but the chromogen tends to diffuse into it from the tissue after several weeks. Alternatively, Crystal Mount provides more permanent preparations.[11]

The PAP method is still widely used, because of its relative simplicity and the low cost of the reagents. However, it does have two potential failings. One relates to a relative insensitivity for low antigen densities, which may be partially overcome by "reiterative" application of the PAP complex.[12] The other problem reflects the need to "quench" endogenous tissue peroxidase in specimens to avoid unwanted background staining.

The Avidin-Biotin-Peroxidase Complex Procedure

Hsu et al[54] introduced the avidin-biotin-peroxidase complex (ABC) method in 1981 as an alternative to the PAP technique. The former procedure employs secondary, generic antispecies antibodies that are labeled by chemical attachment of biotin to their Fc fragments. This provision allows the biotin to bind to commercially synthesized tertiary complexes of avidin, biotin, and horseradish peroxidase. These aggregates contain several-fold more peroxidase molecules than tertiary reagents in the PAP method.

The slightly greater cost of the ABC technique is more than offset by its higher degree of sensitivity relative to PAP. Moreover, "second-generation" ABC kits have now been introduced with even more peroxidase molecules in the tertiary complexes, and the PAP and ABC procedures can be done in sequence (the "ABPAP" method) to further amplify sensitivity.[15] The only real disadvantage of ABC reagents is the continued need to quench endogenous tissue peroxidase, as noted above (Fig. 2-6).

The Alkaline Phosphatase-Anti-Alkaline Phosphatase Method

To avoid the need to inactivate native peroxidase in clinical specimens, the alkaline phosphatase-anti-alkaline phosphatase (APAAP) procedure was developed in the middle 1980s.[55] Its principle is basically the same as that described for the PAP technique, except that the intestinal isozyme of alkaline phosphatase is used as the chromogenic enzyme instead of peroxi-

dase, and Fast Red is substituted for DAB as the chromogen in APAAP. Because intestinal-type AP is not seen in most human tissues (including the skin), background staining is negligible and there is no need to quench endogenous catalytic agents.[15] This is a distinct advantage in certain diagnostic situations. For example, a biopsy specimen containing numerous neutrophils or erythrocytes (with considerable cell-bound peroxidase) would be expected to show high background labeling with the PAP or ABC procedures. By contrast, the APAAP method yields a very crisp result in such samples.

Disadvantages of APAAP are few, but may be troublesome nonetheless. It has been our experience that the reaction steps take longer to complete than those of the ABC or PAP methods, and the eventual precipitate of the Fast Red is not particularly dense. Lastly, APAAP is more expensive than the other techniques.

Choice of an Immunohistologic System

One serious problem confronting pathologists is that which concerns nonuniformity of methodology in immunohistochemistry. It may be safely said that, in general, the overall results of the PAP, ABC, and APAAP procedures should be comparable over a broad range of immunoreactants. Nonetheless, a huge body of disparate, often-contradictory information exists in the literature on immunohistologic findings in human diseases. This has resulted from many idiosyncratic approaches to such specific procedural details as antibody selection, antibody concentration, periods of incubation, and reaction temperatures. Attention to reports emanating from reputable diagnostic immunohistochemistry laboratories shows that they do, in fact, employ similar methods and reagents, with consonant results. Hence, this methodology should be emulated by responsible scientists to ensure reproducibility of the technique. There is no room for "mavericks" in immunohistology.[56]

Figure 2-6. An example of an ABC method immunoperoxidase stain for HMB-45. The melanoma cells are prominently stained against a faintly counterstained pale background. (HMB-45, × 100.)

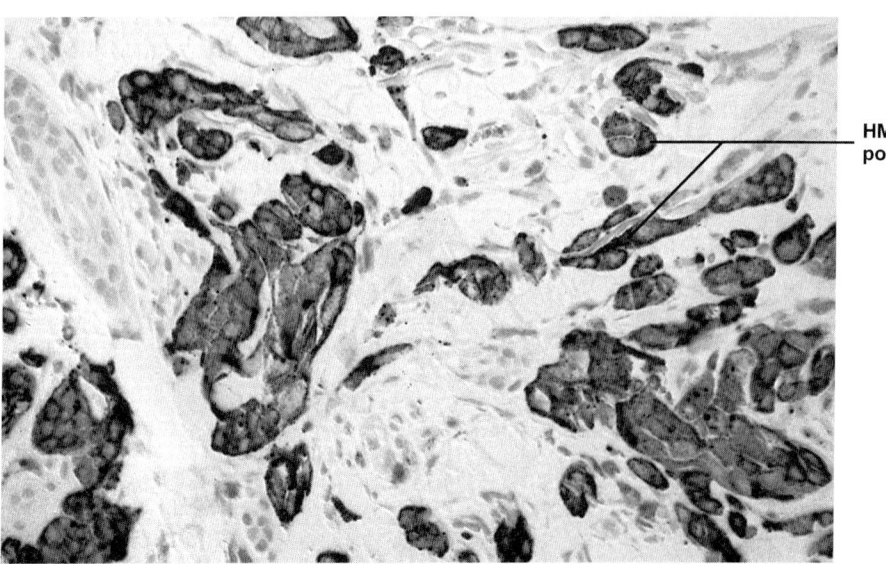

Preprocedural Considerations in Immunohistology

Contrary to what many pathologists prefer to believe, simply changing immunohistologic methods is not the solution for poor results that may be obtained with this technique. Instead, the most common problems in this realm relate to improper handling of specimens before they reach the histology laboratory or to inadequate attention to nonimmunologic reagents that are used in these procedures.[15]

Tissue Procurement

One of the best adages for the budding immunohistochemist to remember is also one of the most banal: "garbage in, garbage out." It is amazing how often pathologists expect immunohistologic studies on "tortured" tissues to yield definitive diagnostic results, even though an interpretation was impossible by routine H&E studies because of processing distortions. Specimens that have been frozen and thawed, crushed, allowed to autolyze, fixed badly, or harshly decalcified are predictably poor substrates for immunologic analysis, and little can be done to retrieve their complete antigenic integrity.

Preservation difficulties are among the most prevalent in this context. Overfixation in formalin (e.g., for more than 24 hours) causes "masking" of many antigens by protein cross-linkage via methylol bonds.[57] Heavy metal solutions, and those containing picric acid, denature many cytoplasmic proteins and severely limit the scope of immunohistologic studies. By contrast, *under*fixation promotes autolysis, with similar loss of antigenicity. The best approach is to carefully control the preparation of NBF that one uses for all specimens, with limitation of the fixation time to under 12 hours whenever possible; formalin-alcohol is also a viable option to improve tissue preservation. Specimens should be prosected so that submitted sections are no more than 3 to 5 mm thick, to allow for optimal penetration of fixatives.

Many immunohistochemists have applied digestion procedures with such enzymes as trypsin, pepsin, or pronase to counter the effects of overfixation in formalin. It is true that these agents (as well as ficin, papain, DNAse, and bromelain) are capable of restoring the immunoreactivity of several cellular markers.[15] These include intermediate filament proteins, factor VIII-related antigen, CD30 molecules, collagen type IV, and others. However, the use of proteases may *damage* other determinants, and it must, in any case, be tailored to the antigens of interest. For example, the exposure of immunoreactive sites in S-100 protein is enhanced by bromelain, but they may be digested entirely by ficin. Obviously, these agents must be applied after careful thought and familiarity with the pertinent literature.[58]

Nonimmunologic Reagents

As mentioned earlier, some clearing agents, even those as "innocuous" as xylene, may *damage* tissue antigens. Embedding procedures with paraffin that have been heated to above 60°C, or the alternative use of Carbowax, also have deleterious effects on immunohistochemistry.

Without any hesitation, we would also note that *buffers* used in this facet of histology are the greatest source of technical difficulty in our experience. These must be scrupulously prepared with respect to ionic constituency and pH, and such factors should be monitored carefully during storage of the solutions. The target value for buffer pH is the narrow physiologic range of 7.2 to 7.4. Inappropriately acid reagents may preclude primary antibody binding totally, and overly basic solutions may result in extreme degrees of background labeling. Buffers with excessive ionic strength commonly cause nonspecific precipitation of DAB and AEC,[15] yielding virtually uninterpretable preparations.

Selection of Primary Antibody Reagents

There are literally hundreds of antibodies in the catalogues of commercial vendors, many of which are applicable to diagnostic immunohistochemistry. However, these "menus" are often fraught with pitfalls for the unwary customer. Several antibodies have been developed for exclusive use in frozen sections, such as those applied to the study of hematolymphoid proliferations (e.g., reagents in the Leu series). Unless one asks for data from the manufacturer on optimal reaction conditions, sensitivity, and specificity, a large sum of money and a great deal of time may be invested in the workup of useless antibodies. Reagents that fail to demonstrate their stated characteristics should be promptly returned to the supplying firm, and payment for them can be appropriately withheld.

Also, an often-asked question concerns the "superiority" of monoclonal antibodies over heteroantisera for use as primary reagents in diagnostic immunohistochemistry. It is true that hybridoma products commonly yield "cleaner" staining results, but this may be at the expense of sensitivity or specificity. All pathologists should attempt to assess the latter performance factors "in house" by studying prior specimens from their own files that have been thoroughly characterized for their spectrum of immunoreactivity. The "sausage block" method is an efficient means of attaining this goal. In this procedure, strips of tissue from 50 to 70 sectioned paraffin blocks are rearranged in a predetermined fashion in one conglomerate block.[59,60] The latter may be structured to contain many examples of one tumor type (e.g., 50 examples of malignant melanoma), or, more commonly, it is configured to include 4 or 5 grouped examples of 10 of 15 neoplasms (e.g., 5 melanomas, 5 basal cell carcinomas, 5 lymphomas). Any new antibody can be applied to sections of the sausage block and "scored" with regard to its specificity and sensitivity for a particular tissue type.

Another caveat pertaining to antibody selection refers to the analysis of any given diagnostic case. In an attempt to save money, many pathologists still attempt to "confirm" an H&E interpretation with *one* immunohistologic reaction. For example, they may study a tumor for its expression of S-100 protein to support a diagnosis of malignant melanoma. This approach is deplorable. As we have learned more and more about the scope of distribution of many antigens, it has become clear that very few are tissue or tumor specific. In the above-cited instance, a poorly differentiated metastatic carcinoma of the breast could also be reactive for S-100 protein, and it could show histologic synonymity with malignant melanoma as well.[61] Thus, immunohistology should always be applied *exclusively* in a multiantibody panel setting. The combinations of reactivity patterns that are expected in dermatologic diseases are impossible to outline here. However, they have been considered in depth in other publications[62–64] and are mentioned in context in the remaining chapters of this text.

Positive and Negative Controls

All immunohistologic techniques must include a positive (method) and negative (tissue) control.[15] Positive controls are, as noted above, archival specimens that have been well characterized immunologically in the past. These serve to ensure that the immunohistochemical procedure, as a unit, has been performed properly on any given day and that antibody reactivities are constant over time. Negative controls are represented by sections of a study case that are stained immunohistologically after substitution of nonimmune sera for primary antibodies. The purpose of this step is to assure oneself that the tissue does not spuriously (nonspecifically) bind immunoglobulin from a particular animal source. Hence, nonimmune rabbit sera are substituted for specific primary rabbit antisera in a properly done negative control. If the negative control looks "positive," a tissue-related problem exists that will interfere with reliable interpretation of results.

In this age of increasing medicolegal accountability, it is highly desirable to keep written records of control reactivities over time in the immunohistochemistry laboratory. This aids in assessing the reagent performance and the competence of technical personnel and in maintaining documentation of quality assurance practices.

ELECTRON MICROSCOPY

Electron microscopy has, in many people's minds, been rendered "obsolete" by the availability of immunohistology and in situ hybridization. This is a fatuous contention. Ultrastructural studies do still have a potentially major role to play in the localization of immune complexes in skin biopsies, the identification of diagnostically helpful cellular constituents, and the detailed localization of antigens (in combination with immunohistology).[65]

Appropriate fixation of tissue for electron microscopy necessitates prompt immersion of carefully handled (uncrushed) specimens in 2% to 4% phosphate-buffered glutaraldehyde; the tissue blocks must be no larger than 2 mm^2.[11] Fixation occurs optimally at 4°C and should be allowed to proceed for a minimum of 2 hours. This step is followed by postfixation in osmium tetroxide, dehydration in graded alcohols, and the embedding of each block in one of a number of polymeric resins. The latter include Epon, Spurr resin, and Lowicryl, which are "cured" by incubation at 60°C for 8 to 10 hours.[66]

Thereafter, "thick" (1-mm) sections are cut, mounted on glass slides, and stained with a polychromatic dye such as methylene blue. The pathologist should review each thick section with the responsible ultrastructural technologist and indicate those that are suitable for further study. These specimens are then subjected to ultrathin (60 to 70 nm) sectioning with a diamond knife microtome, after which they are mounted on round copper grids and stained with uranyl acetate and lead citrate. Formvar (a plastic resin) can be added as a thin coating over the mounted ultrathin grid sections to provide additional support prior to staining.[67]

Proper polymerization of the supporting resin and attention to microtomy technique are crucial to preparation of suitable specimens for electron microscopy. Incomplete resin curing, dull microtome knives, and overly thick ultrathin sections all are responsible for wrinkles in the final tissue preparations. These are even more troublesome in ultrastructural studies than in routine light microscopy, because the electron beam that is used to illuminate the specimen will literally melt grids that have folds in the tissue.

Lowicryl is the resinous mounting medium of choice for immunoultrastructural analysis in which tissue grids are incubated with antibodies that have been labeled with electron-dense gold or ferritin particles.[68] This resin allows immunologic reagents to penetrate the specimen well, whereas Epon and Spurr do not.

IN SITU HYBRIDIZATION

In situ hybridization (ISH) procedures are, in many ways, similar to those used in immunohistochemistry. However, instead of employing antibodies as diagnostic reagents, ISH techniques use segments of single-stranded nucleic acid ("probes") that are carefully prepared in vitro. These are tagged with a radioactive moiety such as tritium or with biotin. The binding of radiolabeled probes to tissue specimens is visualized by autoradiography (a similar process to the development of photographic images), and biotin-labeled reagents are localized via the ABC procedure.[69,70] It should be noted at this point that tissue must be affixed to glass slides with a special adhesive, aminoalkylsilane,[11] to prevent its loss during this "harsh" procedure.

Either DNA or RNA probes can be utilized, depending on whether one wishes to determine the presence of nuclear or cytoplasmic (protein-related) nucleic acids in the target specimen. Prior, controlled heating of the tissue is necessary in DNA ISH techniques to cause denaturation of the double-stranded nucleic acid. RNA ISH is particularly demanding technically, because RNAse is a ubiquitous enzyme that is found in sweat and sebum. Therefore, glassware must be meticulously cleaned, and the technologist must be careful to wear surgical gloves to avoid contact of skin surfaces with the specimens. Strict attention to the ionic strength and chemical constitution of all reagents is required to avoid inactivation of the probes or, alternatively, their nonspecific attachment to the specimen being analyzed.[70]

The sequence of nucleotides in each probe is structured in such a fashion that it is complementary to portions of the target nucleic acid in the tissue sample. If annealing occurs, DNA probes will show nuclear autoradiographic or ABC positivity, whereas RNA reagents label the cytoplasm preferentially.

At present, ISH procedures are limited in their diagnostic applicability. They are most often used to evaluate the presence of viral (e.g., human papillomavirus) nucleic acid sequences in cutaneous biopsy specimens. However, they have substantial research value because ISH is capable of demonstrating the nucleic acid counterparts of cellular protein markers, even if the latter are not being actively synthesized. This technique can therefore be viewed as a definitive confirmatory method grave vis-á-vis immunohistochemistry. As additional practical information accrues on such topics as oncogene amplification and mutation in cutaneous diseases, it is anticipated that ISH will acquire more diagnostic (or prognostic) utility.

REFERENCES

1. Wick MR, Manivel JC, Millns JL: Histopathologic considerations in the management of skin cancer. pp. 246–275. In Schwartz RA (ed): Skin Cancer: Recognition and Management. Springer–Verlag, New York, 1988
2. Banks PM: Lymphoid neoplasms of the skin. pp. 299–356. In Wick MR (ed): Pathology of Unusual Malignant Cutaneous Tumors. Marcel Dekker, New York, 1985
3. Trimble JW, Schwartz RA: Microscopically controlled excision of skin cancer. Am Fam Physician 25:187–190, 1982
4. Swanson NA; Mohs surgery. Arch Dermatol 119:761–773, 1983
5. Bennett RG: The meaning and significance of tissue margins. Adv Dermatol 4:343–357, 1989
6. Huang WM, Gibson SJ, Facer P: Improved section adherence for immunocytochemistry using high molecular weight polymers of L-lysine as a slide coating. Histochemistry 77:275–279, 1983
7. Hopwood D: Fixatives and fixation: a review. Histochem J 1:323–360, 1969
8. Hopwood D: Cell and tissue fixation. Histochem J 17: 389–442, 1985
9. Leatham A, Atkins NJ: Fixation and immunohistochemistry of lymphoid tissue. J Clin Pathol 33:1010–1012, 1980
10. Hopwood D, Yeaman G, Milne G: Differentiating the effects of microwave and heat on tissue proteins and their cross linking by formaldehyde. Histochem J 20:341–347, 1988
11. Carson FL: Histotechnology: A Self-Instructional Text. ASCP Press, Chicago, 1990
12. McLean IW, Nakane PK: Periodate-lysine-paraformaldehyde fixative: a new fixative for immunoelectron microscopy. J Histochem Cytochem 22:1077–1083, 1974
13. NIOSH 85-114: NIOSH Pocket Guide to Chemical Hazards. U.S. Department of Health and Human Services, Washington, DC, 1985
14. Puchtler H, Meloan SN: On the chemistry of formaldehyde fixation and its effects on immunohistochemical reactions. Histochemistry 82:201–204, 1985
15. Reisner HM, Wick MR: Theoretical and technical considerations for the use of monoclonal antibodies in diagnostic immunohistochemistry. pp. 1–50. In Wick MR, Siegal GP (eds): Monoclonal Antibodies in Diagnostic Immunohistochemistry. Marcel Dekker, New York, 1988
16. Luna LG: Specimen preparation. pp. 30–41. In Farmer ER, Hood AF (eds): Pathology of the Skin. Appleton & Lange, East Norwalk, CT, 1990
17. Luna LG: Amorphous bevel surface and moisture: important factors in microtomy. Microviews [Surgpath Medical Industries Newsletter] 4:5–9, 1988
18. Molner LM: Eliminate wrinkles on paraffin section slides. Histology 5:59–62, 1975
19. Thompson SW, Luna LG: An Atlas of Artifacts. Charles C Thomas, Springfield, IL, 1978
20. Bancroft JD, Stevens A: Theory and Practice of Histological Techniques. Churchill Livingstone, New York, 1982
21. McGee-Russell SM: Histochemical methods for calcium. J Histochem Cytochem 6:22–42, 1958
22. Johnson WC: Histochemistry of the cutaneous adnexa and selected adnexal neoplasms. J Cutan Pathol 11:352–356, 1984
23. John WC, Helwig EB: Histochemistry of the cutaneous interfibrillar ground substance. J Invest Dermatol 42:81–85, 1964
24. Luna LG: Manual of Histologic Staining Methods. 3rd Ed. Armed Forces Institute of Pathology, Washington, DC, 1968
25. Vacca LL: Laboratory Manual of Histochemistry. Lippincott-Raven, Philadelphia, 1985
26. Sheehan DC, Hrapchak BB: Theory and Practice of Histotechnology. 2nd Ed. Battelle Press, Columbus, OH, 1980
27. Stoward PJ: Histochemical methods for routine diagnostic histopathology. pp. 13–30. In Filipe MI, Lake BD (eds): Histochemistry in Pathology. Churchill Livingstone, New York, 1990
28. Johnson WC, Helwig ED: Histochemistry of primary and metastatic mucin-secreting tumors. Ann NY Acad Sci 106:794–803, 1963
29. Wick MR, Swanson PE: Cutaneous Adnexal Tumors: A Guide to Pathologic Diagnosis. ASCP Press, Chicago, 1991
30. Wood MG, Beerman H: Necrobiosis lipoidica, granuloma annulare, and rheumatoid nodule. J Invest Dermatol 34:139–147, 1960
31. Panet-Raymond G, Johnson WC: Lupus erythematosus and polymorphous light eruption: differentiation by histochemical procedures. Arch Dermatol 108:785–787, 1973
32. Alroy J, Ucci AA, Pereira MEA: Lectin histochemistry: an update. pp. 93–131. In DeLellis RA (ed): Advances in Immunohistochemistry. Lippincott-Raven, Philadelphia,
33. McNeal JE, Alroy J, Villers A et al: Mucinous differentiation in prostatic adenocarcinoma. Hum Pathol 22:979–988, 1991
34. Ordonez NG, Batsakis JG: Comparison of *Ulex europaeus* I lectin and factor VIII-related antigen in vascular lesions. Arch Pathol Lab Med 108:129–132, 1984
35. Wick MR, Manivel JC: Vascular neoplasms of the skin: a current perspective. Adv Dermatol 4:185–254, 1989
36. Robbins SL, Cotran RS, Kumar V (eds): Pathologic Basis of Disease. 3rd Ed. WB Saunders, Philadelphia, 1984
37. Filipe MI, Lake BD: Appendices. pp. 433–488. In Filipe MI, Lake BD (eds): Histochemistry in Pathology. Churchill Livingstone, New York, 1990
38. Potvin C: A simple, modified methyl green-pyronine Y stain for DNA and RNA in formalin-fixed tissues. Lab Med 10:772–776, 1979
39. Egan MJ, Crocker J: Nucleolar organizing regions in cutaneous tumours. J Pathol 154:247–254, 1988
40. Crocker J, Skilbeck N: Nucleolar organizing region-associated proteins in cutaneous melanotic lesions: a quantitative study. J Clin Pathol 40:885–889, 1987
41. Smith R, Crocker J: Evaluation of nucleolar organizing region-associated proteins in breast malignancy. Histopathology 12:113–123, 1988
42. Gomori G: Aldehyde fuchsin: a new stain for elastic tissue. Am J Clin Pathol 20: 665–672, 1950
43. Holmes W: Silver staining of nerve axons in paraffin sections. Anat Rec 86:157–169, 1943
44. Lack EE, Mercer L: A modified Grimelius argyrophil technique for neurosecretory granules. Am J Surg Pathol 1:275–280, 1977
45. Churukian CJ, Schenk EA: A modification of Pascual's argyrophil method. J Histochem Cytochem 2:102–111, 1979

46. Wick MR: Appendix I. pp. 399–404. In Wick MR (ed): Pathology of Unusual Malignant Cutaneous Tumors. Marcel Dekker, New York, 1985

47. Nelson DA: Leukocytic disorders. pp. 1036–1100. In Henry JB (ed); Clinical Diagnosis and Management by Laboratory Methods. 16th Ed. WB Saunders, Philadelphia, 1979

48. Coons AH, Creech JH, Jones RN: Immunological properties of an antibody containing a fluorescent group. Proc Soc Exp Biol Med 47:200–202, 1941

49. Taylor CR: Immunoperoxidase techniques: practical and theoretical aspects. Arch Pathol Lab Med 102:113–121, 1978

50. Michel B, Milner Y, David K: Preservation of tissue-fixed immunoglobulins in skin biopsies of patients with lupus erythematosus and bullous diseases: a preliminary report. J Invest Dermatol 59:449–452, 1972

51. Collins AB: Immunofluorescence. pp. 421–435. In Colvin RB, Bhan AK, McCluskey RT (eds): Diagnostic Immunopathology. Lippincott-Raven, Philadelphia, 1988

52. Gammon WR, Briggaman RA, Inman MS et al: Differentiating anti-lamina lucida and anti-sublamina densa anti-BMZ antibodies by indirect immunofluorescence on 1.0 M sodium chloride-separated skin. J Invest Dermatol 82:139–144, 1984

53. Sternberger LA, Hardy PH, Cuculis JJ, Meyer HG: The unlabeled antibody enzyme method for immunohistochemistry. Preparation and properties of soluble antigen-antibody complex (horseradish peroxidase-antihorseradish peroxidase) and its use in the identification of spirochetes. J Histochem Cytochem 18:315–333, 1970

54. Hsu SM, Raine L, Fanger H: Use of avidin-biotin-peroxidase complex (ABC) in immunoperoxidase techniques: a comparison between ABC and unlabeled antibody (PAP) procedures. J Histochem Cytochem 29:577–580, 1981

55. Cordell JL, Falini B, Erber W et al. Immunoenzymatic labeling of monoclonal antibodies using complexes of alkaline phosphatase and monoclonal anti-alkaline phosphatase (APAAP complexes). J Histochem Cytochem 32:219–229, 1984

56. Wick MR: Quality control in diagnostic immunohistochemistry: a discipline coming of age. Am J Clin Pathol 92:844, 1989

57. Pinkus GS, O'Connor EM, Etheridge CL, Corson JM: Optimal immunoreactivity of keratin proteins in formalin-fixed, paraffin-embedded tissue requires preliminary trypsinization: an immunoperoxidase study of various tumors using polyclonal and monoclonal antibodies. J Histochem Cytochem 13:465–473, 1985

58. Andrade RE, Hagen KA, Swanson PE, Wick MR: The use of ficin for proteolysis in immunostaining of paraffin sections. Am J Clin Pathol 90:33–39, 1988

59. Battifora H: The multi tumor (sausage) tissue block: novel method for immunohistochemical antibody testing. Lab Invest 55:244–248, 1986

60. Miller RT, Groothuis CL: Multi tumor "sausage" blocks in immunohistochemistry: simplified methods of preparation, practical uses, and roles in quality assurance. Am J Clin Pathol 96:228–232, 1991

61. Drier JK, Swanson PE, Cherwitz DL, Wick MR: S100 protein immunoreactivity in poorly differentiated carcinomas. Arch Pathol Lab Med 111:447–452, 1987

62. Wick MR, Kaye VN: The role of diagnostic immunohistochemistry in dermatology. Semin Dermatol 5:346–358, 1986

63. Wick MR, Swanson PE, Manivel JC: Immunohistochemical findings in tumors of the skin. In DeLellis RA (ed): Advances in Immunohistochemistry. Lippincott-Raven, Philadelphia, 1988

64. Flotte TJ, Margolis RJ, Mihm MC Jr: Skin diseases. pp. 65–85. In Colvin RB, Bhan AK, McCluskey RT (eds): Diagnostic Immunopathology. Lippincott-Raven, Philadelphia, 1988

65. Zelickson AS (ed): Clinical Use of Electron Microscopy in Dermatology, 4th Ed. Bolger Press, Minneapolis, MN, 1985

66. Carlemalm E, Garavito RM, Villiger W: Resin development for electron microscopy and an analysis of embedding at low temperatures. J Microscopy 126:123–143, 1982

67. Pease DC: Histological Techniques for Electron Microscopy, 2nd Ed. Academic Press, San Diego, 1964

68. Warhol MJ: Immunoelectron microscopy. pp. 67–91. In DeLellis RA (ed): Advances in Immunohistochemistry. Lippincott-Raven, Philadelphin, 1988

69. Van der Ploeg T, Landegent JE, Hopman AHN, Raap AK: Non-autoradiographic hybridocytochemistry. J Histochem Cytochem 34:126–133, 1986

70. Lambert WC: Beyond hybridomas: cell identification by in situ nucleic acid hybridization. Am J Dermatopathol 10:144–154, 1988

3

CUTANEOUS REACTION PATTERNS IN INFLAMMATORY DISEASES OF THE SKIN

AN INTRODUCTION TO PATTERN ANALYSIS

Although it is possible to learn dermatopathology by committing to memory the visual image of each inflammatory disease, malformation, and neoplasm that occurs in the skin, this process is tedious and does not provide an overall perspective on the dynamics of pathologic processes in the skin. Moreover, when observers are confronted by a specimen that does not fit into a neat pigeonhole, they may become stalemated. It is better to be able to recognize basic patterns that enable the grouping of conditions that share major histopathologic features and then distinguish among the members of each group by looking for the less obvious features that characterize each of them. This approach is fundamental to all morphologic classifications, and it has as much validity and usefulness in dermatopathology as it does in botany or zoology.

Pattern recognition is a basic neurophysiologic function, and it is evident that most pattern recognition in our everyday lives is by gestalt. That is to say that we do not consciously dissect each image into its component parts for analysis because the whole image is more meaningful than simply a compilation of its parts. Moreover, once we have become intimately familiar with an image, for example, the physiognomy of a family member, it is commonplace to be able to recognize that person at a fleeting glance, even if only from a considerable distance or in profile or in unfavorable lighting. Nevertheless, police artists can often sketch a near likeness of the perpetrator of a crime by having an eyewitness who is an accurate observer describe that person's facial features in detail. That reconstructed image can then be used to apprehend the suspect.

Experienced dermatopathologists usually make most diagnoses instantaneously at scanning magnification without consciously thinking about each morphologic feature of the condition being examined. This is true even though there are hundreds of distinctive skin diseases, and each one looks different at different points in its evolution and resolution. When confronted by an unusual specimen, however, microscopists must take stock of each component feature and accord it a degree of importance. They will integrate this information and come to a reasonable differential diagnosis. Correlation of the microscopic information with the clinical information that has been provided by the physician who performed the biopsy will enable them to select the most likely probability from all the possible choices. Less experienced observers, however, must go through this exercise time and again with each specimen until they develop the pattern recognition skills that enable instantaneous diagnoses to be made. This process is similar to that of the police artist who must piece together facial features in order to synthesize a recognizable image.

The student of skin pathology must be familiar with the microanatomy of the skin and its regional variation as well as the basic structural alterations that occur in pathologic conditions. This information must then be integrated into a framework that facilitates classification of skin diseases. In this regard, it is useful to think in terms of reaction compartments in the skin and how the various pathologic processes may affect them. There are five anatomic units that are important in skin pathology:

1. The epidermis, papillary dermis, and superficial vascular plexus as a mutually dependent unit
2. The reticular dermis and deep vascular plexus
3. The subcutaneous fat
4. The pilosebaceous units and their associated apocrine glands
5. The eccrine glands

REACTION COMPARTMENTS

Epidermis, Papillary Dermis, and Superficial Vascular Plexus

The superficial reaction unit made up by the epidermis, papillary dermis, and superficial vascular plexus is involved in the great majority of common inflammatory diseases of the skin. The earliest changes involve the small blood vessels of the superficial plexus. If the inflammatory stimulus is transient, there may only be a functional change (e.g., hyperemia) that is not apparent microscopically. If the stimulus persists, there will be observable changes, including endothelial swelling, accumulation of inflammatory cells around the vessels, and interstitial edema. Persistence of the inflammation eventually leads to structural changes in the papillary dermis. If the epidermis is the target of the inflammatory reaction, it too will be affected. There can be no change in the epidermis without involvement of the superficial plexus and papillary dermis. Moreover, every architectural alteration of the epidermis is accompanied by an obligatory reciprocal change in the papillary dermis. For example, elongation of the rete ridges in psoriasis is accompanied by equal elongation of the dermal papillae, and effacement of the rete ridges in lichen planus results in accretion of collagen in the papillary dermis between the dermal papillae to compensate for the loss of volume of the rete. Conversely, diseases that affect the papillary dermis will be accompanied by alteration of the epidermis even if it is not the primary target of the inflammatory reaction. A good example is lichen sclerosus et atrophicus in which the papillary dermis is primarily affected but the remodeling of the papillary dermis is accompanied by effacement of the rete ridges of the epidermis.

Reticular Dermis and Deep Vascular Plexus

The reticular dermis and deep vascular plexus, which is situated at the dermal-subcutaneous junction, and the communicating vessels that link it to the superficial plexus comprise another reaction compartment. Conditions that affect this more deeply situated unit often have systemic implications. Deep gyrate erythemas affect the vessels at all levels of the dermis and may occur as a manifestation of systemic infection (erythema chronicum migrans), autoimmune disease (Sjögren syndrome), or adenocarcinoma (erythema gyratum repens).

Granulomatous diseases such as sarcoidosis, leprosy, and necrobiosis lipoidica are mainly situated in the reticular dermis, and the connective tissue diseases, including lupus erythematosus, scleroderma, and dermatomyositis, also affect this compartment. This is not to say that less serious conditions do not affect the reticular dermis because several do, including arthropod bite and sting reactions, granuloma annulare, and polymorphous light eruption, but the spectrum of diseases is different from those that exclusively involve the superficial reaction unit, perhaps because it interfaces directly with the environment.

Subcutaneous Fat

The subcutaneous tissue is rarely involved in dermatologic diseases, although those that involve the reticular dermis and deep dermal plexus sometimes spill over into the fat lobules situated along the dermal-subcutaneous junction. Conversely, the panniculitides do not usually affect the dermis, although there is the potential for cutaneous involvement if the blood supply to the overlying skin is compromised, such as occurs in erythema induratum or if there is severe fat necrosis as happens in the panniculitis associated with a deficiency of α_1-trypsin inhibitor.

Although it can be difficult to determine the etiology of a panniculitis, that a disorder belongs in this general category can usually be discerned easily at scanning magnification provided that the biopsy is sufficient. This is true even though some panniculitides, such as lupus erythematosus profundus, can also involve the dermis and even the epidermis because the bulk of the inflammation is clearly situated in the fat. However, there are a few conditions that involve the dermis and subcutis almost equally such as scleroderma and necrobiosis lipoidica, illustrating that no system of classification is either ideal or foolproof.

Adnexal Structures

The adnexal structures can be the targets of inflammatory reaction. Thus, in conditions such as acne, eosinophilic folliculitis, and tinea capitis the follicular units are the focal points at scanning magnification, whereas in miliaria it is the eccrine units and in Fox-Fordyce disease it is the apocrine units. By contrast, sparing of the adnexal structures can sometimes be a helpful microscopic finding. For example, both granuloma faciale and follicular mucinosis exhibit a dense dermal infiltrate of mononuclear cells and eosinophils. In granuloma faciale, however, the infiltrate characteristically spares the follicles, whereas in follicular mucinosis they are prominently involved by it. Similarly, the lymphocytes of lupus erythematosus characteristically infiltrate and destroy follicular units, whereas the lymphocytes of polymorphous light eruption and Jessner's lymphocytic infiltrate may surround the follicles but do not damage the follicular epithelium.

COMMON HISTOLOGIC REACTIONS OF THE EPIDERMIS

Once the microscopist has scanned the specimen at low magnification and has made the determination that the superficial reaction compartment is involved in the inflammatory process, the next steps are to determine whether the epidermis is involved, and, if so, to identify the nature of the involvement.

The epidermis can be involved in three important ways. The inflammatory reaction may primarily affect the dermoepidermal junction, or it may infiltrate the epidermis and elicit intercellular edema, or it may induce the epidermis to proliferate in response to the inflammatory injury. An uncommon and unwelcome sequel to severe, chronic, involvement of the dermoepidermal junction is epidermal atrophy.

Alterations of the Dermoepidermal Interface

Vacuolar Alteration

The dermoepidermal junction is often the target of inflammatory reactions in the skin. The subepidermal vesiculobullous diseases have provided the impetus for investigators to learn the intricacies of this structurally simple but immunochemically complex zone ever since the discovery of circulating basement membrane zone antibodies in the serum of patients with pemphigoid. In the very earliest lesions of pemphigoid, there is a tendency for inflammatory cells to align themselves sparsely along the dermoepidermal junction interspersed with minute vacuoles of interstitial fluid. This change may be referred to as vacuolar alteration. A similar phenomenon is seen in many other conditions that primarily affect this complex junction, including such diverse conditions as drug and viral exanthems, erythema multiforme, graft-versus-host disease, and lupus erythematosus. In most of these diseases, the vacuoles form both beneath and above the light microscopic basement membrane (Fig. 3-1). Usually, the inflammatory process causes injury to the cells of the basal layer, and this injury can result in cell death. Therefore, vacuolar interface changes are often accompanied by the presence of individual necrotic cells in the basal layer. This pathologic alteration of the basal zone has also been called *hydropic* or *liquefactive degeneration of the basal layer.*

Lichenoid Alteration

Another group of conditions that affects the dermoepidermal junction is characterized by a dense accumulation of inflammatory cells in the papillary dermis, usually lymphocytes and macrophages, that may become so confluent that they obscure the basal zone. This group of conditions is usually referred to as having a "lichenoid" infiltrate by analogy with lichen planus, which is the prototype for this morphologic pattern (Fig. 3-2). The term *lichen,* however, is actually a clinical term that was chosen because the flat-topped, polyangular papules and plaques of this condition resemble lichens on trees and rocks, and it has histopathologic meaning only because it was adapted for this purpose.

The lichenoid tissue reaction also is accompanied by the formation of vacuoles at the dermoepidermal junction, but their presence may not be noticed at first because of the dense cellular infiltrate. Cell injury also occurs in the lower epidermis, resulting in individual cell necrosis. These homogeneous, round, pink bodies have been variously referred to as Civatte bodies, apoptotic cells, colloid bodies, dyskeratotic cells, and individual necrotic keratinocytes. As pointed out by Pinkus,[1] this damage to the basal layer leads to a reproducible series of changes in the epidermis. The keratinocytes in the spinous layer become larger, there are more granular cells, and there is a thickened orthokeratotic cornified layer. This spectrum of changes is seen not only in lichen planus but also in many other etiologically separate conditions, including inflammatory diseases such as lichenoid drug reactions and lupus erythematosus and as a manifestation of the host response to neoplasms, such as solar and seborrheic keratoses, Bowen's disease, and keratoacanthoma.

Figure 3-1. Lupus erythematosus exhibiting vacuolar change at the dermoepidermal junction. The vacuoles are situated both above and below the thickened basement membrane.

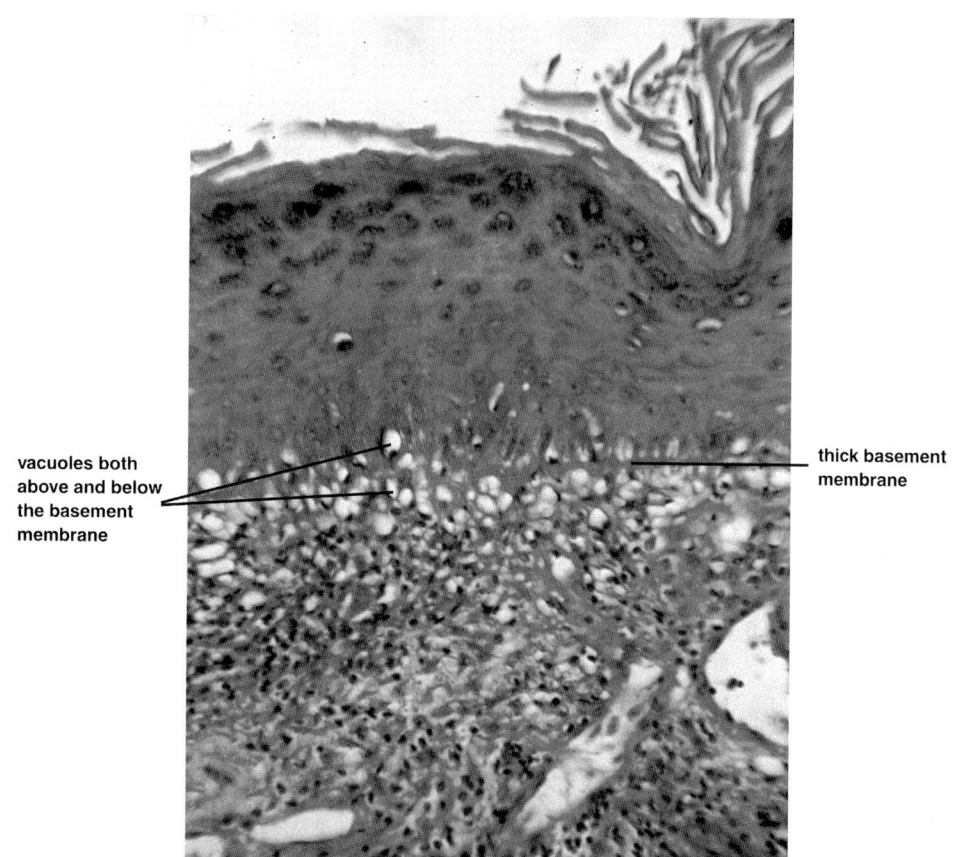

vacuoles both above and below the basement membrane

thick basement membrane

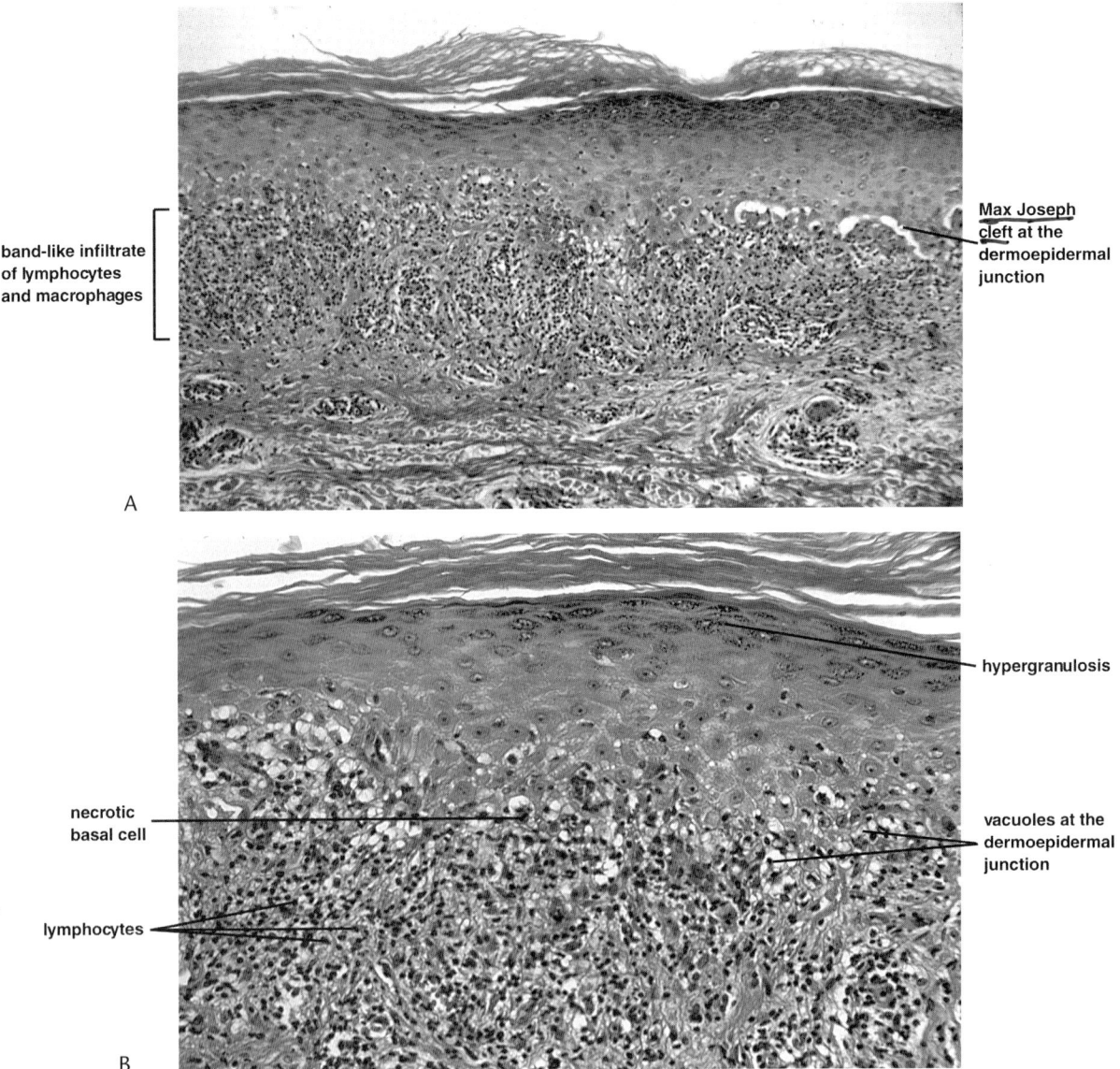

band-like infiltrate
of lymphocytes
and macrophages

Max Joseph
cleft at the
dermoepidermal
junction

hypergranulosis

necrotic
basal cell

vacuoles at the
dermoepidermal
junction

lymphocytes

A

B

Figure 3-2.   (A & B) Lichen planus. A dense infiltrate of lymphocytes and macrophages fills the papillary dermis and obscures the dermoepidermal junction.

Spongiosis

Spongiosis is the most common inflammatory reaction that affects the epidermis. It is the histopathologic correlate of the conditions that are grouped together clinically under the term
eczema, although spongiosis is not limited to this group of diseases because it is also seen in many diverse conditions that
range morphologically from some that are categorized clinically
as papulosquamous diseases, such as pityriasis rosea and seborrheic dermatitis, to annular erythemas and papular reactions to
arthropod bites and stings. Therefore, clinicopathologic correlation is often necessary to distinguish among these disorders.

The spongiotic tissue reaction has two essential epidermal
components, exocytosis of inflammatory cells and intercellular
edema. The inflammatory cells are usually lymphocytes and
monocytes but may be eosinophils or neutrophils depending on

the cause of the condition. The intercellular edema is first seen
as widening of the intercellular spaces and stretching of the intercellular bridges. In time, the spaces enlarge and become confluent with rupture of the desmosomes and cell membranes to
form intraepidermal vesicles (Fig. 3-3). If there are several
small vesicles of varying size separated only by thin walls made
up of the compressed membranes of the admixed keratinocytes
that form a net-like framework, then a multiloculated vesicle is
the end result (Fig. 3-4). This process is referred to as *reticular
degeneration*. Keratinocytes are damaged by the inflammatory
cells or their products, so spongiosis is not simple intercellular
edema; there is also intracellular edema, which may be harder to
detect in cases with slight spongiosis, and there may also be cell
death. The intracellular edema makes the keratinocytes appear
pale and swollen, and the individual dying cells have pyknotic
nuclei and eosinophilic cytoplasm. Acantholysis also may oc-

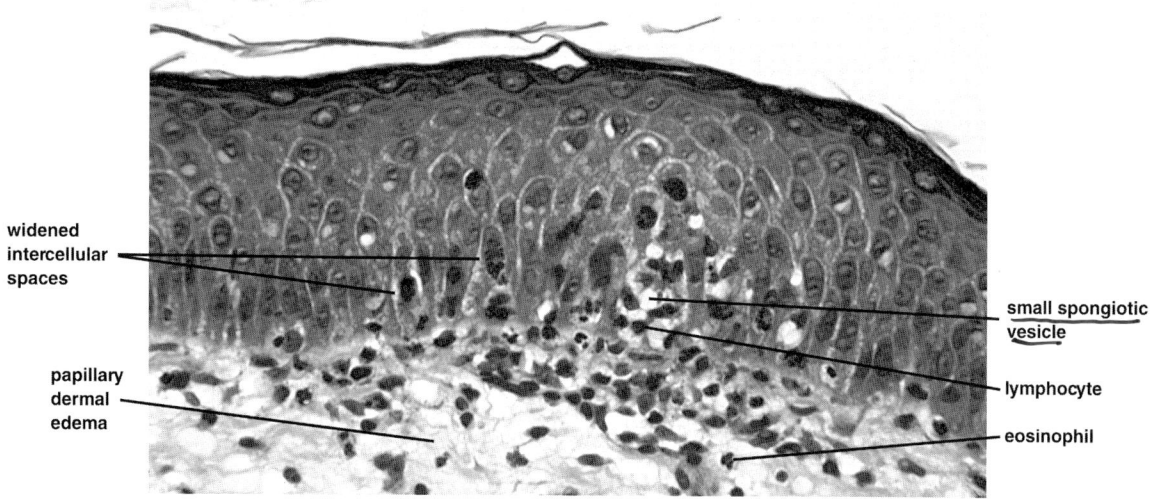

Figure 3-3. Early spongiosis. This evolving spongiotic dermatitis shows intercellular edema and exocytosis of inflammatory cells. There is a small vesicle in the stratum spinosum.

cur, so some of the large cells that resemble enlarged mononuclear cells in spongiotic vesicles are in actuality rounded up keratinocytes.

Although spongiosis usually results from a delayed hypersensitivity reaction as in the case of allergic contact dermatitis, which is the prototype for the spongiotic tissue reaction, there are other inflammatory mediators of spongiosis. This can be deduced from the observations that some spongiotic reactions are associated with exocytosis of eosinophils or neutrophils rather than lymphocytes. These uncommon types of spongiosis have diagnostic importance because only a limited number of diseases are associated with them. The prototype for spongiosis with eosinophils is the precursor lesion of pemphigus vulgaris, a condition of dysadhesion that in some instances begins with intercellular edema and exocytosis of eosinophils rather than the expected suprabasal acantholysis. Since the seminal observation of this phenomenon is pemphigus,[2] several other conditions have also been identified that show this type of spongiotic reaction. The prototype for spongiosis with neutrophils is primary irritant dermatitis, but this histologic feature also occurs in a limited spectrum of other etiologically diverse conditions. Unlike spongiosis with eosinophils, spongiosis with neutrophils

Figure 3-4. Severe spongiosis. The epidermis shows several microvesicles separated by septa formed by compressed squamous cells.

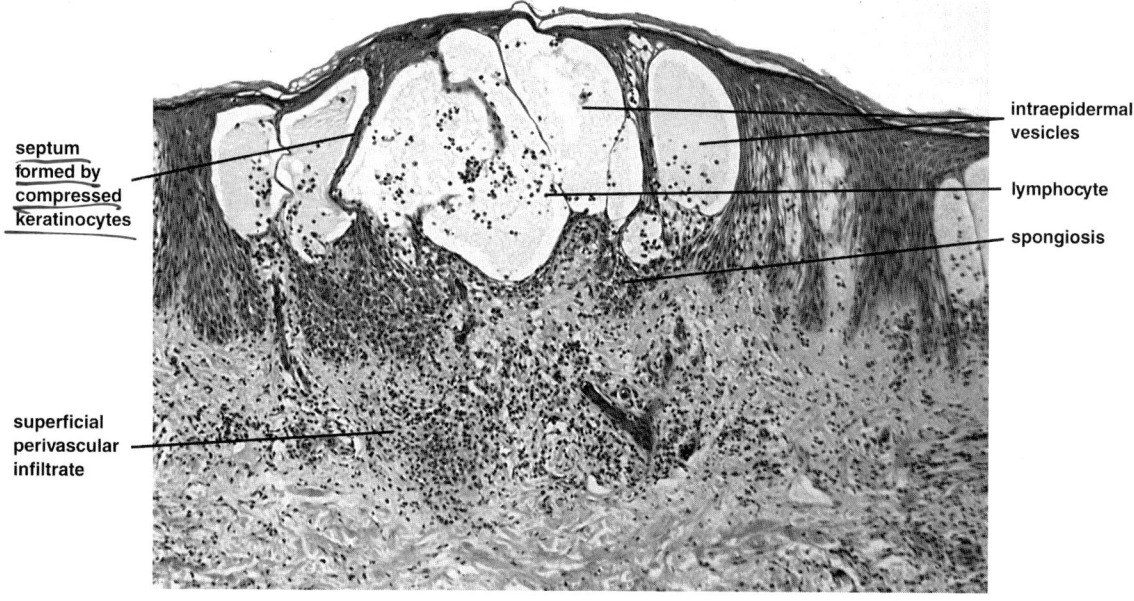

only has significance when the stratum corneum is intact. Once it has lost its integrity, neutrophils may be seen in any type of spongiotic dermatitis. Therefore, it is important to determine the predominant cell type within the epidermis in spongiotic tissue reactions because it may provide a helpful clue for differential diagnosis.

Hyperplasia

Hyperplasia is another basic way that the epidermis responds to exogenous or endogenous trauma. Injury to the epithelial cells induces a repair reaction that requires proliferation to generate new cells. This repair reaction may be self-limited if the injury is of brief duration, or it may be long-lived if the injurious stimulus persists. The prototype for epidermal hyperplasia is psoriasis, so some authors refer to the group of inflammatory dermatoses demonstrating epidermal hyperplasia as the *psoriasiform dermatitides*. This is despite the fact that well-developed plaques of psoriasis have a distinctive histologic picture that permits a specific diagnosis to be made in most instances. That epidermal hyperplasia is a generic response of the epidermis to persistent injury is supported by the observation that conditions that begin as spongiotic reactions, such as nummular dermatitis, eventually evolve into psoriasiform dermatitides if left untreated. Furthermore, chronic external trauma from rubbing or scratching of the skin induces epidermal hyperplasia and papillary dermal fibroplasia in most persons. In most conditions of epidermal hyperplasia, there will be a perturbance of differentiation that results in parakeratosis. The degree of parakeratosis and the distribution of the parakeratotic cells can prove helpful in differential diagnosis. For example, in the typical active lesion of psoriasis, the parakeratosis is confluent, whereas in the herald patch of pityriasis rosea the parakeratotic cells are clustered in mound-like aggregates, and in pityriasis rubra pilaris the parakeratotic cells are distributed haphazardly in an otherwise orthohyperkeratotic stratum corneum.

The architecture of the epidermis and the reciprocal alterations of the papillary dermis are also helpful features in differential diagnosis. In well-developed plaques of psoriasis, the elongated rete ridges are fairly uniform in length. The rete ridges are usually club shaped, and the intervening dermal papillae are narrow (Fig. 3-5). By contrasts in lichen simplex chronicus the rete are markedly irregular in length and width, and the dermal papillae are widened because of deposition of new collagen in concentric lamellae that follow the contour of the hyperplastic rete ridges (Fig. 3-6).

Atrophy

Atrophy is the loss of tissue substance. With regard to the epidermis, it refers to loss of cell layers. Although aging and chronic sun exposure can produce atrophy of the epidermis, it usually occurs as a result of destruction of the basal zone of the epidermis and effacement of the rete ridges by an inflammatory process. The diseases that most commonly produce atrophy of the epidermis are those that affect the dermoepidermal junction. Lupus erythematosus is the classic example of interface dermatitis that results in epidermal atrophy.

Atrophy is an end-stage process, and it may not be possible to make a specific diagnosis of the cause unless the biopsy specimen is obtained while the underlying disease is still in its active phase (Fig. 3-7). The porokeratoses are distinctive in that the epidermis in the center of the lesions is atrophic, and there is centrifugal enlargement of the lesions with a characteristic ridge of scale marking the active margin. The correct histologic diagnosis can be made only if the parakeratotic coronoid lamella at the advancing edge of the expanding clone of altered squamous cells is included in the biopsy specimen.

The poikilodermatous changes that may occur in cutaneous

Figure 3-5. Psoriasis. This well-developed lesion has rete ridges that are equally elongated and bulbous. The intervening dermal papillae are narrow. The epidermis overlying the dermal papillae is not thickened.

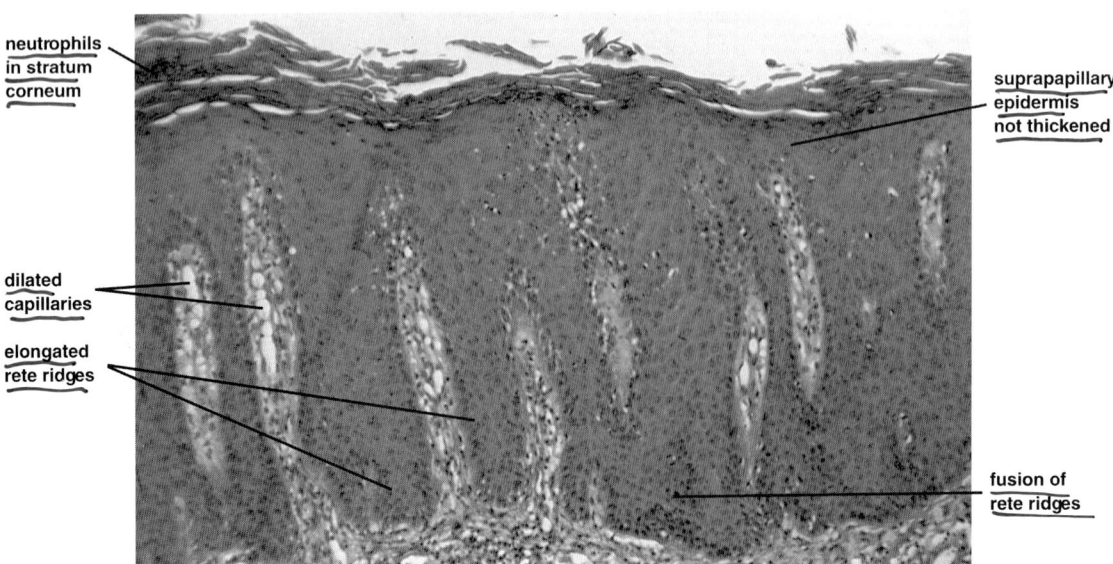

neutrophils in stratum corneum

dilated capillaries

elongated rete ridges

suprapapillary epidermis not thickened

fusion of rete ridges

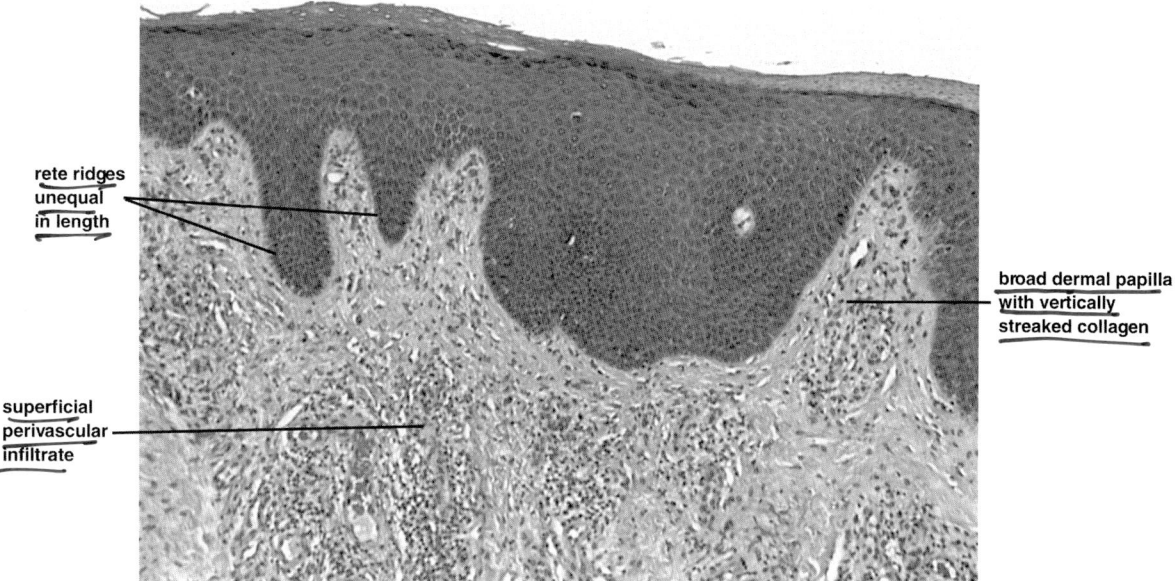

Figure 3-6. Lichen simplex chronicus. The epidermis shows hyperplasia with rete ridges that are unequal in length and width. The dermal papillae are broad and show vertical streaking of the collagen.

T-cell lymphoma, poikiloderma congenitale, hereditary sclerosing poikiloderma, and hereditary acrokeratotic poikiloderma also are associated with destruction of the basal zone and pigmentary incontinence. These conditions must be considered in the differential diagnosis of epidermal atrophy along with the inflammatory diseases that damage the dermoepidermal interface.

DISTRIBUTION PATTERNS OF INFLAMMATORY CELLS IN THE DERMIS

Perivascular Pattern

The cells that mediate inflammatory reactions in the skin are able to attach to the endothelial cells of the cutaneous microvasculature by the action of cell adhesion molecules.[3] There-

Figure 3-7. Lichen sclerosus et atrophicus. The epidermis is thin with effacement of the rete ridges. The thickened, hyalinized papillary dermis is characteristic of lichen sclerosus.

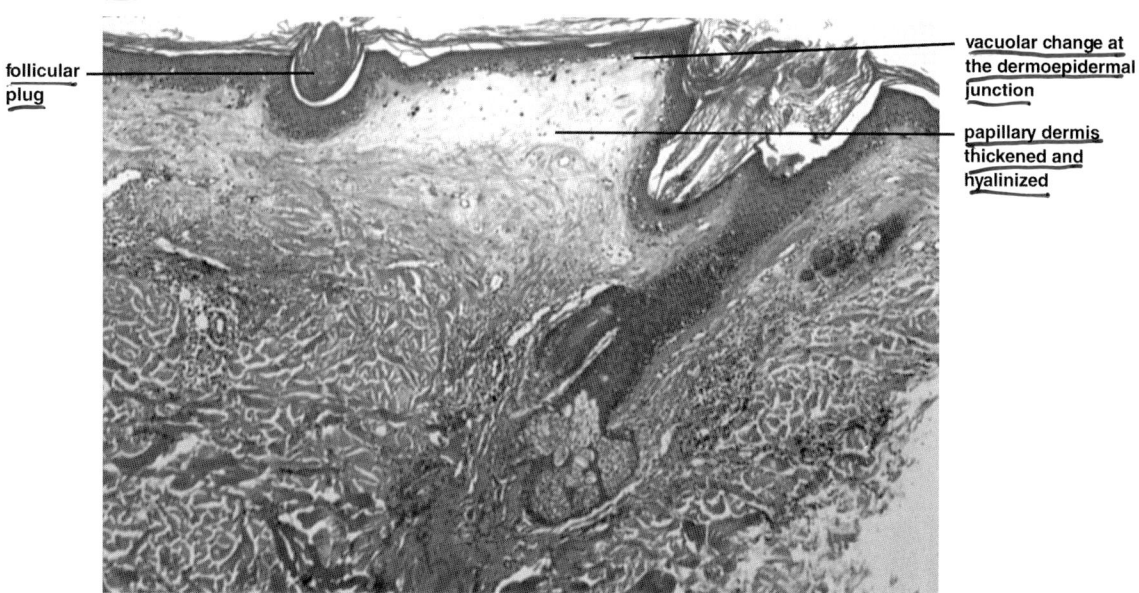

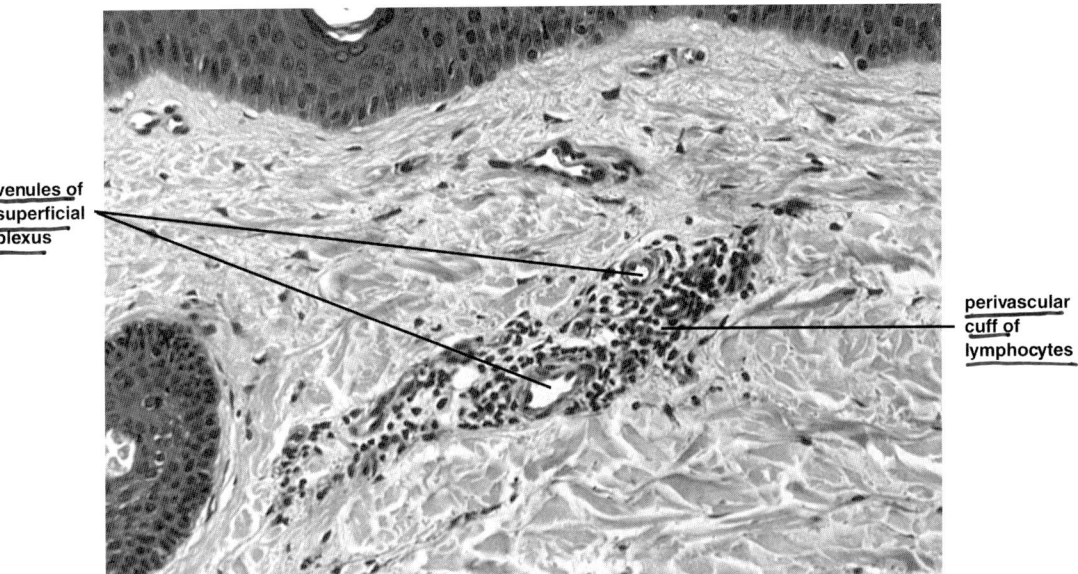

venules of
superficial
plexus

perivascular
cuff of
lymphocytes

Figure 3-8. Erythema annulare centrifugum, advancing edge. There is a moderately dense infiltrate of lymphocytes that is tightly circumscribed around the vessels of the superficial vascular plexus.

fore, they accumulate first around the vessels that brought them there. This accounts for the observation that almost any inflammatory response in the skin has as its earliest microscopic findings a sparse perivascular infiltrate. The types of inflammatory cells involved depend on the nature of the immunologic reaction that underlies the disease. In time, the infiltrate may become more dense and the cells may migrate away from the vessels in response to the chemotaxins that are being elaborated in the microenvironment. They may migrate to the epidermis or into the interstitial spaces among collagen bundles.

In the vast majority of inflammatory dermatoses, the perivascular pattern of infiltrate is the dominating pattern (Fig. 3-8). In some conditions, especially those that involve the deep reaction compartment, there is also a tendency toward interstitial distribution of cells in addition to the perivascular accumulation of them. The lichenoid tissue reaction is associated with a marked tendency for interstitial accumulation of the inflammatory cells throughout the full thickness of the papillary dermis.

Nodular Pattern

In a relatively small number of conditions, the cells of the infiltrate continue to aggregate around the vessels rather than to migrate away from them. These accumulations eventually take the form of small nodular aggregates within the dermis. Granulomas comprise a unique subset of nodular infiltrates in which the blood monocytes differentiate into epithelioid cells[4] (Fig. 3-9). Examination of serial sections often reveals the small blood vessel that lies within the center of each granuloma, although the swollen endothelial cells may themselves closely resemble epithelioid macrophages, making their recognition difficult. In other instances in which there is necrosis in the center of the granuloma, the vessel may be destroyed.

Diffuse Pattern

Rarely, the inflammatory reaction results in an effusive influx of cells that not only accumulate around the vessels but also fill the interstitial spaces to form a massive, diffuse cellular infiltrate in the dermis. Sweet's disease is a good example of the dense, diffuse pattern of infiltrate (Fig. 3-10). Granuloma faciale, nodular scabies, and lepromatous leprosy are other examples of this distribution pattern of inflammatory cells.

Periadnexal Pattern

In diseases that affect the cutaneous adnexal structures, the inflammatory infiltrate is usually most prominent around the structures being affected. For example, in acne the infiltrate surrounds the affected hair follicles and in miliaria rubra, the eccrine ducts. In some conditions, both the epidermis and the adnexal structures derived from it are affected e.g., discoid lupus erythematosus, in which the hair follicles as well as the epidermis are damaged by the inflammatory infiltrate (Fig. 3-11).

OTHER IMPORTANT HISTOLOGIC CHANGES

Vesicle Formation

Intraepidermal Vesicles

Vesicles that arise within the epidermis can form as the result of spongiosis, ballooning of keratinocytes, acantholysis, or cytolysis. Spongiotic vesicles are the most common. Allergic contact dermatitis is the prototype for spongiotic vesiculation, but spongiosis can be caused by many factors. Other types of allergic reactions, toxic reactions, and metabolic disturbances can cause

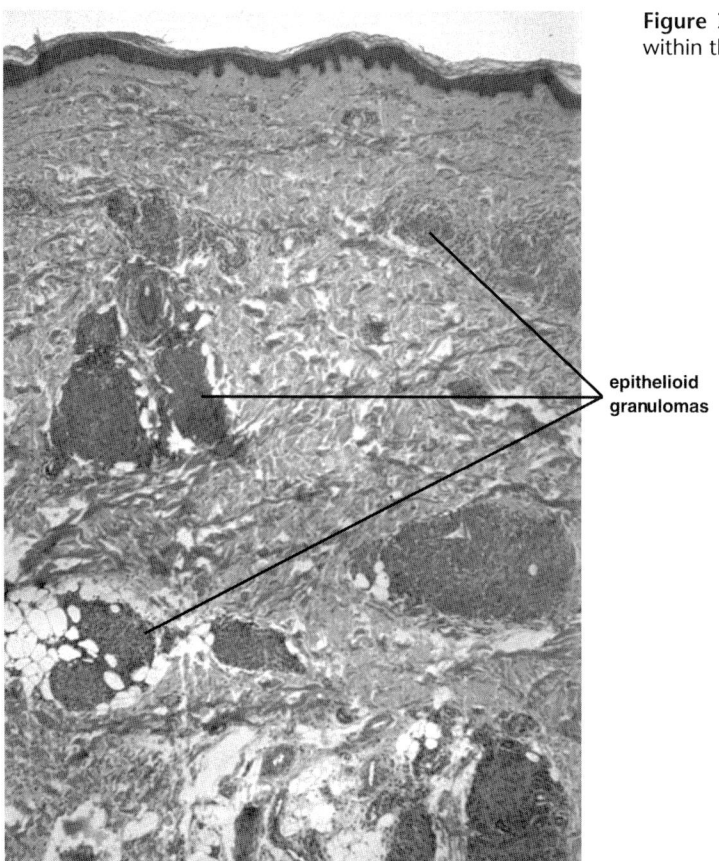

Figure 3-9. **(A & B)** Sarcoid. There are epithelioid tubercles within the reticular dermis.

epithelioid
granulomas

A

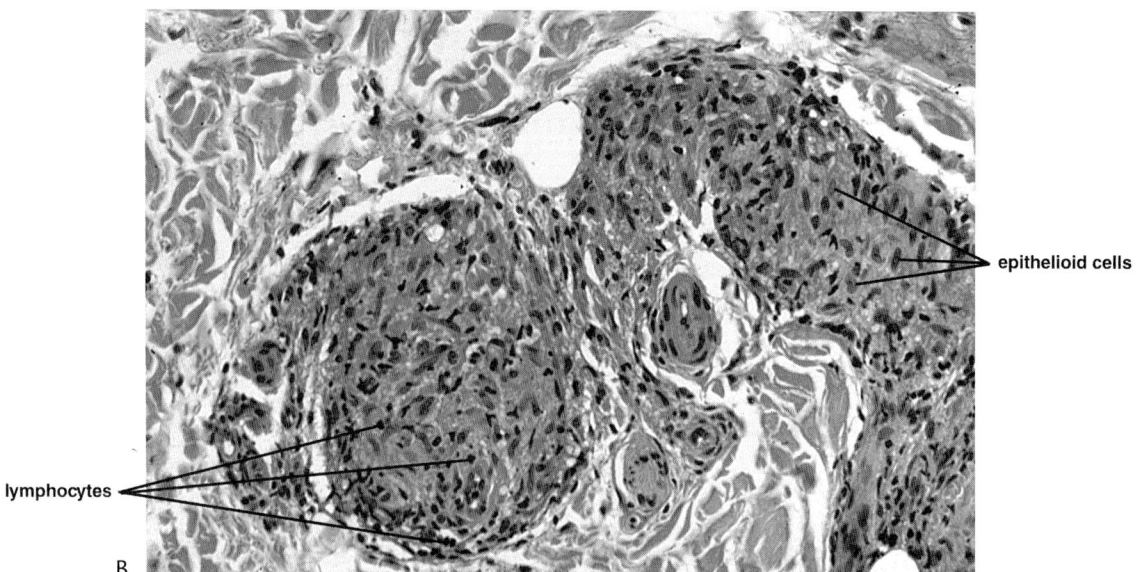

epithelioid cells

lymphocytes

B

spongiotic vesiculation. Being the most common mechanism of intraepidermal vesiculation, spongiosis is also the least specific, so clinicopathologic correlation is often important for identification of the cause.

Ballooning degeneration of keratinocytes is due to intracellular edema. Several viruses can produce intracellular edema, in-cluding the herpesvirus group, the poxviruses, and some enteroviruses. Herpesviruses also cause other cytopathologic changes that permit recognition of them, including intranuclear inclusion bodies, peripheral margination of the nucleoplasm, and formation of multinucleated epidermal giant cells (Fig. 3-12). Likewise, poxviruses often leave a calling card in the

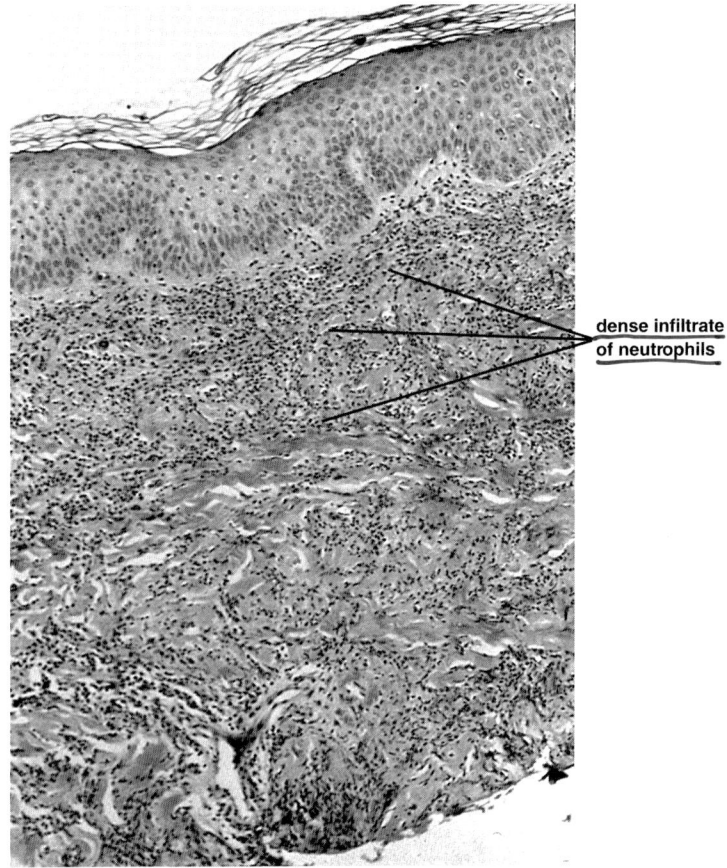

dense infiltrate
of neutrophils

Figure 3-10. Sweet's disease. Within the dermis is a dense infiltrate of neutrophils. The cells are present diffusely among collagen bundles as well as around blood vessels.

Figure 3-11. Chronic cutaneous lupus erythematosus. In addition to interface changes involving the epidermis, there is a prominent infiltrate of lymphocytes around the hair follicles. The hair follicles may be destroyed by the inflammatory process.

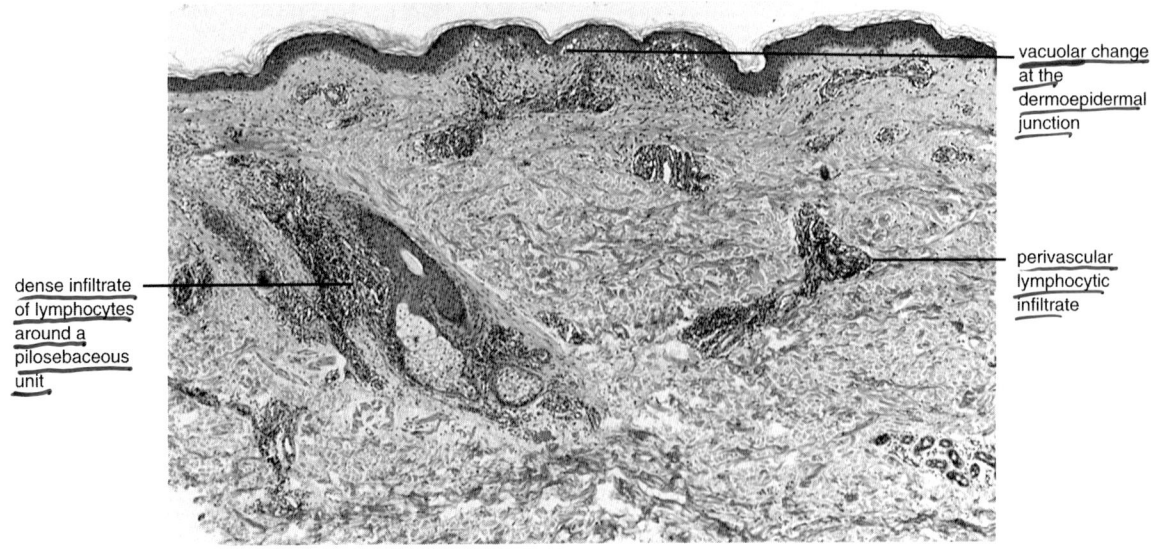

vacuolar change
at the
dermoepidermal
junction

perivascular
lymphocytic
infiltrate

dense infiltrate
of lymphocytes
around a
pilosebaceous
unit

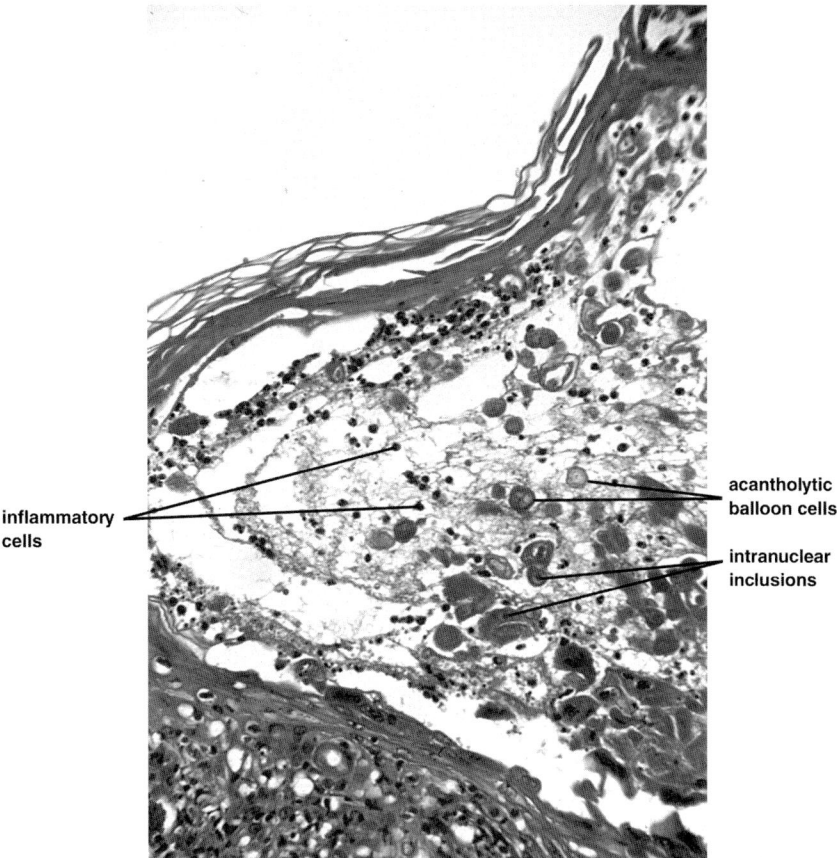

inflammatory cells

acantholytic balloon cells

intranuclear inclusions

Figure 3-12. Herpes simplex. This vesicle demonstrates ballooning change with acantholysis. Characteristic intranuclear inclusion bodies are also present in some cells.

form of intracytoplasmic inclusion bodies. Enteroviruses, such as Coxsackie, however, do not leave "fingerprints." Rupture of the swollen keratinocytes leads to reticular degeneration of the epidermis and thus to intraepidermal vesiculation. Viruses are not the only cause of ballooning, however, as it also occurs in toxic reactions in the skin and in erythema multiforme and fixed drug eruption.

Acantholysis means the dissolution of intercellular adhesion in the epidermis with separation of the spinous cells one from another. The separated keratinocytes loose their polyangular contours and become rounded in shape. This phenomenon occurs in all forms of pemphigus. In pemphigus vulgaris, pemphigus vegetans, and Hailey-Hailey disease, it occurs in the lower epidermis just above the basal cells, which remain attached to the basement membrane zone (Fig. 3-13). In pemphigus erythematosus and foliaceous, the acantholysis occurs in the granular zone. With the exception of Hailey-Hailey disease in which the cause of the acantholysis is genetically determined, although the pathophysiology remains undetermined, the cell dysadhesion is due to the formation of autoantibodies directed against components of the desmosomes. Acantholysis also occurs in the stratum granulosum in impetigo and staphylococcal scalded skin syndrome and in the suprabasal zone in Grover's disease and Darier's disease.

Cytolysis is a peculiar phenomenon that occurs in epidermolysis bullosa simplex and epidermolytic hyperkeratosis due to genetically determined defects in keratin production. In these conditions, friction sets off a reaction in the cytoplasm of the keratinocytes that results in autolysis. In epidermolysis bullosa simplex, this leads to separation of the epidermis from the basement membrane (Fig. 3-14). In epidermolytic hyperkeratosis, bullae form in the stratum spinosum.

Subepidermal Vesicles

Subepidermal vesicles can form at different levels of the basement membrane zone from the basal cells to the anchoring fibrils of the dermis. The causes range from developmental abnormalities of the structural components of the basement membrane zone to immunologic reactions to physical trauma, and the histopathologic picture ranges from subepidermal bullae with no inflammatory infiltrate and no evidence of structural damage to bullae containing a dense infiltrate with massive destruction of the components of the dermoepidermal junction. The differential diagnosis can often be narrowed to a few possibilities by light microscopic examination, the caveats being that the biopsy specimen is taken from an early lesion without ex-

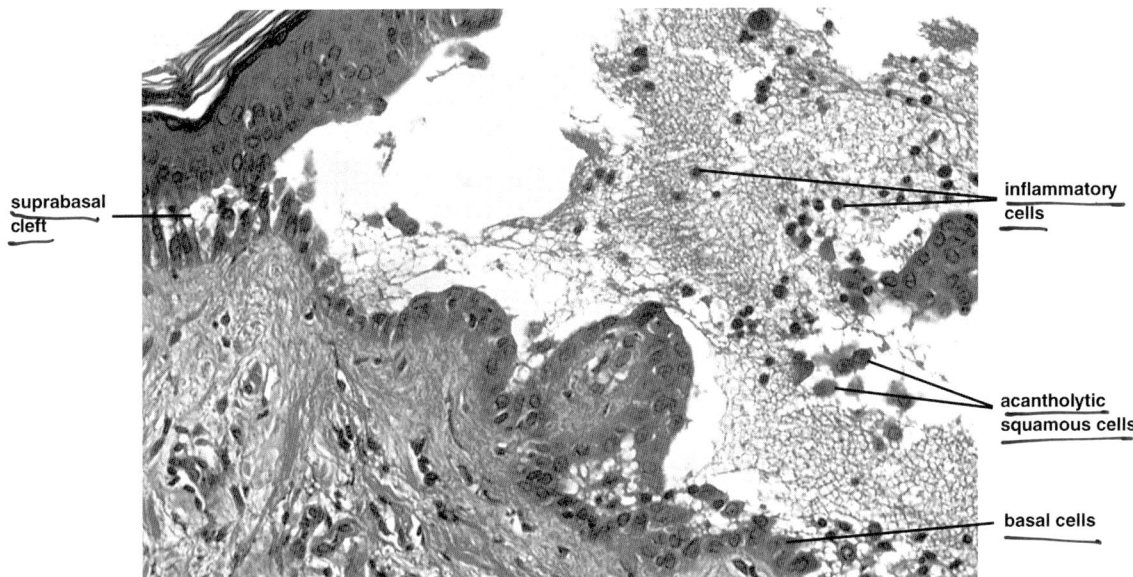

suprabasal cleft

inflammatory cells

acantholytic squamous cells

basal cells

Figure 3-13. Pemphigus vulgaris. There is a suprabasal bulla containing acantholytic squamous cells.

tensive secondary changes and includes the periphery of the bulla. The features that are important are the architecture of the bulla, the presence or absence of an inflammatory cell infiltrate, and the composition of the infiltrate if one is present.

The architectural features of subepidermal bullae are the profiles of the rete ridges in the blister roof and the dermal papillae at the base of the blister and the presence or absence of microabscesses in the dermal papillae adjacent to it. In porphyria cutanea tarda, the intact bullae have no cellular infiltrate, the dermal papillae are preserved, and the epidermal rete in the blister roof are effaced (Fig. 3-15). In dermatitis herpetiformis, both the dermal papillae and the epidermal rete are effaced, and there are neutrophil microabscesses in the dermal papillae adjacent to the bulla (Fig. 3-16). In the subepidermal bullae of pemphigoid, the dermal papillae are preserved and the epidermal rete maintain their configuration in the blister roof. These are but a few examples of the architectural aspects of subepidermal bullous diseases.

Figure 3-14. Epidermolysis bullosa simplex. This lesion demonstrates incipient bulla formation. There are vacuolated cells in the basal layer that represent degenerating basal keratinocytes. This confluent process results in loss of attachment of the epidermis.

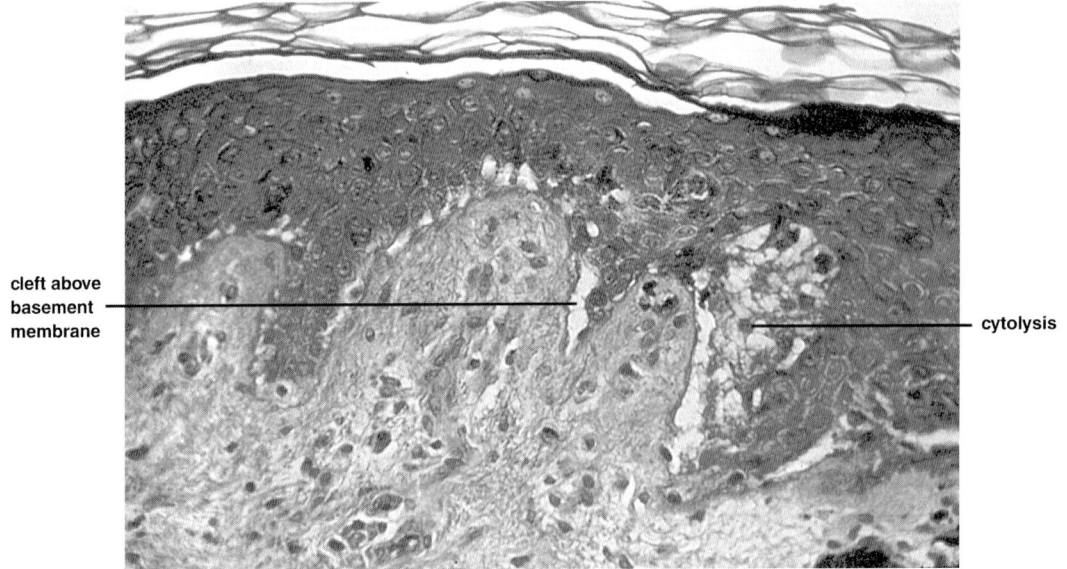

cleft above basement membrane

cytolysis

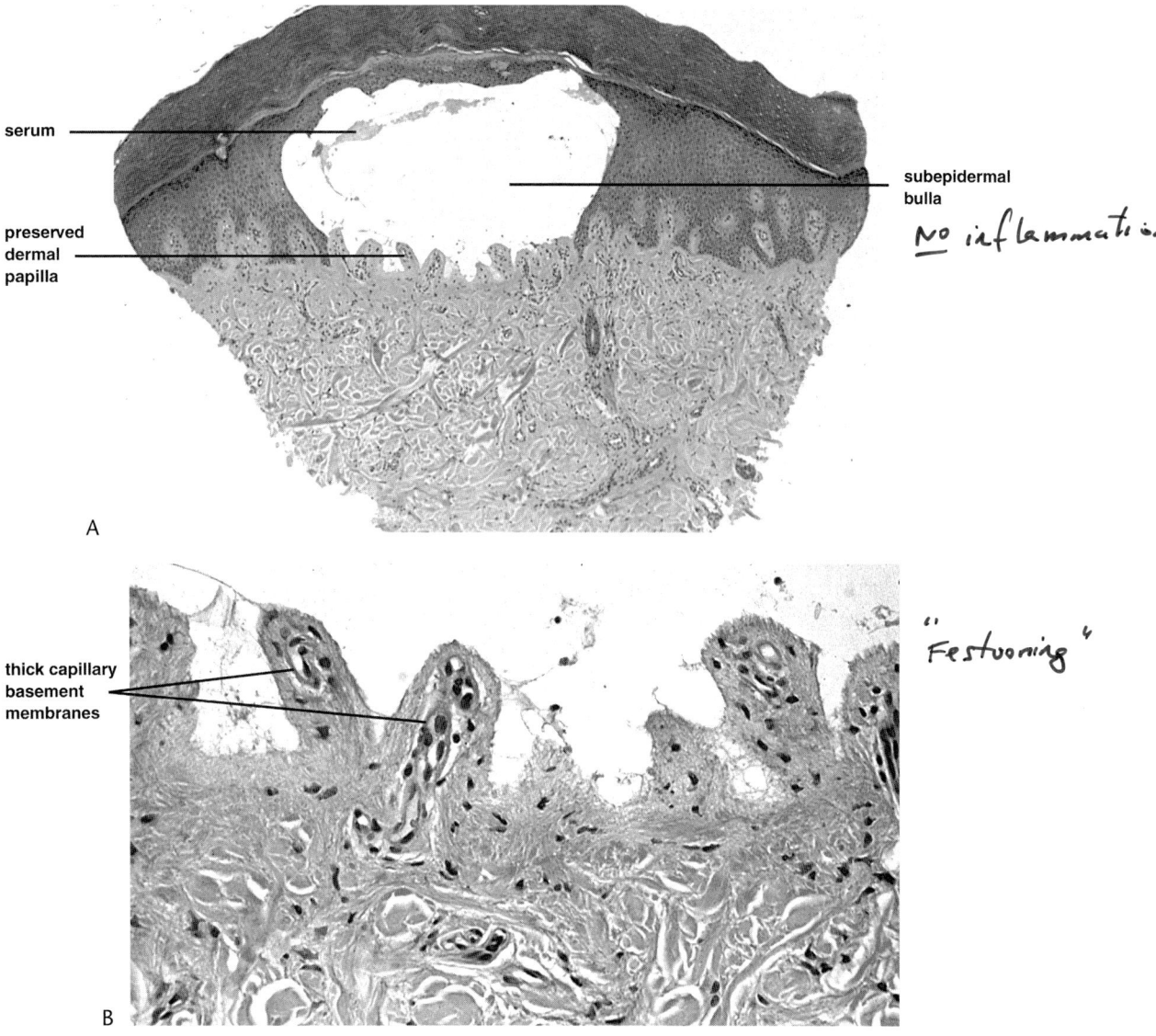

serum

subepidermal
bulla

No inflammation

preserved
dermal
papilla

A

thick capillary
basement
membranes

"Festooning"

B

Figure 3-15. **(A & B)** Porphyria cutanea tarda. There is a subepidermal bulla with preservation of the dermal papillae at the base. Their appearance is reminiscent of a string of leaves and thus has been referred to as "festooning." Some serum is present in the blister space, but no inflammatory cells are present either in the blister or in the dermis.

Some subepidermal bullous diseases are not associated with inflammation as long as the blisters remain intact. Conditions that fall into this category include all the forms of hereditary epidermolysis bullosa, porphyria cutanea tarda, and some cases of epidermolysis bullosa acquisita and toxic epidermal necrolysis. Furthermore, some bullous diseases that usually are associated with a prominent inflammatory infiltrate may on occasion show only a sparse infiltrate. This occurs, for example, in the cell-poor variant of pemphigoid, so the dermis should be carefully examined in every case in which the scanning power view appears to show no inflammatory cells.

In those cases in which there is an easily detectable inflammatory cell infiltrate in the bulla and the dermis, determination of the composition of the infiltrate is often the most helpful feature in differential diagnosis. Pemphigoid is usually associated with a mixed infiltrate in which eosinophils are prominent and neutrophils are either absent or inconspicuous. By contrast, dermatitis herpetiformis is mediated by neutrophils, and there are relatively few eosinophils in most instances. Erythema multiforme bullosa has neither eosinophils nor neutrophils in the infiltrate in most cases, only mononuclear cells.

For every rule there are exceptions; thus, subepidermal bullous diseases may not always show the expected features. Pemphigoid can on occasion have an infiltrate rich in neutrophils, and erythema multiforme may have eosinophils; therefore, it is important to consider all available information in making a diagnosis, including not only the architectural features of the bulla, the presence or absence of an inflammatory infiltrate, and,

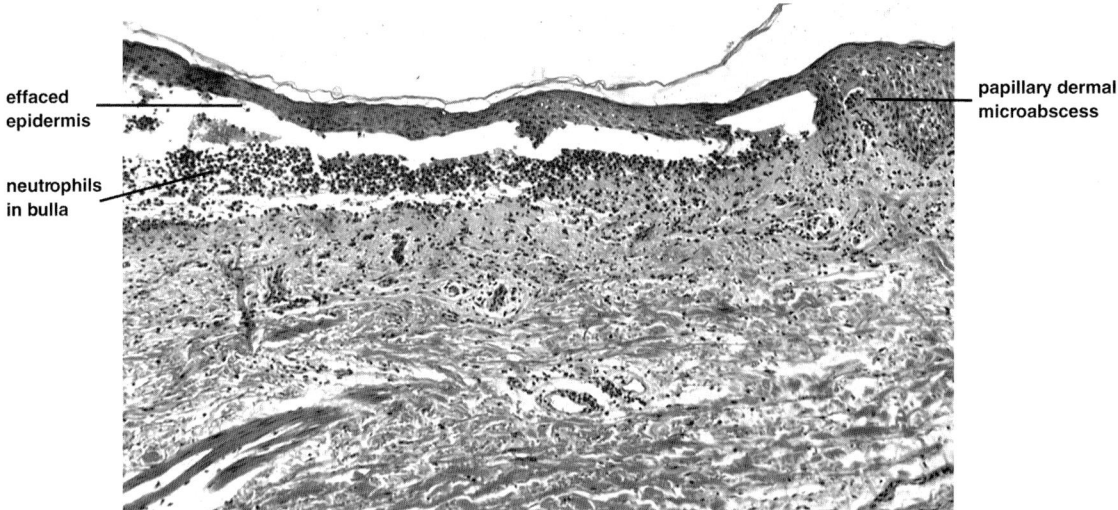

effaced epidermis

neutrophils in bulla

papillary dermal microabscess

Figure 3-16. Dermatitis herpetiformis. There is a subepidermal bullae containing neutrophils. The epidermal rete and the dermal papillae have been effaced. There is a papillary microabscess to the right of the bulla.

if present, its constituent cells, but also the clinical features and immunopathologic findings if available.

Pustule Formation

Whenever a pustule is seen, there is almost a reflex assumption made that it is due to pyogenic infection. Indeed, pyoderma is a common cause of cutaneous pustules, but there are many conditions of the skin that are associated with sterile pustules. The morphology of the pustule and its site of origin relative to the adnexal orifices can be helpful in histologic differential diagnosis. Many types of folliculitis are associated with pustule formation, and the follicular unit should be closely examined for fungi, yeasts, bacteria, and evidence of viral cytopathic changes. If the plane of the tissue section is adjacent to the involved follicle, sometimes an intraepidermal pustule is seen from extension of the inflammatory exudate outward from the follicular orifice, and the follicle itself is not present in the tissue section. The correct diagnosis will not be made unless the pathologist suspects folliculitis and obtains additional tissue sections. The same can occur in miliaria pustulosa.

Spongiform pustules occur only in certain diseases (Fig. 3-17). The spongiform pustule is characteristic of pustular psoriasis and its variants but also can be seen in secondary syphilis, dermatophyte infections, and candidiasis. Keratoderma blenorrhagicum, which occurs in Reiter's disease, also is characterized by spongiform pustules.

Subcorneal pustules are seen in impetigo, but the superficial types of pemphigus may often have an identical histologic picture as may subcorneal pustulosis, so the correct diagnosis may require clinicopathologic correlation and knowledge of the results of bacterial cultures and immunopathologic studies.

Many intraepidermal or subepidermal vesicles due to inflammation that remain intact for more than a few days become pustules due to the influx of leukocytes. Therefore, the differential diagnosis of pustules also includes the various intra- and subepidermal vesicular diseases.

Vasculitis

The blood vessels are usually just the conduits for the leukocytes to make their way to the site of inflammation, but as such they can be affected by the mediators of inflammation that are being released in the area. It is common to see changes in the blood vessels in inflammatory reactions in the skin. Most of the time they are surrounded by inflammatory cells. They may be dilated and congested with red cells or marginating leukocytes. Sometimes, they show swelling of the endothelial cells, almost to the point of obscuring the lumen, and there may be extravasation of red cells. None of these changes, however, signify vasculitis.

Only the blood vessels of the subcutaneous fat are usually large enough to have muscular walls, so vessel wall necrosis is only seen in the types of vasculitis that involve the subcutis such as polyarteritis nodosa and nodular vasculitis. Vasculitis is a distinctive reaction that clearly is different than the constellation of changes that may occur in perivascular inflammation. The typical small vessel vasculitis that involves the skin can only be diagnosed by applying stringent criteria. The most reliable criteria are deposition of fibrin around the affected vessels, leukocytoclasis related to the vessel walls, and formation of thrombi within them (Fig. 3-18).

SCANNING POWER APPROACH TO DIAGNOSIS

Students of dermatology are taught a systematic approach to the morphologic diagnosis of skin diseases. The key features to be observed are the nature of the primary lesion, the evolutionary or secondary changes that have occurred in the lesion(s), the configuration of the lesion(s), and their distribution. Whereas most authors and teachers emphasize the importance of the primary lesion, the distribution of the lesions is equally important if not more so in many cases. For example, if a patient presents with a disease that affects the antecubital and popliteal fossae, the diagnosis most likely is atopic dermatitis. If the condition in-

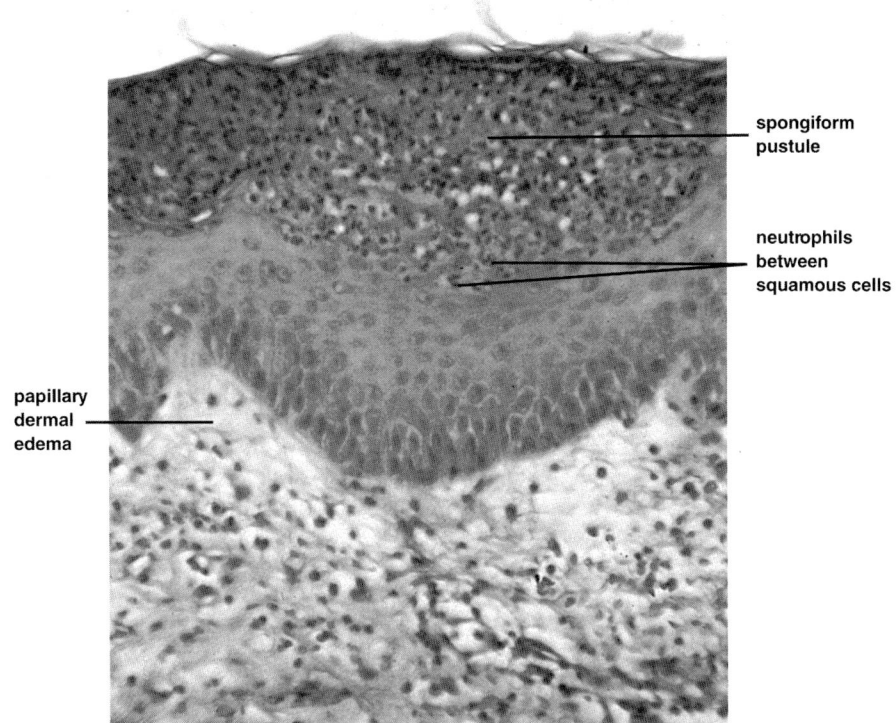

spongiform pustule

neutrophils between squamous cells

papillary dermal edema

Figure 3-17. Pustular psoriasis. There is a characteristic spongiform pustule in the upper epidermis. It is formed by exocytosis of myriad neutrophils that fill the spaces among the compressed keratinocytes, thereby resembling the cut surface of a sponge with neutrophils in the holes.

Figure 3-18. Leukocytoclastic vasculitis. This small blood vessel is ringed by deposits of fibrin. There is prominent leukocytoclasis.

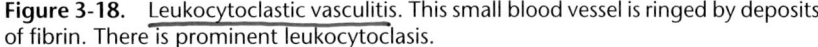

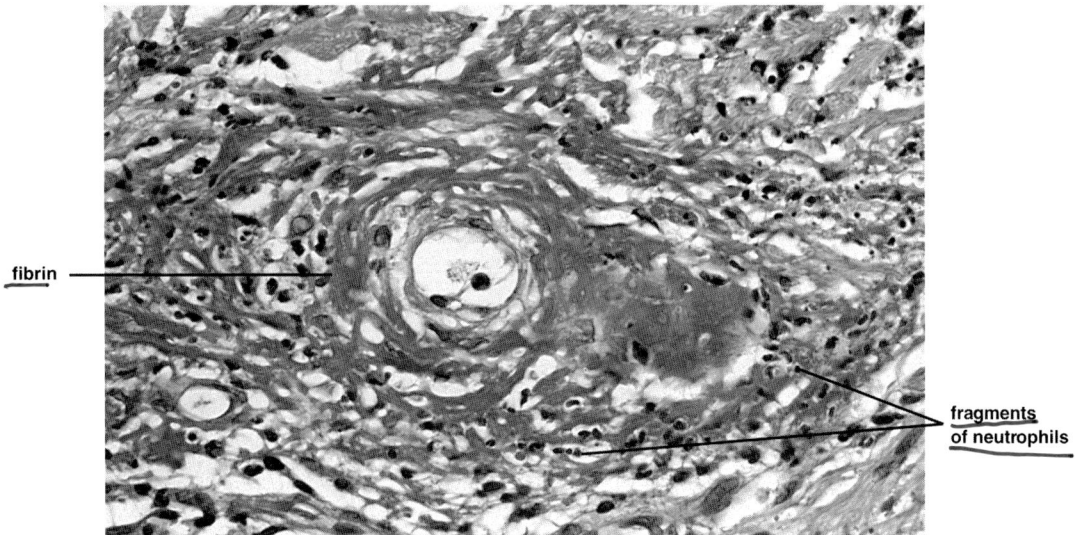

fibrin

fragments of neutrophils

volves the elbows, knees, and scalp, the most likely diagnosis is psoriasis; if it affects the scalp, eyebrows, and nasolabial folds, it most likely is seborrheic dermatitis. These diagnoses can be made with a high degree of assurance without even knowing the nature of the primary lesions. Configuration is also important in differential diagnosis, as there are only a limited number of diseases that are annular or linear or herpetiform or corymbiform and so forth. Once the configuration is known, the differential diagnosis can be further refined by knowing the nature of the primary lesion. For example, if an annular lesion is formed by papules it could be granuloma annulare, sarcoidosis, or lichen planus, but it would not likely be porokeratosis or tinea corporis.

Dermatopathology can be approached in a similar fashion. In microscopic morphology, the primary lesions in inflammatory diseases can be thought of as spongiosis, vacuolar interface change, epidermal hyperplasia, intra- and subepidermal vesicles, vasculitis, and granulomas. Distribution can be regarded as the distribution of the inflammatory cells in the skin (i.e., the superficial reaction compartment, the deep reaction compartment, the panniculus, or the adnexal structures). Configuration pertains to the arrangement of the inflammatory cells, but it also pertains to the architectural features of the lesions. Thus, there are palisaded granulomas as seen in granuloma annulare and necrobiosis lipoidica, wedge-shaped infiltrates as seen in arthropod bite reactions and Mucha-Habermann disease, band-like infiltrates as in lichen planus and lichenoid photodermatitis, nodular infiltrates as in infectious granulomas and pseudolymphomas, and so forth. Finally, there are secondary changes that can be helpful in classification such as colloid bodies in the papillary dermis as a clue to interface pathology, scale-crusts in the stratum corneum as a clue to antecedent spongiosis, or widening and fibrosis of the subcutaneous septa as a clue to septal panniculitis.

The most fruitful approach to the histologic diagnosis of inflammatory skin diseases is to look first with the scanning power objective in a systematic fashion and to answer the following questions. What body site is the biopsy specimen from, and are the microanatomic features normal for that site? Is the epidermis involved? If so, is it by spongiosis, interface changes, hyperplasia, or intraepidermal-subepidermal vesicle formation? Are the adnexal structures or panniculus involved? What is the distribution, density, and configuration of the inflammatory infiltrate?

Once these basic observations have been made, it is usually possible to rapidly assign the condition to one of the major reaction patterns. Then the epidermis, dermis, subcutis, and adnexal structures can be examined at higher magnification for details that may not be apparent at scanning power. These details that are gleaned from closer inspection then can be used to distinguish among the conditions included in the major groups. Finally, the clinical information can be taken into account in determining the most likely probability among the conditions being considered on the basis of the histologic examination.

CLINICAL CORRELATION IN DERMATOPATHOLOGY

Differential diagnosis is often a difficult problem in dermatopathology, most often among inflammatory conditions but also not uncommonly among neoplasms. Astute microscopists can often make the correct diagnosis in difficult cases without knowledge of the clinical features by careful attention to and proper interpretation of subtle changes. More often, however, correlation of the microscopic findings with the clinical features is helpful or even necessary for correct diagnosis. In all cases, however, the histologic specimen should be examined first without knowledge of the clinical features. This will force the observer to search out all the microscopic abnormalities without bias and to formulate an objective opinion before taking into account the clinical description.

Because the potential number of specific examples in which clinicopathologic correlation is helpful in dermatopathology is limitless, not all possibilities can be covered in a brief discussion; however, the most common situations can be divided into several major groups. The following list gives illustrative examples and is not intended to include all possibilities.

1. Conditions that share a discrete, highly characteristic histologic abnormality but are heterogeneous clinically:
   A. *Epidermolytic hyperkeratosis*[5]: a distinctive epithelial alteration that was thought to be specific for *bullous congenital ichthyosiform erythroderma*. Subsequently, it was found to occur in several other conditions, including
      i. Ichthyosis hystrix
      ii. Linear epidermal nevus (some cases)
      iii. Palmoplantar keratoderma (some cases)
      iv. Isolated epidermolytic acanthoma
      v. As an incidental finding in several unrelated pathologic conditions
   B. *Focal acantholytic dyskeratosis*[6]: a descriptive term used for the characteristic epidermal changes of Darier's disease (keratosis follicularis). Identical changes have been found in
      i. Transient acantholytic dermatosis (Grover's disease)
      ii. Systematized epidermal nevus (some cases)
      iii. Isolated dyskeratosis follicularis (warty dyskeratoma)
      iv. As an incidental finding in several unrelated pathologic conditions
   C. *Cornoid lamella formation*[7]: the characteristic feature of the various forms of *porokeratosis*. Cornoid lamellae, however, are not specific for porokeratosis because they are sometimes found in other unrelated conditions, including
      i. Some inflammatory conditions (e.g., psoriasis)
      ii. Benign epithelial proliferations
         a. Seborrheic keratosis
         b. Warts
         c. Cysts
      iii. Premalignant and malignant epithelial proliferations
         a. Solar keratosis
         b. Squamous cell carcinoma in situ
         c. Basal cell carcinoma
      iv. Linear epidermal nevus (some cases)
2. Conditions that show the same general reaction pattern and in which differential diagnosis is facilitated by clinical correlation:
   A. Clinicopathologic correlation is often necessary to distinguish between inflammatory conditions that show the same or very similar histologic features. This applies to

several basic histologic reactions groups. Examples include

    i. *Simple perivascular dermatitis,* viral exanthem vs. Schamberg's disease

    ii. *Lichenoid dermatitis,* lichen planus vs. lichenoid benign keratosis

    iii. *Spongiotic dermatitis,* allergic contact dermatitis vs. nummular dermatitis

    iv. *Psoriasiform dermatitis,* psoriasis vs. Reiter's disease

    v. *Subepidermal vesicular dermatitis,* bullous pemphigoid vs. herpes gestationis

    vi. *Vasculitis,* Henoch-Schönlein purpura vs. erythema elavatum diutinum

    vii. *Panniculitis,* erythema nodosum vs. subacute nodular migratory panniculitis

    viii. *Fibrosing dermatitis,* scleroderma vs. morphea

B. Benign epithelial proliferations

    i. Some epidermal nevi vs. seborrheic keratosis

    ii. Inflammatory linear epidermal nevus vs. lichen simplex chronicus

    iii. Acanthosis nigricans vs. confluent and reticulated papillomatosis

    iv. Dermatosis papulosis nigra vs. seborrheic keratosis

    v. Reticulated pigmentary anomaly of the flexures vs. adenoidal seborrheic keratosis

C. Premalignant and malignant epithelial proliferations

    i. Arsenical keratosis vs. Bowen's disease

    ii. Erythroplasia of Queyrat vs. Bowen's disease

    iii. Epidermotropic metastatic melanoma vs. primary malignant melanoma

    iv. Linear basal cell nevus vs. nevoid basal cell carcinoma syndrome

3. Conditions in which the biopsy shows no apparent abnormality and clinical information provides the key to diagnosis.

Sometimes, without a clinical clue, the microscopist is at a loss as to what the histologic abnormality may be. These are the so-called nothing lesions. They include, for the most part, abnormalities of epidermal pigmentation and connective tissue alterations. The human race has a spectrum of normal melanin pigmentation that ranges from almost none in fair-skinned Scandinavians to black. Therefore, subtle pigmentary changes such as seen in freckles and café-au-lait spots may not be diagnosable unless a portion of the contiguous normal skin is available for comparison. Abnormalities of elastin, such as anetoderma or stria distense, also may escape notice unless an elastin stain is performed. Likewise, changes in tissue mass (e.g., atrophoderma or scleredema), may be undiagnosable unless continuous skin is available for comparison.

4. Instances in which an unintended lesion is biopsied by mistake or the characteristic portion of the lesion is not biopsied:

Sometimes the clinician, in seeking out the "juiciest" papule for biopsy, may inadvertently biopsy an intradermal nevus. A clinically subtle lesion can be obscured by injection of too much local anesthetic or by blanching due to epinephrine in the anesthetic solution causing the clinician to miss the lesion. More commonly, a deep lesion (e.g., erythema nodosum or nodular vasculitis) is missed because the biopsy is too superficial. If the clinical information does not fit with the histologic features, such mistakes must be considered.

5. Instances in which the histologic changes are not specific and the clinical information may enable a more precise differential diagnosis or even a specific diagnosis to be made.

Sometimes, subtle histologic changes are noted by the pathologist, but he is not able to put them into perspective unless the clinical features of the case are known to him. For example, if slight orthohyperkeratosis and slight acanthosis are the only histologic findings, not many pathologists would suspect X-linked ichthyosis unless the clinician suggested that the patient has a type of ichthyosis. Once the pathologist knows that the patient has a form of ichthyosis, the four major forms can be differentiated on histologic grounds.

6. The initial tissue sections do not show histologic evidence of the conditions suspected clinically.

If a disease process is suspected by the clinician that has only focal histologic changes (e.g., folliculitis or Grover's disease), the pathologist must be aware of this in order to know that serial sections must be made to find the characteristic histologic changes.

7. Technical error in the laboratory:

Examples of technical error that can be corrected by attention to clinicopathologic correlation are numerous. Probably most common is the mix-up of specimens by the accession clerk or technician. By comparing the clinical impression to the histologic findings, such mix-ups can usually be unraveled. Another common error is misorientation of the tissue specimen in the paraffin block, causing a spurious appearance of the lesion histologically. This can be corrected by reorientation of the tissue. If a large specimen is received, sampling error in the selection of chips for processing can result in failure to submit the area of maximal involvement.

REFERENCES

1. Pinkus H: Lichenoid tissue reactions: a speculative review of the clinical spectrum of epidermal basal cell damage with special reference to erythema dyschromicum perstans. Arch Dermatol 107:840–846, 1973

2. Emmerson RW, Wilson Jones E: Eosinophilic spongiosis in pemphigus. Arch Dermatol 97:252–257, 1968

3. Garcia-Gonzalez E, Swerlick RA, Lawley TJ: Cell adhesion molecules. Am J Dermatopathol 12:188–192, 1990

4. Hirsh BC, Johnson WC: Concepts of granulomatous inflammation. Int J Dermatol 23:90–100, 1984

5. Ackerman AB: Histopathologic concept of epidermolytic hyperkeratosis. Arch Dermatol 102:253–259, 1970

6. Ackerman AB: Focal acantholytic dyskeratosis. Arch Dermatol 106:702–706, 1972

7. Wade TR, Ackerman AB: Cornoid lamellation—a histologic reaction pattern. Am J Dermatopathol 2:5–15, 1980

4

DERMATITIS WITHOUT EPIDERMAL CHANGES

John S. Metcalf

APPROACH TO DIAGNOSIS

To resolve the histopathologic differential diagnosis of a dermal infiltrate unaccompanied by epidermal change, it is necessary to define the infiltrate further and identify associated dermal changes. Factors to be considered include (1) distribution of the infiltrate (whether it surrounds only the superficial plexus or whether it extends into the lower half of the reticular dermis and to what extent it is localized around vessels), (2) density of the infiltrate and its cellular composition, and (3) the presence or absence of a dermal reaction accompanying the infiltrate (e.g., edema or dermal fibrosis).

Although the pattern of a dermal infiltrate is seldom pathognomonic, certain inflammatory processes such as lymphocytic infiltrate of Jessner, deep gyrate erythema, postinflammatory pigmentary alteration, and urticaria can usually be easily distinguished at scanning magnification by noting the depth of the infiltrate, its distribution with respect to blood vessels, and its density.

At higher magnification the cellular composition of dermal infiltrates can usually be defined. This sometimes enables a specific diagnosis to be made (e.g., mast cell disease), but more frequently this information only serves to narrow the differential diagnosis.

Dermal fibrosis, if present, indicates chronicity and to some extent is associated with those conditions in which there has been a relatively more severe insult to the dermis.

In most cases it is only by combining these features and correlating them with the clinical picture that a specific diagnosis (or a relevant differential diagnosis) can be made.

LYMPHOMONOCYTIC INFILTRATES

Postinflammatory Pigmentary Alteration

Clinical Features

Postinflammatory pigmentary alteration is among the most common "inflammatory" conditions that confront the dermatopathologist. Clinically this appears as either discrete or less

well-defined macules or patches of hyperpigmentation or hypopigmentation. Their location correlates with a previous inflammatory process and is therefore a useful clue to the nature of the precursor, particularly in those instances in which the condition is localized. An example is the postinflammatory hyperpigmentation that frequently follows fixed drug eruption. The hyperpigmented patches correspond in location and shape with the earlier inflammatory process. Phototoxic dermatitis, often caused by oil of bergamot, a component of some fragrances, often results in postinflammatory hyperpigmentation with the same distribution as the application of the causative agent. Reticulated hyperpigmentation of the pretibial areas is suggestive of erythema ab igne caused by prolonged exposure to radiant heat.[1] From a histologic standpoint it is usually impossible to reconstruct the clinical picture completely and determine histologically whether a given lesion is hypopigmented or hyperpigmented.

Histopathologic Features

Histopathologically, postinflammatory pigmentary alteration appears as a superficial perivascular dermatitis often without epidermal changes (Fig. 4-1). The infiltrate is usually sparse and consists chiefly of lymphocytes and variable numbers of melanophages. In such cases, it can be impossible to deduce the nature of the process that led to the pigment incontinence.

In many instances, however, there are epidermal and/or dermal changes that accompany the infiltrate. These clues can help one to understand the pathogenesis of the change. Thus, a compact stratum corneum, with or without parakeratosis, in association with psoriasiform hyperplasia of the epidermis suggests previous spongiotic dermatitis, although there is no current evidence of spongiosis. Effacement of the epidermal rete ridge pattern, frequently with atrophy of the epidermis and sometimes accompanied by papillary dermal fibrosis, usually indicates damage at the dermoepidermal junction, the hallmark of an interface dermatitis. In such cases, there is usually marked

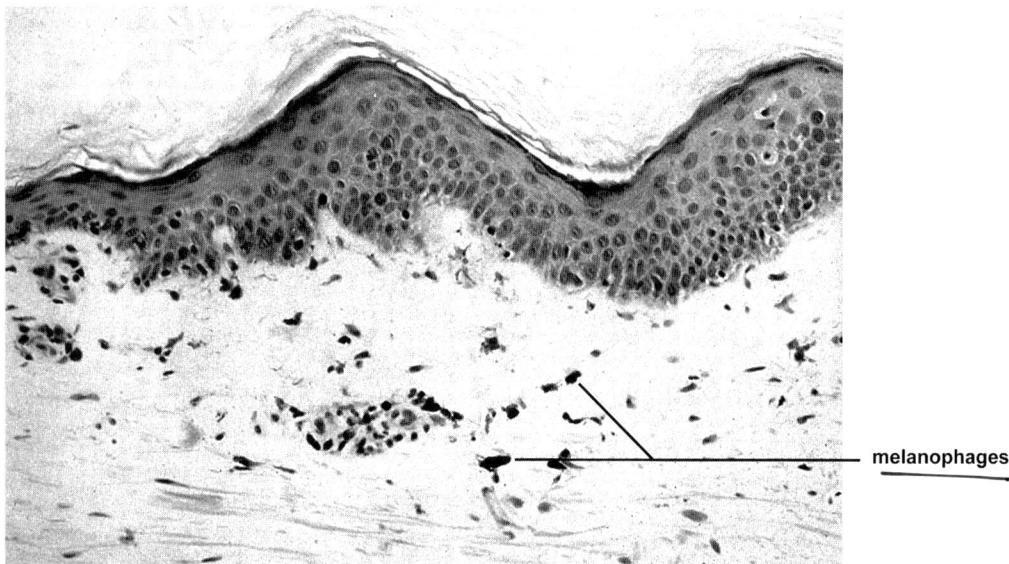
melanophages

Figure 4-1. Postinflammatory pigment alteration. There is a superficial perivascular lymphomononuclear infiltrate with scattered melanophages.

pigment incontinence with numerous heavily pigmented melanophages in the infiltrate.

Differential Diagnosis

When there are no discernible epidermal changes the histopathologic differential diagnosis includes other superficial perivascular dermatitides such as a morbilliform drug eruption or a viral exanthem. Careful evaluation of the basement membrane zone, however, will often reveal mild, focal interface changes in these conditions. Vitiligo can be distinguished from other forms of postinflammatory pigmentary change by the absence of melanin and melanocytes in the basal layer. This can be demonstrated with the Fontana-Masson stain.

When there is evidence of a prior interface dermatitis, the differential diagnosis includes regressed melanocytic lesions, fixed drug eruption, and macular amyloidosis. With regression of a melanocytic neoplasm, there is frequently significant dermal fibrosis, and the previous low power architecture of the lesion is often retained. The diagnosis of macular amyloidosis depends on identification of amyloid deposits in the papillary dermis. Amyloid stains may be required for their recognition.

Pigmented Purpuric Dermatitis

Clinical Features

The idiopathic pigmented purpuric dermatoses, progressive pigmentary dermatosis (Schamberg's disease), purpura annularis telangiectodes (Majocchi), eczematoid-like purpura of Doucas and Kapetanakis, and pigmented purpuric lichenoid dermatosis of Gougerot and Blum possibly represent a single disease process with different clinical manifestations and a spectrum of histopathologic findings.[2,3] Schamberg's disease and Majocchi's disease represent that portion of the spectrum that is apt to

present as a perivascular lymphomonocytic infiltrate without epidermal changes. The eruption, which usually occurs on the lower extremities but may not be confined to them, is characterized by diffuse red-brown oval macules or patches frequently with puncta ("cayenne pepper spots") at their periphery.[2,4] These lesions are usually asymptomatic, and there is no known association with any systemic disease.

Histopathologic Features

There is a sparse to moderate lymphomonocytic infiltrate that surrounds the vessels of the superficial vascular plexus (Fig. 4-2). Although this is usually accompanied by siderophages, hemosiderin deposits are not always present and, even if present, may be difficult to see. There are frequently extravasated erythrocytes in the superficial dermis. This is the histopathologic pattern that corresponds to Schamberg's disease. Sometimes focal vacuolar interface change is present (Fig. 4-3). Pigmented lichenoid purpura of Gougerot and Blum is almost always associated with epidermal alterations and hyperkeratosis, sometimes parakeratosis, and pronounced interface change with obliteration of the normal rete ridge pattern. The dermal infiltrate of lymphocytes and monocytes may be dense and is usually associated with fibroplasia.

Differential Diagnosis

The distinction between Schamberg's disease and other diseases characterized by a similar inflammatory infiltrate is based on the demonstration of hemosiderin-laden macrophages (siderophages) in the upper dermis and/or by the identification of extravasated erythrocytes. The former can usually be distinguished from melanophages by the refractile quality of the pigment or through the use of iron stains.

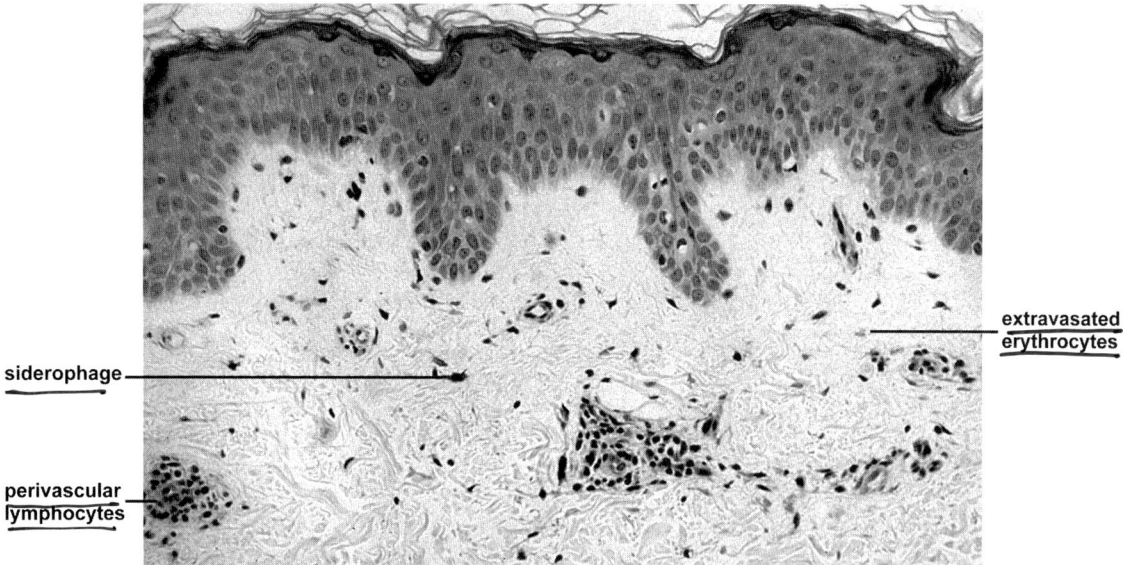

siderophage

extravasated
erythrocytes

perivascular
lymphocytes

Figure 4-2.   Pigmented purpuric dermatosis of Schamberg's type. There is a sparse superficial perivascular lymphomononuclear infiltrate. Extravasated erythrocytes are sometimes seen as are scattered siderophages.

Morbilliform Eruptions

Symmetrically distributed erythematous macules and papules as a reaction to a viral or rickettsial illness or a wide variety of medications are usually described as "morbilliform." As the histologic picture is often nonspecific, the determination of etiology depends largely on clinical factors.

Morbilliform Viral Exanthems

Clinical Features

Many viral illnesses can be associated with a morbilliform eruption. Common causes include the adenoviruses, other respiratory viruses, and the enteroviruses. An exanthem characterized

Figure 4-3.   Pigmented purpuric dermatosis of Schamberg's type. Although there may be no epidermal changes present, often there is focal vacuolar alteration along the basal layer.

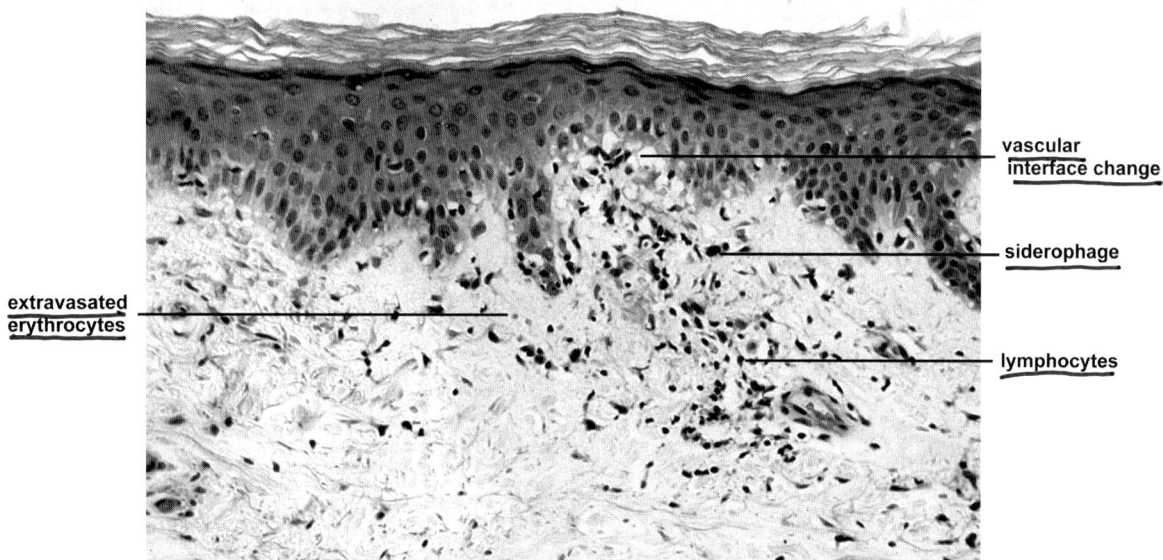

extravasated
erythrocytes

vascular
interface change

siderophage

lymphocytes

Differential Diagnosis

The clinical appearance is critical in distinguishing erythema gyratum repens from the remainder of this group. Erythema chronicum migrans often contains an admixture of plasma cells in the inflammatory infiltrate and may show changes typical of an arthropod bite reaction centrally. Furthermore, its diagnosis can be confirmed by the presence of an elevated serum antibody titer against the causative spirochete *Borrelia burgdorferi*. Sometimes *Borrelia* organisms can be identified in sections stained with the Warthin-Starry stain.

The histopathologic differential diagnosis of the deep gyrate erythemas also includes lymphocytic infiltrate of Jessner, reticular erythematous mucinosis of the plaque type, the tumid form of lupus erythematosus, polymorphous light eruption, and the inflammatory stage of scleroderma. The identification of mucin within the reticular dermis favors a diagnosis of tumid lupus erythematosus or reticular erythematous mucinosis.[15] Although there may be slight papillary dermal edema in deep gyrate erythema, it is seldom as pronounced as in the typical case of papulovesicular polymorphous light eruption. However, nonspecific deep gyrate erythemas and the plaque type of polymorphous light eruption may be indistinguishable. The presence of plasma cells in the infiltrate favors tumid lupus erythematosus, inflammatory scleroderma, and erythema chronicum migrans rather than deep nonspecific gyrate erythema.

Erythema Chronicum Migrans

Clinical Features

Erythema chronicum migrans, the primary cutaneous lesion of Lyme borreliosis, occurs in about one-half the cases of the systemic disease.[16] Developing usually as a single reddish macule and expanding to form a round, oval, irregularly shaped or annular plaque, the primary cutaneous lesion arises within days or several weeks following inoculation of the infectious agent.[16,17] It is frequently accompanied by constitutional symptoms of chills, fever, fatigue, myalgias, arthralgias, and headaches. The responsible organism is *B. burgdorferi,* a spirochete that is transmitted by the hard-bodied tick of genus *Ixodes.*[17,18]

Although erythema chronicum migrans is the usual cutaneous manifestation of Lyme borreliosis in the United States, chronic cutaneous involvement has been frequently reported in Europe. *Borrelia* spp. have been implicated in acrodermatitis chronica atrophicans, morphea, lichen sclerosis, ulnar fibrous nodules, and lymphadenosis benigna cutis.[19]

Histopathologic Features

Biopsies taken from the periphery of cutaneous lesions of erythema chronicum migrans are histologically similar to deep gyrate erythema. However, plasma cells often accompany the lymphocytes in the superficial and deep infiltrate. Less commonly, the infiltrate contains admixed eosinophils. Biopsies taken from the centers of lesions often have characteristic features of arthropod assault reactions with a superficial and deep perivascular and interstitial mixed infiltrate.[17]

The spirochetes can be visualized with the same staining techniques used for *Treponema pallidum* and are usually found in the epidermis and superficial dermis.[17]

Differential Diagnosis

The histologic pattern of a superficial and deep perivascular infiltrate is shared with deep gyrate erythema, Jessner's lymphocytic infiltrate, and tumid lupus erythematosus. The presence of plasma cells is somewhat suggestive of erythema chronicum migrans or tumid lupus erythematosus. Resolution of the differential diagnosis requires clinicopathologic correlation and ultimately serologic confirmation or culture, or both.

[handwritten: Plasma cell]

Polymorphous Light Eruption

Clinical Features

Pruritus, erythema, urticarial plaques, hemorrhagic papules, and eczematous eruption, or papulovesicles that arise after sun exposure comprise the clinical spectrum of polymorphous light eruption. Despite the variability in the clinical presentation in a patient population, the reaction pattern is constant in a given patient.[20]

The plaque form of polymorphous light eruption sometimes presents histopathologically as a perivascular lymphomonocytic infiltrate without significant epidermal change. However, there is a broad spectrum of changes that reflects the diverse clinical presentation, and many, if not most, cases of polymorphous light eruption show epidermal spongiosis in addition to the dermal infiltrate.

Histopathologic Features

The plaque type of polymorphous light eruption is generally characterized by a perivascular lymphomonocytic infiltrate that extends to the mid-reticular dermis[21,22] (Fig. 4-6). This is often accompanied by marked edema of the papillary dermis.[21,22]

Differential Diagnosis

The histologic pattern is similar to that of gyrate erythemas, although papillary dermal edema tends to be more marked in polymorphous light eruption. The clinical distribution of polymorphous light eruption is helpful in distinguishing it from gyrate erythema in that polymorphous light eruption is absolutely dependent on light exposure (usually the sunburn spectrum, 290 to 320 mμ), and the reaction can be reproduced by phototesting.[23]

Jessner's Lymphocytic Infiltrate

Clinical Features

Jessner's lymphocytic infiltrate clinically is manifest as indurated pink to red-brown papules and plaques that are usually located on the face. These lesions persist for weeks, months, or years. They resolve spontaneously without sequelae, but may recur.[24,25]

Histopathologic Features

The skin biopsy shows virtually no epidermal changes. The papillary dermis may be edematous. There is a superficial and deep perivascular dermal infiltrate of lymphocytes and mononuclear cells (Fig. 4-7).

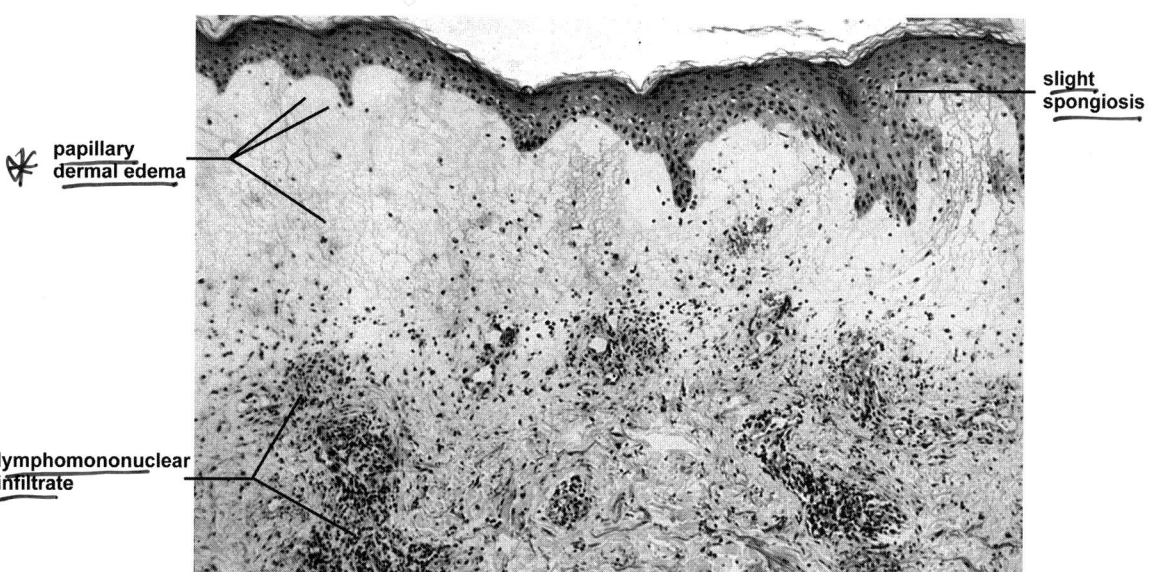

papillary
dermal edema

slight
spongiosis

lymphomononuclear
infiltrate

Figure 4-6. Polymorphous light eruption. The plaque form is characterized by marked papillary dermal edema and a moderately dense perivascular lymphomononuclear infiltrate. This example also shows slight spongiosis.

Figure 4-7. Lymphocytic infiltrate of Jessner. There is a superficial and deep perivascular and periappendageal infiltrate without overlying epidermal changes. The infiltrate is made up of lymphocytes, mononuclear cells, and sometimes plasma cells.

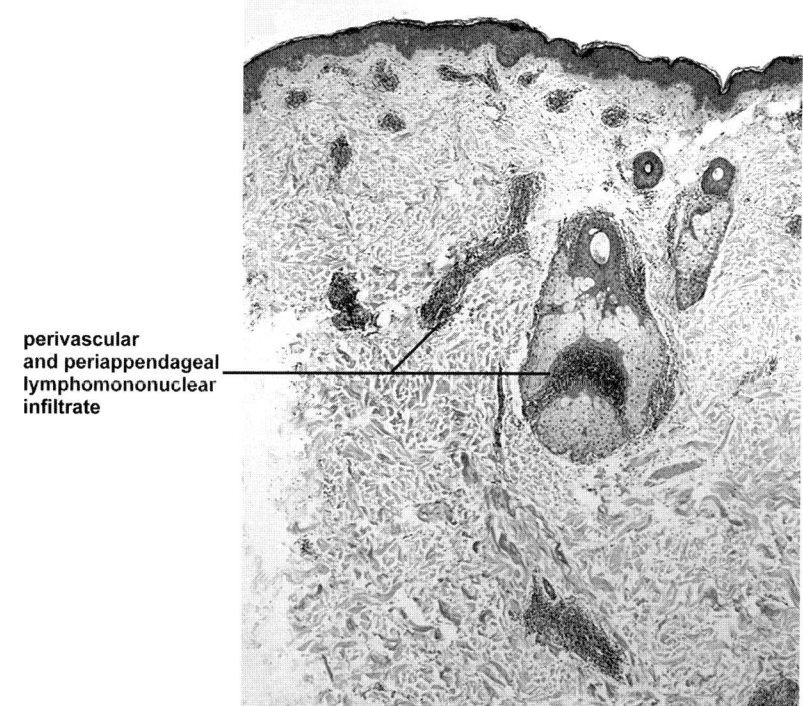

perivascular
and periappendageal
lymphomononuclear
infiltrate

Differential Diagnosis

The differential diagnosis includes lupus erythematosus, polymorphous light eruption, gyrate erythema, *Borrelia* infection, and lymphocytoma cutis.[25] Unlike most cutaneous lesions of lupus erythematosus, Jessner's lymphocytic infiltrate shows no interface damage, and, in contrast to the tumid form of lupus erythematosus, there is no increase in the mucin content of the reticular dermis. Furthermore, the immunofluorescence findings, useful in lupus erythematosus, are negative in this lymphocytic infiltrate.

Polymorphous light eruption is almost identical histologically to Jessner's lymphocytic infiltrate. Resolution of this differential diagnosis requires phototesting. *Borrelia* infection (erythema chronicum migrans) is also similar histologically and should be excluded clinically.[25]

‖ MAST CELL INFILTRATES

Cutaneous mast cell infiltrates take the form of either a nodular aggregate or a perivascular infiltrate. These correspond to lesions that clinically have the appearance of papules or nodules (nodular aggregate) or macules (perivascular infiltrate). Each develops a wheal and flare reaction after mechanical stimulation (Darier's sign). The macular forms of urticaria pigmentosa and telangiectasia macularis eruptiva perstans have histologic features that fall into the differential diagnosis of dermal perivascular infiltrates without epidermal change.

Urticaria Pigmentosa, Macular Lesions

Clinical Features

Urticaria pigmentosa is characterized by multiple pigmented macules, papules, or nodules. This form of mast cell proliferation is divided according to age of onset: (1) those arising in infancy or early childhood and (2) those arising during adolescence or adult life. When the disease is congenital or arises early in childhood, extracutaneous lesions are rare and there is seldom progression to systemic disease, while urticaria pigmentosa

arising later in life can be associated with systemic lesions, which, however, are usually self-limited.[26]

Histopathologic Features

Macular lesions of urticaria pigmentosa are characterized by a perivascular mast cell infiltrate usually limited to the upper dermis (Fig. 4-8). The mast cells may have round or oval nuclei and may be mistaken for lymphocytes on casual inspection or spindle-shaped nuclei, in which case they may be similar in appearance to fibroblasts or pericytes. The characteristic cytoplasmic granules (Fig. 4-9), which can be demonstrated with toluidine blue, Giemsa, or chloroacetate esterase (Leder) stains, can occasionally be seen in hematoxylin and eosin (H&E) sections.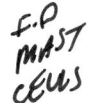

Telangiectasia Macularis Eruptiva Perstans

Clinical Features

Telangiectasia macularis eruptiva perstans (TMEP) probably represents a cutaneous mast cell hyperplasia.[26] It is a disease of adulthood that appears as red to brown oval macules with or without telangiectasias. Systemic involvement is rare.

Histopathologic Features

The mast cell infiltrate is characteristically sparse and closely mimics superficial perivascular lymphomonocytic infiltrates in its appearance. The mast cells are distributed around dilated capillaries and venules in the papillary dermis. When accentuated through histochemical staining techniques, mast cells are usually found to comprise most of the infiltrate.

Differential Diagnosis

To distinguish a macular lesion of urticaria pigmentosa or TMEP from a perivascular lymphomonocytic infiltrate, it is necessary to identify and quantify the number of mast cells in the infiltrate. This usually requires histochemical stains.

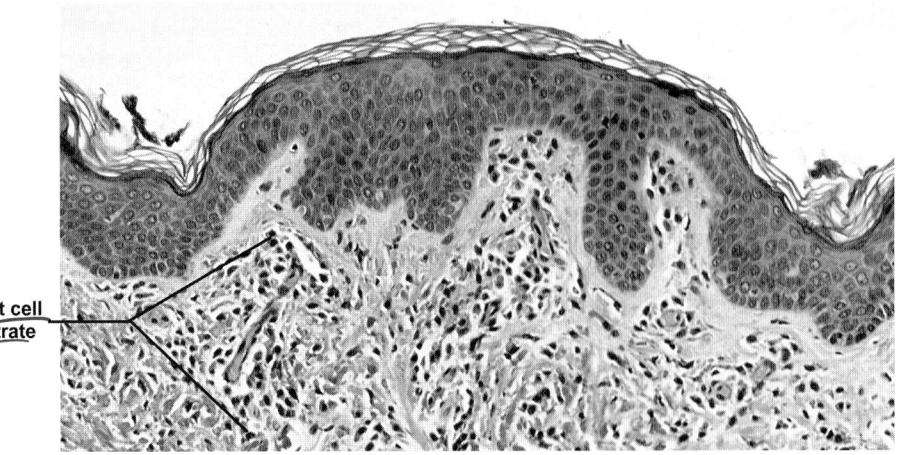

Figure 4-8. Urticaria pigmentosa, macular lesions. The perivascular infiltrate consists chiefly of mast cells, although at low magnification they might be mistaken for lymphocytes.

mast cell infiltrate

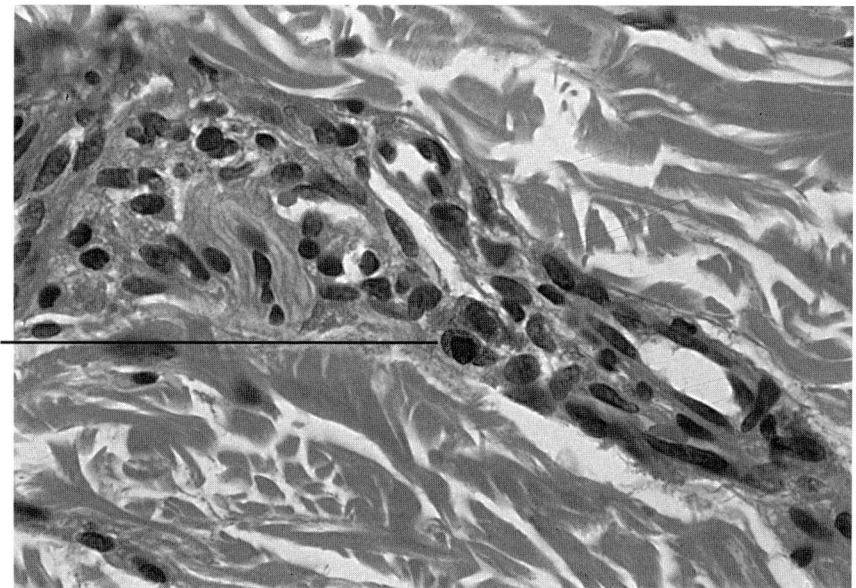

cytoplasmic
granules of
mast cell

Figure 4-9. Urticaria pigmentosa, macular lesions. At higher magnification, even on H&E staining, the cells can frequently be distinguished from lymphocytes and histiocytes by their granular cytoplasm.

NEUTROPHILIC INFILTRATES

Erythema Marginatum

Clinical Features

Erythema marginatum is the pathognomonic cutaneous eruption of acute rheumatic fever[27] and occurs in about 18% of patients with rheumatic fever.[28] Erythema marginatum, along with carditis, arthralgia, chorea, and subcutaneous nodules, can be considered one of the major manifestations of rheumatic fever.[29] It begins as small erythematous macules or papules that rapidly evolve into an annular or polycyclic eruption that changes its configuration rapidly (hourly). It tends to involve the trunk and extremities and sometimes extends to the hands and face.[28]

Histopathologic Features

There is a perivascular infiltrate usually composed of neutrophils confined to the papillary dermis and superficial reticular dermis (Fig. 4-10). Nuclear dust is sometimes identified, but there is neither fibrin deposition nor other evidence of vascular damage.[27] Rarely, the infiltrate can be lymphomonocytic as described in the section on superficial gyrate erythemas.

Differential Diagnosis

The histologic differential diagnosis includes dense infiltrate urticaria from which erythema marginatum can usually be distinguished by a lack of eosinophils. Leukocytoclastic vasculitis, which is also characterized by neutrophils and nuclear dust, usually shows evidence of vascular damage in the form of fibrin deposition and numerous extravasated erythrocytes. Although the cellular composition of the eruption of juvenile rheumatoid

arthritis (Still's disease) is similar, the infiltrate tends to be considerably more dense in erythema marginatum.

Evanescent Eruption of Juvenile Rheumatoid Arthritis

Clinical Features

The cutaneous eruption associated with juvenile rheumatoid arthritis in 33% to 50% of patients[30] consists of small macules that occasionally become confluent on the trunk and extremities. Unlike the lesions of erythema marginatum, there is no tendency to spread but rather a tendency to appear when the patient is febrile, usually in the afternoons, and to disappear when the patient becomes afebrile.

Histopathologic Features

There is a sparse, chiefly neutrophilic infiltrate that surrounds the vessels of the edematous papillary dermis. There is no fibrin deposition or other evidence of vascular damage, although some nuclear dust is present.

Differential Diagnosis

The morphologic picture is similar to that of urticaria, although eosinophils are not a characteristic of Still's disease.

Erythropoietic Protoporphyria

Clinical Features

Erythropoietic protoporphyria, inherited as an autosomal dominant trait, results in acute cutaneous changes of erythema, edema, and a stinging sensation on sun exposure and chronic

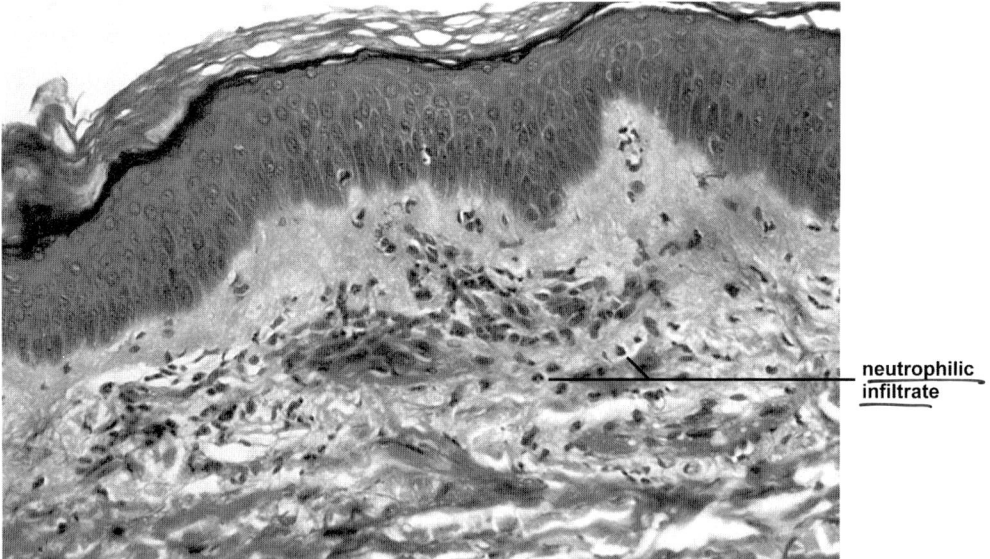

neutrophilic infiltrate

Figure 4-10. Erythema marginatum. There is a sparse superficial perivascular infiltrate of neutrophils.

changes of thickening of sun-exposed skin,[31] particularly on the dorsum of the hands and face. An accumulation of protoporphyrin IX secondary to a deficiency of ferrochelatase is characteristic of the disease.[32] Laboratory studies show elevated protoporphyrin IX in the blood and feces but not in urine.

Histopathologic Features

The histologic picture of a perivascular inflammatory infiltrate corresponds to the edematous reaction after sun exposure. The infiltrate is usually mixed and contains predominantly neutrophils but also mononuclear cells and sometimes eosinophils. There may be a little nuclear dust and a few extravasated erythrocytes. The infiltrate is most prominent in the papillary dermis but can also involve the superficial reticular dermis.

Accompanying the infiltrate is an accumulation of periodic acid–Schiff (PAS)-positive, diastase-resistant, eosinophilic material that rims the capillaries and venules of the papillary dermis. Ultrastructural features include extensive reduplication of the basal lamina of the involved vessels and accumulations of a finely fibrillar material that surround the basement membrane material.[31]

With direct immunofluorescence, IgG deposition in the blood vessel walls and, to a lesser extent, in the basement membrane zone is seen. IgM, in a similar distribution, has been identified in a smaller percentage of patients.[31] These patterns, although more intense, are identical to those observed in porphyria cutanea tarda.

Differential Diagnosis

The distinction between erythropoietic protoporphyria and other superficial neutrophilic or mixed cutaneous infiltrates rests on the identification of the characteristic perivascular cuffing by eosinophilic material that stains with PAS and is resistant

to diastase digestion. To distinguish between the porphyrias requires laboratory measurements of specific heme precursors.

Cellulitis

Clinical Findings

Erythematous, edematous plaques with poorly defined borders in association with a fever in a systemically ill patient characterize cellulitis, an infection of both the dermis and the subcutis by streptococci, staphylococci, *Haemophilus influenzae* (usually in young children), or other bacteria or fungi. Lesions of erysipelas may exhibit an indurated, shelf-like border. Traumatic injury, inflammatory dermatoses, or a burn can provide the entrance for the pathogen. When the infection of the subcutaneous tissues is severe and there is vascular thrombosis, ischemic necrosis can develop. This combination of ischemic necrosis and suppurative inflammation is what is commonly called *necrotizing fasciitis* and is rapidly progressive and potentially fatal.[33]

Histopathologic Features

Although spongiotic vesicles can form in the epidermis, the constant changes are in the dermis and subcutis, which are markedly edematous and infiltrated diffusely by neutrophils and lesser numbers of other inflammatory cells. Causative organisms can usually be identified with tissue Gram stains or the Giemsa stain. However, they are usually few in number.

Differential Diagnosis

The histopathologic differential diagnosis can include reactions to certain arthropod assaults as well as Sweet syndrome, both of which can usually be distinguished clinically. The reaction in cellulitis is usually more diffuse than the reaction to arthropod assault and the infiltrate is usually not so dense as in Sweet's disease. In the latter condition there is no evidence of an infectious process.

Acute Febrile Neutrophilic Dermatosis (Sweet Syndrome)

Clinical Features

In 1964, Sweet[34] described "an acute febrile neutrophilic dermatosis" as a distinctive condition, most commonly of middle-aged women, manifested by "fever, neutrophil polymorphonuclear leukocytosis of the blood, raised painful plaques on the limbs, face and neck and histologically a dense dermal infiltration with mature neutrophil polymorphs."

Although there are usually no epidermal changes, there may be vesicles or sterile pustules. Improvement in response to corticosteroid therapy is the rule, but recurrences are not uncommon. There is no response to antibiotic therapy. Some patients who have the clinical and histologic features of Sweet syndrome either have or eventually develop myelocytic leukemia; however, there are no clinical or histologic criteria that are helpful for distinguishing them from patients with idiopathic neutrophilic dermatosis.[35]

Histopathologic Features

There is characteristically a dense dermal infiltrate that is predominantly neutrophilic with some lymphocytes, eosinophils, and monocytes (Fig. 4-11). Although the infiltrate often shows some aggregation around vessels, there can be marked interstitial involvement as well. Involvement of the subcutis is uncommon. There is papillary dermal edema that is sometimes marked and, rarely, intra- or subepidermal vesicles.[36]

Differential Diagnosis

The histopathologic differential diagnosis includes erythema elevatum diutinum from which it can be distinguished by the lack of vasculitis. The clinical appearance serves to distinguish it from cellulitis and arthropod assaults.

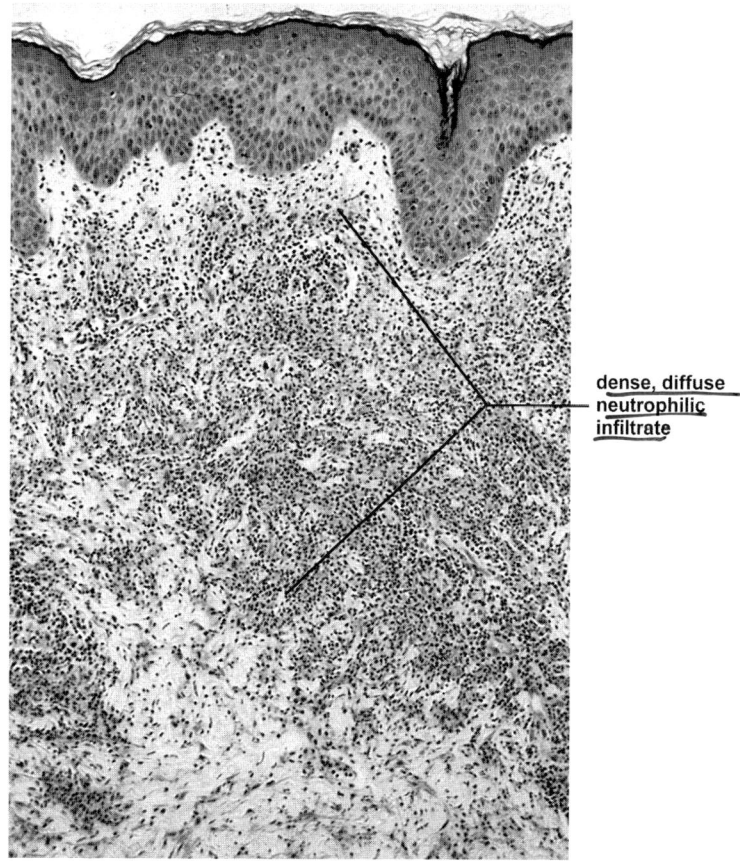

Figure 4-11. Sweet's syndrome. A dense diffuse dermal infiltrate in which neutrophils predominate, but which can also contain eosinophils, lymphocytes, and mononuclear cells.

dense, diffuse neutrophilic infiltrate

MIXED INFILTRATES

Urticaria

Clinical Features

Urticaria is characterized by wheals, elevated areas of dermal edema frequently accompanied by erythema. In most instances, the wheals evolve and resolve in less than 24 hours but may recur. Acute urticaria resolves in less than 1 month. In chronic urticaria, urticarial wheals continue to develop for more than 1 month.[37] The term *urticarial vasculitis* is applied to patients who have the clinical manifestations of urticaria but whose skin biopsy specimens have the histopathologic appearance of leukocytoclastic vasculitis.

Urticaria is thought to result from degranulation of mast cells or basophil leukocytes with the release of vasoactive substances such as histamine.[37] This reaction can be elicited by exposure to various antigens or physical stimuli. In many instances it appears to be IgE-mediated and, in other cases, the activation of complement appears to play a role.[37] Circulating immune complexes are frequently present in patients with dense infiltrate urticaria and urticarial vasculitis. The deposition of immune complexes in vessel walls probably plays a role in the pathogenesis of urticarial vasculitis.[38]

Histopathologic Features

Urticaria is characterized by a mixed inflammatory cell infiltrate (Fig. 4-12). It is usually confined to the upper half of the dermis, surrounds capillaries and venules, and is scattered in the interstitium. Dermal edema can sometimes be visualized microscopically, although evaluation of it tends to be somewhat subjective.

In those instances in which the infiltrate is sparse, it usually consists of lymphocytes admixed with a few eosinophils and rare neutrophils. In so-called dense infiltrate urticaria, eosinophils are usually more numerous, and there may be evidence of their degranulation.[38]

There is a third type of urticaria that is histologically identical to leukocytoclastic vasculitis. It has been postulated that immune complex deposition plays a role in the pathogenesis of these lesions.[38]

Differential Diagnosis

The morphologic appearance of arthropod assault reactions and of the "urticarial phase" of bullous pemphigoid may be virtually identical to urticaria. Clues to pemphigoid are neutrophils and eosinophils lined up along the dermoepidermal junction, slight vacuolar change in the basal layer, and mild spongiosis. These cases are usually easily resolved by clinical correlation. Occasionally, skin adjacent to the diagnostic papillary dermal microabscesses of dermatitis herpetiformis can show similar histopathologic changes.

Arthropod Bites, Stings, and Infestations

Clinical Features

Early reactions to the bites of many common arthropods (e.g., mosquitoes) appear similar to urticarial wheals. It is at these early stages of evolution that the histologic picture is often that of a perivascular inflammatory infiltrate without significant epidermal change. The intensity and components of the infiltrate vary as the lesion evolves and are probably also related to the sensitivity of the victim to the injected toxins or antigenic material.[39]

Infestation by the scabies mite *Acarus scabiei* is characterized clinically by subcorneal burrows on the hands (palmar surfaces, web spaces of the fingers), wrists (flexor surfaces), male genitalia and nipples of women, and as a papular or nodular eruption of buttocks, abdomen, or axillae.

Figure 4-12. Urticaria. A superficial perivascular infiltrate of neutrophils and eosinophils accompanied by dermal edema.

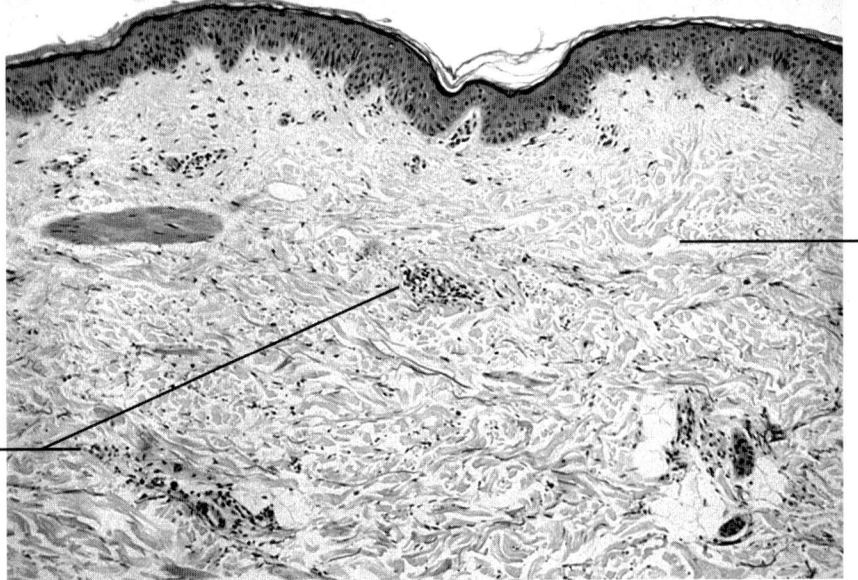

dermal edema

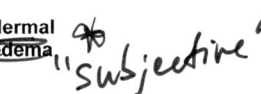

sparse perivascular infiltrate of neutrophils and eosinophils

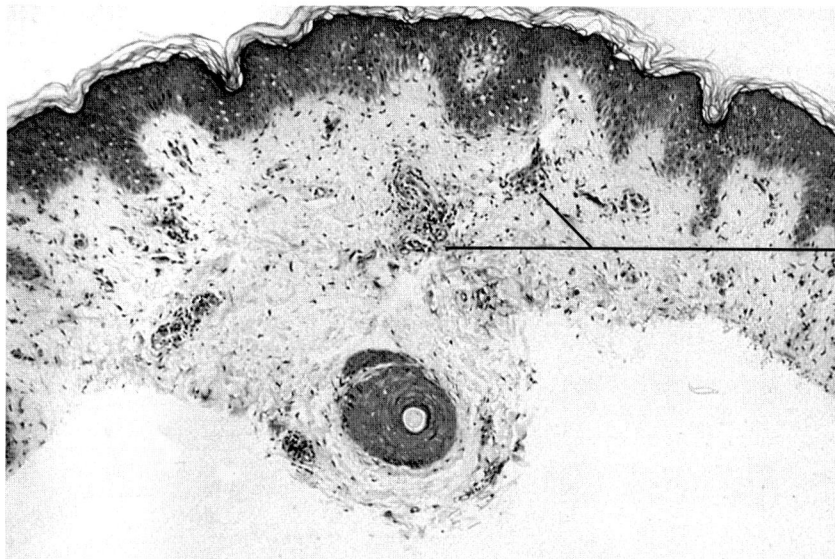

perivascular infiltrate of lymphocytes, mononuclear cells, eosinophils

Figure 4-13. Pruritic urticarial papules and plaques of pregnancy. A superficial perivascular and interstitial mixed infiltrate of lymphocytes, mononuclear cells, and eosinophils. In this example there is focal mild spongiosis.

Histopathologic Features

A perivascular and interstitial infiltrate of a mixture of inflammatory cells that usually extends into the lower half of the reticular dermis is the hallmark of most arthropod bite reactions. The overall configuration of the infiltrate is that of a wedge the apex of which extends deep into the reticular dermis. The epidermis often appears uninvolved, but frequently some focal spongiosis can be discerned. Lymphocytes, neutrophils, and eosinophils are frequent constituents of the infiltrate; the latter are often seen in the interstitium of the reticular dermis between the coarse bundles of collagen. However, the make-up of the infiltrate can vary with the type of "assaulting" creature; the response to some species (fleas) is virtually lacking in eosinophils and contains numerous neutrophils.[40] Occasionally eosinophils are numerous, and flame figures can be identified.

The microscopic appearance of the reaction to scabies mite infestation is identical to other arthropod bite reactions. Chronic nodules often contain an extremely dense lymphomonocytic infiltrate, often with eosinophils, and have the picture of so-called pseudolymphoma. A definitive diagnosis of scabies can only be made by observing mites, fecal deposits, or eggs in or beneath the stratum corneum. This is unusual except in "Norwegian" scabies in which numerous organisms are present. However, if scabies is suspected, it is best to examine multiple histologic sections. Pathognomonic material is occasionally found.

Differential Diagnosis

Although a deep, wedge-shaped mixed infiltrate that is both perivascular and interstitial is highly suggestive of arthropod assault, there are instances in which the infiltrate is confined to the superficial dermis or is more diffuse. The histologic differential diagnosis in these instances includes urticaria, the urticarial phase of bullous pemphigoid, pruritic urticarial papules and plaques of pregnancy, and, particularly if there is spongiosis, allergic contact dermatitis or other acute spongiotic dermatitides. In such cases, the differential diagnosis can usually be resolved by consideration of the clinical history and appearance.

Pruritic Urticarial Papules and Plaques of Pregnancy

Clinical Features

Pruritic urticarial papules and plaques of pregnancy (PUPPP) is a distinctive urticarial and papular eruption of the last trimester of pregnancy that is most often seen in prima gravidas.[41] It begins as erythematous papules that enlarge and coalesce to form edematous plaques. Lesions usually develop first on the abdomen but may spread to involve the proximal lower extremities, anterior chest, upper extremities, and back.[42]

Histopathologic Features

The infiltrate of PUPPP is usually confined to the superficial dermis and can be both perivascular and interstitial. Although lymphocytes and monocytes predominate, scattered eosinophils are usually present. Accompanying this infiltrate is a variable amount of papillary dermal edema, and focal epidermal spongiosis is sometimes present (Fig. 4-13).

Differential Diagnosis

A histologically similar appearance can occur in arthropod bites, common urticaria, the urticarial phase of bullous pemphigoid, and allergic contact dermatitis. Herpes gestationis can also enter into the differential diagnosis, but its urticarial papules are characterized by more pronounced papillary dermal edema that sometimes gives the papilla the profile of a light

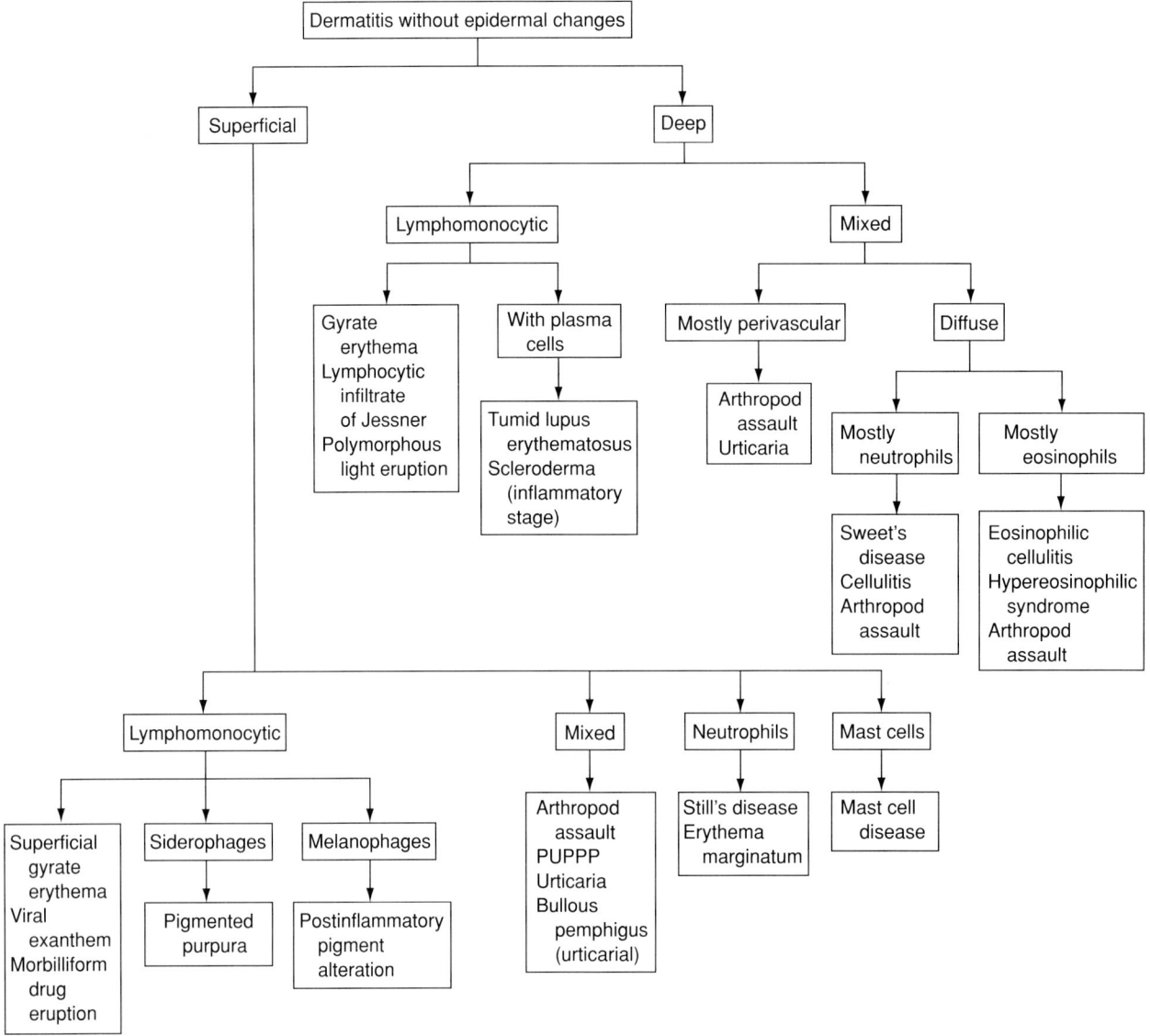

Figure 4-14. Approach to forming a histopathologic differential diagnosis of dermatitis without epidermal changes.

bulb. Eosinophilic spongiosis and necrosis of individual keratinocytes are frequently features of herpes gestationis and are not found in PUPPP.

Hypereosinophilic Syndrome

Clinical Features

The term *hypereosinophilic syndrome* has been applied to a number of diseases that have in common marked blood eosinophilia and eosinophilic infiltrates of parenchymal organs and skin.[43] Some authors have further restricted the term to include only those diseases in which the eosinophilia has no known cause.[44] The relationship between hypereosinophilic syndrome and the recently described tryptophan-induced eosinophilia with associated connective tissue disease[45] has not

been clearly delineated. Scleroderma-like findings have not been described in patients with the hypereosinophilic syndrome.[44,46] However, several patients in one series complained of weakness and arthralgias, and biopsy specimens of skin and skeletal muscle contained interstitial and perivascular infiltrates of eosinophils.[44]

Cutaneous manifestations of hypereosinophilic syndrome are not specific and consist of urticaria or angioedema of the face or extremities (or both) or of pruritic erythematous macules and papules on the trunk and extremities.[46]

Histopathologic Features

Although epidermal vesiculation and even ulceration have been reported in some cases, the consistent findings are a perivascular infiltrate of eosinophils, lymphocytes, histiocytes, and often plasma cells in the dermis. There has been no reported involvement of the subcutis.

Differential Diagnosis

The histologic changes seen in this condition are not pathognomonic and require clinicopathologic correlation. Features may be similar to those observed in arthropod bite reactions, allergic contact dermatitis, and urticaria, all of which are more common.

Eosinophilic Cellulitis

Clinical Features

Several well-demarcated edematous erythematous plaques, usually located on the extremities, but often with involvement of the trunk, are the usual clinical manifestations of eosinophilic cellulitis. However, the disease is polymorphous in its presentation, and papules, vesicles, and bullae may be seen.[47]

This condition represents an unusual reaction pattern that can be the histopathologic manifestation of a variety of inflammatory dermatoses that range from eczematous dermatitis to bullous pemphigoid to a reaction to an arthropod bite.

Histopathologic Findings

The epidermis is often spongiotic, and sometimes vesicles may be present. The dermis is edematous and infiltrated by large numbers of eosinophils and relatively few cells of other types. In some examples, granules from degranulated eosinophils are deposited on collagen bundles and form "flame figures." There is no evidence of vasculitis.[48]

Differential Diagnosis

As the reaction pattern of eosinophilic cellulitis can occur in a variety of diseases, evidence of a primary disorder should be sought both clinically and histopathologically. When there is a dense diffuse infiltrate of predominantly eosinophils in an edematous dermis, often with "flame figures," a diagnosis of eosinophilic cellulitis can be made unless there is clinical or histopathologic evidence of another underlying inflammatory dermatosis.

SUMMARY

Figure 4-14 illustrates an approach to forming a histopathologic differential diagnosis when a dermal inflammatory infiltrate and little or no epidermal change are observed. At scanning magnification, the depth of the infiltrate with respect to anatomic boundaries is determined. A superficial infiltrate is restricted to the papillary dermis and the upper half of the reticular dermis. A deep infiltrate extends into the lower half of the reticular dermis and occasionally into the upper subcutis.

If the infiltrate is confined to the superficial vascular plexus, the next step is to determine its elements. If lymphomonocytic and lacking siderophages and melanophages, the differential diagnosis includes superficial gyrate erythema, a morbilliform drug eruption, and a viral exanthem. If siderophages are present, and particularly if they are accompanied by extravasated erythrocytes, a pigmented purpuric dermatosis should be considered. The presence of melanophages implies release of pigment from the epidermis and that there had been previous epidermal injury. Admixtures of lymphocytes and monocytes with eosinophils and neutrophils are seen in arthropod bite and sting reactions, PUPPP, urticaria, the urticarial phase of bullous pemphigoid, and vasculitis. To prove the latter, evidence of vascular damage manifested by fibrin deposition or necrosis of vessel walls must be identified. Mostly neutrophilic infiltrates characterize Still's disease and erythema marginatum. Predominantly mast cell infiltrates are characteristic of mast cell disease.

When the infiltrate extends deeply to involve the deep reticular dermis, recognition of the distribution of the infiltrate with respect to the vessels of the reticular dermis is helpful. In general, lymphomonocytic infiltrates in the reticular dermis tend to be almost purely perivascular as seen in deep gyrate erythemas and polymorphous light eruption. Plasma cells in the infiltrate suggest the possibility of tumid lupus erythematosus, the inflammatory stage of scleroderma, or erythema chronicum migrans.

When a deep infiltrate is chiefly perivascular and contains eosinophils and/or neutrophils in addition to lymphocytes and monocytes, a reaction to arthropod assault is likely. When there is a diffuse infiltrate composed chiefly of neutrophils, accompanied by dermal edema, cellulitis should be considered. Both Sweet's disease and some arthropod assaults have a similar infiltrate. Diffuse infiltrates with a preponderance of eosinophils are seen in eosinophilic cellulitis, hypereosinophilic syndrome, and some arthropod assaults.

REFERENCES

1. Maize JC, Ackerman ABA: Pigmented Lesions of the Skin. Lea & Febiger, Philadelphia, 1987
2. Randall SJ, Kierland RR, Montgomery H: Pigmented purpuric eruptions. AMA Arch Dermatol 64:177–191, 1951
3. Newton RC, Raimer SS: Pigmented purpuric eruptions. Dermatol Clin 3:165–169, 1985
4. Schamberg JF: A peculiar progressive pigmentary disease of the skin. Br J Dermatol 13:1–5, 1901
5. Balslev E, Thomsen HK, Weismann K: Histopathology of acute immunodeficiency virus exanthema. J Clin Pathol 43:201–202, 1990
6. Mims CA: Pathogenesis of rashes in virus diseases. Bacteriol Rev 30:739–760, 1966
7. Suringa DWR, Bank LJ, Ackerman ABA: Role of measles virus in skin lesions and Koplik's spots. N Engl J Med 283:1139–1142, 1970
8. Pariser RJ: Histologically specific skin lesions in disseminated cytomegalovirus infection. J Am Acad Dermatol 9:937–946, 1983
9. Wintroub BU, Stern R: Cutaneous drug reactions: pathogenesis and clinical classification. J Am Acad Dermatol 13:167–179, 1985

10. Fellner MJ: Adverse effects of drugs on skin. pp. 230–234. In Helwig E, Mostofi FK (eds): The Skin. Williams & Wilkins, Baltimore, 1971

11. Fellner MJ, Prutkin L: Morbilliform eruptions caused by penicillin. J Invest Dermatol 55:390–395, 1970

12. White JW: Gyrate erythema. Dermatol Clin 3:129–139, 1985

13. Ackerman ABA: Histologic Diagnosis of Inflammatory Skin Diseases. Lea & Febiger, Philadelphia, 1978

14. Sahn EE, Maize JC, Silver RM: Erythema marginatum: an unusual histopathologic manifestation. J Am Acad Dermatol 21:145–147, 1989

15. Clark WH, Mihm MC, Reed RJ, Ainsworth AM: The lymphocytic infiltrates of the skin. Hum Pathol 5:25–43, 1974

16. Berger BW: Dermatologic manifestations of Lyme disease. Rev Infect Dis, suppl. 6, 11:1425–1481, 1989

17. Berger BW, Clemmensen OJ, Ackerman AB: Lyme disease is a spirochetosis. Am J Dermatopathol 5:111–124, 1983

18. Scarpa C, Trevisan G, Sinco G: Lyme borreliosis. Dermatol Clin 12:669–685, 1994

19. Duray PH: Histopathology of clinical phases of human Lyme disease. Rheum Clin North Am 15:691–710, 1989

20. Holzle E, Plewig G, Hofmann C, Roser-Maass E: Polymorphous light eruption. J Am Acad Dermatol 7:111–125, 1982

21. Epstein JH: Adverse cutaneous reactions to the sun. pp. 5–43. In Malkinson FD, Pearson RH (eds): Yearbook of Dermatology. Year Book Medical, Chicago, 1971

22. Ackerman ABA: Histologic Diagnosis of Inflammatory Skin Diseases. Lea & Febiger, Philadelphia, 1978

23. Fisher DA, Epstein JH, Kay DN, Tuffanelli DL: Polymorphous light eruption and lupus erythematosus. Arch Dermatol 101:458–461, 1970

24. Jessner M, Kanof N: Lymphocytic infiltration of the skin. Arch Dermatol 68:447–449, 1953

25. Cockerell CJ, Lewis JE: Persistent indurated plaques of the face: a variant of Jessner's lymphocytic infiltrate? Cutis 53:49–52, 1994

26. Mihm MC, Clark WH, Reed RJ, Caruso MG: Mast cell infiltrates of the skin and the mastocytosis syndrome. Hum Pathol 4:231–239, 1973

27. Troyer C, Grossman ME, Silvers DN: Erythema marginatum in rheumatic fever: early diagnosis by skin biopsy. J Am Acad Dermatol 8:724–728, 1983

28. Bywaters EGL: Skin manifestations of rheumatic disease. pp. 1316–1326. In Fitzpatrick T (ed): Dermatology in General Medicine. 2nd Ed. McGraw-Hill, New York, 1979

29. Jones TD: The diagnosis of rheumatic fever. JAMA 126:481–486, 1944

30. Isdale IC, Bywaters EGL: The rash of rheumatoid arthritis and Still's disease. Q J Med 99:377–387, 1956

31. Epstein JH, Tuffanelli DL, Epstein WL: Cutaneous changes in the porphyrias. Arch Dermatol 107:689–698, 1973

32. Elder GH: Metabolic abnormalities in the porphyrias. Semin Dermatol 5:88–98, 1986

33. Braverman IM: Skin Signs of Systemic Disease. 2nd Ed. WB Saunders, Philadelphia, 1981

34. Sweet RD: An acute febrile neutrophilic dermatosis. Br J Dermatol 76:349–356, 1964

35. Cooper PE, Innes DJ, Greer KE: Acute febrile neutrophilic dermatosis (Sweet's syndrome) and myeloproliferative disorders. Cancer 51:1518–1526, 1983

36. Goldman GC, Moschella SL: Acute febrile neutrophilic dermatosis (Sweet's syndrome). Arch Dermatol 103:654–660, 1971

37. Soter NA, Wasserman SI: Urticaria/angioedema: a consideration of pathogenesis and clinical manifestations. Int J Dermatol 18:517–532, 1979

38. Monroe EW, Schulz CI, Maize JC, Jordan RE: Vasculitis in chronic urticaria: an immunopathologic study. J Invest Dermatol 76:103–107, 1981

39. Goldman L, Rockwell E, Richfield DF: Histopathological studies on cutaneous reactions to the bites of various arthropods. Am J Trop Med 1:514–525, 1952

40. Ackerman ABA: Histologic Diagnosis of Inflammatory Skin Diseases. Lea & Febiger, Philadelphia, 1978

41. Yancey KB, Hall RP, Lawley TJ: Pruritic urticarial papules and plaques of pregnancy. J Am Acad Dermatol 10:473–480, 1984

42. Ahmed AR, Kaplan R: Pruritic urticarial papules and plaques of pregnancy. J Am Acad Dermatol 4:679–681, 1981

43. Nir MA, Westfried M: Hypereosinophilic dermatitis. Dermatologica 162:444–450, 1981

44. Chusid MJ, Dale DC, West BC, Wolff SM: The hypereosinophilic syndrome. Medicine (Baltimore) 54:1–27, 1975

45. Silver RM, Heyes MP, Maize JC et al: Scleroderma, fasciitis, and eosinophilia associated with ingestion of tryptophan. N Engl J Med 322:874–881, 1990

46. Kazmierowski JA, Chusid MJ, Parrillo MD et al: Dermatologic manifestations of the hypereosinophilic syndrome. Arch Dermatol 114:531–535, 1978

47. Fisher GB, Greer KE, Cooper PH: Eosinophilic cellulitis (Wells' syndrome). Int J Dermatol 24:101–107, 1985

48. Wells GC, Smith NP: Eosinophilic cellulitis. Br J Dermatol 100:101–109, 1979

5

DERMATITIS INVOLVING THE DERMOEPIDERMAL JUNCTION

Philip LeBoit

An inflammatory skin disease in which the junction between the papillary dermis and epidermis is obscured is termed an *interface dermatitis*. In most of these diseases, T lymphocytes infiltrate the basal layer of the epidermis (and often the lower spinous layer as well) and cause cytotoxic damage to, or kill keratinocytes by, the induction of a form of cell death known as *apoptosis*.[1] Apoptotic keratinocytes become detached from their neighbors, become round, and undergo an orderly sequence of events resulting in the degradation of their nuclear DNA, lysis of their nuclei, and coagulation of proteins in their cytoplasms, without spilling enzymes that could damage adjacent cells. Such keratinocytes have traditionally been referred to as *dyskeratotic cells* and, when they find their way into the papillary dermis, as *colloid, cytoid*, or *Civatte bodies*. The pathophysiologies of many of the diseases in which interface dermatitis occurs are similar and involve not only T-cell-mediated damage to keratinocytes but also remodeling of the basement membrane zone.[2] Injury to basal keratinocytes and other structures produces tiny vacuoles along the dermoepidermal junction, on both sides of the basal lamina, a finding variously known as *vacuolar alteration, vacuolization, vacuolpathy*, and *liquefaction degeneration*. Liquefaction degeneration implies that solid substances turn into fluid, a conclusion not substantiated by scientific evidence.

The clinical lesions produced by an interface dermatitis may be flat or raised, smooth or scaly, depending on the epidermal reaction. Persistent interface reactions often result in loss of pigment from basal cells and their ingestion by melanophages. Hence, postinflammatory pigmentary changes can result from long-standing lesions of an interface dermatitis.

There are several ways in which one can divide the diseases that comprise the interface dermatitides. One can group them into conditions characterized by sparse infiltrates and vacuolar change at the dermoepidermal junction (vacuolar interface der-

matitis) and those that, in addition to vacuolar change, also have denser, band-like infiltrates (lichenoid interface dermatitis). Most commonly, the perivascular infiltrates beneath an interface reaction only involve the superficial vascular plexus. The prototype of a superficial vacuolar interface dermatitis is erythema multiforme and that of a lichenoid interface dermatitis, lichen planus. If both the superficial and deep plexuses are involved, the differential diagnoses are different. Interface reactions can have superimposed psoriasiform epidermal hyperplasia or spongiosis, or both. The interface dermatitides can be divided by this schema into 10 categories with both superficial and superficial and deep versions of vacuolar, lichenoid, psoriasiform lichenoid, spongiotic psoriasiform lichenoid, and spongiotic lichenoid dermatitis.[3]

Another approach to the classification of interface dermatitis is by analysis of the epidermal changes.[4] The epidermal findings in erythema multiforme and lichen planus are morphologically distinct and reflect pathophysiologic differences. The pathologic events in a single lesion of erythema multiforme unfold and resolve over the course of a few days. T cells that infiltrate the basal layer kill keratinocytes and depart so swiftly that cornification is not affected. In erythema multiforme, necrotic keratinocytes are sometimes present in whorled aggregates that are transepidermally eliminated, lymphocytes are often present well above the basal layer, and the interstices between keratinocytes in the superficial spinous zone are often wide, evidence that the epidermis remains permeable. In lichen planus the attack of lymphocytes on the epidermis is more persistent, and chronic changes result. There is continuous disruption of the junctional zone, and, as a result, keratinocytes of the basal layer are often polygonal, with eosinophilic cytoplasms, resembling the cells of the spinous layer rather than those of the normal basal layer. The upper portion of the epidermis changes to resemble volar skin, with a thickened granular and a compact

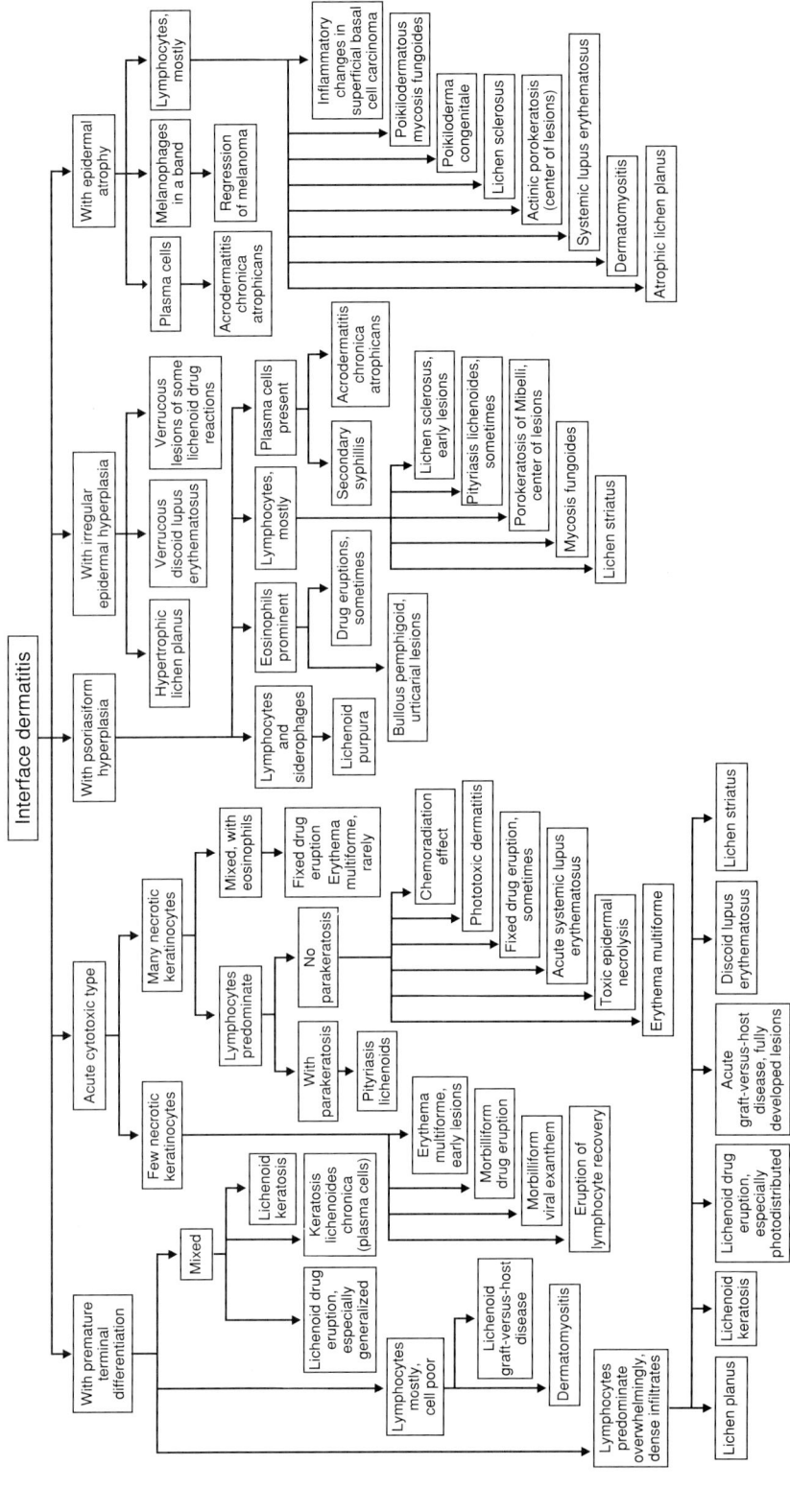

Figure 5-1.   Algorithm for the diagnosis of interface dermatitis.

cornified layer. Just as the epidermis on the volar surfaces of the acra is relatively impermeable, the superficial spinous zone in lichen planus and related conditions is typified by keratinocytes with tightly adherent junctions. Colloid bodies generated by the apoptosis of keratinocytes drop down into the papillary dermis in most examples of these conditions rather than being expelled upward, as they can be in erythema multiforme. The constellation of epidermal changes seen in lichen planus and related conditions can be termed *premature terminal differentiation*, terminal differentiation of epidermal keratinocytes being their maturation into granular and cornified layer cells.

The epidermal reactions in an interface dermatitis often correlate with the density of the subjacent infiltrate. An interface dermatitis with acute cytotoxic changes is usually accompanied by only sparse infiltrates, and premature differentiation of the epidermis is most often the result of dense, band-like lymphocytic infiltrates, but there are many exceptions. Pityriasis lichenoides may have a band-like infiltrate but epidermal findings similar to those of erythema multiforme. Lichenoid lesions of chronic graft-versus-host disease may have epidermal changes indistinguishable from lichen planus but be nearly devoid of lymphocytes. The pattern of inflammatory cells thus correlates imperfectly with epidermal changes.

Aside from the acute cytopathic pattern typified by erythema multiforme and the pattern of chronic injury at the dermoepidermal junction, with resultant alteration of cornification exemplified by lichen planus, there are three other distinct epidermal reactions seen in interface dermatitis. In interface dermatitis with irregular epidermal hyperplasia, the epidermis proliferates in an irregular pattern at the same time as cells of its basal layer are damaged. In interface dermatitis with psoriasiform hyperplasia, rete ridges elongate evenly in response to a milder attack. The last of these is epidermal atrophy, the result of an attack on rete ridges by lymphocytes that outstrips the ability of their basal keratinocytes to replenish themselves.

We have grouped diseases typified by interface dermatitis according to the most characteristic pattern that they take histologically when lesions are at their zeniths and noted other patterns that they can have on occasion. For instance, fully developed papules of lichen planus demonstrate interface dermatitis with premature terminal differentiation, atrophic planus shows interface dermatitis with epidermal atrophy, and hypertrophic lichen planus is marked by an interface dermatitis with irregular epidermal hyperplasia. Early lesions of acute cutaneous graft-versus-host disease can be difficult to distinguish from those of the acute cytotoxic reaction, erythema multiforme, but fully developed ones have squamatization of the basal layer and an altered cornified layer and exemplify interface dermatitis with premature terminal differentiation. Lichen sclerosus et atrophicus begins with psoriasiform hyperplasia and ends with epidermal atrophy. The three conditions that typically have interface dermatitis with irregular epidermal hyperplasia (hypertrophic lichen planus, verrucous lupus erythematosus, and hypertrophic lichenoid drug eruptions) are listed under the pattern that their "parent" diseases assume, namely, interface dermatitis with premature terminal differentiation. An algorithm for the diagnosis of interface dermatitis is shown in Figure 5-1.

DISEASES TYPIFIED BY ACUTE CYTOTOXIC INTERFACE DERMATITIS

Erythema Multiforme and Toxic Epidermal Necrolysis

Erythema multiforme, Stevens-Johnson syndrome, and toxic epidermal necrolysis (TEN) are conditions in which erythematous macules or patches caused by lymphocyte-mediated necrosis of keratinocytes may evolve into bullae with groups of necrotic keratinocytes in their roofs or even necrosis of the entire thickness of the epidermis. Whether all of these conditions are expressions of the same disease process and are part of a spectrum, or whether Stevens-Johnson syndrome and TEN together constitute an entity separate from erythema multiforme is a question under debate. In erythema multiforme, lesions are discrete and often target shaped; less precisely targetoid lesions occur in Stevens-Johnson syndrome along with systemic symptoms and involvement of at least two mucous membranes. The term *toxic epidermal necrolysis* is reserved by most authors for a widespread process involving over 10% of the cutaneous surface.

Clinical Features

Erythema multiforme manifests as erythematous, urticarial papules, papulovesicles, and plaques surmounted by vesicles, sometimes in a targetoid configuration and often favoring the acra. The fully developed centers of targetoid lesions may be gray, reflecting epidermal necrosis. Erythema multiforme has been divided into major and minor forms, depending on the presence of systemic symptoms and the involvement of mucosal surfaces. Some discriminate between erythema multiforme major and Stevens-Johnson syndrome.[5] Like leukocytoclastic vasculitis, erythema nodosum, and erythema annulare centrifugum, erythema multiforme can be the result of a variety of inciting factors and can be considered an inflammatory reaction pattern. The most common association of typical erythema multiforme is pre-existent herpes simplex infection. Both the polymerase chain reaction and the in situ hybridization techniques have demonstrated the herpes simplex virus genome in lesional keratinocytes. Conceivably, drugs, infections, and other triggers can reactivate a latent herpes virus infection that results in a distinctive cell-mediated response.

In Stevens-Johnson syndrome and in TEN, mucosal sites are involved along with cutaneous ones. An acral distribution is seldom present, and the cutaneous lesions are not the classic targetoid ones seen in erythema multiforme. Discrete lesions are often purpuric. In both conditions, a drug is often implicated as the causative factor, although *Mycoplasma pneumoniae* infection is associated with Stevens-Johnson syndrome but only rarely with TEN. TEN is a serious matter, because it can result in denudation of nearly the entire cutaneous surface, with sepsis and death, much as in patients with extensive burns. This variant is sometimes confused with the staphylococcal scalded skin syndrome, which is caused by a toxin produced by the organism and which is manifested histopathologically by intraepidermal, not subepidermal, vesiculation.

Because the histopathologic features of erythema multiforme, Stevens-Johnson syndrome, and TEN overlap to a great degree, they are discussed together, allowing for the possibility that their differing pathogenesis and clinical presentations indicate that they may be separate conditions.

Histopathologic Features

Erythema multiforme is the prototypical acute cytotoxic interface dermatitis. Lymphocytes ascend into the epidermis, kill keratinocytes, and depart, without altering epidermal keratinization.

Early lesions contain lymphocytes around vessels of the superficial plexus and scattered along the dermoepidermal junc-

tion, in association with vacuoles both above and beneath the basal lamina. As lesions evolve, necrotic keratinocytes are seen, initially as single cells and eventually in a whorled array (Fig. 5-2). Necrotic keratinocytes can plug acrosyringia, especially in cases associated with drug ingestion.[6] The preservation of basket-weave orthokeratosis testifies to the acute nature of the process.[7]

In fully developed lesions, subepidermal vesiculation can occur via the confluence of clefts at the dermoepidermal junction (Fig. 5-3). The periphery of some target lesions features marked papillary dermal edema, with only a few lymphocytes in the epidermis (Fig. 5-4). This appearance has in part led to the confusing concept that in addition to "epidermal erythema multi-

Figure 5-2. (A) In erythema multiforme, there are superficial perivascular infiltrates of lymphocytes that ascend to obscure the dermoepidermal junction. **(B)** The papillary dermis is edematous, and many dyskeratotic keratinocytes are present in clusters within the upper spinous zone. **(C)** Note that cornification in erythema multiforme is unaffected; despite the presence of many necrotic keratinocytes, there is a basket-weave cornified layer.

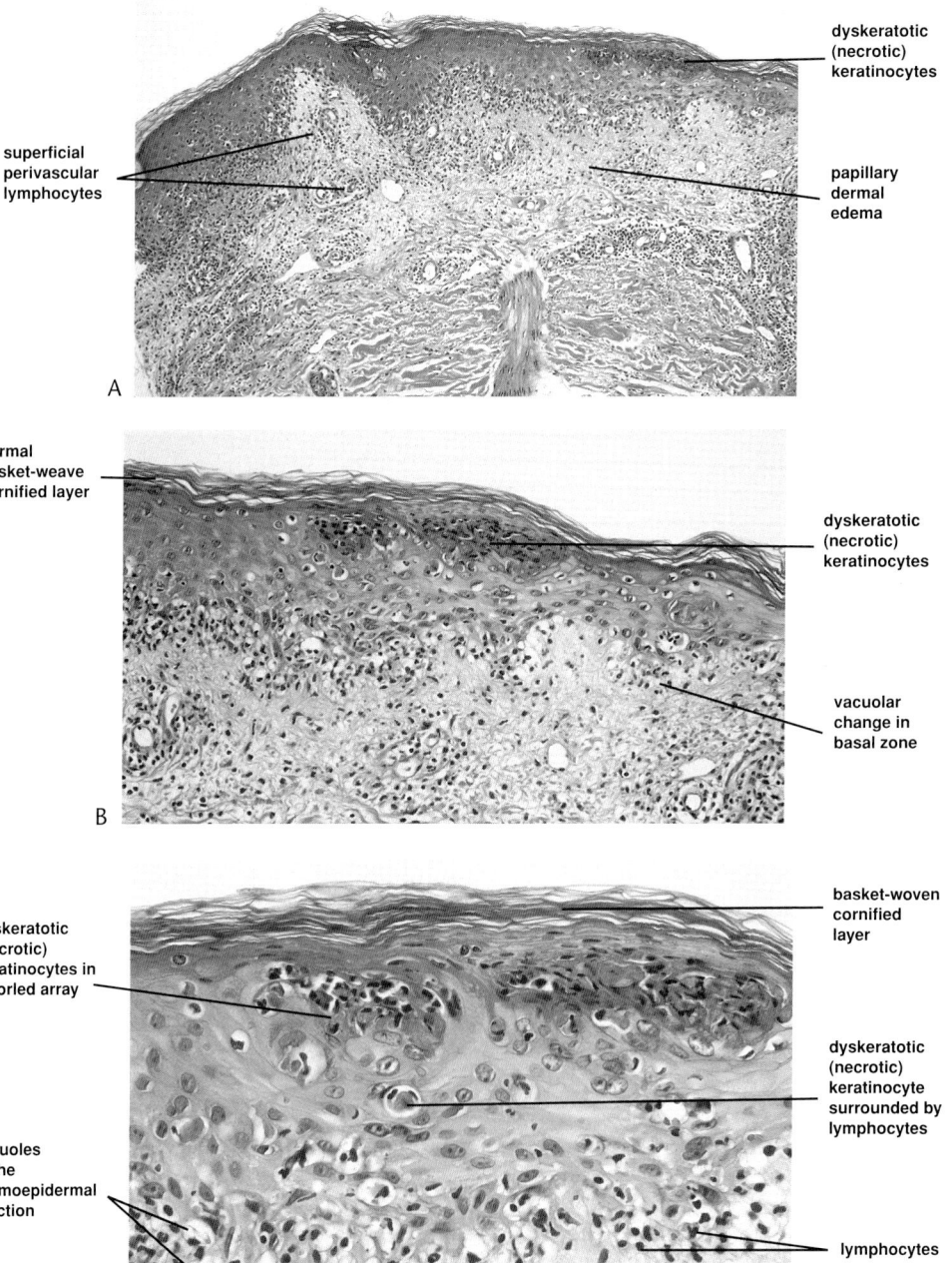

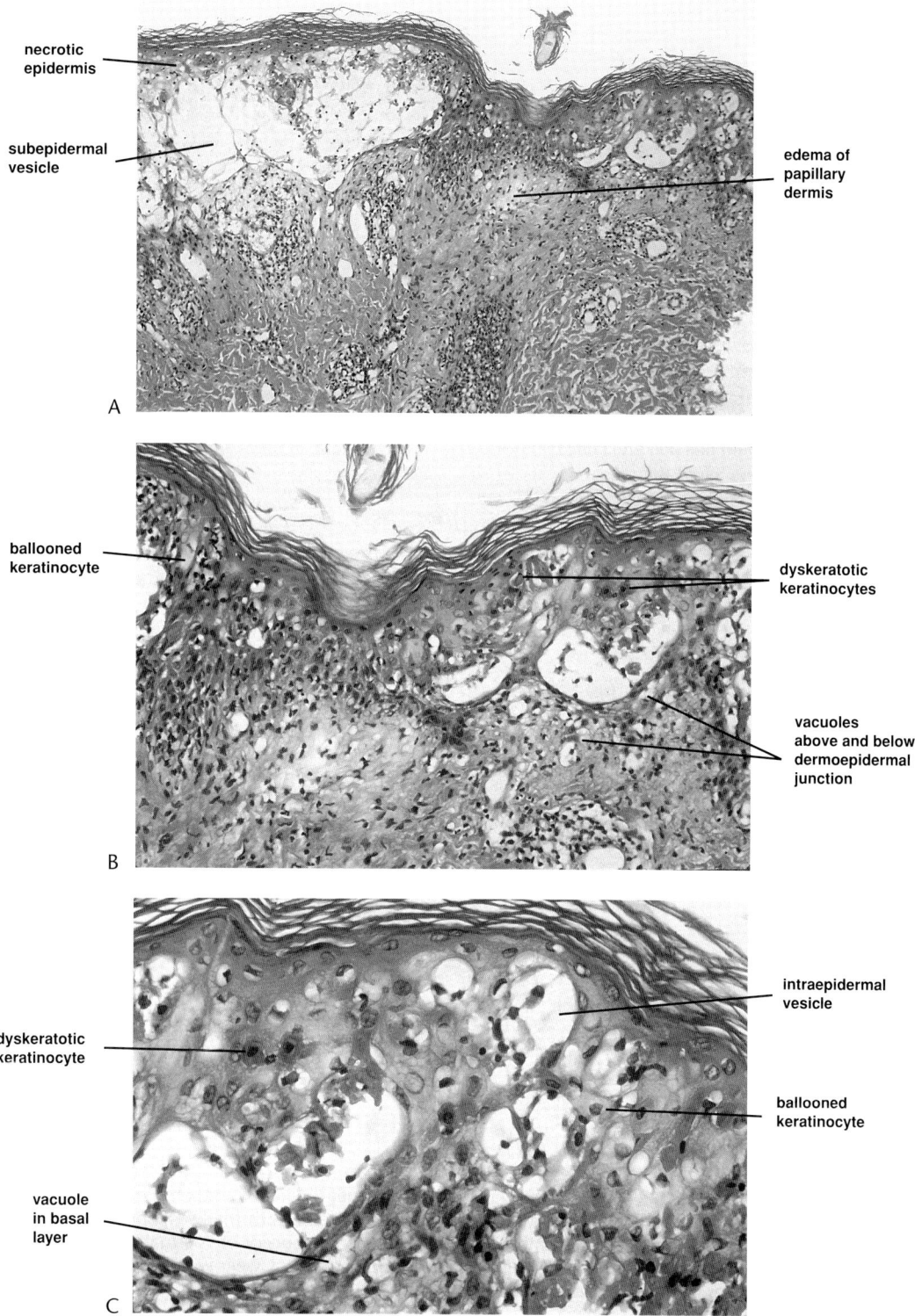

Figure 5-3. **(A)** In this example of erythema multiforme with vesiculation, there is still a central zone with the characteristic findings of an acute cytotoxic interface dermatitis. **(B)** Lymphocytes are distributed on either side of the dermoepidermal junction, where there is vacuolar change with single necrotic keratinocytes. **(C)** Ballooned keratinocytes (recognizable by their abundant pale cytoplasm) and scattered dyskeratotic or apoptotic cells are present, again with a basket-woven cornified layer.

Cytokines such as tumor necrosis factor may be responsible for epidermal necrosis to a greater extent in TEN than in erythema multiforme, where most of the epidermal damage is the result of infiltration by cytotoxic T cells. These cells are present in TEN, although they are fewer in number. The binding of lymphocytes to keratinocytes is also mediated by cytokines. In erythema multiforme, basilar keratinocytes express intercellular adhesion molecule (ICAM)-1, the ligand for lymphocyte function antigen-1. The fusion of this pair is believed to mediate the attachment of lymphocytes to keratinocytes. In contrast to lichen planus, in which only basilar keratinocytes express ICAM-1, there is patchy suprabasilar expression of the molecule in erythema multiforme, perhaps due to its induction by herpes simplex.[12]

Phototoxic Dermatitis

Phototoxic dermatitis is an eruption caused by ultraviolet (UV) radiation–mediated necrosis of keratinocytes. The process is typified by the common sunburn. It occurs at lower dosages of UV in patients who are taking drugs (e.g., tetracycline) and in those exposed topically to photosensitizing agents such as lime juice. Sunburn associated with photosensitizing agents is an example of a phototoxic contact dermatitis. Prior sensitization is not required as it is in photoallergic dermatitis.

Similar histologic changes to those of phototoxic dermatitis occur in acutely irradiated skin and in chronically heat-exposed skin as in erythema ab igne.

Clinical Features

Confluent erythematous patches evolve several hours after exposure and are often sharply delineated by the edges of garments worn during exposure. In phototoxic contact dermatitis, the eruption is confined to sun-exposed areas that the noxious substance contacted. Desquamation occurs in both conditions during recovery.

Histopathologic Features

The so-called sunburn cell is the hallmark of all types of phototoxic dermatitis. Usually located in the midepidermis, it is rounded, often brightly eosinophilic, and anucleate. In phototoxic dermatitis, sunburn cells in the spinous zone are coupled with vacuolar change at the dermoepidermal junction (Fig. 5-5). As lesions evolve, a few lymphocytes may be seen around dilated vessels of the superficial plexus or near the dermoepidermal junction and sometimes within the epidermis adjacent to necrotic keratinocytes.

Clinicopathologic Correlation

As desquamation occurs, an eosinophilic coagulum resulting from the confluence of apoptotic keratinocytes appears beneath the basket-weave pattern of the normal cornified layer with eventual shedding of both. A blistering sunburn is seldom biopsied, but the blisters in a phototoxic dermatitis are subepidermal and are formed via the confluence of vacuoles.

Differential Diagnosis

The clinical differential diagnosis of phototoxic dermatitis is usually photoallergic dermatitis or polymorphous light eruption. Photoallergic dermatitis is characterized by spongiosis with either superficial or superficial and deep perivascular infiltrate and the latter by either a perivascular lymphocytic infiltrate alone or accompanied in edematous papules or papulovesicles by papillary dermal edema and, sometimes, spongiosis. In assessing biopsy specimens of phototest sites where patients have been exposed to high doses of UV, it should be kept in mind that scattered dyskeratotic cells can occur in patients with nearly any of the photodermatitides.

Pathophysiology

Phototoxic dermatitis is initiated by UV alone or by UV in combination with a sensitizing agent. Sensitizing agents may exert their effects through alteration of cell membranes, nuclear DNA, or lysozomes. The result of sufficient doses of UV on the epidermis, or lesser doses augmented by sensitization, is apoptosis of susceptible keratinocytes. The exact roles of such factors as tumor necrosis factor-α, p53, and other proteins that regulate apoptosis and how UV light triggers apoptosis of keratinocytes remains to be determined.

Acute Cytotoxic Interface Dermatitis Secondary to Chemotherapy or Radiotherapy

Both chemotherapeutic agents and radiotherapy can cause erythematous patches through necrosis of keratinocytes and other effects.

Clinical Features

Some chemotherapeutic agents given at high doses may cause an erythematous, sometimes painful, eruption. A characteristic expression of toxicity from chemotherapeutic agents is so-called acral erythema, which affects the skin of the palms and fingers.[13] Acutely irradiated skin usually shows a pattern of injury indistinguishable from phototoxic dermatitis, but in occasional cases there is persistent erythema limited to radiated areas, characterized histologically by vacuolar interface dermatitis, a finding termed *subacute radiation dermatitis.*

Histopathologic Features

Chemotherapeutically induced interface dermatitis demonstrates marked alteration of the normal epidermal architecture. Basal keratinocytes, usually cuboidal, are replaced by cells with a more polygonal appearance and abundant cytoplasm, a change termed *squamatization of the basal layer* (Fig. 5-6). Necrotic keratinocytes may be scattered throughout the entire thickness of the epidermis.[13] The nuclei of keratinocytes may be pleomorphic because of damage to nuclear DNA.[14] Despite cytologic atypia, the granular layer of the epidermis often remains continuous, and cornification is usually normal. In cases in which large amounts of a chemotherapeutic agent are injected, confluent necrosis of the epidermis can occur, simulating TEN or erythema multiforme.[15]

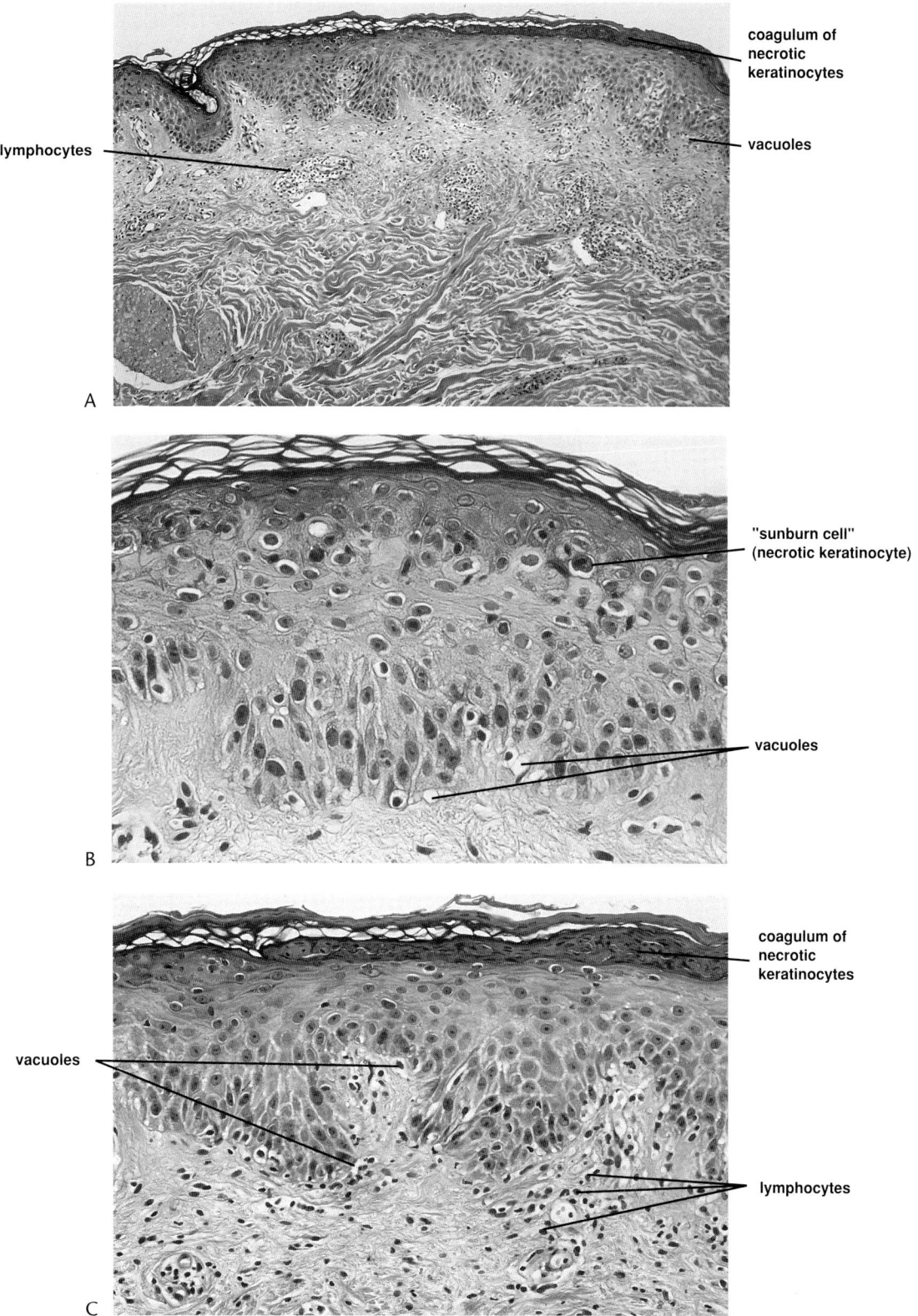

Figure 5-5.   **(A)** Phototoxic dermatitis features vacuolar change along with scattered single dyskeratotic cells. **(B)** At first, single necrotic keratinocytes are present in the superficial spinous zone. **(C)** Later on, necrotic keratinocytes form a coagulum, which is exfoliated.

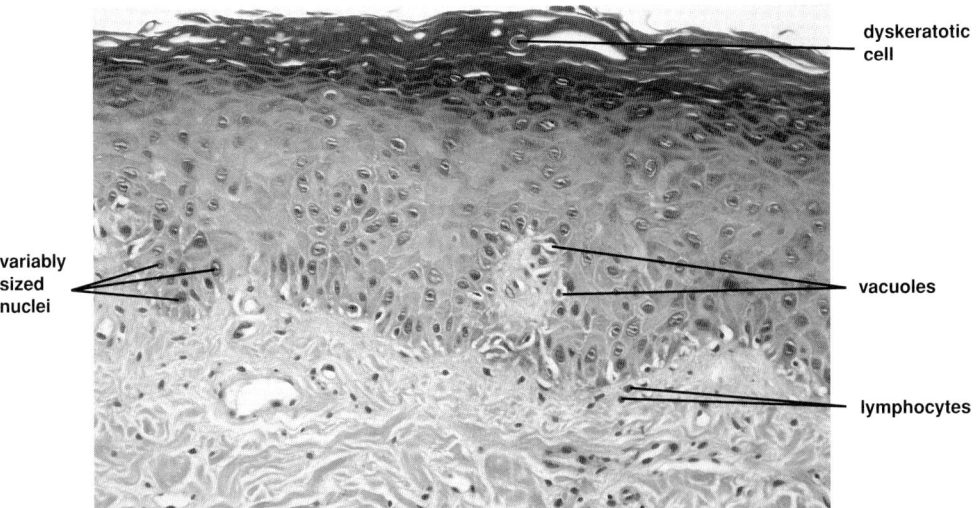

Figure 5-6. In acute cytotoxic interface dermatitis due to antineoplastic drugs, there are sparse lymphocytic infiltrates along with dyskeratotic cells. Abnormal maturation of keratinocytes results in focal crowding of nuclei of variable sizes and shapes.

In subacute radiation dermatitis, a sparse lymphocytic infiltrate obscures the dermoepidermal junction, accompanied by numerous necrotic keratinocytes, some satellited by lymphocytes as in acute graft-versus-host disease.

Clinicopathologic Correlation

The erythematous patches of acute radiation dermatitis may have a weeping appearance clinically, a finding that corresponds to serum in foci of parakeratosis histologically. In subacute radiation dermatitis, there can be mottled hyperpigmentation and hypopigmentation, correlating with melanophages in the papillary dermis and papillary dermal sclerosis, respectively.

Differential Diagnosis

The distinction between chemotherapy- and radiotherapy-induced interface dermatitis and acute cutaneous graft-versus-host disease in transplant recipients may be critical, and is discussed later.

Pathophysiology

Radiation directly induces the apoptosis of keratinocytes through damage to their genomes. In subacute radiation dermatitis there is also a cell-mediated cytotoxic reaction, presumably to altered antigens on the surfaces of cells. Chemotherapeutic agents often affect dividing cells, inducing apoptosis in them. They undoubtedly also trigger the release of many cytokines by susceptible tissues, resulting in altered antigenicity and a T-cell–mediated immune response targeting keratinocytes in some cases.

Fixed Drug Eruption

In a fixed drug eruption, lesions occur repetitively in the same area after each exposure to an offending drug.

Clinical Features

The lesions of fixed drug eruption are often ovoid or round, erythematous patches that sometimes vesiculate. They remain inflamed for up to 10 days after exposure to the inciting agent and resolve as persistent, well-demarcated areas of hyperpigmentation. In rare cases, the agent is never identified. Recrudescent lesions are orange to mercurochrome-like in color. Agents commonly responsible for fixed drug eruption include phenolphthalein, tetracycline, and barbiturates. Usually a patient develops only one lesion or a few. The characteristic sites of lesions include the genitalia, lips, and limbs. When multiple lesions are present, they are distributed asymmetrically. There is a rare, generalized form in which many lesions occur and are widely distributed over the skin surface.

Histopathologic Features

The epidermal changes of most cases of fixed drug eruption are similar to those of erythema multiforme, with vacuolization and necrotic keratinocytes that are disposed singly and in clusters not only near the junction but sometimes within the middle and upper spinous layers as well. The rete ridges tend to be slightly elongated, and dyskeratotic cells in the spinous layer sometimes retain their polygonal shapes. If vacuolar change is extensive, subepidermal vesiculation can result (Fig. 5-7). Spongiosis is more often present in fixed drug eruptions than in erythema multiforme, aside from mucosal lesions of erythema multiforme. In some cases, the epidermis responds with ballooning, reticular alteration, and intraepidermal vesiculation. The lesions of fixed drug eruption evolve and devolve quickly so that corni-

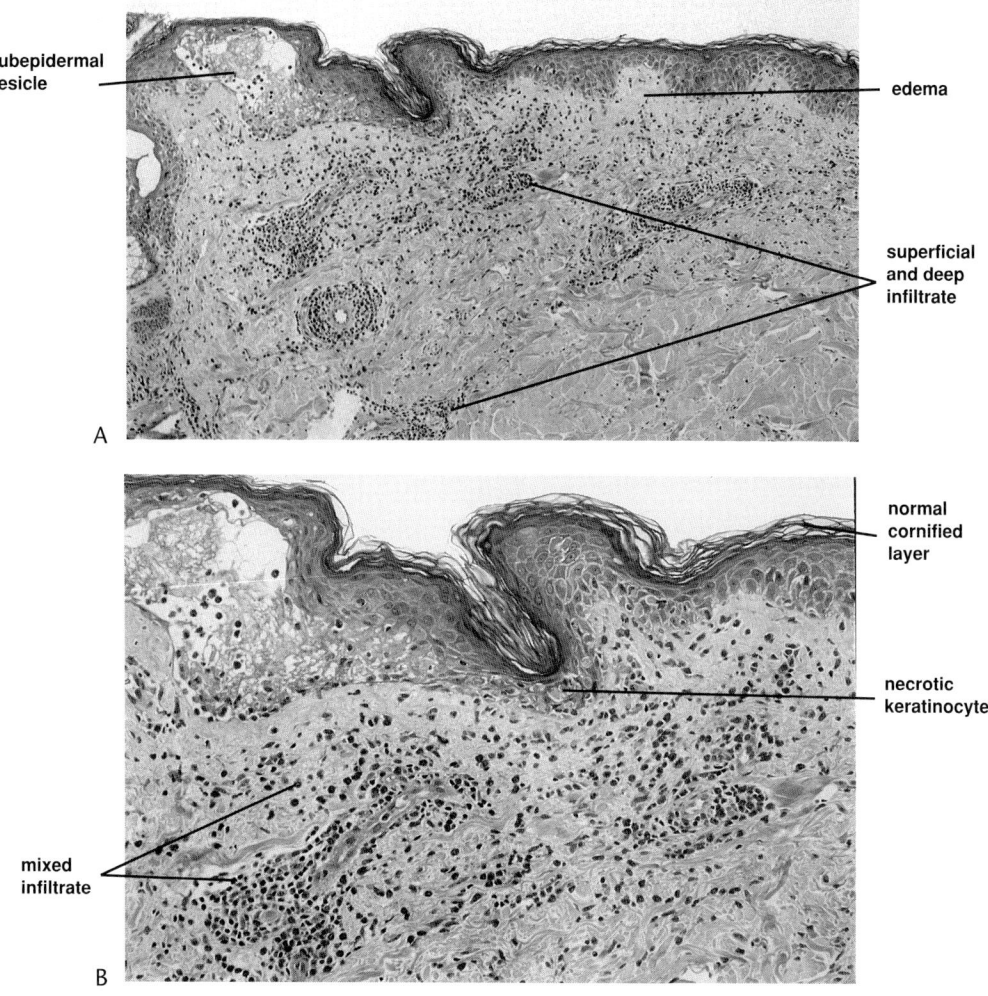

Figure 5-7. **(A)** In the fixed drug eruption, there are epidermal changes similar to those of erythema multiforme in conjunction with infiltrates that often are superficial and deep and have many eosinophils, neutrophils, or both. **(B)** Incipient subepidermal vesiculation.

fication is seldom affected. In some resolving lesions, there can be an eosinophilic coagulum that results from sloughing of confluently necrotic keratinocytes.

The dermis of fixed drug eruptions shows a superficial, or superficial and deep perivascular, and interstitial infiltrate that often includes eosinophils and sometimes neutrophils. Some have described dense infiltrates of neutrophils in the superficial dermis in early, evolving lesions.[16] If previous episodes have occurred in the area of the biopsy specimen, melanophages may be present and may be deeper in the dermis than in other conditions that result in postinflammatory hyperpigmentation.

Clinicopathologic Correlation

The mercurochrome-colored lesions are produced by a combination of erythema from recent inflammation and deeply situated melanophages from prior episodes. The hyperpigmentation of old lesions is caused by epidermal pigmentation and dermal melanophages.

Differential Diagnosis

Erythema multiforme may be difficult to distinguish from fixed drug eruption. Numerous eosinophils, neutrophils, or melanophages and involvement of the deep plexus favor a fixed drug eruption. However, many lesions of fixed drug eruption lack these findings, and a histopathologic picture indistinguishable from erythema multiforme should not be a bar to the diagnosis if the clinical setting is compatible. There are some subtle epidermal signs—slight psoriasiform hyperplasia, polygonally shaped dyskeratotic cells, and many lymphocytes and adjacent dyskeratosis high in the spinous layer that favor a fixed drug eruption over erythema multiforme, even in the absence of a mixed infiltrate or melanophages situated deep in the dermis.

Pathophysiology

The reason that a limited area of the skin becomes inflamed on exposure to a drug is unknown. Interestingly, patch testing with a topically applied drug can result in a flare in the affected area of the skin, with an inert reaction in other areas. As is the case with erythema multiforme, helper (CD4+) cells predominate at the peripheries of lesions, and CD8+ (cytotoxic-suppressor) cells are prominent in the centers of lesions.[17]

Pityriases Lichenoides et Varicoliformis Acuta and Pityriases Lichenoides Chronica

Pityriasis lichenoides is an idiopathic condition in which small papules appear in crops and spontaneously involute in otherwise healthy people. The acute form of the condition features papules that become hemorrhagic in appearance and often ulcerate. In the chronic form, lesions evolve more slowly, and the condition often persists for several years.

Clinical Features

In the acute form (pityriasis lichenoides et varicoliformis acuta [PLEVA]) papules become hemorrhagic and resolve with shallow scars similar to those induced by smallpox. PLEVA usually wanes within a few months, but while they are active, there may be lesions at all stages of evolution at any one time. In the rare, ulceronecrotic form a high fever and constitutional symptoms accompany large necrotic skin lesions.[18] The lesions may be pruritic and can be accompanied by constitutional symptoms. Pityriasis lichenoides chronica (PLC) may eventuate or the eruption may cease, although it may also recur at a later date. PLC can also arise de novo and usually persists for many years with tan to red-brown papules surmounted by scale. Lesions do not usually scar but may leave pigmentary changes on resolution. Lesions of acute and chronic pityriasis lichenoides sometimes occur in the same patient.

The relationship between pityriasis lichenoides and cutaneous T-cell lymphoma is tenuous. Although Brocq classified both forms of parapsoriasis along with parapsoriasis en plaques (considered by most dermatopathologists to be the patch stage of mycosis fungoides), there are only a few reports of PLEVA or PLC eventuating in mycosis fungoides.[19] The finding of clonal T-cell populations in PLEVA by Southern blot analysis and its clinical resemblance to lymphomatosis papulosis, a condition undoubtedly related to mycosis fungoides, gives pause.[20] However, some lesions of lymphomatoid papulosis (termed *type B lesions* by Willemze) are composed of lymphocytes with only moderately enlarged nuclei and can be confused with PLEVA. This may be the explanation for these findings, as a more recent study of PLEVA using the polymerase chain reaction method to study the T-cell receptor γ-chain gene did not find evidence of clonality.

Histopathologic Features

The earliest lesions of PLEVA and PLC all show vacuolar rather than a lichenoid interface dermatitis and may be indistinguishable. As lesions of PLEVA progress, they develop denser papillary dermal infiltrates, slight psoriasiform epidermal hyperplasia, extensive vacuolar change, and necrotic keratinocytes that first appear as single cells and subsequently collect in clusters similar to those seen in erythema multiforme or in the fixed drug eruption (Fig. 5-8). Lymphocytes are often positioned in the middle and upper portions of the spinous zone, with adjacent necrotic keratinocytes. The upper portion of the epidermis is often pallid, due to ballooning of keratinocytes. If ballooning is severe enough, intraepidermal vesiculation can result. Vesiculation is unusual in PLEVA and, when it occurs, is usually subepidermal rather than intraepidermal, although both can occur in the same lesion.

Both ulcerated and intact lesions of pityriasis lichenoides can have parakeratotic mounds that contain inflammatory cells. Some of these are fragmented lymphocytes, whereas others are neutrophils, which are usually layered throughout rather than situated at the summits of the mounds as in psoriasis or dermatophytosis. Extravasated erythrocytes can be numerous and may enter the epidermis. Often, vessels of the deep plexus are involved.

The clinical differential diagnosis of many cases of PLEVA

Figure 5-8. **(A)** The acute form of pityriasis lichenoides often displays a superficial and deep lymphocytic infiltrate that is band-like within the papillary dermis. (*Figure continues.*)

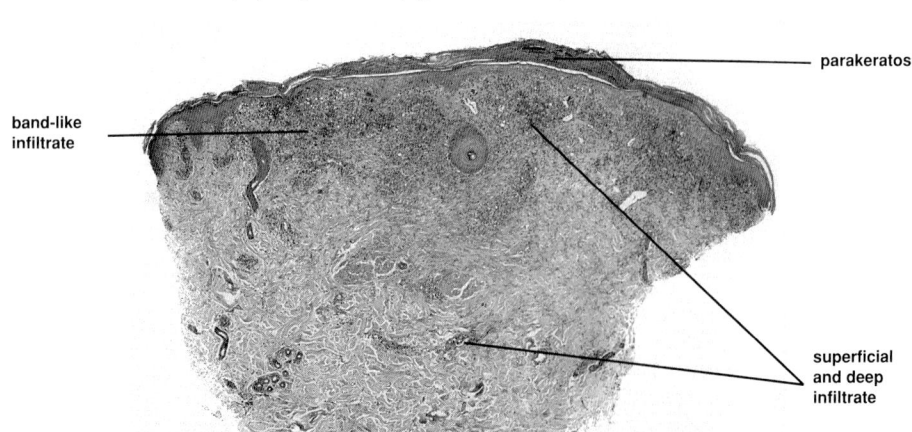

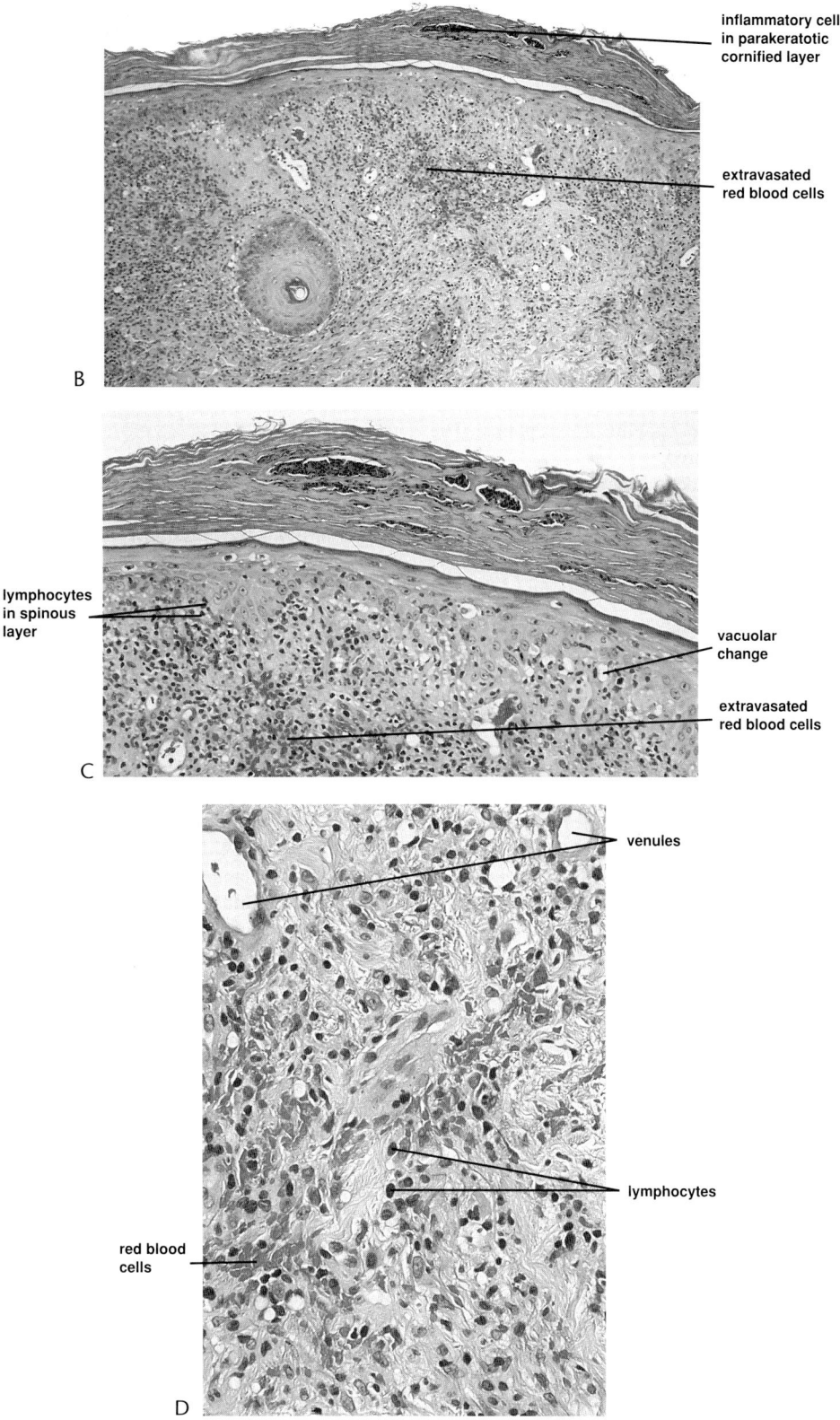

Figure 5-8 *(Continued).* **(B)** The dermoepidermal junction is obscured by lymphocytes, and there are many extravasated erythrocytes in the papillary dermis. **(C)** Lymphocytes frequently ascend into the superficial spinous zone, and some are adjacent to dyskeratotic cells. **(D)** Even though pityriasis lichenoides is considered to be a lymphocytic vasculitis by many observers, extravasated erythrocytes are commonly seen adjacent to venules whose walls are morphologically unaltered (D).

guish some of these lesions from acute cutaneous graft-versus-host disease by microscopic examination, and indeed the acute graft-versus-host reaction in autologous marrow transplant patients may be an example of the eruption of lymphocyte recovery.

INTERFACE DERMATITIS RESULTING IN PREMATURE TERMINAL DIFFERENTIATION

Lichen Planus

Lichen planus is an idiopathic disorder that affects skin and mucous membranes. It is characterized by small, flat-topped papules clinically and a band-like mononuclear cell infiltrate histologically.

Clinical Features

The individual papules often have a polygonal shape, a violaceous to gray-red hue, and a thin, refractile scale. Some macules contain thin white lines (Wickham's striae). Mucous membrane lesions leave a lacy, white appearance. The flexural aspects of arms and legs are among the most frequent sites of involvement, with a particular predilection for wrists and ankles. Occasional patients have isolated genital or oral lesions. Lesions of lichen planus usually erupt over a period of a few weeks and are usually intensely pruritic.

Most patients with lichen planus that affects only the skin will recover entirely in a year or so, while those with mucosal lesions may have a more prolonged course. Relapses occur in about one-fifth of patients with lichen planus of the skin and in a higher percentage of those with mucosal disease.[24]

Lichen planus has a variety of morphologic appearances. Cutaneous lesions may be annular, especially in dark-skinned patients. Linear lesions may occur secondary to the Koebner phenomenon but may also erupt in a dermatomal distribution, often as an episode of herpes zoster.

Lichen simplex chronicus may be superimposed on the pruritic lesions of lichen planus and result in hypertrophic lichen planus. This most frequently occurs on the anterior legs and is characterized by wart-like lesions.

As lesions of lichen planus resolve, the epidermis may thin, resulting in atrophic lichen planus. This variant can be difficult to recognize clinically. Its hallmarks include a dusky purplish gray hue.

Lichen planus may present with vesicles or bullae in two situations. Small vesicles may appear within lesions of ordinary lichen planus. In some patients with lichen planus, vesicles or bullae may arise in clinically uninvolved skin, accompanied by deposition of IgG and C3, a condition termed *lichen planus*

pemphigoides because of its similarity to bullous pemphigoid. However, antigen recognized by the IgG of lichen planus pemphigoides is different from that of ordinary bullous pemphigoid.[25]

Lichen planus actinus occurs mainly in the Middle East but occasionally in dark-skinned persons in other areas. It is characterized by small lichenoid papules in sun-exposed skin. It differs from lichenoid photodermatitis in that there is no known sensitizing drug.

Lichen planopilaris is the term given to lichen planus with substantial follicular involvement. It often presents as patches of scarring alopecia that do not show the surface changes of lichen planus. The diagnosis is often made only when nail or cutaneous lesions are present.

The nails of patients with lichen planus of the skin are involved in roughly 10% of cases but may be the presenting or only manifestation.

The mucous membranes, including the gastrointestinal tract on rare occasions, may be involved by lichen planus, either together with cutaneous lesions or, on occasion, exclusively. Erosive lesions and squamous cell carcinoma can develop in mucosal sites.

Histopathologic Features

In the very earliest macules of lichen planus, there are increased numbers of Langerhans cells in the epidermis, with sparse superficial perivascular infiltrates of lymphocytes.[26] As papules develop, the configuration of the epidermis is affected. Lymphocytes appear on either side of the epidermal basement membrane, and pointed rete ridges rapidly appear as a result of T-cell–mediated necrosis of keratinocytes at the bases of the rete. A thickened granular layer and a compact cornified layer rapidly evolve. Even in a papule less than 1 mm in size, the superficial epidermis is already affected in a stereotypic manner (Fig. 5-10).

As lesions of lichen planus evolve, a band-like infiltrate usually composed exclusively of lymphocytes and macrophages becomes apparent within the papillary dermis. It usually extends across most of the width of a 4-mm punch biopsy specimen. The rete ridges may exhibit small clefts along their sides (Max Joseph spaces). Colloid or Civatte bodies that represent the mummified, anucleate remnants of basal cells are present along with melanophages in the papillary dermis.

A number of changes occur in epidermis affected by lichen planus. The cells of the basal layer change from cuboidal to polygonal, an alteration known as *squamatization of the basal layer*. The cells of the spinous layer become larger than normal and develop a glassy-appearing cytoplasm. Although some intercellular spaces in the lowermost epidermis may be widened,

Figure 5-10. Lichen planus exemplifies interface dermatitis in which there is premature differentiation of keratinocytes. **(A)** Even in this early papule, there are distinctive epidermal changes. The junction between eccrine ducts and the epidermis is often at the center of tiny papules in lichen planus. **(B)** Already, there is a band-like lymphocytic infiltrate, and the granular layer is thickened in a wedged configuration beneath a compact cornified layer. **(C)** A cluster of colloid bodies is present in the papillary dermis. **(D)** The edge of this lesion shows what seem to be even earlier findings, with vacuolar change and only subtle compact hyperkeratosis.

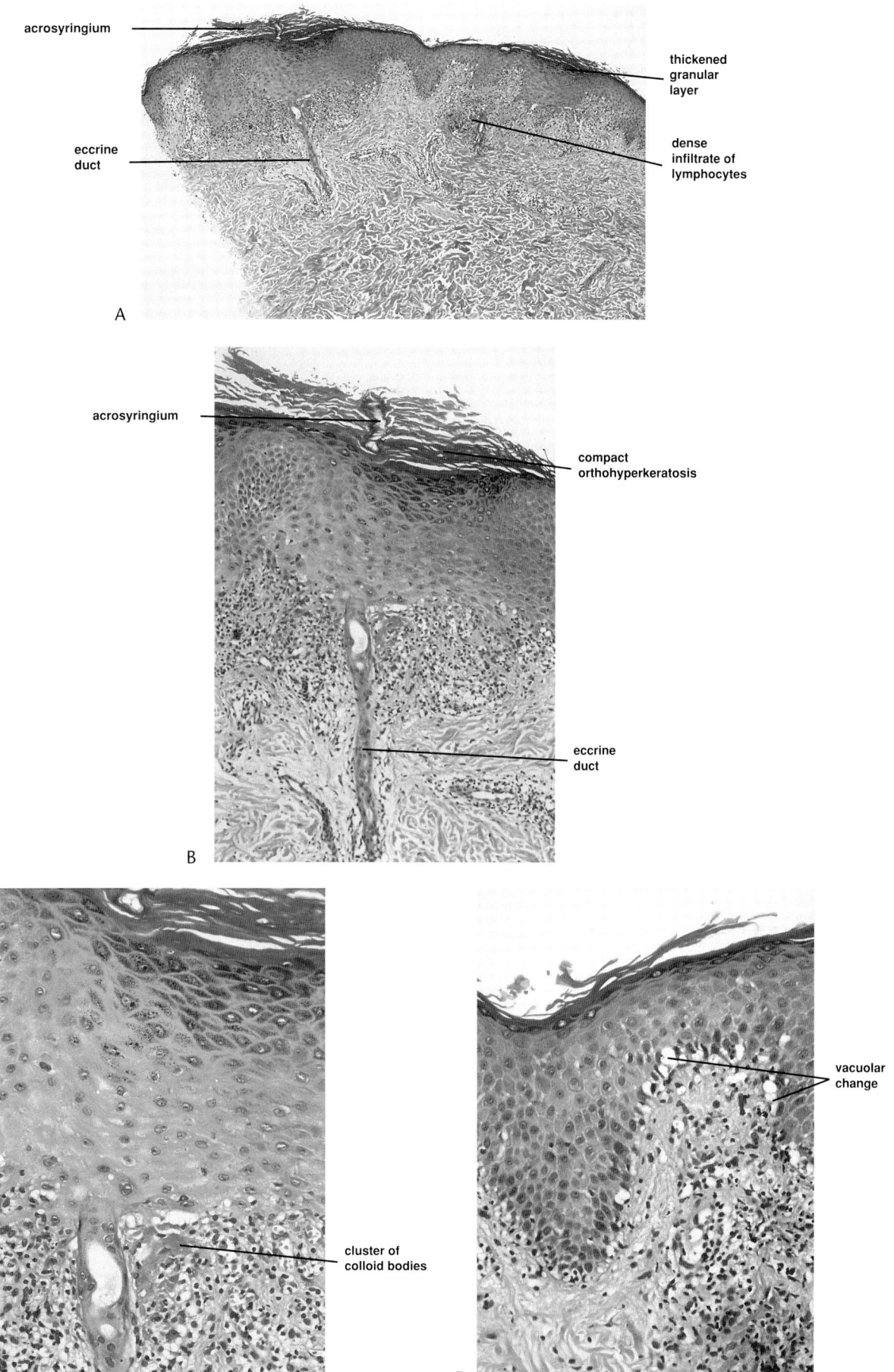

A

acrosyringium

thickened granular layer

eccrine duct

dense infiltrate of lymphocytes

B

acrosyringium

compact orthohyperkeratosis

eccrine duct

C

cluster of colloid bodies

D

vacuolar change

those in the upper spinous layer appear narrowed, and the granular layer is thickened, especially over the orifices of eccrine ducts; this results in foci of wedge-shaped hypergranulosis. In lichen planopilaris, these foci may also be seen in the base of follicular infundibula that have bulbous keratinous plugs. The cornified layer in lesions of lichen planus is generally thickened and compact or lamellar.

As lesions of lichen planus persist, fibrosis may occur at the apices of dermal papillae, separating the epidermis from the underlying band-like infiltrate. Eventually the epidermis may become flattened and thinned, either focally or confluently, in atrophic lesions (Fig. 5-11).

Clinicopathologic Correlations

The classic polygonal papule of lichen planus reflects the way in which the lymphocytic infiltrate and hyperplastic epidermis raise the surface of the skin. The violaceous color is imparted by the hues of inflammatory cells, dilated vessels, and melanophages filtered through a thickened epidermis. The translucent scale is produced by uniform hyperkeratosis without the intracorneal inflammatory cells that would render it opaque.

The variants of lichen planus have distinctive histologic features. In hypertrophic lichen planus the histologic features are those of lichen planus overlain by lichen simplex chronicus (Fig. 5-12). The lesions have verrucous surfaces, compact hyperkeratosis, markedly irregular epidermal and infundibular epithelial hyperplasia and hypergranulosis, and more pronounced and vertically oriented fibrosis of the papillary dermis. If the lesions have been picked as well as scratched, the summits of the papillations may be necrotic or eroded. Although eosinophils are rare in ordinary lesions of lichen planus, it is common to see a few of these cells in hypertrophic ones.

Lichen planus pemphigoides microscopically resembles bullous pemphigoid, with subepidermal vesiculation and sometimes eosinophils in the dermal infiltrate. The band-like

Figure 5-11. Atrophic lichen planus is the result of a sustained attack on the basal layer of the epidermis by T cells, in which keratinocytic replication cannot keep pace. **(A)** A band-like infiltrate of lymphocytes resides beneath an epidermis whose rete ridge pattern is drastically attenuated. **(B)** Note the wedge-shaped foci of hypergranulosis and slight hyperkeratosis.

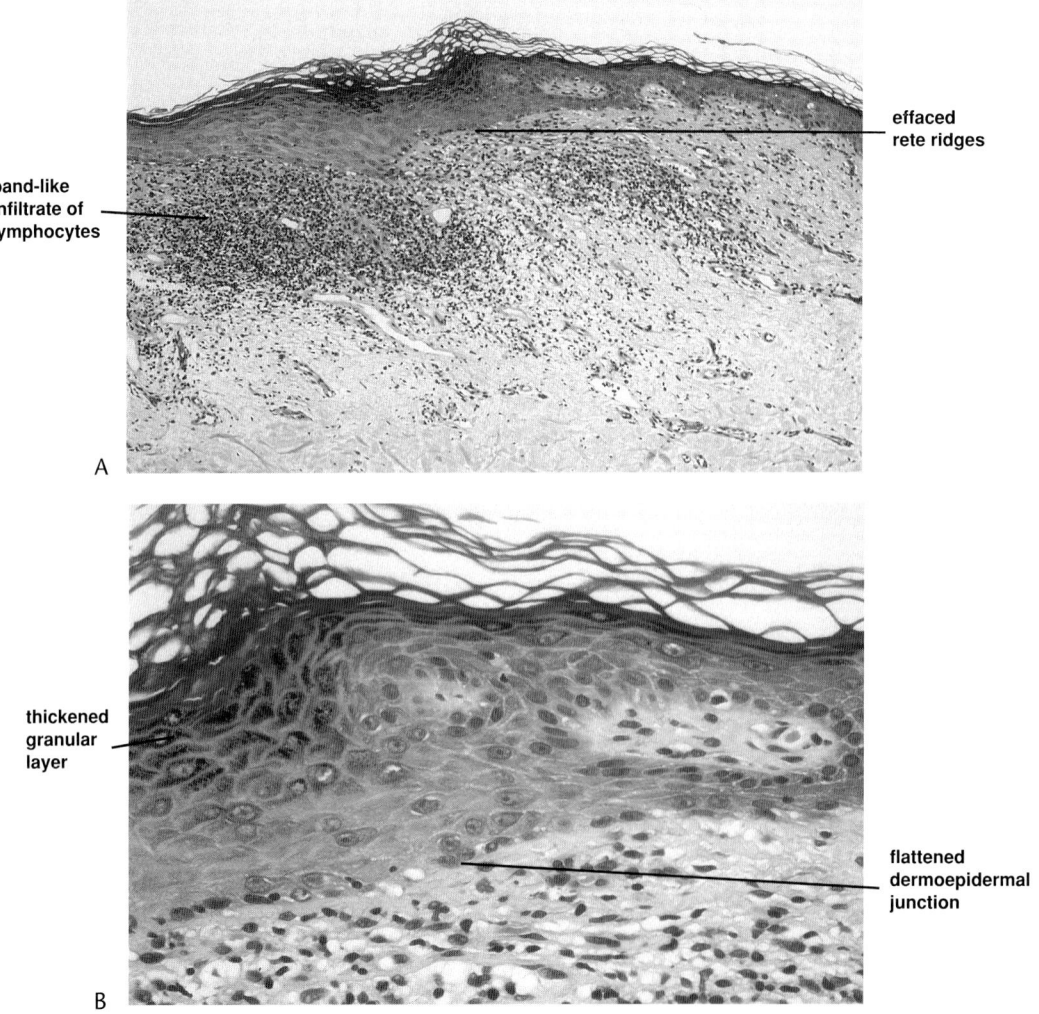

effaced rete ridges

band-like infiltrate of lymphocytes

A

thickened granular layer

flattened dermoepidermal junction

B

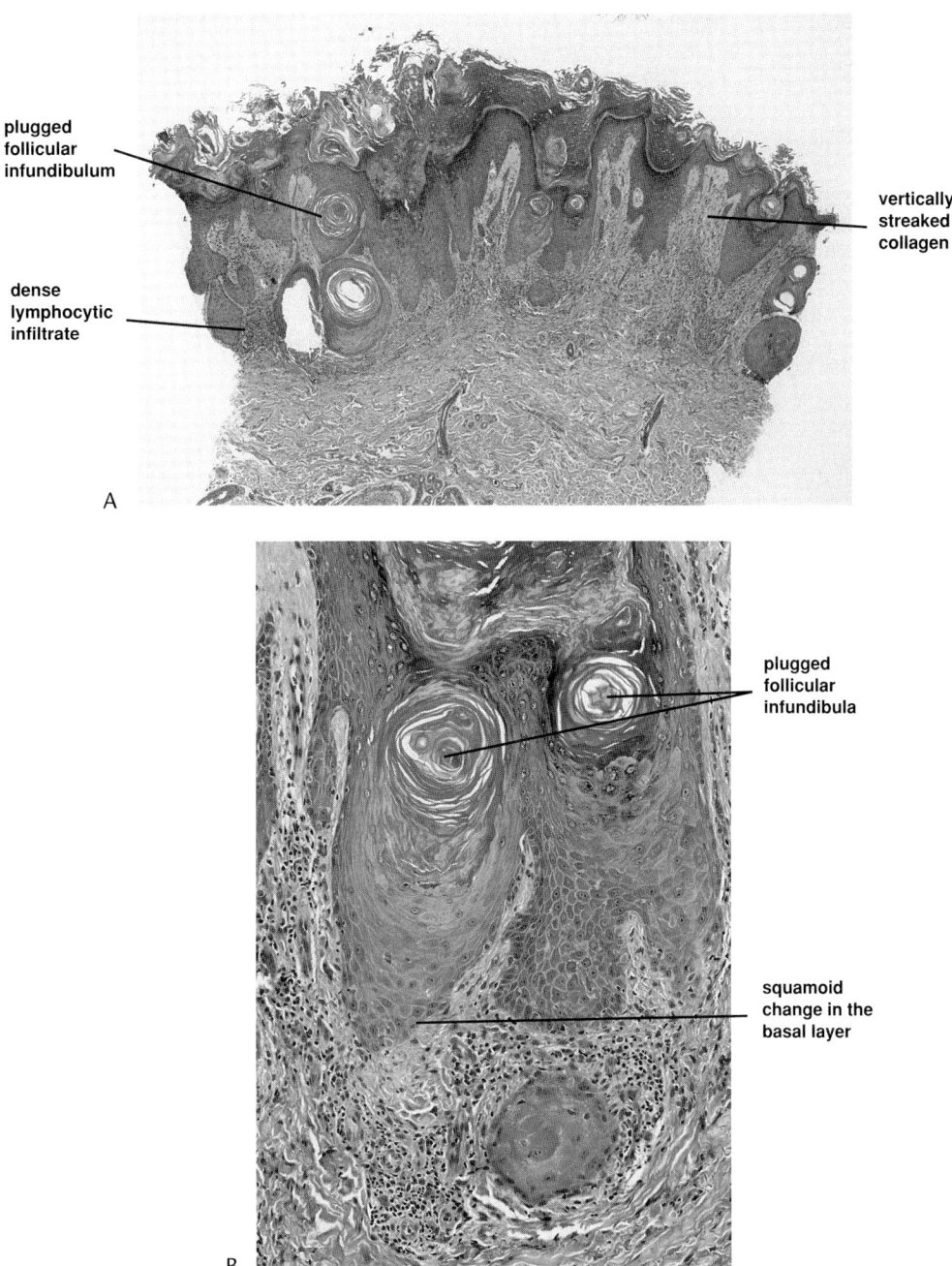

Figure 5-12. In hypertrophic lichen planus, the epidermis is often verrucous and irregularly hyperplastic, with irregular hyperplasia of infundibular epithelium as well. **(A)** Discontinuous bands of lymphocytes that focally abut the bases of jagged rete ridges. **(B)** Plugging of infundibula by compact cornified material is present. (*Figure continues.*)

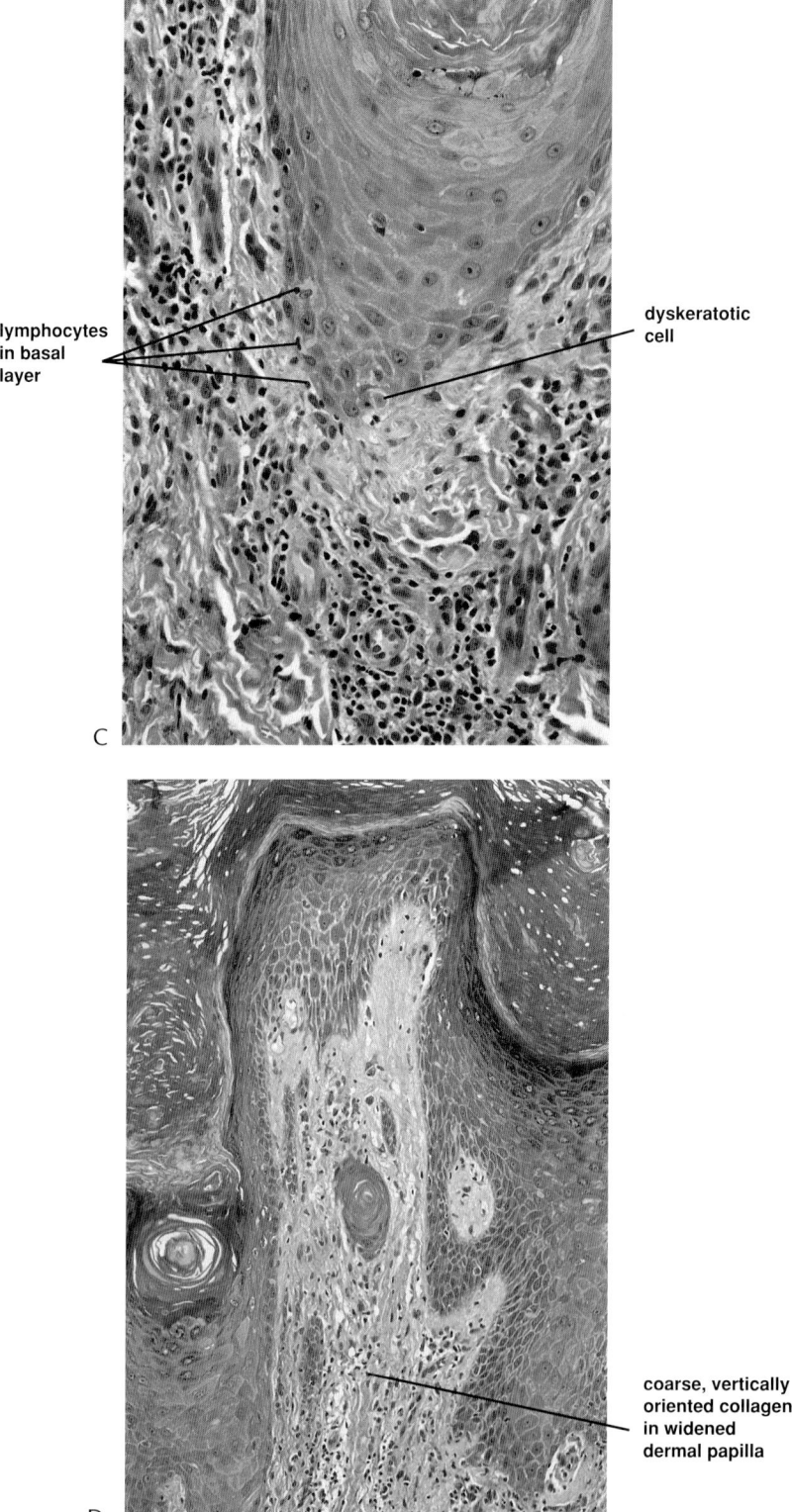

Figure 5-12 *(Continued).* **(C)** A few lymphocytes are evident in the basal zone of the epidermis, along with rare dyskeratotic cells. **(D)** The papillations have only a few lymphocytes, but demonstrate the thick, vertically oriented collagen bundles that characterize chronically rubbed lesions of many conditions, of which hypertrophic lichen planus is one.

mononuclear cell infiltrate seen in other forms of lichen planus is not found.

The lesions of lichen planus actinicus are histologically identical to those of nonactinic lichen planus, except that plasma cells are often present and individual lesions can sometimes be so minute as to simulate lichen nitidus.

The histologic features of lichen planopilaris are those of lichen planus transposed from the epidermis to the upper portion of hair follicles. Although follicular involvement within a lesion of lichen planus often occurs incidentally, in lichen planopilaris, individual follicles are often affected and the infiltrates that surround adjacent affected follicles may not merge. Indeed, some follicles are often entirely spared by the process.[27] A detailed consideration of lichen planopilaris is presented in Chapter 12.

A nail biopsy specimen of lichen planus usually shows changes indistinguishable from those of specimens of glabrous skin.

Lichen planus of the mucous membranes may have some rounded rather than pointed rete and sometimes a greater degree of parakeratosis than is usual for cutaneous lesions (Fig. 5-13). The lacy white streaks, termed *Wickham striae,* correspond to foci of marked epidermal hyperplasia and hypergranulosis.[28]

Differential Diagnosis

Because all lichenoid dermatitides have a band-like infiltrate, each one of them should be considered in the differential diagnosis of lichen planus. Figure 5-1 shows their distinguishing features.

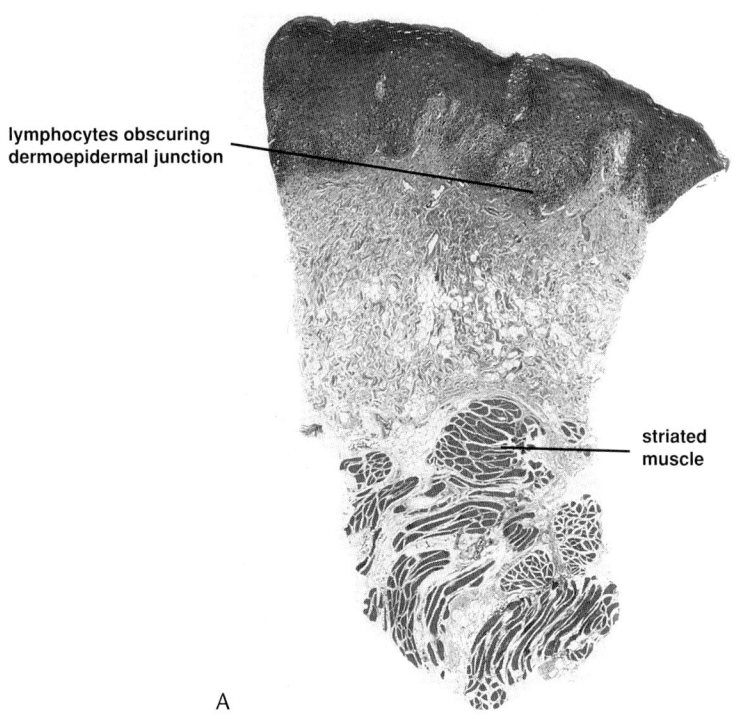

lymphocytes obscuring
dermoepidermal junction

striated
muscle

A

Figure 5-13. Lichen planus of the lip. There are skeletal muscle fibers insinuated into the subcutis, which is a feature of this site. **(A)** Band-like infiltrates of lymphocytes obscure the undersurface of an epidermis whose rete ridges are both rounded and jagged and vary considerably in width. **(B)** The granular layer is practically nonexistent in this example of mucosal lichen planus. (*Figure continues.*)

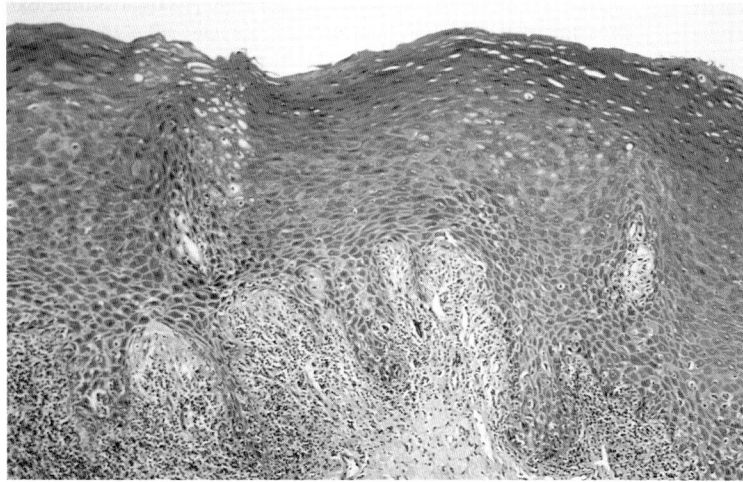

B

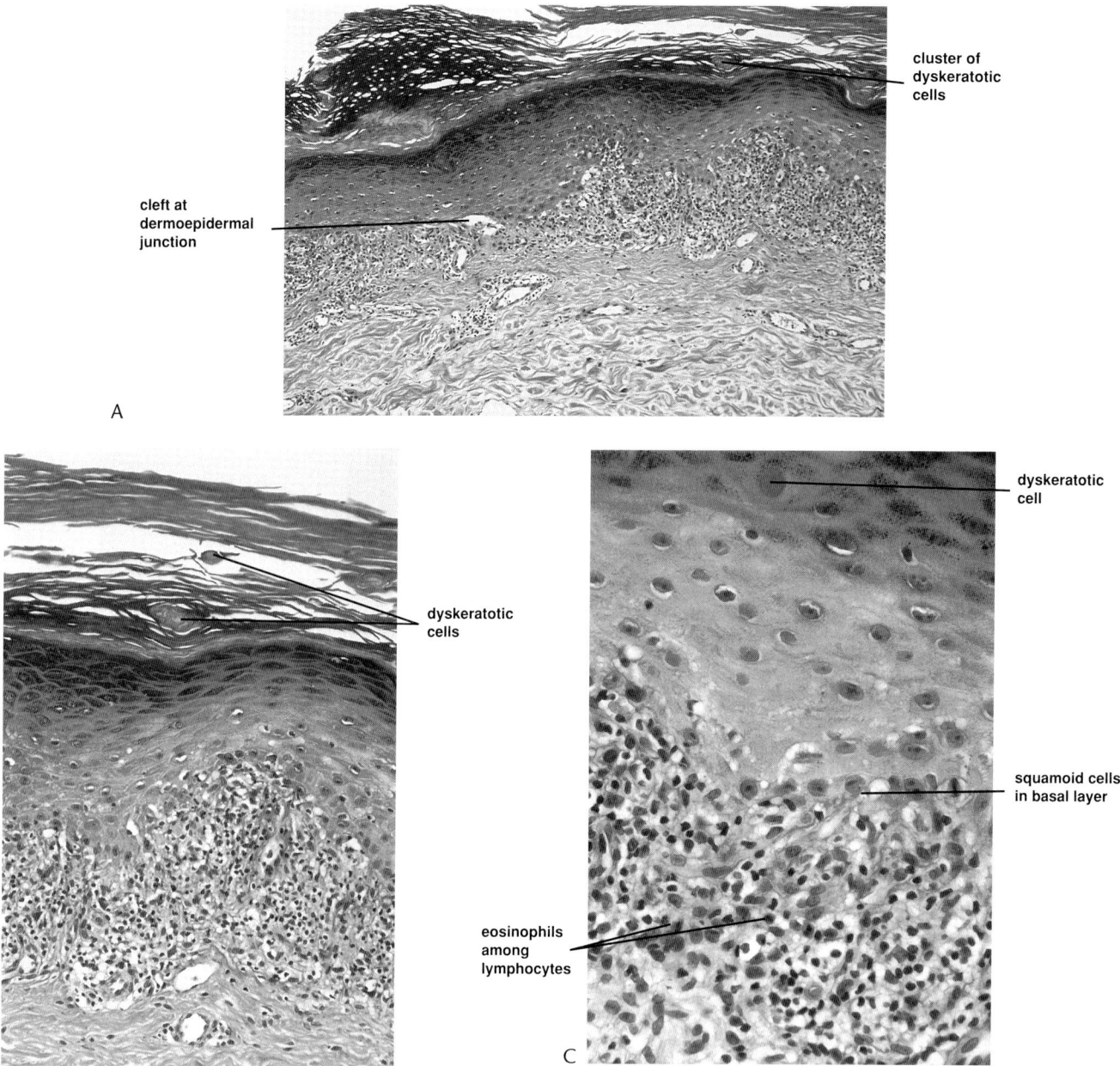

Figure 5-15. **(A)** In many lichenoid drug eruptions, there are only subtle histologic findings that differ from those of lichen planus. **(B)** The infiltrates in this example include eosinophils, and there are clusters of cytoid or colloid bodies in the cornified layer, a finding that is rare in idiopathic lichen planus. **(C)** The basal layer consists of polygonal cells with abundant cytoplasm, as in lichen planus. Note the dyskeratotic cell high up within the spinous zone.

parakeratosis does not favor a lichenoid drug eruption or photodermatitis.

Pathophysiology

The mechanism by which drugs predispose patients to a lichenoid reaction is uncertain. Drugs may alter the antigenicity of basal keratinocytes, or dysregulate the presentation of antigens to lymphocytes by Langerhans cells. In the case of

lichenoid photodermatitis, UV-induced apoptosis of keratinocytes may also play a role.

Acute Cutaneous Graft-Versus-Host Disease

Acute graft-versus-host disease is caused by foreign lymphocytes that have entered the host via transplanted tissue, usually bone marrow. Other transplanted organs or the transfusion of nonirradiated blood into immunocompromised hosts can also be causative. Disease caused by donor lymphocytes is referred to as *acute* when it occurs less than 60 days after transplantation and, arbitrarily, *chronic* thereafter. The histopathologic findings correlated with acute graft-versus-host disease are generally those described below, but many dermatopathologists who practice in medical centers in which bone marrow transplantation is a common procedure have realized that "acute" histopathologic changes can be seen even many months following transplantation in the clinical setting of chronic cutaneous graft-versus-host disease (see later).

Clinical Features

Early lesions of acute graft-versus-host disease are usually erythematous macules that may progress to confluence and involve much of the skin surface. Some early lesions are minute follicular papules that can simulate folliculitis. In severely affected patients, large, confluent areas of erythema develop that can vesiculate.[31]

Because of improved techniques for ridding donor marrow of lymphocytes, such as ricin-tagged, anti-T-cell–antibody treatment, severe acute cutaneous graft-versus-host disease is far less common than it was a decade ago.

Histopathologic Features

Like erythema multiforme, acute graft-versus-host disease is typified by a superficial perivascular lymphocytic infiltrate, vacuolar change at the dermoepidermal junction, and necrotic keratinocytes, individually and clustered, within the epidermis. Unlike the case in erythema multiforme, there is often parakeratosis or compact hyperkeratosis in fully evolved lesions (Fig. 5-16). In patients treated with chemotherapy and radiation before transplantation to rid them of a neoplasm and enable a graft to "take," there may be disorderly maturation and cytologic atypia of keratinocytes in the background.

In the most severe cases, but only rarely seen with current preparatory regimens, clefts may develop at the dermoepidermal junction and progress to vesiculation, and the entire epidermis may become necrotic and slough.

Satellite cell necrosis (i.e., the finding of a necrotic keratinocyte with closely apposed lymphocytes) is sometimes stated to be pathognomonic of acute graft-versus-host disease. Such is not the case because satellite cell necrosis can be seen in almost all conditions discussed in this chapter.

Clinicopathologic Correlation

In early erythematous macules, there is usually minimal vacuolar change and scattered necrotic keratinocytes. The cornified layer is unaffected, corresponding to the smooth surfaces that lesions have initially. By the time that macules become confluent, necrotic keratinocytes are numerous and may be aggregated in whorls similar to those seen in erythema multiforme and Mucha-Habermann disease. In fully developed lesions, the surface is scaly, reflecting hyper- and parakeratosis. Follicular epithelium is often involved, and can be the major site of involvement in small follicular papules.[32]

Differential Diagnosis

Patients who receive allogenic marrow transplants are usually induced with high doses of radiation and chemotherapeutic agents to rid them of residual hematopoietic cells. These agents may cause erythema, especially of the palms and soles. A biopsy specimen demonstrates vacuolization of the dermoepidermal junction, squamatization of the basal layer, and disorderly maturation of keratinocytes. These changes can usually be distinguished clinically from acute graft-versus-host disease because they are diffuse rather than circumscribed and a biopsy specimen contains far fewer lymphocytes. In a few days, the clinical and histologic changes diminish, whereas those of evolving acute graft-versus-host disease will increase in severity, both clinically and histologically.

Viral exanthems and drug eruptions frequently simulate graft-versus-host disease in transplant recipients. Although viral exanthems may have a vacuolar interface change, it is frequently subtle, and necrotic keratinocytes are few. Drug eruptions are a more frequent problem in histopathologic differential diagnosis. Clear-cut histologic criteria to separate drug-induced erythema multiforme in recipients of transplants from early evolving lesions of acute graft-versus-host disease in which the cornified layer has not yet become altered do not exist. Involvement of follicular epithelium is more common in graft-versus-host disease, but is seen in a minority of cases of erythema multiforme. Luckily, acute graft-versus-host disease and erythema multiforme usually have different clinical appearances.

As engraftment occurs in autologous bone marrow transplant patients, the increase in the number of lymphocytes is sometimes paralleled by their efflux into the skin, and erythematous macules result. This so-called eruption of lymphocyte recovery can be confused with acute graft-versus-host disease clinically and histologically. In some examples, the eruption of lymphocyte results in slight spongiosis, or lymphocytes that obscure the basal layer.[33] It may be impossible to distinguish between the eruption of lymphocyte recovery and an acute graft-versus-host reaction in an autologous marrow transplant patient, and indeed the two conditions may be identical.

Herpetic infections are more frequent in transplant recipients than in the immunocompetent population. Although lesions of herpes simplex or varicella-zoster with viral cytopathic changes are easily distinguished from acute graft-versus-host disease, some nonvesicular papules may show an interface reaction with necrotic keratinocytes. The infiltrate is usually denser and more band-like than that of acute graft-versus-host disease, and marked papillary dermal edema, sometimes simulating the edematous papular lesions of polymorphous light eruption, may be present. In such cases, level sections through the specimen may reveal herpetic nuclear changes or inclusions.

Pathophysiology

Many studies have clearly shown that acute graft-versus-host disease is caused by donor lymphocyte cytotoxicity to host epidermal cells. Various authors have postulated that basal keratinocytes, especially the mitotically active population situated at the bases of rete ridges, are the target of this reaction, although Langerhans cells and melanocytes are also damaged.[34] Follicular keratinocytes can also be targeted.[35] In satellite cell

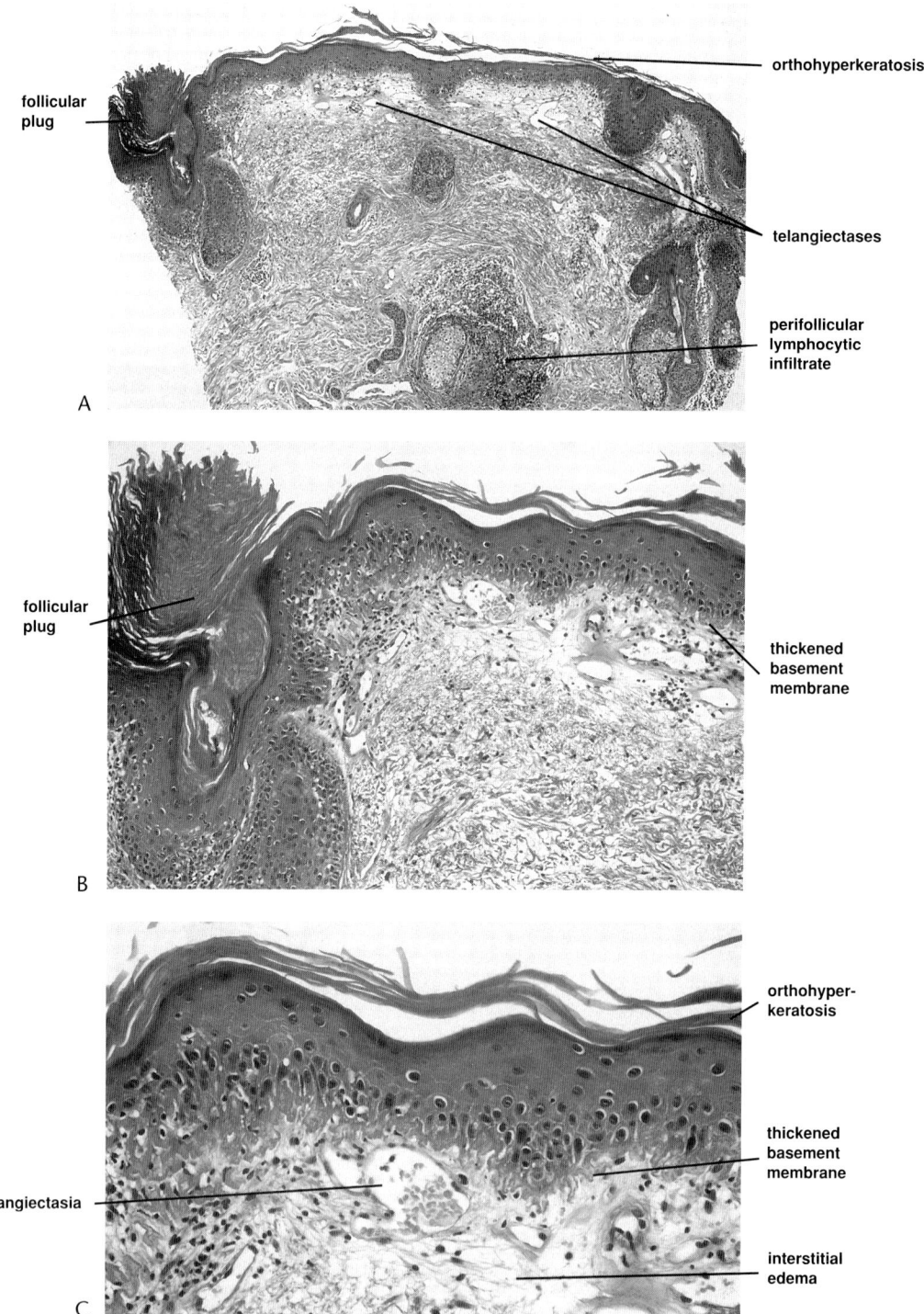

follicular plug

orthohyperkeratosis

telangiectases

perifollicular lymphocytic infiltrate

A

follicular plug

thickened basement membrane

B

orthohyper-keratosis

thickened basement membrane

telangiectasia

interstitial edema

C

Figure 5-19. Fully established lesion of discoid lupus erythematosus. **(A)** There are superficial and deep lymphocytic infiltrates that also surround a follicular unit. **(B)** Plugging of both acrotrychia (shown here) and acrosyringea is a hallmark of this condition. **(C)** Vacuolar change at the dermoepidermal junction is coupled with thickening of the epidermal basement membrane. (*Figure continues.*)

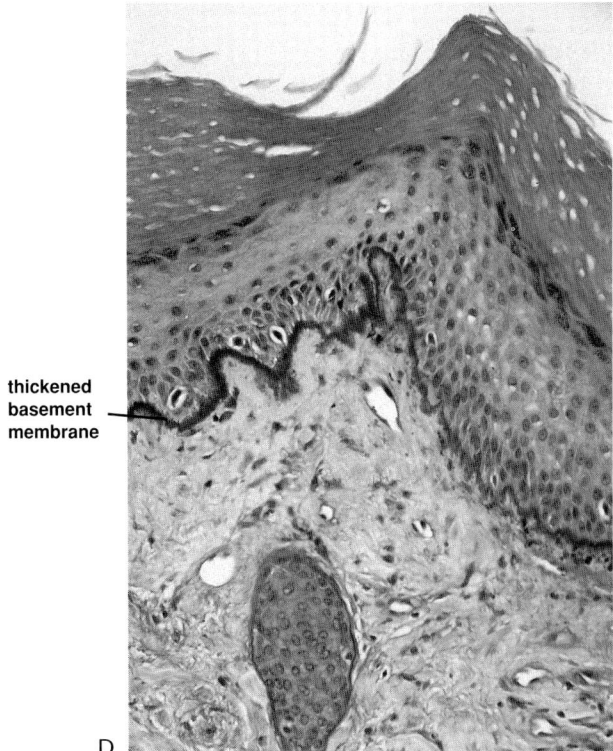

thickened
basement
membrane

D

Figure 5-19. *(Continued).* **(D)** Such change can be highlighted by staining with periodic acid–Schiff.

collagen that intervenes between elastotic material on sun-damaged skin and the epidermis is sometimes mistaken for a thick basement membrane. Necrotic keratinocytes, colloid bodies, and melanophages are found in discoid lupus erythematosus and are evidence of damage to the basal cell layer. Injury of the dermis also occurs in lupus erythematosus, as evidenced by fibrosis in long-standing lesions and connective tissue (acidic) mucin in both early and late lesions.

Lymphocytic infiltrates in both discoid and systemic lupus erythematosus are sometimes accompanied by fibrin thrombi within the lumens of venules or by fibrin deposition within venular walls. These changes indicate a true lymphocytic vasculitis rather than merely perivascular dermatitis, a supposition buttressed by the finding of the terminal components of the complement cascade C5–9 in the walls of venules. The role of lymphocytic vasculitis in the pathogenesis of lupus erythematosus is uncertain.[21]

The hair follicles are affected in discoid lupus erythematosus by vacuolar change at the junction between their epithelium and the perifollicular adventitial dermis and by altered cornification, producing compactly hyperkeratotic follicular plugs. Lesions of discoid lupus erythematosus on hair-bearing skin eventuate in permanent alopecia if they persist long enough because of destruction of the follicular epithelium and replacement of the follicles by vertically oriented fibroid tracts (Fig. 5-20).

In some lesions of discoid lupus erythematosus, the infiltrates extend into the subcutaneous fat, usually involving lobules rather than septa. Fully developed changes of lupus panniculitis can occur beneath typical lesions of discoid lupus erythemato-

sus. Lupus panniculitis features lobular infiltrates of lymphocytes and plasma cells, with foci in which adipocytes undergo necrosis and are replaced by sclerosis. Nuclear dust is often present in such foci. Lupus panniculitis, also known as *lupus profundus* is discussed in detail in Chapter 13.

Verrucous lesions of discoid lupus erythematosus show markedly irregular epidermal hyperplasia with a papillated surface along with marked, compact hyperkeratosis and plugging of follicular ostia (Fig. 5-21). There are patchy lichenoid infiltrates, dermal mucin, and focal thickening of the epidermal basement membrane along with colloid bodies. Elastotic fibers can be present within the hyperplastic epithelium of verrucous discoid lupus erythematosus, a finding also seen in wound-healing reactions involving sun-damaged skin and in keratoacanthoma.[38]

Lesions of chilblain lupus erythematosus have been described as resembling those of discoid lupus erythematosus histopathologically.[41] Such features as perifollicular infiltrates and plugging of acrotrychia cannot be evaluated on the volar skin of acral sites. Some lesions of chilblain lupus erythematosus show superficial and deep lymphocytic infiltrates with papillary dermal edema, as do ordinary chilblains.

The tumid lesions of lupus erythematosus are produced by dermal changes accompanied by only slight epidermal ones (Fig. 5-22). There is a superficial and deep lymphocytic infiltrate, abundant mucin between the collagen bundles of the reticular dermis, slight and focal vacuolar junctional change, and sometimes subtle hyperkeratosis.[42]

Acute erythematous lesions in patients with systemic lupus erythematosus have histologic changes that resemble those of early lesions of discoid lupus erythematosus. The infiltrates can be superficial, rather than superficial and deep, with vacuolar change at the junction and necrotic keratinocytes—in short, the changes can resemble those of erythema multiforme. However, there are usually some distinguishing features such as squamatization of the basal layer, nuclear dust immediately beneath the epidermis, and mucin in the reticular dermis.

Subacute cutaneous lupus erythematosus has histologic changes that resemble those seen in acute erythematous lesions, with superficial perivascular lymphocytes, dermal mucin, loss of normal rete ridge pattern, and slight thickening of the basement membrane (Fig. 5-23). Many necrotic keratinocytes can be present, along with numerous colloid bodies, especially at the edges of lesions.[43] Biopsy material from such an area may be indistinguishable from other forms of interface dermatitis with many necrotic keratinocytes. Findings seen in discoid lupus erythematosus such as plugging of adnexal orifices and epidermal basement membrane thickening, may only be evident in the centers of lesions, an exception to the rule that biopsy specimens should be obtained from the active periphery of lesions. In general, the predictive value of histopathology in differentiating between discoid and subacute cutaneous lupus erythematosus in individual cases is limited, as there is a considerable overlap.[44] Subtle changes similar to those seen in subacute cutaneous lesions characterize neonatal lupus erythematosus.

Bullous systemic lupus erythematosus is a blistering disorder that complicates the course of patients with systemic disease. It presents with subepidermal vesiculation and infiltrates in which neutrophils predominate. It is considered in detail in Chapter 11. The findings of nuclear dust beneath the junction

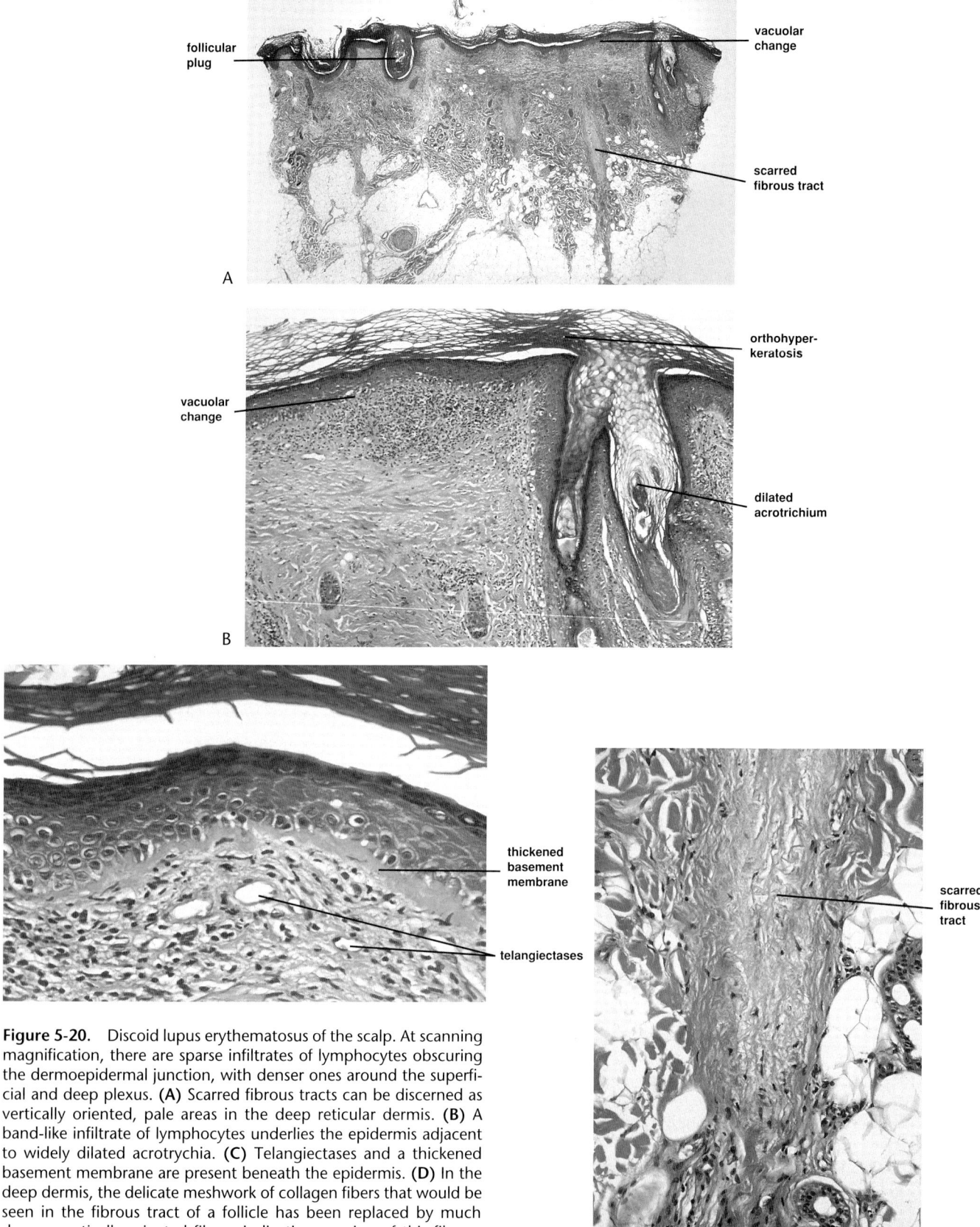

Figure 5-20. Discoid lupus erythematosus of the scalp. At scanning magnification, there are sparse infiltrates of lymphocytes obscuring the dermoepidermal junction, with denser ones around the superficial and deep plexus. **(A)** Scarred fibrous tracts can be discerned as vertically oriented, pale areas in the deep reticular dermis. **(B)** A band-like infiltrate of lymphocytes underlies the epidermis adjacent to widely dilated acrotrychia. **(C)** Telangiectases and a thickened basement membrane are present beneath the epidermis. **(D)** In the deep dermis, the delicate meshwork of collagen fibers that would be seen in the fibrous tract of a follicle has been replaced by much denser, vertically oriented fibers, indicating scarring of this fibrous tract.

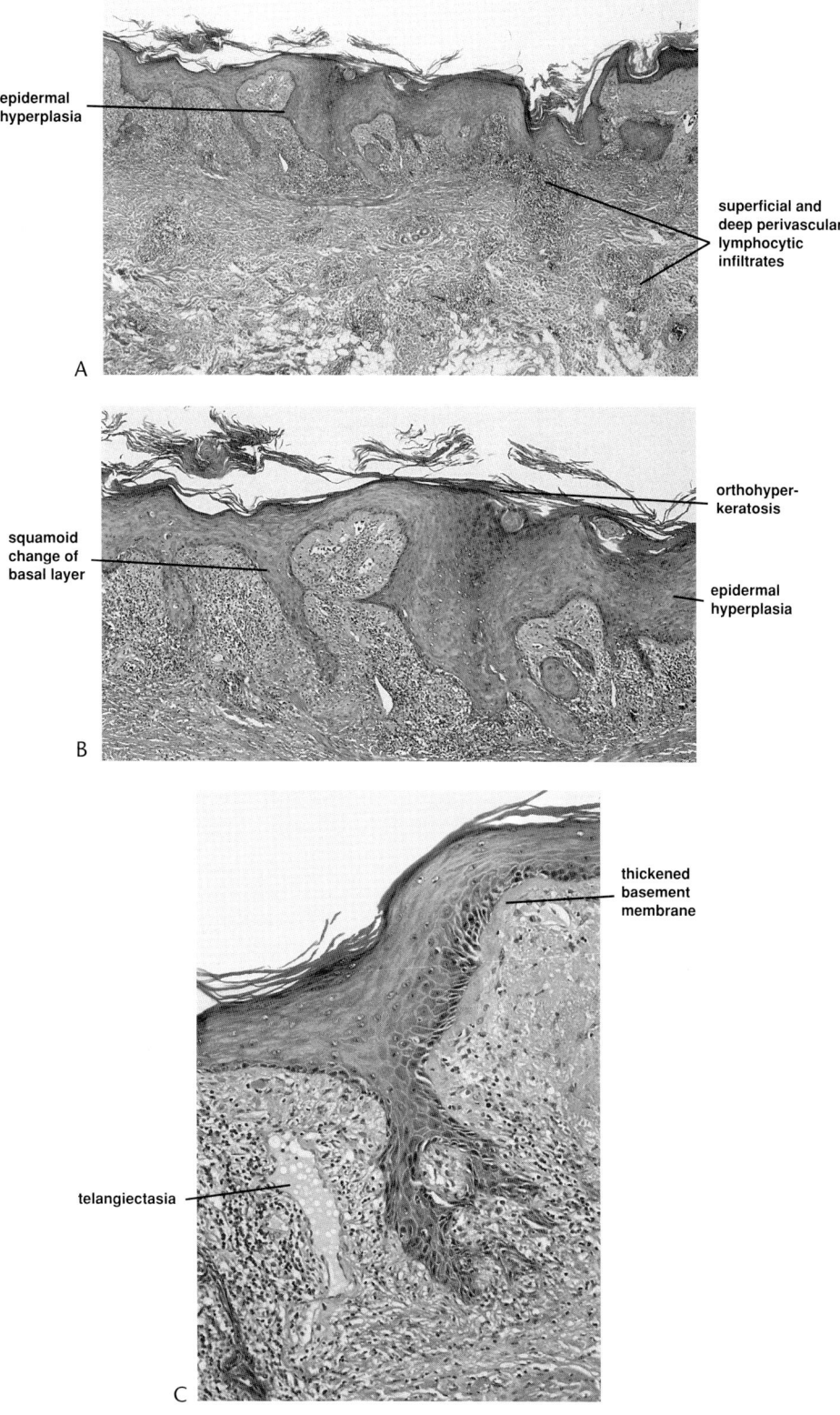

Figure 5-21. Verrucous lesion of discoid lupus erythematosus. An interface dermatitis with striking irregular epidermal hyperplasia can occur in this condition, in verrucous lichen planus, and in some lichenoid drug eruptions. **(A)** In verrucous discoid lupus erythematosus, the deep vascular plexus is usually involved. **(B)** Irregular hyperplasia of both epidermal and adnexal epithelium. **(C)** Telangiectases and a thickened epidermal basement membrane.

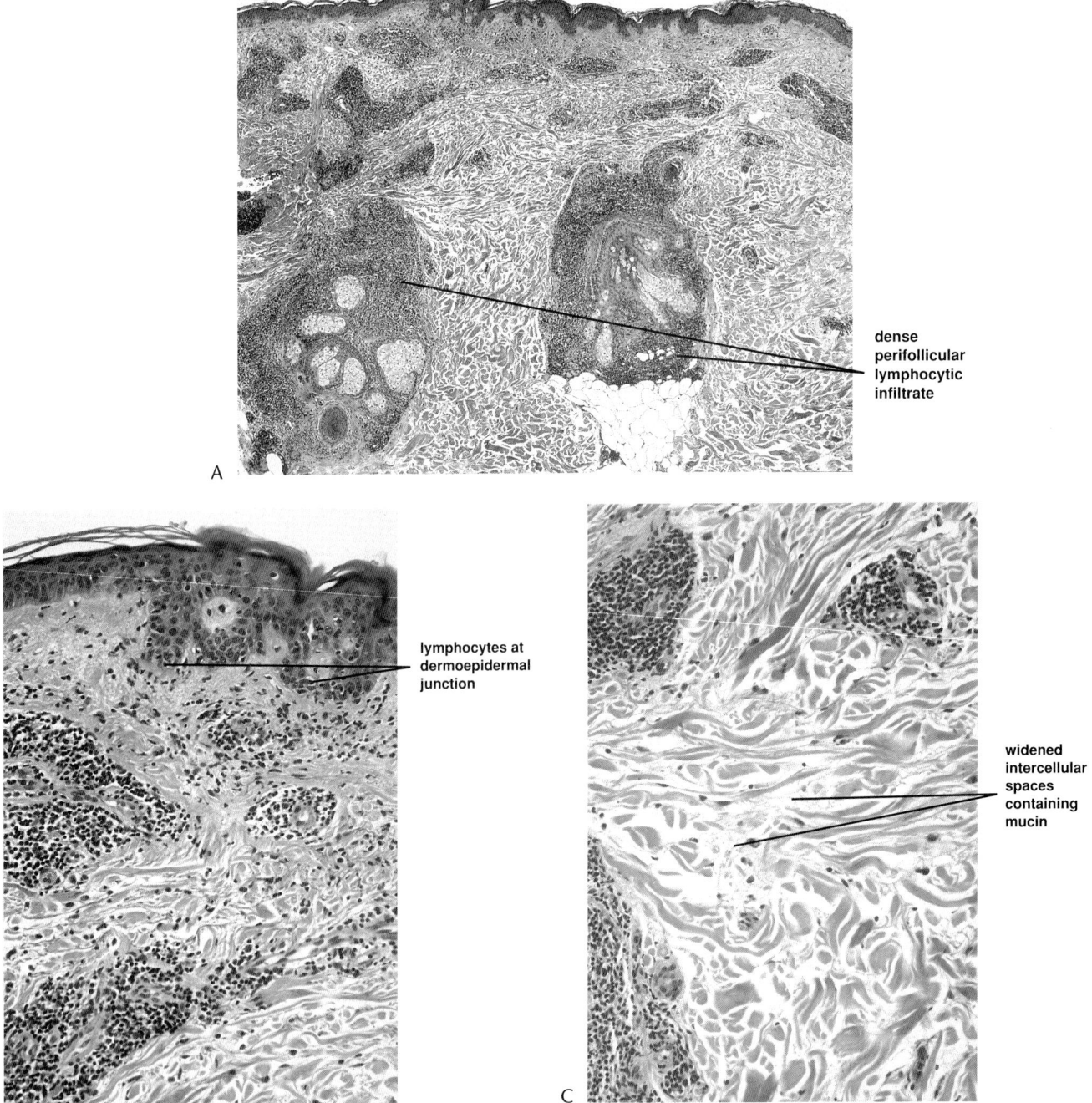

Figure 5-22. Epidermal changes are subtle or absent in tumid lesions of lupus erythematosus, although the dermal lymphocytic infiltrates of classic discoid lesions are present. (A) The infiltrates are densest around follicular epithelium. (B) Only a few lymphocytes are present at the junction. (C) Collagen fibers in the reticular dermis are separated by acid mucopolysaccharides, as in many other cutaneous manifestations of lupus erythematosus.

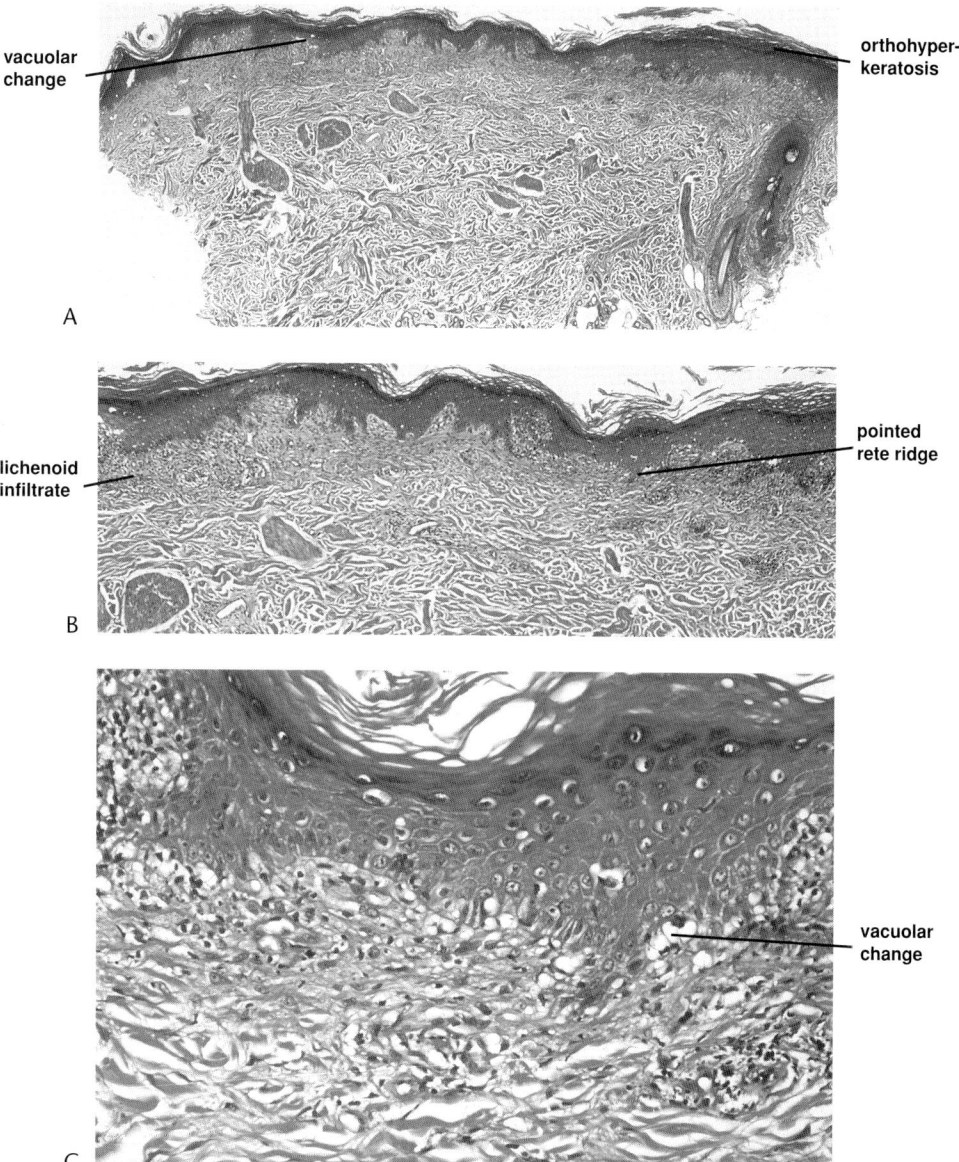

vacuolar change

orthohyper-keratosis

lichenoid infiltrate

pointed rete ridge

vacuolar change

A

B

C

Figure 5-23. In subacute cutaneous lupus erythematosus, the typical features of discoid lupus erythematosus are often present in a muted form. At scanning magnification, there is an interface reaction along with follicular plugging and hyperkeratosis. **(A)** Only slight involvement of the deep plexus is present in many cases. **(B)** Pointed rete ridges and hyperkeratosis are common findings. **(C)** Many cases of lupus erythematosus with lichenoid infiltrates have been reported as exemplifying the "lupus erythematosus–lichen planus overlap syndrome"; the absence of a thickened basement membrane makes this pattern of lupus erythematosus difficult to differentiate from other lichenoid interface reactions, unless there are perifollicular infiltrates, follicular plugging, or mucin in the reticular dermis.

in acute lesions of discoid lupus erythematosus and neutrophils beneath subepidermal vesicles in bullous systemic lupus erythematosus have been used to link the two conditions. Nonetheless, the claim that bullous systemic lupus erythematosus is an exaggeration of acute discoid lupus erythematosus seems improbable, as antibodies against type VII collagen appear to be of great pathogenetic importance in bullous systemic

lupus erythematosus, but are absent in the sera of patients with no systemic disease and only discoid lesions.

Differential Diagnosis

Fully developed lesions of discoid lupus erythematosus have no differential diagnosis–the combination of follicular plugging, epidermal thinning in some areas and irregular hyperplasia in others, telangiectases, marked basement membrane thickening, and a superficial and deep, perivascular and perifollicular lymphocytic infiltrate is not seen in any other disease. Early lesions of discoid lupus erythematosus may be indistinguishable from those of dermatomyositis. Most patients with the heliotrope eruption of dermatomyositis show only subtle smudging of the dermoepidermal junction, however, and not changes that simulate lupus erythematosus.

Several authors have discussed the difficulty of distinguishing lupus erythematosus from lichen planus histologically. Lesions of lupus erythematosus can have a band-like infiltrate and are referred to as *dense infiltrate lupus erythematosus* or *lichenoid lupus erythematosus*. Features that favor lupus erythematosus more than lichen planus include involvement of the deep plexus, dermal mucin deposition, basement membrane thickening, focal atrophy alongside hyperplasia of the epidermis, and follicular plugs with pointed bases. It seems likely that many cases of the so-called lupus erythematosus–lichen planus overlap syndrome, in which lesions of both conditions purportedly occur, are in fact examples of lichenoid lupus erythematosus. In cases in which the conditions cannot be distinguished by conventional histopathology, direct immunofluorescence can be helpful. Lesions of discoid lupus erythematosus that have been present for more than a few months generally have a band-like distribution of granular immunoglobulin(s) and complement, whereas those of lichen planus do not. Some important caveats are that facial skin sometimes has IgG along the junction in normal adults and that nonspecific trapping of immunoglobulin by colloid bodies is not diagnostic of lichen planus, as was once believed.

Tumid lesions of lupus erythematosus can be distinguished from those of polymorphous light eruption, a clinical as well as a histologic simulant, by the presence of mucin in the dermis and vacuolization at the dermoepidermal junction in lupus erythematosus and papillary dermal edema and, rarely, spongiosis in polymorphic light eruption. Some lesions of urticarial drug eruptions and reactions to insect bites also contain superficial and deep infiltrates of lymphocytes, but usually eosinophils are present, the infiltrates are not densest around follicles as they are in tumid lupus erythematosus, and vacuolar change is absent. Patients with either systemic or discoid lupus erythematosus can also develop papules and nodules due to interstitial mucin deposition without lymphocytic infiltrates or accompanied by very sparse ones.[45,46] The dividing line between this variant and tumid lupus erythematosus is unclear at this time.

The question of how to regard superficial and deep perivascular lymphocytic infiltrates that spare the epidermis or cause slight vacuolar change and are accompanied by interstitial dermal mucin deposition is controversial. Some authors consider the conditions described as lymphocytic infiltrate of Jessner and reticular erythematous mucinosis to be variants of lupus erythematosus rather than independent entities. Recent studies have documented cases with superficial and deep dermal perivascular lymphocytic infiltrates, sometimes accompanied by mucin, in patients who do not develop evidence of lupus erythematosus or polymorphous light eruption even when followed for decades.[47] The infiltrates of T cells reportedly differ immunophenotypically from those of lupus erythematosus. In lymphocytic infiltrate of Jessner, the epidermis is usually unaffected as opposed to subtle vacuolar change in tumid lupus erythematosus.

Direct immunofluorescence is often helpful when the diagnosis of lupus erythematosus is in doubt. In more than 90% of lesions of discoid lupus erythematosus that are more than 6 weeks old, positive results are seen with antisera to IgG and C3 and less often with antiserum to IgM or IgA.[48] An important caveat in the interpretation of the results of direct immunofluorescence is that the skin of the face of young adults often has a subepidermal band of IgG. Although at one time many believed that direct immunofluorescence of lesional skin in dermatomyositis did not demonstrate immune reactants, it is clear that there can be similar changes to those seen in lupus erythematosus, and that this test should not be used to tell the two conditions apart. Because patients with systemic lupus erythematosus can have deposition of immunoglobulin and complement beneath the dermoepidermal junction of their entire integument, direct immunofluorescence cannot be used to tell whether a skin lesion in such a patient is due to lupus erythematosus or to another cause.

Clinicopathologic Correlation

Fully developed discoid lesions of lupus erythematosus provide a wealth of correlation between clinical and pathologic findings. The erythema that rings the lesions is produced by a perivascular lymphocytic infiltrate and ectatic vessels. The atrophic centers result from thinning of the epidermis effacement of rete and fibrosis of the dermis. Depigmentation corresponds histologically to melanophages in the papillary dermis that contains clinically visible telangiectatic vessels. The carpet-tack keratinous plugs in the center of lesions are produced by compact keratin in the orifices of hair follicles and sweat ducts. Tumid lesions are smooth surfaced, corresponding to the absence of epidermal changes seen histologically. Subacute cutaneous lupus erythematosus is scaly clinically, reflecting hyperkeratosis, but does not usually demonstrate the other findings seen in fully developed discoid lesions.

Pathophysiology

Discoid lupus erythematosus is produced by the effects of cell-mediated immunity (interface dermatitis) as well as immune complex deposition (basement membrane thickening). The propensity of lesions of discoid lupus erythematosus to occur in sun-exposed skin could be related to UV-induced damage to keratinocyte DNA, resulting in the generation of antinuclear antibodies.[2] DNA is a component of the subepidermal material. Some changes, such as dermal mucinosis, cannot be satisfactorily explained at the current time.

The epidermal changes in discoid lupus erythematosus have been studied with immunohistochemistry, with results that suggest increased proliferation of keratinocytes, with premature terminal differentiation. Premature terminal differentiation is indicated by the expression of involucrin by keratinocytes in the middle and lower spinous layers and by fillagrin in the granular and superficial spinous layers. In the case of both substances, expression is normally found at higher levels of the epidermis. Keratin 16, a species found in the hyperproliferative epidermis of psoriasis, is also found in the epidermis in discoid lupus erythematosus.[49]

Dermatomyositis and Mixed Connective Tissue Disease

Dermatomyositis is an autoimmune disease in which skeletal muscle becomes inflamed and is often accompanied by a cutaneous eruption. In mixed connective tissue disease, signs of both lupus erythematosus and scleroderma may occur. Dermatomyositis can begin at any age, but its onset in adults warrants a search for an underlying malignancy.

Clinical Features

The cutaneous eruption of dermatomyositis has been likened in hue to a flower, the heliotrope. It appears as purple-red discoloration of the eyelids. Another specific manifestation is Gottron sign, papules that are boggy, erythematous, and slightly scaly papules that occur mainly on the knuckles but may involve the exterior surface of other joints. In mixed connective tissue disease, lesions that resemble discoid or systemic lupus erythematosus or scleroderma can occur.

Histopathologic Features

The heliotrope eruption in dermatomyositis has subtle features, with "smudging" of the junctional zone and only rare necrotic keratinocytes. Usually only a few lymphocytes are seen, either around superficial vessels or at the dermoepidermal junction. Mucin may be present in the dermis.

Erythematous, scaling lesions of dermatomyositis may resemble early lesions of discoid lupus erythematosus, but seldom show more than slight thickening of the basement membrane or follicular plugging (Fig. 5-24).

Gottron sign is characterized by sparse superficial perivascular lymphocytic infiltrates, an accumulation of mucin in the superficial dermis, and papillated epidermal hyperplasia (Fig. 5-25). Vacuolar change and basement membrane thickening may be present.[50]

Clinicopathologic Correlation

The heliotrope rash of dermatomyositis is in part due to edema of the dermis, vasodilation, and thinning of the epidermis. Gottron papules derive their appearance from sclerosis of the papillary dermis, papillated epidermal hyperplasia, and hyperkeratosis. The poikilodermatous lesions result from epidermal atrophy, telangiectasia, and the deposition of melanophages.

Differential Diagnosis

Acute lesions of discoid or systemic lupus erythematosus usually demonstrate more necrotic keratinocytes and greater vacuolization than the subtle changes seen in dermatomyositis. Gottron papules can be distinguished from an unrelated entity,

knuckle pads, which are formed by accumulations of fibrous tissue in the dermis and are analogous to superficial fibromatoses at other sites, such as palmoplantar fibromatosis and Peyronie's disease.

Pathophysiology

The cutaneous changes of dermatomyositis appear to be due to mechanisms similar to those at play in lupus erythematosus, namely, a combination of cell-mediated cytotoxicity resulting in necrosis of keratinocytes, with a likely role for autoantibodies reactive to keratinocyte antigens as a co-factor. There have been conflicting studies regarding the prevalence of immune complex deposition in dermatomyositis, but some studies have found a variety of patterns of deposition of antibody and complement, including a granular pattern along the dermoepidermal junction similar to that seen in lupus erythematosus. Damage to superficial vessels by complement may also be important.[51] Close scrutiny of these vessels shows a decrease in their number, necrosis of endothelial cells, and fibrin deposition in their walls. The injury to muscle fibers in dermatomyositis is mediated in part by deposition of the terminal components of the complement cascade (C5–9) in capillaries. Patients with dermatomyositis can have a variety of autoantibodies, the presence of which can indicate a propensity to a specific constellation of disease manifestations.

Other Conditions Featuring Interface Dermatitis with Premature Terminal Differentiation

The most commonly biopsied condition in which there is an interface reaction similar to that seen in lichen planus and related conditions is *lichenoid keratosis,* also known as *lichen planus–like keratosis.* This condition is discussed more fully in the last section of this chapter.

Although lichen striatus is listed in the next section, because specimens of it frequently show psoriasiform epidermal hyperplasia in conjunction with an interface reaction, the condition can have epidermal changes essentially indistinguishable from those of lichen planus.[52]

Keratosis lichenoides chronica is the name now used for a rare and controversial entity that clinically has linear, hyperkeratotic papules often arranged in an intersecting pattern, along with what has been described as a seborrheic dermatitis–like involvement of facial skin. The histopathologic descriptions of the condition vary from report to report, reflecting in part the heterogeneous conditions that these patients had. Irregular epidermal hyperplasia with band-like infiltrates of lymphocytes that sometimes contain plasma cells and columns of parakeratotic cells containing neutrophils are some of the features that deviate from those of authentic lichen planus.[53]

Lichenoid reactions to evolving squamous cell carcinoma in situ of the lip (unfortunately termed *actinic chelitis*) can resemble lichen planus of the lip. Keratinocytes with atypical nuclei and parakeratosis are features that exemplify labial lichenoid solar keratosis, but occasional cases can have wedge-shaped hypergranulosis and mostly orthokeratosis.

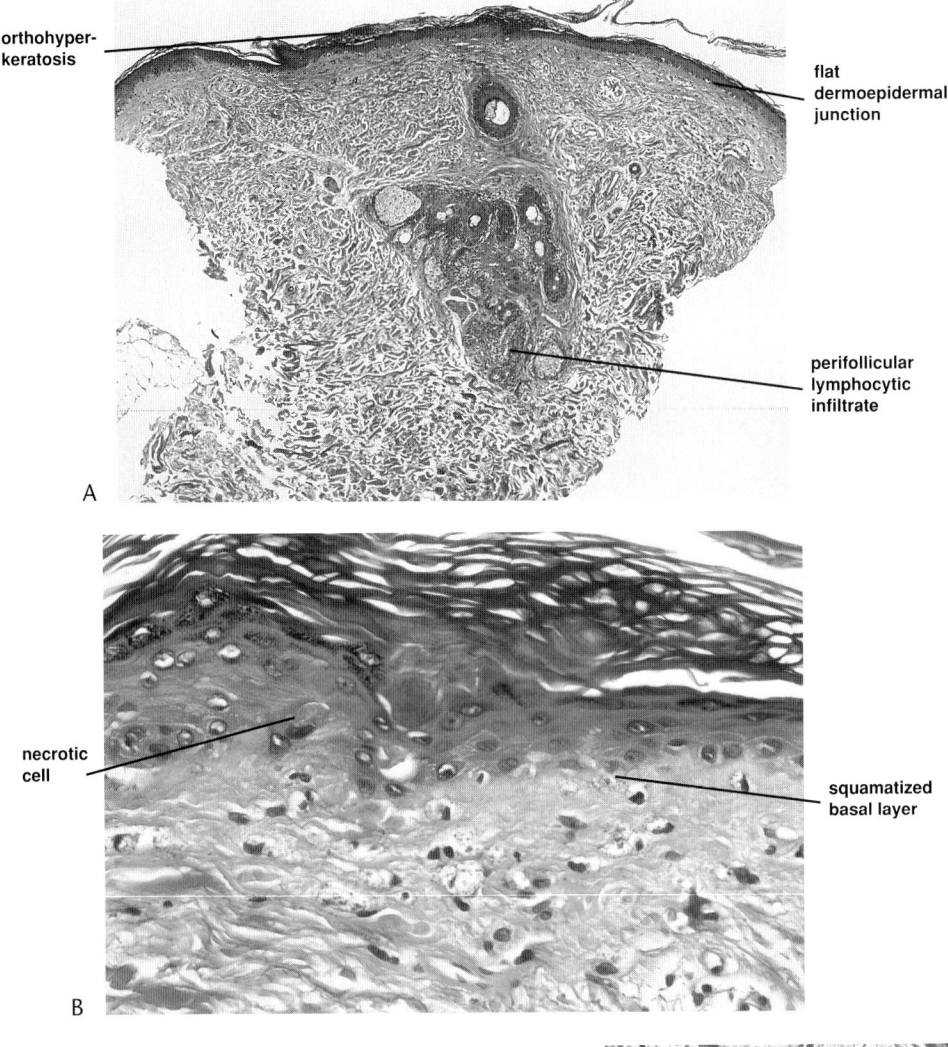

orthohyper-
keratosis

flat
dermoepidermal
junction

perifollicular
lymphocytic
infiltrate

A

necrotic
cell

squamatized
basal layer

B

interstitial
mucin

C

Figure 5-24. A scaly lesion of dermatomyositis. **(A)** At scanning magnification, the epidermis is thinned with loss of the normal rete ridge pattern, and there is slight hyperkeratosis. **(B)** The dermoepidermal junction is "smudged," there is squamatization of basilar keratinocytes, and rare necrotic keratinocytes are present. Note a thickened granular and a compact cornified layer, evidence of premature terminal differentiation of epidermal keratinocytes. **(C)** Collagen bundles in the dermis are widely splayed by acidic mucopolysaccharides, which are out of proportion to the scant lymphocytic infiltrate.

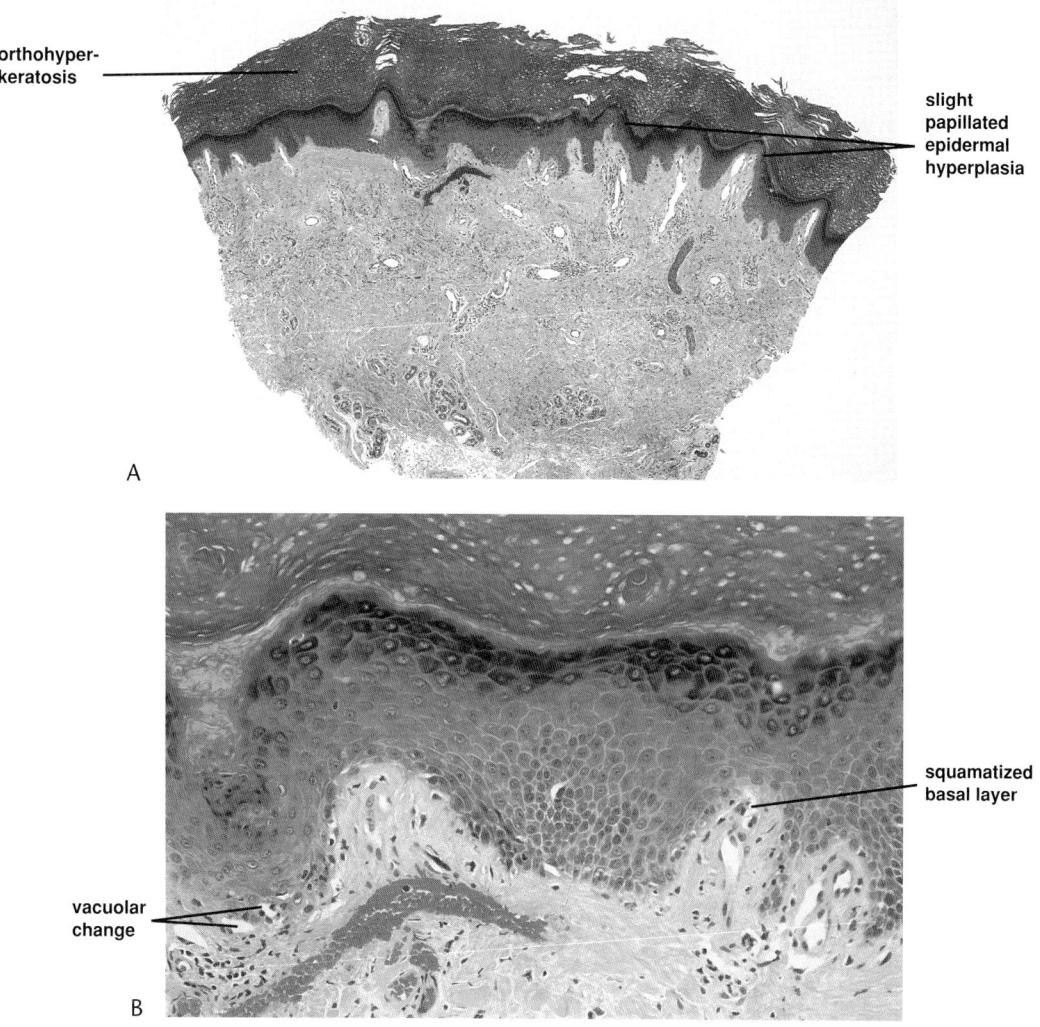

orthohyper-
keratosis

slight
papillated
epidermal
hyperplasia

A

squamatized
basal layer

vacuolar
change

B

Figure 5-25. Gottron papule of dermatomyositis. **(A)** Papillated epidermal hyperplasia and hyperkeratosis coupled with the subtle changes seen in other manifestations of dermatomyositis. **(B)** These can include "smudging" of the junctional zone (seen at left) with squamatization of the basal layer and rare necrotic keratinocytes, as well as mucin deposition in the reticular dermis (not shown here).

INTERFACE DERMATITIS WITH PSORIASIFORM EPIDERMAL HYPERPLASIA

Lichenoid Variants of Persistent Pigmented Purpuric Dermatitis

In persistent pigmented purpuric dermatitis, infiltrates of lymphocytes mediate the extravasation of erythrocytes into the dermis, leading to purpuric lesions. Lichenoid purpura comprises those variants in which there is a band-like lymphocytic infiltrate, resulting in flat-topped papules.

Clinical Features

There are many variants of persistent, pigmented purpuric dermatitis. The two that have band-like infiltrates are the lichenoid purpura of Gougerot and Blum and lichen aureus. The lesions of

lichenoid purpura are in most patients multiple and on the legs but can, albeit rarely, occur above the waist. Those of lichen aureus may be single and are often on the thigh. The cause of either is unknown, but lichen aureus has been attributed to incompetence of perforator veins. Histologically, the two conditions cannot be differentiated, and they can be considered to be part of a spectrum of conditions (Schamberg disease, purpura telangiectoides of Majocchi, and eczematid-like purpura of Doukas and Kapenetakis being the others) in which lymphocytic infiltrates cause venules to leak.

Histopathologic Features

In early lesions of lichenoid purpura, there are perivascular and interstitial infiltrates of lymphocytes, a few of which ascend to the dermoepidermal junction, where they induce slight vacuolar change. The lymphocytic infiltrates in lichenoid purpura quickly become dense and band-like in configuration. Extravasated erythrocytes appear in the papillary dermis, followed within days to a week or two by siderophages. Siderophages are macrophages that have ingested erythrocytes whose hemoglobin has been altered. Siderophages have coarse, golden brown pigment that is often refractile when the condenser of a microscope is lowered. They can have a dendritic appearance and stain with the Prussian blue method or with Perls stain.

Siderophages are often present deep to the band-like infiltrates in lichenoid purpura.

The rete ridges in lichenoid purpura are often slender and elongated, with rounded bases (Fig. 5-26). In long-standing lesions, especially of lichen aureus, many rete disappear and the epidermis has an atrophic appearance. Many lymphocytes can be present in the basal layer of the epidermis in these atrophic lesions. This finding can be coupled with fibrosis of the papil-

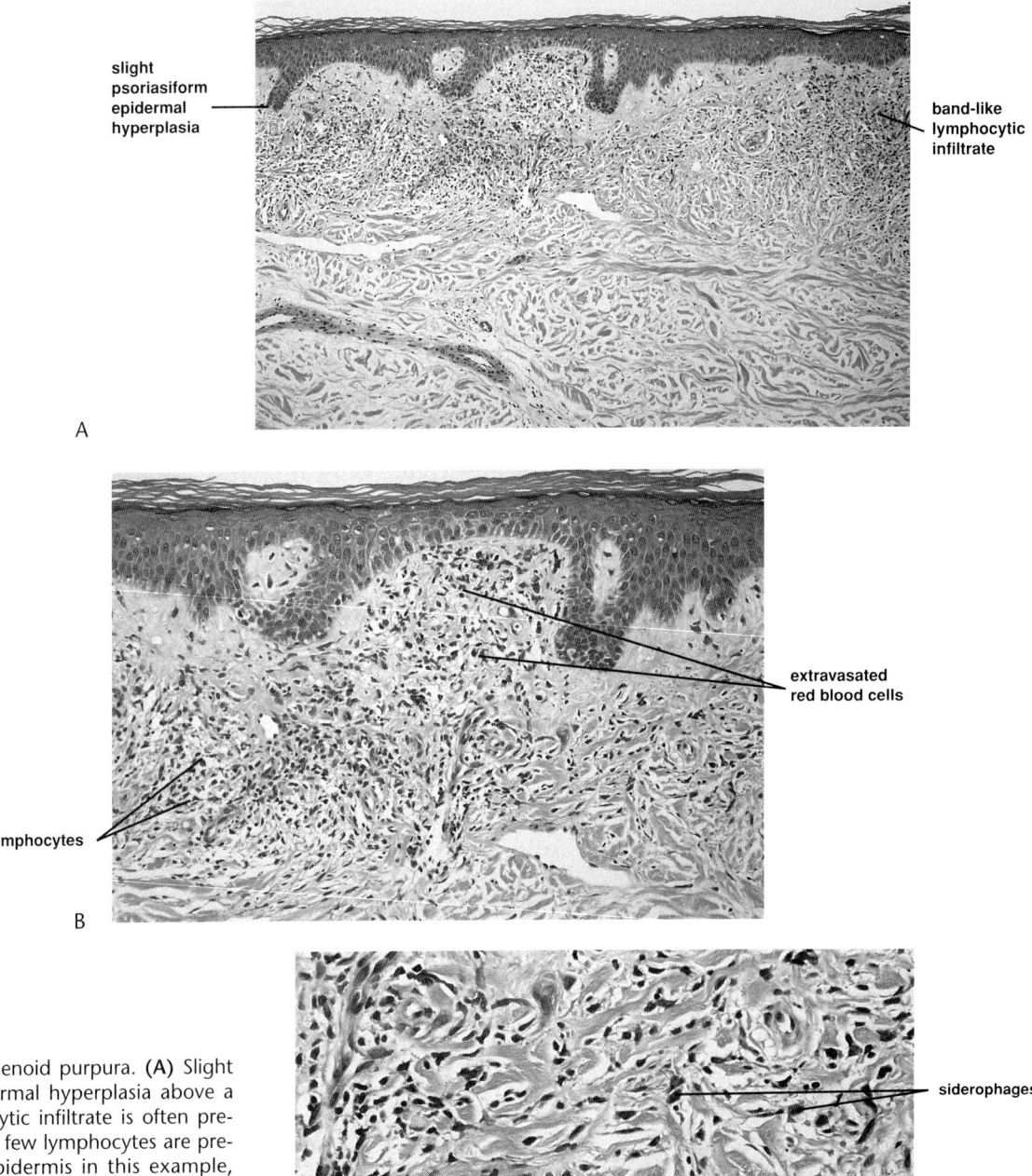

slight
psoriasiform
epidermal
hyperplasia

band-like
lymphocytic
infiltrate

A

extravasated
red blood cells

lymphocytes

B

siderophages

C

Figure 5-26. Lichenoid purpura. **(A)** Slight psoriasiform epidermal hyperplasia above a band-like lymphocytic infiltrate is often present. **(B)** Although few lymphocytes are present within the epidermis in this example, there are many extravasated erythrocytes in the papillary dermis. **(C)** Siderophages are often spindly and can be found deep to lichenoid infiltrates, in contrast to melanophages, which are more superficial. If there is any doubt, the nature of pigmented macrophages can be resolved by Perls and Fontana stains.

lary dermis, resulting in a resemblance to the atrophic patch stage of mycosis fungoides.

Clinicopathologic Correlation

There are many extravasated erythrocytes in lichenoid purpura of Gougerot and Blum, resulting in its purpuric appearance, and more siderophages in lichen aureus but fewer extravasated erythrocytes, resulting in its golden brown color.

Differential Diagnosis

Scant siderophages are sometimes seen in lesions of lichen planus situated on the skin of the legs because of extravasation of erythrocytes due to venous stasis. The two conditions can be easily distinguished in most cases. The rete ridges in lichen planus are pointed, while those in lichenoid purpura are rounded. Many necrotic keratinocytes and perforce colloid bodies are present in lichen planus, whereas few occur in lichenoid purpura. Wedge-shaped hyperkeratosis, emblematic of lichen planus, is not prominent in lichenoid purpura.

Mycosis fungoides often has a psoriasiform lichenoid pattern in which lymphocytes predominate in its patch stage, as do lesions of lichenoid purpura. A curious relationship may exist between lichenoid purpura and mycosis fungoides. The first reported North American case of lichen aureus was discovered in a patient who later developed mycosis fungoides. Several patients with mycosis fungoides have had clinical presentations that simulated persistent pigmented purpuric dermatitis.[54] In many cases of lichenoid purpura, a few lymphocytes are present in the basal layer of the epidermis without much spongiosis, mimicking patch stage mycosis fungoides. If there are lymphocytes with marked nuclear atypia, the diagnosis is mycosis fungoides and not lichenoid purpura. Without that finding, lichenoid purpura tends to have papillary dermal edema rather than fibrosis, and erythrocytes are frequently extravasated into both papillary dermis and epidermis. Some patients seemingly have both conditions (Fig. 5-27). The finding of T-cell–receptor gene rearrangements in lichenoid purpura limits the use of that technique in this differential diagnosis.[55]

Pathophysiology

Lichenoid purpura is clearly, at least in part, a T-cell–mediated process rather than simply the result of the extravasation of erythrocytes.[56] The mechanism by which T cells mediate the efflux of erythrocytes from venules without causing extensive damage to their walls is unclear. Complement has been found in the walls of venules but whether it is of pathogenetic importance or secondarily deposited following cell-mediated damage to vessel walls is not clear.

Secondary Syphilis

Syphilis is a sexually or transplacentally transmitted disease caused by the spirochete *Treponema pallidum*. Secondary syphilis develops weeks to months after infection and represents a reaction to organisms disseminated hematogenously to distant sites. Tertiary syphillis occurs years later and has significant central nervous system and cardiovascular manifestations.

Clinical Features

Cutaneous lesions of secondary syphilis may occur 6 weeks to 6 months after the appearance of a chancre, the ulcer that is the hallmark of primary syphilis. A variety of lesions including macules, papules, follicular papules, plaques, nodules, and condylomata may be seen. Lesions may be smooth, hyperkeratotic, or pustular.

Secondary lesions of syphilis usually resolve spontaneously in several weeks, but relapse, and sometimes multiple relapses because of persistent infection in inadequately treated patients, can occur. Pigmentary alteration and loss of dermal elastic tissue that results in atrophy are possible residua.

Histopathologic Features

Early lesions of secondary syphilis may demonstrate only superficial, or superficial and deep, perivascular lymphocytes and plasma cells, with only negligible epidermal changes. Rarely, plasma cells are absent from early macular lesions.[57,58]

Fully developed lesions of secondary lues usually show superficial and deep plexuses surrounded by lymphocytes, histiocytes, and plasma cells, in addition to a band-like infiltrate of macrophages, plasma cells, and lymphocytes at the dermoepidermal junction (Fig. 5-28). It is worth emphasizing that the infiltrates of secondary syphilis often have a pallid appearance at scanning magnification owing to the abundant pale cytoplasms of plasma cells and to the presence of many histiocytes. Psoriasiform hyperplasia of the epidermis frequently overlies these changes, and a few lymphocytes often obscure the junction.[59] Necrotic keratinocytes are rarely present in number. In lesions with many spirochetes, there are foci of keratinocytes with pale cytoplasms interlaced with neutrophils that form spongiform pustules similar to those of psoriasis.[60] Such foci are among the most fruitful to examine when searching for organisms on silver stain. Neutrophils may be present in zones of parakeratosis in crusted lesions. Although occasional cases of secondary syphilis show extensive vacuolization of the junctional zone and numerous necrotic keratinocytes, most have rounded rate ridges that are sometimes infiltrated by a few lymphocytes. A rare variant demonstrates a dermal neutrophilic infiltrate that can easily be mistaken for that of Sweet syndrome.[61]

The spirochetes of syphilis are demonstrable by a variety of silver stains, including Warthin-Starry silver, Steiner, and Levaditi stains. These stains take considerable technical skill to perform well, requiring clean (preferably acid-washed) glassware and controlling the pH of reagents. Laboratories in which these stains are performed rarely, or with inappropriate control tissues, should consider referring sections to a more proficient laboratory for staining. Immunoperoxidase stains for *T. pallidum* are not commercially available at the time of writing, but are more sensitive than traditional methods. The spirochetes have a helical structure, are roughly equal in length, and are found within foci of epidermal pallor with neutrophilic infiltrates as alluded to above, in the papillary dermis, and around venules in both the superficial and deep dermis.

Many dermatopathology textbooks advocate endothelial swelling and hyperplasia as major criteria of secondary syphilis. Unless truly striking, endothelial swelling is not a feature that

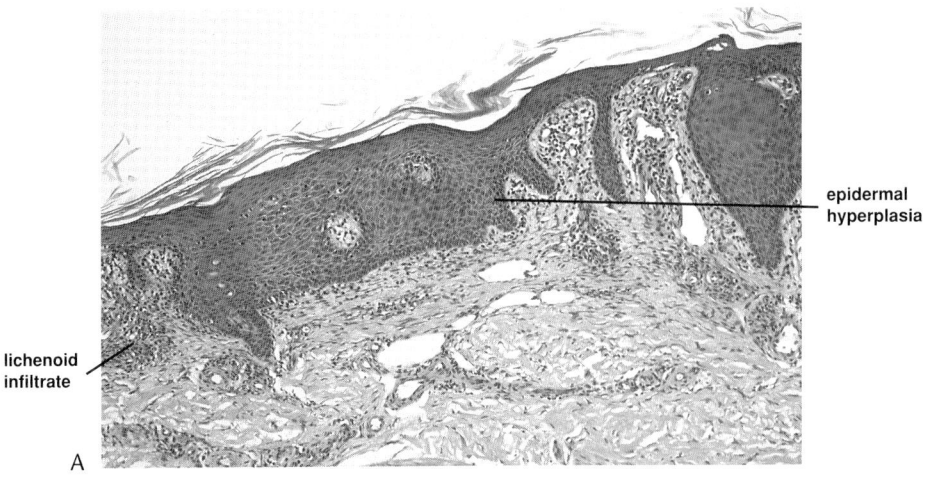

epidermal
hyperplasia

lichenoid
infiltrate

A

Figure 5-27. The differential diagnosis between lichenoid purpura and mycosis fungoides can be extraordinarily difficult, and some patients seem to have both conditions. **(A)** The patient had lesions of conventional mycosis fungoides as well as purpuric lesions such as this one, in which a psoriasiform, lichenoid pattern is present. **(B)** Lymphocytes scattered in the middle and upper spinous zones with enlarged nuclei. **(C)** Subjacent to the epidermis are many spindled siderophages.

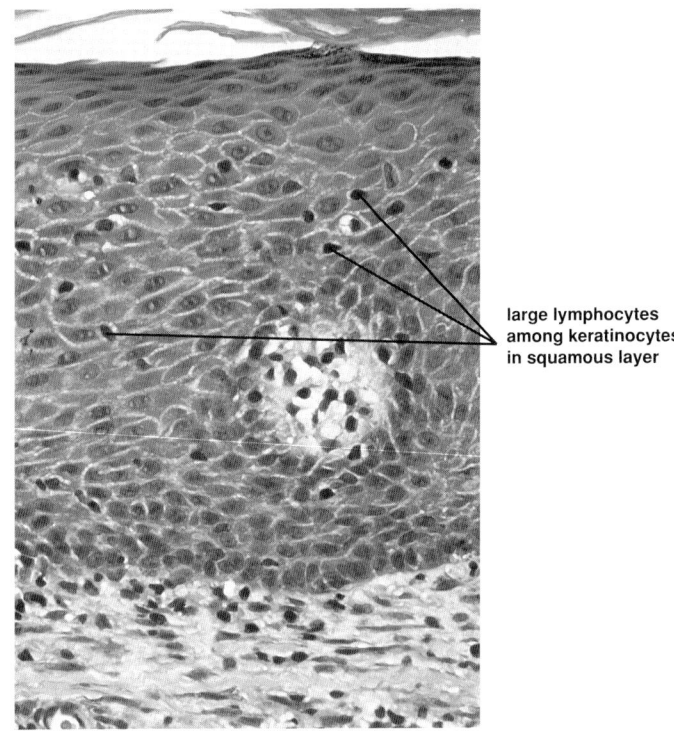

large lymphocytes
among keratinocytes
in squamous layer

B

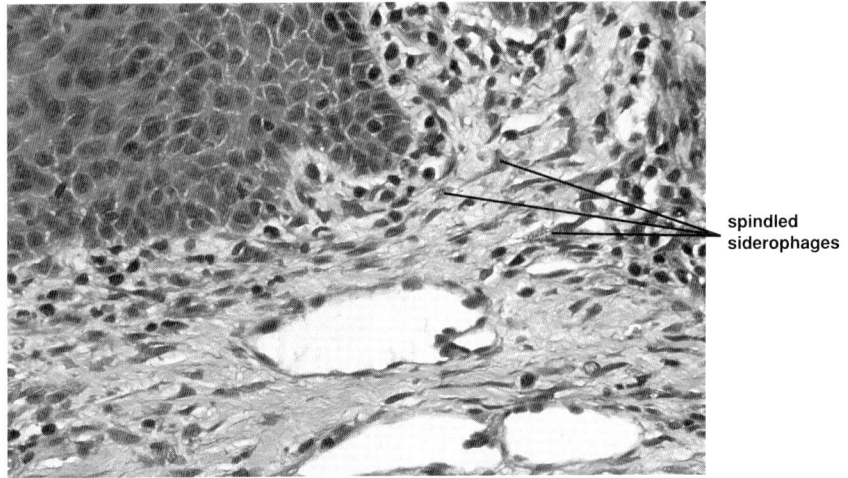

spindled
siderophages

C

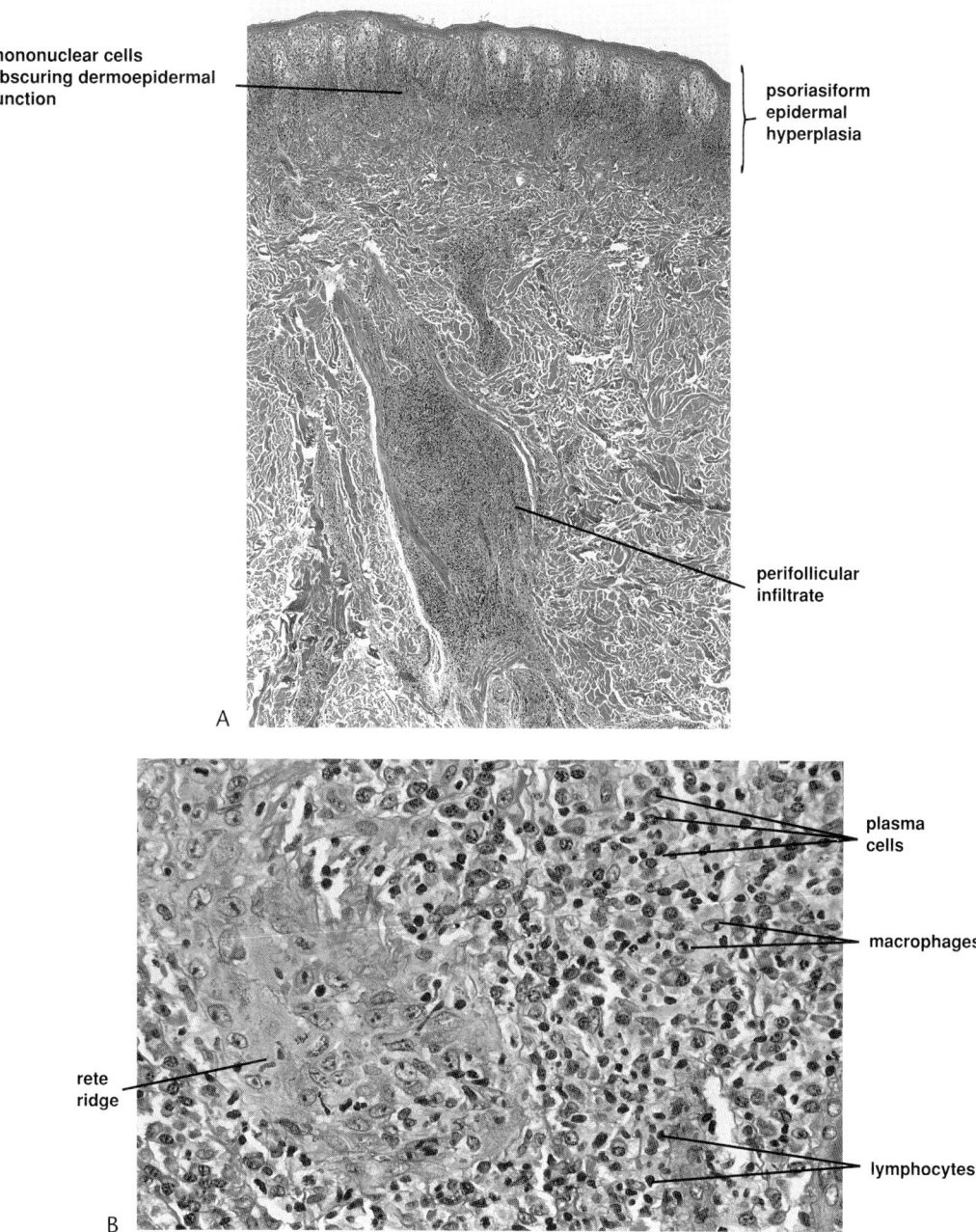

Figure 5-28. **(A)** Lesions of secondary lues are often an interface dermatitis with superficial and deep infiltrates and psoriasiform epidermal hyperplasia. **(B)** Plasma cells are stereotypically present, but there are frequently many macrophages.

strongly favors syphilis, because many other densely cellular inflammatory processes demonstrate it also.

Some lesions of secondary syphilis may develop small or moderately large granulomata over the course of weeks or months. Lesions in which granulomatous inflammation dominates characterize tertiary rather than secondary syphilis. Another change that can occur as secondary lesions age is atrophy of the epidermis.

Condyloma lata are not generally manifestations of interface dermatitis but are included herein for the sake of a complete rendering of the histopathology of secondary syphilis. They appear histologically as papillated epidermal or mucosal epithelial hyperplasia in association with a dense perivascular infiltrate of plasma cells, lymphocytes, and histiocytes (Fig. 5-29). There are usually large numbers of organisms in condyloma lata on silver stain, and foci of epithelial pallor that contain many neutrophils are frequent.

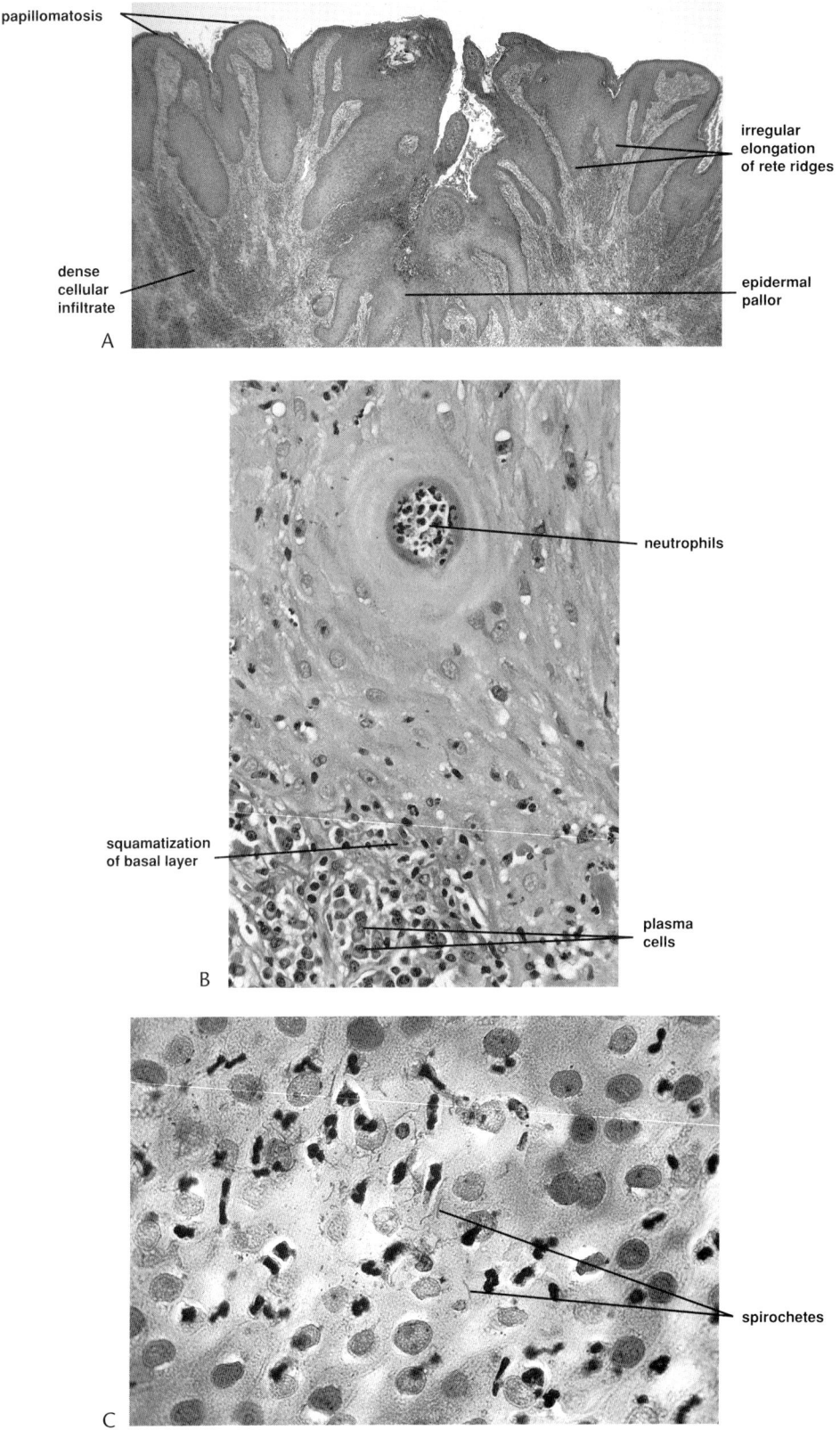

Figure 5-29. **(A)** Condyloma lata are a manifestaton of secondary syphilis resulting from verrucous epithelial hyperplasia at mucosal or juxtamucosal sites. **(B)** The epidermis is pallid in some foci, which often contain neutrophils. **(C)** Spirochetes are evident in this section with Warthin-Starry stain as thin, helical structures.

Differential Diagnosis

The combination of psoriasiform epidermal hyperplasia and superficial and deep lichenoid infiltrates rich in plasma cells and macrophages is essentially pathognomonic of syphilis. Mycosis fungoides may show a nearly identical pattern on low magnification but usually can be distinguished by more numerous intraepidermal lymphocytes and only a few plasma cells. Rare cases of secondary syphilis do contain immunoblasts and can pose a histopathologic problem in their distinction from plaque stage mycosis fungoides.

Lichenoid drug eruptions may have plasma cells in a dense band-like infiltrate with only a few lymphocytes. Occasionally, the deep plexus is involved, which heightens the similarities.

Pityriasis lichenoides et varioliformis acuta shares a superficial and deep lichenoid pattern with secondary syphilis. The lesions of pityriasis lichenoides also can exhibit slight psoriasiform epidermal hyperplasia and scale-crusts containing neutrophils. They lack, however, such features as pallor of the epidermis and significant numbers of either macrophages or plasma cells.[60]

Plaques of mycosis fungoides also can have infiltrates distributed in a pattern similar to those of secondary lues. Some lesions can also have plasma cells, granulomatous foci (so-called granulomatous mycosis fungoides), or both. The lymphocytes in secondary lues seldom infiltrate the epidermis in more than a tentative fashion, and the number of plasma cells in mycosis fungoides is far fewer than in lues.

Acrodermatitis chronica atrophicans (ACA) is a chronic, atrophic condition due to infection with the spirochete *Borrelia burgdorferi*. Although fully developed cases are typified by striking epidermal atrophy, the early stages feature superficial and deep infiltrates rich in plasma cells accompanied by psoriasiform epidermal hyperplasia. There are generally more lymphocytes and fewer histiocytes in ACA. The clinical presentations of the two conditions are different, with widespread discrete plaques in secondary lues and confluent involvement of the skin of the distal limbs and acra in ACA.

If the differential diagnosis cannot be resolved and organisms are not visible in silver- or immunoperoxidase-stained sections, serologic studies can cinch the diagnosis. It should be noted that patients with human immunodeficiency viral infection can have syphilis and have a negative Venereal Disease Research Laboratory (VDRL) test.

Lichen Striatus

Lichen striatus is a condition of unknown cause in which scaly papules due to an interface dermatitis with distinctive features occur in a linear distribution, generally following the lines of Blaschko. The latter are lines that may correspond to the distribution of genetically mosaic keratinocytes.

Clinical Features

Lichen striatus presents in children or young teenagers as linearly distributed papules over an extremity that eventually coalesce. The lesions often regress spontaneously after several months to a year or two. Usually there is only one limb involved by the eruption.

Histopathologic Features

Early lesions of lichen striatus combine the features of a lichenoid interface dermatitis, with or without spongiosis, with slight psoriasiform epidermal hyperplasia. Dyskeratotic cells can be found within the epidermis, and small mounds of parakeratosis are sometimes present (Fig. 5-30).

As lesions of lichen striatus mature, the infiltrates tend to involve both the superficial and deep plexuses and often surround adnexal epithelial structures as well, including both follicles and eccrine coils and ducts (Fig. 5-31). Lymphocytes can be present along the course of eccrine ducts from the secretory coil to the acrosyringium. Macrophages can be present within edematous dermal papillae, and sometimes there are discrete granulomatous foci. The epidermis often shows psoriasiform hyperplasia in fully developed lesions of lichen striatus, although some lesions can show jagged rete ridges and wedge-shaped hypergranulosis, resembling lichen planus in their epidermal changes. The numbers of dyskeratotic cells are greater than in early lesions.[52]

Clinicopathologic Correlation

The scaly appearance of lichen striatus is the result of small foci of parakeratosis. Lesions of lichen striatus are flat-topped papules because of psoriasiform epidermal hyperplasia and band-like lymphocytic infiltrates. The granulomatous foci are generally too small to cause the yellow appearance that characterizes other granulomatous dermatitides.

Differential Diagnosis

Patch and early plaque stage lesions of mycosis fungoides also combine slight psoriasiform epidermal hyperplasia with superficial and deep infiltrates in which lymphocytes predominate and are distributed in a band in the papillary dermis. In some lesions of lichen striatus, lymphocytes can even be present in the basal layer of the epidermis, aligned along the epidermal side of the dermoepidermal junction, just as they are in mycosis fungoides.[52] Patches of mycosis fungoides generally do not feature many necrotic keratinocytes. If granulomatous foci are present in mycosis fungoides, they are situated in the reticular dermis, whereas histiocytes are often present in clusters in the papillary dermis in lichen striatus. Thickened collagen bundles separated by clefts are present in the papillary dermis of mycosis fungoides but only rarely are found in that of lichen striatus. Even cursory attention to the clinical situation can resolve any dilemma in diagnosis, as mycosis fungoides does not present with linear lesions and is rare in children.

Some lesions of lichen striatus have epidermal changes that resemble those of lichen planus, with pointed rete ridges and wedge-shaped foci of hypergranulosis. Lichen planus can present with linear lesions, making this differential diagnosis a realistic one clinically. Lichen planus does not have granulomatous foci, and the finding of dense infiltrates arround eccrine coils and ducts clearly distinguishes the two conditions.

Discoid lesions of lupus erythematosus have irregular epidermal hyperplasia or epidermal atrophy coupled with infiltrates that surround follicular epithelium but not eccrine coils to the extent seen in lichen striatus. Mucin deposition is present in the dermis in lupus erythematosus, but not in lichen striatus, and

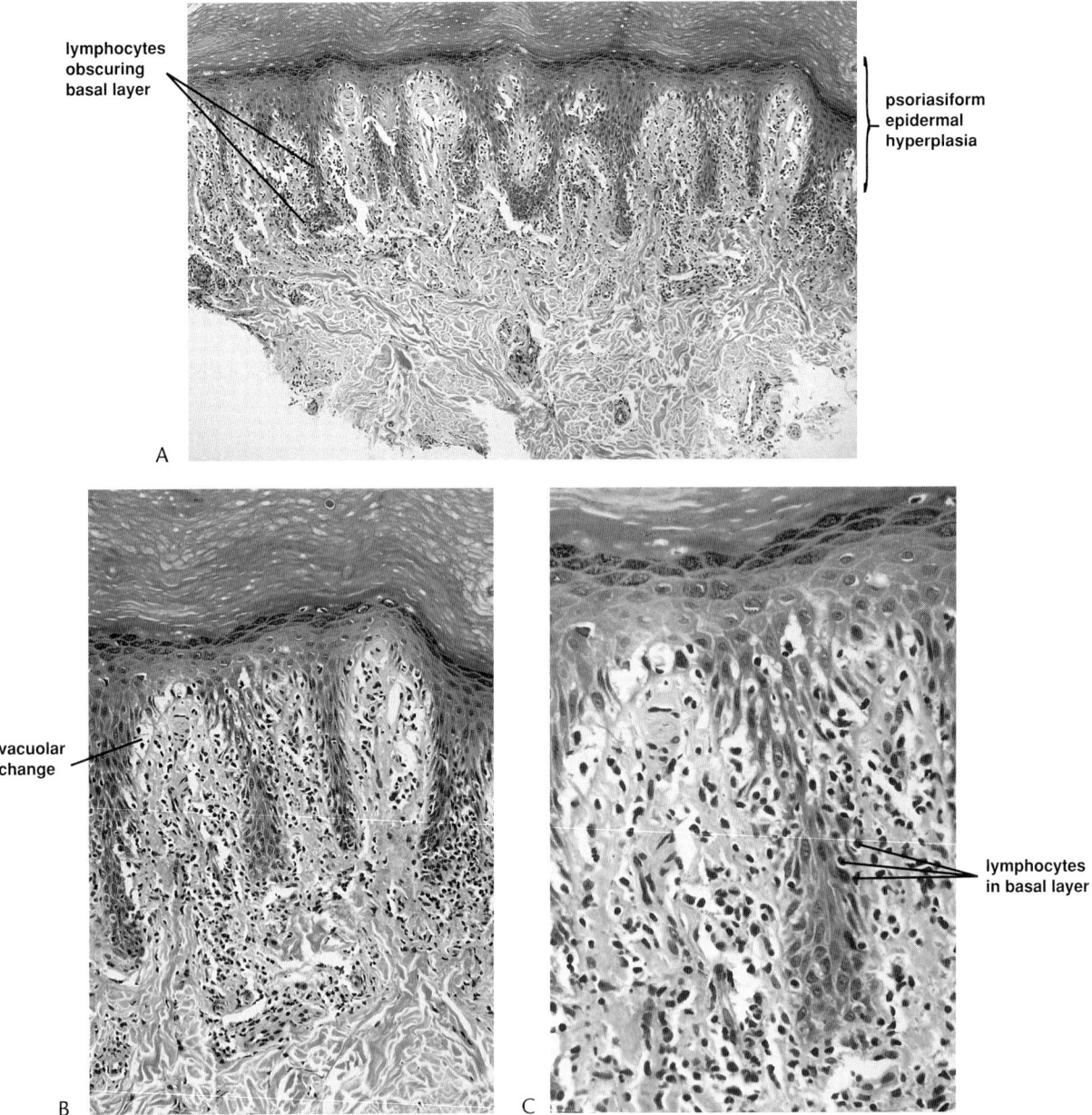

Figure 5-30. Lichen striatus is an interface dermatitis that can show psoriasiform epidermal hyperplasia, irregular epidermal hyperplasia, spongiosis, granulomatous infiltrates, and involvement of eccrine coils and ducts in any combination. **(A)** In this example from acral skin, there is psoriasiform epidermal hyperplasia. **(B)** Lymphocytes obscure the junction along the sides and bases of elongated rete. **(C)** In some examples, many lymphocytes can be present in the basal layer of the epidermis, resulting in a picture simulating the patch stage of mycosis fungoides.

granulomatous foci are practically never seen in lupus erythematosus.

Lichen nitidus (see later) presents with small granulomatous foci that impinge on the dermoepidermal junction, often seen between elongated slender rete ridges that partially enclose them. Evolving lesions of lichen striatus can present with discrete papules, although these papules are larger than those of lichen nitidus. Lichen striatus, unlike lichen nitidus, usually in-

volves the entire width of a punch-biopsied specimen and has infiltrates around the deep vascular plexus and adnexa. Early lesions of lichen striatus can have spongiotic epidermal foci, whereas those of lichen nitidus may thin the epidermis above a tiny granuloma but are not accompanied by spongiosis.

Other linearly distributed conditions such as linear psoriasis and inflammatory linear verrucous epidermal nevus have histologic pictures that in no way resemble those of lichen striatus.

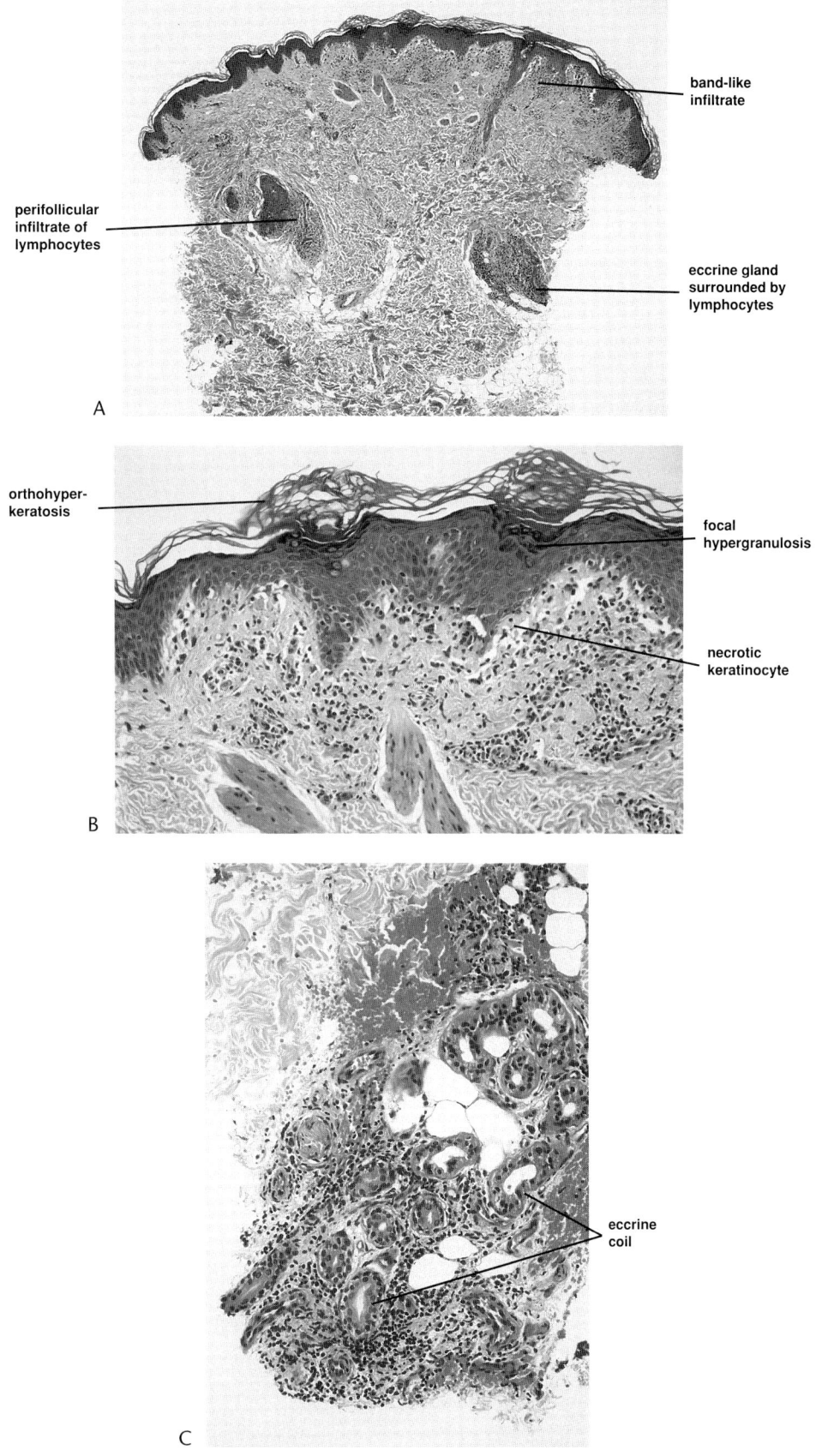

band-like
infiltrate

perifollicular
infiltrate of
lymphocytes

eccrine gland
surrounded by
lymphocytes

A

orthohyper-
keratosis

focal
hypergranulosis

necrotic
keratinocyte

B

eccrine
coil

C

Figure 5-31. Lichen striatus. **(A)** Marked involvement of eccrine epithelium and epidermal changes resembling lichen planus. **(B)** The rete ridges are jagged rather than rounded as in Figure 5-30. **(C)** Dense lymphocytic infiltrates are present around an eccrine coil.

133

Pathophysiology

Because the lesions of lichen striatus follow the lines of Blaschko, many workers have assumed that the condition is a T-cell-mediated reaction to the expression of antigens on keratinocytes of an embryologically mosaic territory that are not present on other keratinocytes. The occurrence of linearly distributed lesions in rare patients with acute cutaneous graft-versus-host reaction may be due to an analogous process in which antigens present on genetically mosaic keratinocytes were tolerated by the immune system of the host prior to transplantation, but not by the engrafted immune system.

Lichen Nitidus

Lichen nitidus is a condition in which many tiny, shiny papules are grouped in one or more of several characteristic locations.

Clinical Features

The papules of lichen nitidus measure from 1 to 2 mm in breadth and have the same color as the surrounding skin. They are asymptomatic. The genitalia, forearms, and sometimes the trunk are sites of predilection.

Histologic Features

Lichen nitidus begins with infiltrates of lymphocytes that fill one or two dermal papillae, accompanied by histiocytes (Fig. 5-32). Rete ridges at the periphery of the infiltrates become slender and elongate. The epidermis overlying the lymphocytic infiltrate often becomes thinned, with overlying foci of parakeratosis.[62]

In more mature lesions of lichen nitidus, there are fewer lymphocytes and larger numbers of macrophages, and a few giant cells are often present. The rete encompassing the granuloma-

Figure 5-32. **(A)** Each papule of lichen striatus is formed by a nodular infiltrate of lymphocytes and macrophages in one or a few contiguous dermal papillae, often with slender rete ridges at each side. **(B)** The junctional zone shows vacuolar change, and there is slight hyperkeratosis. In contrast to lichen planus, there are far many more macrophages, and colloid bodies are infrequent.

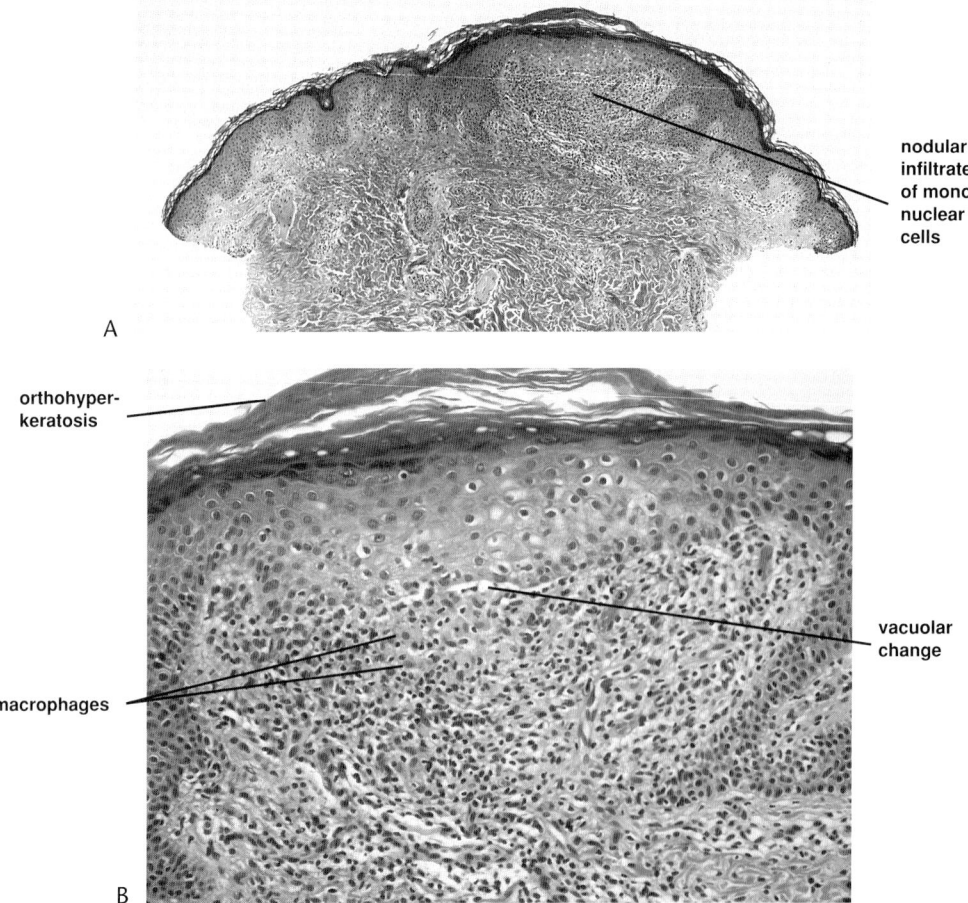

A

nodular infiltrate of mono-nuclear cells

orthohyper-keratosis

macrophages

vacuolar change

B

tous foci often have a bowed appearance, immortalized as resembling a ball and claw, with the granulomatous inflammation being the ball and the elongated rete the claw. As in some early lesions, the epidermis overlying the infiltrate can be thinned, and parakeratosis is commonly present.

Clinicopathologic Correlation

The small bumps of lichen nitidus are caused by dense infiltrates of mononuclear cells in the papillary dermis–mostly lymphocytes in early lesions, and mainly histiocytes in later ones.

Differential Diagnosis

The most important differential diagnoses are lichen planus, sarcoidosis, and lichen striatus. Lichen striatus is discussed in detail in the preceeding section.

Lichen planus can feature small discrete papules involving many of the same sites as lichen nitidus. Because lesions of lichen planus do not contain granulomatous foci, only early lesions of lichen nitidus are likely to be mistaken for lichen planus. Pointed rete ridges, wedge-shaped hypergranulotic foci, and colloid bodies in the papillary dermis, features practically emblematic of lichen planus, are not found in lichen nitidus, and the parakeratosis seen overlying lesions of lichen nitidus is exceptional in lichen planus.

The micropapular form of sarcoidosis can simulate lichen nitidus clinically and pathologically. Both conditions have granulomatous collections in close apposition to the epidermis, which can show vacuolar alteration and thinning above the granuloma and psoriasiform hyperplasia alongside it. In general, lymphocytes are more abundant in lichen nitidus than in sarcoidosis. Slender rete ridges that enfold tiny granulomas only one rete ridge in breadth are not present in sarcoidosis.

Cases reported as lichen nitidus with plasma cells probably represent an unusual form of polymorphous light eruption. These tiny papules are present on the sun-exposed skin of the dorsal limbs and hands, often in immunocompromised patients.

Pathophysiology

The pathophysiology of lichen nitidus is unknown, as is its peculiar clinical distribution. It does not appear to be a variant of lichen planus. Because small, evolving papules of lichen planus can be much the same size as those of lichen nitidus, some authors have considered the two conditions to be related, and they occasionally are discussed in the same chapter in textbooks of clinical dermatopathology. The very different cellular compositions (almost entirely lymphocytic in lichen planus, mostly histiocytic in fully developed lesions of lichen nitidus) and the absence of dyskeratotic cells and colloid bodies in lichen nitidus indicate that the two conditions are not intimately related.

INTERFACE DERMATITIDES THAT COMMONLY RESULT IN EPIDERMAL ATROPHY

Lichen Sclerosus et Atrophicus

Lichen sclerosis et atrophicus (LSA) is a fibrosing and atrophying disease limited to the skin that is characterized by white pru-

ritic plaques. The same condition is termed *balanitis xerotica obliterans* when the glans penis is affected.

Clinical Features

LSA most frequently occurs on the skin of female genitalia and also can affect the mucosal surfaces or extragenital skin. Its onset may be in childhood, but most cases begin in middle age. Genital lesions can grow to confluently involve the perineum and perianal skin in a figure-of-eight-like pattern. The lesions begin as pink macules and eventually become white and atrophic in appearance with wrinkled surfaces and comedo-like follicular plugs. Often an erythematous halo surrounds the depigmented center. There are often secondary changes due to excoriation. Some patients develop vesicles or bullae. In children, lesions may spontaneously involute at puberty, but genital lesions in adults tend to persist and may be the site of eventual squamous cell carcinoma.[63]

Balanitis xerotica obliterans often results in phimosis. The histologic changes of balanitis xerotica are commonly found in foreskins removed for phimosis, even when the diagnosis had not been made before surgery.

Histopathologic Features

The earliest lesions of genital LSA are seldom biopsied, but their histologic changes can be inferred from the findings at the peripheries of large incisional or excisional biopsy specimens. The inflammatory changes to the side of sclerotic zones in LSA have characteristic histopathologic changes (Fig. 5-33). Pink areas at the edges of plaques of LSA and inflamed areas of foreskins affected by balanitis xerotica obliterans demonstrate psoriasiform epidermal hyperplasia and band-like lymphocytic infiltrates with fibrosis of the papillary dermis and compact hyperkeratosis.[64] There are frequently many lymphocytes in the basal zone of the epidermis, on the epidermal side of the basement membrane without either significant spongiosis or more than rare necrotic keratinocytes. The papillary dermis in such areas is often coarsely fibrotic, and often the fine elastic fibers, termed *elaunin* and *oxytalan*, that are ordinarily found in a feltwork beneath the epidermis are destroyed.

In fully developed lesions of LSA, or in foci adjacent to the lichenoid infiltrates there is "edema" of the papillary dermis, which, coupled with a diminution in the diameters of collagen bundles, leads to pallor and homogenization (Fig. 5-34). The papillary dermal edema of LSA is actually due to the deposition of acidic mucopolysaccharides.[65] Although most inflammatory infiltrates in the papillary dermis replace its normally delicate collagen pattern with coarse bundles, LSA eventually leaves in its wake edema and a dense meshwork of even thinner bundles that are at times indistinct. The infiltrate of lymphocytes that is present in a band-like pattern in early lesions is seen beneath the thickened papillary dermis. As the edematous, homogenized papillary dermis expands to many times its normal width, it depresses the conspicuously interstitial mononuclear cell infiltrate seen beneath it so that the inflammatory cells that surround the superficial plexus appear to be mid-dermal in location. In fully developed lesions of LSA the rete ridge pattern is effaced, and in some cases, the epidermis becomes extraordinarily thinned. Rubbing caused by the pruritus may

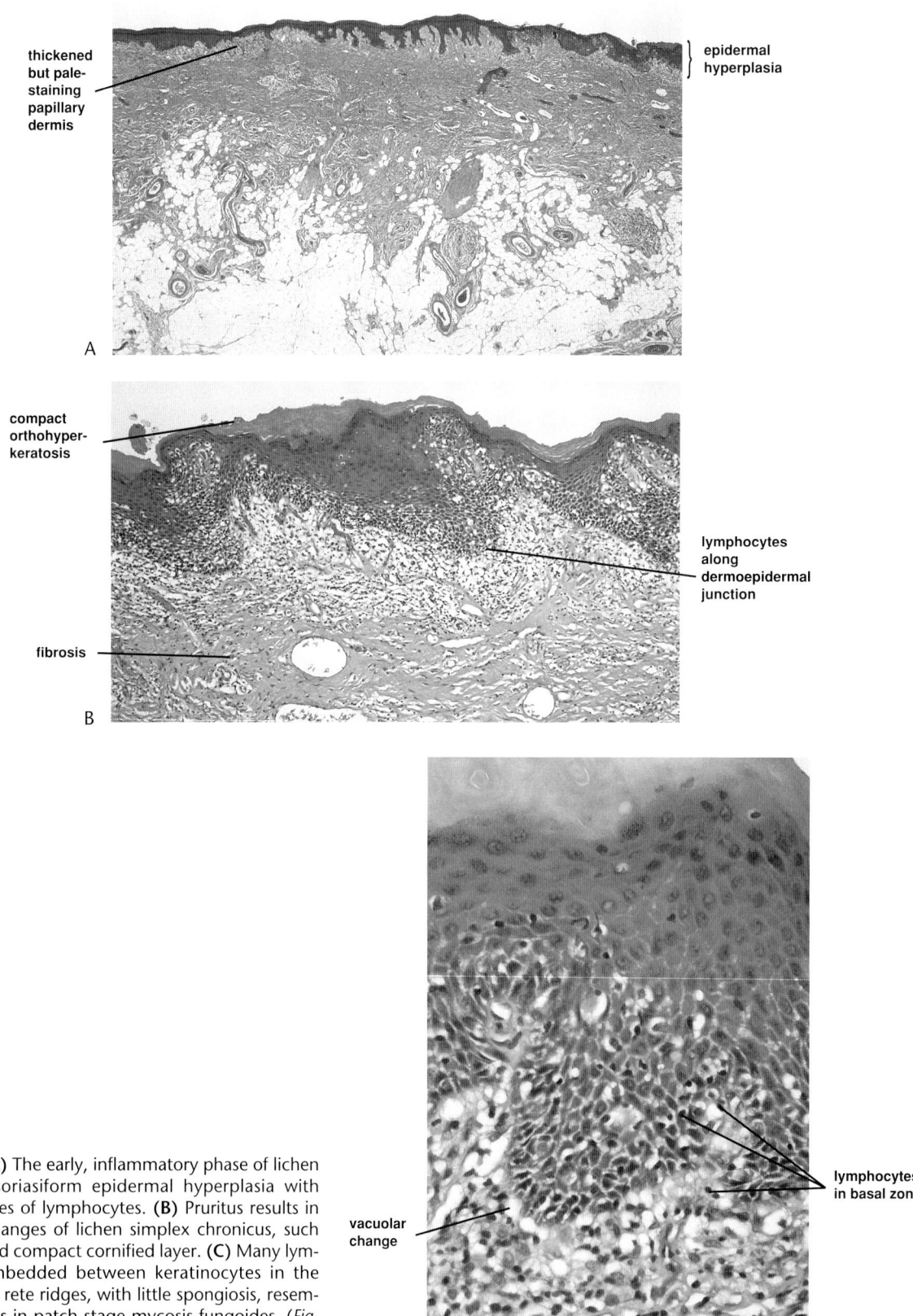

Figure 5-33. **(A)** The early, inflammatory phase of lichen sclerosus has psoriasiform epidermal hyperplasia with lichenoid infiltrates of lymphocytes. **(B)** Pruritus results in superimposed changes of lichen simplex chronicus, such as a thickened and compact cornified layer. **(C)** Many lymphocytes are embedded between keratinocytes in the lower portions of rete ridges, with little spongiosis, resembling the changes in patch stage mycosis fungoides. (*Figure continues.*)

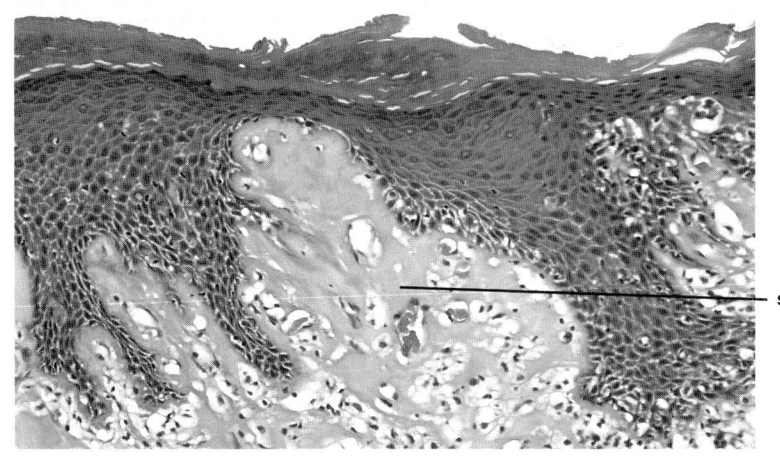

sclerosis

D

Figure 5-33 *(Continued).* **(D)** Adjacent to these changes is a zone in which the papillary dermis is thickened, pale, and sclerotic, as is typical of fully evolved lesions of lichen sclerosus.

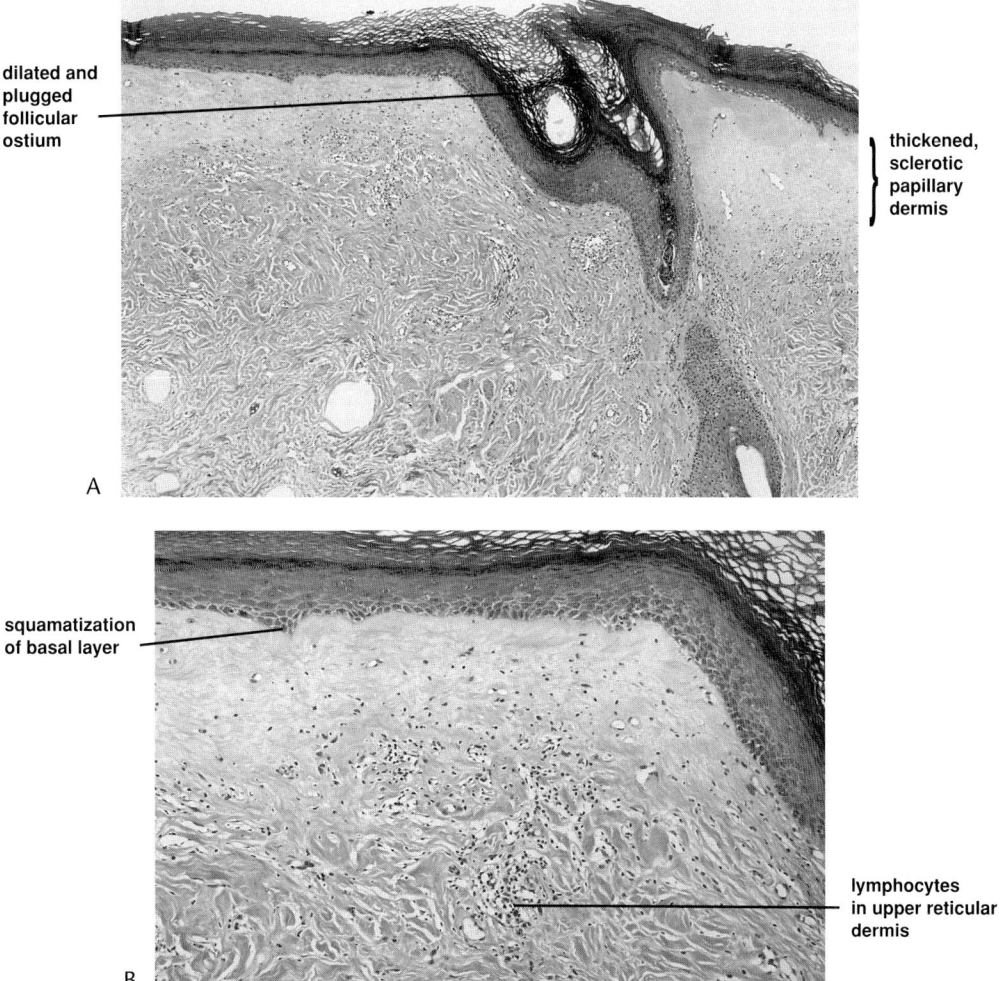

dilated and plugged follicular ostium

thickened, sclerotic papillary dermis

A

squamatization of basal layer

lymphocytes in upper reticular dermis

B

Figure 5-34. **(A)** In fully evolved lesions of lichen sclerosus, the papillary dermis is conspicuous at low magnification as a thickened, pale-staining zone beneath an epidermis whose rete ridge pattern is flattened. **(B)** The lymphocytic infiltrates that are present in a band in early lesions are now found in an interstitial pattern in the superficial reticular dermis. *(Figure continues.)*

Figure 5-34 *(Continued).* **(C)** The papillary dermal collagen fibers are so fine as to be barely discernible at high magnification. Note the presence of a few lymphocytes in the basal layer of the epidermis.

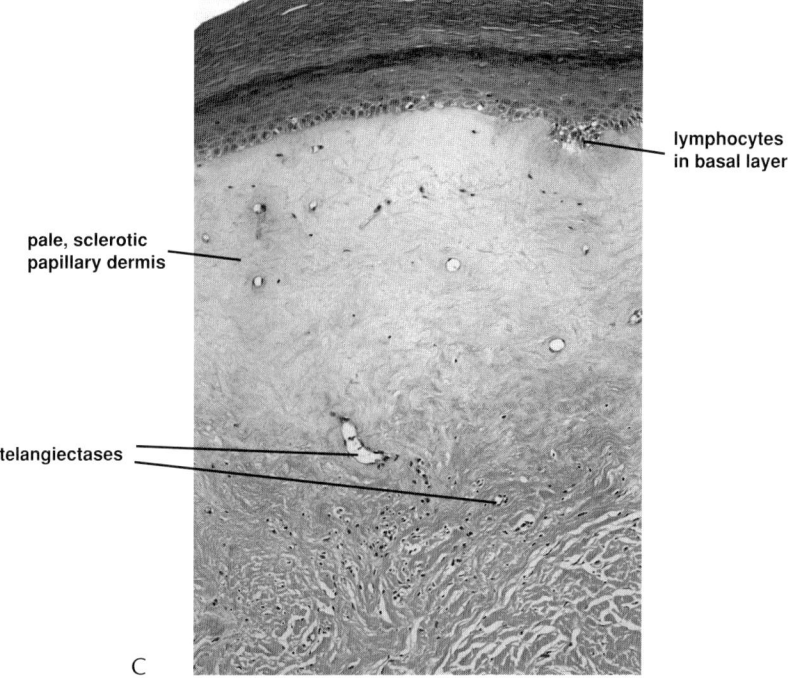

lymphocytes in basal layer

pale, sclerotic papillary dermis

telangiectases

C

result in compact hyperkeratosis and epidermal hyperplasia. The orifices of adnexal structures are plugged, as they are in lupus erythematosus.

Owing to extreme edema and the shearing forces of rubbing, subepidermal bullae, sometimes hemorrhagic, may occur. Some blisters result from marked dilation of lymphatic vessels, which may "blow out."

Papillary dermal sclerosis similar to that of lichen sclerosus, although without its characteristic pallor, is sometimes seen in morphea, where these findings occur above thickened and closely apposed collagen bundles in the reticular dermis.

Clinicopathologic Correlation

Depigmentation of LSA is a consequence of damage to the basal layer and its melanocytes and is accompanied by numerous dermal melanophages. The wrinkled surfaces of lesions reflect the destruction of rete ridges and dermal papillae and the nearly complete loss of papillary dermal elastic tissue, as well as the marked thinning of the epidermis in LSA. The fibrosing character of the disease is apparent in its destruction of genital topography, suggested by the disquieting term *obliterans* in reference to the penile form of the disease.

Differential Diagnosis

Fully formed lesions of LSA are distinctive by virtue of pallor and homogenization of the papillary dermis, a set of features otherwise only seen in LSA-like lesions of borreliosis, in some cases of morphea, and in radiation sclerosis (usually termed *chronic radiation dermatitis*). The elastic tissue of the papillary dermis is destroyed in LSA but not in the LSA-like changes of morphea. Early lesions of LSA that have a band-like infiltrate may be difficult to distinguish from lichen planus, especially at

periorificial locations. Findings such as pointed rete ridges, squamatization of the basal layer, wedge-shaped hypergranulosis, and preservation of superficial elastic tissue favor lichen planus, whereas rounded rete, basilar epidermotropism of lymphocytes, and destruction of the superficial elastic tissue network favor LSA. Lesions that seem indistinguishable from those of idiopathic LSA are sometimes seen in patients with borreliosis.

In radiation sclerosis, the epidermis can be atrophic, with compact hyperkeratosis and loss of the rete ridge pattern, and the papillary dermis may be thickened, with only fine collagen fibers forming a homogeneous-appearing band. Both conditions can have areas in which keratinocytes have abnormal nuclei, with overlying parakeratosis. Lichen sclerosus can have such zones, because its lesions seem predisposed to the development of squamous cell carcinoma, perhaps because of an aberrant mesenchymal-epithelial interface. In radiation sclerosis, one can occasionally observe areas of radiation keratosis, a form of evolving squamous cell carcinoma in situ. Endothelial cells or fibroblasts with atypical or multiple nuclei, perivascular deposits of fibrin, and elastotic material admixed with zones of sclerosis are helpful features that enable one to make a specific diagnosis of radiation sclerosis.

Pathophysiology

The occurrence of LSA in European and in Japanese patients with borreliosis, who can also develop morphea and ACA, suggests that the conditions are pathogenetically linked. There have been conflicting studies regarding the presence of spirochetal DNA in lesional skin using the polymerase chain reaction and silver stains to demonstrate spirochetes in lichen sclerosus are usually negative. Some differences may reflect the prevalence of *B. burgdorferi afzelii* and *B. garinii* in Europe. These strains, which are also associated with ACA, are rarely found in North America.

Some authors regard lichen sclerosus as the superficial expression of morphea, explaining both the coincidence of these diseases in patients with borreliosis and the occurrence of lichen sclerosus–like changes in the papillary dermis in otherwise typical lesions of morphea.

Poikilodermatous Conditions

A number of different diseases result in the clinical appearance of poikiloderma, literally meaning *variable skin*, but specifically characterized by hypopigmentation and hyperpigmentation, atrophy, and telangiectasia.

Clinical Features

Poikiloderma congenitale of Rothmund and Thomson is an autosomal recessive disease in which cataracts, abnormal dentition, skeletal defects, and hypogonadism may also occur.[66] Poikiloderma can also occur in dermatomyositis, an occurrence termed *poikilodermatomyositis*. It may also occur as a sequela to systemic lupus erythematosus. The rippled hyperpigmentation in *dyskeratosis congenita*, a condition also characterized by reticulate hyperpigmentation, nail dystrophy and hyperkeratosis of mucosal surfaces, is accompanied by epidermal atrophy.

Poikiloderma can occur along the sides of the neck in sun-damaged skin, a condition called *poikiloderma of Civatte*. Radiotherapy or topical chemotherapy, most often topical nitrogen mustard or BCNU prescribed for mycosis fungoides, can produce poikiloderma.

Histopathologic Features and Clinicopathologic Correlation

Regardless of cause, the poikilodermas all show loss of the normal rete ridge pattern and thinning of the epidermis, accompanied by fibrosis of the papillary dermis that results in the atrophic, wrinkled clinical appearance (Fig. 5-35). Melanophages are present in the papillary dermis and correspond to the mottled pigmentation. Telangiectases are apparent both clinically and histopathologically.

Poikilodermatous lesions of mycosis fungoides may pose a problem when only the changes that are noted earlier are seen. Usually, there are foci in which sufficient numbers of lymphocytes are present within the epidermis to enable a diagnosis to be made, although several biopsy procedures may be necessary.

Differential Diagnosis

One commonly encountered histologic simulant of the poikilodermatous conditions listed earlier is a specimen taken from the atrophic center of a lesion of actinic porokeratosis often when that diagnosis is not suspected. Only on level sections does the cornoid lamella, which is evidence of porokeratosis, occur, and sometimes not at all. Regressed lesions of malignant melanoma often have band-like infiltrates of melanophages at the base of the fibrotic papillary dermis.

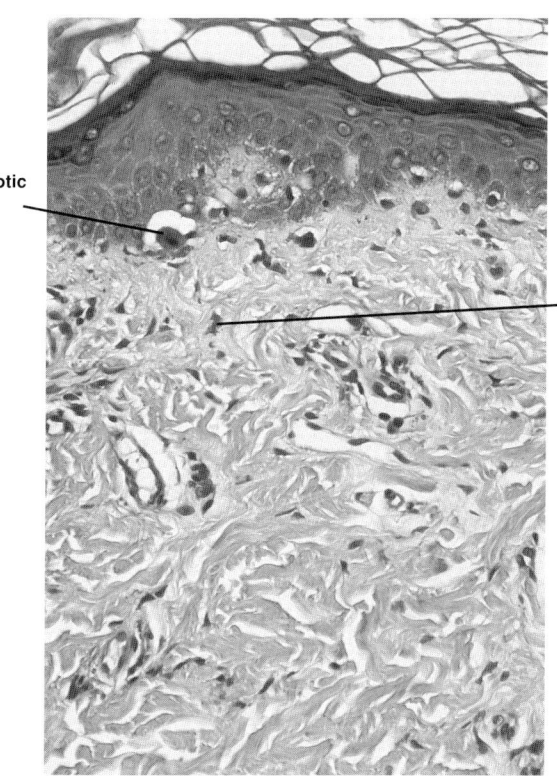

necrotic cell

melanophage

Figure 5-35. In this example of poikiloderma congenitale, the normal rete ridge pattern is effaced, and vacuolar change with rare necrotic keratinocytes is evident along the junctional zone. Melanophages are present in the papillary dermis, a finding in keeping with the mottled pigmentation evident clinically.

Pathophysiology

With regard to the hereditary conditions associated with poikiloderma, there may be a state in which keratinocyte antigens are constitutively perceived as foreign.[67]

Acrodermatitis Chronica Atrophicans

ACA is an inflammatory reaction to chronic infection with the spirochete *B. burgdorferi* that results in cutaneous atrophy, sometimes accompanied by neurologic or musculoskeletal disease.

Clinical Features

ACA follows the initial infection by *B. burgdorferi* by months to years. The initial changes are often diffuse erythema and edema of distal extremities, sometimes with more central lesions that resemble LSA. Eventually there is marked dermal atrophy with a wrinkled surface. Arthritis, subcutaneous fibrous bands, and deformities of the joints that underlie involved skin are often present. The disease responds to antibiotic therapy.

Histopathologic Features

The inflammatory stage of ACA may show a band-like lymphocytic infiltrate, most often with numerous plasma cells in both the superficial and deep dermis. In early lesions, there is psoriasiform epidermal hyperplasia, whereas in later lesions, marked thinning of the epidermis eventuates (Fig. 5-36). Late lesions have sparser papillary dermal infiltrates and show marked loss of reticular dermal collagen, along with profound thinning of the epidermis.

Spirochetes can be found by silver staining in the majority of lesions.[68]

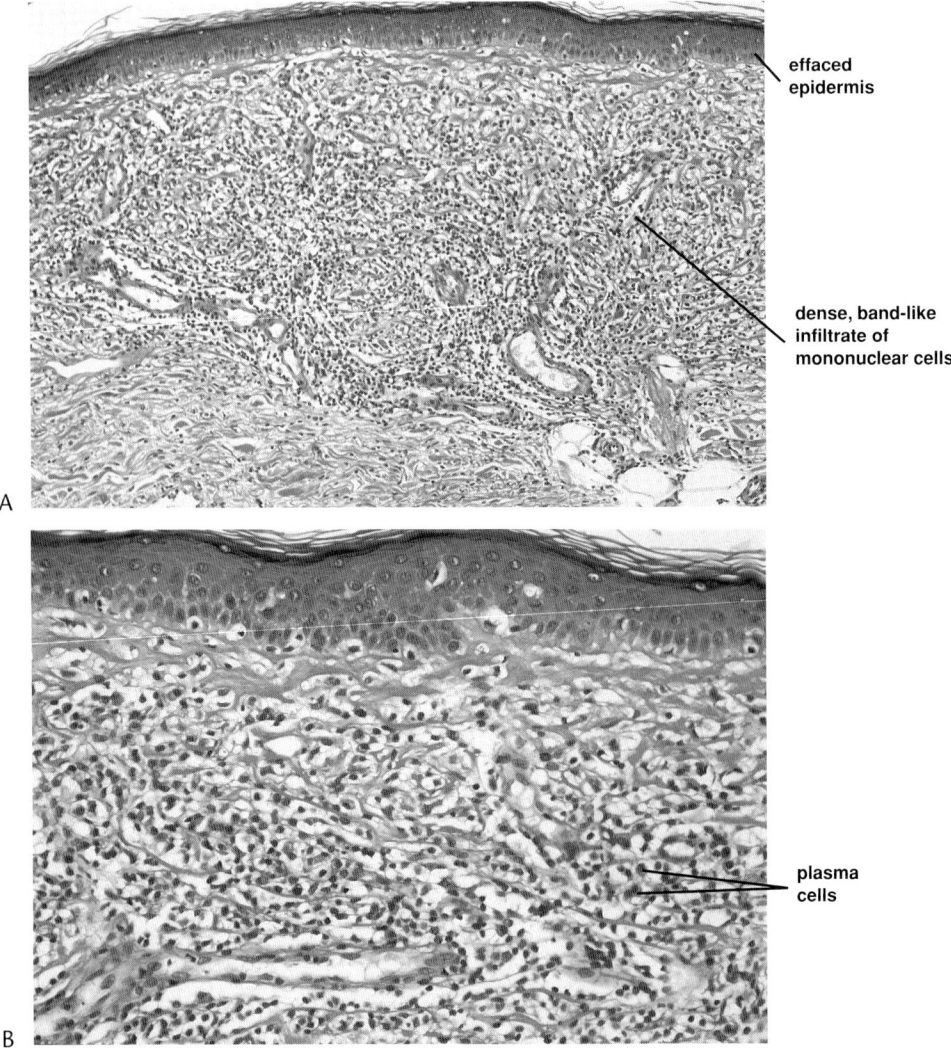

effaced epidermis

dense, band-like infiltrate of mononuclear cells

plasma cells

Figure 5-36. **(A)** Acrodermatitis chronica atrophicans is a complication of borreliosis in which an interface dermatitis with psoriasiform hyperplasia evolves into one with marked epidermal atrophy. **(B)** Lymphocytes and plasma cells are present throughout the superficial dermis (courtesy of Dr. Peter Kind, Dept. of Dermatology, Maximillien–Ludwig University, Munich, Germany).

Clinicopathologic Correlation

The remarkable thinning of the epidermis and dermis in ACA produces the atrophic clinical lesions. The fine elastic fibers of the papillary dermis called elaunin and oxytalan are destroyed by the inflammatory cell infiltrate. Although early lesions are often strikingly edematous clinically, reticular dermal edema is difficult to appreciate histologically. Lesions that simulate morphea or LSA that occur concurrently with ACA have the histopathologic appearance of those diseases.

Differential Diagnosis

The superficial and deep, plasma cell–rich infiltrate of ACA is reminiscent of secondary syphilis. Atrophy only rarely supervenes in syphilis, and granulomas or numerous macrophages, both of which are common in syphilis, are rare in ACA. An occasional biopsy specimen of early ACA may contain numerous intraepidermal lymphocytes that simulate mycosis fungoides.

Pathophysiology

ACA indicates active infection with *B. burgdorferi*. Spirochetes can be identified by culture and by silver stain. Both syphilis and ACA are examples of spirochetoses in which plasma cells are prominent, but the reason for their presence is unknown.

NEOPLASTIC DISEASES IN WHICH LICHENOID INFILTRATES CAN OCCUR

Band-like infiltrates of lymphocytes can be seen in several neoplasms that can be mistaken for inflammatory conditions. Infiltration of the basilar epidermis and resultant necrosis of keratinocytes can occur in any of these.

A *lichen planus–like keratosis* is solitary, occasional multiple lesions that frequently begin as a T-cell-mediated reaction to a solar lentigo. It is caused by a lichenoid interface reaction to either a solar lentigo or seborrheic keratosis (Fig. 5-37). Lichenoid keratoses are frequently found as red-brown flat-topped papules on the arms and chest, usually as solitary le-

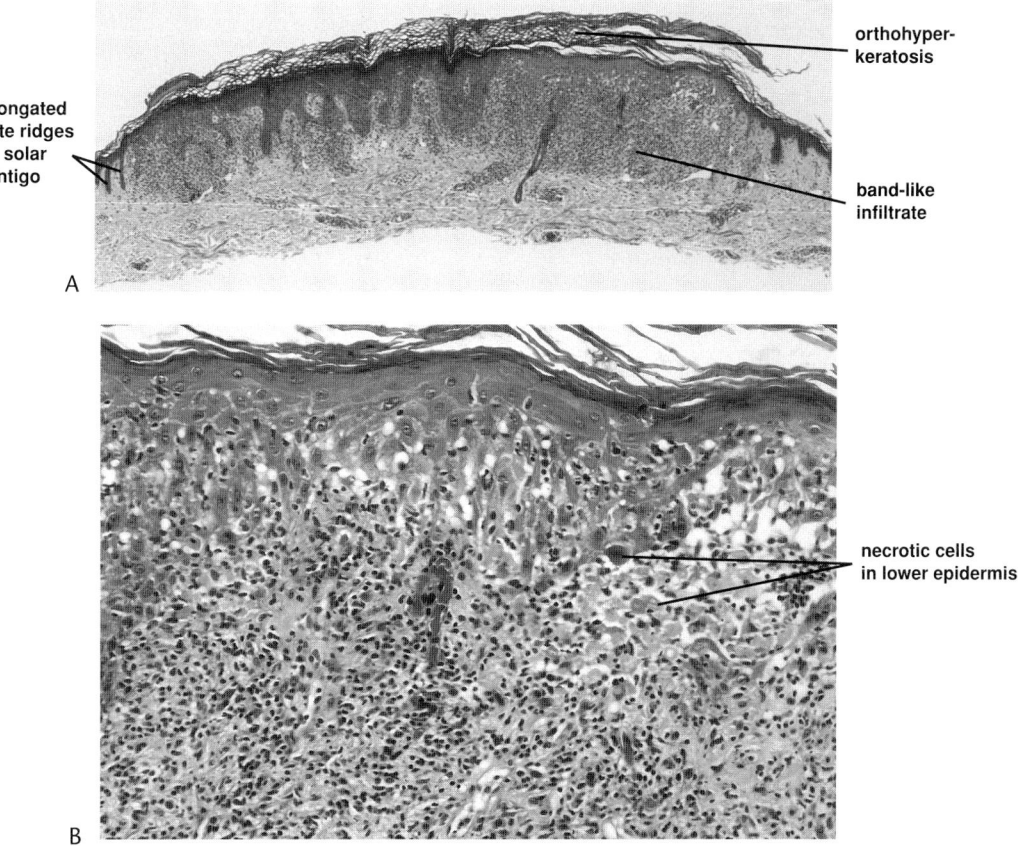

Figure 5-37. A lichenoid or lichen planus–like keratosis. There is a band-like infiltrate of lymphocytes along with pointed, elongated rete ridges and hyperkeratosis. **(A)** The solar lentigo that incited the cell-mediated reaction is evident at extreme left. **(B)** Lymphocytes obscure the junction, there is squamatization of the basal layer, and vacuolar change is accompanied by many dyskeratotic cells. In this particular example, the changes strikingly resemble those of lichen planus, but this need not be the case. (*Figure continues.*)

Figure 5-37 *(Continued).* **(C)** At the edge of the lesion are club-shaped rete with basilar hyperpigmentation typical of a solar lentigo.

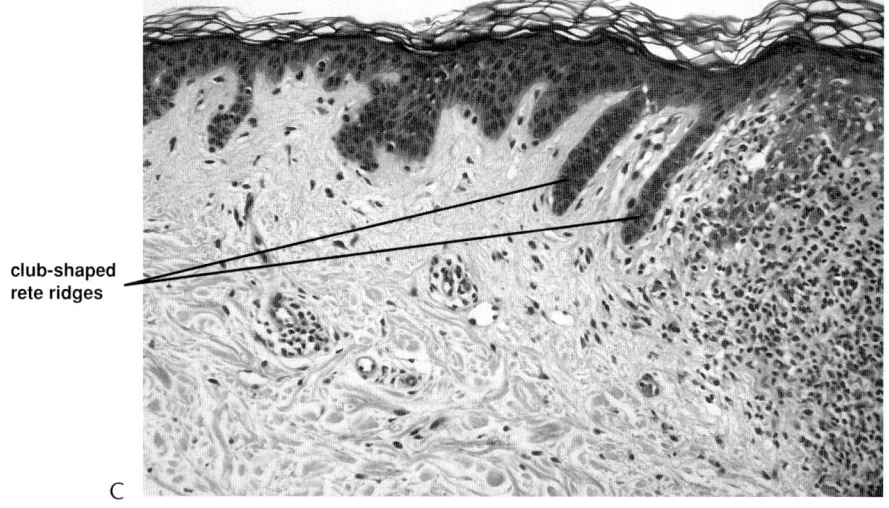

club-shaped
rete ridges

C

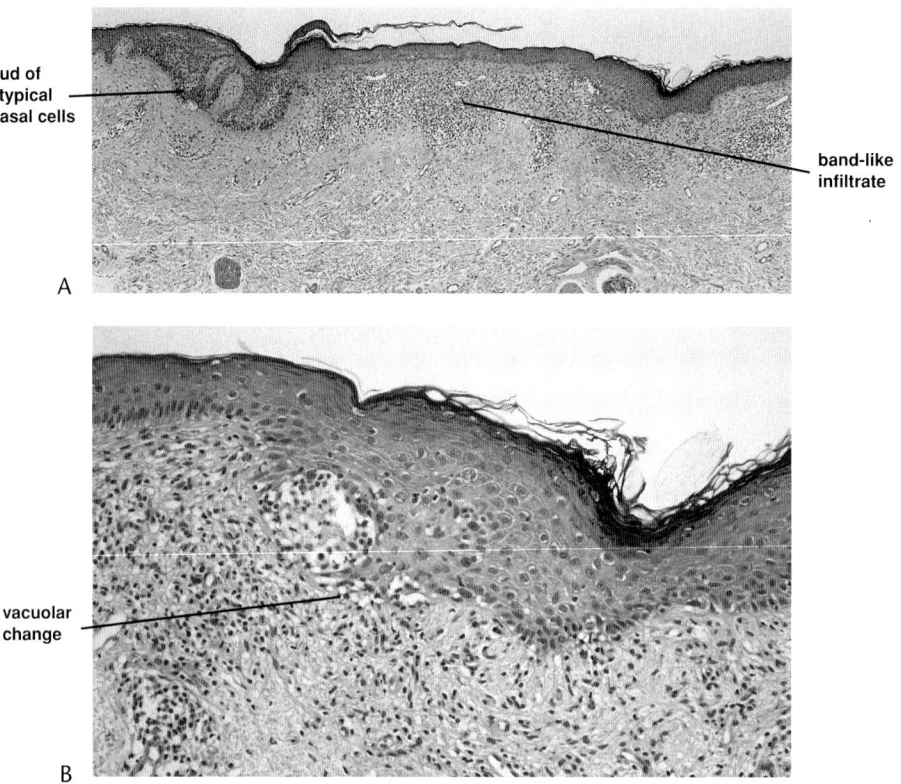

bud of
atypical
basal cells

band-like
infiltrate

A

vacuolar
change

B

Figure 5-38. Superficial basal cell carcinoma is often accompanied by a lymphocytic host response that results in an interface dermatitis. **(A)** Nests of basal cell carcinoma attached to the undersurface of the epidermis at left, and band-like lymphocytic infiltrates beneath a thinned epidermis at center and right. **(B)** If a small punch biopsy had only included this part of the lesion, the differential diagnosis would plausibly be between various forms of interface dermatitis. *(Figure continues.)*

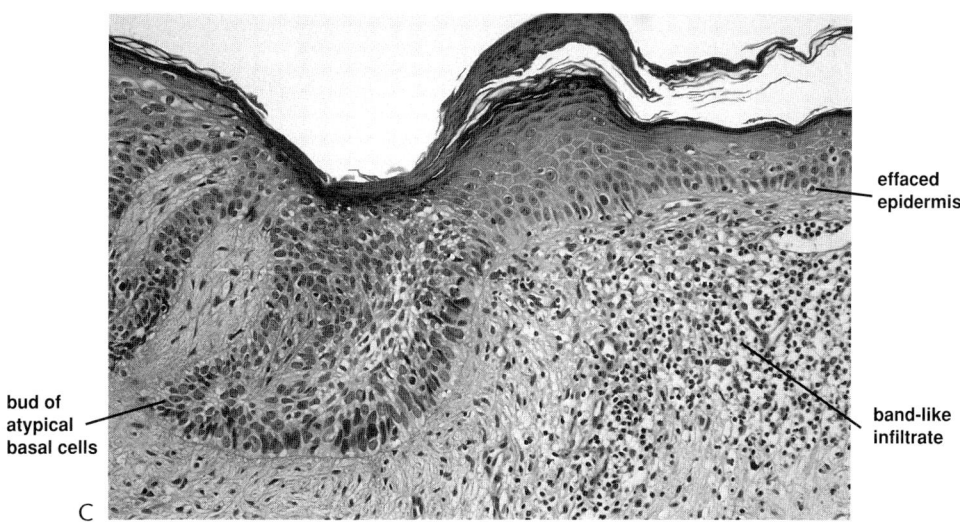

effaced
epidermis

bud of
atypical
basal cells

band-like
infiltrate

C

Figure 5-38 *(Continued).* **(C)** Peripherally palisaded basaloid cells in nests abut the zone of interface dermatitis. If the clinical history implies a solitary lesion, and histopathologic examination shows an interface reaction with features not typical of a lichenoid keratosis, the dermatopathologist should consider the possibility of superficial basal cell carcinoma and obtain level sections.

sions. Rarely, a patient will have several such lesions simultaneously, mimicking a photodermatitis.[69] Although it was initially termed *lichen planus–like*, it only mimics lichen planus in less than half of cases.[70] Features such as extensive spongiosis, parakeratosis, eosinophils in the dermal infiltrate, and marked edema of the papillary dermis, all of which are exceptional in authentic lichen planus, can be seen in lichenoid keratoses. Often, a remnant of the solar lentigo that provoked the reaction can be discerned at the edge of the infiltrate.[71]

Both *porokeratosis of Mibelli* and *disseminated superficial actinic porokeratosis* may have a lichenoid reaction in the center of recent lesions. If the diagnosis is not suspected and the specimen is oriented in such a way that the diagnostic cornoid lamellation is obscured, the diagnosis may be missed. A lichenoid infiltrate beneath an atrophic epidermis in sun-damaged skin is a clue to the diagnosis of actinic porokeratosis, which requires either level sections or rebiopsy to show the cornoid lamella.

Regression in malignant melanoma, and occasionally in melanocytic nevi, is mediated by a lichenoid infiltrate. In active areas of regression, there are usually some persistent melanoma cells, which permits identification even in a partial biopsy specimen. Old regressed areas may contain scattered melanophages, papillary dermal fibrosis, and an altered rete ridge pattern.

Superficial basal cell carcinoma often has a lichenoid infiltrate of lymphocytes, melanophages, and sometimes plasma cells between the nests of basaloid cells, coupled with loss of the normal rete ridge pattern (Fig. 5-38). On occasion, a biopsy specimen shows only the lichenoid infiltrate and not the nests, which appear on level sections in most biopsy specimens.

Mycosis fungoides often has a band-like infiltrate composed largely of small lymphocytes. The differential diagnosis between mycosis fungoides with a lichenoid histologic pattern and an interface dermatitis can be extraordinarily difficult and sometimes insoluable by microscopy alone. Clues that such an infiltrate signifies mycosis fungoides and not a lichenoid dermatitis include foci in which disproportionate numbers of lymphocytes are present within the epidermis, markedly atypical lymphocytes, and rounded rather than pointed rete in a lesion of long enough duration for the papillary dermis to become fibrotic.

REFERENCES

1. Langley RG, Walsh N, Nevill T et al: Apoptosis is the mode of keratinocyte death in cutaneous graft-versus-host disease. J Am Acad Dermatol 35:187–190, 1996

2. Patterson JW: The spectrum of lichenoid dermatitis. J Cutan Pathol 18:67–74, 1991

3. Ackerman AB: Supplement to the Fourth Printing of Histologic Diagnosis of Inflammatory Skin Diseases. Lea & Febiger, Philadelphia, 1988

4. LeBoit PE: Interface dermatitis. How specific are its histopathologic features? [editorial]. Arch Dermatol 129:1324–1328, 1993

5. Cote B, Wechsler J, Bastuji-Garin S et al: Clinicopathologic correlation in erythema multiforme and Stevens-Johnson syndrome. Arch Dermatol 131:1268–1272, 1995

6. Zohdi-Mofid M, Horn TD: Acrosyringeal concentration of necrotic keratinocytes in erythema multiforme: a clue to drug etiology. J Cutan Pathol 24:235–240, 1997

7. Ackerman AB, Ragaz A: Erythema multiforme. Am J Dermatopathol 7:133–139, 1985

8. Bedi TR, Pinkus H: Histopathological spectrum of erythema multiforme. Br J Dermatol 95:243–250, 1976

9. Darragh TM, Egbert BM, Berger TG, Yen TS: Identification of herpes simplex virus DNA in lesions of erythema multiforme by the polymerase chain reaction. J Am Acad Dermatol 24:23–26, 1991

10. Imamura S, Horio T, Yanase K et al: Erythema multiforme: pathomechanism of papular erythema and target lesion. J Dermatol 19:524–533, 1992

11. Kazmierowski JA, Wuepper KD: Erythema multiforme: immune complex vasculitis of the superficial cutaneous microvasculature. J Invest Dermatol 71:366–369, 1978

12. Bennion SD, Middleton MH, David-Bajar KM et al: In three types of interface dermatitis, different patterns of expression of

intercellular adhesion molecule-1 (ICAM-1) indicate different triggers of disease. J Invest Dermatol (suppl. 1) 105:71S–79S, 1995

13. Crider MK, Jansen J, Norins AL, McHale MS: Chemotherapy-induced acral erythema in patients receiving bone marrow transplantation. Arch Dermatol 122:1023–1027, 1986

14. Fitzpatrick JE: The cutaneous histopathology of chemotherapeutic reactions. J Cutan Pathol 20:1–14, 1993

15. Arias D, Requena L, Hasson A et al: Localized epidermal necrolysis (erythema multiforme-like reaction) following intravenous injection of vinblastine. J Cutan Pathol 18:344–346, 1991

16. Van Voorhees A, Stenn KS: Histological phases of Bactrim-induced fixed drug eruption. The report of one case. Am J Dermatopathol 9:528–532, 1987

17. Murphy GF, Guillen FJ, Flynn TC: Cytotoxic T lymphocytes and phenotypically abnormal epidermal dendritic cells in fixed cutaneous eruptions. Hum Pathol 16:1264–1271, 1985

18. Warshauer BL, Maloney ME, Dimond RL: Febrile ulceronecrotic Mucha-Habermann's disease. Arch Dermatol 119:597–601, 1983

19. Fortson JS, Schroeter AL, Esterly NB: Cutaneous T-cell lymphoma (parapsoriasis en plaque). An association with pityriasis lichenoides et varioliformis acuta in young children. Arch Dermatol 126:1449–1453, 1990

20. Weiss LM, Wood GS, Ellisen LW et al: Clonal T-cell populations in pityriasis lichenoides et varioliformis acuta (Mucha-Habermann disease). Am J Pathol 126:417–421, 1987

21. Carlson JA, Mihm MC Jr, LeBoit PE: Cutaneous lymphocytic vasculitis: a definition, a review, and a proposed classification. Semin Diagn Pathol 13:72–90, 1996

22. Longley J, Demar L, Feinstein RP et al: Clinical and histologic features of pityriasis lichenoides et varioliformis acuta in children. Arch Dermatol 123:1335–1339, 1987

23. Horn TD, Redd JV, Karp JE et al: Cutaneous eruptions of lymphocyte recovery. Arch Dermatol 125:1512–1517, 1989

24. Boyd AS, Neldner KH: Lichen planus [see comments]. J Am Acad Dermatol 25:593–619, 1991

25. Davis AL, Bhogal BS, Whitehead P et al: Lichen planus pemphigoides: its relationship to bullous pemphigoid. Br J Dermatol 125:263–271, 1991

26. Ragaz A, Ackerman AB: Evolution, maturation, and regression of lesions of lichen planus. New observations and correlations of clinical and histologic findings. Am J Dermatopathol 3:5–25, 1981

27. Mehregan DA, Van Hale HM, Muller SA: Lichen planopilaris: clinical and pathologic study of forty-five patients. J Am Acad Dermatol 27:935–942, 1992

28. Rivers JK, Jackson R, Orizaga M: Who was Wickham and what are his striae? Int J Dermatol 25:611–613, 1986

29. West AJ, Berger TG, LeBoit PE: A comparative histopathologic study of photodistributed and nonphotodistributed lichenoid drug eruptions. J Am Acad Dermatol 23:689–693, 1990

30. Van den Haute V, Antoine JL, Lachapelle JM: Histopathological discriminant criteria between lichenoid drug eruption and idiopathic lichen planus: retrospective study on selected samples. Dermatologica 179:10–13, 1989

31. Farmer ER: Human cutaneous graft-versus-host disease. J Invest Dermatol (suppl. 1) 85:124s–128s, 1985

32. Friedman KJ, LeBoit PE, Farmer ER: Acute follicular graft-vs-host reaction. A distinct clinicopathologic presentation. Arch Dermatol 124:688–691, 1988

33. Bauer DJ, Hood AF, Horn TD: Histologic comparison of autologous graft-vs-host reaction and cutaneous eruption of lymphocyte recovery. Arch Dermatol 129:855–858, 1993

34. Sale GE, Shulman HM, Gallucci BB, Thomas ED: Young rete ridge keratinocytes are preferred targets in cutaneous graft-versus-host disease. Am J Pathol 118:278–287, 1985

35. Murphy GF, Lavker RM, Whitaker D, Korngold R: Cytotoxic folliculitis in GvHD. Evidence of follicular stem cell injury and recovery. J Cutan Pathol 18:309–314, 1991

36. Sale GE, Anderson P, Browne M, Myerson D: Evidence of cytotoxic T-cell destruction of epidermal cells in human graft vs-host disease. Immunohistology with monoclonal antibody TIA-1. Arch Pathol Lab Med 116:622–625, 1992

37. Favre A, Cerri A, Bacigalupo A et al: Immunohistochemical study of skin lesions in acute and chronic graft versus host disease following bone marrow transplantation. Am J Surg Pathol 21:23–34, 1997

38. Uitto J, Santa-Cruz DJ, Eisen AZ, Leone P: Verrucous lesions in patients with discoid lupus erythematosus. Clinical, histopathological and immunofluorescence studies. Br J Dermatol 98:507–520, 1978

39. Millard LG, Rowell NR: Chilblain lupus erythematosus (Hutchinson). A clinical and laboratory study of 17 patients. Br J Dermatol 98:497–506, 1978

40. Clark WH, Reed RJ, Mihm MC: Lupus erythematosus. Histopathology of cutaneous lesions. Hum Pathol 4:157–163, 1973

41. Su WP, Perniciaro C, Rogers R Sr, White JW Jr: Chilblain lupus erythematosus (lupus pernio): clinical review of the Mayo Clinic experience and proposal of diagnostic criteria. Cutis 54:395–399, 1994

42. Kind P, Lehmann P, Plewig G: Phototesting in lupus erythematosus. J Invest Dermatol 100:53S–57S, 1993

43. Herrero C, Bielsa I, Font J et al: Subacute cutaneous lupus erythematosus: clinicopathologic findings in thirteen cases. J Am Acad Dermatol 19:1057–1062, 1988

44. Jerdan MS, Hood AF, Moore GW, Callen JP: Histopathologic comparison of the subsets of lupus erythematosus [see comments]. Arch Dermatol 126:52–55, 1990

45. Lowe L, Rapini RP, Golitz LE, Johnson TM: Papulonodular dermal mucinosis in lupus erythematosus. J Am Acad Dermatol 27:312–315, 1992

46. Rongioletti F, Parodi A, Rebora A: Papular and nodular mucinosis as a sign of lupus erythematosus. Dermatologica 180:221–223, 1990

47. Toonstra J, Wildschut A, Boer J et al: Jessner's lymphocytic infiltration of the skin. A clinical study of 100 patients. Arch Dermatol 125:1525–1530, 1989

48. Farmer ER, Provost TT: Immunologic studies of skin biopsy specimens in connective tissue diseases. Hum Pathol 14:316–325, 1983

49. de Jong EM, van Erp PE, Ruiter DJ, van de Kerkhof PC: Immunohistochemical detection of proliferation and differentiation in discoid lupus erythematosus. J Am Acad Dermatol 25:1032–1038, 1991

50. Hanno R, Callen JP: Histopathology of Gottron's papules. J Cutan Pathol 12:389–394, 1985

51. Crowson AN, Magro CM: The role of microvascular injury in

the pathogenesis of cutaneous lesions of dermatomyositis. Hum Pathol 27:15–19, 1996

52. Gianotti R, Restano L, Grimalt R et al: Lichen striatus–a chameleon: an histopathological and immunohistological study of forty-one cases. J Cutan Pathol 22:18–22, 1995

53. Masouye I, Saurat JH: Keratosis lichenoides chronica: the centenary of another Kaposi's disease. Dermatology 191: 188–192, 1995

54. Barnhill RL, Braverman IM: Progression of pigmented purpura-like eruptions to mycosis fungoides: report of three cases. J Am Acad Dermatol 19:25–31, 1988

55. Toro JR, LeBoit PE: Persistent pigmented purpuric dermatitis and mycosis fungoides. Precursor, simulant, or both? Am J Dermatopathol 19:108–118, 1997

56. Aiba S, Tagami H: Immunohistologic studies in Schamberg's disease. Evidence for cellular immune reaction in lesional skin. Arch Dermatol 124:1058–1062, 1988

57. Abell E, Marks R, Jones EW: Secondary syphilis: a clinicopathological review. Br J Dermatol 93:53–61, 1975

58. Alessi E, Innocenti M, Ragusa G: Secondary syphilis. Clinical morphology and histopathology. Am J Dermatopathol 5:11–17, 1983

59. Jordaan HF: Secondary syphilis. A clinicopathological study. Am J Dermatopathol 10:399–409, 1988

60. Jeerapaet P, Ackerman AB: Histologic patterns of secondary syphilis. Arch Dermatol 107:373–377, 1973

61. Jordaan HF, Cilliers J: Secondary syphilis mimicking Sweet's syndrome. Br J Dermatol 115:495–496, 1986

62. Lapins NA, Willoughby C, Helwig EB: Lichen nitidus. A study of forty-three cases. Cutis 21:634–637, 1978

63. Meffert JJ, Davis BM, Grimwood RE: Lichen sclerosus. J Am Acad Dermatol 32:393–418, 1995

64. Clemmensen OJ, Krogh J, Petri M: The histologic spectrum of prepuces from patients with phimosis. Am J Dermatopathol 10:104–108, 1988

65. Mihara Y, Mihara M, Hagari Y, Shimao S: Lichen sclerosus et atrophicus. A histological, immunohistochemical and electron microscopic study. Arch Dermatol Res 286:434–442, 1994

66. Vennos EM, Collins M, James WD: Rothmund-Thomson syndrome: review of the world literature. J Am Acad Dermatol 27:750–762, 1992

67. Person JR, Bishop GF: Is poikiloderma a graft-versus-host-like reaction? Am J Dermatopathol 6:71–72, 1984

68. de Koning J, Tazelaar DJ, Hoogkamp-Korstanje JA, Elema JD: Acrodermatitis chronica atrophicans: a light and electron microscopic study. J Cutan Pathol 22:23–32, 1995

69. Barranco VP: Multiple benign lichenoid keratoses simulating photodermatoses: evolution from senile lentigines and their spontaneous regression. J Am Acad Dermatol 13:201–206, 1985

70. Frigy AF, Cooper PH: Benign lichenoid keratosis. Am J Clin Pathol 83:439–443, 1985

71. Berger TG, Graham JH, Goette DK: Lichenoid benign keratosis. J Am Acad Dermatol 11:635–638, 1984

6

DERMATITIS WITH SPONGIOSIS

DEFINITION AND CONCEPT OF SPONGIOSIS

The term *spongiosis* is usually used to describe intercellular edema of the stratified squamous epithelium of the skin and mucous membranes. This concept is not completely accurate because intercellular edema is only one component of spongiosis, albeit an important one. Spongiosis is not simply due to the passive diffusion of water into the extracellular space of the epidermis, but rather it is a manifestation of a complex inflammatory reaction that is taking place there. Trafficking of lymphocytes occurs continuously in the epidermis as part of immune surveillance. In allergic contact dermatitis, the prototype of spongiotic reactions, the primary effector cell is the sensitized T lymphocyte. Therefore, there can be no spongiosis without lymphocytes in the epidermis to initiate the reaction. Once this reaction has been initiated, various cytokines are secreted by leukocytes and epithelial cells that augment the inflammatory reaction and can damage epithelial cells. As the spongiotic reaction evolves, there is not only intercellular edema but also exocytosis of leukocytes and intracellular edema because of injury to keratinocyte membranes.

In the early stages of spongiosis, the epidermal cells are separated by interstitial fluid. Their desmosomes initially remain intact so intercellular bridges appear more prominent. At this stage, few leukocytes are present, but, in time, they become numerous. With increasing severity, the intercellular spaces widen, and eventually the desmosomes rupture. Some keratinocytes become acantholytic, whereas others swell because of damage to their cell walls and may even burst. This combination of inter- and intracellular edema, cell separation, and cell rupture leads to the formation of vesicles within the epidermis (Fig. 6-1). Coalescence of small vesicles leads to the formation of larger unilocular or multilocular spaces that contain interstitial fluid, leukocytes, Langerhans cells, and keratinocytes. In the multiloculated vesicles, the various-sized spaces are separated by the compressed cell walls of ruptured keratinocytes (Fig. 6-2). This gives them a net-like appearance referred to as *reticular degeneration.*

Spongiosis is most commonly seen in the dermatitis reaction. Although the term *dermatitis* can legitimately be applied to almost any inflammation of the skin, it is usually reserved for those pruritic eruptions that begin with erythematous, edematous papules and plaques in which vesicles develop. This group of conditions is also often confusingly and inconsistently referred to as *eczema* or *eczematous dermatitis.* Whereas many dermatologists use the words *dermatitis* and *eczema* interchangeably, *eczema* conjures up different concepts and images to different dermatologists depending on their school of thought. Therefore, it seems more appropriate to use *dermatitis* as a generic term for this set of inflammatory dermatoses and to use modifiers to designate the specific type of dermatitis (e.g., allergic contact dermatitis, stasis dermatitis, nummular dermatitis).

EVOLUTIONARY CHANGES

The spectrum of the clinical manifestations of dermatitis ranges from acute to chronic. In acute dermatitis, all cardinal signs and symptoms of inflammation are present, such as erythema, edema, local warmth, and pain or itching. The spongiotic reaction is manifested initially as minute papules, then as papulovesicles, and ultimately as vesicles and/or bullae that usually break and exude fluid. If the stimulus that caused the dermatitis (e.g., an allergen applied to the skin of a sensitized person) is only transient, the edema and erythema resolves and leaves collarettes of scale and small crusts as residue. If the stimulus persists, then the dermatitis evolves through the subacute to the chronic stage. This phenomenon is called *hardening* in the case of allergic contact dermatitis. The affected skin remains erythematous and becomes progressively thickened. Weeping vesicles are superseded by crust and scales, and eventually the skin becomes lichenified from chronic rubbing.

These evolutionary changes have histopathologic correlates. As the dermatitis reaction persists, the epidermis responds by proliferating and becomes increasingly more hyperplastic. The stratum corneum is also thickened and demonstrates orthokeratosis, parakeratosis, and scale-crusts. Spongiosis diminishes as

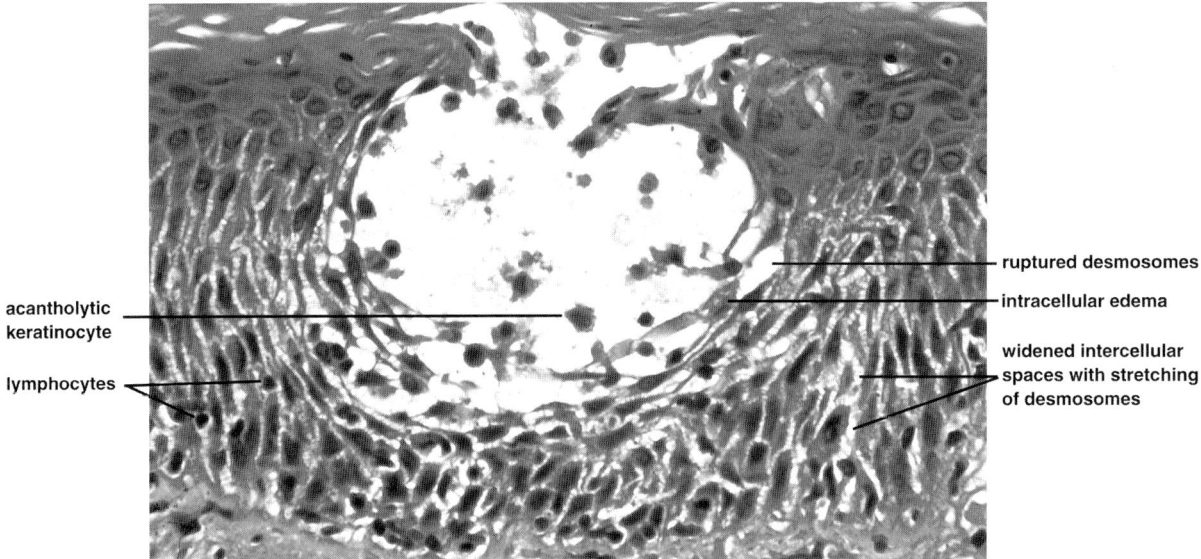

Figure 6-1. Acute spongiotic vesicle. Within the vesicle there are mononuclear inflammatory cells and acantholytic squamous cells. Immediately adjacent to the vesicle, there is prominent intercellular edema indicated by the widening of the intercellular spaces with stretching of the desmosomes. Eventual rupture of the desmosomes can lead to acantholysis.

the epidermis proliferates and may be slight or absent in long-lived lesions. Thus, the acute spongiotic picture that is typical of acute dermatitis changes to the psoriasiform picture seen in chronic dermatitis.

CONTACT DERMATITIS

Contact dermatitis is an inflammatory skin response to substances in the environment. There are two types of contact dermatitis, primary irritant and allergic. Primary irritant dermatitis is caused by the direct noxious effect of a chemical such as an acid, alkali, or organic solvent on the epidermis. All persons exposed to these agents in sufficient concentration for an adequate time subsequently develop an inflammatory response. In allergic contact dermatitis, a person must first be sensitized to an allergen before any inflammatory reaction is mediated by the mechanism of delayed hypersensitivity. Systemic allergic contact-type dermatitis can occur if a person who has become sensitized to an allergen by external exposure subsequently has the same or an immunochemically similar allergen administered systemically.

Phototoxic dermatitis occurs when a chemical substance contacts the skin that, on exposure to the proper wavelength of ultraviolet light, causes damage to the epidermal cells. Phototoxic dermatitis, therefore, is similar to primary irritant contact dermatitis in that both result in epidermal necrosis. Photoallergic dermatitis, by contrast, is pathogenically similar to allergic contact dermatitis, but the antigen must be acted on by the appropriate wavelength of ultraviolet light before it becomes an allergen. As in the case of systemic contact-type dermatitis, both phototoxic and photoallergic dermatitis can be secondary to the systemic administration of the phototoxin or photoallergin.

Allergic Contact Dermatitis
Clinical Features

In acute allergic contact dermatitis there are multiple tiny vesicles at the site(s) of contact with the allergen. The involved areas are red, swollen, and warm. The diagnosis is often suggested by the distribution or configuration of the eruption. The distribution is often characteristic (e.g., a band around the waist from allergy to the elastic material in underwear). The lesional configuration can also be an important clue, such as in the case of poison ivy dermatitis in which there are linear streaks of vesicles on exposed areas. A history of possible contact with the suspected offending substance can often be obtained and the diagnosis confirmed by patch testing. Sometimes, however, clinical acumen must be used to suspect the cause; for example, eyelid dermatitis is often due to touching the periorbital skin with an allergen on the hands. The allergen may not be potent enough to cause inflammation on the thick volar skin but can on the thin skin of the eyelids.

If the diagnosis is quickly made and contact with the offending agent is avoided, the dermatitis resolves spontaneously. If the diagnosis is delayed and contact with the allergen persists, then the clinical features evolve to those of subacute and, ultimately, chronic dermatitis in which the early features of edema and vesiculation are replaced by crusting, scaling, and thickening of the erythematous skin.

In systemic contact-type dermatitis that results from systemic administration of an allergen to which a person has previously been sensitized by external exposure, the cutaneous reaction has a characteristic distribution pattern. There is a symmetric eruption of macules, papules, and papulovesicles with predilection for the antecubital fossae, axillae, eyelids, sides of the neck, and genitalia. This eruption can progress to exfoliative dermatitis.

Histopathologic Features

Allergic contact dermatitis is the prototype of spongiotic reactions. Because it can be induced in animal models as well as in humans, detailed studies of all phases of the reaction have been made. The earliest histopathologic changes occur in the papillary dermis. There is a moderately dense infiltrate, predominantly of lymphocytes and macrophages, around the vessels of the superficial plexus that is associated with interstitial edema of the papillary dermis. Eosinophils are often present at the site of reaction.

The earliest epidermal changes are intracellular edema and slight exocytosis of lymphocytes. Intercellular edema develops after intracellular edema, but it is limited by the desmosomes. Rupture of the keratinocyte membranes leads to widening of the extracellular spaces, cell death, and spongiotic vesiculation. Exocytosis of mononuclear cells increases with time. The vesicles contain interstitial fluid, inflammatory cells, and individual epidermal cells (Fig. 6-3). The stratum corneum maintains its normal basket-weave appearance in the acute phase of the reaction. The volume of the epidermis expands due to the intra- and intercellular edema.

In the subacute phase of the reaction, the epidermis becomes progressively more hyperplastic, and some spongiotic foci are pushed up into the stratum corneum where they form scale-crusts composed of parakeratotic squamous cells, pyknotic in-

Figure 6-2. Acute spongiotic vesicle showing reticular degeneration. **(A)** There are numerous vesicles within the epidermis that are separated by septa that vary in thickness. Some show rupture resulting in fusion of the microvesicles. Within the dermis is a moderately dense superficial perivascular inflammatory infiltrate of lymphocytes and eosinophils. **(B)** At higher magnification, exocytosis of inflammatory cells and intercellular edema in the lower epidermis are prominent. The microvesicles contain inflammatory cells and acantholytic squamous cells in addition to serum.

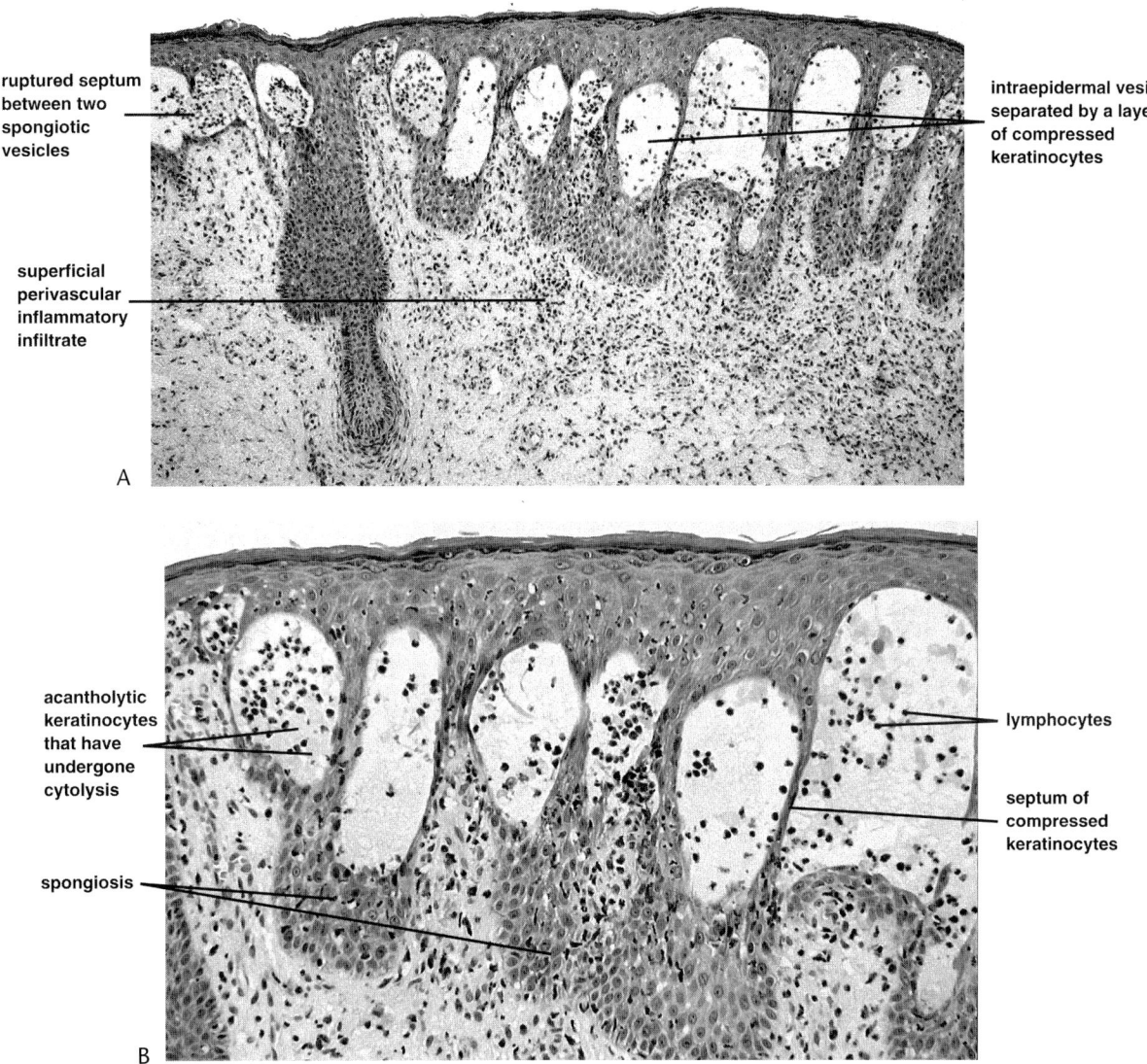

ruptured septum between two spongiotic vesicles

intraepidermal vesicle separated by a layer of compressed keratinocytes

superficial perivascular inflammatory infiltrate

A

acantholytic keratinocytes that have undergone cytolysis

lymphocytes

septum of compressed keratinocytes

spongiosis

B

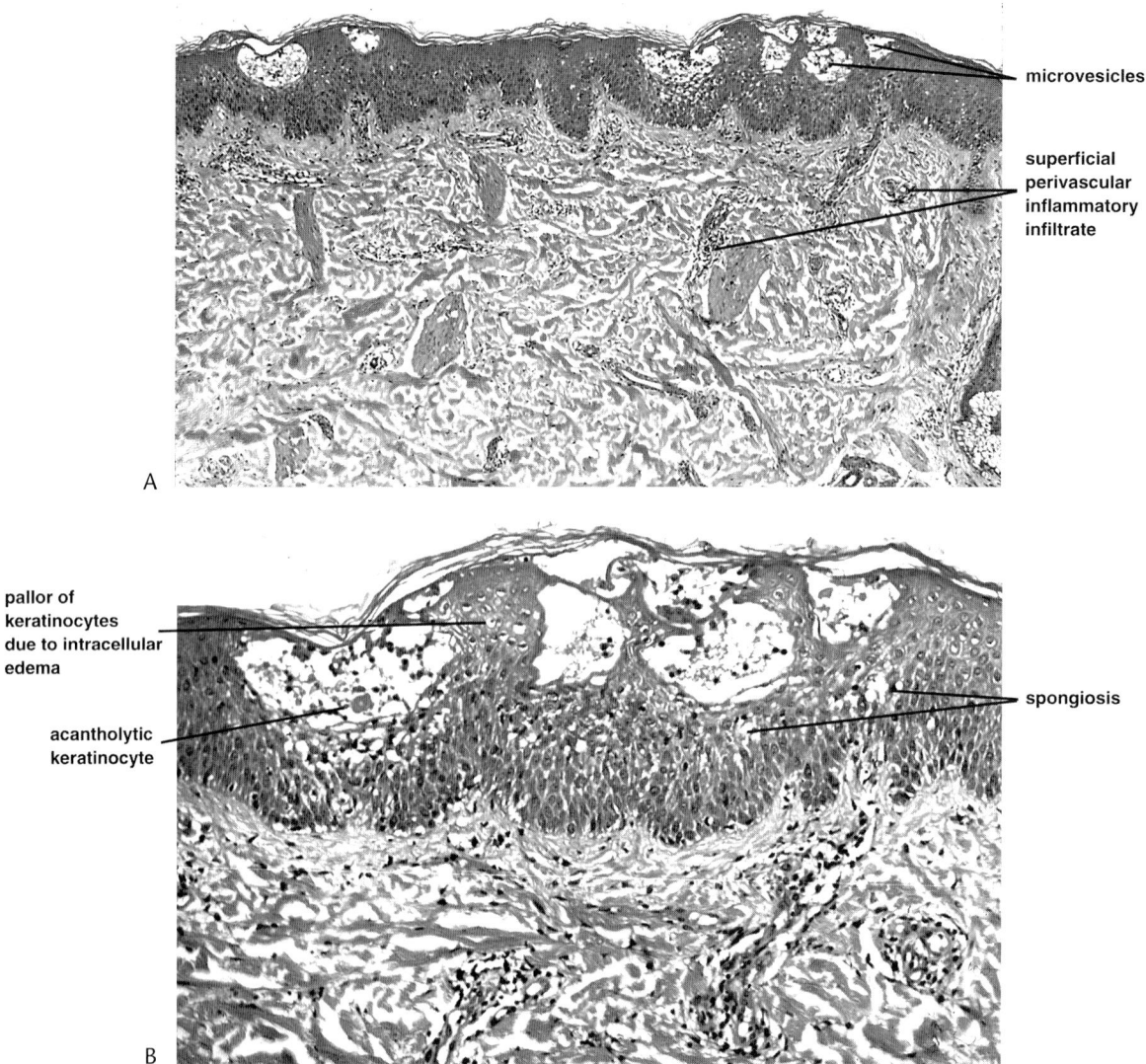

Figure 6-3. Acute allergic contact dermatitis. **(A)** At scanning magnification, several microvesicles are present within the upper half of the epidermis. There is a sparse superficial perivascular inflammatory cell infiltrate in the dermis. **(B)** At higher magnification, spongiosis is evident in the mid and lower epidermis below the vesicles. In addition to intercellular edema, many of the keratinocytes also demonstrate intracellular edema, which results in pallor of the cells. This is most evident in the squamous cells between the microvesicles.

flammatory cells, and interstitial fluid (Fig. 6-4). With the passage of time, if the allergen remains in contact with the skin, epidermal hyperplasia becomes the dominant histopathologic feature, and the amount of spongiosis diminishes. The cornified layer also becomes thickened, and there are foci of parakeratosis and some scale-crusts irregularly dispersed in the predominantly orthokeratotic stratum corneum. The papillary dermis also becomes hyperplastic. The tendency of the newly formed collagen bundles to follow the contour of the rete ridges gives the appearance of concentric lamellae. Their vertical orientation in the widened and elongated dermal papillae is often striking. Unlike psoriasis, the rete ridges in the hyperplastic epidermis are characteristically irregular in length and width.

Clinicopathologic Correlation

The initial clinical findings in allergic contact dermatitis are erythema and edema that are the result of vasodilation, hyperemia, and interstitial edema in the papillary dermis. This is followed by minute agminated vesicles and papulovesicles that result from spongiosis. Merging of the small vesicles can lead to large vesicles and bullae that may rupture and release their contents onto the surface. The scale-crusts and thickening of the skin during the subacute phase correlate with the elimination of the spongiotic foci into the stratum corneum and the reactive hyperplasia of the epidermis. The chronic phase of allergic contact dermatitis is characterized by scaling, fissuring, and increased thickening of the skin. This is due to ortho- and parakeratosis, progressively more marked epidermal hyperplasia, and papillary dermal fibrosis.

Pathophysiology

Allergic contact dermatitis is mediated by cellular immunity. It involves the presentation of an exogenous antigen by cutaneous Langerhans cells to primed T lymphocytes.[1] Keratinocytes, once thought to be immunologically irrelevant, also contribute actively to the inflammatory response. Keratinocytes bear receptors for many cytokines, including interleukin-1 (IL-1), tumor necrosis factor, interferon-γ, and intercellular adhesion molecules and are also capable of producing immunologically active cytokines that bind to receptors on target cells and mediate cell-specific events in the skin. The evolution of these immunologic processes that produce spongiosis is not known, but it can be presumed that a complex interaction of Langerhans cells, T lymphocytes, and keratinocytes is involved in epidermotropic T-cell diseases, and it is likely that endothelial cells, fibroblasts, and other immunologically active cells participate in the inflammatory process.[2]

Primary Irritant Dermatitis

Clinical Features

Primary irritant dermatitis usually cannot be distinguished from allergic contact dermatitis by inspection of the eruption. Red-

Figure 6-4. Subacute allergic contact dermatitis. **(A)** At scanning magnification, there are scale-crusts in the stratum corneum. The epidermis shows moderate but irregular hyperplasia with focal spongiosis. No spongiotic microvesicles are present. Within the dermis is a superficial perivascular inflammatory cell infiltrate. **(B)** At higher magnification, the inflammatory cells, serum and colonies of bacteria are present in the scale-crust. There is focal moderate spongiosis in the hyperplastic epidermis.

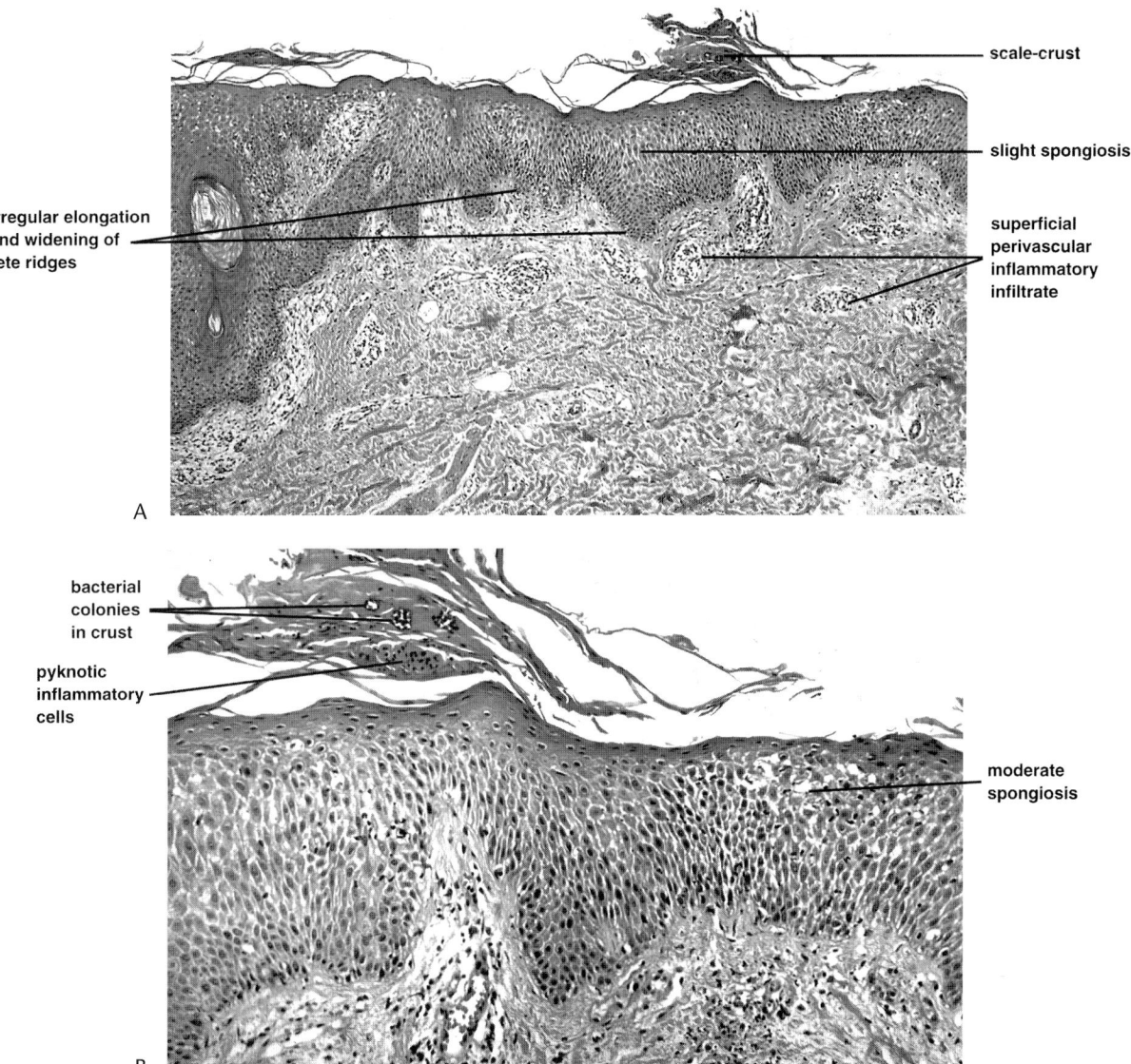

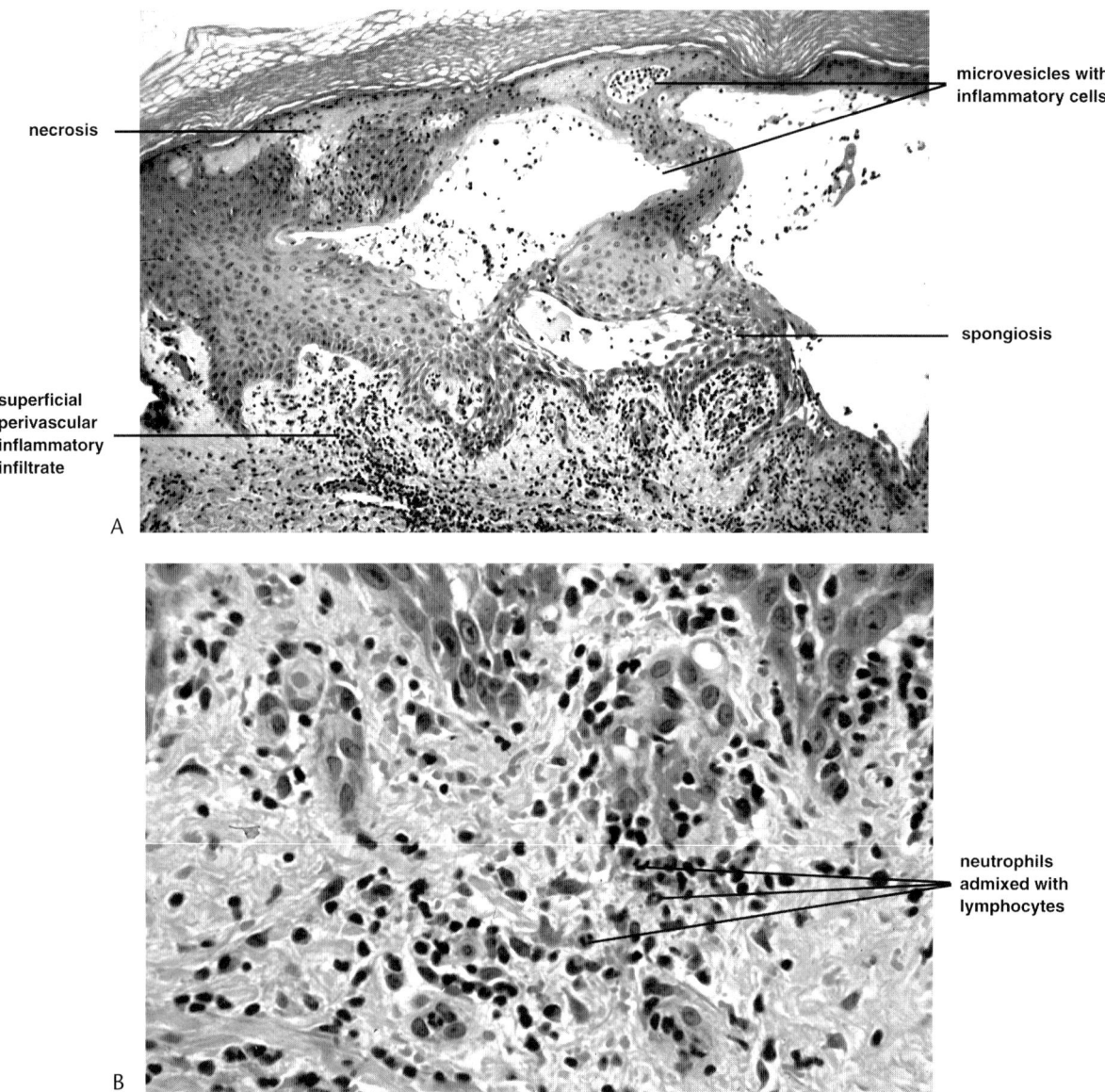

Figure 6-5. Primary irritant dermatitis. **(A)** This specimen from volar skin shows necrosis of keratinocytes in the superficial portion of the epidermis. There are spongiotic microvesicles in the stratum spinosum containing inflammatory cells, some of which are neutrophils. The papillary dermis shows prominent interstitial edema and there is a moderately dense superficial perivascular inflammatory cell infiltrate. **(B)** At higher magnification, the infiltrate consists predominantly of lymphocytes but also contains occasional neutrophils.

ness, edema, vesicles, and sometimes bullae are present, with a variable amount of pain or itching. The reaction occurs quickly after exposure, unlike allergic contact dermatitis, in which the onset is usually delayed for 1 or more days after exposure. The eruption is usually self-limited and disappears promptly if it results from a single exposure to an offending agent. Recurrence can be prevented, once the irritant is identified, by means of protective gloves or clothing, barrier creams, and washing after exposure. Soaps, detergents, acids, alkalis, and petroleum distillates such as kerosene and gasoline are common causes. The hands are most commonly involved.

Histopathologic Features

The most important aspect of irritant dermatitis is that the offending agent produces direct injury to the epidermis. An acid or alkali in sufficient concentration causes simple necrosis of the epidermis. Other less potent chemicals cause less severe degrees of damage. Sequential studies of primary irritant reactions in animal models have yielded different results depending on the agent used to incite the reaction and its concentration. Dinitrochlorobenzene at a relatively high concentration of 10% produces epidermal necrosis and subepidermal vesiculation with a dermal inflammatory infiltrate of neutrophils.[3] A 5% concentration produces intracellular and intercellular edema from the basal layer to the granular layer.[4]

In humans, depending on the chemical nature of the chemical applied, there are varying degrees of keratinocyte necrosis, intracellular and intercellular edema, and exocytosis of inflammatory cells, including neutrophils, lymphocytes, and macrophages[5] (Fig. 6-5). The dermis contains a superficial perivascular infiltrate of similar composition, interstitial edema, and vasodilation.

Photoallergic Dermatitis

Clinical Features

Photoallergic dermatitis is similar to allergic contact dermatitis except that the exogenous drug or chemical must be acted on by ultraviolet or visible light to produce a cutaneous immunologic response. Contact photoallergy occurs when the photoallergen is applied directly to the skin, whereas systemic photoallergy develops when the photoallergen, which in most instances is a drug, is administered parenterally. The cutaneous manifestations include acute, subacute, or chronic dermatitis with involvement of the hands and V-area of the neck and the face, but sparing the submental area, the upper eyelids, and the postauricular area. Occasionally, generalized erythroderma may result and the eruption may persist, although there is no further exposure to the causative allergen persistent light reaction (PLR).

Histopathologic Features

Photoallergic dermatitis has the same histopathologic features as allergic contact dermatitis at comparable points in its evolution and resolution (Fig. 6-6). In some instances, the inflammatory infiltrate is limited to the superficial reaction unit,[6] whereas

in others it extends into the lower reticular dermis.[7] Because ordinary allergic contact dermatitis only occasionally involves the middle or deep reticular dermis by an inflammatory cell infiltrate, a deep infiltrate favors photoallergy but cannot be considered a pathognomonic feature.

Phototoxic (Photoirritation) Dermatitis

Clinical Features

Light-induced damage to the skin that is not dependent on an allergic mechanism can be considered phototoxic. Theoretically, these reactions will occur in essentially anyone if the skin is exposed to enough light energy of the proper wavelength and enough molecules that absorb these wavelengths are present. Phototoxic reactions are characterized by erythema and edema that occurs within a few minutes to several hours after exposure followed by desquamation and pigmentary changes confined to the light-exposed areas. Sunburn is the prototype for phototoxic reactions, as it will occur in anyone exposed to a sufficient amount of ultraviolet B. Phototoxic reactions can be considered to be the light-induced equivalent of primary irritant dermatitis.

Histopathologic Features

The histopathologic features of acute phototoxic dermatitis may resemble those of acute primary irritant dermatitis. The epidermis shows intracellular and intercellular edema, nuclear pyknosis, and individual cell necrosis (sunburn cells) (Fig. 6-7). The extent of the epithelial cell degeneration is proportional to the severity of the reaction. In mild cases, there may only be haphazardly scattered necrotic cells in the spinous layer, whereas in severe cases there may be full thickness coagulation necrosis that simulates toxic epidermal necrolysis. There is a sparse to moderate superficial dermal infiltrate that may contain neu-

Figure 6-6. Photoallergic dermatitis. Photoallergic dermatitis, whether due to ingestion of a sensitizing medication or application of one to the skin, shows histopathologic features similar to those of allergic contact dermatitis. The epidermis shows spongiosis and spongiotic microvesicle formation. Within the dermis is a perivascular inflammatory cell infiltrate that extends into the reticular dermis and may involve the deep plexus in some cases.

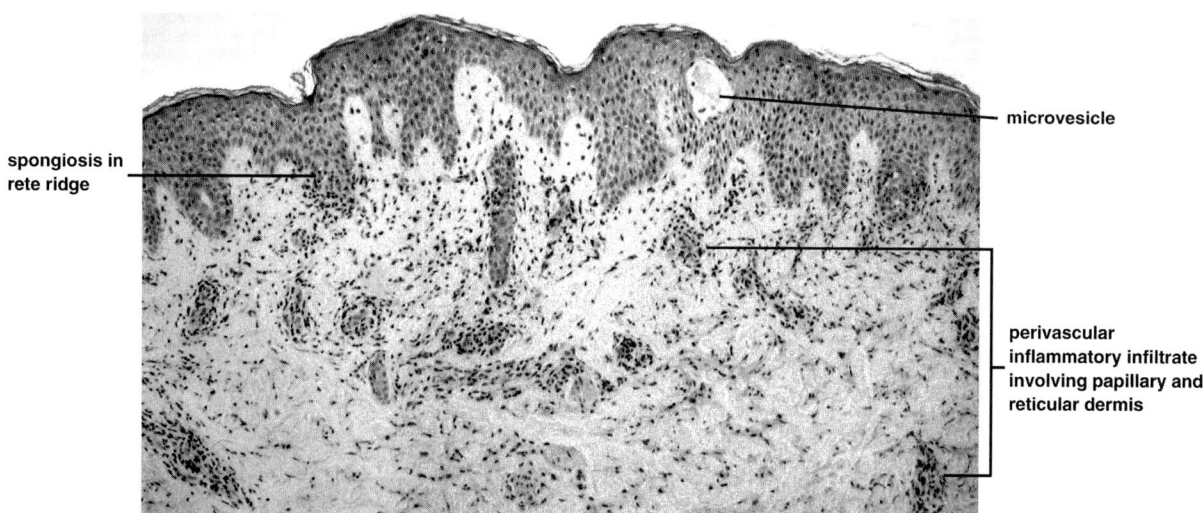

spongiosis in rete ridge

microvesicle

perivascular inflammatory infiltrate involving papillary and reticular dermis

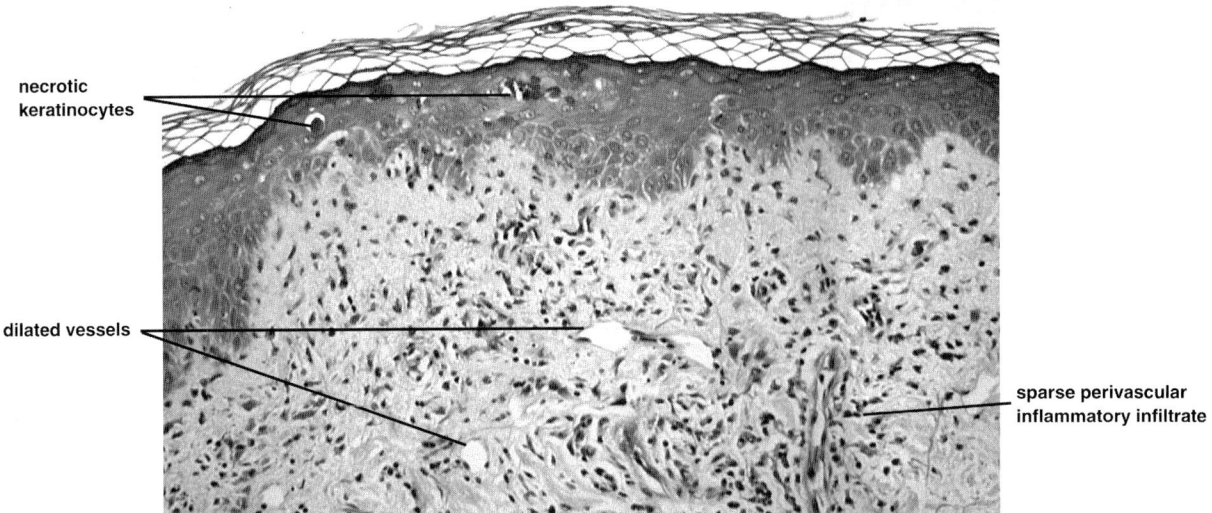

necrotic
keratinocytes

dilated vessels

sparse perivascular
inflammatory infiltrate

Figure 6-7. Phototoxic dermatitis. Within the epidermis there are numerous individual necrotic keratinocytes. These cells have dark-staining cytoplasm and pyknotic or absent nuclei. In the lower epidermis there is mild intercellular edema and slight exocytosis of inflammatory cells focally. The papillary dermis shows a sparse inflammatory cell infiltrate, vascular dilation, and interstitial edema.

trophils in addition to mononuclear cells. In a few days, regenerative changes begin in the lower epidermis, and the damaged epidermis is eventually cast off. Spongiosis may be seen in the regenerating epidermis.

NONCONTACT DERMATITIDES

Atopic Dermatitis

Clinical Features

Atopic dermatitis is a disorder of unknown etiology, but it is related to allergic rhinitis and asthma as approximately 50% of patients have allergic respiratory disease. In infancy, the face is almost always involved, and the diaper area and extensor surfaces of the extremities are frequently affected. The disease in infants is characterized by plaques of erythema, edema, small vesicles, crusts, and occasional pustules. There is circumoral sparing and pallor. In later childhood, the classic sites of involvement include the antecubital and popliteal fossae, the volar aspect of the wrist, and the neck. Some areas become lichenified, and excoriations and crusted papules are often present. In adults, the distribution is the same but lichenification is the characteristic clinical manifestation and weeping, crusted lesions are rare. Severe pruritus is the hallmark of atopic dermatitis at any age. About 80% of affected persons have an elevated IgE level; thus, an elevated IgE level is a helpful but not a specific finding. Hanifin and Rajka[8] have proposed diagnostic criteria for diagnosis.

Histopathologic Features

The histopathologic features depend on the type of lesion that is biopsied. The disease begins as an acute spongiotic process that progresses into subacute and eventually chronic stages as in other types of persistent spongiotic dermatitis. Hurwitz and Detrana[9]

studied the evolution of lesions in adult patients. The early, eruptive lesions were 1 to 2 mm erythematous, dome-shaped papules. These papules coalesced to form lichenified plaques. The early edematous papules exhibited basket-weave orthokeratosis and spongiosis in the epidermis and a superficial perivascular and interstitial infiltrate of mononuclear cells, eosinophils, and neutrophils. The lichenified plaques showed the typical changes of lichen simplex chronicus (Fig. 6-8), and the intermediate lesions showed psoriasiform hyperplasia of the epidermis with prominent spongiosis and frequent microvesiculation. One of 16 patients also had lichenoid papules that histopathologically exhibited interface changes, a change noted previously by Prose and Sedlis.[10] Mihm et al[11] studied the clinically normal skin of persons with atopic dermatitis in addition to lesional skin by use of 1-μm sections of plastic-embedded tissue. They found that the normal-appearing skin showed minimal epidermal hyperplasia, intercellular edema, and dermal cellular infiltrates that reflected either subclinical disease or residual involvement. Their findings in lesional skin were similar to those of others.[9,10]

Nummular Dermatitis

Clinical Features

The classic lesions of nummular eczema are coin-shaped, well-demarcated, erythematous plaques that may be vesicular and edematous or dry and scaly depending on the stage of the disease. They begin as papules and papulovesicles that coalesce to form plaques. The vesicles burst, leaving scale-crusts. Older lesions may exhibit a peripheral collarette of scale. There may be only one or two lesions, but some persons develop many. The dorsum of the forearms and hands and the anterior thighs and legs are most commonly affected. Nummular dermatitis occurs in middle-aged and older persons, especially those with dry skin, and pursues a torpid course. The cause is unknown.

Histopathologic Features

The histopathologic picture of nummular dermatitis mimics allergic contact dermatitis at comparable points in its evolution. These conditions can be differentiated only by clinical correlation.

Pityriasis Alba

Clinical Features

Pityriasis alba is a distinctive discoid dermatitis that occurs in children and occasionally in adolescents and young adults. There is no gender predilection. There are usually only one or two lesions, but some persons have many. The initial lesion is a faintly erythematous round macule with indistinct borders. As the erythema fades, the involved skin becomes lighter than the adjacent skin, and a fine branny scale develops on its surface. The lesions measure about 0.5 to 3 cm in diameter and are usually asymptomatic but may be slightly pruritic. Lesions most often occur on the face, although any body area can be affected. The lesions gradually improve and eventually become repigmented in most persons. Pityriasis alba may or may not be associated with an atopic diathesis.

Histopathologic Features

Pityriasis alba is a mild form of spongiotic dermatitis. Well-developed lesions show mild to moderate orthokeratosis, and

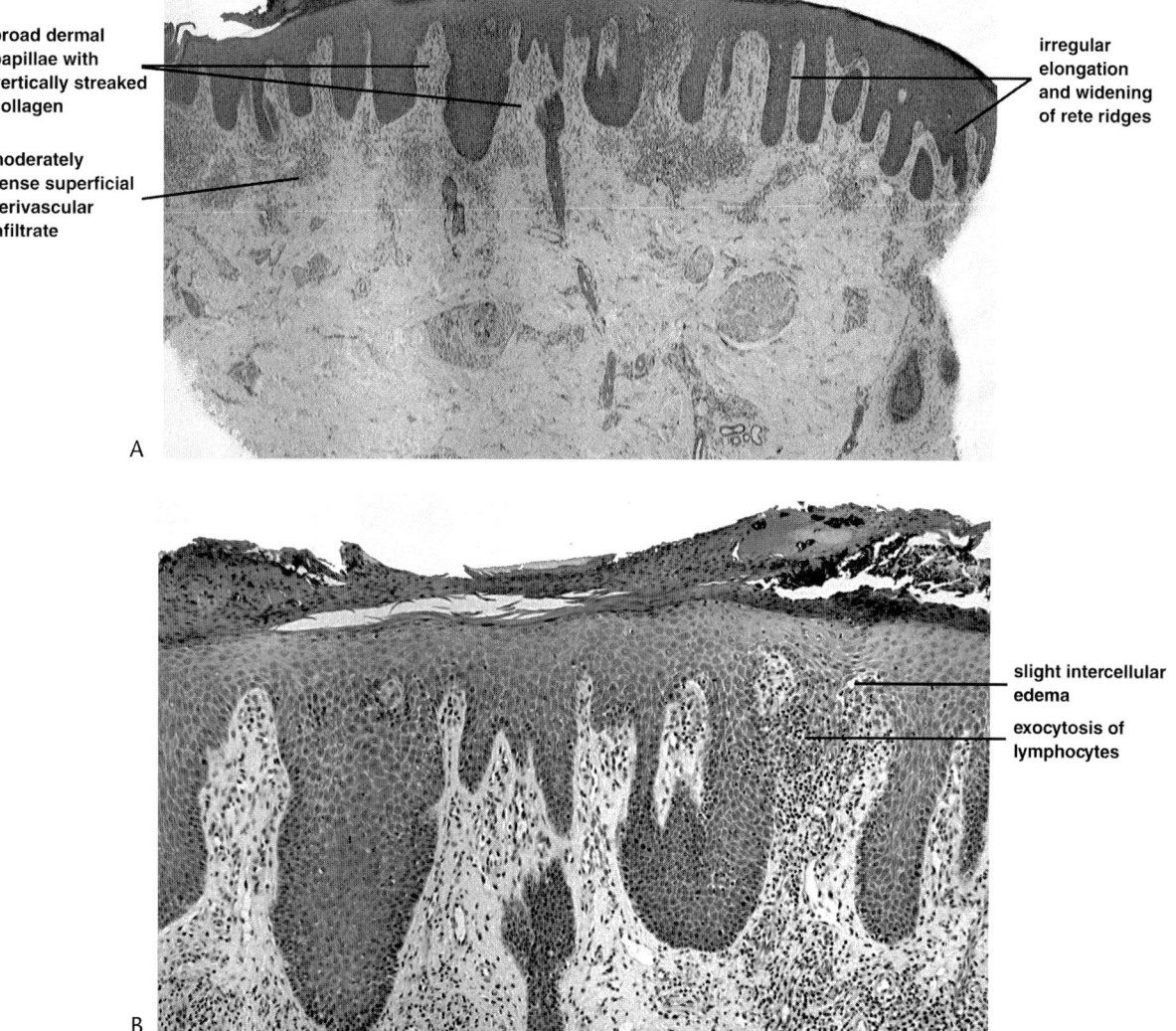

Figure 6-8. Atopic dermatitis. **(A)** At scanning magnification, the epidermis shows prominent but somewhat irregular hyperplasia. There is extensive scale-crust formation on the surface. The papillary dermis is altered as evidenced by widening of dermal papillae with vertical streaking of the collagen due to chronic rubbing. There is a moderately dense superficial perivascular infiltrate of lymphocytes and eosinophils. **(B)** At higher magnification, fairly prominent exocytosis of lymphocytes and slight intercellular edema are evident.

scale-crust

broad dermal papillae with vertically streaked collagen

irregular elongation and widening of rete ridges

moderately dense superficial perivascular infiltrate

A

slight intercellular edema

exocytosis of lymphocytes

B

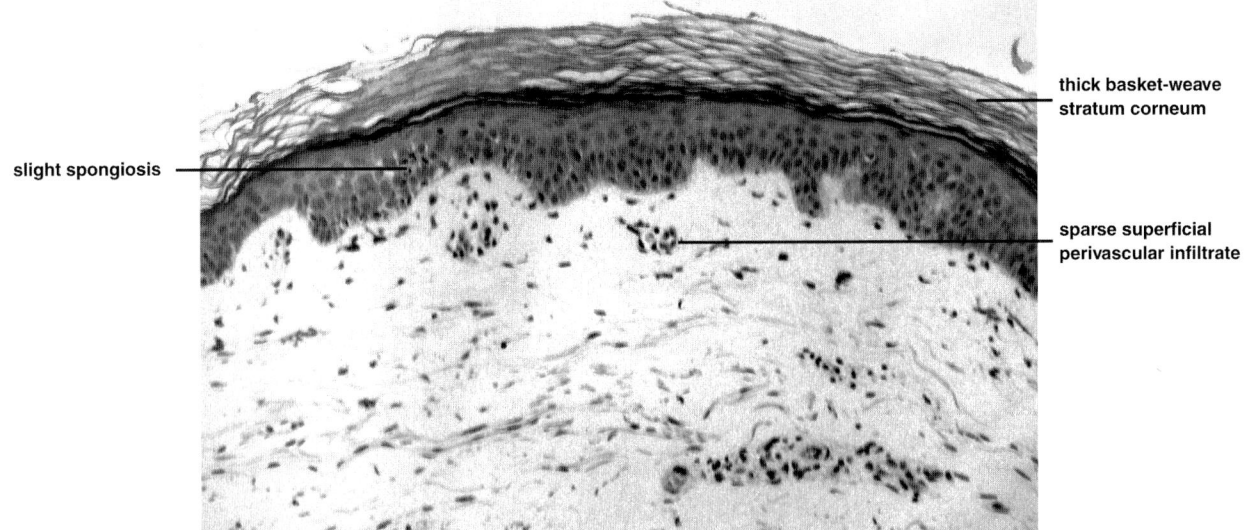

slight spongiosis

thick basket-weave stratum corneum

sparse superficial perivascular infiltrate

Figure 6-9. Pityriasis alba. Pityriasis alba is a mild spongiotic dermatitis that usually exhibits basket-weave orthohyperkeratosis. Note that in this specimen, the stratum corneum is approximately the same thickness as the viable epidermis. This type of stratum corneum may also be seen in tinea versicolor, which also has a branny scale. There is mild focal spongiosis in the lower epidermis, and there is a sparse superficial perivascular mononuclear cell inflammatory infiltrate in the dermis.

some show focal parakeratosis. There is slight spongiosis, mild papillary dermal edema, and a sparse superficial perivascular mononuclear cell infiltrate (Fig. 6-9). A few melanophages may be present in the papillary dermis, and the amount of pigment in the basal layer is less than in the normal adjacent epidermis. In extensive cases there is a reduced number of functionally active melanocytes in the basal layer in affected areas, but there does not appear to be a problem in melanosome transfer.[12]

Dyshidrotic Dermatitis

Clinical Features

This condition is characterized by an acute or subacute dermatitis localized to the hands or feet, or both. The sides of the fingers, the palms, and the soles are affected. The primary lesions are discrete whitish vesicles, and the surrounding skin appears normal. Once the vesicles rupture, brownish scales or collarettes develop. Most patients complain of itching and burning as the vesicles erupt. The lesions tend to come in crops, and the condition waxes and wanes, sometimes for decades.

The cause of dyshidrotic dermatitis is not known. It often is associated with hyperhidrosis, and, in some persons, with emotional upsets. Although clinically associated with hyperhidrosis, the acrosyringium is not histologically involved in the vesicular process, so the term *dyshidrosis* is a misnomer. Oral provocation with nickel in some patients suggests that dyshidrotic dermatitis may represent a form of systemic contact-type dermatitis in some persons who have become sensitized to nickel by prior topical exposure.[13]

Histopathologic Features

The clue to the diagnosis of dyshidrotic dermatitis is a spongiotic reaction in volar skin. The spongiotic reaction is morphologically the same as in allergic contact dermatitis (Fig. 6-10), but it is unusual for allergic contact dermatitis to occur on volar skin because of the barrier to penetration of allergens that is provided to these areas by their thick compact stratum corneum. The intraepidermal portion of the eccrine ducts is not altered by spongiosis.[14]

Id Reaction

Clinical Features

Id reactions characteristically occur on the hands of persons who have inflammatory tinea pedis. It is manifested as discrete vesicles and papulovesicles on the palms, sides of the fingers, and commonly on the dorsum of the hands. When present, involvement of the dorsum of the hands is a useful clue to distinguish id reactions from dyshidrosis. There is usually little, if any, erythema surrounding the papules and vesicles.

Histopathologic Features

Id reactions are histologically identical to dyshidrosis and to allergic contact dermatitis. Dermatophyte organisms are not present in the epidermis; this distinguishes id reactions from vesicular dermatophyte infections.

Stasis Dermatitis

Clinical Features

Stasis dermatitis involves the legs of persons with chronic venous insufficiency, especially those who have had deep venous thrombosis or chronic edema from other causes. Women are affected much more often than men. The legs are edematous and usually show hemosiderin staining. The dermatitis is usually situated on the medial aspect of the leg above the malleolus. It begins as poorly marginated areas of erythema that become scaly, fissured, and crusted. Ulcers may develop secondary to scratching or other trauma. In patients with severe disease, particularly those who have ulcers and superimposed infection, autosensitization dermatitis can develop. This condition morphologically resembles nummular dermatitis.[15] It first appears on the leg around the area affected by stasis, but it can spread to other areas of the body. In exceptional cases it progresses to exfoliative dermatitis. Another unusual condition that may develop in persons with venous insufficiency is acroangiodermatitis.[16,17] It has also been observed in persons with arteriovenous malformations of the leg and in paralyzed limbs. In this disorder there are purple papules and nodules on the extensor surface of the foot or toes. The lesions can resemble the nodules of Kaposi's sarcoma, and, because both conditions are associated with edema, examination of a biopsy specimen may be necessary to distinguish between them. A helpful clinical clue is that Kaposi's sarcoma exhibits polymorphous lesions (i.e., patches, plaques, and nodules), whereas acroangiodermatitis consists only of papules and occasional nodules.

Histopathologic Features

The most important histopathologic features of stasis dermatitis are found in the dermis. The vessels of the leg have thicker walls than those on the nondependent areas of the body. In persons with venous stasis, the persistent venous hypertension produces additional thickening of the walls of the small veins and venules. Moreover, the vessels become tortuous and form glomerular tufts that, when viewed in two-dimensional tissue sections, appear as clusters of thick-walled venules in the subepidermal region (Fig. 6-11). There usually are extravasated red blood cells and siderophages in the edematous papillary and upper reticular dermis in addition to a perivascular inflammatory infiltrate of variable density. The infiltrate consists of lymphocytes and macrophages unless there is epidermal ulceration or secondary infection (or both). Eosinophils are not present unless there is a coincidental allergic contact dermatitis to a topical medication used to treat the dermatitis.

The epidermis may exhibit a spectrum of changes. In relatively early lesions, there may be spongiosis and variable epidermal hyperplasia with parakeratosis or scale-crusts. In persistent lesions, there may be erosions or ulcers, and there may be superimposed lichen simplex chronicus from chronic rubbing. The ulcers may heal and leave fibrosis and siderosis in the dermis. In acroangiodermatitis, the most striking feature is clusters of thick-walled vessels in the upper and middle dermis. This is actually an accentuation of the vascular changes that occur in all persons with chronic venous insufficiency. The other histopathologic features are identical to stasis change. The vessels maintain regular round to oval contours, which is the most helpful feature to distinguish acroangiodermatitis from early lesions of Kaposi's sarcoma in which the vessels have irregular, jagged shapes.[17]

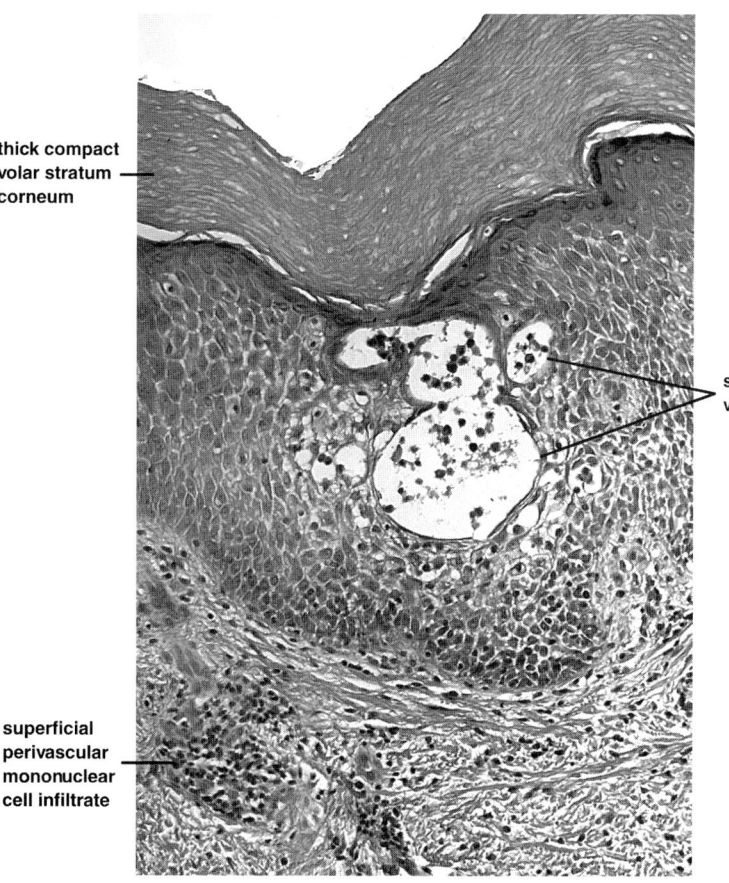

thick compact volar stratum corneum

spongiotic vesicles

superficial perivascular mononuclear cell infiltrate

Figure 6-10. Dyshidrotic dermatitis. The major histopathologic clue to the diagnosis of dyshidrotic dermatitis is recognizing the volar stratum corneum. The resistance to breakage of the vesicles is due to the thick compact stratum corneum. Otherwise, the spongiotic reaction within the epidermis is similar to that seen in allergic contact dermatitis, although eosinophils are usually not present in the infiltrate.

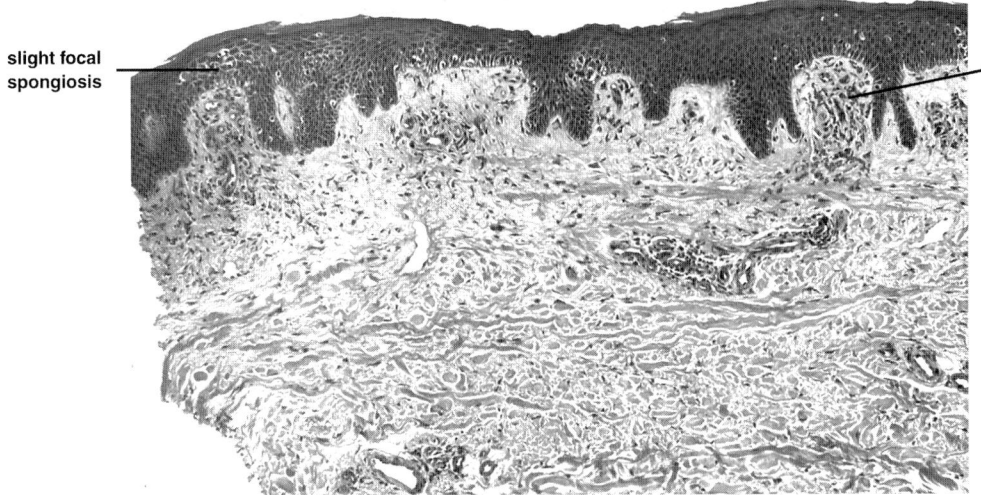

slight focal spongiosis

thick-walled tortuous capillaries in widened dermal papilla

Figure 6-11. Subacute stasis dermatitis. The epidermis shows irregular hyperplasia with mild focal spongiosis. The major clue to the diagnosis of stasis dermatitis is the presence of clusters of thick-walled capillaries and venules in the expanded dermal papillae. This results from venous hypertension in the lower extremities. Extravasation of erythrocytes and the presence of siderophages may also be helpful features.

Seborrheic Dermatitis

Clinical Features

Seborrheic dermatitis is the most common of the papulosquamous diseases, although paradoxically it has the histopathologic features of a spongiotic process. Its etiology is unknown, but it occurs in the areas of the skin that have the greatest number of and most active sebaceous glands (i.e., scalp, face, chest, back, axillae, and anogenital area). This suggests an abnormality of sebaceous gland metabolism, but other factors, possibly microbial, are almost surely involved. Severe, recalcitrant seborrheic dermatitis is a common cutaneous finding in acquired immunodeficiency syndrome.

The primary lesion is a papule with a pink or slightly yellow color. The papules may become confluent, forming plaques that

Figure 6-12. Acute seborrheic dermatitis. The focus of pathology is the epithelium surrounding the ostia of the pilosebaceous units. There is spongiosis at the edges of the follicular openings. The stratum corneum surrounding the ostia shows scale-crust formation. There are usually numerous neutrophils in the scale-crust. Within the dermal papillae there is vasodilation, and there is a sparse superficial perivascular infiltrate of lymphocytes and occasional neutrophils.

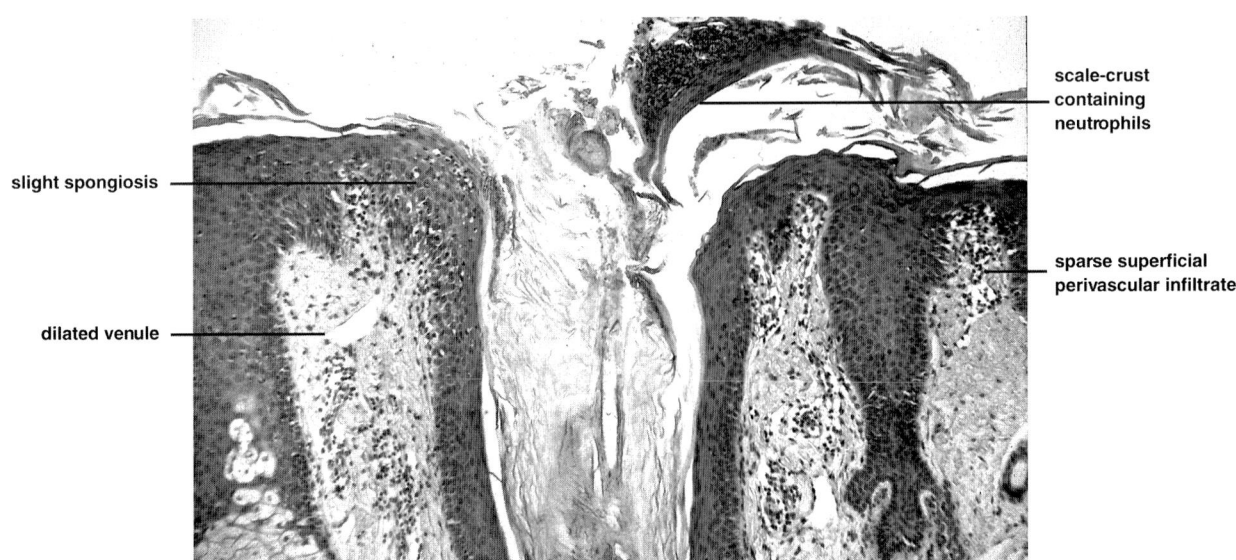

slight spongiosis

dilated venule

scale-crust containing neutrophils

sparse superficial perivascular infiltrate

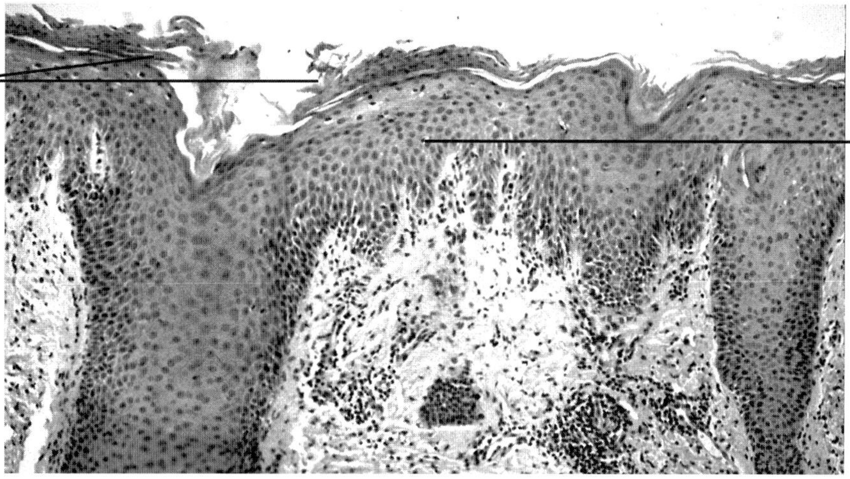

Figure 6-13. Subacute seborrheic dermatitis. In addition to the spongiosis and scale-crust surrounding the openings of the hair follicles, there may also be slight epidermal hyperplasia in the interfollicular regions of the epidermis with mild spongiotic change.

sometimes are polycyclic. The amount of scale is variable, and it usually has a greasy texture. Pityriasis capitis, a fine branny scaling of the scalp, commonly accompanies seborrheic dermatitis. Blepharitis may also be present.

Histopathologic Features

The earliest histopathologic manifestation of seborrheic dermatitis is dilation of the vessels of the superficial plexus and a sparse perivascular inflammatory cell infiltrate of lymphocytes, monocytes, and occasional neutrophils. It is not diagnosable at this stage. Eventually spongiosis develops in the epithelium of the upper portion of the follicular infundibula and the adjacent epidermis followed by the appearance of scale-crusts around the follicular openings (Fig. 6-12). Neutrophils are commonly present in the scale-crusts and in the spongiotic foci. This predilection for involvement of the upper follicular epithelium and perifollicular epidermis and the presence of neutrophils in the scale-crusts characterize seborrheic dermatitis.

In time, the interfollicular epidermis becomes irregularly thickened (Fig. 6-13). In the subacute and chronic phases, the parakeratosis and scale-crusts may also be present in the interfollicular epidermis. The neutrophils in the scale-crusts and the epidermal hyperplasia suggest psoriasis, but the irregular rather than regular elongation of the rete ridges, the tendency for the scale-crusts to be situated primarily around the follicular ostia, and the follicular and epidermal spongiosis distinguish seborrheic dermatitis from psoriasis.

Seborrheic dermatitis often accompanies acne vulgaris and rosacea. Dilation and keratin plugging of the follicular infundibula characterize acne vulgaris. The early histopathologic changes of rosacea are quite similar to those of early seborrheic dermatitis. In more advanced lesions of rosacea there are follicular pustules and perifollicular granulomas. Concomitant seborrheic dermatitis is indicated by the presence of scale-crusts around the follicular ostia.

Persons with acquired immunodeficiency syndrome may de-velop a seborrheic-like dermatitis that histopathologically differs from ordinary seborrheic dermatitis in a few important ways.[18] Individual necrotic keratinocytes are haphazardly scattered in the epidermis in early lesions. In later lesions, there is a tendency for more pronounced epidermal hyperplasia and more extensive parakeratosis and scale-crusts not necessarily limited to the parafollicular areas. Furthermore, the dermal infiltrate often contains numerous plasma cells, and the walls of the small blood vessels are thickened.

Pityriasis Rosea

Clinical Features

Pityriasis rosea is a papulosquamous disease of unknown etiology that, as in the case of seborrheic dermatitis, has spongiotic changes in the epidermis. It occurs with increasing frequency in the fall and the spring. Pityriasis rosea begins abruptly and resolves spontaneously after 6 to 12 weeks. Children and young adults are most often affected, but it can occur at any age; recurrences are rare.

Pityriasis rosea starts with a single red, scaly plaque called the *herald* or *mother* patch. A week or so later there is a secondary eruption of crops of scaly papules. The papules are oval and are distributed on the trunk and proximal extremities. Their long axes follow the lines of cleavage of the skin (so-called Christmas tree distribution). The papules typically have a collarette of scale near their margins with the free edge of the scale on the inner aspect. This scale is similar to the scale of erythema annulare centrifugum, both of which are due to the spongiotic reaction within the epidermis.

Histopathologic Features

Histopathologically there is focal mound-like parakeratosis, focal spongiosis (usually beneath the parakeratotic foci), slight epidermal hyperplasia, and a superficial perivascular infiltrate

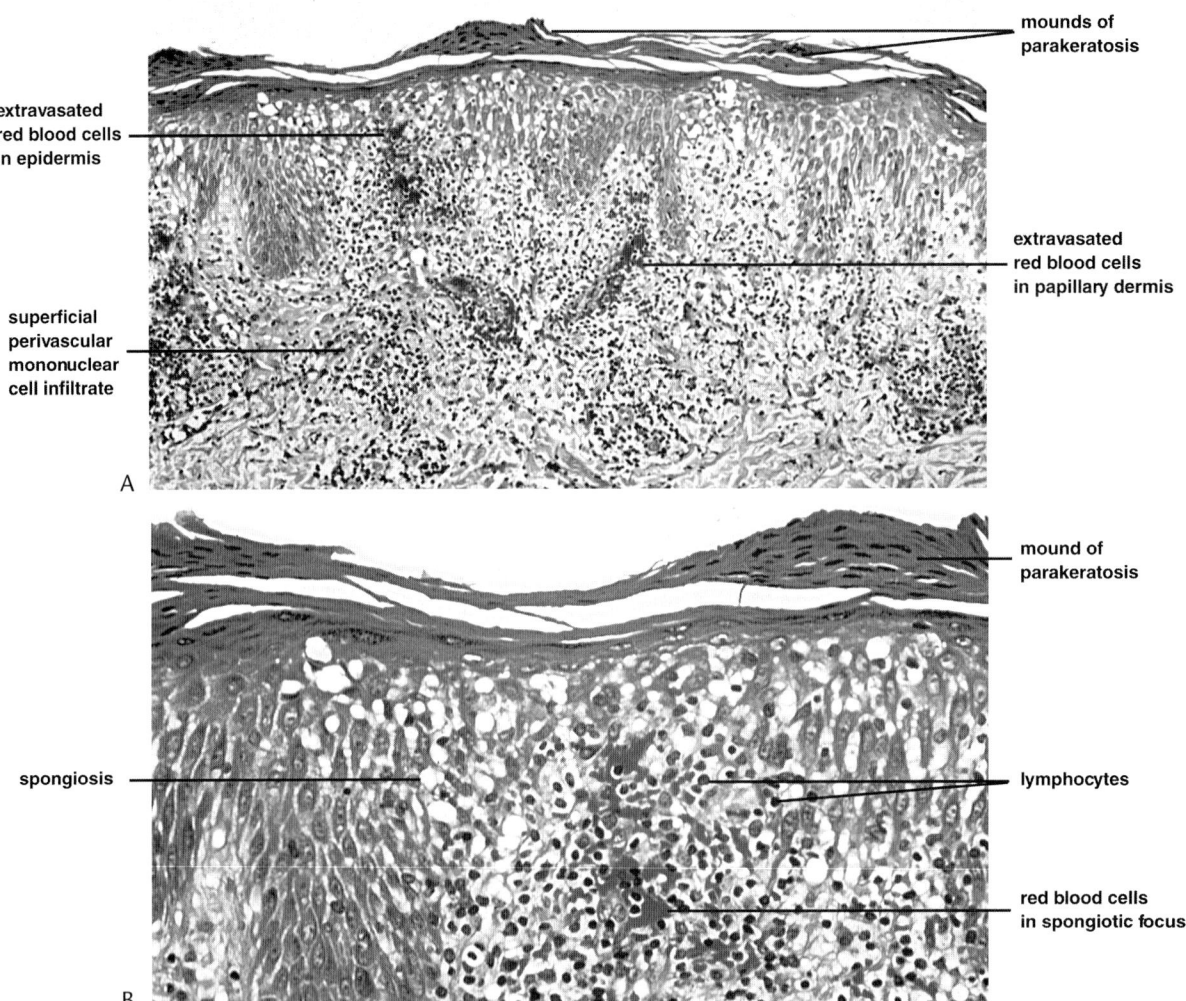

extravasated
red blood cells
in epidermis

mounds of
parakeratosis

superficial
perivascular
mononuclear
cell infiltrate

extravasated
red blood cells
in papillary dermis

A

spongiosis

mound of
parakeratosis

lymphocytes

red blood cells
in spongiotic focus

B

Figure 6-14. Pityriasis rosea. **(A)** At low magnification, the most characteristic feature of pityriasis rosea is the presence of mounds of parakeratosis in the stratum corneum. Another fairly constant feature of pityriasis rosea is the tendency toward extravasation of erythrocytes around vessels of the superficial plexus. Some of the extravasated erythrocytes may also be seen within the spongiotic foci in the slightly hyperplastic epidermis. **(B)** At higher magnification, prominent intercellular edema and exocytosis of lymphocytes are evident in addition to the mounds of parakeratosis. Microvesicles, however, are usually not present.

of lymphocytes and macrophages (Fig. 6-14). Occasional eosinophils may be present, but numerous eosinophils would militate against pityriasis rosea. Extravasated red blood cells are often found in the dermal papillae and the lower epidermis above the affected papillae. The constellation of histopathologic features noted above enable a definitive diagnosis to be made in most cases, especially if a small lesion is biopsied so that the microscopist can determine that these changes are occurring in a well-demarcated papule. Identical changes are seen in pityriasis rosea-like drug eruptions.[19]

Erythema Annulare Centrifugum (Superficial Gyrate Erythema)

The clinical and histopathologic features of the gyrate erythemas are discussed in Chapter 5. Erythema annulare centrifugum is characterized by an expanding erythematous, raised border and a trailing collarette of scale on the inside edge of the raised border. This scale is caused by the spongiosis that accompanies the superficial perivascular inflammatory cell infiltrate of lymphocytes and then is pushed up into the stratum corneum as the

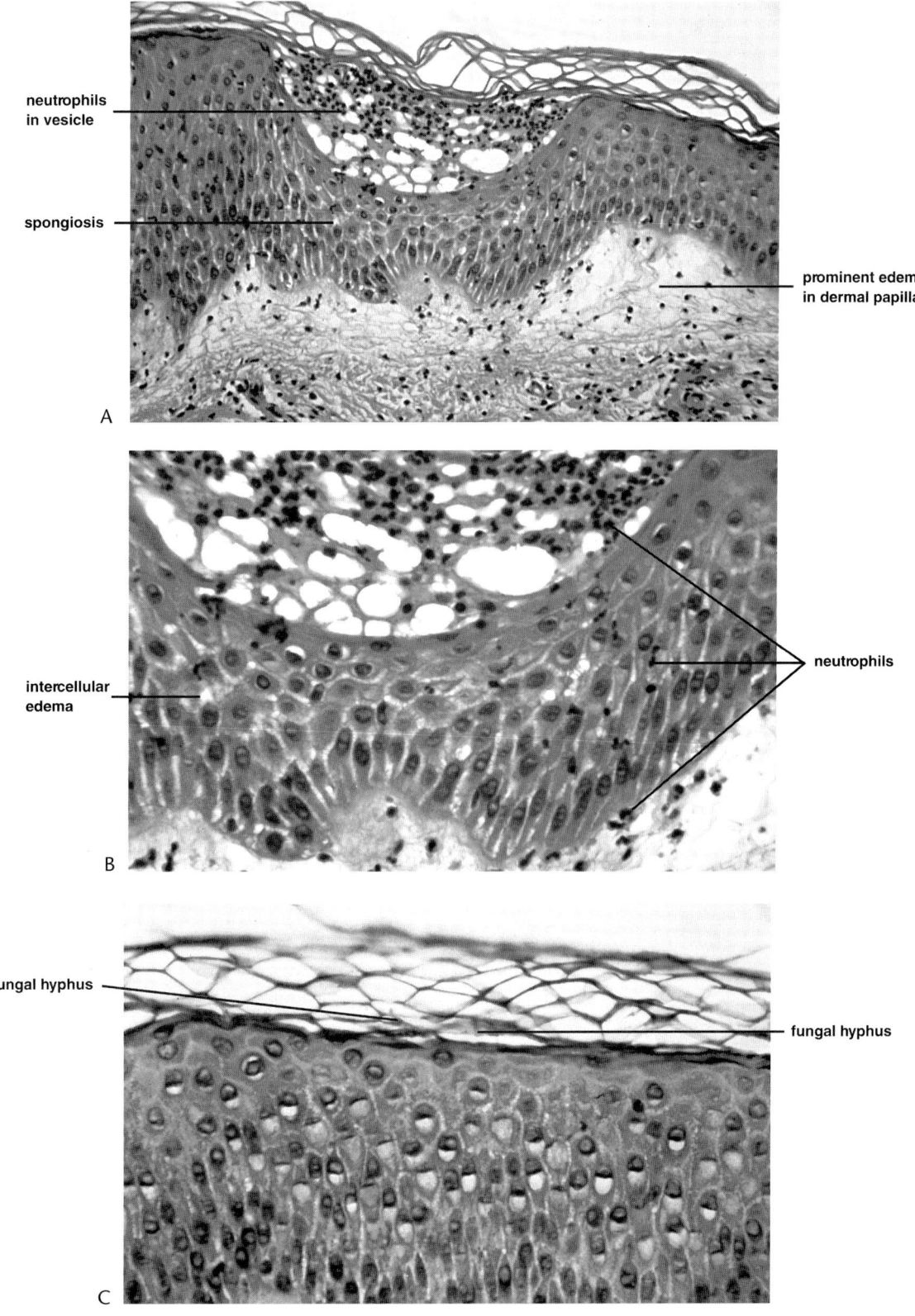

neutrophils
in vesicle

spongiosis

prominent edema
in dermal papilla

A

intercellular
edema

neutrophils

B

fungal hyphus

fungal hyphus

C

Figure 6-15. Acute dermatophytosis. **(A)** Acute dermatophyte infections, especially when due to zoophilic organisms, show a spongiotic reaction in the epidermis with exocytosis of neutrophils. **(B)** At higher magnification, neutrophils can be seen among keratinocytes in the spongiotic epithelium as well as within the microvesicle. **(C)** A PAS-stained section shows fungal hyphae in the stratum corneum. The basket-weave character of the stratum corneum indicates the acuteness of the process, since there has not yet been time for transition to hyperkeratosis or parakeratosis.

epidermis heals behind the outwardly migrating wave of inflammation.

Dermatophytosis (Tinea)

Clinical Features

The most important superficial fungi are the dermatophytes that infect the skin, hair, and nails. There are three genera of dermatophytes: *Trichophyton, Microsporum*, and *Epidermophyton*. Dermatophyte infections can take many forms and involve many different anatomic sites (e.g., tinea pedis, tinea corporis, tinea facie, and tinea cruris). Most commonly, dermatophyte infections present either as a papulosquamous or spongiotic condition. In dermatophyte infections due to *Trichophyton mentagrophytes* var *granulosum* or to zoophilic fungi such as *Microsporum canis* or *M. gypseum*, the lesions are characteristically dermatitic. They begin as erythematous edematous papules that expand outward with vesicles and pustules in the advancing borders. As they expand outward, they resolve in the center, thereby forming arcs and/or rings. The arciform and annular configurations distinguish tinea from nummular dermatitis, which is coin shaped but does not resolve centrally.

Histopathologic Features

The early lesions of dermatophytosis have a sparse superficial or superficial and deep perivascular infiltrate of lymphocytes, neutrophils, and sometimes occasional eosinophils. There are variable amounts of papillary dermal interstitial edema and epidermal spongiosis with exocytosis of neutrophils (Fig. 6-15). In time, the epidermis becomes hyperplastic and the stratum corneum may show compact orthokeratosis or parakeratosis, or a combination of both. Compact orthokeratosis and neutrophils in the stratum corneum are indications to search for fungal hyphae in the cornified layer of a spongiotic process.[20,21] Gottlieb and Ackerman[22] have also called attention to the "sandwich sign" of early evolving dermatophytosis. This refers to the compact orthokeratosis or parakeratosis that develops beneath the normal basket-weave stratum corneum; the fungal hyphae are found "sandwiched" between the two layers of cornified cells. Although this finding is not specific for dermatophytosis, as it also occurs in guttate psoriasis, pityriasis lichenoides et varioliformis acuta, and pityriasis rubra pilaris, its frequency in dermatophytosis should alert the microscopist to perform a periodic acid-Schiff stain to identify occult hyphae.

Papular Acrodermatitis of Childhood (Gianotti-Crosti Syndrome)

Clinical Features

Papular acrodermatitis of childhood is usually associated with hepatitis B infection, but several other viral infections, including Epstein-Barr virus, Coxsackie virus, and parainfluenza virus, have been implicated in some patients.[22,23] The condition is characterized by a symmetric eruption of nonpruritic, edematous, erythematous papules on the face, extremities, and buttocks.[24] The papules may show slight scaling or crusting. The skin eruption is often accompanied by lymphadenopathy, mainly affecting the axillary and inguinal lymph nodes, and constitutional symptoms of malaise and low grade fever. Liver dysfunction can often be detected by laboratory studies, but it is not usually severe enough to cause jaundice. The disease resolves spontaneously in a few weeks or months.

Histopathologic Features

The histopathologic features are variable from case to case. All patients have a superficial perivascular mononuclear cell infiltrate as in typical morbilliform viral exanthems (Fig. 6-16). There may be endothelial cell swelling and focal extravasation of red blood cells. Spongiosis and slight epidermal hyperplasia are present in some cases.[23,25] Occasionally there is a more dense perivascular and interstitial mononuclear cell infiltrate in the papillary dermis that may focally obscure the dermoepidermal junction.[26]

Miliaria Rubra (Prickly Heat)

Clinical Features

Miliaria rubra is a common problem that results from occlusion of the eccrine sweat ducts. It is especially common in infants and children who are overly dressed in warm, humid weather. It is also commonly seen in persons with febrile illnesses. Prickly heat develops most often on covered or occluded areas. The eruption consists of pruritic erythematous papules. In some patients, pustules develop on the erythematous papules (miliaria pustulosa). Miliaria rubra clears quickly if the skin is kept dry and cool.

Histopathologic Features

Blockage of the acrosyringium gives rise to miliaria. In miliaria crystallina, the blockage occurs in the stratum corneum, whereas in miliaria rubra the blockage develops in the viable portion of the epidermis.[27] In acute lesions, there is spongiosis in the stratum spinosum around the occluded acrosyringium, and there is edema and an inflammatory infiltrate of lymphocytes and macrophages in the papillary dermis beneath the spongiotic focus surrounding the involved duct (Fig. 6-17). In some lesions, the continued influx of leukocytes into the spongiotic epidermis results in pustule formation (miliaria pustulosa). Eventually in the subacute phase, the spongiotic focus is eliminated and results in scale-crust formation (Fig. 6-18). There is no chronic phase of individual lesions of miliaria rubra.

Incontinentia Pigmenti (Bloch-Sulzberger Syndrome)

Clinical Features

Incontinentia pigmenti is a rare hereditary disorder that affects not only the skin but also the teeth, bones, central nervous system, and eyes.[28] Data regarding the genetic features of incontinentia pigmenti suggest that it is an X-linked dominant trait that is lethal in utero in almost all male fetuses. The skin lesions are

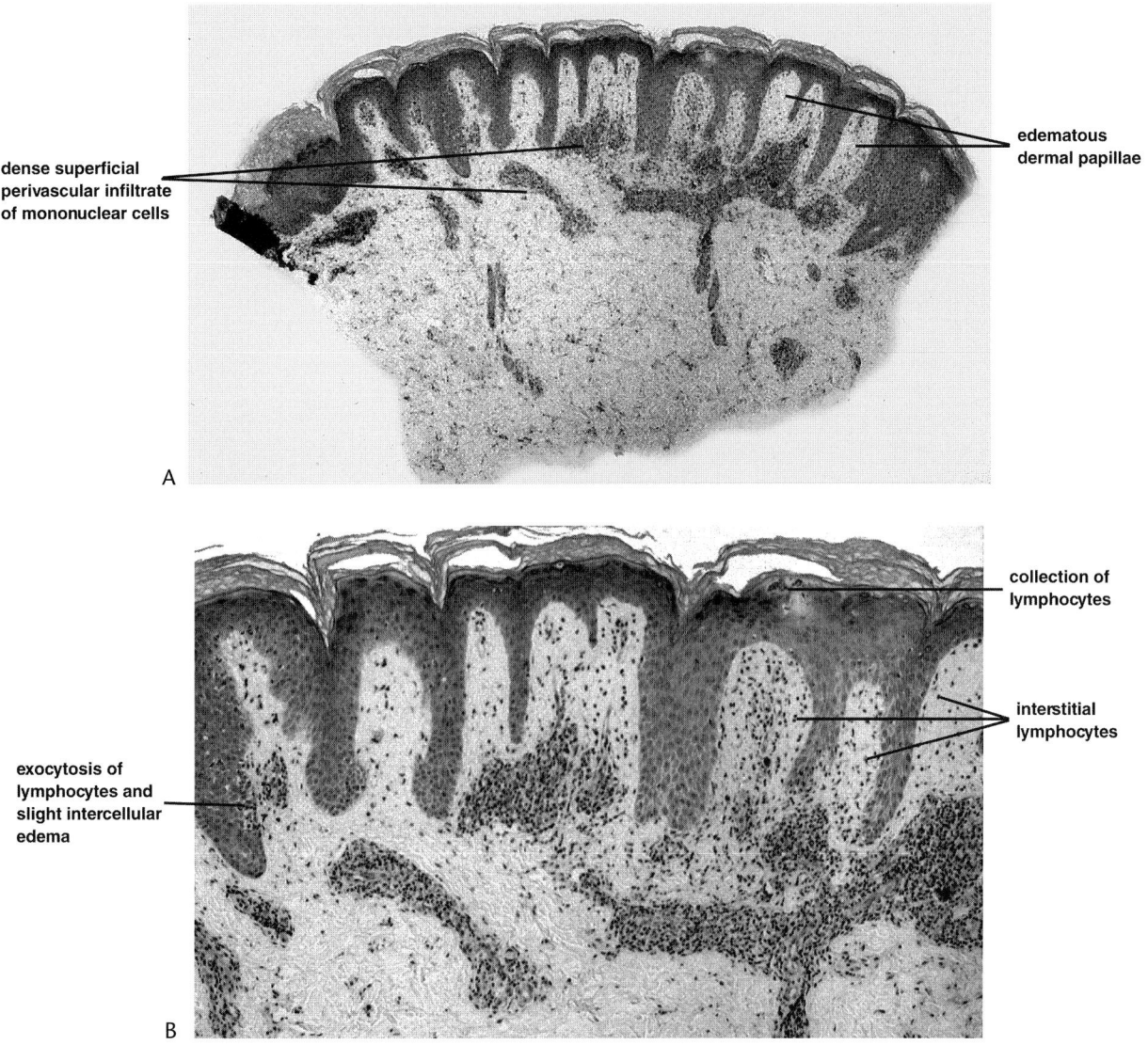

dense superficial
perivascular infiltrate
of mononuclear cells

edematous
dermal papillae

A

collection of
lymphocytes

interstitial
lymphocytes

exocytosis of
lymphocytes and
slight intercellular
edema

B

Figure 6-16. Papular acrodermatitis of childhood. **(A)** At scanning magnification, the papular nature of the lesion is evident. There is a dense superficial perivascular and interstitial mononuclear cell inflammatory infiltrate. The papillary dermis shows prominent edema. There is elongation of the rete ridges and the dermal papillae. **(B)** At higher magnification, small foci of spongiosis and exocytosis of lymphocytes can be seen in the epidermis, especially at the tips of the rete ridges.

usually present at birth or begin in the neonatal period. There are three morphologically different types of lesions. The first are vesicles that are often arranged in linear groups. These are often superseded by verrucous papules and lichenoid plaques that develop in the same areas. They may resemble linear epidermal nevi. The third phase consists of linear and whorled macules and patches of hyperpigmentation that may eventually resolve spontaneously. The cutaneous lesions occur on the trunk and extremities, and there is a broad range in their extent and severity. Lesions of all three types may be present concomitantly. Anomalies of the teeth, hair, and eyes are the most common ex-

tracutaneous lesions. Hypereosinophilia is common during the inflammatory stage of the disease.

Histopathologic Features

The early vesicular lesions result from marked spongiosis. In addition to spongiosis, there are individual necrotic cells within the stratum spinosum, and squamous eddies may also be present (Fig. 6-19). There are numerous eosinophils within the dermal infiltrate and also within the spongiotic foci in the epidermis.

One hypothesis regarding the inflammatory features of in-

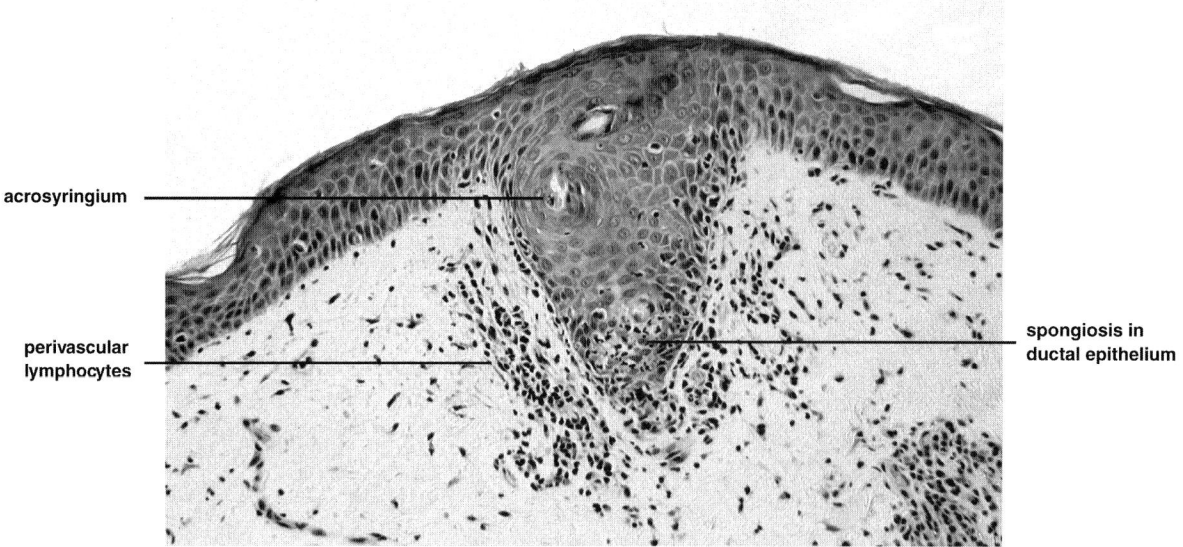

acrosyringium

perivascular
lymphocytes

spongiosis in
ductal epithelium

Figure 6-17. Miliaria rubra. There is spongiosis with exocytosis of lymphocytes surrounding an acrosyringium. Within the dermis there is a moderately dense perivascular mononuclear cell inflammatory infiltrate.

continentia pigmenti is that incontinentia pigmenti may be analogous to graft-versus-host disease with an immunologic response directed at a mutant clone of epidermal cells.[29] Basophils have been demonstrated in the epidermis in one case of incontinentia pigmenti, and it is known that basophil granules contain eosinophil chemotactic factor of anaphylaxis.[30] Eosinophil chemotactic factor of anaphylaxis has also been detected in blister fluid in incontinentia pigmenti. These isolated findings must be confirmed and must be subjected to study by modern molecular methods to define further the nature of the inflammatory reaction in incontinentia pigmenti.

Larva Migrans (Creeping Eruption)

Clinical Features

Larva migrans is an infestation of the skin with larvae of the dog and cat hookworms, *Ancylostoma braziliensis* and *A. caninum.*

Figure 6-18. Resolving lesion of miliaria rubra. Later in the evolution of the lesions of miliaria rubra, there may be parakeratosis and scale-crust formation within the ostium of the involved acrosyringium. The lumen of the acrosyringium is dilated and plugged.

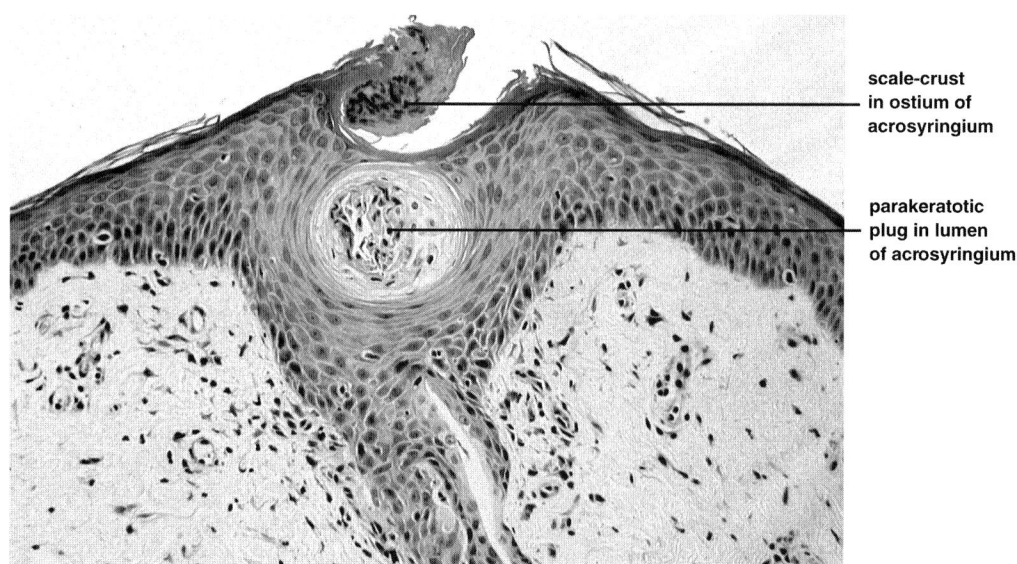

scale-crust
in ostium of
acrosyringium

parakeratotic
plug in lumen
of acrosyringium

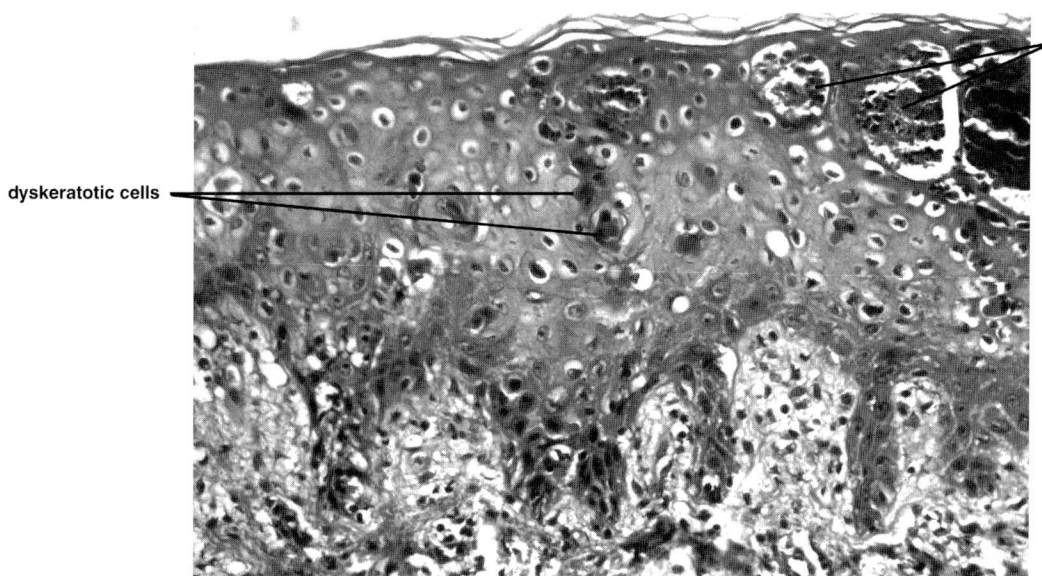

Figure 6-19. Incontinentia pigmenti. Incontentia pigmenti is the prototype for eosinophilic spongiotic dermatitis. In this biopsy specimen from a newborn infant with incontentia pigmenti, there are several microvesicles within the upper portion of the epidermis that are packed with eosinophils. Both intra- and intercellular edema are also present within the epidermis. A notable feature is the presence of individual dyskeratotic cells, which helps to distinguish incontentia pigmenti from other conditions that also show spongiosis with exocytosis of eosinophils.

It is most common in tropical and subtropical regions. In the United States, the highest incidence is in the Southeast. The larvae are present in soil contaminated by the feces of dogs or cats.

The earliest lesion of larva migrans is an erythematous, pruritic papule that resembles an arthropod bite reaction. As the larva tunnels aimlessly outward from the papule, a serpiginous track develops, and it may extend 1 cm or more per day. The skin adjacent to the track is usually inflamed, and the associated pruritus is intense. If untreated, lesions may persist for months. However, because the organisms cannot complete their life cycle in humans, the disease is self-limited.

Histopathologic Features

Larvae burrow in the spinous layer of the surface epidermis or follicular infundibula (Fig. 6-20), but most biopsy specimens of larva migrans do not contain larvae. The larvae are more likely to be found if the specimen is taken from the normal-appearing skin ahead of the advancing ends of the tract. The burrow may contain desquamated keratinocytes and debris. Even if the larva is present in the burrow, identification of the species of the parasite is not possible.[31] The epidermis adjacent to the burrow often exhibits slight spongiosis and exocytosis of inflammatory cells. The dermis contains a superficial and deep perivascular and interstitial inflammatory infiltrate of lymphocytes, macrophages, and eosinophils. The follicular units are also often surrounded by an infiltrate of similar cells. There is usually moderate to marked interstitial edema, especially in the papillary dermis.

Radiation Dermatitis

Clinical Features

Acute dermatitis from ionizing radiation can almost always be diagnosed clinically by history and its appearance, which, as in contact dermatitis, has an unnatural configuration and distribution. The severity of radiation dermatitis depends predominantly on the total dosage but also on how it is administered (i.e., the size and frequency of the fractions). The acute changes resolve relatively quickly but inevitably lead to variable degrees of atrophy, pigmentary alterations, and telangiectasia.

Histopathologic Features

The histopathologic features of acute radiation dermatitis resemble those of phototoxic dermatitis; however, the damage is not limited to the surface epidermis because of the deeper penetration of the ionizing rays that also damage the epithelial structures of adnexa.[32] The epithelial cells are swollen and pale staining with pyknotic nuclei, and some are necrotic. There is often spongiosis with exocytosis of inflammatory cells. Intraepidermal vesiculation, erosion, and even ulceration may occur. The dermis shows edema and some vascular dilation. Some vessels may be thrombosed. A perivascular infiltrate of mononuclear cells and neutrophils is present. The changes of late radiation dermatitis are more characteristic and have features of a poikilodermatous reaction.

Figure 6-20. Larva migrans. **(A)** At scanning magnification, a portion of the track of a larva can be seen in the epidermis on the right-hand side of the picture. A curled up larva is present in the follicular epithelium in the dermis. The follicle is surrounded by an inflammatory cell infiltrate. **(B)** Within the follicular epithelium there is a larva of *Ancylostoma* spp. cut in longitudinal section. The follicular epithelium shows exocytosis of inflammatory cells and intercellular edema.

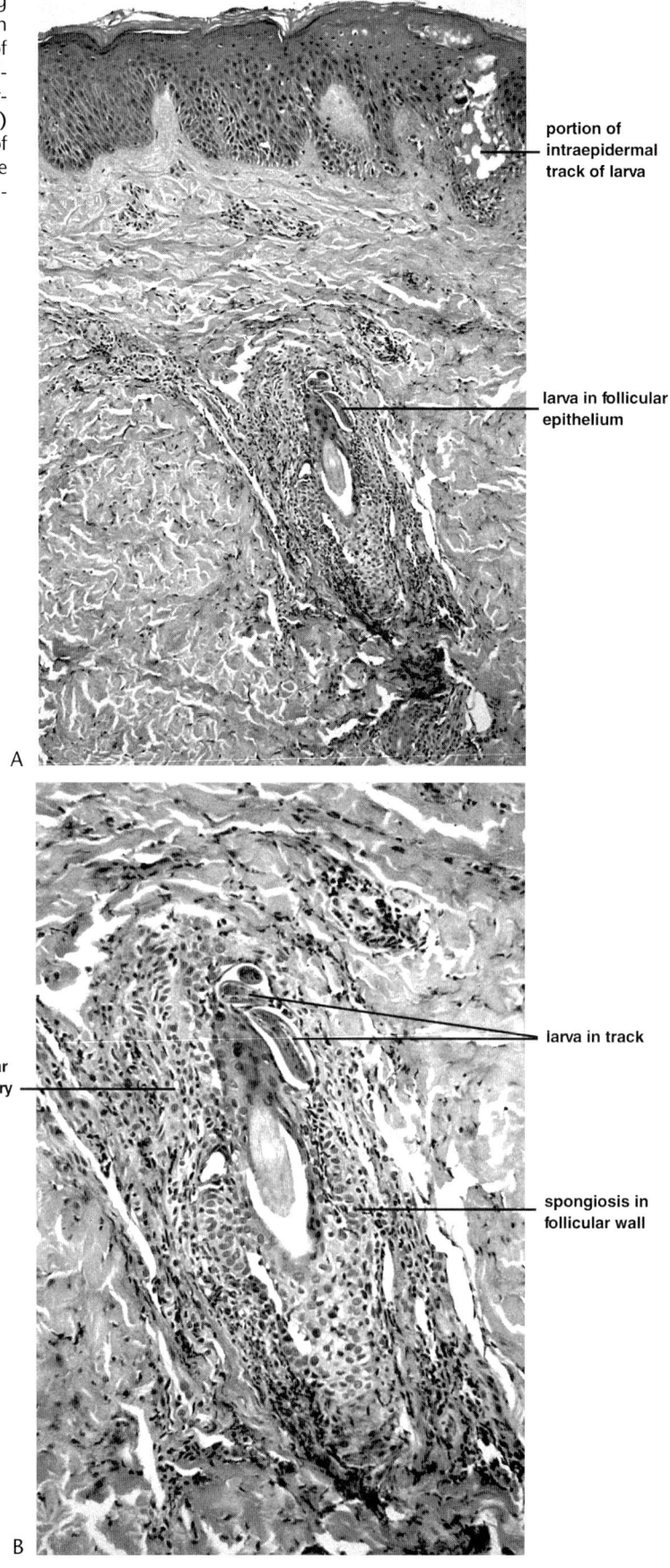

portion of intraepidermal track of larva

larva in follicular epithelium

A

larva in track

perifollicular inflammatory infiltrate

spongiosis in follicular wall

B

DERMATITIDES THAT SOMETIMES ARE SPONGIOTIC

There are several conditions that usually do not exhibit spongiosis, but may do so more frequently than can be accounted for simply by chance (Table 6-1). In these conditions, spongiosis is a variable feature and is neither necessary for making the histopathologic diagnosis nor a feature that argues against a diagnosis if all other appropriate features are present. For example, polymorphous light eruption is characterized by a superficial and deep perivascular mononuclear cell infiltrate with prominent papillary dermal edema often to the point of incipient subepidermal vesiculation. Some persons, however, have lesions with spongiosis in addition to the aforementioned features.[33] The presence of spongiosis is not necessary to make the diagnosis nor does it argue against the diagnosis. In Grover's disease, by contrast, there is a variant that typically exhibits a combination of spongiosis and acantholysis.[34]

Drug reactions do not usually take the form of a spongiotic dermatitis. This occurs most frequently in systemic contact dermatitis. Some drug-induced cases of exfoliative dermatitis, pityriasis rosea-like eruption, and morbilliform eruptions may exhibit slight spongiosis. Fixed drug reactions typically show both spongiosis and marked vacuolar interface changes, intracellular edema, and keratinocyte necrosis.[35]

Of this group of conditions, exfoliative dermatitis merits special comment. Generalized redness and scaling is the final common pathway for several cutaneous diseases. Conditions as diverse as pediculosis corporis, pemphigus foliaceus, pityriasis rubra pilaris, and Sézary syndrome can present as exfoliative erythroderma. As a rule, most diseases maintain their characteristic histopathologic features when they become generalized. In primary spongiotic diseases such as allergic contact dermatitis, seborrheic dermatitis, and stasis dermatitis, the exfoliative erythroderma shows the features of a subacute spongiotic process. However, exfoliative erythroderma from other causes may exhibit identical features. Cases due to drug hypersensitivity, a reaction to an occult or overt lymphoma, carcinoma, or other systemic disease and so-called idiopathic or essential exfoliative erythroderma are characterized histologically by reactive epidermal hyperplasia, mild to moderate spongiosis, and a mononuclear or mixed inflammatory infiltrate. Therefore, the patient's history, physical findings, and laboratory studies must be taken into account. At least three biopsy specimens should be obtained in cases of exfoliative erythroderma to avoid sampling error. The major purpose of the biopsy procedure in assessing exfoliative erythrodermas is to rule out cutaneous T-cell lymphoma or other dermatoses with specific histopathologic features.

CLUES TO DIFFERENTIAL DIAGNOSIS OF SPONGIOTIC DERMATITIDES

In assessing spongiotic dermatitides every clue must be used. Histopathologic features that may be helpful include the type of leukocytes present in the spongiotic foci, the distribution of the spongiotic foci relative to the adnexal orifices, and the distribution of the cellular infiltrate in the dermis (Table 6-2).

In regard to the type of leukocytes present within the spongiotic foci, only eosinophils and neutrophils are significant in as much as lymphocytes are almost always found. Neutrophils are only important in the differential diagnosis when there is no erosion or ulceration of the epidermis. By contrast, eosinophils within spongiotic foci are significant even if the epithelium has lost its integrity.

Table 6-1. Dermatitides That Sometimes Are Spongiotic

Arthropod bite/sting reactions and infestations
Polymorphous light eruption
Grover's disease
Pruritic urticarial papules and plaques of pregnancy
Measles and some other viral exanthems
Pigmented purpuric dermatoses
Drug reactions
Eruptive psoriasis
Exfoliative dermatitis
Precursor lesions to certain vesiculobullous diseases
  Pemphigus (spongiosis with eosinophils)
  Pemphigoid (urticarial lesions)
  Herpes gestations (urticarial lesions)

Table 6-2. Clues to Differential Diagnosis of Spongiotic Dermatitides

Spongiosis with eosinophils
  Incontinentia pigmenti (first stage)
  Pemphigus
  Pemphigoid
  Herpes gestationis
  Allergic contact dermatitis
  Arthropod bites/stings/infestations
  Hypereosinophilic syndrome
  Eosinophilic cellulitis (Wells syndrome)
Spongiosis with neutrophils in the intact epithelium
  Dermatophytosis
  Seborrheic dermatitis
  Eruptive psoriasis
  Incipient intraepidermal pustular diseases (i.e., impetigo)
  Primary irritant contact dermatitis
Acrosyringeal spongiosis
  Miliaria rubra
Parafollicular spongiosis
  Seborrheic dermatitis
Spongiosis with superficial and deep perivascular infiltrates
  Photoallergic dermatitis
  Polymorphous light eruption (some cases)
  Arthropod bites/stings/infestations
  Larva migrans (creeping eruption)
  Dermatophytosis (some cases)

REFERENCES

1. Silberberg I, Baer RI, Rosenthal SA: The role of Langerhans cells in allergic contact hypersensitivity. A review of findings in man and guinea-pigs. J Invest Dermatol 66:210–217, 1976
2. Kupper TS: Mechanisms of cutaneous inflammation: interactions between epidermal cytokines, adhesion molecules and leukocytes. Arch Dermatol 125:1406–1412, 1989
3. Medenica M, Rostenberg A: A comparative light and electron microscopic study of primary irritant contact dermatitis and allergic contact dermatitis. Invest Dermatol 56:259–271, 1971
4. Hall JB, Smith JG Jr, Burnett SC: The lysosome in contact dermatitis: a histochemical study. J Invest Dermatol 49:590–594, 1967
5. Willis CM, Stephens CJM, Willeinson JD: Differential pattern of epidermal leukocyte infiltration in patch test reactions to structurally unrelated chemical irritants. J Invest Dermatol 101:364–370, 1993
6. Robinson HN, Morison WL, Hood AF: Thiazide diuretic therapy and chronic photosensitivity. Arch Dermatol 121:522–524, 1985
7. Epstein JH: Adverse cutaneous reactions to the sun. pp. 5–43. In Malkinson FD, Pearson RW (eds): Year of Dermatology. Yearbook Medical, Inc, Chicago, 1971
8. Hanifin JM, Rajka G: Diagnostic features of atopic dermatitis. Acta Dermatovener 92:44–47, 1980
9. Hurwitz RM, Detrana C: The cutaneous pathology of atopic dermatitis. Am J Dermatopathol 12:544–551, 1990
10. Prose PH, Sedlis E: Morphologic and histochemical studies of atopic eczema in infants and children. J Invest Dermatol 34:149–165, 1960
11. Mihm MC Jr, Soter NA, Dvorak HF, Austen KF: The structure of normal skin and the morphology of atopic eczema. J Invest Dermatol 67:305–312, 1976
12. Zaynoun ST, Aftimos BG, Tenekjian KK et al: Extensive pityriasis alba: a histological, histochemical, and ultrastructural study. Br J Dermatol 108:83–90, 1983
13. Veien NK, Kaaber K: Nickel, cobalt, and chromium sensitivity in patients with pompholyx (dyshidrotic eczema). Contact Derm 5:371–374, 1979
14. Kutzner H, Wurzel RM, Wolff HH: Are acrosyringia involved in the pathogenesis of "dyshidrosis"? Am J Dermatopathol 8:109–116, 1986
15. Bendl BJ: Nummular eczema of stasis origin. Int J Dermatol 18:129–131, 1979
16. Mali JWH, Kuiper JP, Hamers AA: Acro-angiodermatitis of the foot. Arch Dermatol 92:515–518, 1965
17. Strutton G, Weed D: Acro-angiodermatitis: a stimulant of Kaposi's sarcoma. Am J Dermatopathol 9:85–89, 1987
18. Soeprono FF, Schinella RA, Lockerell CJ, Comite SL: Seborrheic-like dermatitis of acquired immunodeficiency syndrome: a clinicopathologic study. J Am Acad Dermatol 14:242–248, 1986
19. Maize JC, Tomecki KJ: Pityriasis rosea-like drug eruption secondary to metronidazole. Arch Dermatol 113:1457–1458, 1977
20. Ackerman AB: Neutrophils within the cornified layer are clues to infection by superficial fungi. Am J Dermatopathol 1:69–75, 1979
21. Ollague J, Ackerman AB: Compact orthokeratosis as a clue to dermatophytosis and candidiasis. Am J Dermatopathol 4:355–363, 1982
22. Gottlieb GJ, Ackerman AB: The "sandwich sign" of dermatophytosis. Am J Dermatopathol 8:347–350, 1986
23. Raimer S: Gianotti-Crosti syndrome. Unit 7–21. In Demis DJ, Thiers BT, Smith ER (eds): Clinical Dermatology. 15th Rev. Lippincott-Raven, Philadelphia, 1988
24. Gianotti F: Popular acrodermatitis of childhood and other papulovesicular acro-located syndromes. Br J Dermatol 100:49–59, 1979
25. Taieb A, Plantin P, Du Pasquier P et al: Gianotti-Crosti syndrome: a study of 26 cases. Br J Dermatol 115:49–59, 1986
26. Spear KL, Winkelmann RK: Gianotti-Crosti syndrome: a review of ten cases not associated with hepatitis B. Arch Dermatol 120:891–896, 1984
27. Dobson RL, Lobitz WC Jr: Some histochemical observations on the human eccrine sweat glands. II. The pathogenesis of miliaria. Arch Dermatol 75:653–666, 1957
28. Carney RG Jr: Incontinentia pigmenti: a worldwide statistical analysis. Arch Dermatol 112:535–542, 1976
29. Person JR: Incontinentia pigmenti: a failure of immune tolerance? J Am Acad Dermatol 13:120–123, 1985
30. Schmalstieg FC, Jorizzo JL, Tschen J, Subet P: Basophils in incontinentia pigmenti. J Am Acad Dermatol 10:362–364, 1984
31. Meyers WM, Neafie RC: Creeping eruption. pp. 437–439. In Binford DH, Connor DH (eds): Pathology of Tropical and Extraordinary Diseases. Armed Forces Institute of Pathology, Washington, DC, 1976
32. Van Scott EJ, Reinertson RP: Detection of radiation effects on hair root of the human scalp. Invest Dermatol 29:205–212, 1957
33. Holzle E, Plewig G, Jofmann C, Roser-Maass E: Polymorphous light eruption: experimental reproduction of skin lesions. J Am Acad Dermatol 7:111–125, 1982
34. Chalet M, Grover R, Ackerman AB: Transient acantholytic dermatosis. Arch Dermatol 113:431–435, 1977
35. Van Voorhees A, Stenn KS: Histologic phases of Bactrim-induced fixed drug eruption: the report of one case. Am J Dermatopathol 9:528–532, 1987

7

DERMATITIS WITH EPIDERMAL HYPERPLASIA

DEFINITION AND CONCEPT

There are only a few ways in which the epidermis can respond to tissue injury of inflammation. These include cell death, atrophy, cellular hypertrophy, and cellular proliferation. Cell death and atrophy usually occur when the inflammatory response severely injures the germinative cells in the basal layer. This is best exemplified in those conditions that microscopically exhibit lichenoid or vacuolar changes (or both) at the dermoepidermal junction. Cell hypertrophy in the stratum spinosum is less common than cellular proliferation as a cause of acanthosis. However, it is important to recognize it and to realize that it often does not occur in concert with hyperplasia. In lichen planus, lichen planus-like keratosis, keratoacanthoma, and other conditions in which there is a cell-mediated immune response that results in persistent damage to the basal layer, the keratinocytes in the spinous layer increase in volume and their cytoplasm takes on a pale glassy, eosinophilic tinctorial quality in hematoxylin and eosin-stained sections. Thus, in lichen planus, the epidermis becomes thickened because of an increase in cell size not because of an increase in the number of cells.

In many diseases of the skin there is stimulation of the germinative cells to divide more rapidly, and the epidermis becomes increased in thickness because of accretion of cells. This type of acanthosis is appropriately called *epidermal hyperplasia*. The prototype of epidermal hyperplasia is psoriasis, so some pathologists characterize inflammatory dermatoses that exhibit epidermal hyperplasia as psoriasiform dermatitides. However, the epidermis in a well-developed plaque of psoriasis has characteristic architectural features that include (1) elongation of the rete ridges to a fairly uniform length, (2) clubbing (i.e., widening of the lower portion of the rete), (3) reciprocal elongation of the dermal papillae that are narrow at the base and wider at the top, and (4) apparent thinning of the epidermis above the dermal papillae (see below). Furthermore, there is usually confluent loss of the granular layer and parakeratosis. Because most conditions associated with epidermal hyperplasia

do not exhibit the same histopathologic features, the term *psoriasiform* applies only in a general sense.

For the purpose of differential diagnosis, it is useful to think in terms of a prototype for each reaction pattern and then to compare the case in question to the prototype. Once it is determined that the most important histopathologic feature of an inflammatory dermatosis is epidermal hyperplasia, the next step is to determine whether it is psoriasis. If all of the other architectural features are consistent with psoriasis, a diagnosis can be made. If not, the specimen must be examined for other features that enable either a definitive diagnosis (e.g., hyphae in the stratum corneum in tinea corporis) or a pertinent differential diagnosis to be established (e.g., lichen simplex chronicus vs. inflammatory linear epidermal nevus that can be resolved by clinicopathologic correlation).

PSORIASIS AND ITS VARIANTS

Psoriasis Vulgaris

Clinical Features

Genetic predisposition to psoriasis has been well established, but pedigree analysis has not shown a constant genetic pattern.[1] Approximately 30% of family members with the genetic predisposition will express the disease. It affects about 1% to 2% of the population. Psoriasis usually appears in the second or third decade of life and pursues an unpredictable course of remissions and exacerbations. The skin of psoriatics is vulnerable to injury, and psoriatic lesions may develop in areas of cutaneous trauma (Koebner phenomenon). A small percentage of persons, usually children, develop an acute outbreak of small, red, nonconfluent papules (guttate psoriasis) after a β, hemolytic streptococcal infection of the oropharynx. Compared with the general population, an increased number of psoriatics have seronegative, rheumatoid-like arthritis.

The individual lesions of psoriasis are sharply demarcated

papules or plaques. They have a beefy red color and are covered by fine, silvery (micaceous) scales. If the scales are removed, small bleeding points may be produced (Auspitz sign). However, this phenomenon is not specific for psoriasis.[2] The distribution of the lesions is as characteristic as their morphologic features. They are most commonly situated on the scalp, elbows, and knees. The extensor surfaces of the arms and legs are also commonly involved. The gluteal folds and umbilicus are less frequently involved, although these sites are quite distinctive for psoriasis.

The nails are often affected. Involvement of the nail matrix leads to tiny pits on the nail surface. Involvement of the nail bed leads to "oil spots" and onycholysis. Late changes include nail plate dystrophy and accumulation of keratinous debris beneath the free edge of the nails. There is a close correlation between psoriatic arthritis of the distal interphalangeal joints and severe nail involvement.

In addition to the usual papules and plaques of psoriasis, some persons may express atypical forms of the disease. These variants fall into two general categories, abnormal distribution and unusual lesions. The lesions may be confined to flexural areas such as the groin and axillae in so-called inverse psoriasis or to palms and soles in volar psoriasis. In occasional instances of erythrodermic psoriasis, the disease may involve the entire skin. Rarely the lesions are pinpoint papules distributed around follicular units. Unusual lesions include the geographic, ostraceous, and rupial forms. Geographic plaques can be subdivided into annular, figurate, linear, and polycyclic types. Ostraceous lesions have laminated, heaped-up scale resembling the outer surface of an oyster shell. The term *ostraceous lesions* is sometimes used incorrectly as a synonym for *rupial lesions,* which

have an unusually dirty appearance due to purulence in addition to accumulated scale. Pustular psoriasis is discussed below.

Histopathologic Features

The early lesions of psoriasis exhibit slight epidermal hyperplasia, papillary dermal edema, and dilated, tortuous capillaries in the dermal papillae. The epidermis shows increased mitotic activity, slight exocytosis of inflammatory cells, mild spongiosis, and focal loss of the granular layer.[3] The most characteristic feature is the development of small lentil-shaped mounds of parakeratosis that contain neutrophils (Fig. 7-1). Whereas pityriasis rosea and the trailing border of superficial gyrate erythema also exhibit mound-like aggregates of parakeratotic cells, they do not contain the tell-tale neutrophils of psoriasis. Furthermore, it is not uncommon to find evidence of episodic activity in early psoriasis, with collections of parakeratotic cells and neutrophils haphazardly distributed at various levels in the predominantly orthokeratotic stratum corneum[4] (Fig. 7-2). The dilated capillaries in the dermal papillae are tortuous and are often congested with erythrocytes. There is a sparse superficial perivascular infiltrate of mononuclear cells and occasional neutrophils. Eosinophils are not usually present. These histopathologic features are seen in all early lesions of psoriasis regardless of their extent. Thus, eruptive guttate lesions cannot be distinguished from evolving erythrodermic psoriasis. Similar changes also occur in the so-called hot spots of plaque-type psoriatic lesions.

Established plaques of psoriasis show prominent hyperplasia that involves primarily the rete ridges and spares the epidermis over the dermal papillae (Fig. 7-3). This pattern of epidermal hyperplasia is characteristic of psoriasis. The rete are elongated

Figure 7-1. Guttate psoriasis. This small papule is approximately six rete ridges in width. There are mounds of parakeratosis that contain neutrophils. The epidermis shows irregular hyperplasia with somewhat club-shaped rete alternating with elongated dermal papillae. There are dilated capillaries in the dermal papillae and a sparse superficial perivascular inflammatory infiltrate.

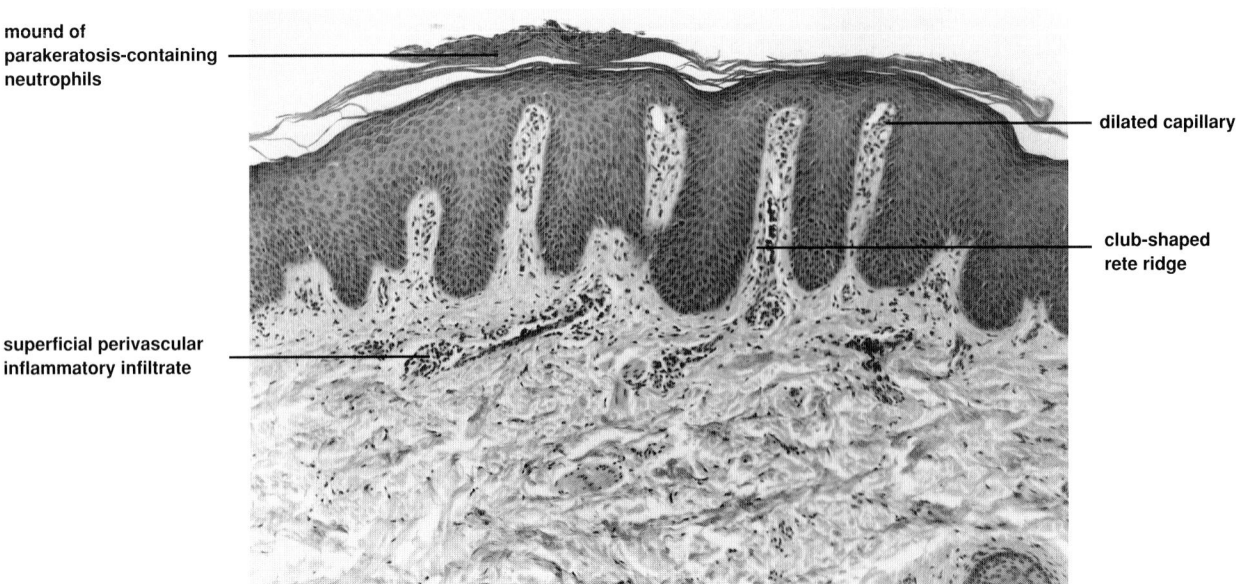

mound of parakeratosis-containing neutrophils

dilated capillary

club-shaped rete ridge

superficial perivascular inflammatory infiltrate

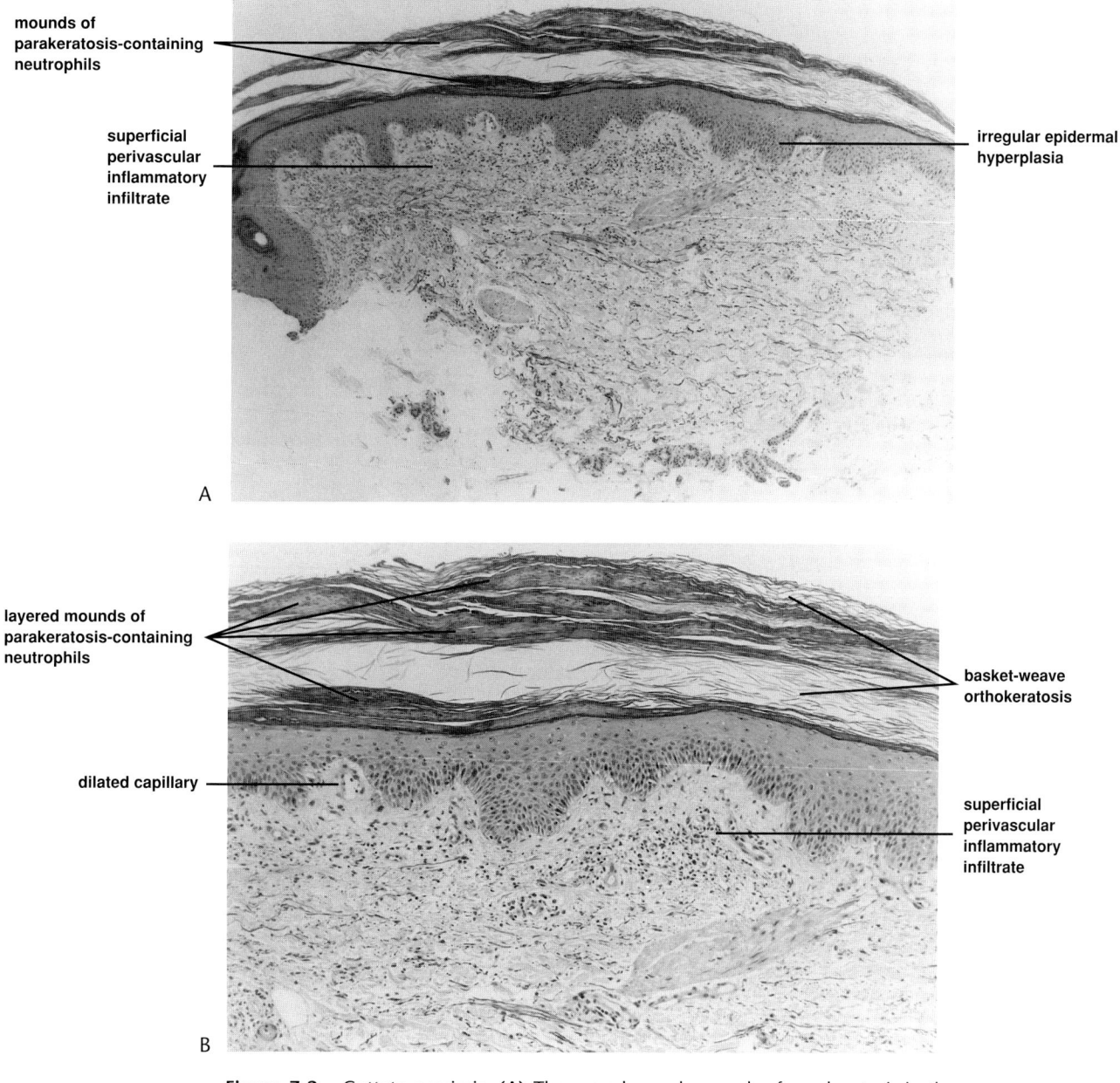

mounds of parakeratosis-containing neutrophils

superficial perivascular inflammatory infiltrate

irregular epidermal hyperplasia

A

layered mounds of parakeratosis-containing neutrophils

basket-weave orthokeratosis

dilated capillary

superficial perivascular inflammatory infiltrate

B

Figure 7-2. Guttate psoriasis. **(A)** There are layered mounds of parakeratosis in the basket-weave stratum corneum due to episodic bursts of activity. The epidermis shows slight irregular hyperplasia, and there is a sparse superficial perivascular inflammatory infiltrate in the papillary dermis. **(B)** Neutrophils are present in the parakeratotic mounds, and there is absence of the granular layer beneath the parakeratin.

to a fairly uniform length and show bulbous enlargement of their tips. The bases of the rete are usually narrow. There may be anastomoses of the tips of some adjacent rete even in properly oriented specimens. The sparing of the epidermis above the dermal papillae creates the optical illusion of thinning of these segments.[5] The stratum corneum, and stratum granulosum show different changes depending on the state of evolution of the lesion. There also can be significant intralesional variation because there may be a "hot spot" of activity in otherwise stable plaques. In active areas there is confluent parakeratosis and ab-

sence of the granular layer. These foci also usually exhibit collections of neutrophils (Munro microabscesses) at the level of the junction of the spinous layer with the parakeratotic stratum corneum (Fig. 7-4). These foci usually are situated above the dermal papillae. They are eventually pushed up into the parakeratotic stratum corneum, where they take the form of flat layers of crenated neutrophils among the parakeratotic cells. The dermal papillae are thin and tall with delicate, fibrillary collagen and contain dilated, tortuous capillaries. There is a sparse perivascular mononuclear cell infiltrate. The papillary dermis

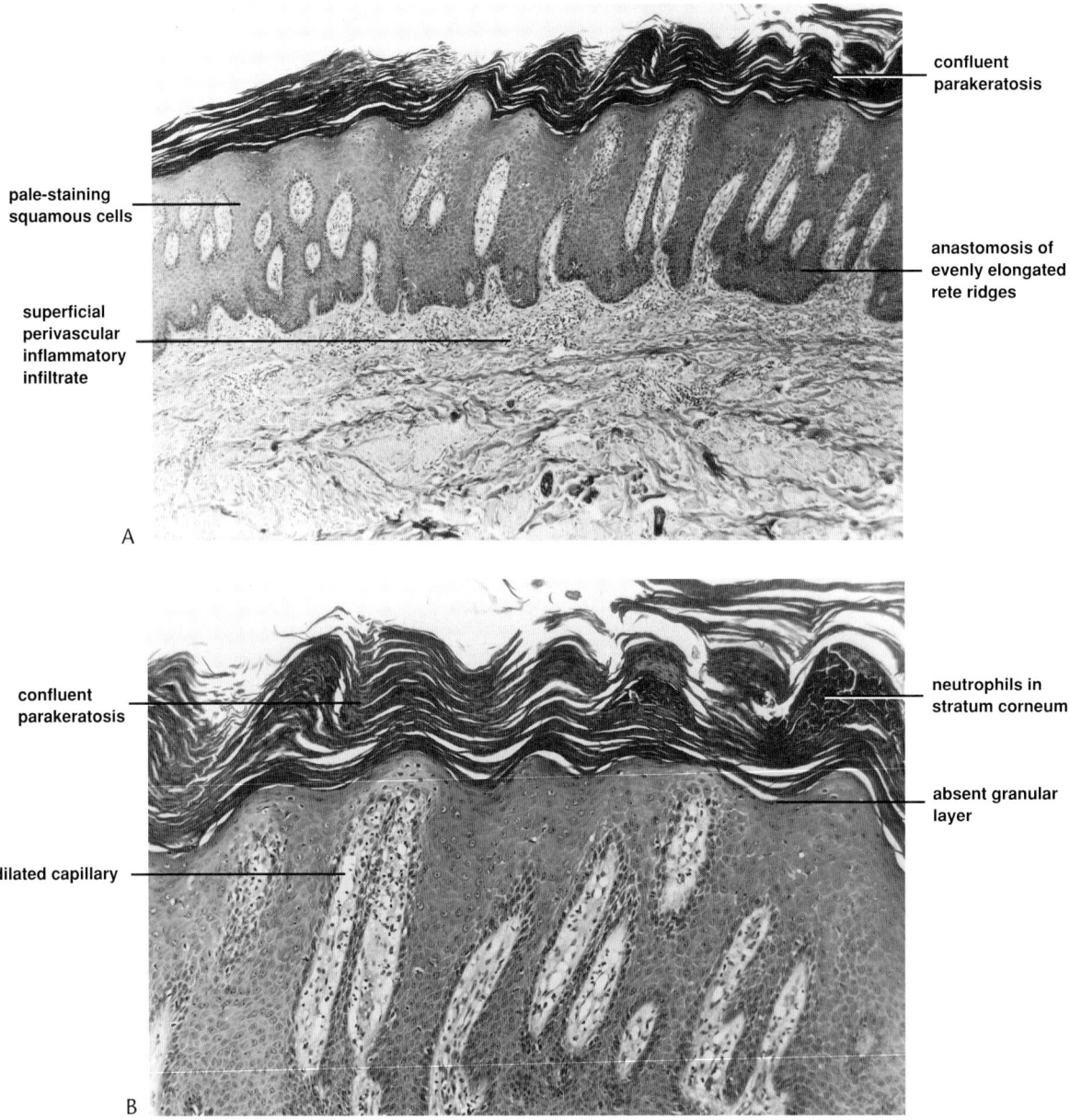

pale-staining
squamous cells

superficial
perivascular
inflammatory
infiltrate

confluent
parakeratosis

anastomosis of
evenly elongated
rete ridges

A

confluent
parakeratosis

dilated capillary

neutrophils in
stratum corneum

absent granular
layer

B

Figure 7-3. Plaque of psoriasis. **(A)** At scanning magnification, the most striking feature is the prominent elongation at the rete ridges to a uniform length. There is no increase in the thickness of the epidermis above the dermal papillae. **(B)** The stratum corneum demonstrates confluent parakeratosis with focal collections of neutrophils. The granular layer is absent. There is a sparse perivascular infiltrate around the dilated capillaries in the dermal papillae.

beneath the hyperplastic epidermis usually shows a more dense inflammatory infiltrate of lymphocytes, macrophages, and occasional neutrophils. The presence of more than an occasional plasma cell should arouse suspicion of human immunodeficiency virus infection.[6]

Involvement of the nail matrix and nail bed (Fig. 7-5) accounts for the changes in the nail plate. Exfoliation of the parakeratotic foci in the nail plate because of involvement of the ma-

trix leads to the formation of pits, and involvement of the nail bed leads to onycholysis and subungual debris.[7]

In quiescent plaques of psoriasis there is return to a more normal type of keratinization with re-formation of the granular layer and orthokeratosis[3] (Fig. 7-6). In the absence of neutrophils and confluent parakeratosis in the cornified layer, the most suggestive features of psoriasis are the distinctive epidermal architecture and the tortuous capillaries in the dermal

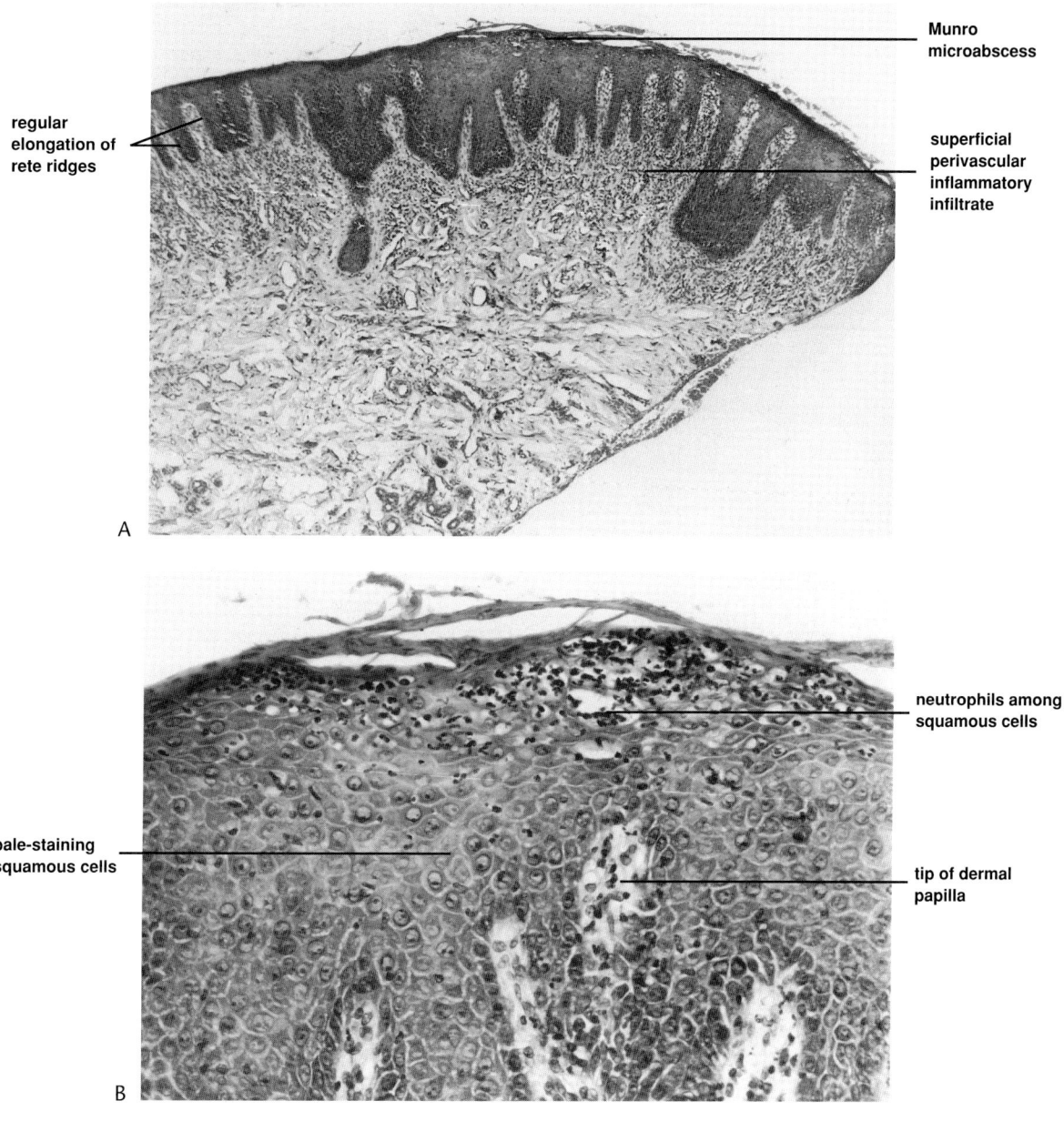

regular
elongation of
rete ridges

Munro
microabscess

superficial
perivascular
inflammatory
infiltrate

A

pale-staining
squamous cells

neutrophils among
squamous cells

tip of dermal
papilla

B

Figure 7-4. "Hot spot" in a plaque of psoriasis. **(A)** Near the middle of the field is a Munro microabscess in the upper spinous layer. **(B)** The microabscess is formed by neutrophils that fill the spores between keratinocytes. It is situated above the tip of a dermal papilla.

papillae. However, these too eventually disappear in resolving lesions.

Clinicopathologic Correlation

The silvery scale of psoriasis correlates histologically with the confluent parakeratosis in the cornified layer. The elevation of the plaques is due primarily to the elongation of the rete ridges and the reciprocal hypertrophy of the dermal papillae, although the interstitial edema associated with the dermal inflammatory response may contribute to the elevation. The beefy red color of the lesions is produced by the reactive hyperemia and vasodilation of the vessels of the superficial plexus.

In the ostraceous lesions of psoriasis the stratum corneum is markedly thickened compared with ordinary lesions. In rupial lesions there is not only piling up of the parakeratotic cell, but also numerous and large collections of degenerating neutrophils, other cell debris, bacterial colonies, and sometimes serum in the cornified layer.

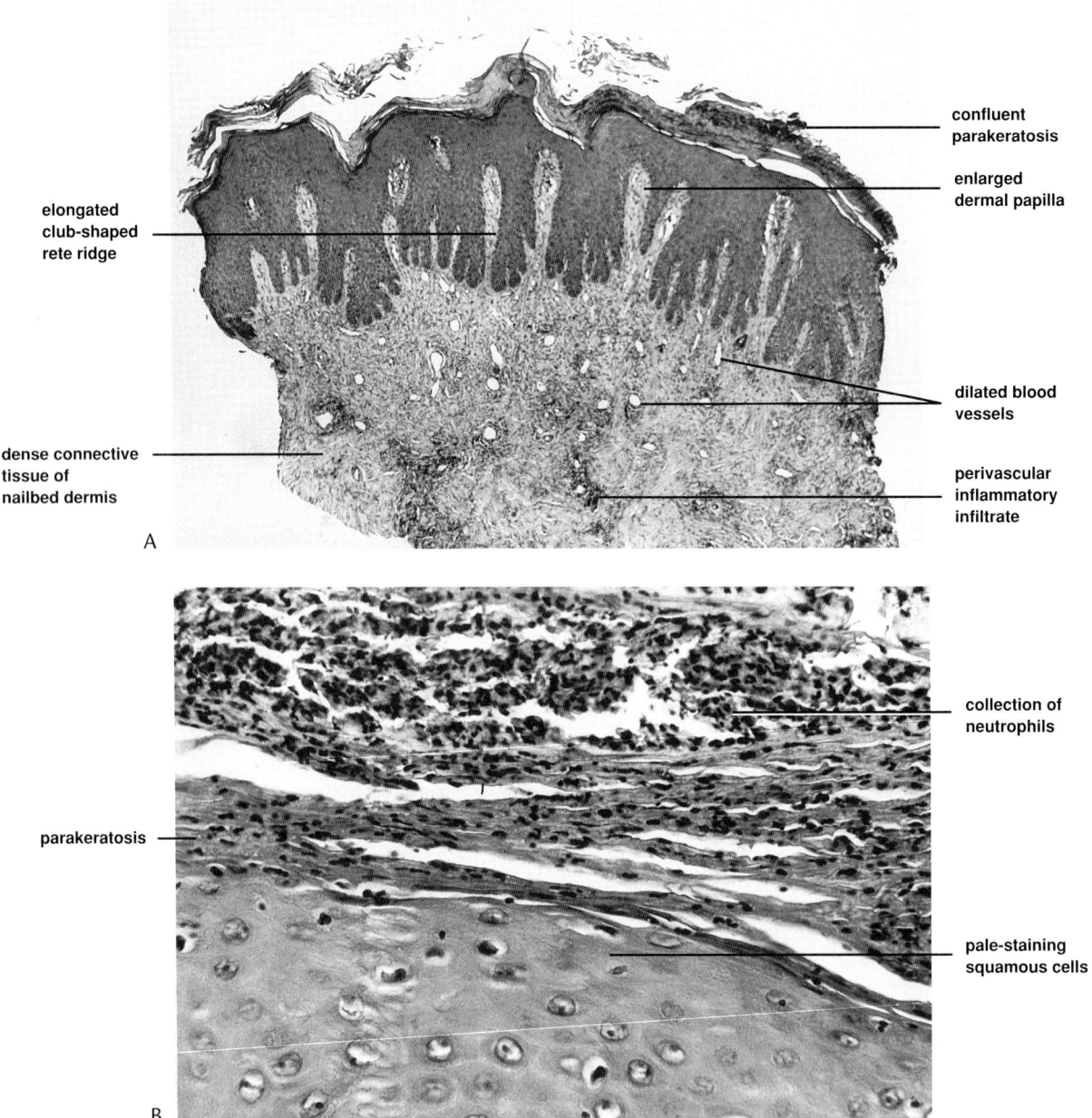

Figure 7-5. Psoriasis involving nail bed. **(A)** The architecture of the epidermis is identical to psoriasis on glabrous skin. The parakeratosis results in onycholysis. **(B)** The parakeratotic layer contains abundant neutrophils due to movement of a Munro microabscess up into the stratum corneum.

Pathophysiology

Although the cause of psoriasis is unknown, there is no doubt that genetic factors play an important role in the development of the disease. Approximately 20% to 30% of persons with psoriasis have a positive family history. Furthermore, psoriatics have an increased prevalence of certain class I MHC antigens of the B group, especially HLA-B13, B17, B37, B39, and Cw6 and the class II MHC antigen HLA-DR7.[8] Systematic analysis of the fa-

milial segregation of psoriasis in regard to the inheritance of HLA antigens suggests that one or more HLA-linked genes are implicated in the development of psoriasis.[1] Incomplete concordance among identical twins indicates that environmental factors influence the expression of the disease.

Much attention has been paid to the kinetics of the epidermal hyperplasia in psoriasis. Early observations noted that there is an increased mitotic rate in psoriatic lesions and a direct proportional relationship between the size of the dermal papillae

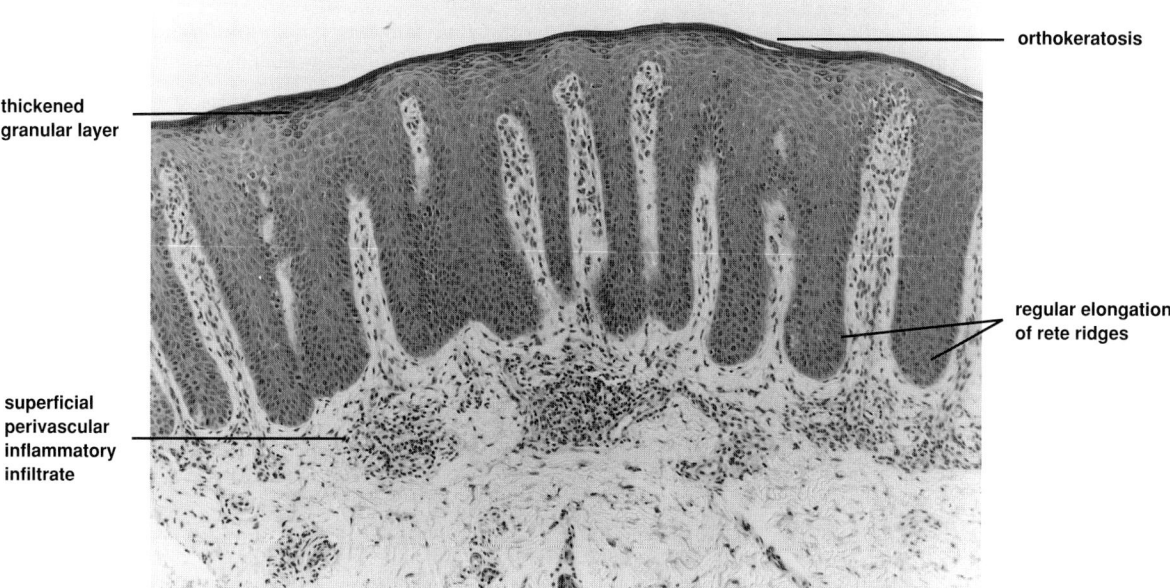

thickened
granular layer

orthokeratosis

regular elongation
of rete ridges

superficial
perivascular
inflammatory
infiltrate

Figure 7-6. Quiescent plaque of psoriasis. The earliest change in healing is return to the normal mode of keratinization. This plaque shows orthokeratin and a well-developed granular layer. The epidermal architecture is typical of a plaque of psoriasis.

and the size of the population of germinative cells they support. Cell kinetic studies demonstrated a 7-fold increase in the transit time of psoriatic epidermal cells accompanied by 12-fold decrease in the cell cycle time of the germinative cells.[9] There is also evidence that more epidermal cells are in the germinative pool than in normal epidermis.[10] This enhanced proliferation occurs in a milieu in which there are elevated levels of cyclic guanosine monophosphate (cGMP), certain prostaglandins (especially PGE_2), and polyamines in the epidermis.[11] However, it is not known whether the biochemical alterations are the cause of the increased proliferative activity or are epiphenomena.

A unifying theory of psoriasis must also account for the inflammatory changes that occur in the skin in addition to the proliferative activity.[8] The influx of inflammatory cells is undoubtedly due to the production of inflammatory mediators that are chemotactic for inflammatory cells. The recent observation that cyclosporine has dramatic therapeutic benefit in recalcitrant psoriasis has stimulated interest in the immunopathology of psoriasis.[12] Although various aberrations of the humoral and cellular immune systems have been noted, no global theory has emerged that solves the pathophysiologic riddle of psoriasis.

Pustular Psoriasis

Clinical Features

Pustular psoriasis is a generic term that encompasses a heterogenous group of conditions. Some persons with typical plaque-type psoriasis may experience the development of numerous pustules superimposed on their plaques. Their course, however, does not otherwise differ from psoriasis vulgaris. Another form primarily involves the palms and soles and is ac-

companied by typical plaque-type psoriasis elsewhere. This is called the *Barber* type. The *von Zumbusch* form presents as an acute generalized eruption of pustules on tender erythematous skin accompanied by fever, anemia, leukocytosis, and debilitation. Affected persons may or may not have had pre-existent psoriasis vulgaris. Generalized pustular psoriasis can be precipitated by withdrawal of systemic corticosteroid therapy or by administration of lithium carbonate to persons with psoriasis vulgaris. It can evolve into erythroderma. Absolute lymphopenia has been found at the onset of the flares of generalized pustular psoriasis.[13] This "lymphocyte eclipse" is a harbinger of impending relapse of pustular activity.

In addition to these three variants of pustular psoriasis, there are other pustular dermatoses that are now generally regarded as clinical variants of pustular psoriasis. These include acropustulosis (acrodermatitis continua of Hallopeau and dermatitis repens of Crocker) and impetigo herpetiformis.

Acrodermatitis continua is an inflammatory dermatosis that affects the hands and feet and sometimes the forearms and legs. It has the appearance of an intractable pyoderma or purulent psoriasis. It usually begins adjacent to the nail of one or more fingers and slowly extends proximally. The nails are severely dystrophic and may be shed because of an accumulation of pus beneath them.

The term *dermatitis repens* means a creeping dermatitis. It has been applied to a recalcitrant pustular eruption of the hands and feet. It is characterized by erythematous plaques with small pustules on the volar skin. It is not associated with typical plaques elsewhere, which distinguishes it from pustular psoriasis of Barber. It does not evolve into generalized pustular psoriasis.

Impetigo herpetiformis is a rare, sometimes fatal eruption of pregnancy in which the lesions tend to cluster and enlarge centrifugally. The onset is usually in the last trimester. It begins in the genitocrural region and other flexural areas. The lesions come in waves as in von Zumbusch psoriasis and are accompanied by severe constitutional symptoms.

Histopathologic Features

In acute pustular psoriasis the histopathologic features are not reminiscent of ordinary psoriasis. The exocytosis of neutrophils occurs at such a rapid rate that they form collections within the epidermis before it has time to proliferate. The pustules begin as focal collections beneath the stratum corneum that enlarge by expansion and coalescence. The neutrophils push aside the keratinocytes as they accumulate to form small pockets separated by the compressed remnants of the keratinocytes. This gives the appearance of the cut surface of a sponge in which the holes are packed with neutrophils (spongiform pustules of Kogoj) (Fig. 7-7). The stratum corneum, if intact, shows a normal delicate basket-weave appearance. In time, there is slight to moderate but irregular hyperplasia of the subjacent epidermis, and, eventually, the pustule is pushed up into the stratum corneum where it forms a purulent scale-crust.

In cases in which pustules develop within plaques of psoriasis, there is simply an expansion of the Munro microabscesses into spongiform pustules large enough to be apparent clinically. The other characteristic histologic features of psoriasis are present.

Spongiform pustules are not specific for the pustular forms of psoriasis. They also may be seen in geographic tongue (Fig. 7-8), dermatophyte and *Candida* infections, seborrheic dermatitis (at the edges of follicular orifices), secondary syphilis (especially condyloma latum), and Reiter syndrome (which may or may not be etiologically related to psoriasis). Clinicopathologic correlations and appropriate special stains for infectious organisms can usually distinguish among these entities.

Reiter Syndrome

Clinical Features

Reiter syndrome is a symptom complex that consists of nongonorrheal urethritis that may be associated with *Chlamydia trachomatis* plus conjunctivitis, arthritis, and mucocutaneous lesions. There are two forms of the illness, an epidemic type that occurs after outbreaks of dysentery and a sporadic type. The epidemic form of the disease follows bacillary, amebic, or nonspecific dysentery. The sporadic form occurs almost exclusively in sexually active men. The incidence of Reiter syndrome is unknown.

The initial episode usually occurs between the ages of 20 and 40 years. The first manifestation is usually urethritis, which may precede the other symptoms by several weeks. Conjunctivitis is the only common eye manifestation, but iridocyclitis, keratitis, and retrobulbar neuritis also occur. The skin, oral cavity, and penis are affected, singly or in combination, in almost all cases. The penile lesions consist of moist eroded papules that coalesce to form circinate and serpiginous patches on the glans (circinate balanitis). The cutaneous lesions develop on the palms and soles but can occur elsewhere. They begin as pustules on erythematous macules that become crusted and keratotic and can merge to form fissured, purulent plaques resembling rupial psoriasis (keratoderma blenorrhagica). Subungual keratoses and paronychia also may occur, but nail pits do not develop. The oral le-

Figure 7-7. Pustular psoriasis. Because the spongiform pustules form very rapidly, there is no alteration of the stratum corneum. At the superior margins of the pustule, neutrophils are seen in small collections among the compressed squamous cells.

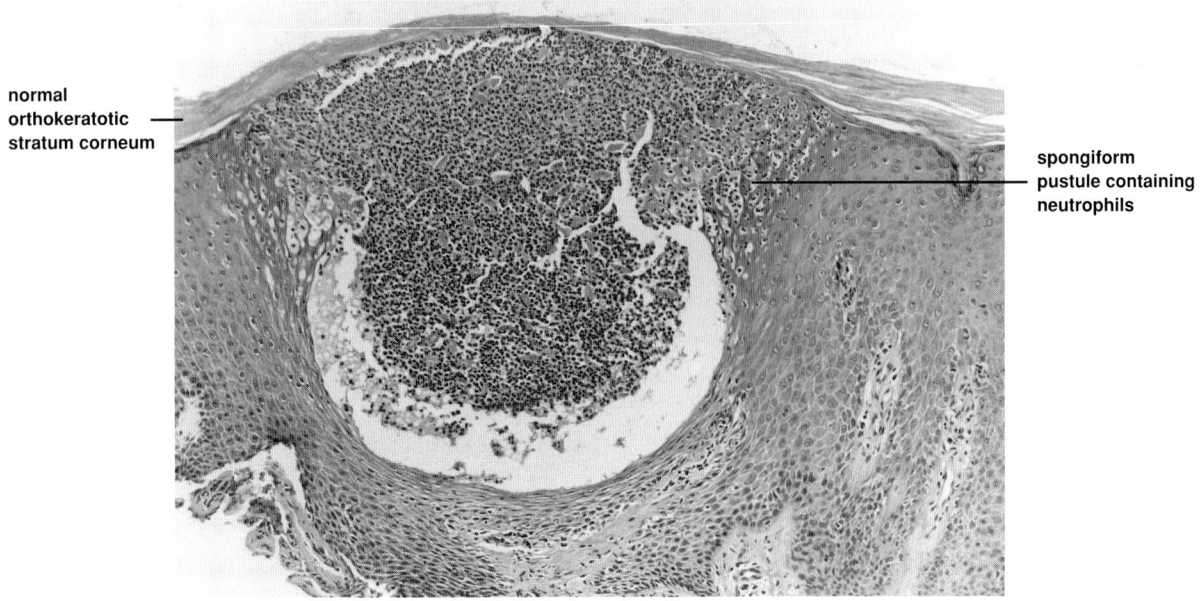

normal orthokeratotic stratum corneum

spongiform pustule containing neutrophils

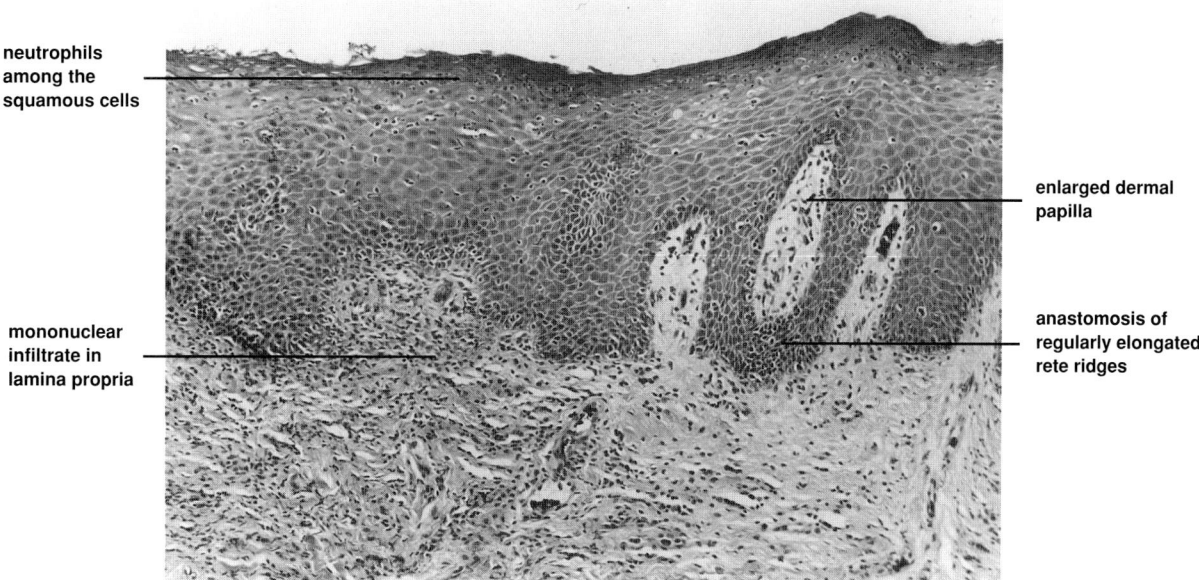

neutrophils
among the
squamous cells

enlarged dermal
papilla

mononuclear
infiltrate in
lamina propria

anastomosis of
regularly elongated
rete ridges

Figure 7-8.   Geographic tongue. The epithelium shows hyperplasia resembling psoriasis. There is a microabscess in the superficial spinous layer near the middle of the field. Within the lamina propria is a superficial perivascular inflammatory infiltrate.

sions consist of nondescript erythematous erosions and shallow ulcers.

The most disabling feature is arthritis, which has a striking resemblance to psoriatic arthritis. It involves only a few joints and tends to be asymmetric. Sacroileitis is common and is frequently associated with the HLA-B27 haplotype, as is psoriatic arthritis.[14]

Most patients have constitutional symptoms of malaise, low-grade fever and loss of appetite. Electrocardiographic changes are noted in about one-third of cases during an acute attack, and some patients develop pericarditis, myocarditis or aortic insufficiency due to inflammation of the aortic root. Recurrent attacks occur in 75% of patients, some of whom develop chronic arthritis.

The arthritis of Reiter syndrome resembles psoriatic arthritis. Both conditions are frequently associated with HLA-B27, and the acral lesions of Reiter syndrome look like rupial psoriasis. Therefore, it has been suggested that Reiter syndrome could be an atypical form of psoriasis. Because the cause of neither is known and because Reiter syndrome includes several components not found in psoriasis, they should be regarded as separate conditions until more is known about their pathogenesis.

Histopathologic Features

The early lesions are indistinguishable from pustular psoriasis. More long-standing lesions show varying degrees of epidermal hyperplasia, parakeratosis, and scale-crust formation, which may reach impressive proportions in palmoplantar lesions (Fig. 7-9). The dermal papillae are edematous, and there is a superficial perivascular inflammatory infiltrate. These lesions mimic rupial psoriasis.

NONPSORIATIC DERMATOSES WITH EPIDERMAL HYPERPLASIA

Pityriasis Rubra Pilaris

Clinical Features

Pityriasis rubra pilaris (PRP) is an uncommon chronic disease that is characterized clinically by pink follicular papules that become agminated to form well-demarcated, often salmon-colored plaques. As the plaques enlarge and coalesce, there are often noninvolved patches of skin among the confluent plaques. This "island sparing" also occurs in mycosis fungoides and occasionally in psoriasis, but it is most common in PRP. PRP usually begins on the scalp and the dorsal extremities, especially the extensor aspects of the fingers between the joints (Devergie's sign). The whole body may eventually become involved in the erythrodermic form. The skin of the palms and soles becomes thickened, hyperkeratotic, and shiny. This peculiar appearance on the soles is referred to as *keratodermic sandals.* It is sharply demarcated at the juncture of the volar and glabrous skin. The volar skin loses its pliability. This makes it susceptible to fissuring that can be extremely painful and even disabling. The nails are thickened and demonstrate longitudinal ridging but do not show pitting or onycholysis.

PRP may be familial or acquired. Griffiths[15] has defined five types based on age of onset and family history. Type I is the common acquired type that accounts for the great majority of cases. It usually begins in middle-aged adults and is self-limited in 3 to 5 years. The three juvenile types have a poor prognosis.

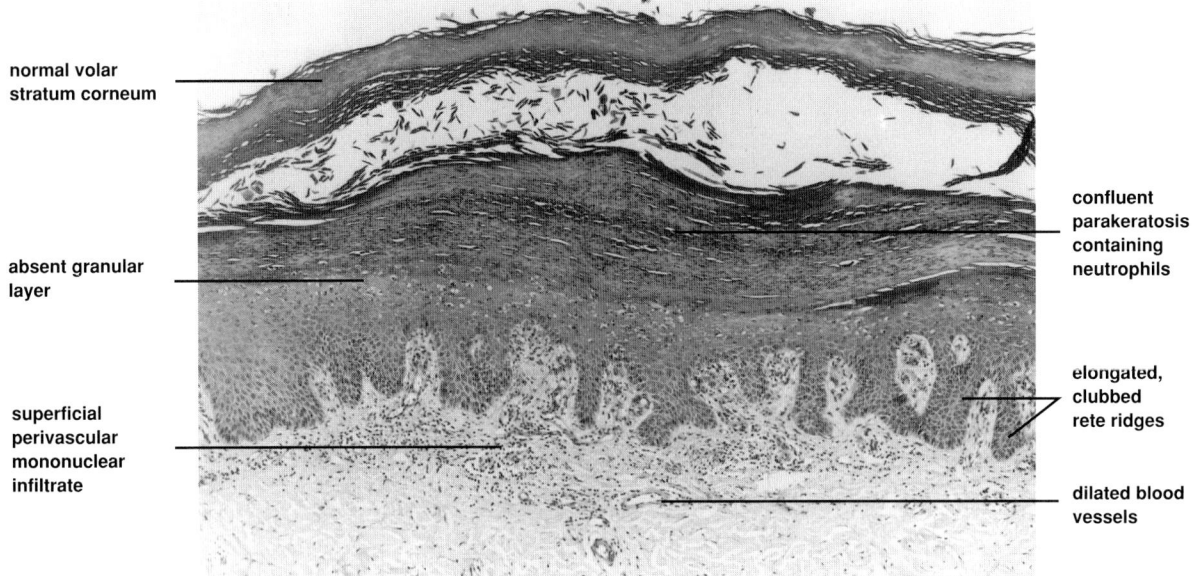

normal volar
stratum corneum

absent granular
layer

superficial
perivascular
mononuclear
infiltrate

confluent
parakeratosis
containing
neutrophils

elongated,
clubbed
rete ridges

dilated blood
vessels

Figure 7-9. Reiter syndrome. An early plantar lesion demonstrating confluent parakeratosis beneath the normal volar stratum corneum, loss of the granular zone, somewhat irregular epidermal dysplasia, and exocytosis of neutrophils. The dermal papillae contain dilated, tortuous capillaries, and there is a superficial perivascular inflammatory infiltrate.

Histopathologic Features

PRP shows slight to moderate epidermal hyperplasia with broad rete ridges and thickening of the suprapillary plates (Fig. 7-10). The granular layer is thickened, and the stratum corneum shows alternating foci of ortho- and parakeratosis.[16] The stratum corneum consists mainly of laminated or compact orthokeratin with foci of parakeratosis alternating haphazardly in both the vertical and horizontal planes. There may or may not be follicular plugs, but perifollicular parakeratosis is common.[17] Mitoses may be seen in the basal zone but are less numerous than in psoriasis.

There is a consistent but not a conspicuous inflammatory component. The epidermis may contain foci of slight spongiosis with exocytosis of a few lymphocytes. These foci are usually in the lower epidermis and differ from interface dermatitis in that there is no evidence of cell damage in the form of necrotic keratinocytes. There is vasodilation in the papillary dermis and a sparse superficial perivascular infiltrate of lymphocytes and macrophages. Neutrophils are not found in the epidermis or dermis in PRP.

Clinicopathologic Correlation

The follicular papules that characterize PRP are probably the result of two phenomena, follicular plugging and perifollicular parakeratosis. The red plaques result from interfollicular epidermal hyperplasia and vasodilation. The adherent scale is the result of the predominantly orthokeratotic changes that occur in the stratum corneum.

Pathophysiology

Virtually nothing is known about the pathogenesis of this condition. The occurrence of both familial and acquired types suggests that there may be more than one abnormality that can produce the same phenotypic changes. Low serum levels of retinol-binding protein have been found in some patients, but some of their unaffected relatives had similarly low levels.[18] Elevated proliferative indices similar to psoriasis have been found in PRP.[19]

Lichen Simplex Chronicus, Prurigo Nodularis, and Picker's Nodule

Clinical Features

Lichen simplex chronicus is characterized by a pruritic, discrete, lichenoid papular eruption usually confined to a localized area, especially the anogenital region, back of the neck, knee or elbow flexure, ankle, or dorsum of the hand or foot. These morphologic features are due to chronic rubbing and scratching.

Lichenification is a thickening of the epidermis with exaggeration of its normal markings so that the lines form a crisscross pattern enclosing flat-topped, often shiny, smooth quadrilateral facets between them. The localized condition without an antecedent cause is labeled *lichen simplex chronicus*. The disseminated form that characteristically affects flexural areas such as the antecubital and popliteal fossae is a major component of atopic dermatitis. Lichenification may be superimposed on numerous pruritic diseases, including arthropod reactions,

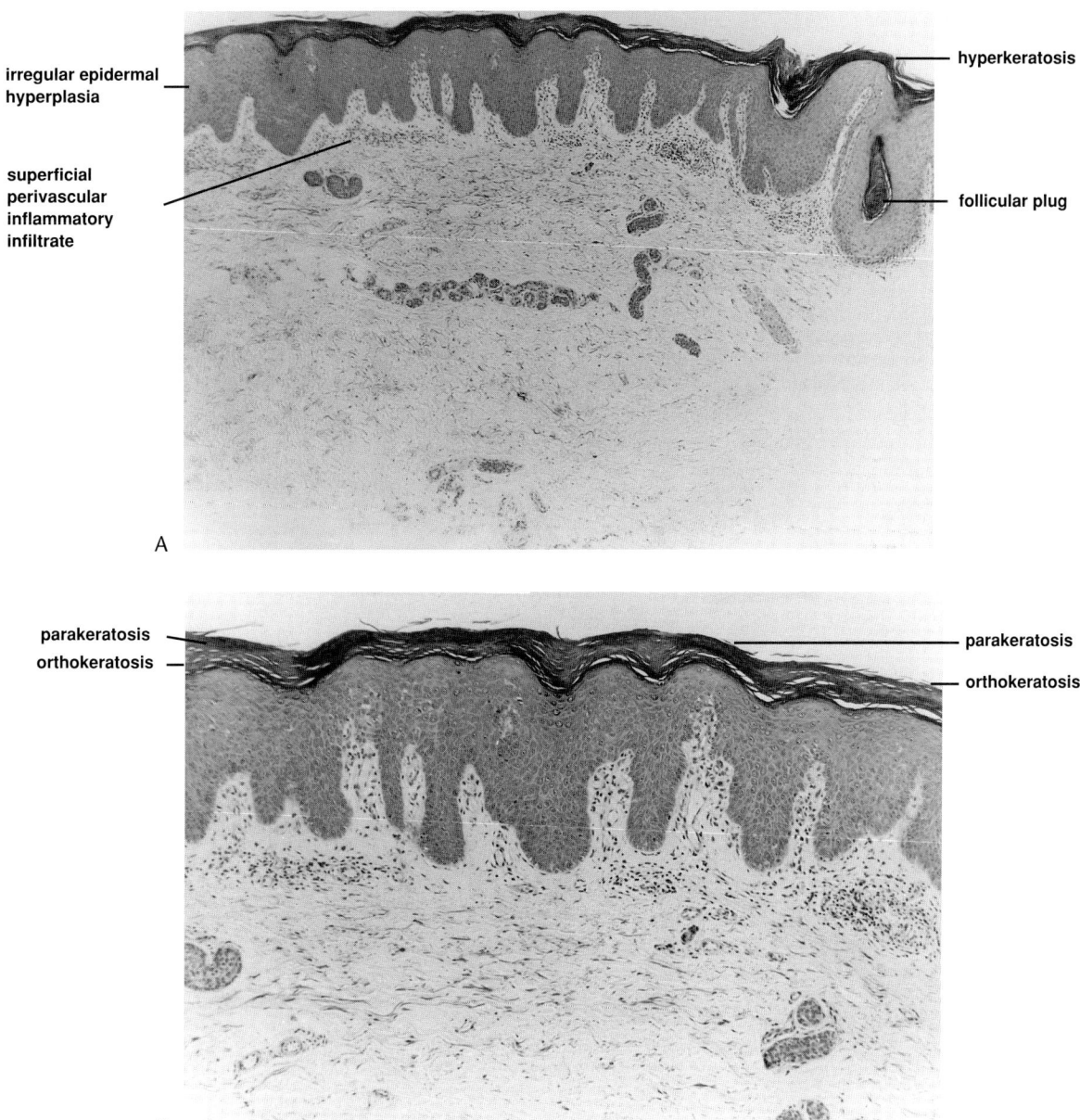

irregular epidermal
hyperplasia

superficial
perivascular
inflammatory
infiltrate

hyperkeratosis

follicular plug

A

parakeratosis
orthokeratosis

parakeratosis
orthokeratosis

B

Figure 7-10. Pityriasis rubra pilaris. **(A)** At scanning power, there is moderate, slightly irregular epidermal hyperplasia with thickening of the epidermis over the tips of the dermal papillae. The stratum corneum is hyperkeratotic, and the follicle at the right shows plugging of the infundibulum. **(B)** At higher power, the stratum corneum shows foci of dark parakeratin alternating both horizontally and vertically with lighter orthokeratin. There is a sparse superficial perivascular mononuclear cell infiltrate in the papillary dermis.

allergic contact dermatitis, stasis dermatitis, dermatophyte infections, lichen planus, linear epidermal nevus, and mycosis fungoides. Therefore, it is necessary to exclude a preceding or concomitant disease process before making a diagnosis of lichen simplex chronicus.

Prurigo nodularis refers to a condition in which there are one or more well-defined pruritic nodules with a hyperkeratotic, sometimes verrucous surface. It usually occurs on the extremi-

ties, especially the lower. Picker's nodule is a similar condition in which the surface is crusted and eroded due to picking with a fingernail rather than rubbing.

Histopathologic Features

Lichen simplex chronicus shows dense orthohyperkeratosis that can be striking (Fig. 7-11). Parakeratosis and scale-crust formation is usually focal and limited to excoriated foci. The

Figure 7-11. Lichen simplex chronicus. **(A)** The epidermis shows marked hyperplasia with unequal elongation of the rete ridges. There is prominent orthohyperkeratosis. **(B)** The dermal papillae are broad and demonstrate lamellar fibrosis with vertically oriented coarse collagen bundles. There is a perivascular and interstitial infiltrate of mononuclear cells.

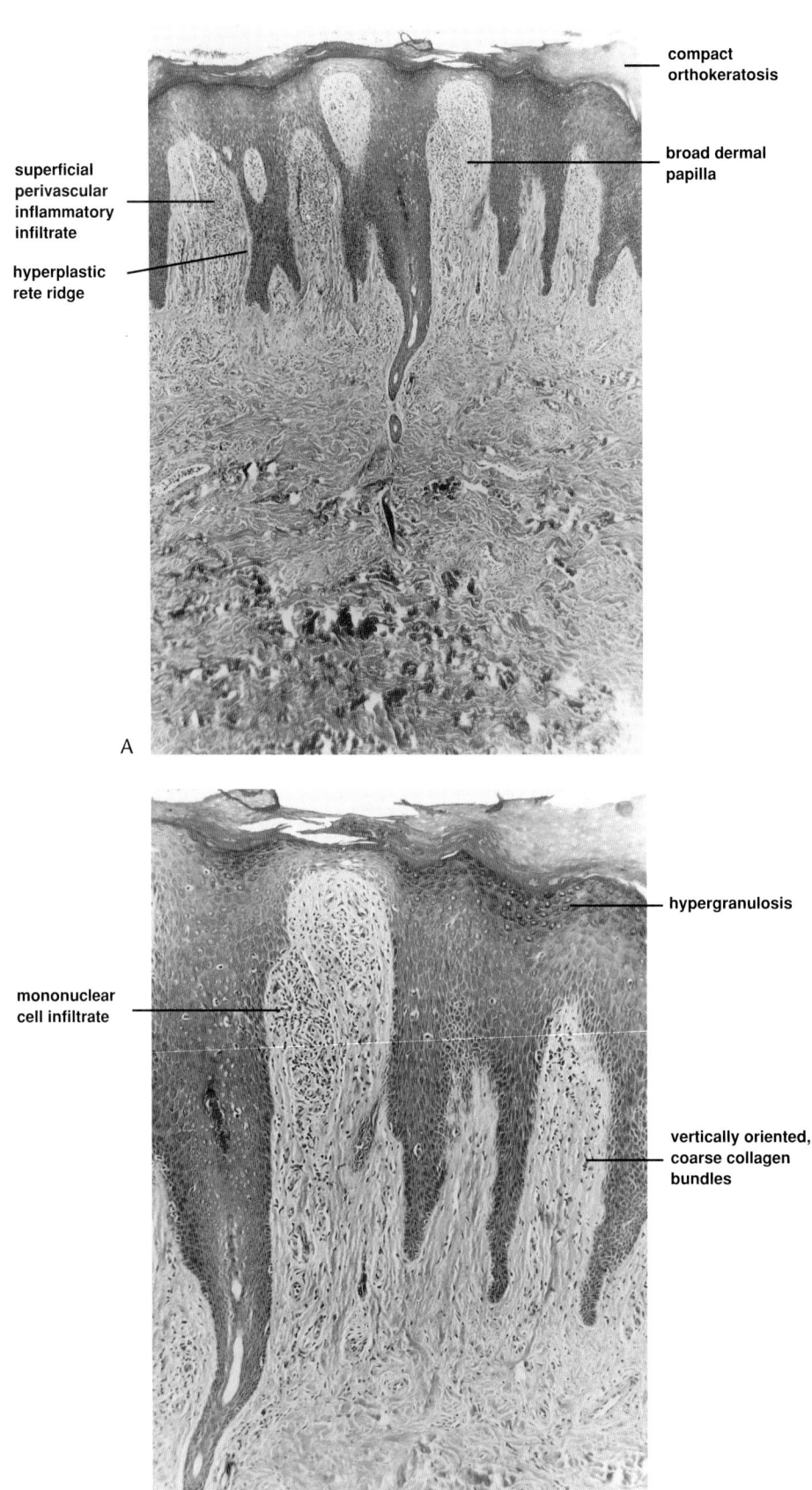

compact orthokeratosis

broad dermal papilla

superficial perivascular inflammatory infiltrate

hyperplastic rete ridge

A

mononuclear cell infiltrate

hypergranulosis

vertically oriented, coarse collagen bundles

B

stratum corneum often simulates that of volar skin and may be the most conspicuous feature of lichen simplex chronicus, especially on the skin of the scalp and genitalia. The granular layer is usually thickened, and acanthosis with irregular elongation of the rete ridges is present. An important aspect of the altered rete is that they vary not only in length but also in width. The rete tend to be broad rather than narrow, as in psoriasis. The papillary dermis is hyperplastic. The coarse collagen bundles follow the profile of the rete ridges, giving them a vertical orientation in the widened dermal papillae. Plump and sometimes stellate fibroblasts are present among the thickened collagen bundles. A sparse to moderate inflammatory cell infiltrate of lymphocytes and monocytes with rare or no eosinophils is present around the vessels of the superficial plexus.

Identical histopathologic changes occur in the lichenified lesions of atopic dermatitis. Furthermore, lichenification may be superimposed on chronic dermatitides of various etiologies. Therefore, it is worthwhile to look for clues to the cause of the histopathologic changes. If there are abundant eosinophils around the superficial plexus, chronic allergic contact dermatitis or nummular dermatitis should be considered. If there is a superficial and deep perivascular and interstitial mixed infiltrate that contains eosinophils, chronic arthropod reaction is a consideration. The stratum corneum should be examined for fungal hyphae to exclude dermatophytosis. The tips of the rete ridges show interface changes and obscuration by lymphocytes in hypertrophic lichen planus.

Prurigo nodularis can be considered to be hypertrophic lichen simplex chronicus (Fig. 7-12). The microscopic changes in this condition are only quantitatively different. If the entire nodule is excised, the chief clue to the differential diagnosis from lichen simplex chronicus is its dome shape rather than the flatter profile of the plaque of lichen simplex chronicus. Picker's nodule is identical to prurigo nodularis but has the added features of erosions covered by scale-crusts due to excoriation. Granuloma fissuratum is also a variation on this theme. In this disorder, the epidermal reaction is caused by pressure or friction generated by the frames of glasses on the nose or in the post auricular sulcus.

Clinicopathologic Correlation

The firm, elevated plaque of lichen simplex chronicus is due to alterations in both the epidermis and dermis. The often smooth surface is due to orthohyperkeratosis in which the corneocytes are tightly adherent. The epidermal hyperplasia and fibroplasia of the dermal papillae account for the elevation and mammillation of the plaques. There is usually only minimal erythema in idiopathic lichen simplex chronicus, which correlates with the sparse superficial perivascular inflammation.

Pathophysiology

Lichenification is due to persistent rubbing and scratching of the skin. Some observers have noted prominence of nerves in lichenified skin and have postulated that neural hyperplasia leads to the itch-scratch-itch cycle that perpetuates the disease. This lends support to the concept of neurodermatitis. It seems more likely that the neural changes are secondary to cytokine growth factors elaborated in the area to promote healing of the chronically traumatized skin. Increased synthesis of growth factors such as epidermal growth factor and nerve growth factor could account for the hyperplasia of the epidermis, papillary dermis, and nerves. This hypothesis has not been scientifically tested.

Figure 7-12. Prurigo nodularis. The histologic changes are similar to lichen simplex chronicus but even more marked. This dome-shaped nodule has markedly hyperplastic rete ridges and very broad dermal papillae with vertically streaked collagen.

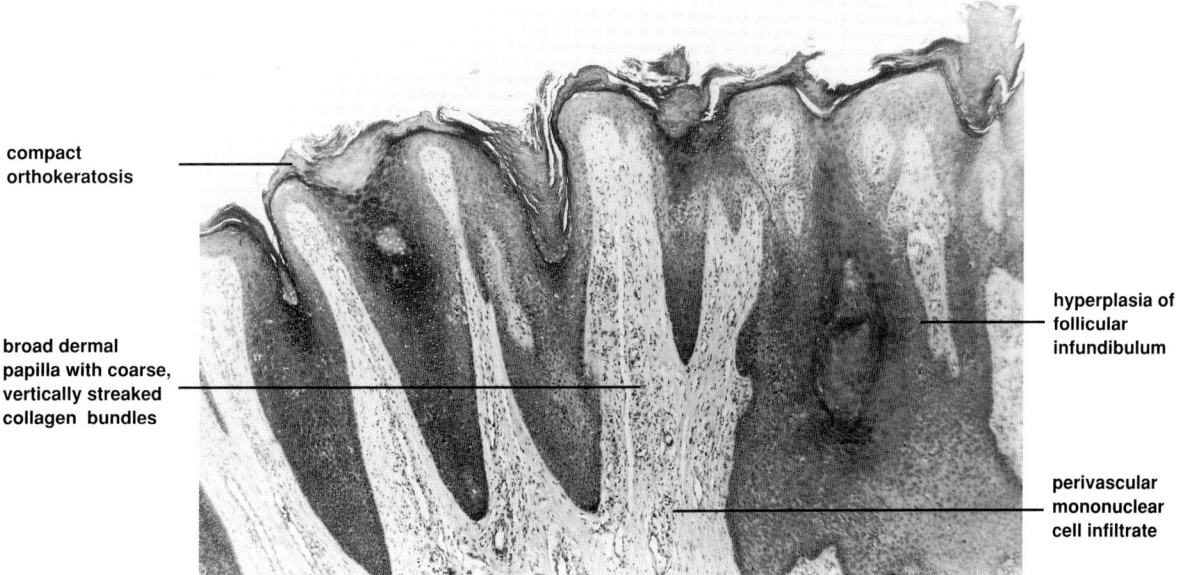

compact orthokeratosis

broad dermal papilla with coarse, vertically streaked collagen bundles

hyperplasia of follicular infundibulum

perivascular mononuclear cell infiltrate

Pellagra

Clinical Features

In the early stage of pellagra there is symmetric erythema and sometimes vesiculation on sun-exposed areas, including the face, ears, V-area of the neck, and the dorsum of the hands and wrists. The acute vesicular stage gives way to the chronic phase of erythema, scaling, and fissuring. A broad collar-like band of erythema and scaling around the neck known as Casal's "necklace" is a clinical hallmark of pellagra. Dull erythema and fine, branny scaling of the bridge of the nose is also characteristic. In addition to the dermatitis, there is also diarrhea and dementia in more advanced cases. Less frequent signs and symptoms include angular cheilitis and glossitis, loss of appetite, cachexia, and insomnia. Pellagra occurs in malnourished persons secondary to poverty, malabsorption, or alcoholism. After restoration of adequate nutrition and niacin supplementation, the cutaneous changes resolve and leave prominent postinflammatory hyperpigmentation.

Histopathologic Features

Early in the course of the disease, there may still be basket-weave orthokeratin above foci of parakeratosis. The squamous cells in the stratum spinosum usually are pale staining (Fig. 7-13). Ballooning change may lead to intraepidermal vesiculation.[20] Later, the epidermis shows variable hyperplasia and less pallor. The stratum corneum shows confluent hyperkeratosis and parakeratosis.[21] The capillaries in the papillary dermis are dilated. There is a sparse superficial perivascular infiltrate of lymphocytes and monocytes, and there may be focal extravasation of erythrocytes. The lipocytes in the subcutis may appear shrunken.

Clinicopathologic Correlation

The early vesicular stage of the disease is due to ballooning change in the stratum spinosum. The scale seen later correlates with the broad foci of parakeratosis. The epidermal hyperplasia accounts for the thickening of the skin, and the superficial perivascular inflammation and vasodilation are responsible for the erythema.

Pathophysiology

Pellagra is caused by a deficiency of niacin in the diet. Tryptophan can be converted to niacin, so dietary deficiency of tryptophan may contribute to the development of pellagra. A pellagra-like state can develop in persons who have a carcinoid tumor or Hartnup syndrome in which niacin synthesis is impeded by a diversion of tryptophan metabolism.[22] Pellagra has also been associated with isoniazid therapy in high doses.[23] Pyridoxine (vitamin B_6) is a coenzyme in tryptophan metabolism, and isoniazid competitively inhibits the conversion of pyridoxal phosphate to pyridoxine by the enzyme apotryptophanase. There is a striking association of the dermatitis with sun exposure, but the action spectrum is not known.

Acrodermatitis Enteropathica

Clinical Features

Acrodermatitis enteropathica is a disease mainly of infancy. It is closely associated with persistent diarrhea and failure to thrive, which are clues to the etiology of the skin involvement. There is a weeping vesiculobullous eruption characteristically distributed around the mouth, in the diaper area, and on the distal extremities that evolves to crusted papulopustular and psori-

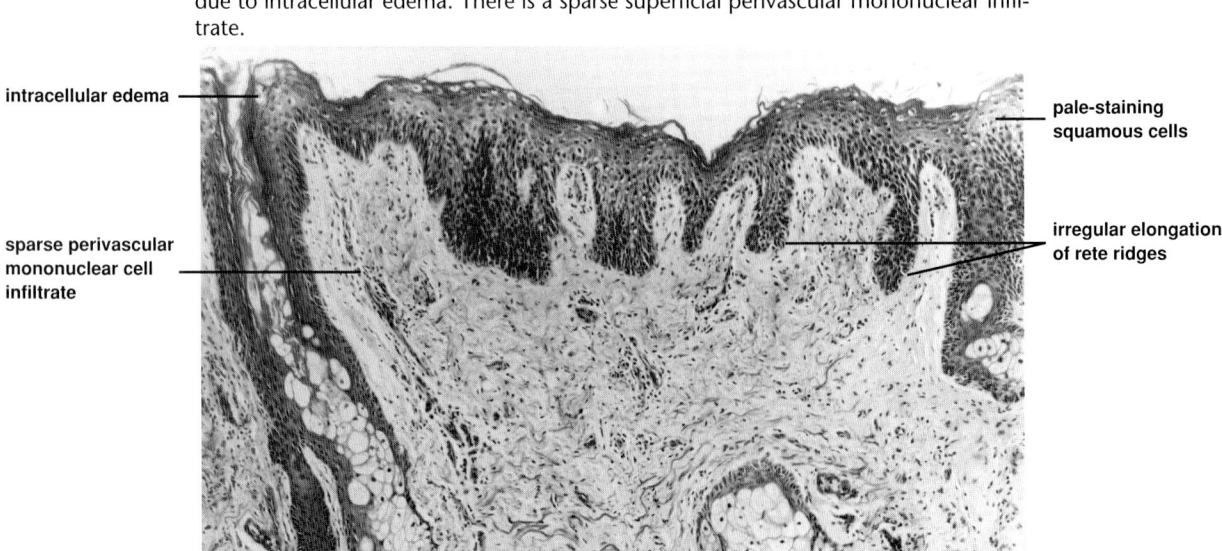

Figure 7-13. Pellagra, early lesion. There is moderate but irregular epidermal hyperplasia. The keratinocytes in the spinous layer are pale staining. Some cells are swollen due to intracellular edema. There is a sparse superficial perivascular mononuclear infiltrate.

intracellular edema

sparse perivascular mononuclear cell infiltrate

pale-staining squamous cells

irregular elongation of rete ridges

asiform lesions. Nail dystrophy is common as is secondary infection by *Candida albicans*. Glossitis, stomatitis, and hair loss also occur. Similar clinical findings may be seen in adults with acquired zinc deficiency.

Histopathologic Features

Acrodermatitis enteropathica demonstrates different features at each point in its evolution.[24,25] The chronic psoriasiform lesions may show either confluent parakeratosis or orthokeratosis with focal parakeratosis and irregular epidermal hyperplasia. The granular zone is diminished in the regions of parakeratosis. Tortuous capillaries that resemble those of psoriasis are present in the dermal papillae. The dermis shows a moderately dense superficial perivascular infiltrate of mononuclear cells. Superimposed candidiasis is suggested by spongiform pustules and neutrophils in the papillary dermis.

The early lesions are more characteristic because they show prominent pallor of the keratinocytes caused by intracellular edema that may progress to ballooning change. Focal spongiosis may be present. The stratum corneum shows confluent parakeratosis over the zone of epidermal pallor. The parakeratosis may be covered by the residual normal basket-weave stratum corneum. In subacute lesions, a subcorneal vesicle with features of reticular degeneration may develop (Fig. 7-14). The dermis shows vascular dilation and tortuosity, interstitial edema, and a sparse perivascular mononuclear cell infiltrate.

Clinicopathologic Correlation

The early vesicles that may occur in acrodermatitis enteropathica are the result of ballooning and lysis of keratinocytes in the upper layers of the stratum spinosum. The psoriasiform plaques are caused by reactive epidermal hyperplasia that evolves as the condition persists. It is not known whether the parakeratosis is the result of hyperproliferation or a failure of differentiation. Secondary changes such as pustule formation, erosions, and crusts are often caused by superimposed infection with bacteria or *C. albicans*.

Pathophysiology

Acrodermatitis enteropathica is caused by zinc deficiency and can be inherited or acquired. The inherited type is thought to be transmitted as an autosomal dominant trait.[26] Acquired zinc deficiency has been found in adult patients who are receiving zinc-deficient hyperalimentation, in alcoholics, in patients with various chronic illnesses, and in persons with disease-induced or surgically induced malabsorption. Zinc is essential for homeostasis because of the many zinc metalloenzymes that are important in the metabolism of proteins, fat, and carbohydrates in addition to maintaining numerous cell functions, including cellular immunity.[27]

Necrolytic Migratory Erythema (Glucagonoma Syndrome)

Clinical Features

Necrolytic migratory erythema is a distinctive eruption that is a cutaneous marker for a glucagon-secreting tumor of the pancreatic alpha cells. These tumors are uncommon and occur mainly in women around and after menopause. They are associated with mild diabetes, weight loss, depression, and normocytic anemia in addition to the cutaneous eruption. Plasma glucagon levels are elevated, there is hyperglycemia, and fasting amino acid levels are significantly decreased. Pancreatic computed tomography scans and celiac arteriography may be helpful in establishing the diagnosis. A similar eruption has also been observed in patients with intestinal malabsorption and normal glucagon levels.[28]

The cutaneous lesions usually involve the face, perineum, and lower abdomen but may occur on the proximal extremities. They appear as figurate erythematous patches and plaques with central flaccid bullae that rupture, leaving an eroded surface and a peripheral scale. This cycle of events may be repeated at 1- to 2-week intervals. Scaling macules and papules may also be seen. Mucositis may also occur, involving the angles of the mouth, tongue, vagina, and perianal area. These lesions resemble the changes seen in acrodermatitis enteropathica.

Patients who have a benign, functioning α-cell tumor experience rapid and complete remission after resection of the neoplasm. About one-half the patients with necrolytic migratory erythema have malignant glucagonomas that have already metastasized to regional lymph nodes and liver by the time the diagnosis is made.[29] These patients may experience relief of symptoms after a debulking procedure but will have recurrence of symptoms as the metastases grow in size.

Histopathologic Features

The histopathologic features of the early lesions are usually characteristic enough to enable a definitive diagnosis. Beneath the normal basket-weave stratum corneum there is a broad, confluent zone of necrosis marked by flattened keratinocytes with eosinophilic cytoplasm and degeneration of nuclei overlying a zone of pallid keratinocytes that demonstrate prominent intracellular edema and pyknotic nuclei[30,31] (Fig. 7-15). Clefts often occur in this zone. There is papillary dermal edema, vasodilation, and sometimes angioplasia of the superficial plexus and a sparse perivascular infiltrate of mononuclear cells and sometimes neutrophils. Some early lesions show only scattered individual necrotic keratinocytes in the mid to upper stratum spinosum, spongiosis, and variable parakeratosis.[32] Later lesions are not specific as they demonstrate psoriasiform epidermal hyperplasia, focal to confluent parakeratosis, and a superficial perivascular mononuclear cell infiltrate.

Clinicopathologic Correlation

The flaccid bullae that developed in necrolytic migratory erythema correlate with the superficial epidermal necrosis that evolves into clefts in the stratum granulosum or upper stratum spinosum. The peeling stratum corneum at the edges of the subsequent erosions, therefore, is similar to the peripheral scale of pemphigus foliaceous.

Pathophysiology

The pathogenesis of the epidermal necrosis in necrolytic migratory erythema is unclear, because not every person who has a glucagon-secreting tumor develops skin lesions. Because of the correlation with decreased serum amino acids and improvement

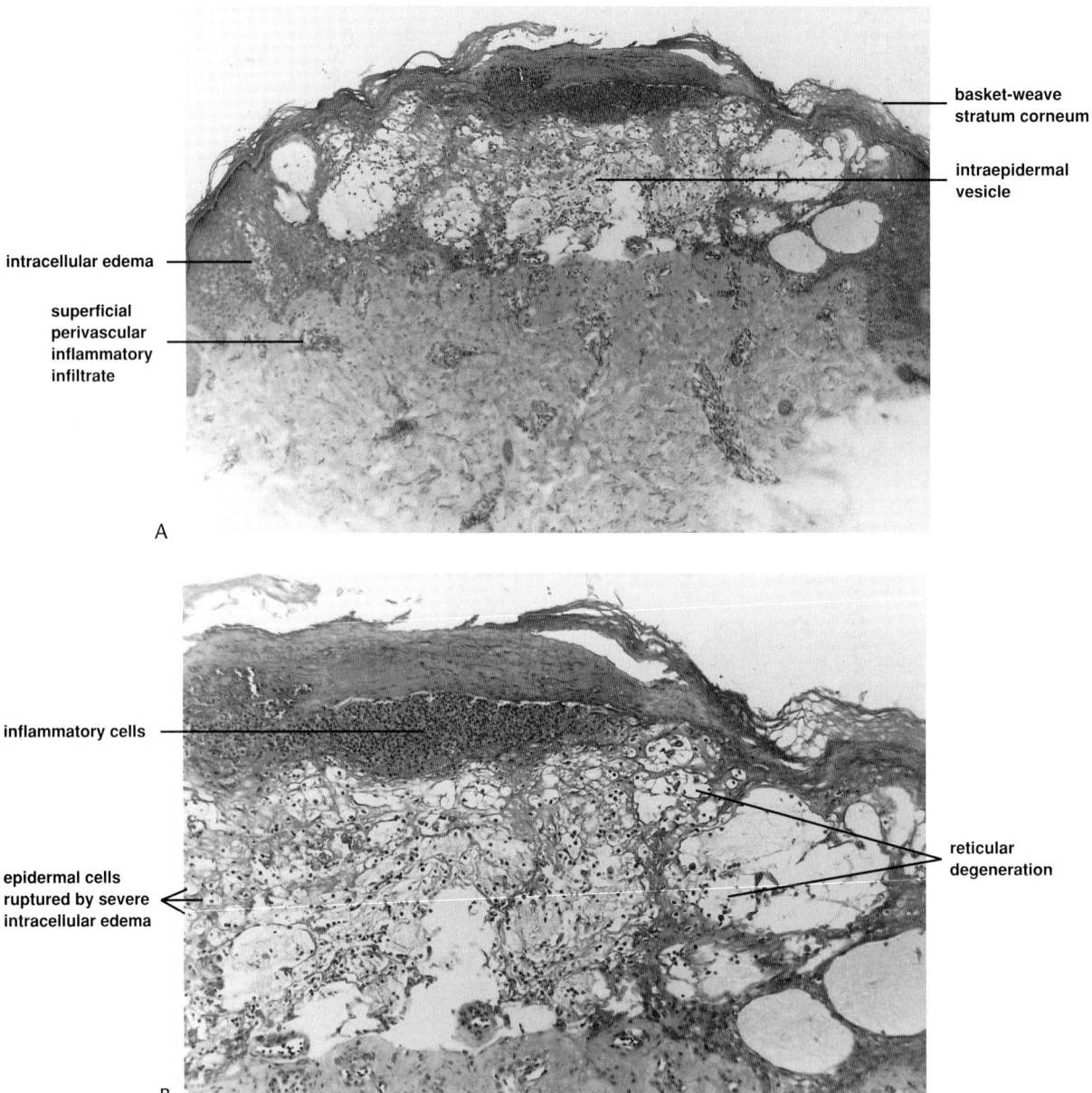

Figure 7-14. Acrodermatitis enteropathica, subacute lesion. **(A)** There is prominent reticular degeneration of the epidermis with formation of a multiloculated intraepidermal vesicle. The dermis shows a relatively sparse perivascular mononuclear infiltrate. **(B)** At higher power, there is a scale-crust beneath the basket-weave stratum corneum. Note the severe intracellular edema with rupture of the keratinocytes.

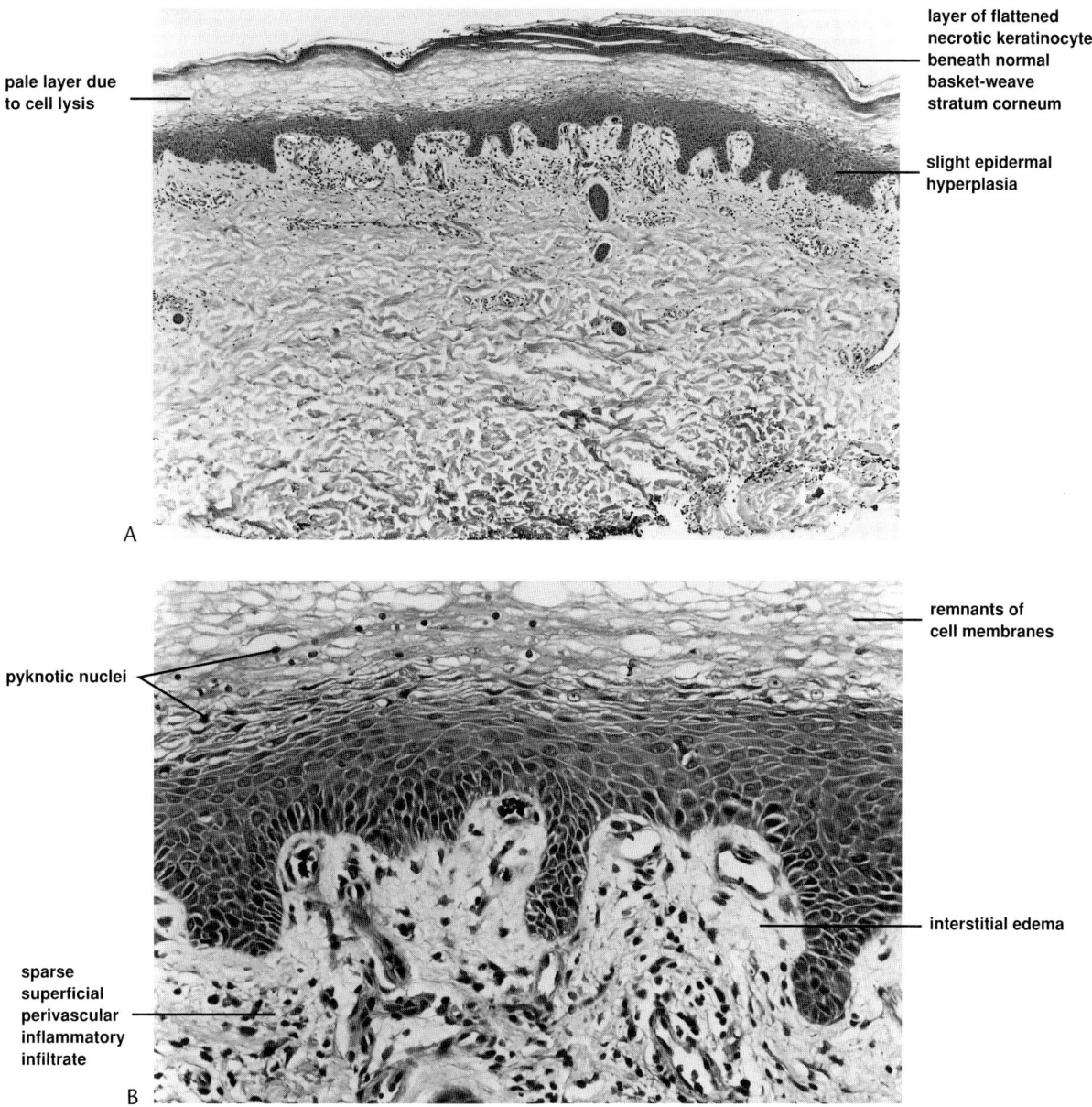

pale layer due to cell lysis

layer of flattened necrotic keratinocytes beneath normal basket-weave stratum corneum

slight epidermal hyperplasia

A

remnants of cell membranes

pyknotic nuclei

interstitial edema

sparse superficial perivascular inflammatory infiltrate

B

Figure 7-15. Necrolytic migratory erythema, early lesion. **(A)** Beneath the normal basket-weave stratum corneum there is a broad zone of pallor due to intracellular edema and necrosis of the upper spinous layer. **(B)** Pyknotic nuclei are present in the necrotic cells in the upper spinous layer. There is edema in the dermal papillae, and there is a sparse mononuclear cell infiltrate around the dilated capillaries of the papillary dermis.

with intravenous amino acid supplementation, amino acid catabolism may play a role in the epidermal damage. An abnormality of zinc metabolism, as in acrodermatitis enteropathica, has also been postulated but is inconsistently found in glucogonoma syndrome.

OTHER DERMATOSES THAT DEMONSTRATE EPIDERMAL HYPERPLASIA

Subacute and Chronic Spongiotic Dermatitides

Nummular, allergic contact, and other spongiotic dermatitides show a progression of epidermal hyperplasia and decreasing spongiosis in persistent lesions (Fig. 7-16). Nummular and al-

lergic contact dermatitis also show thickening of the papillary dermis with vertical streaking of the collagen that simulates lichen simplex chronicus and atopic dermatitis. The frequent presence of eosinophils in the dermal infiltrate, the coarse, rather than delicate, fibrillary collagen in the dermal papillae, and the irregular hyperplasia of the epidermis distinguish these spongiotic conditions from psoriasis.

Pityriasis Rosea (Herald Patch)

The herald patch of pityriasis rosea is not only larger than the secondary lesions but also is often thicker. The histologic correlates are more prominent epidermal hyperplasia than in the secondary lesions and sometimes a deeper dermal infiltrate

Figure 7-16. Chronic allergic contact dermatitis. **(A)** The epidermis shows hyperkeratosis, irregular epidermal hyperplasia, and focal spongiosis. The papillary dermis is increased in thickness, and there is vertically streaked coarse collagen due to persistent rubbing. A moderately dense superficial perivascular and interstitial inflammatory infiltrate is present. **(B)** There is predominant orthokeratosis with focal parakeratosis. Focal slight spongiosis is present in the epidermis above the dermal papillae.

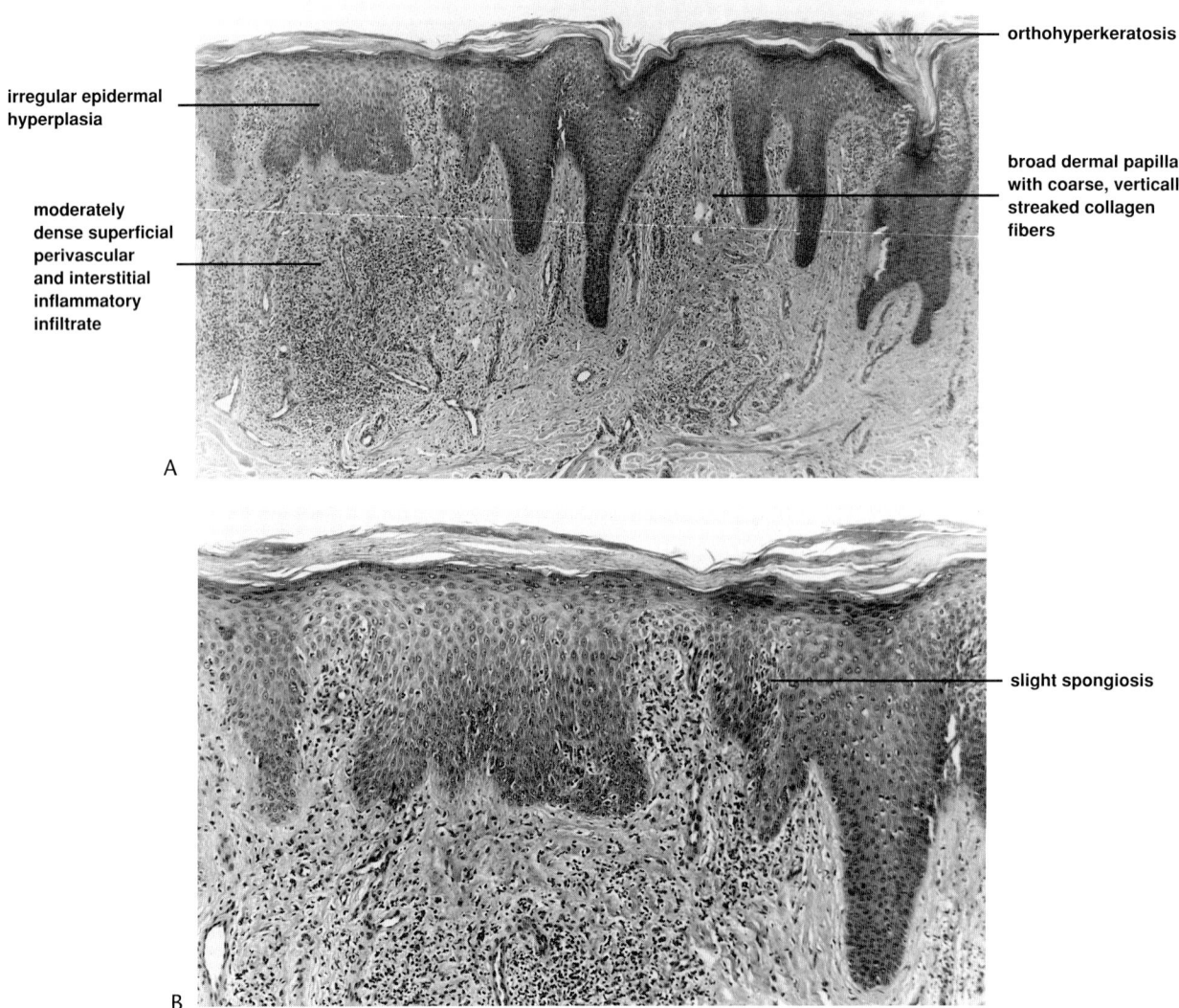

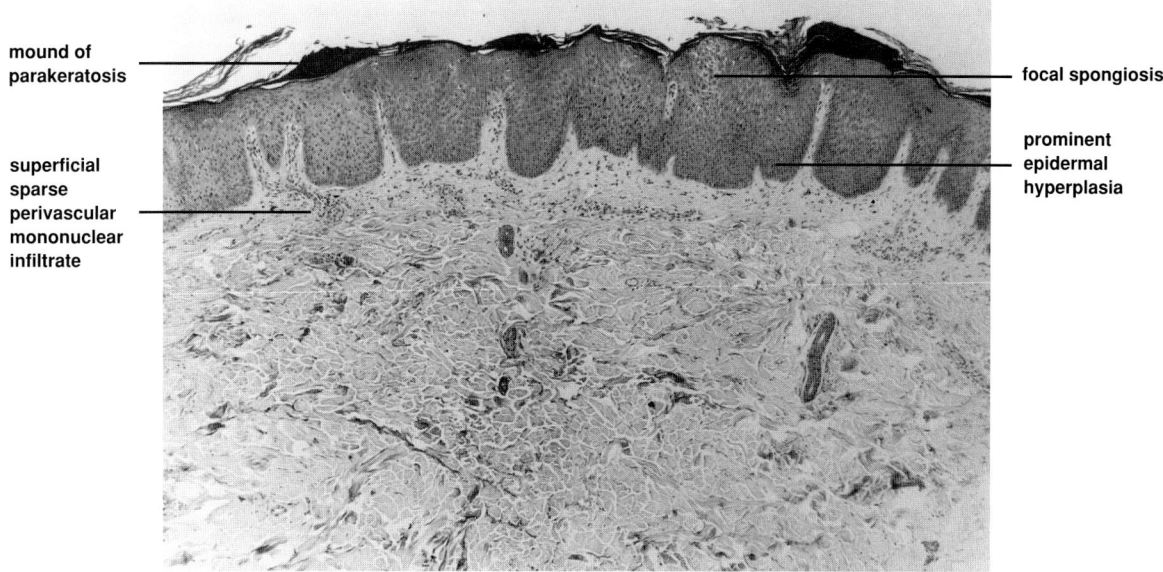

mound of
parakeratosis

focal spongiosis

superficial
sparse
perivascular
mononuclear
infiltrate

prominent
epidermal
hyperplasia

Figure 7-17. Herald patch of pityriasis rosea. The epidermis exhibits prominent hyperplasia with broad rete ridges, narrow dermal papillae, and no apparent thinning of the epidermis above the dermal papillae as in psoriasis. Characteristically, there are mounds of parakeratosis as in the secondary lesions of pityriasis rosea, and focal spongiosis may be present. This example shows only a sparse superficial perivascular mononuclear cell infiltrate, but some lesions may also show involvement of the deep plexus.

(Fig. 7-17). The parakeratotic foci may also be more prominent. An unusual cytolytic change has been noted in keratinocytes adjacent to Langerhans cells in herald patches in some cases.[33]

Hypertrophic Lichen Planus

Lichen planus is noted for its intense pruritus. Most affected persons do not rub or scratch the lesions because the scratching produces pain. However, some persons tolerate the pain better than the pruritus, so they compulsively traumatize the lesions and thereby superimpose the changes of lichen simplex chronicus on the papules of lichen planus. This occurs usually on the shins.

Histologically such lesions show more pronounced epidermal hyperplasia than ordinary lichen planus. The interface changes are localized to the tips of the elongated rete ridges (Fig. 7-18). The dermal papillae are widened and show vertical lamellae of coarse collagen. Some lesions also show crusted erosions or ulcers.

Secondary Syphilis

The early lesions of secondary syphilis are erythematous macules that evolve into papulosquamous plaques. The papulosquamous lesions may be relatively smooth surfaced as in lichen planus or scaly as in pityriasis rosea or psoriasis. The rupial lesions have a thick, dirty-appearing scale.

Secondary syphilis regularly shows the histopathologic pattern of an interface dermatitis with a superficial and deep perivascular infiltrate of lymphocytes, macrophages, and

plasma cells. In the papulosquamous lesions there is variable epidermal hyperplasia that can resemble psoriasis in more advanced lesions (Fig. 7-19). The keratinocytes are often pale staining. There may be confluent parakeratosis with concomitant loss of the granular zone. To complete the comparison with psoriasis, there may also be exocytosis of neutrophils with formation of microabscesses in the upper stratum spinosum, which are then pushed up into the parakeratotic stratum corneum by epidermal proliferation. This occurs particularly in rupial lesions.

Subacute and Chronic Candidiasis and Dermatophytosis

Persistent infection with *Candida* spp. and dermatophytes leads to reactive epidermal hyperplasia. This phenomenon occurs most commonly in the moccasin type of tinea pedia caused by chronic *Trichophyton rubrum* infection. The skin becomes thickened, erythematous, and scaly. Persons with chronic mucocutaneous candidiasis associated with an endocrinopathy or an immune deficiency also usually demonstrate clinical lesions that simulate psoriasis and appear as rather well-marginated, erythematous plaques with superimposed scale.

Persistent candida and dermatophyte infections histologically show mild to moderate epidermal hyperplasia that does not show the even elongation of rete ridges that characterized the well-developed plaque of psoriasis (Fig. 7-20). There is exocytosis of inflammatory cells with slight spongiosis. Spongiform pustules may form and are identical to those seen in psoriasis. The stratum corneum in a *Candida* infection generally shows

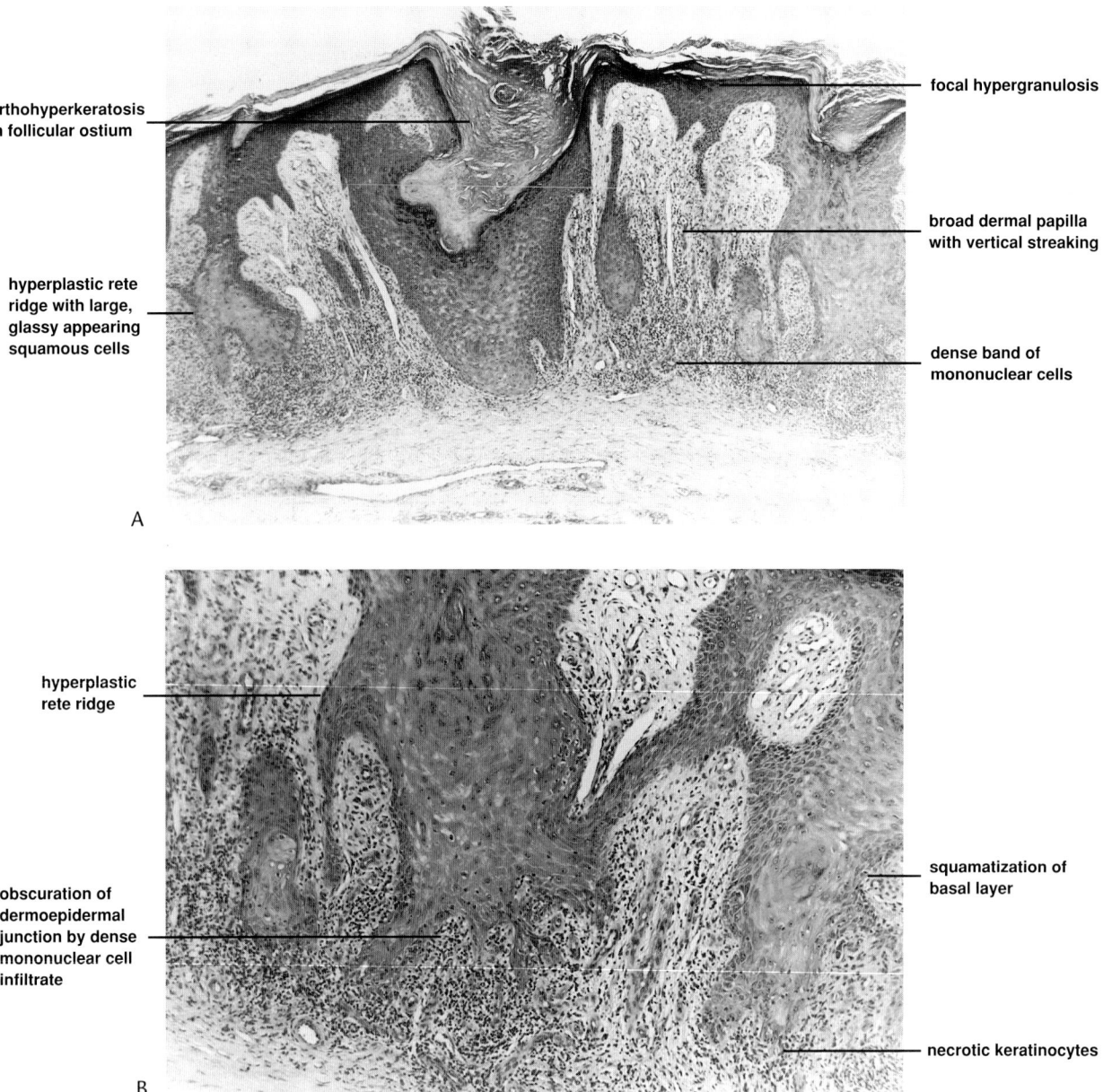

orthohyperkeratosis
in follicular ostium

focal hypergranulosis

hyperplastic rete
ridge with large,
glassy appearing
squamous cells

broad dermal papilla
with vertical streaking

dense band of
mononuclear cells

hyperplastic
rete ridge

squamatization of
basal layer

obscuration of
dermoepidermal
junction by dense
mononuclear cell
infiltrate

necrotic keratinocytes

A

B

Figure 7-18. Hypertrophic lichen planus. **(A)** There is compact orthohyperkeratosis, focal hypergranulosis, marked hyperplasia of some rete ridges, and wide dermal papillae with coarse, vertically streaked collagen fibers owing to persistent rubbing. There is a band-like mononuclear cell infiltrate that spares the upper papillary dermis but obscures the dermoepidermal junction around the bases of the rete ridges. **(B)** The keratinocytes in the spinous layer are large and have abundant, pale-staining cytoplasm. The dense inflammatory infiltrate obscures the dermoepidermal junction of the rete ridges. There is squamatization of the epidermal basal layer.

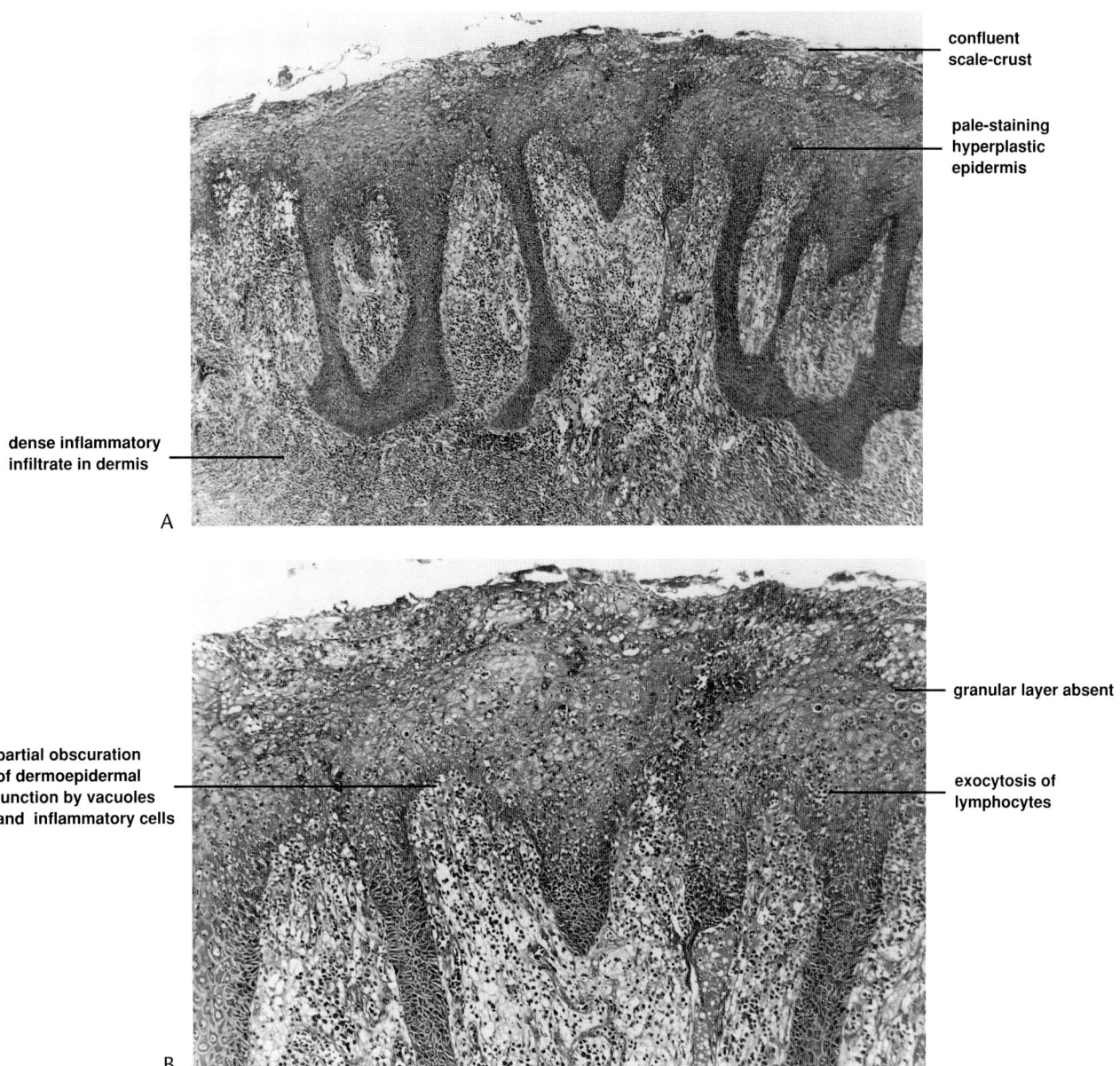

Figure 7-19. Condyloma lata of secondary syphilis. **(A)** There is markedly irregular epidermal hyperplasia with elongation and anastomosis of rete ridges. The stratum corneum shows diffuse parakeratosis and accumulation of inflammatory cell debris. A dense diffuse infiltrate of lymphocytes, macrophages, neutrophils, and plasma cells is present in the papillary and upper reticular dermis. **(B)** The squamous cells are pale staining, and there is diffuse exocytosis of inflammatory cells.
(Figure continues.)

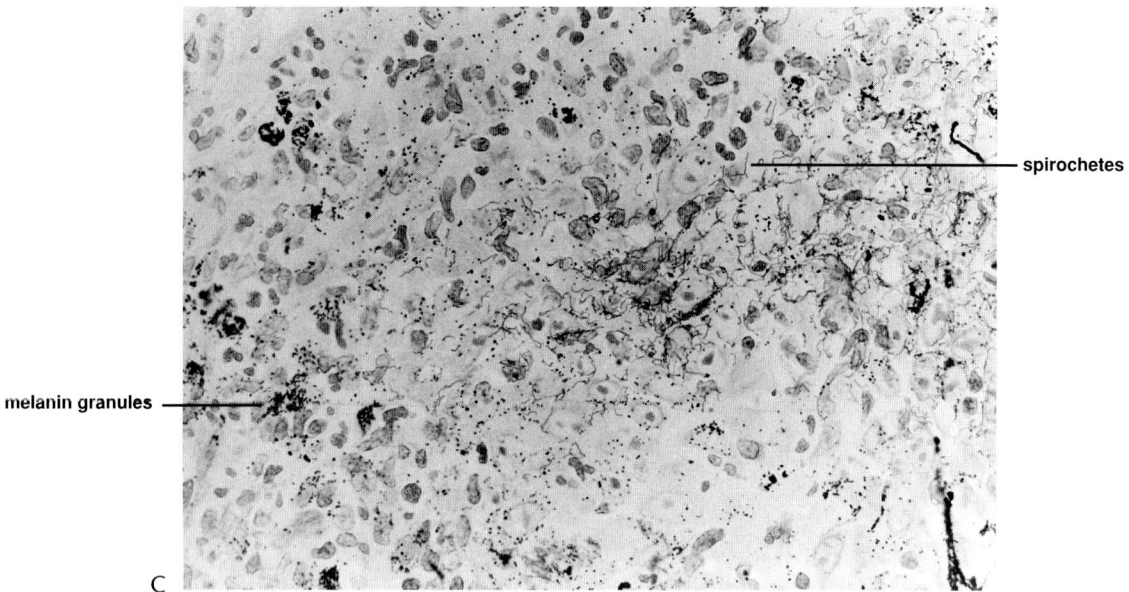

C

Figure 7-19 *Continued.* **(C)** Warthin-Starry silver stain. Many spirochetes are present in the papillary dermis among the inflammatory cells.

confluent areas of parakeratosis and scale-crust. Chronic dermatophyte infections are more apt to show predominant compact orthohyperkeratosis with focal parakeratosis (Fig. 7-21). Dermatophyte infections may sometimes display the "sandwich" sign in which there is a parakeratotic or compact orthokeratotic layer that contains the fungal hyphae sandwiched between the viable epidermis beneath it and the normal stratum corneum above it.

The dermal infiltrate is usually situated around the vessels of the superficial plexus but can extend to the middle or deep reticular dermis. It consists mainly of lymphocytes and macrophages but often contains neutrophils. The presence of neutrophils is a clue to search the cornified layer for fungal organisms. The periodic acid-Schiff stain and methenamine silver stain are helpful for identifying fungal organisms.

Hyperkeratotic Scabies

In fastidious persons who have contracted scabies, it is often difficult to confirm the diagnosis because their attention to hygiene keeps the number of organisms at a minimum. At the opposite end of the spectrum are individuals who, because of mental retardation, a psychiatric illness, or immune deficiency, are unable to control the proliferation of the scabies mites. These persons develop thickened, hyperkeratotic, crusted plaques that teem with scabies mites.

Histologically, there is prominent orthohyperkeratosis with foci of parakeratosis and scale-crust. The thickened stratum corneum contains numerous scabies mites, larvae, and ova (Fig. 7-22). The epidermis shows prominent hyperplasia, usually with only slight spongiosis and exocytosis of inflammatory cells. The inflammatory dermal infiltrate is of variable density and usually contains eosinophils.

Inflammatory Linear Verrucal Epidermal Nevus

This entity is mentioned here for completeness. Epidermal nevi are discussed in depth in Chapter 16. Clinically, these lesions are red-brown, scaly, slightly verrucous papules that tend to coalesce and form a linear streak. They occur most commonly on the leg, thigh, or buttock. Because they are pruritic, they are usually rubbed or scratched, which superimposes the changes of lichen simplex chronicus on the epidermal malformation. As with other hamartomas, they may be evident at birth or develop in early childhood.

Histologically, the epidermis shows papillated epidermal hyperplasia (Fig. 7-23). There are sharply demarcated foci of parakeratosis situated above the epidermal spires. There is hypogranulosis in the regions of parakeratosis, and, on occasion, slight spongiosis is present in the spinous layer. Between the papillations there is orthohyperkeratosis and hypergranulosis. The dermis shows vertically streaked, coarse collagen bundles in the dermal papillae and a sparse superficial perivascular infiltrate of mononuclear cells.

Some Ichthyoses

Certain types of ichthyosis demonstrate epidermal hyperplasia with inflammation. Lamellar ichthyosis is usually mentioned in this context, but nonbullous congenital ichthyosiform erythroderma, epidermolytic hyperkeratosis, and ichthyosis linearis circumflexa also show both. These conditions are discussed in Chapter 16.

Text continued on p. 195

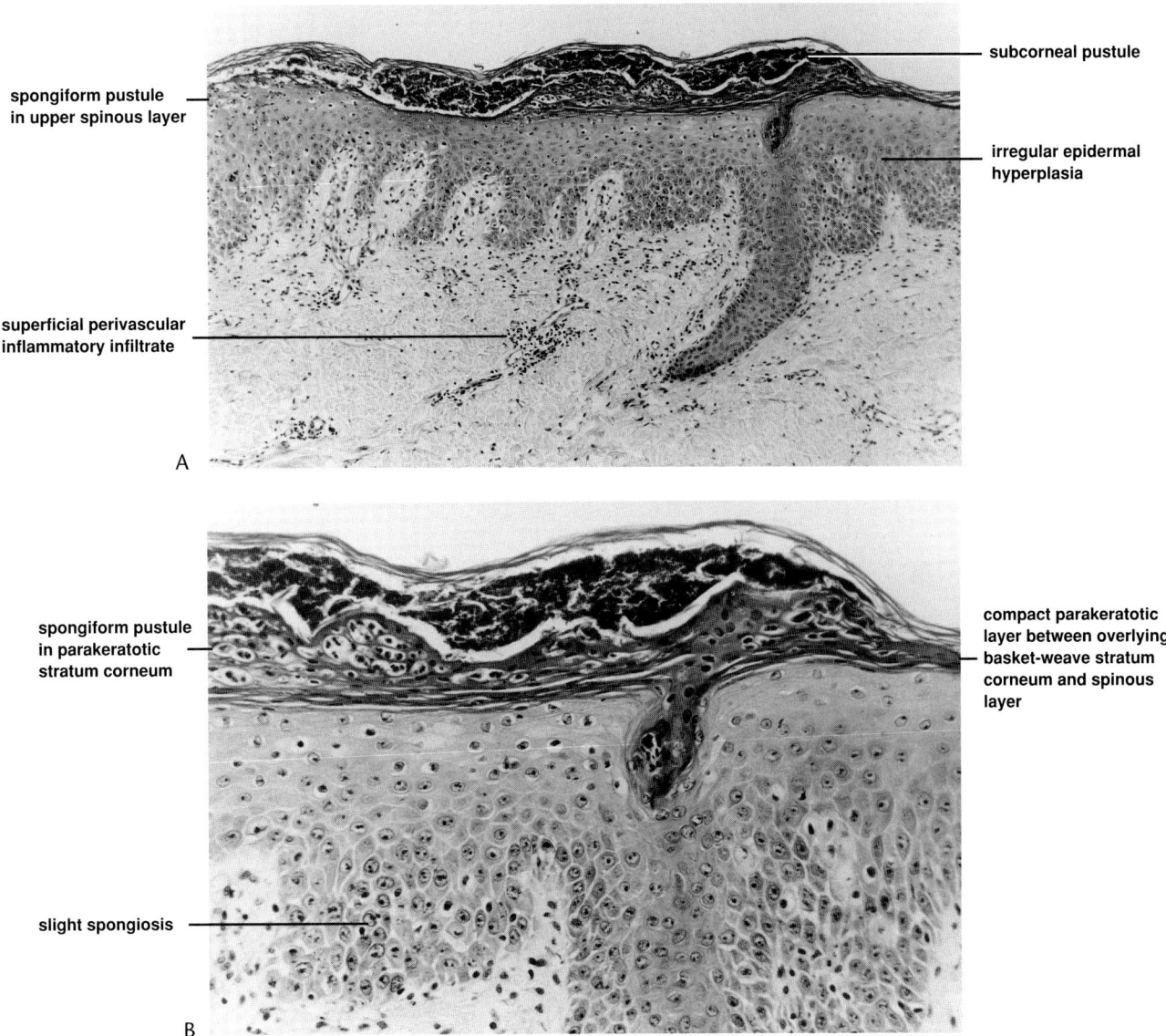

spongiform pustule
in upper spinous layer

subcorneal pustule

irregular epidermal
hyperplasia

superficial perivascular
inflammatory infiltrate

A

spongiform pustule
in parakeratotic
stratum corneum

compact parakeratotic
layer between overlying
basket-weave stratum
corneum and spinous
layer

slight spongiosis

B

Figure 7-20. Subacute dermatophyte infection (tinea corporis). **(A)** There is slightly irregular epidermal hyperplasia that involves both the rete ridges and the epidermis above the dermal papillae. Neutrophils are present within the parakeratotic zone beneath the basket-weave stratum corneum. There is slight spongiosis and a moderately dense superficial perivascular inflammatory infiltrate. **(B)** Cell debris is evident between the basket-weave stratum corneum and the parakeratotic zone. Numerous neutrophils are found among the parakeratotic squames resembling a spongiform pustule of psoriasis. Spongiosis is present in the lower epidermis. At the far right, there is a layer of parakeratin "sandwiched" between orthokeratin and the squamous layer; dermatophyte organisms are often found in this layer.

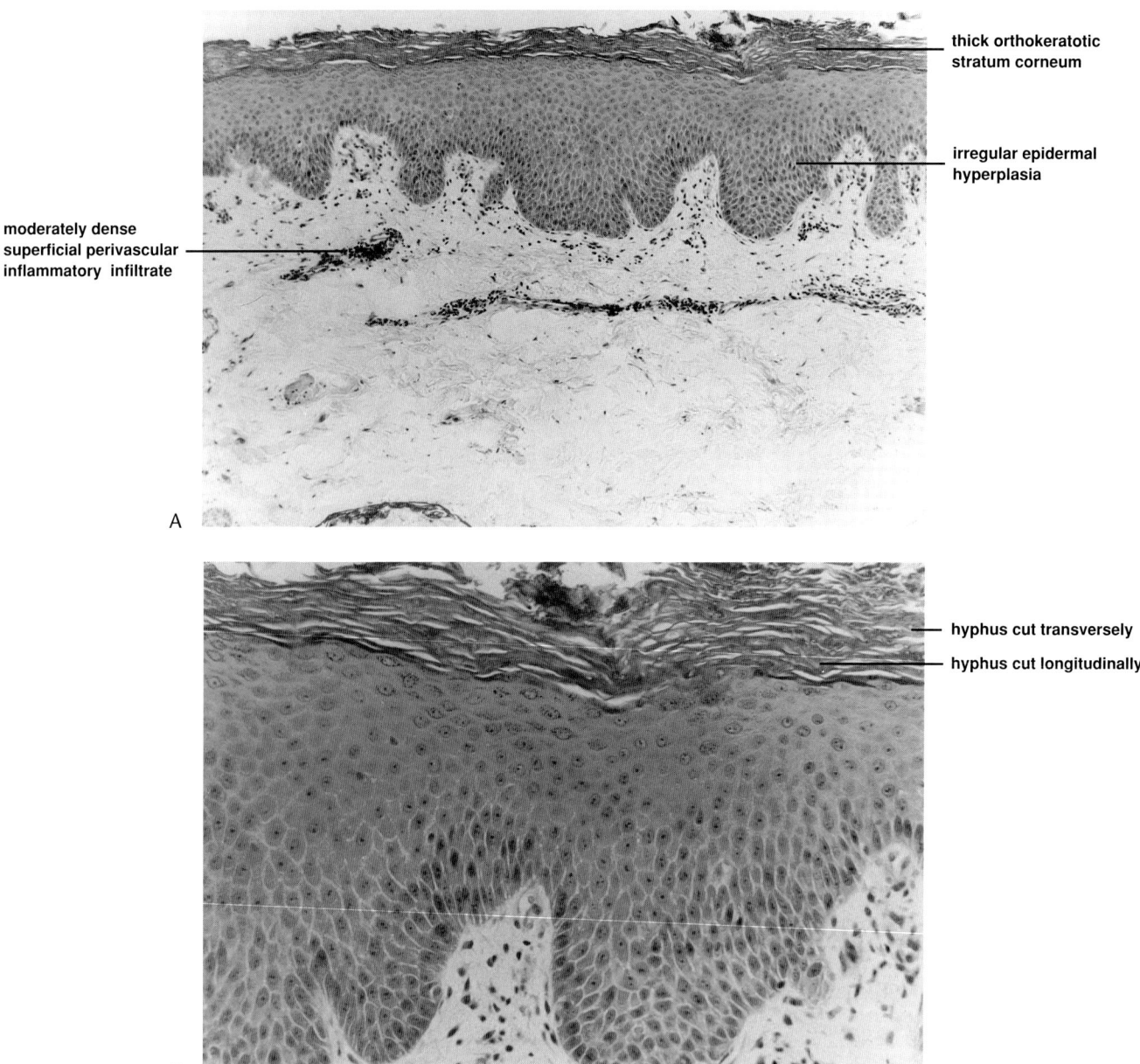

thick orthokeratotic
stratum corneum

irregular epidermal
hyperplasia

moderately dense
superficial perivascular
inflammatory infiltrate

A

hyphus cut transversely

hyphus cut longitudinally

B

Figure 7-21. Chronic dermatophyte infection. **(A)** The epidermis shows irregular hyperplasia and orthohyperkeratosis. There is a sparse perivascular inflammatory infiltrate in the dermis. **(B)** Fungal hyphae are readily apparent in the stratum corneum. Slight spongiosis is present in the lower epidermis.

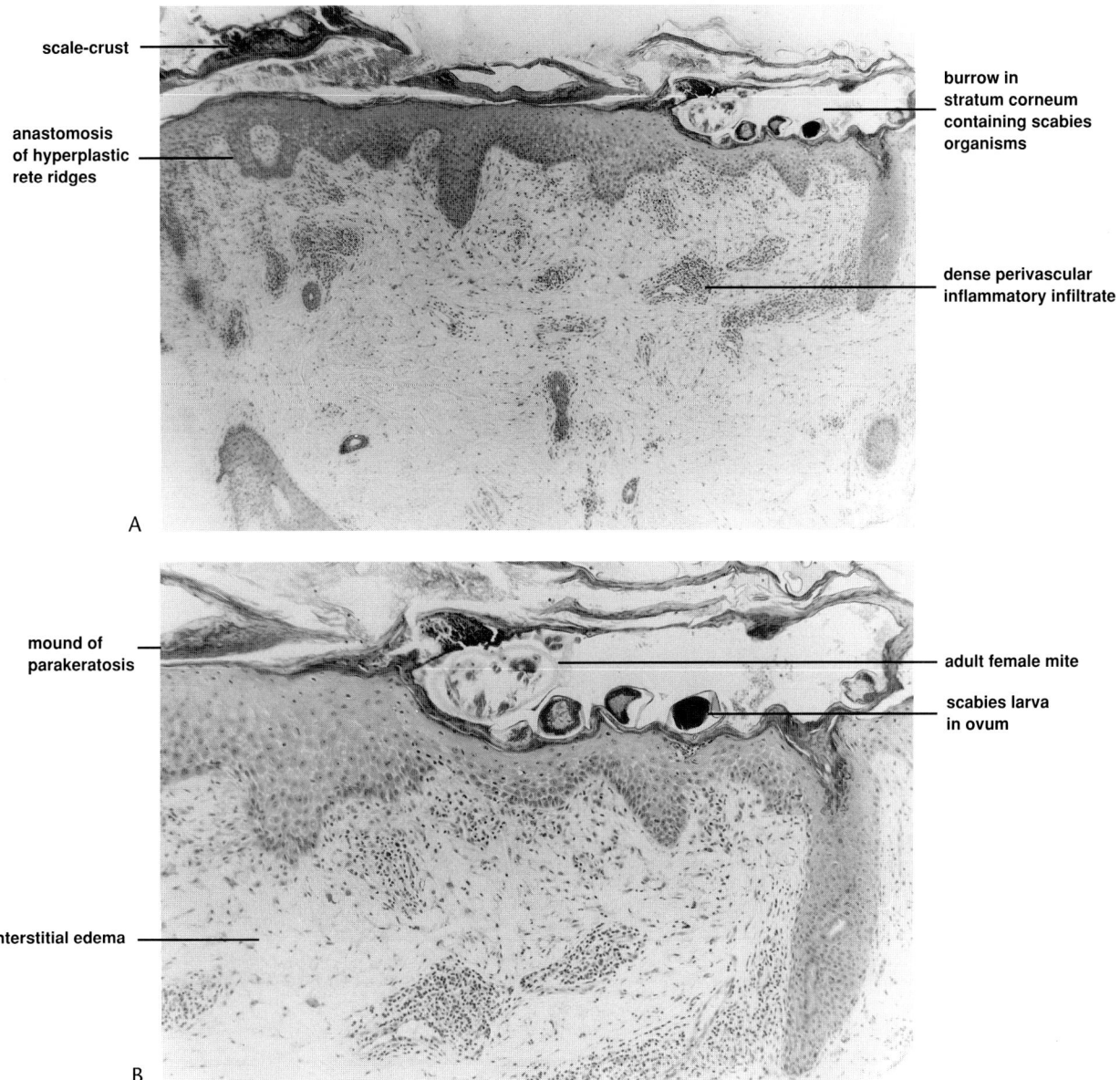

scale-crust

anastomosis
of hyperplastic
rete ridges

burrow in
stratum corneum
containing scabies
organisms

dense perivascular
inflammatory infiltrate

A

mound of
parakeratosis

adult female mite

scabies larva
in ovum

interstitial edema

B

Figure 7-22. Hyperkeratotic scabies. **(A)** The epidermis exhibits orthokeratosis, para-keratosis, scale-crusts, and irregular hyperplasia. There is a burrow that contains several scabies mites. **(B)** There is spongiosis in the epidermis beneath the burrow. Within the dermis is a perivascular and interstitial mixed inflammatory infiltrate.

orthohyperkeratosis

rete ridges
elongated to
fairly uniform
length

parakeratosis above
tip of papillomatous
projection

broad dermal papilla
with vertically
streaked collagen

moderately dense
superficial perivascular
inflammatory infiltrate

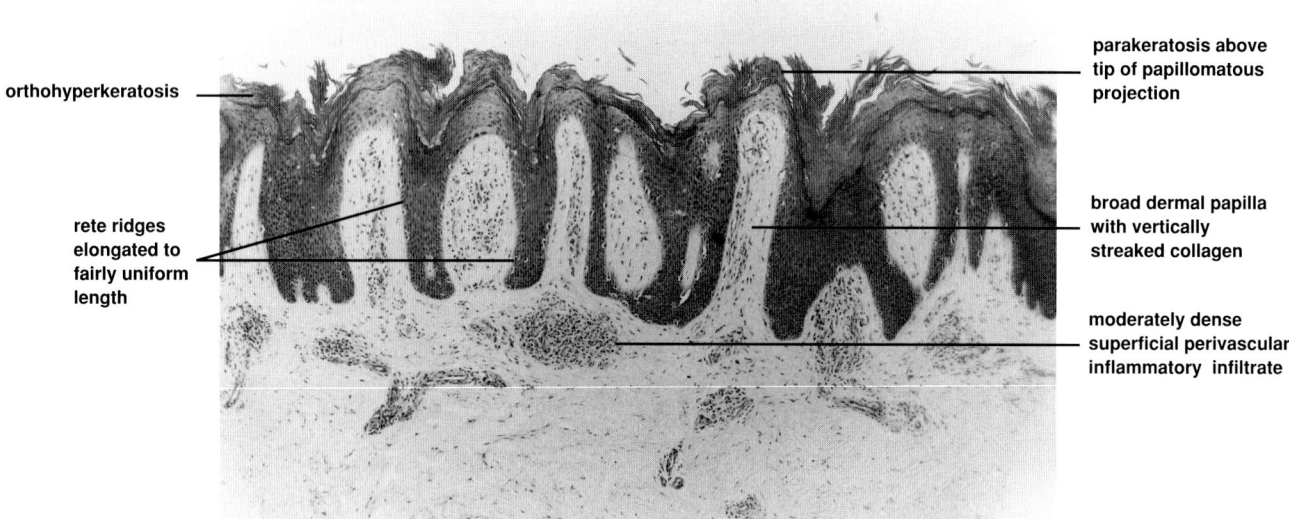

Figure 7-23. Inflammatory linear verrucal epidermal nevus. There is fairly regular elongation of rete ridges with focal anastomosis of them. The surface shows papillomatosis. There is orthohyperkeratosis with focal parakeratosis above the papillomatous projections. The dermis shows vertical streaking of collagen in the broad dermal papillae and a moderately dense superficial perivascular mononuclear infiltrate.

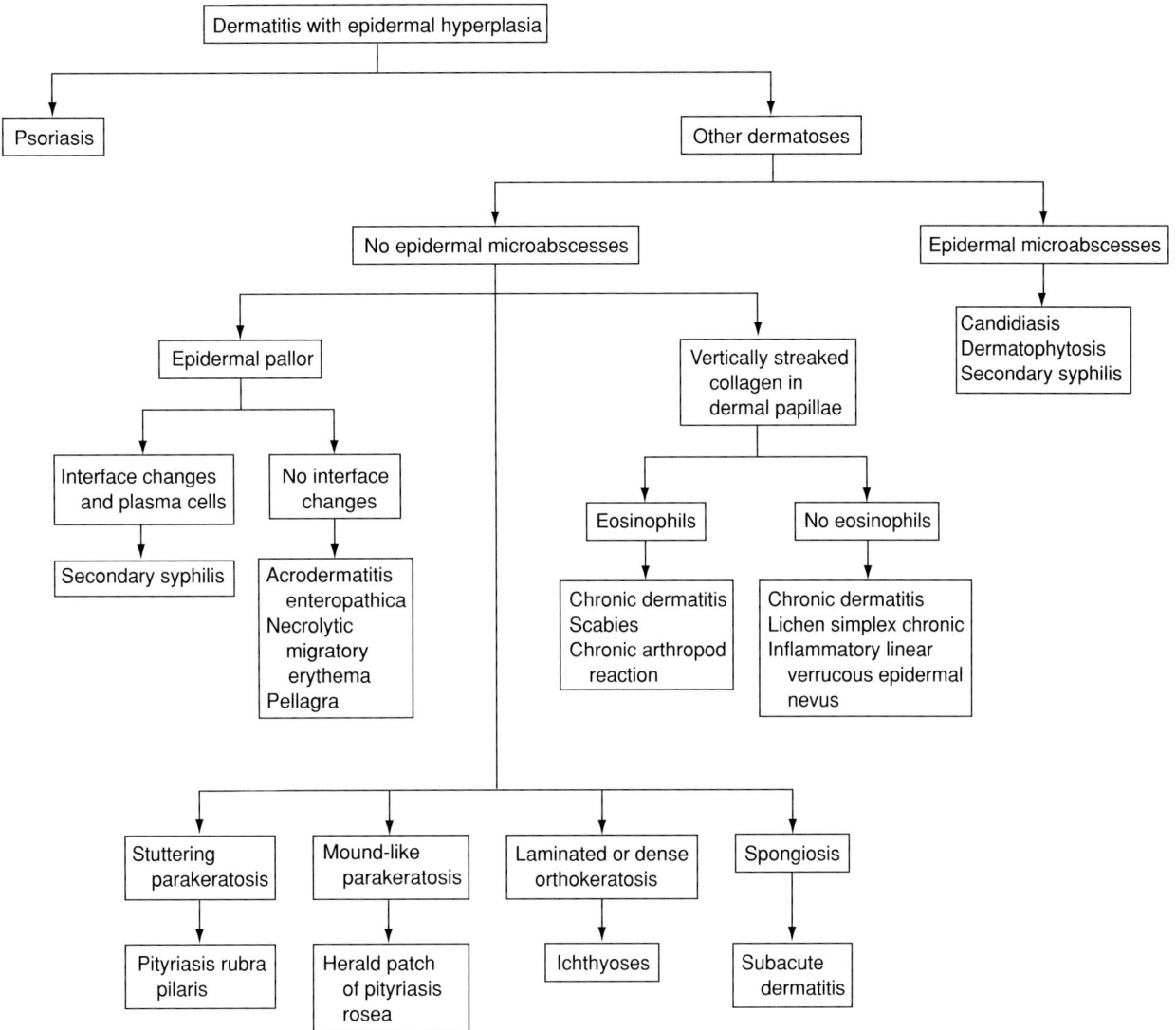

Figure 7-24. Algorithm for the classification of dermititis with epidermal hyperplasia.

CLUES TO THE DIFFERENTIAL DIAGNOSIS OF DERMATITIDES WITH EPIDERMAL HYPERPLASIA

The histologic differential diagnosis of dermatitides with epidermal hyperplasia can be challenging. Although it is often possible to make a definitive diagnosis if the clinician has selected the appropriate representative site for biopsy and the technical quality of the sections is good, it is sometimes possible to give only a relevant differential diagnosis. For example, the histopathologic features of acrodermatitis enteropathica, necrolytic migratory erythema, and psoriasis are similar. Given this limited differential diagnosis, the clinician can usually discriminate among these possibilities by taking into consideration the clinical features of the eruption, the age of the patient, and the results of laboratory studies. In other cases, it may only be possible to suggest a group of diseases, and the clinician then must use other means to make the correct diagnosis. This per-

tains especially to the chronic spongiotic dermatitides in which the histologic differential diagnosis could include allergic contact dermatitis, nummular dermatitis, asteatotic dermatitis, autosensitization dermatitis, exfoliative dermatitis, atopic dermatitis, photoallergic dermatitis, seborrheic dermatitis, ichthyosis linearis circumflexa, and lichen simplex chronicus.

The basic approach that is most fruitful is to first decide whether the histopathologic features of the case under consideration are those of psoriasis. In most cases of psoriasis, this is possible because the architectural features of the epidermis are so characteristic even when there are no neutrophil microabscesses. If the features are not suggestive of psoriasis, then other dermatoses with epidermal hyperplasia must be considered in an orderly fashion. Figure 7-24 is an algorithm that is often helpful in arriving at the correct diagnosis. It is always necessary to be sure that the proposed histopathologic diagnosis is compatible with the clinical data obtained from the clinician.

REFERENCES

1. Suarez-Almazur ME, Russell AS: The genetics of psoriasis: haplotype sharing in siblings with the disease. Arch Dermatol 126:1040–1042, 1990
2. Bernhard JD: Auspitz sign is not sensitive or specific for psoriasis. J Am Acad Dermatol 22:1079–1081, 1990
3. Ragaz A, Ackerman AB: Evolution, maturation, and regression of lesions of psoriasis: new observations and correlation of clinical and histologic findings. Am J Dermatopathol 1:199–214, 1979
4. Cox AJ, Watson W: Histologic variations in lesions of psoriasis. Arch Dermatol 106:503–506, 1972
5. Soltani K, VanScott EJ: Patterns and sequence of tissue changes in incipient and evolving lesions of psoriasis. Arch Dermatol 106:484–490, 1972
6. Horn TD, Herzberg GZ, Hood AF: Characterization of the dermal infiltrate in human immunodeficiency virus-infected patients with psoriasis. Arch Dermatol 125:1462–1465, 1990
7. Zaias N: Psoriasis of the nail: a clinical pathologic study. Arch Dermatol 99:567–579, 1969
8. Gottlieb AB, Krueger JG: HLA region genes and immune activation in pathogenesis of psoriasis. Arch Dermatol 126:1083–1086, 1990
9. Weinstein GD, Frost P: Abnormal cell proliferation in psoriasis. J Invest Dermatol 50:254–259, 1968
10. Gelfant S: The cell cycle in psoriasis: a reappraisal. Br J Dermatol 95:577–590, 1976
11. Voorhees JJ: Polyamines and psoriasis. Arch Dermatol 115:943–944, 1979
12. Bos JD: The pathomechanisms of psoriasis: the skin immune system and cyclosporin. Br J Dermatol 118:141–155, 1988
13. Sauder Db, Steck WD, Bailin PD et al: Lymphocyte kinetics in pustular psoriasis. J Am Acad Dermatol 4:458–460, 1981
14. Butler MJ: A follow-up study of 48 patients with Reiter's syndrome. Am J Med 67:808, 1979
15. Griffiths WAD: Pityriasis rubra pilaris. Dermatology 5:105–112, 1980
16. Soeprono FF: Histologic criteria for the diagnosis of pityriasis rubra pilaris. Am J Dermatopathol 8:277–283, 1986
17. Niemi KM, Kousa M, Storgards K et al: Pityriasis rubra pilaris. Dermatologica 152:109–118, 1976
18. Finzi AF, Altomare GF, Bergamaschini L et al: Pityriasis rubra pilaris and retinol binding protein. Br J Dermatol 104:253–256, 1981
19. Ralfs IG, Dawbar RPR, Ryan TJ et al: Pityriasis rubra pilaris: epidermal cell kinetics. Br J Dermatol 104:249–252, 1981
20. Ackerman AB: Histologic Diagnosis of Inflammatory Skin Diseases. Lea & Febiger, Philadelphia, 1978, pp. 269, 512, 828
21. Moore RA, Spies TD, Cooper K: Histopathology of the skin in pellagra. Ann Dermatol Venereol 46:100–106, 1942
22. Castiello RJ, Lynch PJ: Pellagra and the carcinoid syndrome. Arch Dermatol 105:574–577, 1972
23. Cohen LK, George W, Smith R: Isoniazid-induced acne and pellagra. Arch Dermatol 109:377–381, 1974
24. Gonzalez JR, Botet VM, Sanchez J: The histopathology of acrodermatitis enteropathica. Am J Dermatopathol 4:303–311, 1982
25. Ackerman AB: Histologic Diagnosis of Inflammatory Skin Diseases. Lea & Febiges, Philadelphia, 1978, pp. 274, 512, 828
26. Moynahan EJ: Acrodermatitis enteropathica: a lethal inherited human zinc deficiency disorder. Lancet 2:399–400, 1974
27. Norris D: Zinc and cutaneous inflammation. Arch Dermatol 121:985–989, 1985
28. Ranchoff RE, Kantor GR, Slugg PH et al: Necrolytic migratory erythema-like dermatitis with malabsorption. Cleve Clin Q 52:81–85, 1985
29. Vandersteen PR, Scheithauer BW: Glucagonoma syndrome: a clinicopathologic, immunocytochemical, and ultrastructural study. J Am Acad Dermatol 12:1032–1039, 1985
30. Kheir SM, Omura EF, Grizzle WE et al: Histologic variation in the skin lesions of the glucagonoma syndrome. Am J Surg Pathol 10:445–53, 1986
31. Ackerman AB: Histologic Diagnosis of Inflammatory Skin Diseases. Lea & Febiger, Philadelphia, 1978 pp. 512, 514, 828
32. Hunt SJ, Navus VT, Abell E: Necrolytic migratory erythema: dyskeratotic dermatitis, a clue to early diagnosis. J Am Acad Dermatol 24:473–77, 1991
33. Takaki Y, Miyazaki H: Cytolytic degeneration of keratinocytes adjacent to Langerhan's cells in pityriasis rosea (Gilbert). Acta Dermatovener 56:99, 1976
34. Gottlieb G, Ackerman AB: The "sandwich sign" of dermatophytosis. Am J Dermatopathol 8:347–350, 1986

8

VASCULITIS AND VASCULOPATHY

Vasculitis is defined as inflammation of blood vessels.[1–3] Strict adherence to this definition is important in the microscopic approach to vasculitis, because a perivascular inflammatory cell infiltrate is found in many inflammatory diseases. Complete or partial destruction of blood vessels is essential to make an unequivocal diagnosis of vasculitis. Two patterns of vasculitis are generally recognized in the skin—leukocytoclastic and granulomatous. Leukocytoclastic vasculitis primarily affects the capillaries, arterioles, and venules of the dermis and subcutis, whereas granulomatous vasculitis is essentially limited to the larger vessels (i.e., the arteries and veins).[4,5] A third pattern of vessel-based inflammation, sometimes referred to as *lymphocytic vasculitis,* is exemplified by diseases such as pityriasis lichenoides et varioliformis acuta and erythema multiforme.[6] Not all authors accept the premise that lymphocytes alone can effect a true vasculitis. These diseases are discussed in other chapters.

Vasculitis is a difficult subject made more so by the extensive, frequently contradictory literature that attempts to classify these diseases and elucidate their mechanisms. In addition, the cutaneous vasculitides are in many aspects a unique subset of vasculitis. Careful clinicopathologic correlation has led to the delineation of a diverse group of diseases, all of which show vasculitis microscopically. Although the main emphasis of this chapter is an approach to the diagnostic microscopic features of cutaneous vasculitis, a brief discussion of current concepts about the pathogenesis of this process helps one to understand many of the microscopic findings.

The sequence that leads to vessel damage has been most extensively studied in small vessel vasculitis (i.e., vasculitis that affects capillaries, venules, and arterioles)[4] (Fig. 8-1). Circulating, soluble immune complexes (i.e., antigen complexed with antibody) become bound to endothelial cells directly or to platelets that then adhere to endothelial cells.[7] The adherent immune complex activates the complement cascade. Terminal complement components, C5b through C9, form the membrane attack complex that can cause lysis of endothelial cells. Another component of complement, C5a, is a potent chemotactic agent that recruits neutrophils, eosinophils, and monocytes. Proteolytic lysosomal enzymes released by these cells, especially neutrophils, result in further damage to endothelial cells and, if unchecked, lead to vessel wall necrosis, activation of clotting factors, and ultimately thrombus formation. The end results of this cumulative damage are loss of integrity of the blood vessel with extravasation of erythrocytes, leakage of plasma, and migration of inflammatory cells into the dermis around the vessel, the adventitial dermis.

The inflammatory cells, especially neutrophils, are eventually destroyed by these proteolytic enzymes and possibly other inflammatory cell mediators such as the prostaglandins and cytokines.[7–9] This results in pyknosis, karyorrhexis, and total cellular disintegration (leukocytoclasis). Fibrin deposition in and around the blood vessel walls imparts a smudgy, eosinophilic character to the affected vessels (fibrinoid necrosis). Leukocytoclastic neutrophils and fibrinoid necrosis are the microscopic hallmarks of leukocytoclastic vasculitis. Other terms that have been used for this process include *neutrophilic vasculitis* or *venulitis, allergic vasculitis, hypersensitivity vasculitis,* and *necrotizing vasculitis.*

A variant of leukocytoclastic vasculitis characterized by the microscopic and clinical features of urticaria has been described.[10–13] Aptly named *urticarial vasculitis,* this pattern of vasculitis is frequently associated with low levels of the early components of the classic complement pathway, especially C1q. Immune complexes have also been identified in this type of vasculitis. Urticarial vasculitis appears to be a variant of leukocytoclastic vasculitis from a mechanistic as well as a morphologic point of view.

The pathogenic mechanisms of granulomatous vasculitis are much less clear.[4] As in leukocytoclastic vasculitis, immune complexes may initiate the vasculitis, but for some reason lymphocytes, monocytes, and macrophages eventually predominate rather than neutrophils. Monocytes and macrophages have Fc receptors on their cell surfaces so that it is possible that immune complexes attract these cells directly. Alternatively, sensitized lymphocytes, especially T lymphocytes, may release a number

Both type I (monoclonal) and type II (polyclonal) cryoglobulinemia can induce leukocytoclastic vasculitis.[36,37] In type II cryoglobulinemia (mixed cryoglobulinemia), polyclonal IgG is complexed to monoclonal IgM with rheumatoid factor (anti-Fc) activity.[4,5,37,38] Both IgG and the IgM components frequently have anti-hepatitis B surface antigen specificity. IgG, IgM, and frequently C3 deposits can be present in affected vessels.[4,5,37,38]

Leukocytoclastic Vasculitis Without Palpable Purpura

A pustule, rather than palpable purpura, is the clinical lesion of pustular vasculitis.[39,40] The pustules may be as large as the primary lesion, or they may be small and superimposed on palpable purpura. The lesions of the bowel bypass syndrome typify the former, whereas the eruption of meningococcemia and gonococcemia are characteristic of the latter.[41] A mixture of pustules and palpable purpura may occur in rheumatoid disease.[42,43] Pustular vasculitis in Behçet's disease may occur spontaneously after trauma or histamine injection (pathergy).[44] Secondary leukocytoclastic vasculitis may be found in vesicular and pustular phases of herpes simplex or varicella-zoster eruptions.[45] Pustulosa acuta generalisata is a pustular eruption associated with streptococcal tonsillitis. The pustules are less than 1 cm in diameter and tend to be acral.

Erythema elevatum diutinum is a rare form of leukocytoclastic vasculitis limited to the skin. Erythematous papules and nodules coalesce to form large plaques that tend to be symmetrically located on the arms and legs, especially on the dorsal surface or over large joints such as the elbow or knee.[46] Pustules may form on the plaques in early lesions. The plaques are at first soft and even fluctuant. Older, resolving plaques turn dark red to brown and become quite firm. Erythema elevatum diutinum is most common in middle-aged adults. It has also been described in patients with acquired immunodeficiency syndrome (AIDS), ulcerative colitis, pyoderma gangrenosum, Wegener's granulomatosis, hypergammaglobulinemia, relapsing polychondritis, and several hematologic disorders, including chronic lymphocytic leukemia, monoclonal gammopathies, multiple myeloma, and myelodysplasia.[47–60]

As the name implies, granuloma faciale is usually, but not always, limited to the face.[61,62] In a pattern similar to erythema elevatum diutinum, erythematous papules coalesce to form large plaques.[63,64] Telangiectasia and dilation of the follicular orifices may be evident. As they age, the plaques turn red-brown. In contrast to erythema elevatum diutinum, the plaques remain soft and pustule formation is rare.

Urticarial vasculitis (hypocomplementemic vasculitis) is frequently associated with depression of the early components of the classic complement pathway.[65–70] The clinical lesion of urticarial vasculitis resembles urticaria, but differs in that the individual lesions are present for more than 24 hours.[69] The urticarial plaques may also be painful. Arthralgia, abdominal pain, central nervous system symptoms, and glomerulonephritis may accompany the cutaneous lesions.[70] When these features are present, the patient should be evaluated for systemic lupus erythematosus because lupus may present with urticarial vasculitis.[66,67,71] Most patients have only cutaneous disease, which is self-limited but frequently recurrent.

Histopathologic Features

As might be expected from the numerous clinical presentations of leukocytoclastic vasculitis, the microscopic findings are variable and highly dependent on the stage of development of the sampled lesion.[1,2,12] The affected vessels are capillaries, small arterioles, and venules. The vessels of the superficial vascular plexus are most frequently involved, but in severe cases vessels at all levels of the reticular dermis and even the subcutis are affected.

The first diagnostic microscopic finding in leukocytoclastic vasculitis is a neutrophilic infiltrate around and within the affected blood vessel.[1,2,12,72] In early, evolving lesions the density of the neutrophilic infiltrates may be sparse with minimal karyorrhexis (fragmentation of nuclei) and extravasation of erythrocytes (Fig. 8-2).

As the lesion progresses, the neutrophilic infiltrates increase in density. As the number of neutrophils increases, endothelial cell swelling and necrosis develop. Next, fibrin deposition (i.e., brightly eosinophilic deposits in the wall of the affected vessel)

Figure 8-2. Early leukocytoclastic vasculitis (margination). Intact neutrophils are present at the periphery of small dermal blood vessels. (× 400.)

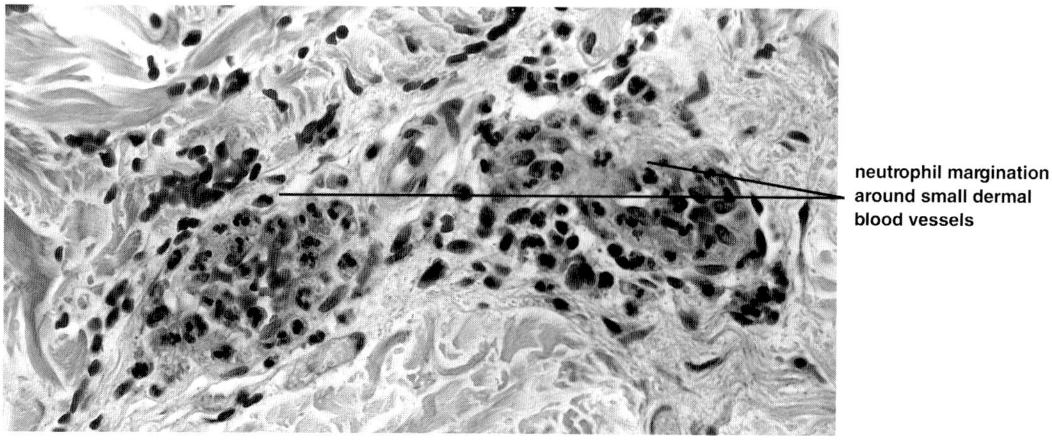

neutrophil margination around small dermal blood vessels

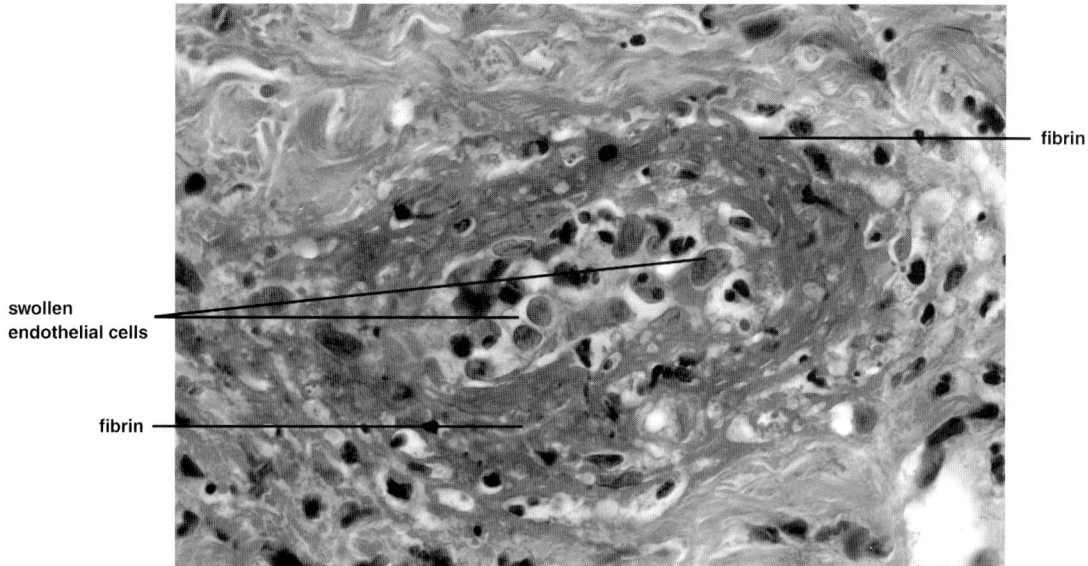

fibrin

swollen
endothelial cells

fibrin

Figure 8-3. Early leukocytoclastic vasculitis (fibrin deposition). Deposition of fibrin imparts a smudged indistinct border to the affected vessel wall. Endothelial cell swelling is prominent in this vessel. (× 400.)

is apparent. This produces a smudgy, indistinct appearance of the vessel wall (Fig. 8-3). Fibrin deposition is an important finding. When it is present in conjunction with neutrophil karyorrhexis, the diagnosis of leukocytoclastic vasculitis is ensured (Fig. 8-4). Unfortunately, fibrin is not always present, especially in very early or late lesions. Small focal areas of fibrin deposition may be difficult to recognize with certainty. In the absence of fibrin, leukocytoclastic vasculitis can usually be recognized by other features such as the density of the neutrophilic infiltrate, neutrophil karyorrhexis, and extravasation of erythrocytes. Often the vessels are completely destroyed so that the only clue to their prior existence is the inflammatory cell infiltrate that outlines their prior location (Fig. 8-5).

As the vasculitis resolves, endothelial cells regenerate. The neutrophilic infiltrate decreases in density. Lymphocytes emerge within the perivascular infiltrates and gradually increase

Figure 8-4. Late leukocytoclastic vasculitis (vessel destruction). The vessel walls are completely necrotic. Fibrin deposition is evident. Karyorrhectic neutrophils are present at the periphery of the vessel. (× 200.)

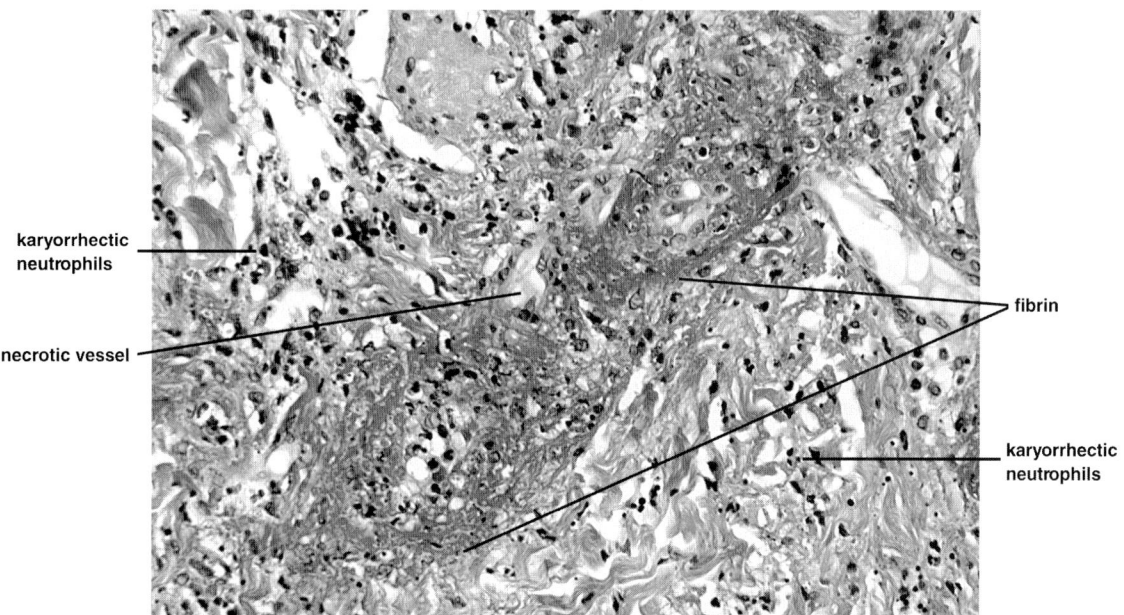

karyorrhectic
neutrophils

necrotic vessel

fibrin

karyorrhectic
neutrophils

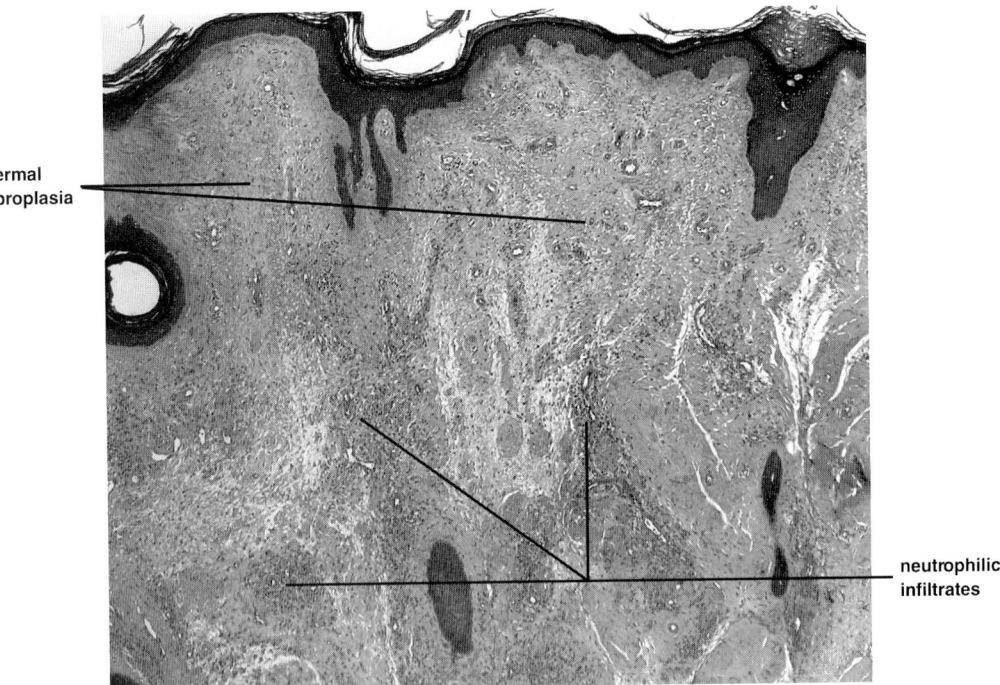

dermal
fibroplasia

neutrophilic
infiltrates

Figure 8-8. Erythema elevatum diutinum (late phase). Dermal fibroplasia is extensive. Neutrophilic infiltrates are less dense than in the early phase lesions. Leukocytoclastic vasculitis may not be present or only minimal and focal. (× 40.)

Figure 8-9. Urticarial vasculitis. Focal leukocytoclastic vasculitis is present within a sparse, diffuse infiltrate of neutrophils in the reticular dermis. (× 80.)

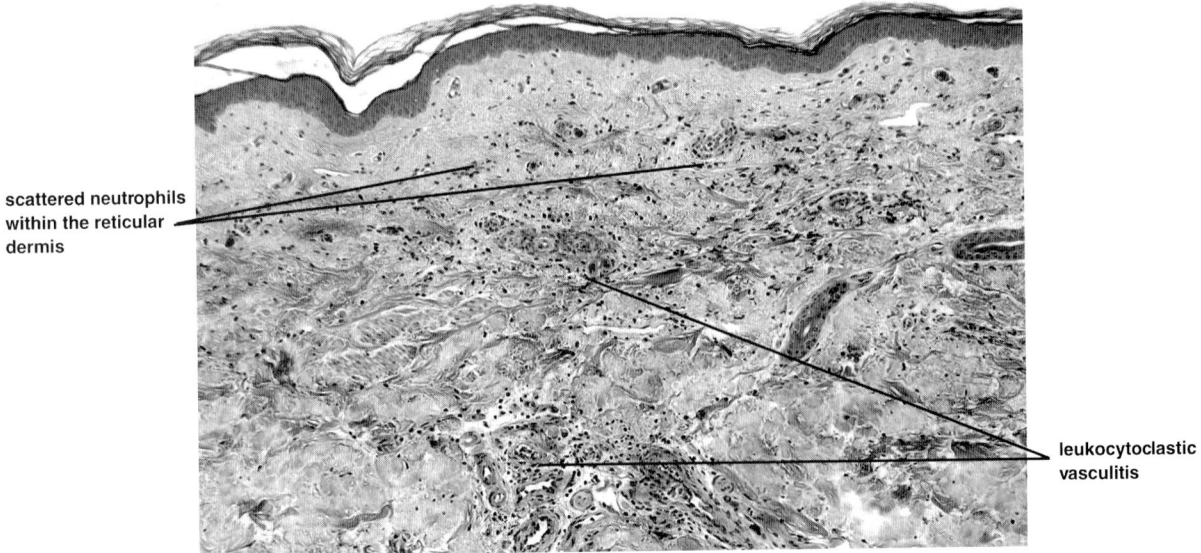

scattered neutrophils
within the reticular
dermis

leukocytoclastic
vasculitis

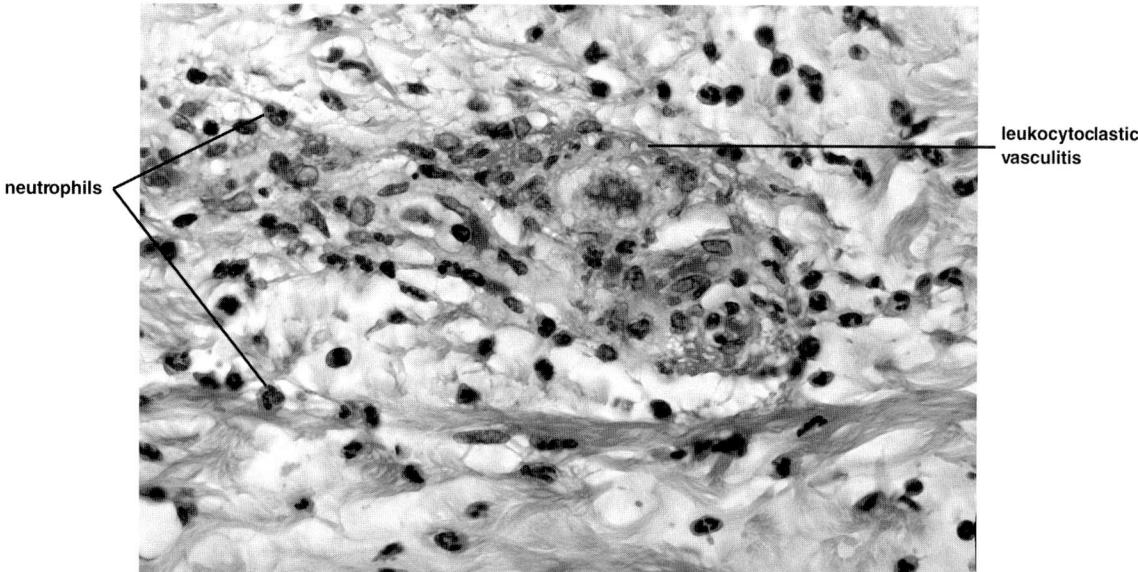

Figure 8-10. Urticarial vasculitis. Vessel wall destruction is less extensive, and only minimal fibrin deposition is present. (× 400.)

GRANULOMATOUS VASCULITIS

Clinical Features

The three main forms of cutaneous granulomatous vasculitis are Wegener's granulomatosis, allergic granulomatosis of Churg-Strauss, and lymphomatoid granulomatosis.[80,81]

Wegener's granulomatosis characteristically involves the upper respiratory tract and kidneys. The skin is involved in approximately one-half of patients.[82–85] A necrotizing granulomatous vasculitis is the primary abnormality in all the affected organs. The patient may present with cutaneous vasculitis that appears clinically as punched out ulcers and erythematous, painful, subcutaneous nodules.

Pulmonary symptoms predominate in allergic granulomatosis of Churg-Strauss.[86–88] As in Wegener's granulomatosis, approximately one-half of patients have cutaneous lesions at some time during their disease.[89] Large subcutaneous nodules that may ulcerate are most common. Some patients develop ulcers as well as nodules and plaques.

Lymphomatoid granulomatosis is a rare multiorgan disease that may have extensive cutaneous involvement. As in Wegener's and allergic granulomatosis, cutaneous lesions may precede visceral manifestations or occur simultaneously with them.[90–94] Approximately 40% of patients with lymphomatoid granulomatosis have skin disease that consists primarily of ulcerating erythematous to violaceous papules, plaques, and nodules.[93,95] Although the early literature suggested that only a portion of patients with lymphomatoid granulomatosis evolve into frank lymphoma, more recent investigations indicate that lymphomatoid granulomatosis is a T-cell lymphoma from the onset.[90–94]

Histopathologic Features

A distinct morphologic form of vessel destruction, necrotizing granulomatous vasculitis, is found in all three diseases. The vessels of the deep reticular and retinacular dermis are most commonly involved.[80] The vasculitis preferentially affects arterioles and small muscular arteries. These vessels are characterized by fibrinoid necrosis, neutrophilic infiltrates with leukocytoclasis, and accumulations of epithelioid histiocytes within the vessel wall and in the surrounding adventitial dermis (Fig. 8-11). Multinucleate cells may be present or even abundant. The granulomatous change occurs after, and perhaps as a reaction to, the fibrinoid necrosis. Lymphocytes and plasma cells are variably present. Thrombus formation is common, and extravasation of erythrocytes may be extensive. The vessels heal with fibrosis. This leads to complete or partial lumen occlusion. A characteristic finding in Wegener's granulomatosis is the presence of vessels at different stages of involvement in the same lesion.[82,84,85] Extravascular necrotizing granulomas may also be present.

The presence of eosinophils, typically in large numbers, superimposed on the necrotizing granulomas is characteristic of allergic granulomatosis.[86–88] Fibrinoid necrosis and leukocytoclasis may be extreme. The destruction and subsequent disintegration of eosinophils result in the deposition of myriad eosinophilic granules within dermis adjacent to the vasculitis. As in Wegener's granulomatosis, extravascular necrotizing granulomas may be present.

Atypical lymphocytes characterized by large, hyperchromatic, irregular nuclei infiltrate the granulomatous vasculitis in lymphomatoid granulomatosis.[90–96] Mitoses may be abundant. The number of atypical lymphocytes is variable; there may be a

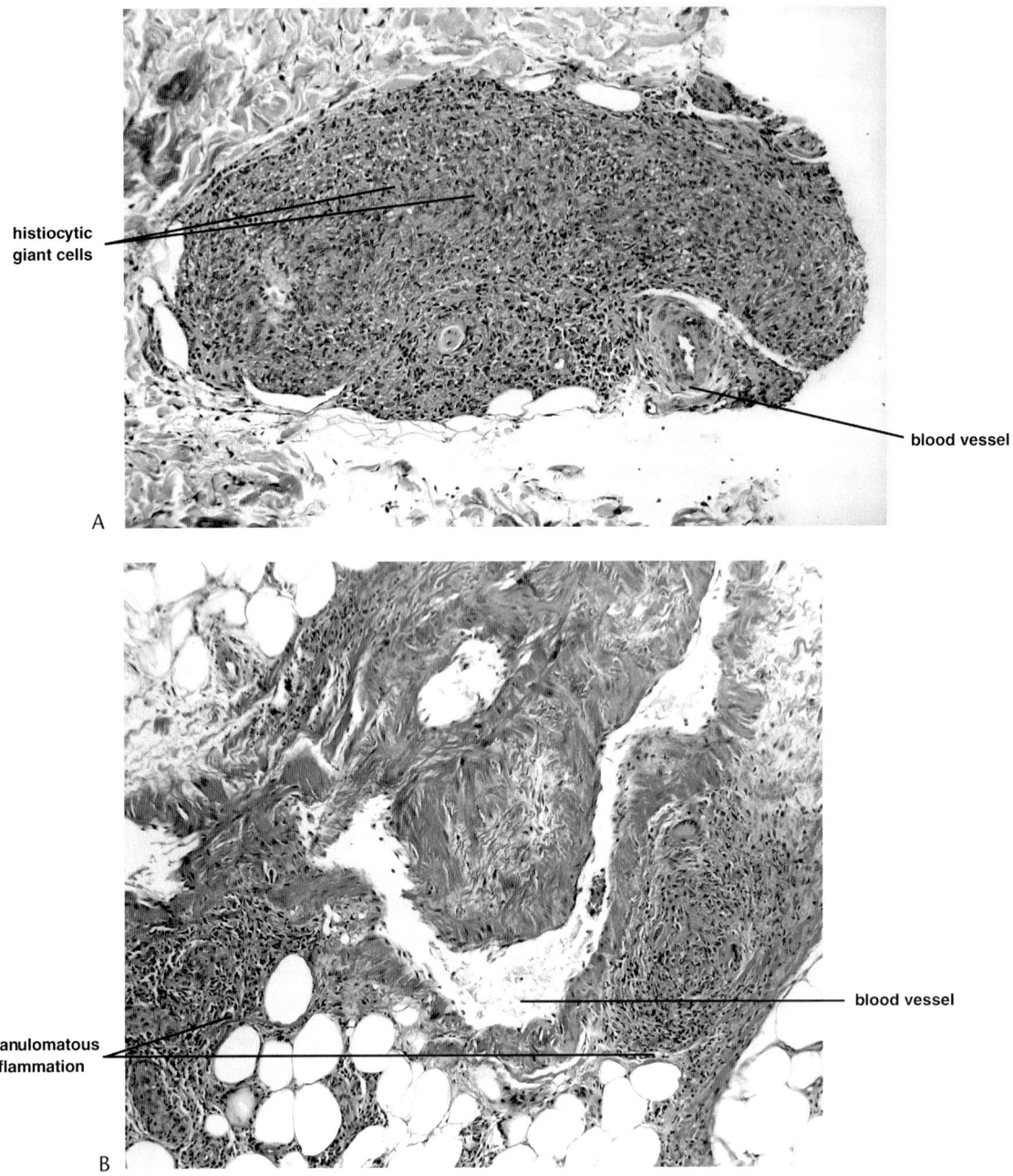

Figure 8-11. (A) Granulomatous vasculitis (transverse section). A dermal vessel is encompassed by granulomatous inflammation, including multinucleate giant cells. (× 80.) (B) Granulomatous vasculitis (longitudinal section). A dermal vessel is encompassed by granulomatous inflammation, including multinucleate giant cells. (× 80.)

few atypical lymphocytes that are difficult to recognize because of the extent of vascular destruction. These cells can also massively infiltrate the lower dermis and subcutis and obscure the vasculitic component. Rarely, the lymphomatous infiltrate is diffuse with only small, focal areas of vasculitis.

Differential Diagnosis

The necrotizing granulomas of Wegener's and allergic granulomatosis may be confused with infectious diseases such as deep fungal and atypical mycobacterial infections. Although the vasculitis of musculocutaneous PAN involves vessels of similar size and location, extravascular granuloma formation is not a feature of PAN (Fig. 8-12). Histiocytes and multinucleate giant cells tend to remain within the vessel walls in PAN and are especially prominent near the internal elastic lamina. They are limited in extent and typically eccentric rather than circumferential in distribution. The massive infiltration of vessel walls in erythema induratum (nodular vasculitis) is limited to the lobules of the subcutis. Neutrophils and fibrinoid necrosis are not as prominent in erythema induratum, but fat necrosis is more extensive. Superficial migratory thrombophlebitis involves the

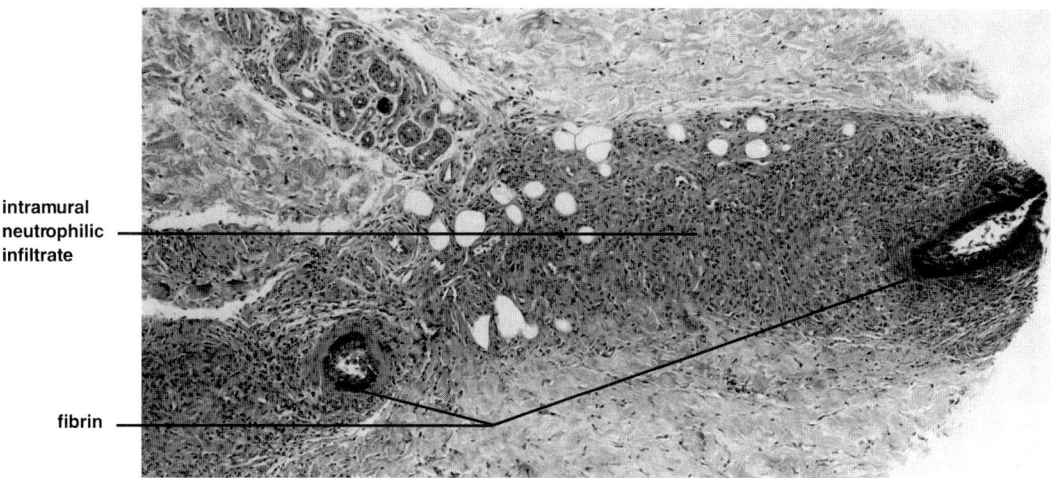

intramural
neutrophilic
infiltrate

fibrin

Figure 8-12. Polyarteritis nodosa. Fibrin deposition and inflammatory cell infiltrates are present in and around large dermal blood vessels. ($\times$ 50.)

relatively large veins of the subcutis. Neutrophils, not histiocytes, are characteristic. As in polyarteritis nodosa, these cells are limited to the vessel wall with no extravascular granuloma formation.

The eosinophilic necrosis of the extravascular granulomas of allergic granulomatosis may resemble rheumatoid nodules and deep dermal or subcutaneous granuloma annulare. Other types of lymphoma may permeate vessels, yet rarely as prominently as lymphomatoid granulomatosis. An exuberant arthropod bite reaction may show dense accumulations of large reactive lymphocytes centered around the deep dermal and subcutaneous vessels in a pattern similar to lymphomatoid granulomatosis. Eosinophils, plasma cells, and an admixture of smaller lymphocytes suggest an arthropod bite reaction. The cobblestone-like epithelioid endothelial cells of angiolymphoid hyperplasia with eosinophilia are diagnostic.

NEUTROPHILIC VASCULAR REACTIONS (DIFFUSE NEUTROPHILIC DERMAL INFILTRATES)

The term *neutrophilic vascular reaction* has been used to describe several neutrophil dominate diseases that do not satisfy strict criteria for the diagnosis of vasculitis (i.e., fibrinoid necrosis and leukocytoclasia are absent).[40,97] Both pyoderma gangrenosum and acute febrile neutrophilic dermatosis can be placed within this category.

Pyoderma Gangrenosum

Clinical Features

Pyoderma gangrenosum begins as a small papulopustule that expands to form nodules and plaques. Early in its evolution, the lesion ulcerates.[40] Eventually large ulcers with a characteristic undermined edge develop. The skin over the undermined area has a violaceous hue. The ulcers are typically painful and may be either single or multiple. A characteristic feature is the pathergy phenomenon (i.e., preferential formation of ulcers at sites of mechanical trauma such as debridement). The ulcers

heal, leaving an irregular, frequently stellate, dermal scar. Pyoderma gangrenosum is frequently associated with inflammatory bowel or rheumatoid disease, but in approximately one-half of patients with pyoderma gangrenosum no associated disease is found.[98] Pyoderma gangrenosum has recently been reported in patients with AIDS.[99] Pyoderma gangrenosum rarely affects children.[100,101] Some patients with idiopathic pyoderma gangrenosum develop systemic manifestations including liver dysfunction, respiratory failure, and aseptic meningeal reaction.[102]

Histopathologic Features

The early appearance of pyoderma gangrenosum that corresponds to the nonulcerated papulopustule is characterized by a diffuse mixed inflammatory cell infiltrate primarily in the upper and middle reticular dermis (Fig. 8-13). Neutrophils predominate, but lymphocytes and eosinophils are also present.[40] The inflammation may initially be centered around a hair follicle.[103] Edema forms in the upper dermis before ulceration occurs. Extensive necrosis of the epidermis and adnexae along with smudgy basophilic alteration of the dermal collagen characterize the later ulcerated stage. If the specimen includes part of the undermined edge of the ulcer, intact epidermis and superficial dermis are found over the dermal necrosis (Fig. 8-14). Histiocytes, including multinucleate cells, are present in late stages. Eventually granulation tissue develops in the ulcer bed, and the epidermis reforms over a dermal scar.

Leukocytoclastic vasculitis and immunoglobulin and complement deposition have been reported in pyoderma gangrenosum but are not consistently present. The rather extensive neutrophilic infiltrates and frequently prominent neutrophil karyorrhexis simulate leukocytoclastic vasculitis.[40]

Differential Diagnosis

Sporotrichosis and atypical mycobacterial infections are characterized by microscopic findings virtually identical to those of pyoderma gangrenosum. Special stains such as the PAS and Fite stains along with culture of excised tissue in appropriate

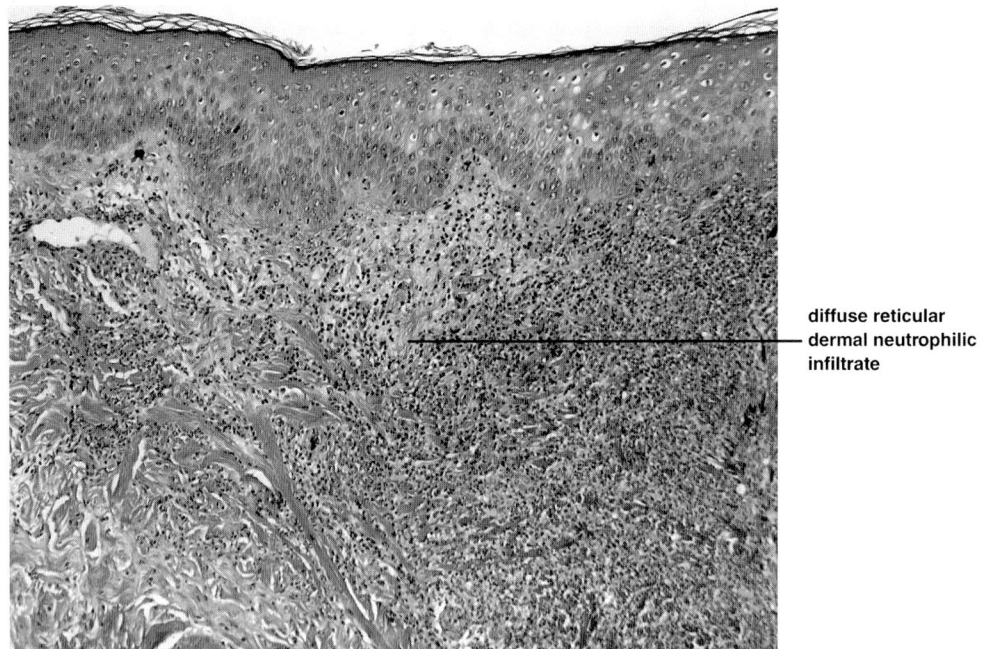

diffuse reticular
dermal neutrophilic
infiltrate

Figure 8-13. Pyoderma gangrenosum, early lesion. A diffuse neutrophilic infiltrate is present in the upper and middle reticular dermis. (× 40.)

Figure 8-14. Pyoderma gangrenosum, late lesion. The infiltrate is more extensive and deeper in the dermis. The intact epidermis correlates with the clinical finding of an undermined ulcer. (× 40.)

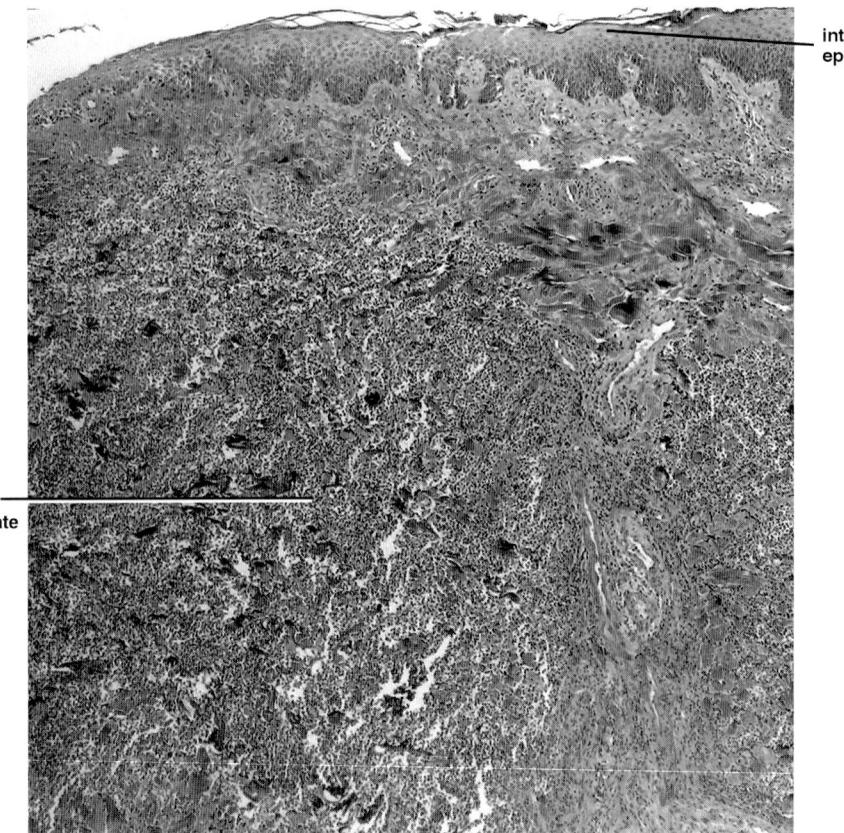

intact
epidermis

extensive diffuse
reticular dermal
neutrophilic infiltrate

media are frequently necessary to eliminate the possibility of an infectious etiology. Severe leukocytoclastic vasculitis, especially pustular vasculitis, may lead to ulceration and extensive necrosis, yet definite vasculitis can be identified in nonulcerated lesions or at the periphery of the ulcer. The histologic features of pyoderma gangrenosum overlap with those of acute febrile neutrophilic dermatosis, especially with the bullous pyoderma gangrenosum variant (see below).

Bullous Pyoderma Gangrenosum (Neutrophilic Dermatosis of Myeloproliferative Disorders)

Clinical Features

A bullous variant of pyoderma gangrenosum may occur in association with myeloproliferative diseases.[104-108] The bullous plaques tend to be acral. This eruption shares many clinical and histologic features with acute febrile neutrophilic dermatosis. The term *neutrophilic dermatosis of myeloproliferative disorders* better describes this entity and would eliminate the need to differentiate between bullous pyoderma gangrenosum and acute febrile neutrophilic dermatosis.[97,109-113]

Histopathologic Features

Prominent subepidermal pustules and bullae are superimposed on the diffuse dermal neutrophilic infiltrate of acute febrile neutrophilic dermatosis[104-108] (Fig. 8-15) (see below).

Differential Diagnosis

The same diseases that can be confused with pyoderma gangrenosum and acute febrile neutrophilic dermatosis should be considered in the differential diagnosis of the bullous variant of pyoderma gangrenosum.

Acute Febrile Neutrophilic Dermatosis (Sweet Syndrome)

Clinical Features

Crops of large erythematous plaques, which begin with an urticarial appearance, erupt primarily over the arms, chest, back, and face.[114] Small or large pustules may develop on the surface of the plaques. Untreated individual lesions resolve in 1 to 2 months and, in contrast to pyoderma gangrenosum, heal without scarring.[115] Systemic manifestations are common and include fever, malaise, arthralgias, and conjunctivitis. Viscera, such as the lung and lymph nodes, can be involved.[116,117] Acute febrile neutrophilic dermatosis is an important diagnosis because it may precede or occur at the onset of myelogenous leukemia in approximately 10% of cases.[110,118-122] Other diseases associated with acute febrile neutrophilic dermatosis include multiple myeloma, lymphoma, AIDS, solid tumors, ulcerative colitis, regional enteritis, lupus erythematosus, and rheumatoid arthritis.[123-132] Acute febrile dermatosis occurs most commonly in middle-aged women after a nonspecific infection of the respiratory or gastrointestinal tract, but men and children may also be affected.[121, 133]

Histopathologic Features

Diffuse neutrophilic infiltrates are found in the upper and middle reticular dermis.[114,121,122] The inflammatory cell infiltrate is accompanied by edema and leukocytoclasis, yet definite leukocytoclastic vasculitis is not a prominent feature[121,122,134,135] (Figs. 8-16 and 8-17). Lymphocytes and occasional eosinophils may be present.[136] Pustules may form from collections of neutrophils in the superficial dermis. In later lesions exocytosis of neutrophils, intraepidermal necrosis, and abscess formation may also occur.

Figure 8-15. Bullous pyoderma gangrenosum. Subepidermal pustules are present in the bullous variant. ($\times$ 80.)

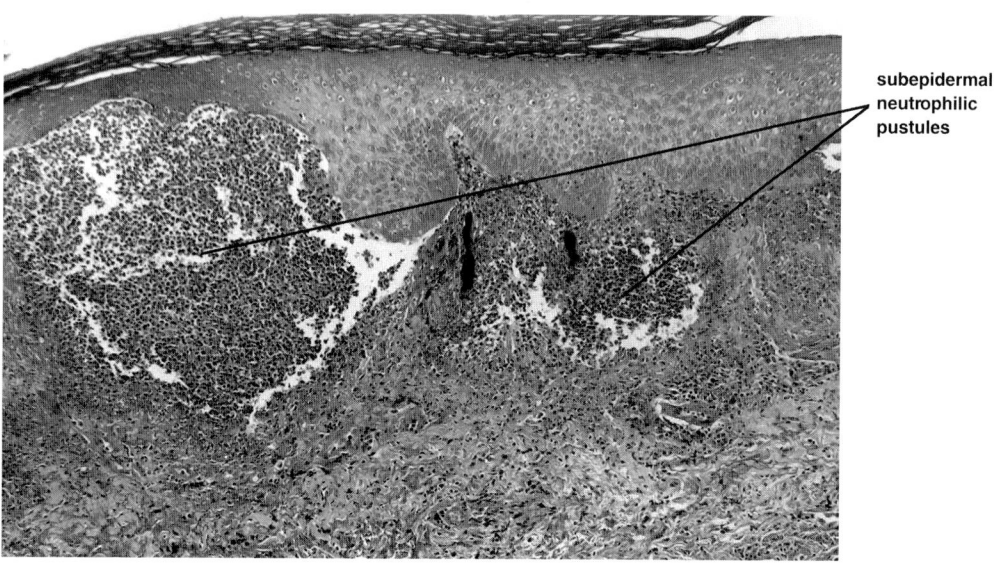

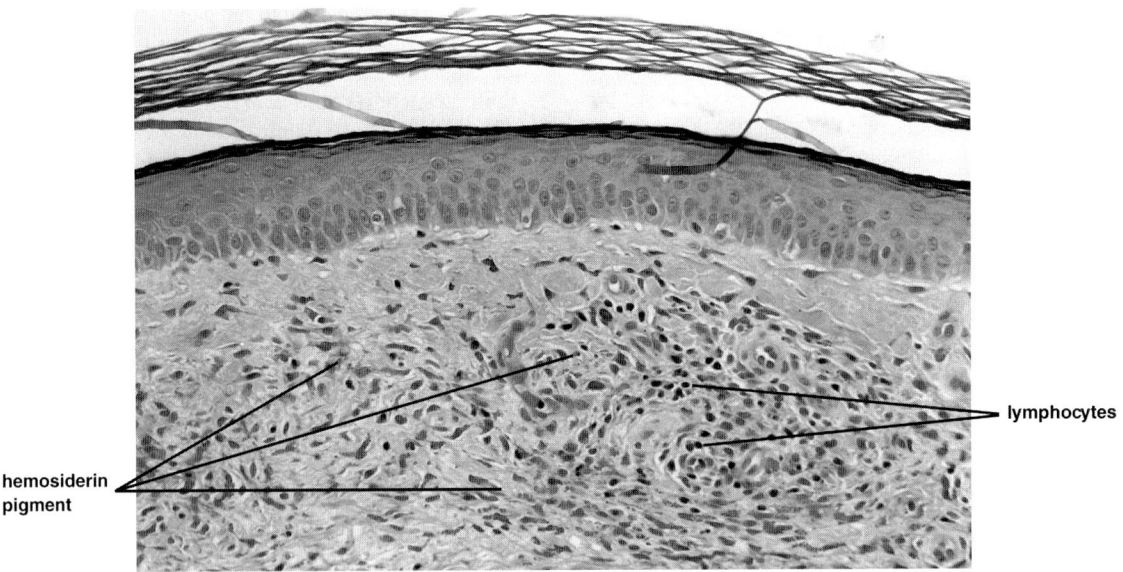

Figure 8-19. Lichen aureus. Hemosiderin pigment deposition is evident within the papillary dermal lymphocytic infiltrate. (× 200.)

Lividoid Vasculitis (Atrophie Blanche, Segmental Hyalinizing Vasculitis)

Clinical Features

The multiple names used to describe this vasculopathy reflect the different stages of its evolution. The disease most commonly affects middle-aged women who develop recurrent painful ulcers that heal with irregular, stellate, atrophic hypopigmented scars on the legs, ankles, and feet bilaterally.[140–142] Although usually idiopathic, associated conditions include systemic lupus erythematosus, γ-heavy chain disease, essential cryoglobulinemia, Raynaud's phenomenon, and PAN.[143–145]

Histopathologic Features

The characteristic microscopic finding of lividoid vasculitis is complete or partial occlusion of the small vessels of the papillary and reticular dermis by brightly eosinophilic, PAS-positive, diastase-resistant thrombi[140,141] (Fig. 8-21). Extravasated erythrocytes surround the thrombosed vessels and indicate loss of integrity of the vessel wall. In older lesions similar-appearing hyaline material is deposited in vessel walls. Both the thrombi and the intramural deposits may be extensive so that vessels appear smudged and thickened, or they may be focal and minimal. In older lesions the adjacent reticular dermis is fibrotic and eventually sclerotic. Throughout the evolution of the vascu-

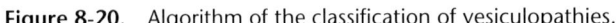

Figure 8-20. Algorithm of the classification of vesiculopathies.

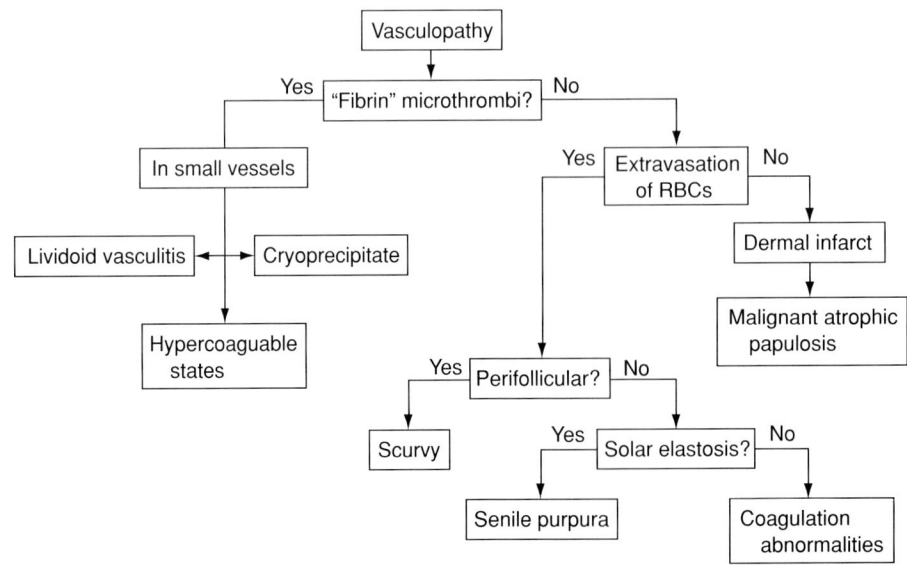

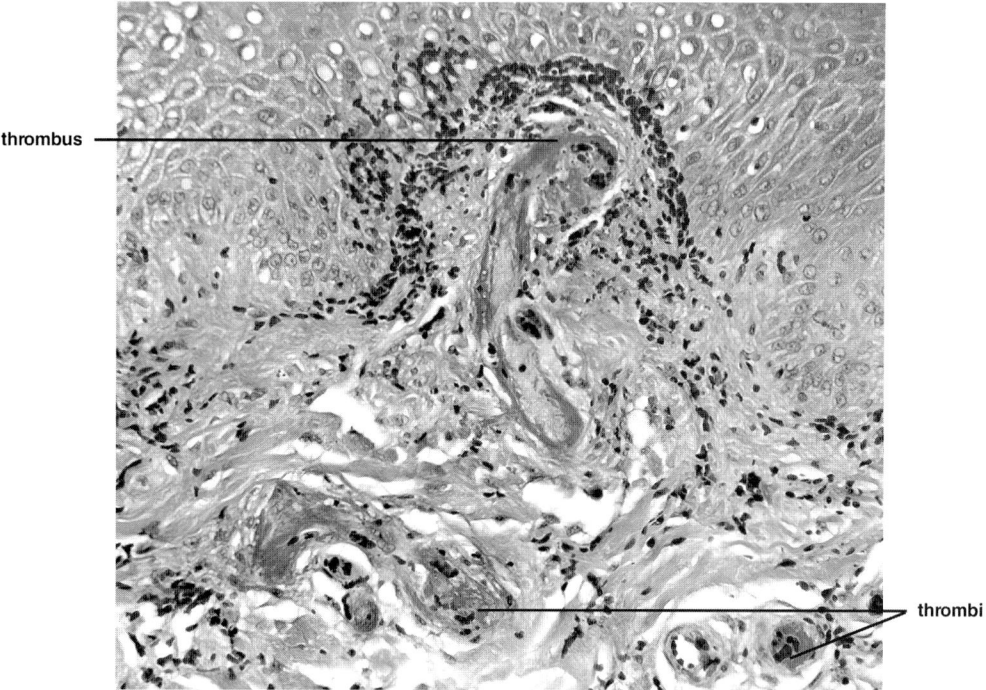

thrombus

thrombi

Figure 8-21. Lividoid vasculitis. Brightly eosinophilic thrombi occlude small vessels. No leukocytoclastic vasculitis is present. (× 200.)

lopathy, inflammation is minimal and no true leukocytoclastic vasculitis is seen. The few inflammatory cells present are primarily lymphocytes.

Differential Diagnosis

A variable degree of thickening of the walls of the small vessels of the dermis occurs with age presumably as a result of vascular stasis. This process may be greatly exaggerated in patients with diabetes mellitus, but thrombi are not present. Both thickened small vessel walls and surrounding dermal fibrosis are found in stasis dermopathy (the dermal changes of stasis dermatitis), but thrombosis is not a feature.

Malignant Atrophic Papulosis (Degos' Disease)

Clinical Features

Malignant atrophic papulosis is included under vasculopathy by default.[146–149] The mechanism responsible for the development of the characteristic dermal infarcts remains elusive, but the disease is not a form of leukocytoclastic vasculitis.[150,151] In fact, inflammatory cell infiltrates of any type are scant in malignant atrophic papulosis.[152] Different abnormalities of the small blood vessels of the dermis have been described, including the enigmatic "endovasculitis." This term was coined to describe an hypothesized subintimal fibrosis that supposedly leads to occlusion and thrombosis of small dermal vessels. However, this change has not been verified in the more recent literature.

Lately, investigators suggested a relationship to the antiphospholid syndrome.[153, 154]

Classic malignant atrophic papulosis is a uniformly fatal disease.[150, 151] The cutaneous lesions are distinctive and are usually present well in advance of the visceral changes. Crops of asymptomatic erythematous macules evolve into depressed macules with diagnostic porcelain white centers. The eruption occurs at any location but tends to spare the face and distal extremities. Within a few months after the onset of the cutaneous eruption, symptoms that result from bowel and brain infarcts complete the triad. Patients die from either gastrointestinal bleeding or cerebral infarcts.[155] To date no treatment has altered the course of the disease.

Histopathologic Features

No consistent vessel abnormality is found. As discussed above, observers have claimed that various combinations of endothelial cell hypertrophy, subintimal fibrosis and thrombosis are present.[150–152] Inflammation is not a consistent feature. In essence, both the small and large dermal vessels appear normal at the light microscopic level. The characteristic porcelain white papules are formed by a wedge-shaped dermal infarct pointing toward the deep dermis (Fig. 8-22). Hyperkeratotic, thinned epidermis is present over the broad base of the wedge-shaped infarct. Focal interface change is present. The infarcted dermis is paucicellular and fibrotic. Mucin is relatively abundant. Mucin stains may help to delineate the infarcted area from the adjacent normal dermis.

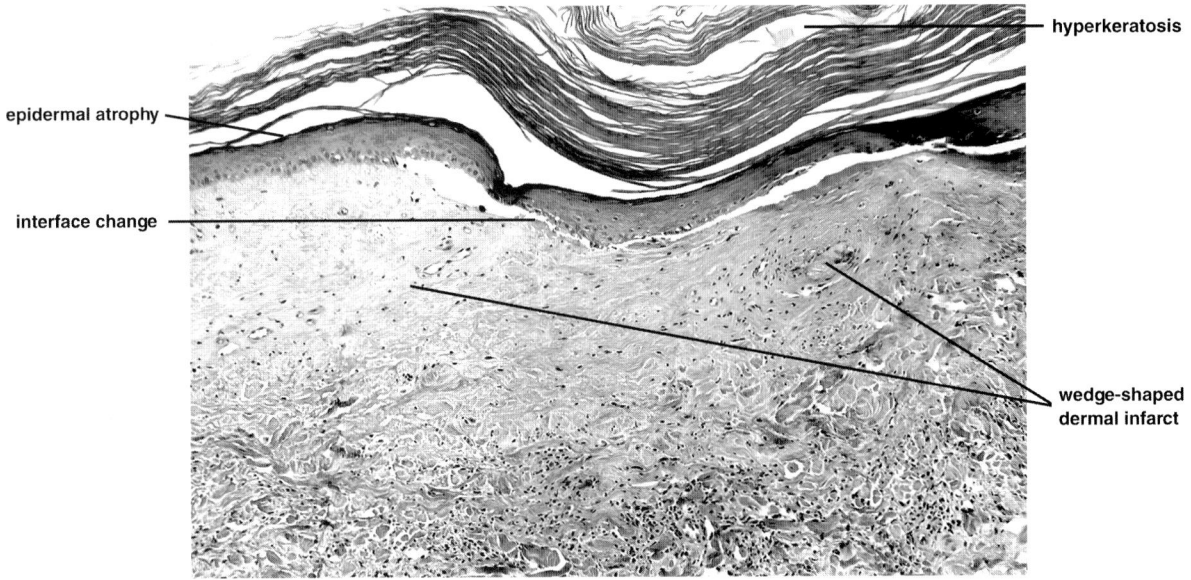

Figure 8-22. Malignant atrophic papulosis. Hyperkeratotic, atrophic epidermis with interface change overlies a pale wedge-shaped infarct. Mucin is present within the infarcted area. Leukocytoclastic vasculitis is not a feature. (× 80.)

Differential Diagnosis

The pale, homogeneous altered collagen of the upper dermis that is characteristic of lichen sclerosus et atrophicus may closely mimic the dermal infarct of malignant atrophic papulosis. The zone of altered collagen is only rarely wedge shaped in lichen sclerosus et atrophicus; a linear configuration is typical. Vacuolar interface change at the dermoepidermal junction over the homogenized collagen and lymphocytic infiltrates at the advancing edge of the altered collagen also help to differentiate lichen sclerosus et atrophicus from malignant atrophic papulosis. An increase in dermal mucin is also found in systemic lupus

erythematosus and dermatomyositis, but the wedge-shaped dermal infarct of malignant atrophic papulosis is not present.

NONINFLAMMATORY PURPURA

Clinical Features

In addition to vasculitis and other inflammatory diseases, defects in the blood vessels themselves and abnormalities of the blood coagulation process can both produce cutaneous hemorrhage and/or infarctive necrosis of the dermis and subcutis. The loss of blood vessel integrity with resultant hemorrhage is par-

Figure 8-23. Noninflammatory purpura, lupus anticoagulant. A relatively large vessel is occluded by a thrombus. Inflammation is minimal. (× 200.)

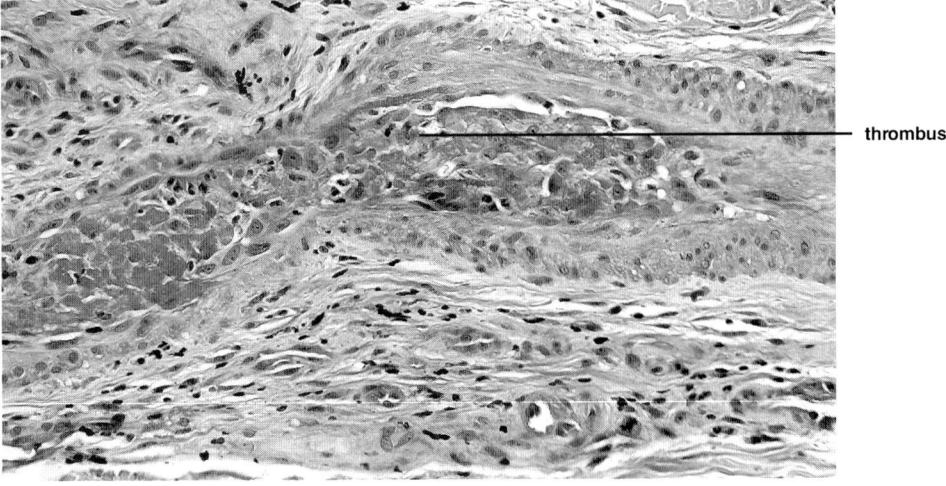

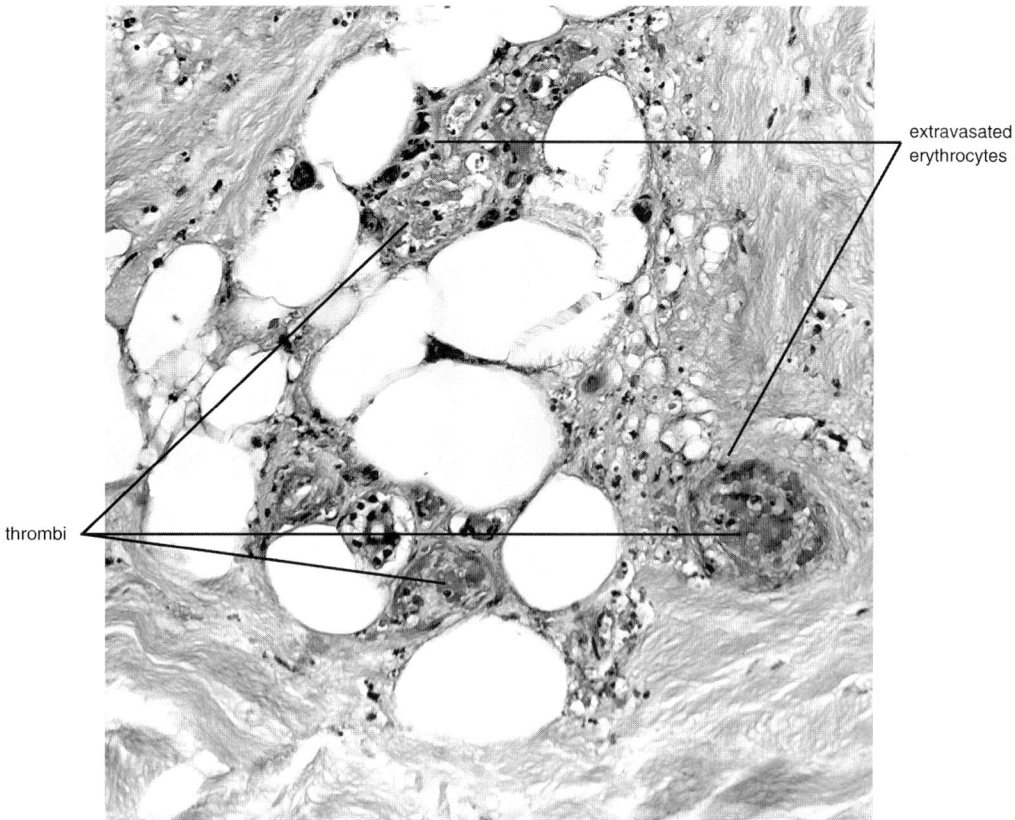

extravasated erythrocytes

thrombi

Figure 8-24. Noninflammatory purpura, cryoglobulinemia. Small vessels within the superficial subcutis are occluded by thrombi formed from cryoprecipitate. Extravasated erythrocytes are present adjacent to the affected vessels. (× 200.)

tially dependent on the inherent capacity of blood to clot. Coagulation is a complex sequence regulated by coordinated interaction of circulating plasma proteins (coagulation factors), platelets, and endothelial cells.[156] If either of these components is deficient or nonfunctional, hemorrhage may result. Conversely, hypercoaguable states and thrombocytosis can lead to occlusion of cutaneous vessels with secondary infarction and necrosis.[157, 158] Defects of vessel walls or the supporting adventitial collagen can also result in loss of vessel integrity and hemorrhage. Clinically, all these abnormalities manifest as purpura.

Coagulopathies may be either inherited such as hemophilia or acquired as in disseminated intravascular coagulation and the lupus anticoagulant syndrome (Sneddon syndrome).[159–164] Thrombocytopenia may be secondary to drug therapy, bone marrow abnormalities, or consumption states such as disseminated intravascular coagulation.[165] Patients who receive large, loading doses of coumarin may develop hemorrhage and necrosis.[166–173] Thrombotic thrombocytopenia purpura is characterized by widespread petechia due to microthrombi.[174] In scurvy, lack of ascorbic acid results in deficient synthesis of collagen in both the vessel walls and supporting dermis.[175] Replacement of normal dermal collagen by solar elastosis and aging leads to loss of support for the small dermal vessels so that minimal trauma results in loss of vessel integrity and hemorrhage.[176] This process has been termed *senile* or *Bateman's purpura.*

Histopathologic Features

Extravasation of erythrocytes alone is found in those abnormalities in which blood clotting is deficient. If a hypercoaguable state is present, then hemorrhage is accompanied by fibrin thrombi[156,158,165,166,174] (Figs. 8-23 and 8-24). Small vessels tend to be affected more than larger ones. Inflammation is not a feature. Hemosiderin deposits, both intra- and extracellular, are present in older, resolving lesions.

The hemorrhage in scurvy tends to be perifollicular.[175] Extravasated erythrocytes, frequently in massive numbers, blend into the elastotic dermis in senile purpura.[176]

Differential Diagnosis

Hemorrhage into the biopsy site may simulate noninflammatory purpura. In operative hemorrhage, the erythrocytes tend to be at the specimen edges. Hemosiderin pigment will not be present. Lividoid vasculitis is virtually limited to the legs and ankles. In addition to small vessel occlusion by fibrin thrombi, the dermis is diffusely fibrotic or sclerotic.

REFERENCES

1. Smoller BR, McNutt NS, Contreras F: The natural history of vasculitis. What the histology tells us about pathogenesis. Arch Dermatol 126:84–89, 1990
2. Jennette CJ, Milling DM, Falk RJ: Vasculitis affecting the skin. A review, editorial. Arch Dermatol 130:899–906 1994
3. Hiltz RE, Cupps TR: Cutaneous vasculitis. Curr Opin Rheumatol 6:20–24, 1994
4. Cupps TR, Fauci AS: pp. 6–19. In The Vasculitides. Vol 21. WB Saunders, Philadelphia, 1981
5. Swerlick RA, Lawley TJ: Cutaneous vasculitis: its relationship to systemic disease. Med Clin North Am 73:1221–1235, 1989
6. Massa MC, Su WP: Lymphocytic vasculitis: is it a specific clinicopathologic entity? J Cutan Pathol 11:132–139, 1984
7. Kerdel FA, Soter NA: Cutaneous inflammation. Prog Dermatol 20:1–12, 1986
8. Swerlick RA: Cytokines in dermatology. Semin Dermatol 10:260–267, 1991
9. Zachariae CO: Chemotactic cytokines and inflammation: biological properties of the lymphocyte and monocyte chemotactic factors ELCF, MCAF and IL-8. Acta Derm Venereol Suppl (Stockh) 181:1–37, 1993
10. Soter NA: Chronic urticaria as a manifestation of necrotizing vasculitis. N Engl J Med 296:1440, 1977
11. Monroe EW, Schulz CI, Maize JC, Jordon RE: Vasculitis in chronic urticaria: an immunopathologic study. J Invest Dermatol 76:103–107, 1981
12. Sanchez NP, Van HHM, Su WP: Clinical and histopathologic spectrum of necrotizing vasculitis: report of findings in 101 cases. Arch Dermatol 121:220–224, 1985
13. Berg RE, Kantor GR, Bergfeld WF: Urticarial vasculitis. Int J Dermatol 27:468–472, 1988
14. Cochrane CG, Koffler D: Immune complex disease in experimental animals. Adv Immunol 16:185, 1973
15. Ekenstam E, Callen JP: Cutaneous leukocytoclastic vasculitis. Clinical and laboratory features of 82 patients seen in private practice. Arch Dermatol 120:484–489, 1984
16. Mullick FG, McAllister HAJ, Wagner BM, Fenoglio JJJ: Drug related vasculitis: clinicopathologic correlations in 30 patients. Hum Pathol 10:313–325, 1979
17. Fauci AS, Haynes BF, Katz P: The spectrum of vasculitis: clinical, pathologic, immunologic and therapeutic considerations. Ann Intern Med 89:660–676, 1978
18. DeSpain JD, Swinfard RW: Collagen vascular disease. Dermatol Clin 10:1–18, 1992
19. Cupps TR, Springer RM, Fauci AS: Chronic, recurrent small-vessel cutaneous vasculitis: clinical experience in 13 patients. JAMA 247:1994–1998, 1982
20. Smith ML, Jorizzo JL, Semble E et al: Rheumatoid papules: lesions showing features of vasculitis and palisading granuloma [see comments]. J Am Acad Dermatol 20:348–352, 1989
21. Finan MC: Rheumatoid papule, cutaneous extravascular necrotizing granuloma, and Churg-Strauss granuloma: are they the same entity? letter; comment. J Am Acad Dermatol 22:142–143, 1990
22. Higaki Y, Yamashita H, Sato K et al: Rheumatoid papules: a report on four patients with histopathologic analysis. J Am Acad Dermatol 28:406–411, 1993

23. Greer JM, Longley S, Edwards NL et al: Vasculitis associated with malignancy: experience with 13 patients and literature review. Medicine (Baltimore) 67:220–230, 1988
24. Kois JM, Sexton FM, Lookingbill DP: Cutaneous manifestations of multiple myeloma. Arch Dermatol 127:69–74, 1991
25. Kurzrock R, Cohen PR, Markowitz A: Clinical manifestations of vasculitis in patients with solid tumors: a case report and review of the literature. Arch Intern Med 154:334–340, 1994
26. Goodless DR, Dhawan SS, Alexis J, Wiszniak J: Cutaneous periarteritis nodosa. Int J Dermatol 29:611–615, 1990
27. Homas PB, David-Bajar KM, Fitzpatrick JE et al: Microscopic polyarteritis: report of a case with cutaneous involvement and antimyeloperoxidase antibodies. Arch Dermatol 128:1223–1228, 1992
28. Chiu G, Rajapakse CN: Cutaneous polyarteritis nodosa and ulcerative colitis. J Rheumatol 18:769–770, 1991
29. Grana Gil J, Alonso Aquirre P, Yebra Pimental MT et al: Cutaneous polyarteritis nodosa and Crohn's disease. Clin Rheumatol 10:196–200, 1991
30. Siberry GK, Cohen BA, Johnson B: Cutaneous polyarteritis nodosa: reports of two cases in children and review of the literature. Arch Dermatol 130:884–889, 1994
31. Mankowitz G, Smoller BR, McNutt NS: Benign cutaneous polyarteritis nodosa: relationship to systemic polyarteritis nodosa and to hepatitis B infection. Arch Dermatol 127:1520–1523, 1991
32. Ilan Y, Naparstek Y: Schonlein-Henoch syndrome in adults and children. Semin Arthritis Rheum 21:103–109, 1991
33. Robson WL, Leung AK: Henoch-Schonlein purpura. Adv Pediatr 41:163–194, 1994
34. Raimer SS: Controversies in pediatric dermatology. Adv Dermatol 9:193–203, 1994
35. Cream JJ, Gumpel JM, Peachey RDG: Schönlein-Henoch purpura in the adult: a study of seventy-seven adults with anaphylactoid or Schönlein-Henoch purpura. Q J Med 39:461–484, 1970
36. Cohen SJ, Pittelkow MR, Su WP: Cutaneous manifestations of cryoglobulinemia: clinical and histopathologic study of seventy-two patients. J Am Acad Dermatol 25:21–27, 1991
37. Dupin N, Chosidow O, Lunel F et al: Essential mixed cryoglobulinemia: a comparative study of dermatologic manifestations in patients infected or noninfected with hepatitis C virus. Arch Dermatol 131:1124–1127, 1995
38. Ellis FA: The cutaneous manifestations of cryoglobulinemia. Arch Dermatol 89:690–697, 1964
39. Jorizzo JL, Schmalstieg FC, Dinehart SM et al: Bowel-associated dermatosis-arthritis syndrome: immune complex-mediated vessel damage and increased neutrophil migration. Arch Intern Med 144:738–740, 1984
40. Jorizzo JL, Solomon AR, Zanolli MD, Leshin B: Neutrophilic vascular reactions. J Am Acad Dermatol 19:983–1005, 1988
41. Jorizzo JL: Pustular vasculitis: an emerging disease concept. J Am Acad Dermatol 9:160–162, 1983
42. Scott DG, Bacon PA, Tribe CR: Systemic rheumatoid vasculitis: a clinical and laboratory study of 50 cases. Medicine (Baltimore) 60:288–297, 1981

43. Jorizzo JL, Daniels JC: Dermatologic conditions reported in patients with rheumatoid arthritis. J Am Acad Dermatol 8:439–457, 1983

44. Jorizzo JL, Solomon AR, Cavallo T: Behçet's syndrome: immunopathologic and histopathologic assessment of pathergy lesions is useful in diagnosis and follow-up. Arch Pathol Lab Med 109:747–751, 1985

45. Cohen C, Trapuckd S: Leukocytoclastic vasculitis asociated with cutaneous infection by herpesvirus. Am J Dermatopathol 6:561–565, 1984

46. Katz SI, Gallin JI, Hertz KC et al: Erythema elevatum diutinum: skin and systemic manifestations, immunologic studies, and successful treatment with dapsone. Medicine (Baltimore) 56:443–455, 1977

47. Buahene K, Hudson M, Mowat A et al: Erythema elevatum diutinum–an unusual association with ulcerative colitis. Clin Exp Dermatol 16:204–206, 1991

48. Cockerell CJ: Noninfectious inflammatory skin diseases in HIV-infected individuals. Dermatol Clin 9:531–541, 1991

49. Requena L, Sanchez Yus E, Martin L et al: Erythema elevatum diutinum in a patient with acquired immunodeficiency syndrome: another clinical simulator of Kaposi's sarcoma. Arch Dermatol 127:1819–1822, 1991

50. Wilkinson SM, English JS, Smith NP et al: Erythema elevatum diutinum: a clinicopathological study. Clin Exp Dermatol 17:87–93, 1992

51. Bernard P, Bedane C, Delrous JL et al: Erythema elevatum diutinum in a patient with relapsing polychondritis. J Am Acad Dermatol 26:312–315, 1992

52. Yiannias JA, el-Azhary RA, Gibson LE: Erythema elevatum diutinum: a clinical and histopathologic study of 13 patients. J Am Acad Dermatol 26:38–44, 1992

53. Planaguma M, Puig L, Alomar A et al: Pyoderma gangrenosum in association with erythema elevatum diutinum: report of two cases. Cutis 49:261–266, 1992

54. Kavanagh GM, Colaco CB, Bradfield JW, Archer CB: Erythema elevatum diutinum associated with Wegener's granulomatosis and IgA paraproteinemia. J Am Acad Dermatol 28:846–849, 1993

55. LeBoit PE, Cockerell CJ: Nodular lesions of erythema elevatum diutinum in patients infected with the human immunodeficiency virus. J Am Acad Dermatol 28:919–922, 1993

56. McDonagh AJ, Colver GB: Ulcerated nodules on the elbows, fingers, and knees: erythema elevatum diutinum (EED). Arch Dermatol 129:1043–1044, 1046–1047, 1993

57. Hansen U, Haerslev T, Knudsen B, Jacobsen GK: Erythema elevatum diutinum: case report showing an unusual distribution. Cutis 53:124–126, 1994

58. Farella V, Lotti T, Difonzo EM, Panconesi EX: Erythema elevatum diutinum. Int J Dermatol 33:638–640, 1994

59. Delaporte E, Aleandari S, Fenaux P et al: Erythema elevatum diutinum and chronic lymphocytic leukemia, letter. Clin Exp Dermatol 19:188, 1994

60. Aractingi S, Bachmeyer C, Dombret H et al: Simultaneous occurrence of two rare cutaneous markers of poor prognosis in myelodysplastic syndrome: erythema elevatum diutinum and specific lesions. Br J Dermatol 131:112–117, 1994

61. Kolbusz RV, Pearson RW: A solitary plaque of the cheek–granuloma faciale. Arch Dermatol 129:634–635, 637, 1993

62. Konohana A: Extrafacial granuloma faciale. J Dermatol 21:680–682, 1994

63. Johnson WC, Higdon RS, Helwig EB: Granuloma faciale. 79: 42–52, 1959

64. Pedace FJ, Perry HO: Granuloma faciale: a clinical and histopathologic review. Arch Dermatol 94:387–395, 1966

65. Monroe EW: Urticarial vasculitis: an updated review. J Am Acad Dermatol 5:88–95, 1981

66. Asherson RA, Sontheimer R: Urticarial vasculitis and syndromes in association with connective tissue diseases. Ann Rheum Dis 50:743–744, 1991

67. Asherson RA, D DC, Stephens CJ et al: Urticarial vasculitis in a connective tissue disease clinic: patterns, presentations, and treatment. Semin Arthritis Rheum 20:285–296, 1991

68. Mehregan DR, Hall MJ, Gibson LE: Urticarial vasculitis: a histopathologic and clinical review of 72 cases. J Am Acad Dermatol 26:441–448, 1992

69. Sanchez JL, Benmaman O: Clinicopathological correlation in chronic urticaria. Am J Dermatopathol 14:220–223, 1992

70. Wisnieski JJ, Baer AN, Christensen J et al: Hypocomplementemic urticarial vasculitis syndrome: clinical and serologic findings in 18 patients. Medicine (Baltimore) 74:24–41, 1995

71. O'Loughlin S, Schroeter AL, Jordon RE: Chronic urticaria-like lesions in systemic lupus erythematosus. Arch Dermatol 114:879–883, 1978

72. Zax RH, Hodge SJ, Callen JP: Cutaneous leukocytoclastic vasculitis: serial histopathologic evaluation demonstrates the dynamic nature of the infiltrate. Arch Dermatol 126:69–72, 1990

73. Chen KR, Pittelkow MR, Su WPD et al: Recurrent cutaneous necrotizing eosinophilic vasculitis: a novel eosinophil-mediated syndrome. Arch Dermatol 130:1159–1166, 1994

74. Chen KR, Su WP, Pittelkow MR, Leiferman KM: Eosinophilic vasculitis syndrome: recurrent cutaneous eosinophilic necrotizing vasculitis. Semin Dermatol 14:106–110, 1995

75. McNeely MC, Jorizzo JL, Solomon AR Jr et al: Primary idiopathic cutaneous pustular vasculitis. J Am Acad Dermatol 14:939–944, 1986

76. Jorizzo JL, Schmalsteig FC, Solomon AR Jr et al: Thalidomide effects in Behçet's syndrome and pustular vasculitis. Arch Intern Med 146:878–881, 1986

77. Shapiro L, Teisch JA, Brownstein MH: Dermatohistopathology of chronic gonococcal sepsis. Arch Dermatol 107: 403–406, 1973

78. LeBoit PE, Yen TS, Wintroub B: The evolution of lesions in erythema elevatum diutinum. Am J Dermatopathol 8:392–402, 1986

79. Peteiro C, Toribio J: Incidence of leukocytoclastic vasculitis in chronic idiopathic urticaria: study of 100 cases. Am J Dermatopathol 11:528–533, 1989

80. Yevich I: Necrotizing vasculitis with granulomatosis. Int J Dermatol 27:540–546, 1988

81. Churg J, Churg A: Idiopathic and secondary vasculitis: a review. Mod Pathol 2:144–160, 1989

82. Hu CH, O'Loughlin S, Winkelmann RK: Cutaneous manifestations of Wegener granulomatosis. Arch Dermatol 113: 175–182, 1977

83. Le T, Pierard GE, Lapiere CM: Granulomatous vasculitis of Wegener. J Cutan Pathol 8:34–39, 1981
84. Frances C, Du LT, Piette JC et al: Wegener's granulomatosis: dermatological manifestations in 75 cases with clinicopathologic correlation. Arch Dermatol 130:861–867, 1994
85. Barksdale SK, Hallahan CW, Kerr GS et al: Cutaneous pathology in Wegener's granulomatosis: a clinicopathologic study of 75 biopsies in 46 patients. Am J Surg Pathol 19:161–172, 1995
86. Crotty CP, DeRemee RA, Winkelmann RK: Cutaneous clinicopathologic correlation of allergic granulomatosis. J Am Acad Dermatol 5:571–581, 1981
87. Calonje JE, Greaves MW: Cutaneous extravascular necrotizing granuloma (Churg-Strauss) as a paraneoplastic manifestation of non-Hodgkin's B-cell lymphoma. J R Soc Med 86:549–550, 1993
88. Abe-Matsuura Y, Fujimoto W, Arata J: Allergic granulomatosis (Churg-Strauss) associated with cutaneous manifestations: report of two cases. J Dermatol 22:46–51, 1995
89. Chanda JJ, Callen JP: Necrotizing vasculitis (angiitis) with granulomatosis. Int J Dermatol 23:101–107, 1984
90. Churg A: Pulmonary angiitis and granulomatosis revisited. Hum Pathol 14:868–883, 1983
91. Carlson KC, Gibson LE: Cutaneous signs of lymphomatoid granulomatosis. Arch Dermatol 127:1693–1698, 1991
92. Rimsza LM, Rimsza ME, Gilbert-Barness E: Pathological cases of the month: lymphomatoid granulomatosis. Am J Dis Child 147: 693–694, 1993
93. Tawfik NH, Magro CM, Crowson AN, Maxwell I: Lymphomatoid granulomatosis presenting as a solitary cutaneous lesion. Int J Dermatol 33:188–189, 1994
94. Magro CM, Tawfik NH, Crowson AN: Lymphomatoid granulomatosis. Int J Dermatol 33:157–160, 1994
95. Wood ML, Harrington CI, Slater DN et al: Cutaneous lymphomatoid granulomatosis: a rare cause of recurrent skin ulceration. Br J Dermatol 110:619–625, 1984
96. Macdonald DM, Sarkany I: Lymphomatoid granulomatosis. Clin Exp Dermatol 1:163–173, 1976
97. Vignon-Pennamen MD, Wallach D: Cutaneous manifestations of neutrophilic disease. A study of seven cases. Dermatologica 183:255–264, 1991
98. Duguid CM, Powell FC: Pyoderma gangrenosum. Clin Dermatol 11:129–133, 1993
99. Clark HH, Cohen PR: Pyoderma gangrenosum in an HIV-infected patient. J Am Acad Dermatol 32:912–914, 1995
100. Venkateswaran S, Garg BR, Reddy BS, Ratnakar C: Pyoderma gangrenosum in childhood: case report. J Dermatol 21:670–673, 1994
101. Graham JA, Hansen KK, Rabinowitz LG, Esterly NB: Pyoderma gangrenosum in infants and children. Pediatr Dermatol 11:10–17, 1994
102. Urano S, Kodama H, Kato K, Nogura K: Pyoderma gangrenosum with systemic involvement. J Dermatol 22: 515–519, 1995
103. Hurwitz RM, Haseman JH: The evolution of pyoderma gangrenosum: a clinicopathologic correlation. Am J Dermatopathol 15:28–33, 1993
104. Perry HO, Winkelmann RK: Bullous pyoderma gangrenosum and leukemia. Arch Dermatol 106:901–905, 1972
105. Helm KF, Peters MS, Tefferi A, Leiferman KM: Pyoderma gangrenosum-like ulcer in a patient with large granular lymphocytic leukemia. J Am Acad Dermatol 27:868–871, 1992
106. Ho KK, Otridge BW, Vandenberg E, Powell FC: Pyoderma gangrenosum, polycythemia rubra vera, and the development of leukemia. J Am Acad Dermatol 27:804–808, 1992
107. Duguid CM, O'Loughlin S, Otridge B, Powell FC: Paraneoplastic pyoderma gangrenosum. Australas J Dermatol 34: 17–22, 1993
108. Koester G, Tarnower A, Levisohn D, Burgdorf W: Bullous pyoderma gangrenosum. J Am Acad Dermatol 29:875–878, 1993
109. Klock JC, Oken RL: Febrile neutrophilic dermatosis in acute myelogenous leukemia. Cancer 37:922–927, 1976
110. Caughman W, Stern R, Haynes H: Neutrophilic dermatosis of myeloproliferative disorders: atypical forms of pyoderma gangrenosum and Sweet's syndrome associated with myeloproliferative disorders. J Am Acad Dermatol 9:751–758, 1983
111. Davies MG, Hastings A: Sweet's syndrome progressing to pyoderma gangrenosum–a spectrum of neutrophilic skin disease in association with cryptogenic cirrhosis. Clin Exp Dermatol 16:279–282, 1991
112. Aractingi S, Mallet V, Pinquier L et al: Neutrophilic dermatoses during granulocytopenia. Arch Dermatol 131: 1141–1145, 1995
113. Wong TY, Suster S, Bouffard D et al: Histologic spectrum of cutaneous involvement in patients with myelogenous leukemia including the neutrophilic dermatoses. Int J Dermatol 34:323–329, 1995
114. Kemmett D, Hunter JA: Sweet's syndrome: a clinicopathologic review of twenty-nine cases. J Am Acad Dermatol 23:503–507, 1990
115. Storer JS, Nesbitt LTJ, Galen WK, Deleo VA: Sweet's syndrome. Int J Dermatol 22:8–12, 1983
116. Bourke SJ, Quinn AG, Farr PM et al: Neutrophilic alveolitis in Sweet's syndrome. Thorax 47:572–573, 1992
117. Itoh H, Shimasaki S, Nakashima A et al: Sweet's syndrome associated with subacute necrotizing lymphadenitis. Intern Med 31:686–689, 1992
118. Gonzalez-Castro U, Julia A, Pedragosa R et al: Sweet syndrome in chronic myelogenous leukemia. Int J Dermatol 30:648–650, 1991
119. Feliu E, Cervantes F, Ferrando J et al: Neutrophilic pustulosis associated with chronic myeloid leukemia: a special form of Sweet's syndrome. Report of two cases. Acta Haematol 88:154–157, 1992
120. Watanabe R, Iijima M, Otsuka F: A case of neutrophilic dermatosis (ND) complicated by cryofibrinogenemia (CFGN) and myelodysplastic syndrome (MDS). J Dermatol 19: 181–185, 1992
121. von den Driesch P: Sweet's syndrome (acute febrile neutrophilic dermatosis). J Am Acad Dermatol 31:535–560, 1994
122. Su WP, Fett DL, Gibson LE, Pittelkow MR: Sweet syndrome: acute febrile neutrophilic dermatosis. Semin Dermatol 14:173–178, 1995
123. Krolikowski FJ, Reuter K, Shultis EW: Acute febrile neutrophilic dermatosis (Sweet's syndrome) associated with lymphoma. Hum Pathol 16:520–522, 1985

124. Goette DK: Sweet's syndrome in subacute cutaneous lupus erythematosus. Arch Dermatol 121:789–791, 1985
125. Harary AM: Sweet's syndrome associated with rheumatoid arthritis. Arch Intern Med 143:1993–1995, 1983
126. Beitner H, Nakatani T, Hammar H: A case report of acute febrile neutrophilic dermatosis (Sweet's syndrome) and Crohn's disease. Acta Derm Venereol 71:360–363, 1991
127. Hilliquin P, Marre JP, Cormier C et al: Sweet's syndrome and monarthritis in a human immunodeficiency virus-positive patient. Arthritis Rheum 35:484–486, 1992
128. Barnadas MA, Sitjas D, Brunet S et al: Acute febrile neutrophilic dermatosis (Sweet's syndrome) associated with prostate adenocarcinoma and a myelodysplastic syndrome. Int J Dermatol 31:647–648, 1992
129. Cohen PR, Holder WR, Tucker SB et al: Sweet syndrome in patients with solid tumors. Cancer 72:2723–2731, 1993
130. Cohen PR, Kurzrock R: Sweet's syndrome and cancer. Clin Dermatol 11:149–157, 1993
131. Chan HL, Lee YS, Kuo TT: Sweet's syndrome: clinicopathologic study of eleven cases. Int J Dermatol 33:425–532, 1994
132. Berger TG, Dhar A, McCalmont TH: Neutrophilic dermatoses in HIV infection. J Am Acad Dermatol 31:1045–1047, 1994
133. Boatman BW, Taylor RC, Klein LE, Cohen BA: Sweet's syndrome in children. South Med J 87:193–196, 1994
134. Cooper PH, Innes DJJ, Greer KE: Acute febrile neutrophilic dermatosis (Sweet's syndrome) and myeloproliferative disorders. Cancer 51:1518–1526, 1983
135. Su WP, Liu HN: Diagnostic criteria for Sweet's syndrome. Cutis 37:167–174, 1986
136. Masuda T, Abe Y, Arata J, Nagao Y: Acute febrile neutrophilic dermatosis (Sweet's syndrome) associated with extreme infiltration of eosinophils. J Dermatol 21:341–346, 1994
137. Randall SJ, Kierland RR, Montgomery H: Pigmented purpuric eruptions. Arch Dermatol Syph 64:177–191, 1951
138. Wilkinson SM, Smith AG, Davis M, Dawes PT: Capillaritis: a manifestation of rheumatoid disease. Clin Rheumatol 12:53–56, 1993
139. Waisman M: Lichen aureus. Int J Dermatol 24:645–646, 1985
140. Winkelmann RK, Schroeter AL, Kierland RR, Ryan TM: Clinical studies of livedoid vasculitis (segmental hyalinizing vasculitis). Mayo Clin Proc 49:746–750, 1974
141. Stiefler RE, Bergfeld WF: Atrophie blanche. Int J Dermatol 21:1–7, 1982
142. Milstone LM, Braverman IM, Lucky P, Fleckman P: Classification and therapy of atrophie blanche. Arch Dermatol 119:963–969, 1983
143. Cooper DL, Bolognia JL, Lin JT: Atrophie blanche in a patient with gamma-heavy-chain disease [letter]. Arch Dermatol 127:272–273, 1991
144. Elisaf M, Nikou-Stefanaki S, Drosos AA, Moutsopoulos HM: Atrophie blanche: clinical diagnosis and treatment. Ann Med Interne (Paris) 142:415–418, 1991
145. Yang LJ, Chan HL, Chen SY et al: Atrophie blanche: a clinicopathological study of 27 patients. Chang Keng I Hsueh 14:237–245, 1991
146. Burrow JN, Blumbergs PC, Iyer PV, Hallpike JF: Kohlmeier-Degos disease: a multisystem vasculopathy with progressive cerebral infarction. Aust NZ J Med 21:49–51, 1991
147. Demitsu T, Nakajima K, Okuyama R, Tadaki T: Malignant atrophic papulosis (Degos' syndrome). Int J Dermatol 31:99–102, 1992
148. Bulengo-Ransby SM, Burns MK, Taylor WB et al: Peristomal atrophic papules: Degos' disease (malignant atrophic papulosis). Arch Dermatol 128:256–257, 259–260, 1992
149. Snow JL, Muller SA: Degos' syndrome: malignant atrophic papulosis. Semin Dermatol 14:99–105, 1995
150. Degos R: Malignant atrophic papulosis. Br J Dermatol 100:21–35, 1979
151. Tribble K, Archer ME, Jorizzo JL et al: Malignant atrophic papulosis: absence of circulating immune complexes or vasculitis. J Am Acad Dermatol 15:365, 1986
152. Muller SA, Landry M: Malignant atrophic papulosis (Degos' disease): a report of two cases with clinical and histological studies. Arch Dermatol 112:357–363, 1976
153. Grattan CE, Burton JL: Antiphospholipid syndrome and cutaneous vasoocclusive disorders. Semin Dermatol 10:152–159, 1991
154. Asherson RA, Cervera R: Antiphospholipid syndrome. J Invest Dermatol 100:21S–27S, 1993
155. Casparie MK, Meyer JW, van Huystee BE et al: Endoscopic and histopathologic features of Degos' disease. Endoscopy 23:231–233, 1991
156. Auletta MJ, Headington JT: Purpura fulminans: a cutaneous manifestation of severe protein C deficiency. Arch Dermatol 124:1387–1391, 1988
157. Wyshock E, Caldwell M, Crowley JP: Deep venous thrombosis, inflammatory bowel disease, and protein S deficiency. Am J Clin Pathol 90:633–635, 1988
158. Smith KJ, Skelton HGd, James WD et al: Cutaneous histopathologic findings in "antiphospholipid syndrome": correlation with disease, including human immunodeficiency virus disease. Arch Dermatol 126:1176–1183, 1990
159. Stephansson EA, Niemi KM, Jouhikainen T et al: Lupus anticoagulant and the skin: a long-term follow-up study of SLE patients with special reference to histopathological findings. Acta Derm Venereol 71:416–422, 1991
160. Stephens CJ: The antiphospholipid syndrome: clinical correlations, cutaneous features, mechanism of thrombosis and treatment of patients with the lupus anticoagulant and anticardiolipin antibodies. Br J Dermatol 125:199–210, 1991
161. Sempere AP, Martinez B, Bermejo F et al: Sneddon's syndrome: its clinical characteristics and etiopathogenic factors. Rev Clin Esp 191:3–7, 1992
162. Naldi L, Locati F, Marchesi L et al: Cutaneous manifestations associated with antiphospholipid antibodies in patients with suspected primary antiphospholipid syndrome: a case-control study. Ann Rheum Dis 52:219–222, 22, 1993
163. Kampe CE: Clinical syndromes associated with lupus anticoagulants. Semin Thromb Hemost 20:16–26, 1994
164. Bick RL, Baker WF: Antiphospholipid and thrombosis syndromes. Semin Thromb Hemost 20:3–15, 1994
165. Robboy SJ, Mihm MC, Colman RW, Minna JD: The skin in disseminated intravascular coagulation: prospective analysis of thirty-six cases. Br J Dermatol 88:221–229, 1973
166. Russell-Jones R, Cunningham J: Warfarin skin necrosis. Br J Dermatol 101:561–565, 1979
167. Goldberg SL, Orthner CL, Yalisove BL et al: Skin necrosis following prolonged administration of coumarin in a patient

with inherited protein S deficiency. Am J Hematol 38:64–66, 1991

168. Cucuianu M, Hagau N, Cotul M et al: Heterozygous protein C deficiency and coumarin necrosis of the skin. Rom J Intern Med 30:105–111, 1992

169. Hartman EH, Coosemans JA, Tan P: Skin necrosis, a rare complication of coumarin therapy. Acta Chir Plast 34:224–230, 1992

170. Comp PC: Coumarin-induced skin necrosis: incidence, mechanisms, management and avoidance. Drug Saf 8:128–135, 1993

171. Griffin JP: Anticoagulants and skin necrosis. Adverse Drug React Toxicol Rev 13:157–167, 1994

172. Wattiaux MJ, Herve R, Robert A et al: Coumarin-induced skin necrosis associated with acquired protein S deficiency and antiphospholipid antibody syndrome. Arthritis Rheum 37:1096–1100, 1994

173. Balestra B: Skin necrosis: a paradoxical complication of anticoagulation. Schweiz Med Wochenschr 125:361–364, 1995

174. Luttgens WF: Thrombotic thrombocytopenic pupura with extensive hemorrhagic gangrene of the skin and subcutaneous tissue. Ann Intern Med 46:1207–1212, 1957

175. Reuler JB, Broudy VC, Cooney TG: Adult scurvy. JAMA 253:805–807, 1985

176. Feinstein RJ, Halprin KM, Penneys NS et al: Senile purpura. Arch Dermatol 108:229–232, 1973

9

GRANULOMATOUS DERMATITIS

Granulomatous inflammation is a distinctive form of chronic inflammation characterized by clustered modified tissue macrophages called *histiocytes*. Granulomatous dermatitis can be classified by etiology or morphology, the latter system being useful as a diagnostic tool (Fig. 9-1). Location and distribution of histiocytes, their appearance, the presence or absence of necrosis, and the identification of infectious organisms or foreign debris are important factors in arriving at an accurate and specific diagnosis.

Epithelioid granulomas are groups of histiocytes that have assumed an epithelioid appearance. These modified macrophages have abundant cytoplasm and cluster tightly together with little or no intervening stroma.

It is useful to subdivide epithelioid granulomas according to the presence or absence of necrosis. Discrete non-necrotizing granulomas are characteristic of sarcoidosis, Crohn's disease, and certain foreign body reactions. The granulomas of tuberculoid leprosy take this form, but are unusual because of their peculiar relationship to nerves. Because some examples of tuberculosis and fungal infections can result in the same morphologic pattern, all such granulomas should be subjected to stains for acid-fast bacteria and fungi unless the pathogenesis can be determined with hematoxylin and eosin (H&E). Less well-organized epithelioid granulomas can be seen in granulomatous secondary syphilis and indeterminate leprosy.

Conspicuous necrosis at the center of epithelioid granulomas is unusual in sarcoidosis, Crohn's disease, and tuberculoid leprosy. When necrosis is prominent in epithelioid granulomas, tuberculosis and fungal infections should be considered and appropriate stains and cultures performed. Suppurative granulomatous reactions are also seen surrounding keratin liberated from a ruptured follicular cyst or destroyed follicle as in the case of granulomatous rosacea. Halogenodermas can also result in necrotizing granulomatous reactions frequently associated with epidermal hyperplasia. The morphologic picture closely mimics that seen in deep fungal infections.

The term *palisade* as in *palisaded granuloma* refers to an arrangement of histiocytes around a central focus of altered collagen, focus of necrosis, or deposits of crystalline material. These cells tend to be elongate, with their long axis pointing toward the area of injury. Granuloma annulare is the prototype of palisaded granuloma in the skin, but frequently the palisaded arrangement of cells is poorly organized. It is usually located in the dermis with the palisaded cells surrounding an area of altered collagen. Hyaluronic acid (connective tissue mucin) can often be demonstrated within the granuloma by the colloidal iron or Alcian blue stain. Annular elastolytic granuloma (actinic granuloma) is similar to granuloma annulare except that there is no mucin accumulation. Elastic stains show an abrupt loss of elastic fibers within the granuloma and fragments of elastin within giant cells. Asteroid bodies, which are frequently prominent, also stain for elastin.

When palisaded granulomas occur in the subcutis, the differential diagnosis includes rheumatoid nodule and gouty tophus, as well as deep granuloma annulare. Central fibrinoid degeneration is often seen in rheumatoid nodule. Gouty tophi are characterized by urate crystals, which can be demonstrated if the tissue is preserved and processed in nonaqueous fixatives. Even if the tissue is processed conventionally, the deposits within the palisaded granuloma frequently are morphologically distinctive enough to enable the diagnosis to be made. Necrobiosis lipoidica tends to be a more diffuse process than granuloma annulare, rheumatoid nodule, or gouty tophus. It tends to involve both the subcutaneous tissue and the dermis. Large areas of collagen degeneration are usually present as are plasma cells. It is important to remember that epithelioid sarcoma can mimic the morphology of palisaded granuloma and must be recognized.

Xanthogranulomas are granulomatous reactions in which the histiocytes instead of being epithelioid or elongate have abundant foamy cytoplasm. These granulomas frequently contain multinucleate giant cells, often of Touton type. In juvenile xanthogranuloma, there is usually an accompanying infiltrate of eosinophils, lymphocytes, and plasma cells. These findings and the clinical setting usually enable the diagnosis to be made without difficulty. Infiltrates of foamy histiocytes that lack Touton giant cells and eosinophils characterize xanthelasmas and xanthomas. In lepromatous leprosy, foamy histiocytes resemble xanthoma cells, but numerous acid-fast bacilli can be identified within these cells where they often cluster in large clumps, called *globi*. In reticulohistiocytosis, large histiocytes, many of them multinucleate, are

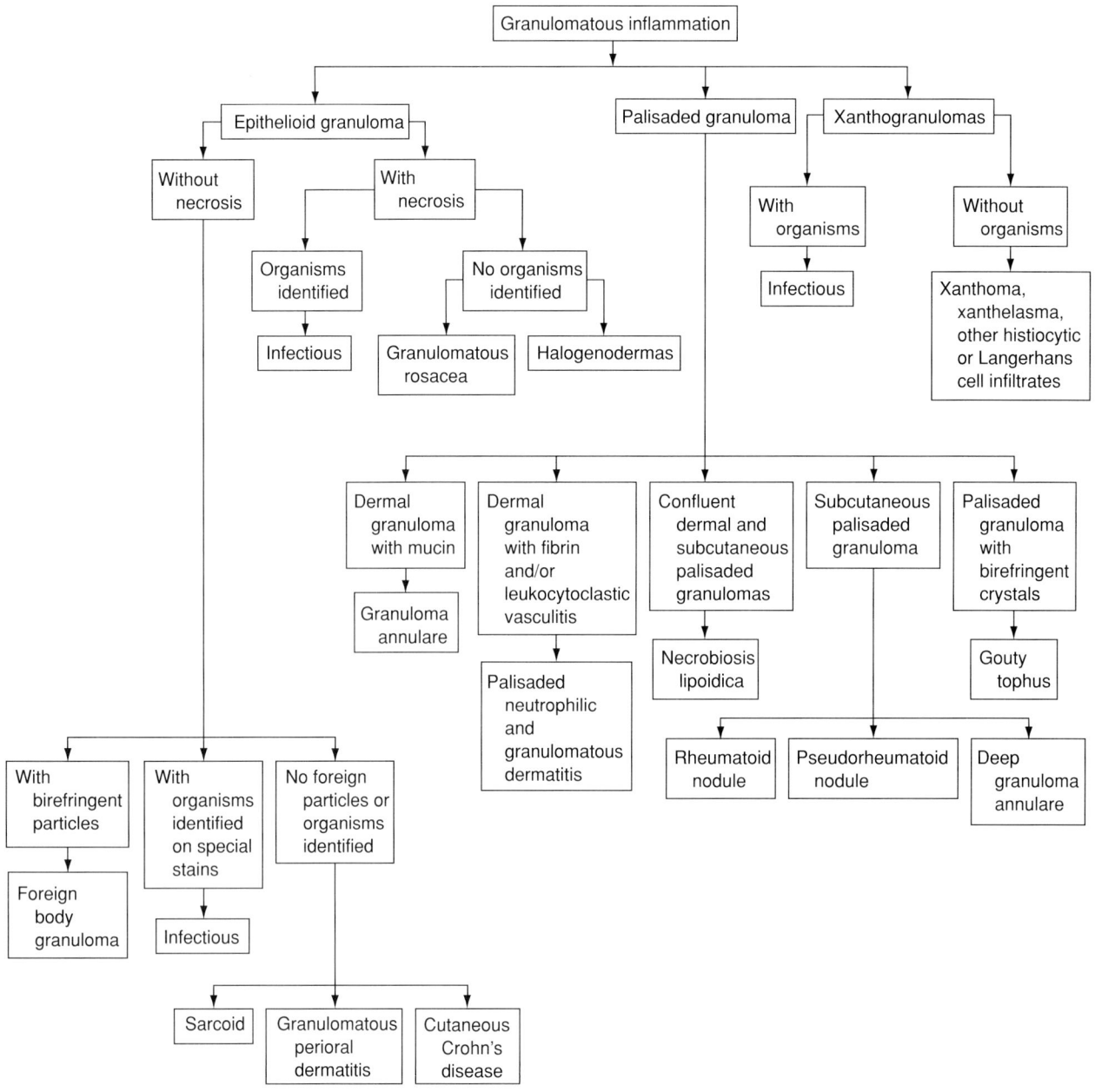

Figure 9-1. Algorithm of the morphologic classification of granulomatous dermatitis.

found to have a "ground-glass" cytoplasm rather than a truly foamy cytoplasm. The cytoplasm stains strongly with periodic acid–Schiff (PAS) even after diastase digestion.

EPITHELIOID GRANULOMAS WITHOUT NECROSIS

Sarcoidosis

Clinical Features

Sarcoidosis is a common granulomatous condition of unknown etiology that can affect many organs and tissues. In the United States its incidence is much higher in American blacks than in whites and higher in women than men. The disease is more prevalent in the southeastern states. Cutaneous lesions are reported to develop in up to 25% of patients with systemic sarcoidosis[1] and are said to portend a poor prognosis. Cutaneous sarcoidal granulomas can also occur in the absence of systemic disease. Sarcoidosis confined to the skin often runs an indolent course without development of lesions elsewhere.[2]

The clinical manifestations of cutaneous sarcoidosis are protean, although papules, plaques, and nodules are the more common presentations. When the granulomas are chronic and occur on the nose, cheeks, or ears, the term *lupus pernio* has been applied, and there is an association between this form and sarcoidosis of the respiratory tract.

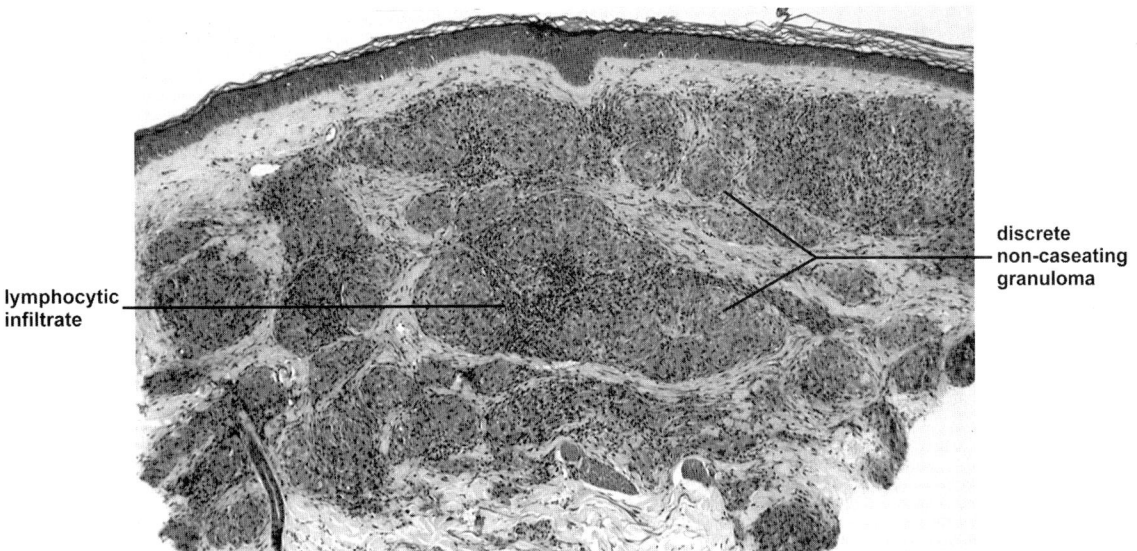

Figure 9-2. Sarcoidosis. There are discrete non-necrotizing granulomas within the dermis. In this example, there is an infiltrate of lymphocytes surrounding several of the granulomas, while several others are "naked."

There is an association between erythema nodosum and systemic sarcoidosis. Most of these patients have a transient disease and show resolution of both their cutaneous and systemic lesions.[3]

Histopathologic Features

There are certain morphologic characteristics that favor the diagnosis of sarcoidosis. The granulomas, which are usually located in the dermis, tend to be discrete, well-formed collections of epithelioid histiocytes with little tendency to undergo central necrosis. Often the granulomas are "naked" with few surrounding lymphocytes, although the density of the accompanying infiltrate is quite variable (Fig. 9-2). Asteroid bodies, stellate eosinophilic inclusions located within cytoplasmic vacuoles of multinucleate giant cells and Schaumann bodies, cytoplasmic laminated calcified structures are sometimes present. However, they are not pathognomonic of sarcoidosis. Polaroscopy occasionally reveals LCRTs (little crystalline refractile things) within the granulomas.

Subcutaneous sarcoidosis is rare and is usually a manifestation of systemic sarcoidosis. This variant was originally described by Darier and Roussy, but the term *sarcoid of Darier-Roussy* has been applied to other granulomatous processes as well as to the subcutaneous granulomas of Boeck's disease.[4,5]

Differential Diagnosis

Sarcoidosis is a diagnosis of exclusion. The evaluation of cutaneous or subcutaneous granulomas requires clinicopathologic correlation and systematic search for etiologic agents. Sections should be polarized in the search for foreign particles and special stains for acid-fast bacilli and fungi carefully examined. Mycobacterial infections, although usually resulting in necrotizing granulomas, sometimes elicit granulomatous reactions indistinguishable from sarcoidosis. Tuberculoid leprosy, in which organisms are often sparse, can sometimes be suspected based on the involvement of nerves in the granulomatous process.

Granulomatous rosacea, a granulomatous reaction associated with folliculitis, can be difficult to distinguish from lupus pernio, but the granulomas often show areas of necrosis. Granulomatous reactions to beryllium and zirconium require a high index of clinical suspicion and spectrographic analysis to enable the diagnosis to be made.

Granulomatous Perioral Dermatitis in Children

Clinical Features

Granulomatous perioral dermatitis is an uncommon condition of children and seen even more rarely in adults characterized by perioral, perinasal, and periorbital papules.[6,7] Unlike granulomatous rosacea, the papules do not appear inflammatory and the background erythema of rosacea is not present. Although its etiology often remains obscure, it has been associated with topical corticosteroid use and sometimes can represent an unusual response to contact allergens. It is self-limited.

Differential Diagnosis

The differential diagnosis includes sarcoidosis, which can usually be ruled out clinically. Unlike most children with sarcoidosis, these patients are generally in good health, without systemic symptoms, with a normal physical examination and chest films. The angiotensin-converting enzyme test is negative.

Histopathologic Features

The microscopic appearance is of noncaseating sarcoidal granulomas surrounded by lymphocytes. Although some of the granulomas may be adjacent to ruptured follicles, they are also found in the interfollicular dermis, away from destroyed follicles (Fig. 9-3).

Although the granulomas are sarcoidal in appearance, the

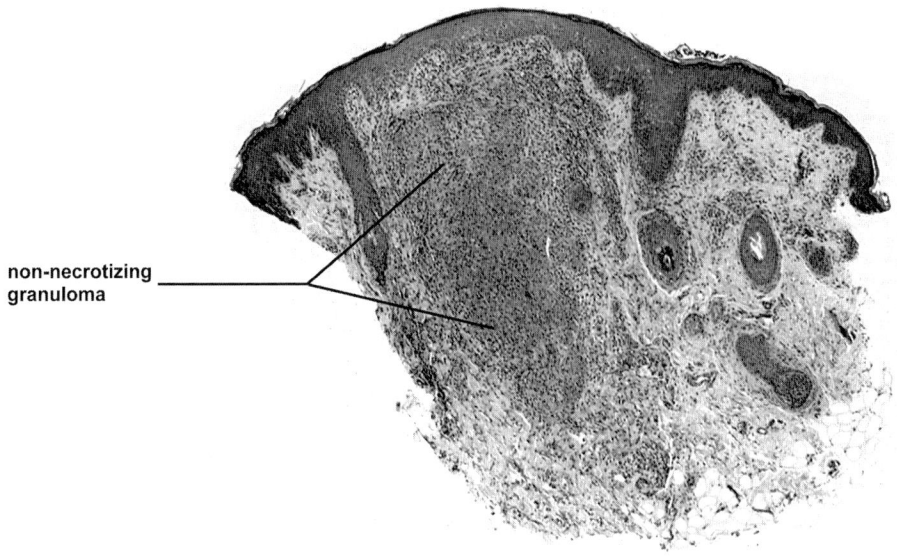

Figure 9-3. Granulomatous perioral dermatitis. There is a non-necrotizing granuloma in the superficial dermis. It is located between hair follicles and is not associated with a destroyed follicle.

lymphocytic component of the infiltrate is said to be more prominent in granulomatous perioral dermatitis.

Cutaneous Crohn's Disease

Clinical Features

The most common presentation of cutaneous Crohn's disease is as perianal fissures, erythema, edema, fistulas, and skin tags in patients with colonic or rectal involvement by regional enteritis.

These lesions can also involve the groin, vulva, buttocks, anterior abdominal wall, and submammary areas.[8–11] Metastatic Crohn's disease is extremely rare, refers to widely disseminated granulomatous lesions, and has only been seen in association with colonic or rectal involvement.[12,13]

Histopathologic Features

The cutaneous granulomas in Crohn's disease are indistinguishable microscopically from those of sarcoidosis consisting of non-

Figure 9-4. Granulomatous reaction to a ruptured follicular cyst. The granulomatous response to liberated keratinous debris is similar to the response to many foreign materials. In this example, remnants of the cyst wall are seen centrally. Multinucleate giant cells and epithelioid histiocytes surround flakes of keratin.

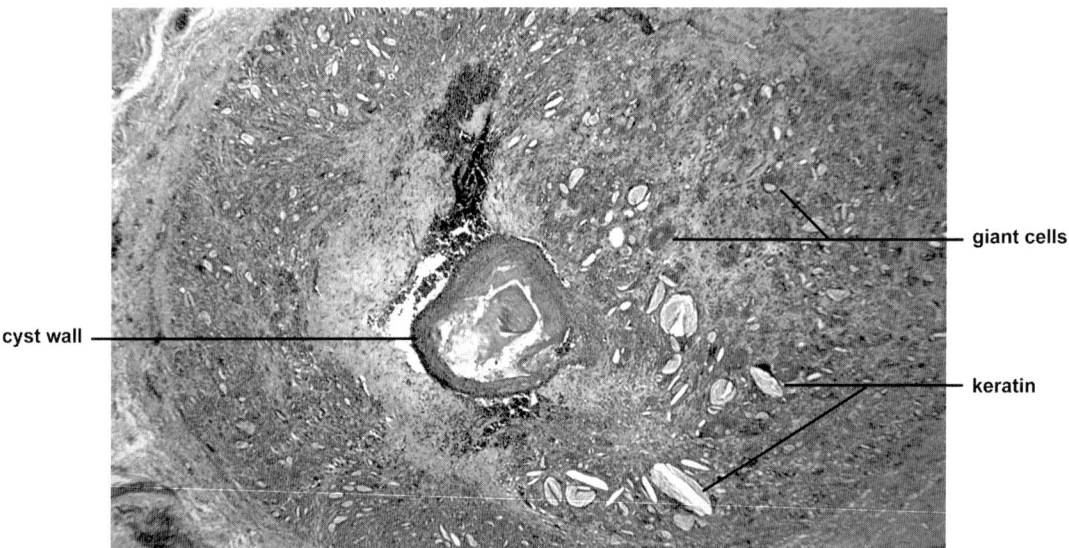

necrotizing discrete granulomas composed of epithelioid histiocytes. They are frequently associated with fistulas or fissures.

Differential Diagnosis

The differential diagnosis includes sarcoidosis, granulomatous reactions to foreign particles, and infectious granulomas. Clinicopathologic correlation is often necessary to resolve the differential diagnosis. Polaroscopy and special stains are useful in identifying foreign body reactions and infections.

Foreign Body Granulomas
Clinical Features

Granulomatous reactions to foreign matter take a variety of forms clinically. The presentation is usually that of a nodule or nodules at the site of inoculation. Granulomatous reactions to follicle contents usually occur in the setting of a folliculitis or rupture of a follicular cyst.

Cutaneous granulomatous reactions to beryllium can occur after direct inoculation[14] and following respiratory exposure. The latter is often associated with dyspnea, cough with hilar adenopathy, and less commonly by musculoskeletal symptoms, nephrolithiasis, and pulmonary osteoarthropathy.[15]

Zirconium, an ingredient in several topical medications, once used in the treatment of poison ivy, has been implicated in cutaneous granulomatous eruptions. Thought to enter the skin through sites of epidermal injury,[16] the reaction takes the form of persistent papular lesions.[17]

Histopathologic Features

Granulomatous reactions to foreign substances can take several forms. Some, such as reactions to silica, beryllium, and zirconium, are virtually indistinguishable from sarcoid granulomas, while others can result in suppurative or caseous necrosis (Fig. 9-4).

Differential Diagnosis

Clinical correlation is often required to distinguish granulomas resulting from reactions to foreign matter from infectious granulomas or from sarcoidosis.

Leprosy

Clinical Features

The clinical presentations of leprosy are extremely varied, depending on the patients' immunologic response to the infectious agent, the acid-fast bacillus *Mycobacterium leprae*. It has proved useful to classify leprosy according to its clinical and immunologic characteristics. At opposite ends of the spectrum are the "polar forms," tuberculoid leprosy and lepromatous leprosy. Host resistance is the highest in tuberculoid leprosy, and the disease presents as a single cutaneous lesion, an erythematous plaque with a raised margin or a thickened nerve, or both. There is frequently sensory or motor dysfunction. Host resistance is the lowest in lepromatous leprosy in which there are multiple erythematous plaques, nodules, or papules that are symmetric in distribution. Polar forms of leprosy tend to remain stable.

Between the two poles is a continuum of disease that has been subdivided into a varying number of compartments depending on the application to which the classification is being applied. The five-group classification proposed by Ridley and Jopling[18] has been the basis for most other classifications. In this system, the spectrum between tuberculoid leprosy and lepromatous leprosy is subdivided into three parts: borderline tuberculoid, borderline, and borderline lepromatous. Classification of leprosy requires, in addition to clinical assessment, histologic evaluation, assessment of bacterial load, and assessment of the cell-mediated response (lepromin skin test). An additional term, *indeterminate leprosy,* is applied to early lesions in which the full immunologic and morphologic features of the disease have yet to develop.

While the polar forms of leprosy tend to remain stable, the intermediate forms are labile and the clinical and immunologic states of these patients are apt to change, with untreated patients undergoing "downgrading" with movement toward the lepromatous end of the spectrum and patients undergoing treatment experiencing "reversal" with movement toward the tuberculoid end of the spectrum. These changes, brought about by alterations in cell-mediated immunity, comprise the type I (lepra) reaction. The clinical appearances of both downgrading and reversal reactions are similar with pronounced erythema of skin lesions, swelling and tenderness of nerves, fever, malaise, and edema. Nerve damage resulting from disease progression or from the intensified immunologic reaction (in reversal) can cause severe morbidity. Histopathology and assessment of immunity are required to determine the direction of the reaction.

The type II reaction (erythema nodosum leprosum) is usually seen in patients with lepromatous leprosy undergoing sulfone therapy, but can also be seen in the absence of therapy. It is thought to result from the release of soluble antigenic material into the circulation that combines with humoral antibodies to form circulating immune complexes. The clinical manifestation is of evanescent crops of tender erythematous papules or nodules located on interlesional skin. These are associated with fever and malaise. Edema, neuritis, arthralgias, arthrosis, rhinitis, epistaxis, epididymo-orchitis, proteinuria, iridocyclitis, and lymphadenopathy can also occur.[19] Lucio's phenomenon, a variant of type II reaction, occurs in Central America and Mexico and is the result of cutaneous infarcts complicating the vasculitis.

Histopathologic Features

The histopathologic appearance is as varied as the clinical presentation. Not only does the morphology of the inflammatory infiltrate vary with the immune state of the patient, but there is marked variation in the number of *M. leprae* bacilli. The number of organisms can be graded using a logarithmic scale termed the bacterial index, the density of organisms using the × 100 oil immersion objective, and the morphologic index, which represents the percentage of bacilli that appear viable.

Indeterminate leprosy represents the earliest skin lesion and predates the formation of recognizable granulomas. Although the inflammatory infiltrate is nonspecific, bacilli can be recognized if the proper histochemical stains are performed. These are usually located in small nerves. The infiltrate, which is mild, consists of lymphocytes, macrophages, and sometimes plasma

inoculation and consists of a verrucous papule *(tuberculosis cutis verrucosa)* or "prosector's wart."

Histopathologic Features

Tuberculosis is characterized by a granulomatous inflammatory reaction. Although the character of the granulomas can vary, in general they are less discrete, are associated with a greater lymphocytic infiltrate, and have more of a tendency to undergo necrosis than the granulomas of sarcoid.

Primary inoculation tuberculosis refers to infection, acquired percutaneously, in a patient never before exposed to the organism. The initial inflammatory reaction is often associated with cutaneous ulceration and is nonspecific, with the infiltrate consisting of neutrophils, lymphocytes, and plasma cells. Granulomatous inflammation replaces the neutrophilic infiltrate of the initial suppurative inflammatory reaction at about the same time that regional lymph nodes become enlarged.[25] The purified protein derivative skin test becomes positive about the time the inflammatory reaction becomes granulomatous.[26,27] The Ghon complex refers to the cutaneous lesion and associated involved lymph nodes. This corresponds to the Ghon complex of primary pulmonary tuberculosis. With time and increasing host resistance, the primary cutaneous lesion can come to resemble secondary inoculation tuberculosis.

In a patient who has previously developed resistance to tuberculosis, inoculation and infection result in a rapidly developing granulomatous reaction, often with marked caseous necrosis *(secondary inoculation tuberculosis).* Clinically this can take the form of "apple jelly nodules" similar to those seen in lupus vulgaris or result in tuberculosis cutis verrucosa (prosector's wart) in which there is marked verrucous hyperplasia of the epidermis.[25]

Orificial tuberculosis results from autoinoculation of periorificial skin or mucous membranes by infectious body secretions or feces. This characteristically occurs in patients with advanced disease and defective immunity.[28] Clinically the lesions can be ulcers or plaques, which may at times be verrucous. In some instances, the inflammatory reaction is nonspecific, while in other patients there is formation of tubercles.[25]

In *scrofuloderma,* the cutaneous infection is the result of direct extension from an underlying site.[28] This can manifest itself as sinus and/or abscess formation. There are often associated caseating granulomas.[25]

Lupus vulgaris is chronic cutaneous tuberculosis characterized by plaques and nodules, frequently located on the face or neck, and usually in women. It is thought to result from hematogenous spread.[28] Histologically, there is tubercle formation, but often with inconspicuous necrosis.[25]

Acute miliary tuberculosis is a fulminant form of the disease, resulting from hematogenous dissemination. It most commonly occurs in infants and children,[28] although it has recently been reported in an adult with acquired immunodeficiency syndrome.[29] There may be only a slight perivascular lymphocytic infiltrate and sometimes focal necrosis, abscess formation, or small granulomas. Acid-fast bacilli are numerous and are found within vessels and in the perivascular interstitium.[25,29]

Occasionally, patients will present with multiple cutaneous tuberculous abscesses resembling acute pyogenic infections.[28]

Papulonecrotic tuberculid, although not a tuberculous infection, is thought to represent an immunologic host response to circulating bacterial antigens. These symmetric papulopustular lesions, which usually occur acrally, are histologically characterized by an area of coagulation necrosis involving the dermis and sometimes the subcutis as well. The necrotic area is surrounded by histiocytes, sometimes in a palisaded arrangement. Vascular changes sometimes include fibrinoid necrosis and thrombosis. Epithelioid tubercles are not usually encountered.[30]

Erythema induratum is a lobular panniculitis having the microscopic appearance of nodular vasculitis from which it is distinguished by its association with tuberculosis. Like papulonecrotic tuberculid, it is not thought to be a tuberculous infection, but an immunologic reaction to an underlying tuberculous infection.

Differential Diagnosis

Because the histologic appearance of cutaneous tuberculosis can be so varied, it is prudent to routinely stain examples of granulomatous dermatitis for acid-fast bacteria unless the pathogenesis is certain. In some situations (e.g., miliary tuberculosis, acute primary inoculation tuberculosis) the absence of granulomas and the nonspecific nature of the inflammatory reaction make it difficult to initially consider a tuberculous etiology without clinical history. If tuberculosis is suspected clinically, the histopathologist should not hesitate to perform the necessary stains, even in the absence of granulomas.

Deep Fungal Infections

Clinical Features

Deep fungal infections are clinically characterized by plaques with pustules. Their surfaces are often verrucous or vegetating. They can be classified according to the route of infection. Some, such as sporotrichosis, are usually contracted by direct inoculation. Others, such as histoplasmosis, represent cutaneous manifestations of a systemic disease process and usually affect immunocompromised hosts.

Histopathologic Features

The microscopic morphology is extremely variable, as dermal fungal infections can result in sarcoidal granulomas, necrotizing granulomas, palisaded granulomas, and diffuse granulomatous inflammation, depending on the immune response of the host to the fungus. Frequently there is marked epidermal hyperplasia corresponding to the vegetating plaques seen clinically. Often the granulomatous inflammation is diffuse with numerous histiocytes and scattered giant cells, lymphocytes, and plasma cells. There are often abscesses with accumulation of neutrophils and their remnants. These sometimes open to the surface via sinus tracts.

Differential Diagnosis

The morphology of the inflammatory reaction varies more with the immune status of the patient than with the specific fungal organism, the identification of which depends on its morphology or culture characteristics, or both. Special stains (Gomori silver

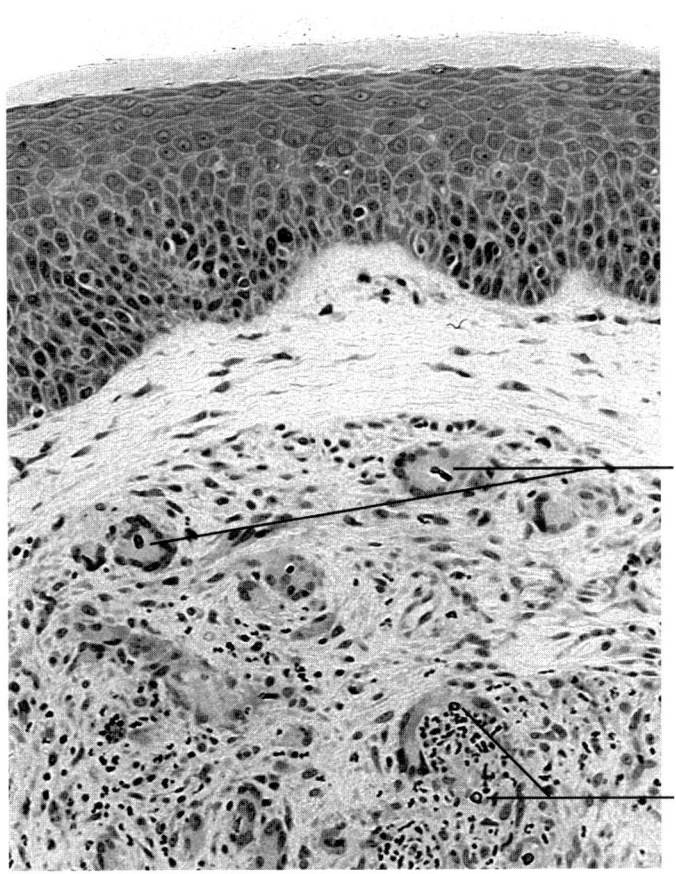

Figure 9-7. Phaeohyphomycosis. Pigmented yeast forms and pseudohyphae are identified within giant cells of this dermal granuloma. (H&E.)

pigmented hyphae
within giant cells

pigmented
yeast forms

stain and PAS) are often required. Mycobacterial infections can exhibit identical clinical and morphologic features, and stains for them should be included in the examination unless fungal structures can be clearly identified. Even with stains, culture of infected material is often required for diagnosis.

Localized Infections

Sporotrichosis

Clinical Features. Cutaneous lesions of sporotrichosis, infection by the dimorphic fungus *Sporothrix schenkii,* result, in most cases, from traumatic inoculation. Less commonly the route of infection is believed to be the respiratory tract through inhalation of spores. The primary cutaneous lesion varies in size from 1 to 5 cm and begins as a small erythematous papulonodule that enlarges and sometimes ulcerates. Over one-half of the patients develop lymphangitic spread.[31,32]

Hematogenous dissemination is generally associated with alcoholism or immune suppression. This mode of spread is probably responsible for most cases of sporotrichal polyarthritis, which presents as a nonspecific inflammatory arthritis.[32,33]

Histopathologic Features. At the site of cutaneous inoculation there is usually hyperkeratosis and parakeratosis in association with pseudoepitheliomatous hyperplasia. There are often intraepidermal pustules. The dermal infiltrate is granulomatous with the clustered histiocytes, and scattered giant cells commonly surrounding a neutrophilic abscess within which may be found asteroid bodies, a manifestation of the Splendore-Hoeppli phenomenon. Budding fungal cells, which stain with PAS, are found within the asteroid bodies. The Gomori methenamine silver stain (GMS) is useful in identification of characteristic "cigar" forms, yeast, and budding forms.[34,35] Granulomas are surrounded by a mixed cellular infiltrate of lymphocytes, plasma cells, and usually eosinophils. Secondary nodules show similar features but frequently are larger, although without epidermal hyperplasia.[35]

Chromomycosis

Clinical Features. The primary cutaneous lesion of chromomycosis is usually located on the lower extremity and begins as an erythematous papule. The process usually remains localized, but evolves into a verrucous plaque. It is initiated by penetrating trauma with implantation of soil or decaying plant material. The responsible organisms are *Fonsecaea pedrosoi, Fonsecaea compactum, Phialophora verrucosa, Cladosporium carroni,* and *Rhinocladiella aquaspersa.*[36-39]

Histopathologic Features. There is, in the vast majority of cases, marked epidermal hyperplasia with intraepidermal neutrophilic abscesses. The dermal infiltrate contains a mixture of histiocytes, giant cells, lymphocytes, plasma cells, and small clusters of neutrophils. Organisms are gold-brown, round to oval, 8 to 15 μm in diameter, with thick refractile cell walls.

They are located within giant cells, within the pus in the center of abscesses, or free in the tissues. They reproduce by cell division, and some of the "Medlar bodies" appear septate. Specific identification requires culture.[34,40,41]

Phaeohyphomycosis

Clinical Features. Primary cutaneous phaeohyphomycosis is caused by those dematiaceous fungi that produce yeast forms, pseudohyphae, and true hyphae, most commonly *Exophiala jeanselmei* and *Wangiella dermatitidis*. The disease affects healthy as well as immunocompromised patients and presents as nodules, which may be cystic, as well as hyperkeratotic plaques. The route of infection is via penetrating injury and inoculation of contaminated vegetable matter or soil.

Histopathologic Features. Those lesions that evolve as verrucous plaques show epidermal pseudoepitheliomatous hyperplasia with microabscesses. There is a granulomatous reaction in the dermis with suppurating granulomas containing pigmented fungal organisms in the form of yeast-like cells, hyphae, and/or pseudohyphae (Fig. 9-7). The brown pigment may be inconspicuous, however, and melanin stains can prove useful in its demonstration. Nodular lesions are frequently cystic and located in the dermis or subcutis. There is usually no overlying epidermal reaction. The cysts, which may contain pus, are surrounded by a granulomatous infiltrate. Sometimes fragments of vegetable matter can be identified.[42,43]

Lobomycosis

Clinical Features. First described in 1930 at the Hospital of Recife (Brazil) by Jorge Lobo, who considered it an attenuated form of paracoccidioidomycosis, it was labeled "Lobo's disease" in 1938 by Fialho, who believed it to be a distinct entity.[44–46] It is a chronic skin disease found chiefly in the Amazon regions of Brazil and Colombia. The mode of infection is thought to be via direct inoculation, which results in slowly enlarging nodules or plaques, sometimes verrucous, which can ulcerate. They are usually located on cooler parts of the body such as the ear lobes or lower extremities.[44,47] The infection may remain localized or spread over wide areas of the skin surface by contiguity, lymphatics, or through autoinoculation.[44]

Histopathologic Features. Nodular, nonulcerated lesions are covered by an attenuated epidermis. There is a diffuse dermal infiltrate of foamy histiocytes and multinucleate giant cells, which are sometimes numerous. The organisms, which are located mostly intracellularly, are characteristically numerous, appearing as rounded, 6- to 12-μm, thick-walled cells that bud to form short chains. Although they can be visualized with H&E, the PAS with diastase and GMS stains are useful in their identification and examination. Ulcerated lesions frequently exhibit adjacent pseudoepitheliomatous hyperplasia.[44,47]

Zygomycosis

Clinical Features. Zygomycosis (cutaneous mucormycosis) is an uncommon cutaneous infection by fungi, class Zygo-

mycetes, order Mucorales. Most patients are immunocompromised and have diabetes mellitus or chronic renal failure, but zygomycosis has also been described in burn and trauma patients with open wounds.[48,49] The clinical picture is described as a necrotic ulceration, a necrotizing cellulitis, or a primary gangrenous cutaneous infection.[48,50,51]

Histopathologic Features. There is frequently ulceration of the epidermis with necrosis of the dermis and subcutis in those cases where vessels are invaded by the fungus.[52,53] The perivascular infiltrate consists of lymphocytes, with neutrophils being found in areas of necrosis. Organisms are identifiable as broad-branching nonseptate hyphae.[48]

Eumycetoma

Eumycetoma refers to a mycetoma caused by true fungi, the best known of which are *Madurella* sp. and *Allescheria boydii*.

Clinical Features. Eumycetoma (mycetoma) is characterized by an inflammatory mass that develops at the site of traumatic injury (scratch or puncture wound). Sinus tracts develop within the mass. Grains or clusters of fungal elements are found within the mucopurulent discharge. The grains may appear black (usually *Madurella*) or pale. The infection slowly invades and destroys adjacent soft tissues and bone.

Although the disease has a worldwide distribution, it is most frequent in the tropics. Those parts of the body most susceptible to traumatic implantation of the organism (feet and hands) are most commonly affected.[54,55]

Histopathologic Features. Eumycetoma is diagnosed microscopically by the identification of fungal colonies (grains) within abscesses and sinus tracts in the setting of a granulomatous mass.

Aspergillosis

Clinical Features. *Aspergillus* is an opportunistic fungus that not only grows in soil and organic material but also colonizes skin and gut, usually without causing infection. Infection (aspergillosis) is usually seen in the immunocompromised patient and most frequently involves the lung, gastrointestinal tract, and central nervous system. The skin is rarely involved in either disseminated disease or primarily.

Primary cutaneous aspergillosis has been reported in immunocompromised patients in the setting of acquired immunodeficiency syndrome, underlying hematologic malignancy, organ transplantation, and diabetes. Sometimes lesions are localized beneath adhesive tape near the sites of intravenous catheters. They can take the form of erythematous papules that are sometimes umbilicated, plaques, subcutaneous nodules, or, when resulting in tissue necrosis, present as black eschar. Invasion of *Aspergillus* into the deep tissues sometimes complicates burn wounds, necrotizing fasciitis, or other conditions resulting in devitalized tissues. When this occurs, the prognosis is grave.[53,56–58]

Histopathologic Features. The microscopic appearance of primary cutaneous aspergillosis can be similar to that of an invasive dermatophyte infection with the organisms colonizing the keratinous contents of a hair follicle and invading the adjacent der-

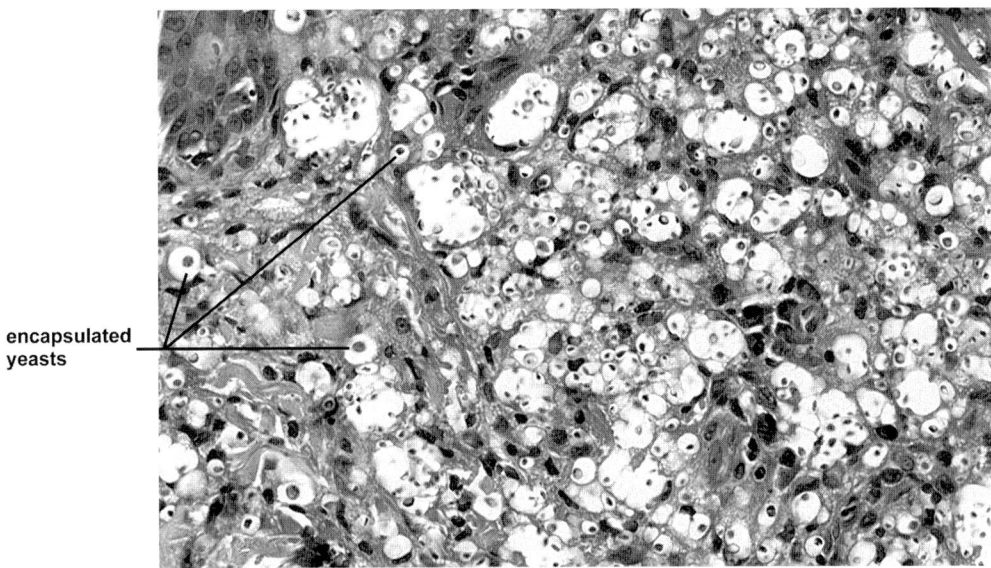

encapsulated
yeasts

Figure 9-8. Cryptococcosis. In this lesion from an immunocompromised patient, there are myriad organisms, most having thick capsules. There is little inflammatory response. (H&E.)

mis.[59] Invasion of *Aspergillus* into deep tissues is often accompanied by invasion of blood vessels with thrombosis and results in ischemic necrosis and gangrene. Wide excision or amputation is the primary mode of therapy for this form of the infection.

Systemic Infections

Histoplasmosis

Clinical Features. *Histoplasma capsulatum* is a dimorphic fungus with a practically worldwide distribution contaminating and growing in bird and bat droppings. Infection is usually via inhalation. Cutaneous lesions are seen almost exclusively in immunocompromised patients and present as a maculopapular eruption. Ulcerations may occur in more advanced lesions.

Histopathologic Features. The host response varies. In aquired immunodeficiency syndrome patients, skin biopsy can show only a sparse perivascular infiltrate with neutrophils, lymphocytes, and histiocytes. There may be prominent leukocytoclasia and dermal necrosis, with the morphology being somewhat suggestive of leukocytoclastic vasculitis.[60] In other examples there may be sheets of histiocytes laden with fungal organisms that can impart a foamy appearance to their cytoplasm.[61]

The organisms can be found either intra- or extracellularly and can usually be demonstrated with the GMS stain (please note modification). They must be distinguished morphologically from *Blastomyces dermatitidis* and *Cryptococcus neoformans.*[62]

Cryptococcosis

Clinical Features. *C. neoformans* is found in soil and contaminated pigeon droppings. Infection is almost invariably via the pulmonary route. Meningitis is the most common site of sys-

temic spread. When cutaneous lesions occur, they are usually the result of vascular dissemination; however, there have been rare instances of direct transmission via cutaneous inoculation. Cutaneous manifestations may precede signs of central nervous system disease.

Disseminated infections (and cutaneous lesions) usually occur in immunocompromised patients, but there is not always immunosuppression or apparent underlying disease process.[40,63–65]

Cutaneous lesions are polymorphous, taking the form of papules, nodules, pustules, and vegetating plaques. Erythematous tender plaques of sudden onset can give the appearance of cellulitis. These may vesiculate and ulcerate.[66] Papular lesions may resemble molluscum contagiosum.[67]

Histopathologic Features. *C. neoformans* is an encapsulated yeast, 5 to 10 μm in diameter, that exhibits narrow-based budding. If numerous, they can usually be tentatively identified on H&E stain as round to oval bodies surrounded by a clear halo (Fig. 9-8). The mucicarmine and GMS stains are useful in demonstrating their cell walls and cytoplasm, while the gelatinous capsule can be demonstrated by the Alcian blue–PAS stain.

The tissue reaction to the organism is variable, sometimes even within the same lesion. In some instances, numerous encapsulated organisms fill the dermis, and there is very little inflammatory response. The organism can also elicit a granulomatous reaction, sometimes with areas of necrosis. This can take the form of a palisaded granuloma.[68,69]

Coccidioidomycosis

Clinical Features. Coccidioidomycosis, caused by *Coccidioides immitis,* results in no apparent clinical symptoms in about two-thirds of patients, but can develop into a severe or even fatal mycosis. Also known as "valley fever" or "desert rheumatism,"

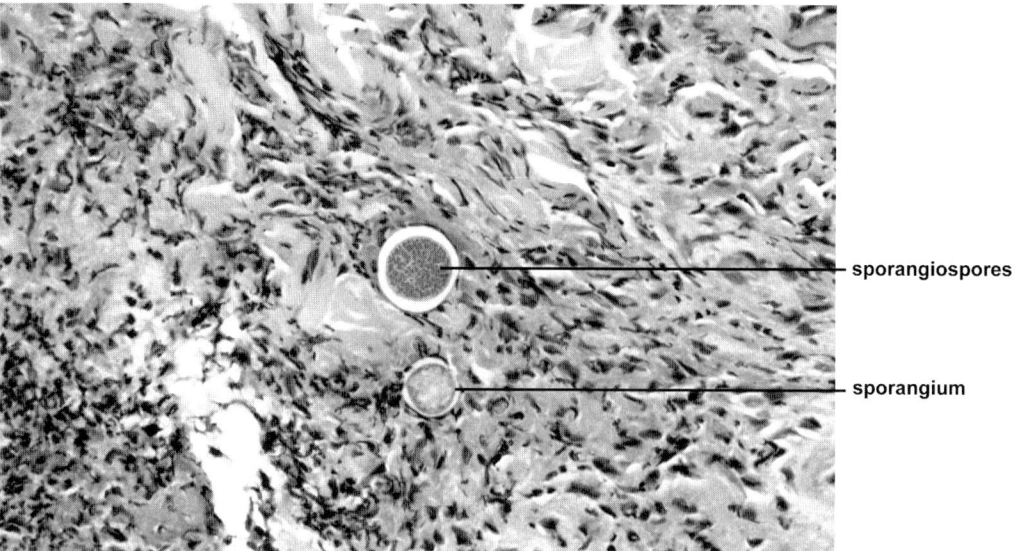

Figure 9-9. Coccidioidomycosis. Cutaneous coccidioidomycosis with a sporangium containing sporangiospores. (H&E.)

this highly infectious mycosis is endemic in areas of the southwestern United States (California, Arizona, New Mexico, Texas) and focally in hot dry regions of Central and South America.[34,40] The primary infection is almost exclusively located in the lungs, with initial complaints of dry cough and pleuritic chest pain accompanied by fever, night sweats, headache, and arthralgias. Erythema nodosum and erythema multiforme, nonspecific cutaneous immune reactions, sometimes develop.[70] Disseminated disease occurs in less than 1% of white men and slightly more frequently in black men. It is less common in women. Spread can be to almost any visceral organ, with the skin, meninges, bones, and joints being common sites. Extrapulmonary disease should prompt a thorough evaluation of the patient's immune status, though it can occur in immunocompetent individuals.

Primary cutaneous coccidioidomycosis is extremely rare and is contracted through inoculation. Criteria for diagnosis include (1) no history of recent pulmonary infection, (2) history of traumatic injury (or inoculation), (3) incubation period of 1 to 3 weeks, (4) chancriform nearly painless nodule or plaque that may be ulcerated, and (5) regional lymphadenopathy limited to region of drainage.[71]

Histopathologic Features. Cutaneous lesions are characterized by epidermal hyperplasia, sometimes adjacent to an ulcer. There is a suppurative and granulomatous dermal infiltrate of epithelioid histiocytes, multinucleate giant cells, and plasma cells. This reaction often surrounds neutrophilic abscesses. The sporangia of *C. immitis* are large, measuring up to 60 μm in diameter. These often contain numerous sporangiospores, which are released when the mature sporangia rupture (Fig. 9-9). Although organisms are easily seen with conventional H&E stains, GMS and PAS sometimes prove useful in identifying them.

Paracoccidioidomycosis

Clinical Features. Paracoccidioidomycosis is a chronic systemic mycosis that infects millions of inhabitants within its en-

demic areas, which include subtropical regions of Central and South America and Mexico.[72] The strong male predominance is thought to result from the organism's sensitivity to estrogen, which apparently inhibits the transformation from mycelial to yeast forms.[73] It is rarely seen in the United States, and the few cases reported are thought to represent reactivation of disease contracted in an endemic area.[40] Such reactivation can occur following a latent asymptomatic period of up to several decades.[74]

The disease is caused by *Paracoccidioides brasiliensis,* a dimorphic fungus that, in nature, forms mycelia and, in living mammalian tissue, yeast-like forms. It is thought that infection results from inhalation of conidia produced by the hyphae.[75]

Chest pain, cough, dyspnea with fever, fatigue, and weight loss often accompany active pulmonary disease. Dissemination from the lungs is the usual pathogenesis of cutaneous and mucous membrane lesions, with primary cutaneous disease being very rare.[72]

Cutaneous lesions usually occur on the face as verrucous plaques, which may be ulcerated, papulonodules, or pustules.[40]

Histopathologic Features. The cutaneous reaction to *P. brasiliensis* is similar to that described in many other deep fungi. There is frequently epidermal hyperplasia with intraepidermal neutrophilic abscesses adjacent to areas of ulceration. The dermis contains a granulomatous and suppurative infiltrate, which heals with fibrosis.[40]

The organisms are characteristic in appearance. The structure is yeast-like and 15 to 30 μm in diameter, from which grow multiple 5- to 10-μm buds in a "pilot wheel" pattern.[72]

Blastomycosis

Clinical Features. Blastomycosis, also known as *North American blastomycosis* or *Gilchrist's disease,* is endemic to the southeastern, south central, and midwestern United States.[76]

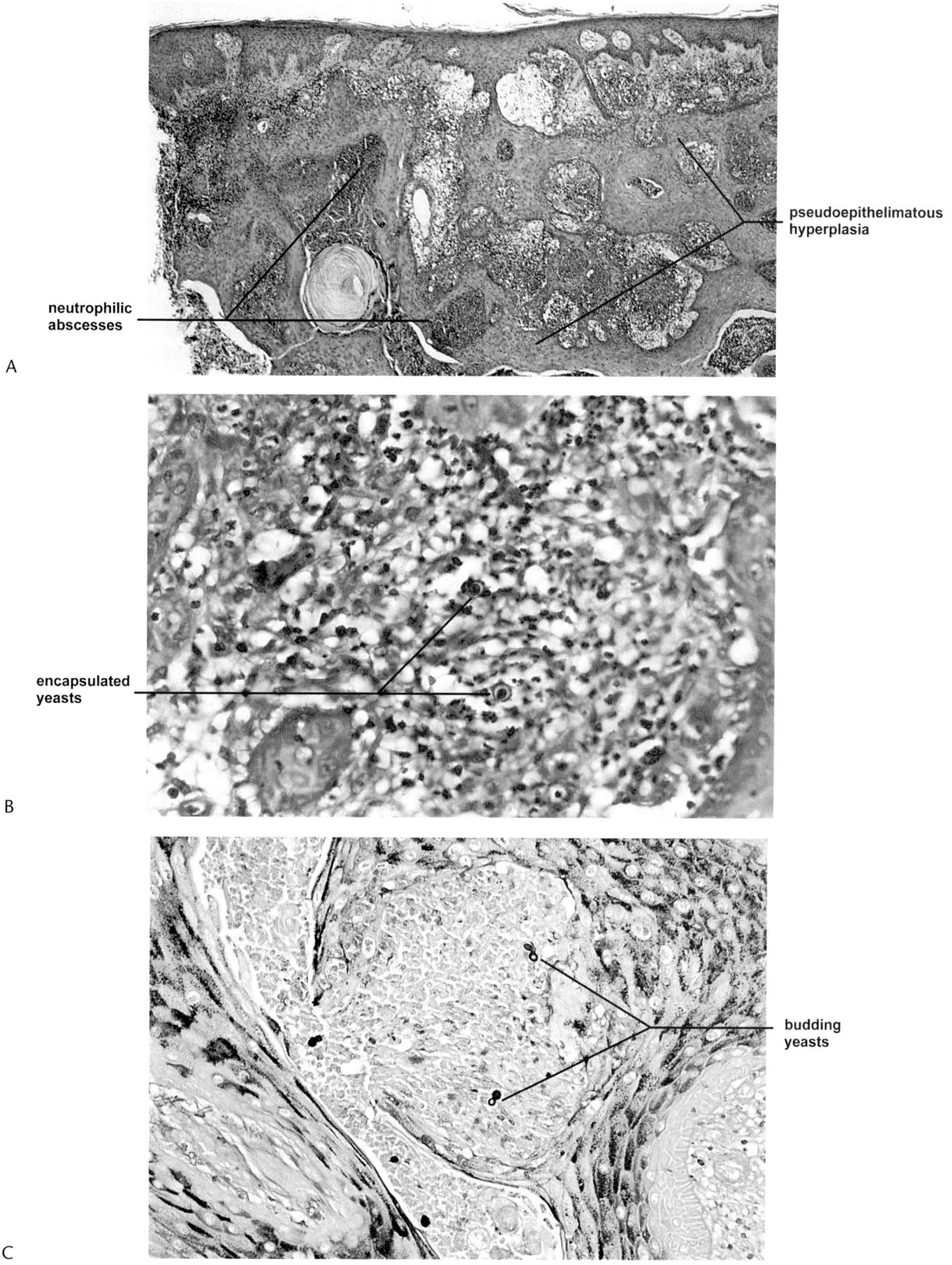

Figure 9-10. Blastomycosis. **(A)** There is massive pseudoepitheliomatous hyperplasia with intraepithelial neutrophilic microabscesses. (H&E.) **(B)** Thick-walled yeasts can often be identified without special stains, but they are often few in number. (H&E.) **(C)** The budding yeasts are more easily identified on silver stains. (GMS.)

Labels in figure:

neutrophilic abscesses

pseudoepithelimatous hyperplasia

encapsulated yeasts

budding yeasts

A

B

C

The organism *Blastomyces dermatitidis (Ajellomyces dermatitidis)* is a dimorphic soil saprophyte that grows as a budding yeast in tissue. Infection is almost always via the pulmonary route resulting from inhalation of oval conidia, with acute disease developing 21 to 106 days following exposure.[76–78]

Systemic dissemination almost always involves the skin, and cutaneous lesions may develop following spontaneous resolution of the pulmonary focus.[77] These lesions are frequently located on the face, mucous membrane, or exposed areas and take the form of verrucous papules, plaques, nodules, and ulcers.[79]

Although there are reports of cutaneous disease acquired by primary inoculation, well-documented cases are rare.

Histopathologic Features. Pseudoepitheliomatous epidermal hyperplasia with neutrophilic microabscesses in the epidermis and dermis are the usual findings. The budding yeasts are usually scarce, intra- or extracellular, 8 to 15 μm in diameter, and characteristically have a thick wall. When well preserved, several nuclei can be seen. Single broad-based buds can sometimes be found. Because there are usually few organisms, the GMS or PAS stain can be useful in their identification[40] (Fig. 9-10).

Granulomatous Rosacea

Clinical Features

Rosacea is a syndrome of chronic or recurring episodes (or both) of facial erythema. It is most prevalent in the fourth to sixth decades and affects women about three times more frequently than men. However, it occasionally develops during adolescence.[80] This erythema is sometimes accompanied by pustules and follicular papules.

Similar papulonodular lesions have been described in a child infected with human immunodeficiency virus.[81] In this case, the granulomas were said to contain *Demodex* mites.

Histopathologic Features

The usual histologic findings in rosacea include solar elastosis and vascular ectasia or dilation. There is usually a dermal lymphomononuclear infiltrate and sometimes a folliculitis, the histologic correlate to the follicular papules and pustules. In some cases, there is a granulomatous dermal infiltrate characterized by epithelioid granulomas sometimes with caseous necrosis.[82] The granulomas are usually seen in close proximity to hair follicles, and sometimes remnants of follicular epithelium or follicle contents can be seen within the granuloma. In some instances, dermal elastosis might play a role in the pathogenesis of the granulomatous reaction,[83] and other authors have postulated a role for *Demodex folliculorum*.[84]

Differential Diagnosis

The differential diagnosis includes sarcoidosis, tuberculosis, and epithelioid granulomas. In resolving the differential diagnosis, it is helpful if a relationship between the infiltrate and destroyed follicle can be identified. Stains for acid-fast bacilli and fungi should be routinely performed unless such a relationship

Figure 9-11. Granuloma annulare. There is a dermal histiocytic infiltrate that surrounds hypocellular areas. The collagen bundles within the hypocellular areas are separated by deposits of connective tissue mucin (hyaluronic acid).

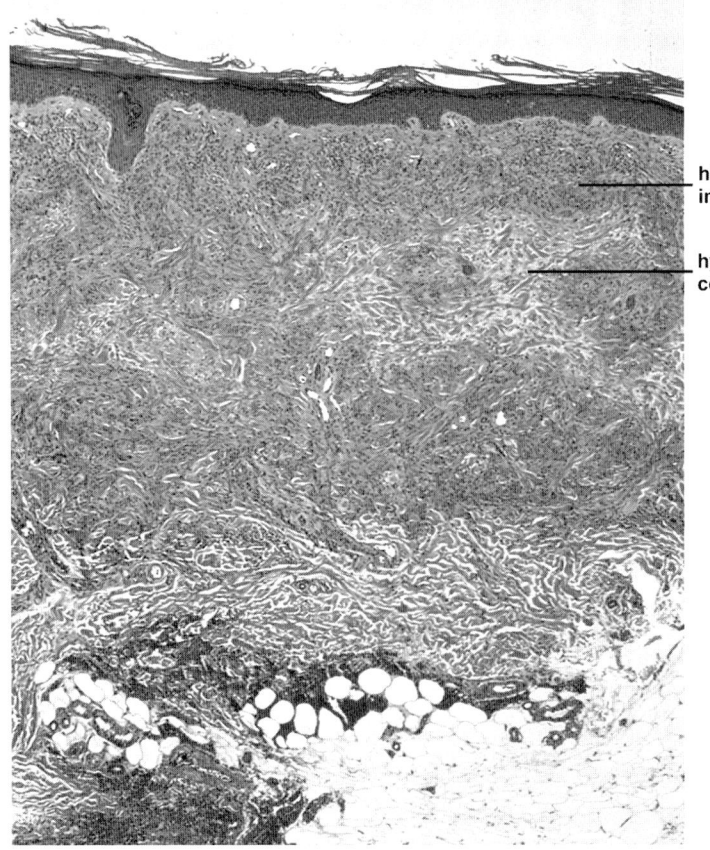

histiocytic infiltrate

hypocellular area containing mucin

can be clearly established microscopically and the clinical presentation is characteristic for the disease.

Halogenodermas

Clinical Features

Cutaneous eruptions due to bromides, iodides, and fluoride clinically and histologically have many features in common with deep fungal and mycobacterial infections. They are, however, unlikely to be confused with other drug eruptions.[85] The lesions begin as pustules or vesicles and progress to form vegetative plaques and nodules that frequently ulcerate. The lesions of iododerma and fluoroderma usually occur on the face, scalp, and neck, although they are occasionally widespread, while those of bromoderma usually appear on the lower extremities.[86] Conjunctival involvement can occur in patients with iododerma.[87]

Histopathologic Features

There is striking pseudoepitheliomatous hyperplasia and ulceration, with the former said to be most pronounced in bromoderma and the latter in iododerma.[86,87] There is exocytosis of neutrophils into the epidermis, sometimes with abscess formation, and a dense mixed dermal infiltrate of neutrophils, eosinophils, lymphocytes, plasma cells, and occasional multinucleate giant cells. There is often abundant leukocytoclysis.

Differential Diagnosis

The histologic differential diagnosis includes deep fungal and mycobacterial infections, which tend to result in striking epidermal hyperplasia. The resolution of the differential diagnosis requires a history of halogen ingestion and, of course, the absence of infectious agents.

PALISADED GRANULOMAS

Granuloma Annulare

Clinical Features

Granuloma annulare can occur at any age, but more often in young people. There is a female preponderance. The condition presents as rings of firm papules up to 5 cm in size, with intact surface epithelium. They may be single or multiple, with multiple lesions being more frequent in younger patients. There is a predilection for extensor surfaces of the extremities, particularly the backs of the hands, but they may be found anywhere. The lesions develop and resolve slowly, with the course often lasting 1 year or longer.

Closely related conditions include actinic granuloma,[88] Miescher's granuloma of the face,[89] and necrobiosis lipoidica of the face and scalp.[90] These entities have been grouped together as "annular elastolytic giant cell granuloma" by Hanke et al.[91]

Histopathologic Features

The morphology of granuloma annulare is quite variable. Granulomas range from well-formed discrete palisades of histiocytes

surrounding a zone of degenerating collagen fibers between which there are frequently deposits of connective tissue mucin (hyaluronic acid) to a sparse infiltrate of histiocytes interposed between collagen bundles (Fig. 9-11). In the last instance, a stain for acid mucin (Alcian blue or colloidal iron) can be particularly useful in delineating the lesion. Although usually located in the reticular dermis, they can be quite superficial and even lead to perforation of the epidermis. Occasionally the lesion is located within the subcutaneous fat. This is termed *deep granuloma annulare* or *pseudorheumatoid nodule.*

Annular elastolytic giant cell granuloma often occurs on sun-damaged skin. The granulomatous infiltrate often contains numerous multinucleate giant cells, in addition to histiocytes (sometimes epithelioid) and lymphocytes. Asteroid bodies are sometimes seen within the giant cells. Elastolysis can be identified within the zone of granulomatous inflammation and within the confines of the granulomatous ring; at the center of the lesion there is dense collagenous tissue devoid of elastic fibers.

Differential Diagnosis

The microscopic appearance of granuloma annulare is often characteristic. However, the histiocytic infiltrate can be extremely sparse and diagnosis can depend on the demonstration of mucin between the collagen bundles (Figs. 9-12 and 9-13). Annular elastolytic granuloma can lead to fibrosis and mimic a scar with surrounding foreign body reaction. We have encountered a lesion in which squamous syringometaplasia in such a setting suggested squamous cell carcinoma morphologically. Clinicopathologic correlation, identification of residual remnants of eccrine ducts, and the pattern of elastolysis as demonstrated by elastic tissue stain helped to resolve the differential diagnosis.

Palisaded Neutrophilic and Granulomatous Dermatitis

Clinical Features

Symmetrically distributed erythematous papules on the extremities of patients with collagen-vascular disease have been described under a variety of terms: *Churg-Strauss granuloma* (cutaneous extravascular necrotizing granuloma),[92] *rheumatoid papules, superficial ulcerating rheumatoid necrobiosis,*[93,94] and *interstitial granulomatous dermatitis with arthritis.*[95] The term *palisaded neutrophilic and granulomatous dermatitis in patients with collagen vascular disease,* coined by Chu et al,[96] describes the clinical and morphologic manifestations of the condition.

Histopathologic Features

These lesions may prove to be the dermal equivalent of rheumatoid nodules. Histologically the papules appear to progress through several stages. Early changes are of a diffuse pandermal neutrophil-rich infiltrate in association with leukocytoclastic vasculitis. Involved vessels are surrounded by cuffs of fibrin. The adjacent reticular dermis contains strands of basophilic material, and the papillary dermis is edematous. Epidermal changes include hyperplasia and/or ulceration.

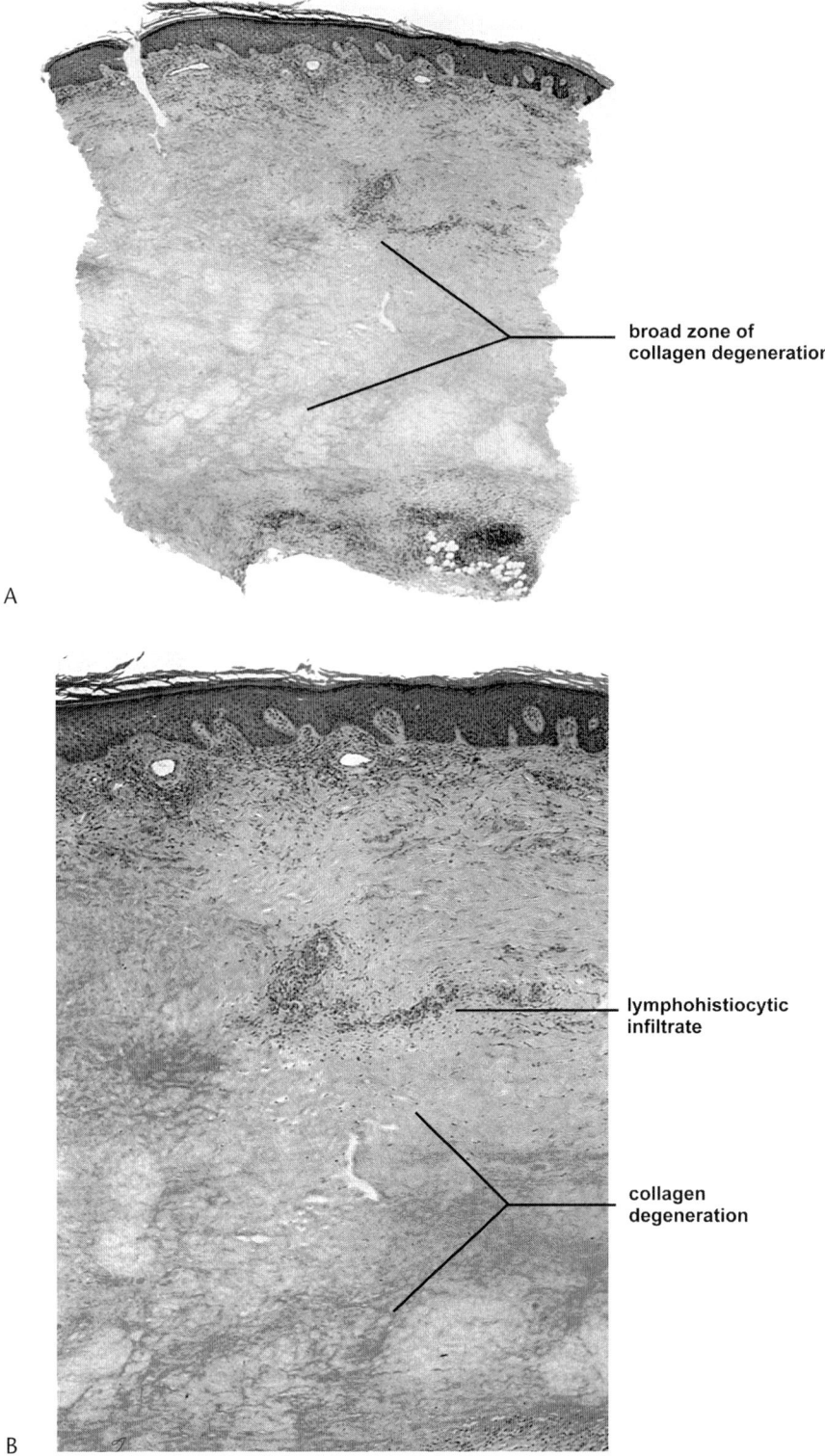

broad zone of
collagen degeneration

A

lymphohistiocytic
infiltrate

collagen
degeneration

B

Figure 9-14. Necrobiosis lipoidica. **(A)** A broad zone of collagen degeneration is seen that involves, confluent fashion, the dermis as well as the superficial subcutis. The collagen appears smudged, similar to the changes in ischemic necrosis. **(B)** The lymphohistiocytic infiltrate, sparse in this example, partially surrounds the zone of collagen degeneration.

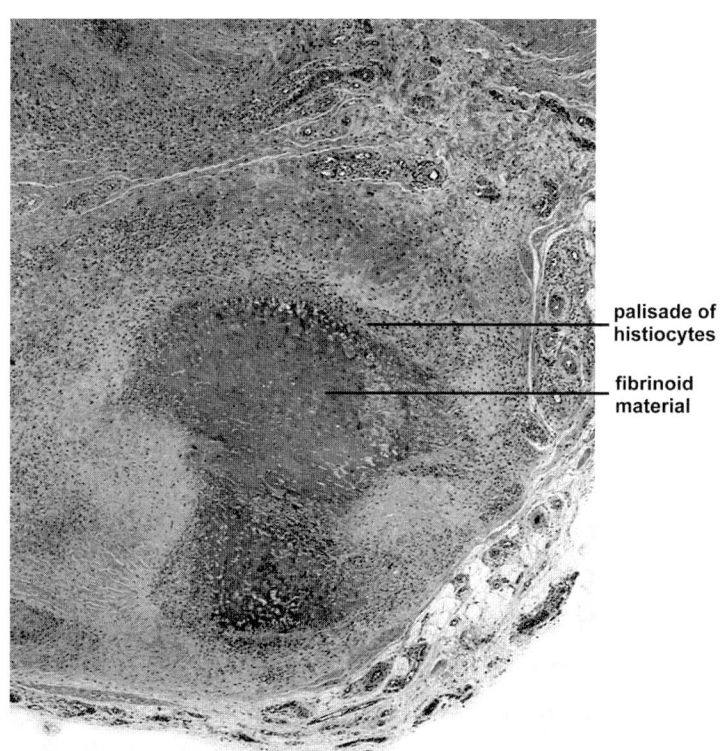

Figure 9-15. Rheumatoid nodule. This palisaded granuloma is located at the interface of the reticular dermis and the subcutis. Centrally there is an accumulation of fibrinoid material that is surrounded by palisaded histiocytes.

palisade of histiocytes

fibrinoid material

sis of the dermis and a thinned epidermis are changes seen in the centers of resolving plaques.

Vascular changes may not be conspicuous in established lesions, but sometimes small and large vessels adjacent to the zone of collagen degeneration have thick walls and show intimal proliferation.

Differential Diagnosis

Granuloma annulare has many features in common with NL. The differential diagnosis can usually be resolved at scanning magnification on H&E-stained tissue. The collagen change in NL is usually confluent and often involves the subcutis as well as the deep reticular dermis. In granuloma annulare, the changes usually have a patchy distribution and do not extend to involve both the dermis and the subcutis.

In those instances where the diagnosis is uncertain, stains for hyaluronic acid (Alcian blue or colloidal iron) are often useful to document accumulation of this connective tissue mucin between the collagen bundles in granuloma annulare.

Rheumatoid Nodule

Clinical Features

Of patients with rheumatoid arthritis (RA) about 20% develop nodules on extensor surfaces and areas sensitive to pressure. The ulnar aspect of the forearms, dorsal hands, feet, and knees are sites of predilection. They are also frequently located over the scapulae and on the ears. Although usually associated with more severe forms of RA, they may precede onset of RA by sev-

eral years.[99] An uncommon variant, rheumatoid nodulosis, is characterized by extensive involvement of the skin and subcutis in the absence of systemic disease and severe arthritis despite the presence of rheumatoid factor in high titer.[100] Subcutaneous nodules can also be seen in patients with juvenile rheumatoid arthritis (Still's disease), though less frequently than in the adult form of RA.[101]

Histopathologic Features

Rheumatoid nodules are palisaded granulomas that are located in the subcutaneous tissue or deep reticular dermis and that are similar histologically to granuloma annulare except for their location. The fully formed granuloma consists of a central zone of fibrinoid material surrounded by a palisade of macrophages positive for either CD68 or nonspecific esterase, the latter resembling synovial intimal macrophages (Fig. 9-15). There are also admixed fibroblasts that stain for prolyl hydrolase.[102] Granulation tissue comprises the center of developing lesions, which resemble the nodules of rheumatic heart disease.[103,104]

Differential Diagnosis

The differential diagnosis includes granuloma annulare and palisaded granulomas associated with other connective tissue diseases–rheumatic fever and lupus erythematosus. In otherwise clinically healthy children such a nodule likely represents a benign localized reaction to trauma and rarely is associated with either RA or rheumatic fever.[105,106] Nearly all subcutaneous nodules associated with rheumatic fever are preceded by other signs and symptoms of that disease.

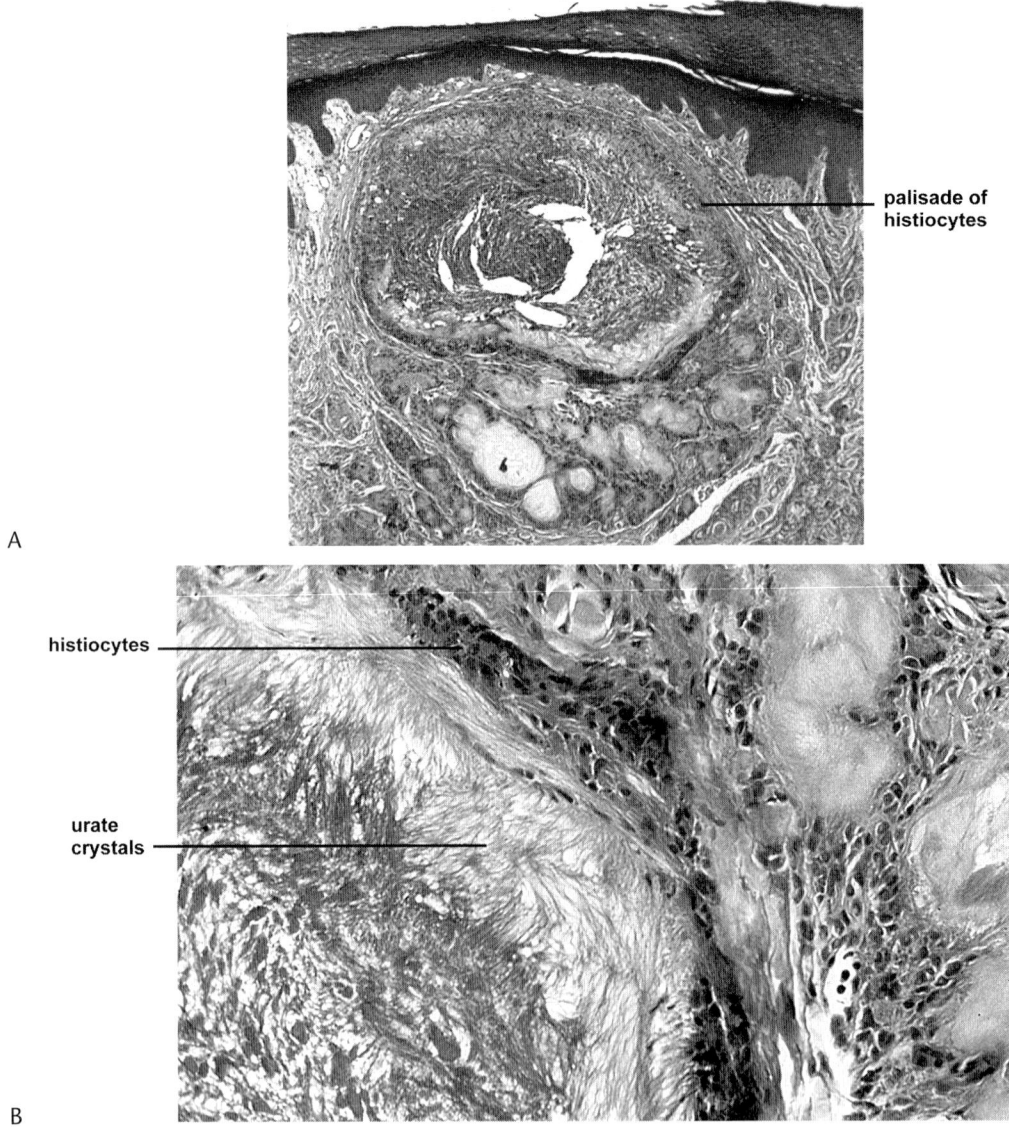

A

B

palisade of
histiocytes

histiocytes

urate
crystals

Figure 9-16. Gouty tophus. **(A)** Masses of urate crystals are surrounded by palisades of histiocytes. **(B)** Crystals are usually dissolved during conventional fixation and processing. They are preserved when fixed and processed in nonaqueous solutions.

In adults, the development of such lesions can precede the development of RA. Reports of such nodules in adults in the absence of connective tissue disease or RA are rare.

Gouty Tophi

Clinical Features

Gout is a disease characterized by chronic hyperuricemia, acute inflammatory arthritis, and sometimes, usually after a course of years and following episodes of gouty arthritis, deposition of monosodium urate crystals in the soft tissues. These deposits are termed *tophi* and are usually located on the extremities near joints, particularly the articular cartilage and other periarticular structures or subcutis, the cartilaginous pinna of the ear, and the interstitium of the kidney.[107,108]

Histopathologic Features

Although gouty tophi usually form in the periarticular soft tissues, in some cases, urate crystals are deposited en masse in the dermis or subcutis where they are surrounded by a granulomatous infiltrate that tends to palisade around the densely packed crystals (Fig. 9-16). Multinucleate giant cells of foreign body type are frequently admixed with the mononuclear histiocytes.

The urate crystals are water soluble and dissolve when aqueous fixatives such as formalin are used. In such instances, the diagnosis must be based on the nature of the granulomatous reaction surrounding amorphous debris, correlated with clinical findings. When tissue is preserved and processed in nonaqueous solutions, the crystals remain and can be visualized as closely packed needle-like structures using conventional light microscopy. They are birefringent and are dramatically demonstrable by polaroscopic examination.

XANTHOGRANULOMATOUS INFLAMMATION

Cutaneous Leishmaniasis

Clinical Features

Leishmaniasis is a protozoan infection, the causative agent being of the genus *Leishmania,* transmitted by the sandflies *Lutzomyia* (New World) and *Phlebotomus* (Old World).[34] Localized cutaneous leishmaniasis (tropical sore) develops at the site of inoculation as a pruritic papule that ulcerates and that is surrounded by a zone of erythematous induration. Lymphatic drainage may result in the development of satellite lesions. The disease is self-limited, but heals slowly over the course of months, resulting in depressed scars.

Mucocutaneous leishmaniasis is distinguished clinically from the localized form by the development of late secondary mucosal lesions, which occur near mucocutaneous junctions. Symptoms of centrofacial fullness, pain, enlargement of lips, mucosal dryness, and epistaxis are common, and in late stages there can be extensive soft tissue destruction, often with septal perforation, and destruction of the vocal cords.[109]

Diffuse (anergic) cutaneous leishmaniasis also begins as a single nodule, but there is progression of the disease with formation of other nodules and slow spread until the disease involves large areas of the integument. The leishmanin test remains negative.[34]

Histopathologic Features

Primary lesions show epidermal hyperplasia and areas of ulceration. Although earlier lesions show a nodular or diffuse mixed infiltrate with easily identifiable parasites, in later stages the infiltrate becomes granulomatous with numerous histiocytes, multinucleate giant cells, and sometimes tuberculoid granulomas. Organisms are less common in this phase. In anergic patients there is a diffuse infiltrate of foamy histiocytes containing numerous organisms.

The mucocutaneous form of the disease is similar microscopically to the primary lesion, with pseudoepitheliomatous hyperplasia, a mixed infiltrate, and often a granulomatous infiltrate. There are sometimes concomitant infections by such organisms as *Candida* sp. and other infections such as tuberculosis.[109]

Differential Diagnosis

The histologic diagnosis depends on the demonstration of the leishmanias (amastigotes), which multiply within the cytoplasm of histiocytes. Although the morphology is sufficiently distinctive to enable identification on routinely stained slides, the Giemsa stain is often useful when organisms are difficult to find.[34]

REFERENCES

1. James DG, Siltzbach LE, Sharma OP, Carstairs LS: A tale of two cities–a comparison of sarcoidosis in London and New York. Arch Intern Med 123:187–191, 1969
2. Hanno R, Needleman A, Eiferman RA, Callen JP: Cutaneous sarcoidal granulomas and the development of systemic sarcoidosis. Arch Dermatol 117:203–207, 1981
3. Sharma OP: Cutaneous sarcoidosis: clinical features and management. Chest 61:320–325
4. Lever WF, Freiman DG: Sarcoidosis: report of an atypical case with erythrodermic lesions, subcutaneous nodes and asteroid inclusion bodies in giant cells. Arch Dermatol 57:639–654, 1948
5. Vainsencher D, Winkelmann RK: Subcutaneous sarcoidosis. Arch Dermatol 120:1028–1031, 1984
6. Frieden IJ, Prose NS, Fletcher V, Turner ML: Granulomatous perioral dermatitis in children. Arch Dermatol 125:369–373, 1989
7. El-Rifaie M El-Saad: Perioral dermatitis with epithelioid cell granulomas in a woman: a possible new etiology. Acta Derm Venereol 60:359–360, 1980
8. Macallum DI, Kinmont PDC: Dermatologic manifestations of Crohn's disease. Br J Dermatol 80:1–8, 1968
9. Burgdorf W: Cutaneous manifestations of Crohn's disease. J Am Acad Dermatol 5:689–695, 1981
10. Parks AG, Morson BC, Pegum JS: Crohn's disease with cutaneous involvement. Proc R Soc Med 58:241–242, 1965
11. Kao M-S, Paulson JD, Askin FB: Crohn's disease of the vulva. Obstet Gynecol 46:329–333, 1975
12. Lebwohl M, Fleischmajer R, Janowitz H et al: Metastatic Crohn's disease. J Am Acad Dermatol 10:33–38, 1984
13. Peltz S, Vestey A, Ferguson A et al: Disseminated metastatic cutaneous Crohn's disease. Clin Exp Dermatol 18:55–59, 1993
14. Neave HJ, Frank SB, Tolmach JA: Cutaneous granuloma following laceration by fluorescent light bulbs. Arch Dermatol 61:401–406, 1950
15. Stoeckle JD, Hardy HL, Weber AL: Chronic beryllium disease: long-term follow-up of sixty cases and selective review of the literature. Am J Med 46:545–557, 1967
16. Baler GR: Granulomas from topical zirconium in poison ivy dermatitis. Arch Dermatol 91:145–148, 1965
17. Williams RM, Skipworth GB: Zirconium granulomas of glabrous skin following treatment of rhus dermatitis. Arch Dermatol 80:273–276, 1959
18. Ridley DS, Jopling WH: Classification of leprosy according to immunity. Int J Leprosy 34: 255–273, 1966
19. Jollieffe DS: Leprosy reactional states and their treatment. Br J Dermatol 97:345–352, 1977
20. Liu TC, Yen LZ, Ye GY, Dung GJ: Histology of indeterminate leprosy. Int J Leprosy Mycobacterial Dis 50:172–176, 1982
21. Ridley DS: Histological classification and the immunological spectrum of leprosy. Bull WHO 51:451–465, 1974
22. Abell E, Marks R, Wilson-Jones E: Secondary syphilis: a clinico pathological review. Br J Dermatol 93:53–61, 1975
23. Jeerapaet P, Ackerman AB: Histologic patterns of secondary syphilis. Arch Dermatol 107:373–377, 1973
24. Kahn LB, Gordon W: Sarcoid-like granulomas in secondary syphilis–a clinical and histopathologic study of five cases. Arch Pathol 92:334–337, 1971

25. Montgomery H: Histopathology of various types of cutaneous tuberculosis. Arch Dermatol Syph 35:698–715, 1937
26. Santa Cruz DJ, Strayer DS: The histologic spectrum of cutaneous tuberculosis. Hum Pathol 13:485–495, 1982
27. O'Leary PA, Harrison MW: Inoculation tuberculosis. Arch Dermatol Syph 44:371–373, 1941
28. Beyt BE, Ortbals DW, Santa Cruz DJ et al: Cutaneous mycobacteriosis: analysis of 34 cases with a new classification of disease. Medicine 60:95–109, 1980
29. Rohatgi PK, Palazzolo JV, Saini NB: Acute miliary tuberculosis of the skin in acquired immunodeficiency syndrome. J Am Acad Dermatol 26:356–359, 1992
30. Wilson-Jones E, Winkelmann RK: Papulonecrotic tuberculid: a neglected disease in Western countries. J Am Acad Dermatol 14:815–826, 1986
31. Fetter BF: Human cutaneous sporotrichosis. Arch Pathol 71:416–419, 1961
32. Winn RE: Sporotrichosis. Infect Dis Clin North Am 2:899–911, 1988
33. Purvis RS, Diven DG, Drechsel RD et al: Sporotrichosis presenting as arthritis and subcutaneous nodules. J Am Acad Dermatol 28:879–884, 1993
34. Binford CH, Connor DH: pp. 258–272. In: Pathology of Tropical and Extraordinary Disease. Armed Forces Institute of Pathology, Washington, DC, 1976
35. Lurie HI: Histopathology of sporotrichosis. Arch Pathol 75:421–437, 1963
36. Rubin HA, Bruce S, Rosen T, McBride ME: Evidence for percutaneous inoculation as the mode of transmission for chromoblastomycosis. J Am Acad Dermatol 25:951–954, 1991
37. Tschen JA, Knox JM, McGavran MH, Duncan WC: Chromomycosis: the association of fungal elements and wood splinters. Arch Dermatol 120:107–108, 1984
38. Milam CP, Fenske NA: Chromoblastomycosis, review. Dermatol Clin 7:219–225, 1989
39. Wiss K, McNeely MC, Solomon AR, Jr: Chromoblastomycosis can mimic keratoacanthoma. Int J Dermatol 25:385–386, 1986
40. Hirsh BC, Johnson WC: Pathology of granulomatous diseases. Int J Dermatol 23:585–597, 1984
41. Faabio Uribe J, Zuluaga AI, Leon W, Restrepo A: Histopathology of chromoblastomycosis. Mycopathologia 105:1–6, 1989
42. Ronan SG, Uzoaru I, Nadimpalli V et al: Primary cutaneous phaeohyphomycosis: report of seven cases. J Cutan Pathol 20:223–228, 1993
43. Fader RC, McGinnis MR: Infections caused by dematiaceous fungi: chromoblastomycosis and phaeohyphomycosis. Infect Dis North Am 2:925–938, 1988
44. Rodrigez-Toro G: Lobomycosis. Int J Dermatol 32:324–332, 1993
45. Lobo J: Um caso de blastomicose produzido por uma especie nova encontrada em Recife. Rev Med Pernambucana 1:763–775, 1931
46. Fialho A: Blasomicose du tipo "Jorge Lobo." O Hospital 14:903, 1938
47. Restrepo A: Treatment of tropical mycoses. J Am Acad Dermatol 31:S91–S102, 1994
48. Umbert IJ, Su WPD: Cutaneous mucormycosis. J Am Acad Dermatol 21:1232–1234, 1989
49. Cocanour CS, Miller Crotchett P, Reed RL II et al: Mucormycosis in trauma patients. J Trauma 32:12–15, 1992
50. Bearer EA, Nelson PR, Chowers MY, Davis CE: Cutaneous zygomycosis caused by Saksenaea vasiformis in a diabetic patient. J Clin Microbiol 32:1823–1824, 1994
51. Sanchez MR, Ponge-Wilson I, Moy JA, Rosenthal S: Zygomycosis and HIV infection. J Am Acad Dermatol 30:904–908, 1994
52. Clark R, Greer DL, Carlisle T, Carroll B: Cutaneous zygomycosis in a diabetic HTLV-1-seropositive man. J Am Acad Sci 22:956–959, 1990
53. Khardori N, Hayat S, Rolston K, Bodey GP: Cutaneous Rhizopus and Aspergillus infections in five patients with cancer. Arch Dermatol 125:952–956, 1989
54. McElroy JA, de Almeida Prestes C, Su WPD: Mycetoma: infection with tumefaction, draining sinuses, and grains. Cutis 49:107–110, 1992
55. Hay RJ, Mackenzie DWR: The histopathologic features of pale grain eumycetoma. Trans R Soc Trop Med Hyg 76:839–844, 1982
56. Hunt SJ, Nagi C, Gross KG et al: Primary cutaneous aspergillosis near central venous catheters in patients with the acquired immunodeficiency syndrome. Arch Dermatol 128:1229–1232, 1992
57. Greenbaum RS, Roth JS, Grossman ME: Subcutaneous nodule in a cardiac transplant. Cutaneous aspergillosis. Arch Dermatol 129:1191–1194, 1993
58. Falsey AR, Goldsticker RD, Ahern MJ: Fatal subcutaneous aspergillosis following necrotizing fasciitis: a case report. Yale J Biol Med 63:9–13, 1990
59. Googe PB, DeCoste SD, Herold WH, Mihm MC, Jr: Primary cutaneous aspergillosis mimicking dermatophytosis. Arch Pathol Lab Med 113:1284–1286, 1989
60. Eidbo J, Sanchez RL, Tsschen JA, Ellner KM: Cutaneous manifestations of histoplasmosis in the acquired immune deficiency syndrome. Am J Surg Pathol 17:110–116, 1993
61. Goodwin RA, Shapiro JL, Thurman SS, Des Prez RM: Disseminated histoplasmosis: clinical and pathologic correlations. Medicine 59:1–33, 1980
62. Hay RJ: Histoplasmosis. Semin Dermatol 12:310–314, 1993
63. Glaser JB, Garden A: Inoculation of cryptococcosis without transmission of the acquired immunodeficiency syndrome. N Engl J Med 313:266, 1985
64. Barfield L, Iacobelli D, Hashimoto K: Secondary cutaneous cryptococcosis: case report and review of 22 cases. J Cutan Pathol 15:385–392, 1988
65. Hernandez AD: Cutaneous cryptococcosis. Dermatol Clin 7:269–274, 1989
66. Hall JC, Brewer JH, Crouch TT, Watson KR: Cryptococcal cellulitis with multiple sites of involvement. J Am Acad Dermatol 17:329–332, 1987
67. Durden FM, Elewski B: Cutaneous involvement with Cryptococcus neoformans in AIDS. J Am Acad Dermatol 30:844–848, 1994
68. Baker RD, Haugen RK: Tissue changes and tissue diagnosis in cryptococcosis. Am J Clin Pathol 25:14–24, 1955
69. Leidel GD, Metcalf JS: Formation of palisading granulomas in a patient with chronic cutaneous cryptococcosis. Am J Dermatopathol 11:560–562, 1989
70. Knoper SR, Galgiani JN: Coccidioidomycosis. Infect Dis Clin North Am 2:861–873, 1988

71. Wilson JW, Smith CE, Plunkett OA: Primary cutaneous coccidioidomycosis. The criteria for diagnosis and a report of a case. Calif Med 79:233–239, 1953

72. Sugar AM: Paracoccidioidomycosis. Infect Dis Clin North Am 2:913–924, 1988

73. Restrepo A, Salazar ME, Cano LE et al: Estrogens inhibit mycelium-to-yeast transformation in the fungus *Paracoccidioides brasiliensis:* implications for resistance of females to paracoccidioidomycosis. Infect Immun 46:346, 1984

74. Murray HW, Littman ML, Roberts RB: Disseminated paracoccidioidomycosis (South American blastomycosis) in the United States. Am J Med 56:209–220, 1974

75. Giraldo R, Restrepo A, Gutierrez F et al: Pathogenesis of paracoccidioidomycosis: a model based on the study of 46 patients. Mycopathologia 58:63, 1976

76. Klein BS, Vergeront JM, Davis JP: Epidemiologic aspects of blastomycosis, the enigmatic systemic mycosis. Semin Respir Infect 1:29–39, 1986

77. Mercurio MD, Elewski BE: Cutaneous blastomycosis. Cutis 50:422–424, 1992

78. Leet NA, Parker CM: Multiple verrucous skin lesions: North American blastomycosis. Arch Dermatol 127:723–726, 1991

79. Helm TN, Tomecki KJ: Respiratory dimorphic fungal infections. pp. 166–171. In: Elewski BE (ed): Cutaneous Fungal Infections. Igaku-Shoin, New York, 1992

80. Marks R: Rosacea, flushing and perioral dermatitis. pp. 1851–1859. In: Champion RH, Burton JL, Ebling FJG (eds): Rook/Wilkinson/Ebling Textbook of Dermatology. Blackwell Scientific, London, 1992

81. Sanchez-Viera M, Hernanz JM, Sampelayo T et al: Granulomatous rosacea in a child infected with the human immunodeficiency virus. J Am Acad Dermatol 27:1010–1011, 1992

82. Helm KF, Menz J, Gibson LE, Dicken CH: A clinical and histopathologic study of granulomatous rosacea. J Am Acad Dermatol 25:1038–1043, 1991

83. Ramelet AA, Perroulaz G: Rosaceé: étude histopathologique de 75 cas. Ann Dermatol Venereol 115:801–806, 1988

84. Grosshans EM, Kremer M, Maleville J: Demodex folliculorum und die histogenese der granulomatösen rosacea. Hautarzt 25:166–177, 1974

85. Rosenberg FR, Einbinder J, Walzer RA, Nelson CT: Vegetating iododerma–an immunologic mechanism. Arch Dermatol 105:900–905, 1972

86. Teller H: Bromoderma und Jododerma tuberosum. Dermatol Wochenschr 143:273–282, 1961 as cited in Lever WF, Schaumburg-Lever G: Histopathology of the Skin. 7th Ed. Lippincott-Raven, Philadelphia, 1990

87. Kincaid MC, Green WR, Hoover RE, Farmer ER: Iododerma of the conjunctiva and skin. Ophthalmology 88:1216–1220, 1981

88. O'Brien JP: Actinic granuloma: an annular connective tissue disorder affecting sun and heat-damaged (elastotic) skin. Arch Dermatol 111:460–466, 1975

89. Mehregan AH, Altman J: Miesher's granuloma of the face. Arch Dermatol 107:62–64, 1973

90. Dowling GB, Wilson-Jones E: Atypical (annular) necrobiosis lipoidica of the face and scalp. Dermatologica 135:11–26, 1967

91. Hanke CW, Bailin PI, Roenigk HH: Annular elastolytic giant cell granuloma: a clinicopathologic study of five cases and a review of similar entities. J Am Acad Dermatol 1:413–421, 1979

92. Finan MC, Winkelmann RK: The cutaneous extravascular necrotizing granuloma (Churg-Strauss granuloma) and systemic disease: a review of 27 cases. Medicine (Baltimore) 62:142–158, 1983

93. Jorizzo JL, Olansky AJ, Stanley RJ: Superficial ulcerating necrobiosis in rheumatoid arthritis. Arch Dermatol 118:255–259, 1982

94. Patterson JW, Demos PT: Superficial ulcerating rheumatoid necrobiosis, a perforating rheumatoid nodule. Cutis 35:323–325, 1985

95. Ackerman AB, Guo Y, Vitale P, Vorsaert K: pp. 309–312. In: Clues to Diagnosis in Dermatopathology. Vol. 3. ASCP Press, Chicago, 1993

96. Chu P, Connolly K, LeBoit PE: The histopathologic spectrum of palisaded neutrophilic and granulomatous dermatitis in patients with collagen vascular disease. Arch Dermatol 130:1278–1283, 1994

97. Muller SA, Winkelmann RK: Necrobiosis lipoidica diabeticorum: histopathologic study of 98 cases. Arch Dermatol 94:1–10, 1966

98. Ackerman AB: Histologic Diagnosis of Inflammatory Skin Diseases: A Method by Pattern Analysis. 1st Ed. Lea & Febiger, Philadelphia 1978

99. Lowney FD, Simons HM: "Rheumatoid" nodules of the skin. Arch Dermatol 88:853–858, 1963

100. Wisnieski JJ, Askari AD: Rheumatoid nodulosis: a relatively benign variant. Arch Intern Med 141:615–619, 1981

101. Sibbitt WL, Jr, Williams RC, Jr: Cutaneous manifestations of rheumatoid arthritis. Int J Dermatol 21:563–572, 1982

102. Edwards JCW, Wilkinson LS, Pitsillides AA: Palisading cells of rheumatoid nodules: comparison with synovial intimal cells. Ann Rheum Dis 52:801–805, 1993

103. Sokoloff L, McCluskey RT, Bunim JJ: Vascularity of the early subcutaneous nodule of rheumatoid arthritis. AMA Arch Pathol 55:475–495, 1953

104. Bywaters EGL, Glynn LE, Zeldis A: Subcutaneous nodules of Still's disease. Ann Rheum Dis 17:278–285, 1958

105. Beatty EC, Jr: Rheumatic-like nodules occurring in nonrheumatic children. AMA Arch Pathol 68:154–159,1959

106. Lowney ED, Simons HM: "Rheumatoid" nodules of the skin: their significance as an isolated finding. Arch Dermatol 88:853–858, 1963

107. Wyngaarden JB: Gout. pp. 1132–1142. In Wyngaarden JB, Smith LH, Jr (eds): Cecil Textbook of Medicine. 6th Ed. WB Saunders, Philadelphia, 1985

108. Seymore CA: Disorders of amino acid metabolism. pp. 2356–2357. In: Champion RH, Burton JL, Ebling FJG (eds): Rook/Wilkinson/Ebling Textbook of Dermatology. Blackwell Scientific, London, 1992

109. Sangueza OP, Sangueza JM, Stiller MJ, Sangueza P: Mucocutaneous leishmaniasis: a clinicopathologic classification. J Am Acad Dermatol 28:927–932

10

INTRAEPIDERMAL VESICULAR AND PUSTULAR DISEASES

ACANTHOLYTIC BULLOUS DISEASES

Intraepidermal vesicles and pustules are found in a diverse group of diseases with equally diverse etiologies. One way to approach these diseases from a diagnostic point of view is to subclassify them on the basis of the presence or absence of acantholysis (i.e., acantholytic and nonacantholytic diseases) (Table 10-1 and Figs. 10-1, 10-2). Acantholysis must be differentiated from spongiosis. Acantholysis is characterized by lack of cohesion between adjacent keratinocytes. The separated keratinocytes are rounded in shape and usually have a brightly eosinophilic band of keratin beneath the cell membrane. Intercellular bridges are lost. This latter finding is helpful in distinguishing acantholysis from spongiosis, since in the latter intercellular bridges are augmented and made more prominent by extracellular edema. Few or no inflammatory cells are present in vesicles; inflammation, usually neutrophilic, is more or less abundant in pustules.

Pemphigus

Until recently, four clinicopathologic subtypes of pemphigus were generally recognized: pemphigus vulgaris, pemphigus vegetans, pemphigus foliaceus, and pemphigus erythematosus. A fifth subtype, pemphigus neoplastica, appears to have clinical, histologic, and immunopathologic features that are sufficiently characteristic to warrant designation as a separate entity. Although each subtype has distinctive features, acantholysis is the common denominator and essential microscopic feature of pemphigus.

Pemphigus Vulgaris

Clinical Features

Pemphigus vulgaris is by far the most common subtype and encompasses approximately 80% of patients.[1] Patients are typically middle-aged or older, but the disease may present in childhood.[2] Men and women are equally affected. More than one-half of the patients with pemphigus vulgaris present with oral lesions.[1,3] In most cases, the disease then progresses to involve glabrous skin, especially the scalp and trunk. The mucosae of the upper airway and esophagus, the conjunctiva, and the urogenital and rectal mucosae may also be involved.[4–7]

The primary lesion of pemphigus vulgaris is a superficial, flaccid bulla.[1] Bullae may be solitary or grouped, numerous or few. They occur on previously normal skin without underlying erythema. Because the cleavage plane is within the epidermis, the bullae are fragile and readily rupture to leave erosions. Healing occurs without scarring. Intact bullae are rarely found on the oral mucosa, because the mechanical trauma of mastication leads to early rupture. The painful erosions commonly lead to an aversion to eating, weight loss, and inanition, a major contributing factor to morbidity and mortality.[4]

Histopathologic Features

Suprabasal acantholysis, the histologic hallmark of pemphigus vulgaris, results from loss of the intercellular bridges between keratinocytes of the lower epidermis and the follicular infundibula[1,8] (Fig. 10-3). After loss of cohesion, the cells lose their normal angular contours and become rounded. The basal keratinocytes remain attached to the epidermal basement membrane. These conspicuous attached basal cells highlight the undulating rete ridges. Rounded, acantholytic keratinocytes with condensed, hyperchromatic nuclei and brightly eosinophilic cytoplasm float in the bullae formed between the basal keratinocytes and the remainder of the epidermis. Only rare acantholytic cells are found in higher levels of the epidermis. Extension of suprabasal acantholysis into follicular infundibula is an important diagnostic finding.[8] Occasionally, acantholysis is present in eccrine ducts. Neither dyskeratosis nor nuclear atypia are features of pemphigus vulgaris.

Table 10-1. Acantholytic Dermatoses

Name	Predominant Site of Acantholysis	Dyskeratosis	Inflammation	Comments
Pemphigus vulgaris	Suprabasal	No	Eosinophils, lymphocytes	Minimal acanthosis
Pemphigus vegetans	Suprabasal	No	Eosinophilic pustules	Acantholysis may be minimal
Paraneoplastic pemphigus	Suprabasal	Yes	Eosinophils, lymphocytes	Vacuolar interface change, dyskeratosis
Pemphigus foliaceus	Subcorneal	Minimal	Lymphocytes, eosinophils	Intact bulla may not be present
Pemphigus erythematosus	Subcorneal	Minimal	Lymphocytes, eosinophils	Intact bulla may not be present
Transient acantholytic dermatosis	Variable	Variable	Lymphocytes	Five different patterns
Benign familial pemphigus	Full thickness of epidermis	Minimal	Lymphocytes	Combination of free and cohesive keratinocytes
Keratosis follicularis	Suprabasal and above	Prominent	Lymphocytes	Dyskeratosis is extreme
Papular acantholytic dyskeratosis of the genitalia	Variable	Variable	Lymphocytes	Genital site in the absence of other disease
Warty dyskeratoma	Full thickness of epidermis	Prominent	Lymphocytes	Cup-shaped configuration
Herpesvirus infection	Variable	Prominent, in addition to necrosis	Neutrophils	Diagnostic nuclear changes
Linear epidermal nevus	Variable	Variable	Lymphocytes or none	Verrucous acanthosis
Bullous impetigo	Sub- or intracorneal	Minimal	Neutrophils	Few acantholytic cells

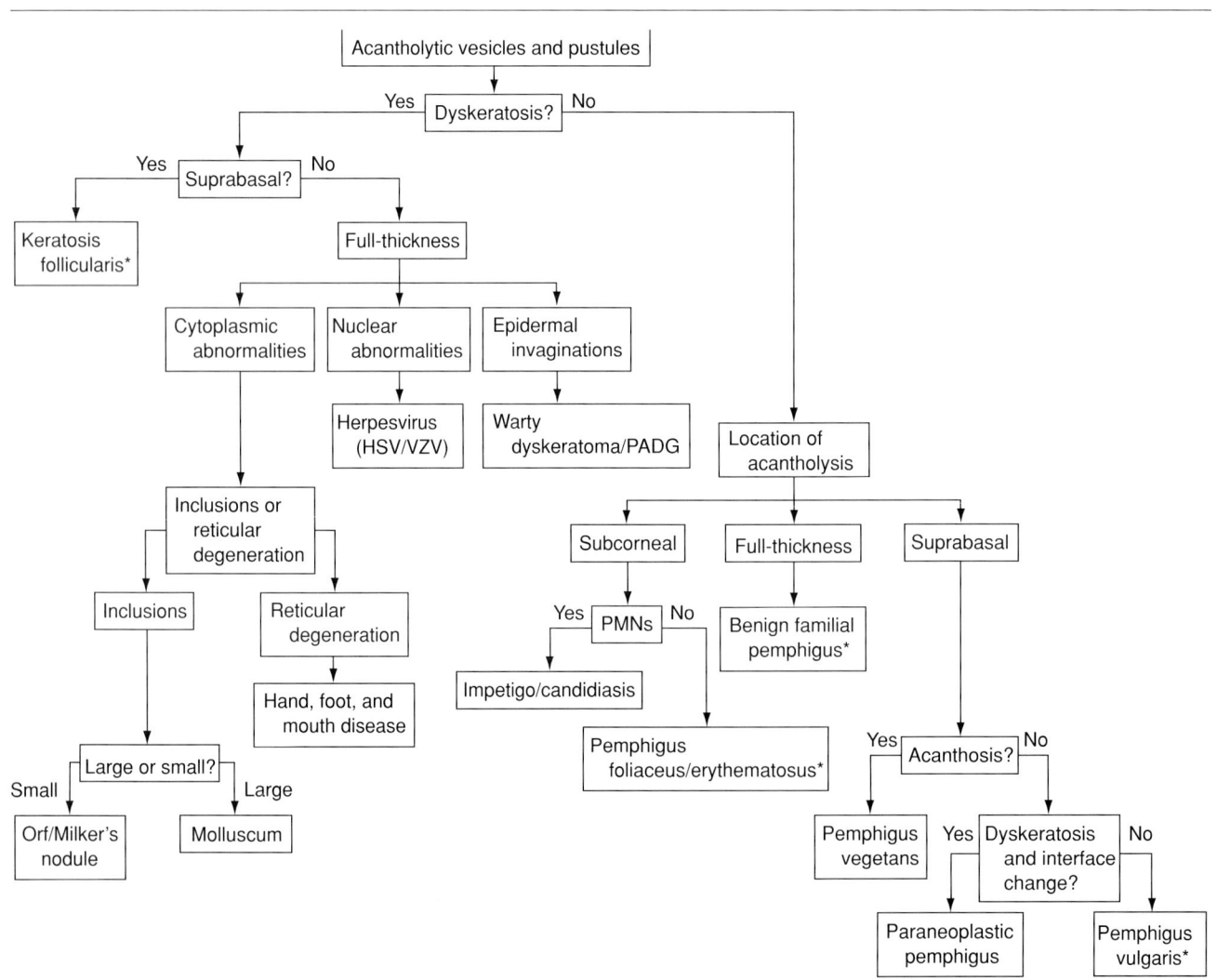

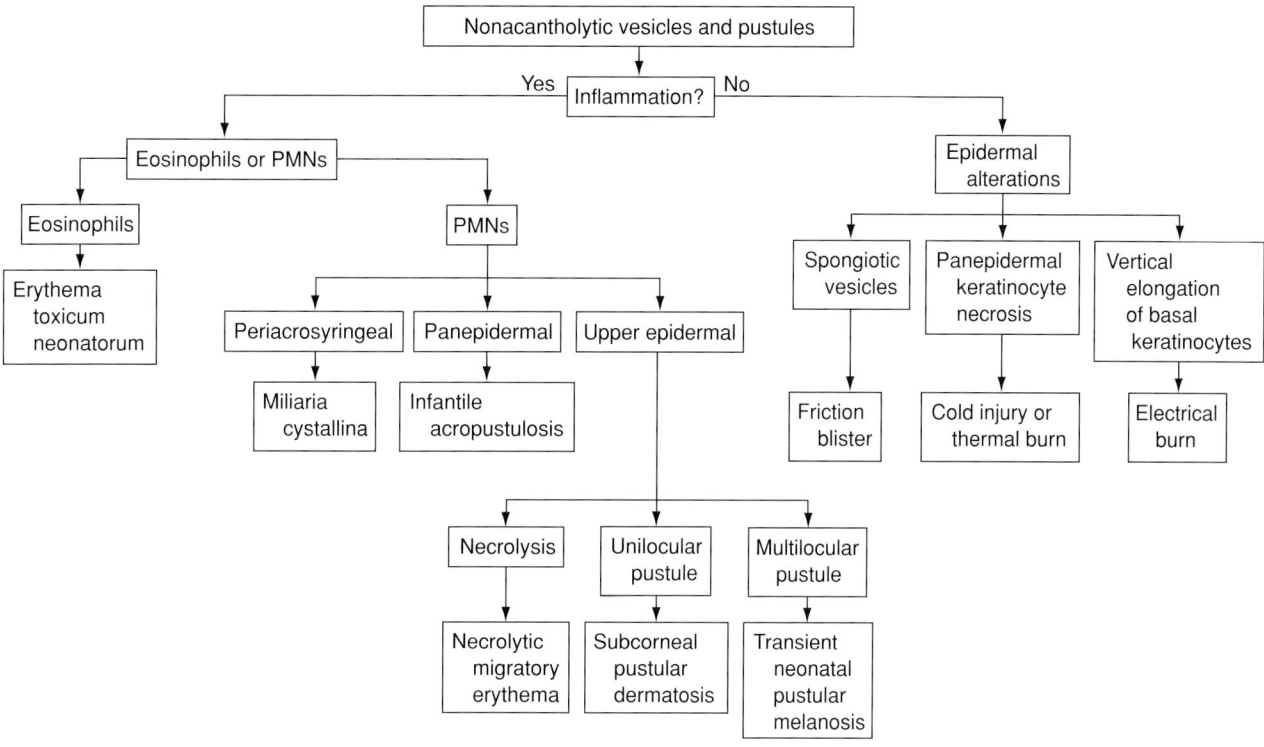

Figure 10-2. Classification of nonacantholytic vesicles and pustules. PMNs, polymorphonuclear neutrophils.

Figure 10-3. Pemphigus vulgaris. Acantholysis is the defining feature of pemphigus. In pemphigus vulgaris the acantholysis is most prominent in the basal and suprabasal epidermal layers. Sparse lymphocytic infiltrates with admixed eosinophils are present in the superficial dermis. (× 200.)

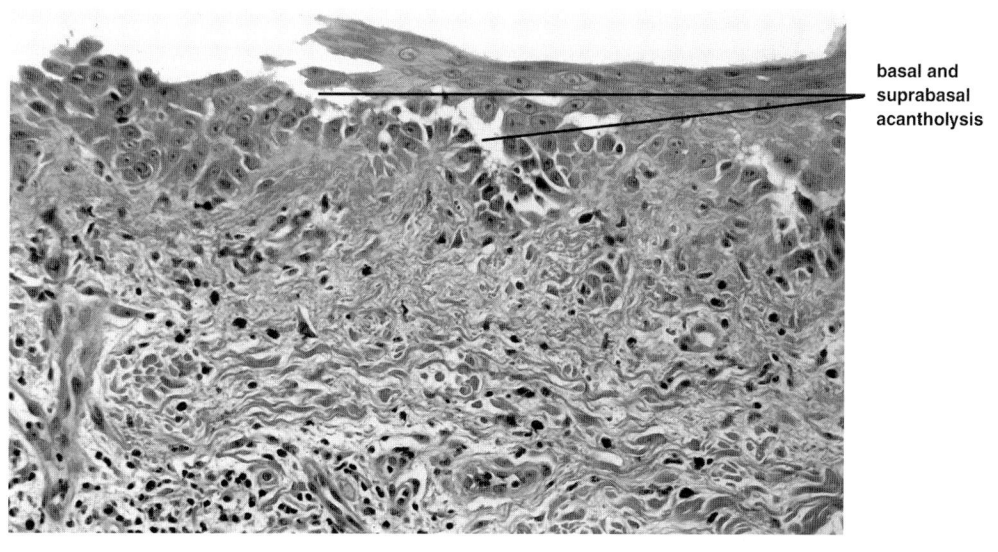

basal and
suprabasal
acantholysis

Figure 10-1. Classification of acantholytic vesicles and pustules. *Similar microscopic changes are present in transient acantholytic dermatosis, but they are limited in extent. HSV, herpes simplex virus; VZV, varicella-zoster virus; PADG, papular acantholytic dyskeratosis of the genitalia; PMNs, polymorphonuclear neutrophils.

Inflammation is variable in pemphigus vulgaris. Eosinophils and lymphocytes are the most common cells and are found in the epidermis, both around and within bullae, and in the subjacent dermis. An incresed number of mast cells has been reported in the dermis of pemphigus lesions.[9] Eosinophilic infiltration of the epidermis either in early, evolving lesions in which no bullae are present or at the periphery of fully developed bullae has been termed *eosinophilic spongiosis*[10,11] (Fig. 10-4).

Differential Diagnosis

The absence of nuclear atypia in keratinocytes distinguishes pemphigus vulgaris from acantholytic actinic keratosis. The acantholysis in the pemphigus vulgaris-like subtype of transient acantholytic dermatosis is rarely as extensive as in true pemphigus vulgaris. In addition, eosinophils and intrafollicular acantholysis are not present. Acantholysis limited to the suprabasal zone of the epidermis and the lack of dyskeratosis differentiate pemphigus vulgaris from benign familial pemphigus and keratosis follicularis, respectively. No interface change and minimal or no dyskeratosis are present in pemphigus vulgaris, unlike paraneoplastic pemphigus, especially the oral lesions of the latter. As bullae heal, they move progressively higher within the epidermis. Older bullae at the level of the granular layer may be confused with pemphigus foliaceus or erythematosus. Identification of additional suprabasal bullae is needed to diagnose pemphigus vulgaris in older, resolving lesions.

Pemphigus Vegetans

Clinical Features

Two variants of this rare form of pemphigus have been described.[12] The transient bullae of the Hallopeau subtype are followed by erythematous, papillomatous, or vegetating plaques studded with pustules of varying size. The plaques have a predilection for flexural surfaces and the oral mucosa.[13,14] These patients have a benign course and suffer only from the more or less recalcitrant plaques and pustules.[15] By contrast, patients with the Neumann type of pemphigus vegetans frequently develop bullae similar to those of pemphigus vulgaris in addition to the plaques and may have the same mucosal complications. Some authors believe that the Neumann type of pemphigus vegetans is simply a variant of pemphigus vulgaris.[12]

Histopathologic Features

Although, as in pemphigus vulgaris, acantholysis is most prominent in the basal and suprabasal zones of the epidermis, marked acanthosis is characteristic of pemphigus vegetans.[12] The rete ridges expand and proliferate downward into the papillary dermis to form bulbous lobules separated by narrow elongated dermal papillae (Fig. 10-5). Acantholytic cells are usually few, and multiple sections may have to be examined to find them.

Eosinophils permeate the epidermis and form large intraepidermal abscesses composed almost exclusively of these cells.[11] Acantholytic keratinocytes are usually evident in the abscesses.[16] Eosinophils are also present in the underlying superficial dermis in a diffuse pattern.

The Hallopeau and Neumann types of pemphigus vegetans cannot be reliably separated solely on the basis of histopathology; clinical findings are essential.[12]

Differential Diagnosis

In the presence of acanthosis combined with a paucity of acantholytic cells, pemphigus vegetans must be differentiated from diseases characterized by pseudoepitheliomatous hyperplasia such as fungal infections, halogenodermas, and the perforating

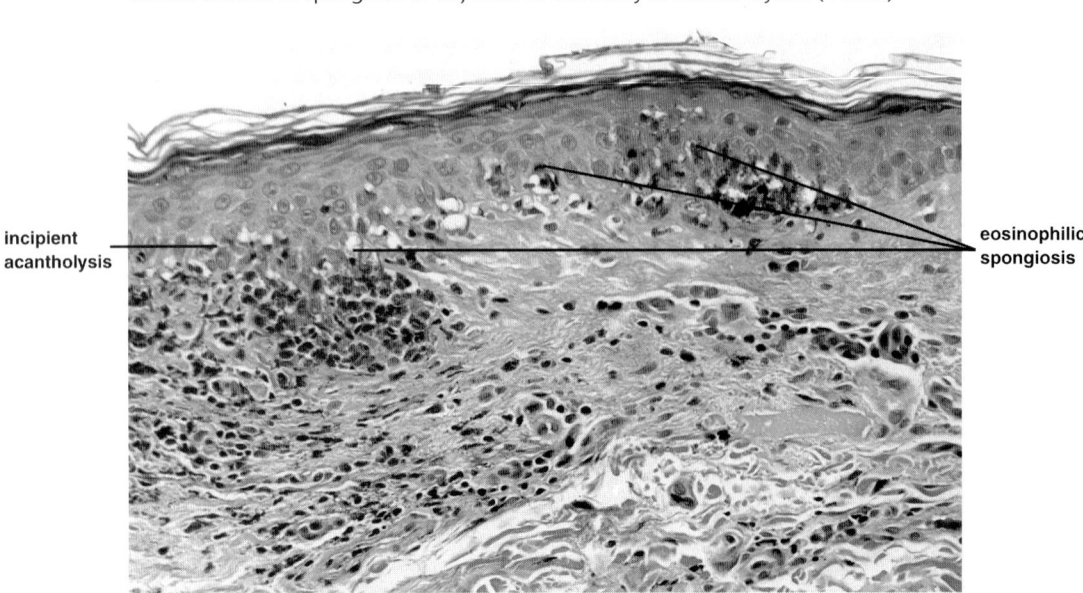

Figure 10-4. Pemphigus vulgaris, early lesion. Eosinophils are present within the epidermis in areas of spongiosis or adjacent to acantholytic keratinocytes. (× 200.)

incipient acantholysis

eosinophilic spongiosis

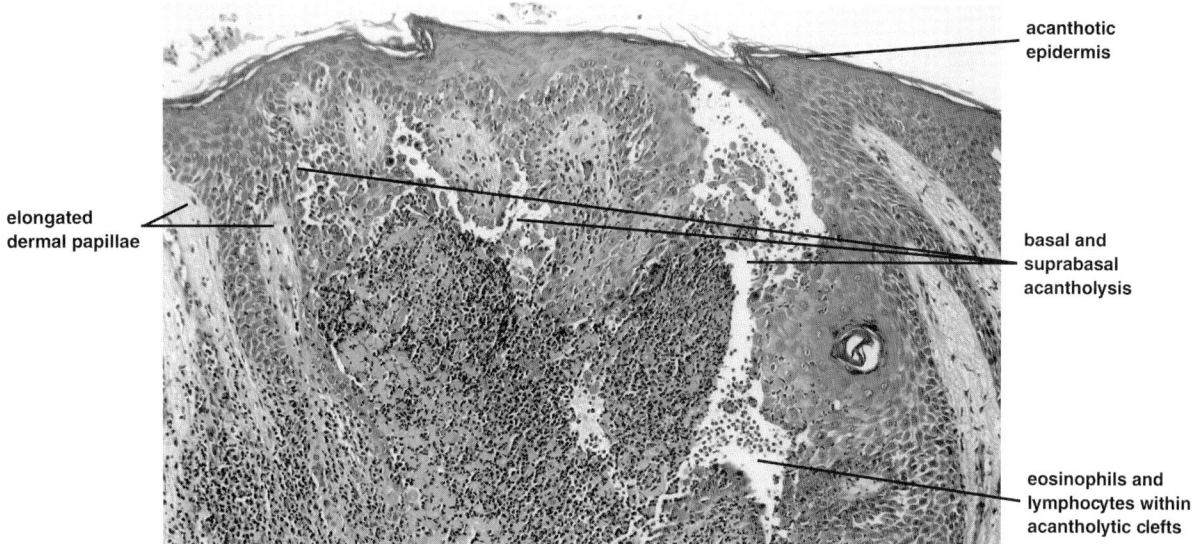

elongated
dermal papillae

acanthotic
epidermis

basal and
suprabasal
acantholysis

eosinophils and
lymphocytes within
acantholytic clefts

Figure 10-5. Pemphigus vegetans. In contrast to pemphigus vulgaris, the epidermis is markedly acanthotic in pemphigus vegetans. The dermal papillae are elongated. Acantholytic keratinocytes form clefts that contain eosinophils and lymphocytes. (× 80.)

diseases. A diligent search for acantholytic keratinocytes is required in many cases. Pyoderma vegetans (blastomycosis-like pyoderma), a disease with virtually identical clinical and histologic features as the Hallopeau type of pemphigus vegetans, can be differentiated by its negative immunofluorescence.

Paraneoplastic Pemphigus

Clinical Features

Although patients with coexistent pemphigus and various neoplasms have been recognized for years, Anhalt and co-workers delineated the clinical, histologic, and immunopathologic features of this unique subtype of pemphigus in 1990.[17–21] Patients with paraneoplastic pemphigus typically present with mucocutaneous lesions, but the oral lesions are usually the most prominent. Oral ulcers are the most common manifestation. The cutaneous lesions are polymorphous, consisting of bullae and erythematous macules, resembling erythema multiforme.[17,19,20] The conjunctival mucosa may be involved.[22] Paraneoplastic pemphigus may present as a lichen planus pemphigoides-like eruption with clinical lesions resembling both pemphigus and lichen planus.[23] Paraneoplastic pemphigus develops most commonly, but not only, in patients with lymphoreticular neoplasms.[17,19,20]

Histopathologic Features

In addition to suprabasal acantholysis, dyskeratosis, vacuolar interface change, suprabasal cleft formation, and inflammatory cell (lymphocyte and/or eosinophil) exocytosis are present in paraneoplastic pemphigus.[17–20] Any of the above findings may be only focally present. adding to the difficulty of histologic interpretation. The combination of suprabasal acantholysis and

dyskeratosis should prompt additional clinical or immunologic evaluation (or both) for paraneoplastic pemphigus.[18]

Differential Diagnosis

Although suprabasal acantholysis is usually not as prominent in erythema multiforme, the microscopic findings of paraneoplastic pemphigus are similar enough to those of erythema multiforme to require immunologic tests (see below) to reliably differentiate between the two diseases. Neither dyskeratosis nor vacuolar interface change is usually present in pemphigus vulgaris. Parakeratosis and a more extensive lymphocytic infiltrate are typically found in pityriasis lichenoides acuta and chronica.

Pemphigus Foliaceus (Fogo Selvagem)

Clinical Features

Pemphigus foliaceus rarely presents with obvious bullae. The superficial location of acantholysis results in early rupture of bullae to form erythematous erosions that ooze and crust.[24] The face, scalp, chest, and back are the most common sites. The combination of crusted papules and anatomic location may suggest the clinical diagnosis of seborrheic dermatitis unless an intact bulla is found. Pemphigus foliaceus usually results in a milder illness than the other types of pemphigus, and patients respond to lower doses of corticosteroids. Persons treated with penicillamine have developed an illness identical to naturally occurring pemphigus foliaceus. Fogo selvagem, a disease essentially limited to Brazil and spread by an insect vector, is also similar, if not identical, to pemphigus foliaceus.[25,26] Pemphigus foliaceus may rarely present in childhood.[27] Although the clinical, microscopic, and immunopathologic features allow separation of pemphigus vulgaris from pemphigus foliaceus, transition from the former to the latter has been reported.[28,29]

Histopathologic Features

In contrast to pemphigus vulgaris and pemphigus vegetans, the acantholysis in pemphigus foliaceus occurs in the upper malpighian layers of the epidermis immediately below the granular layer[30] (Fig. 10-6). Consequently, the bulla is subcorneal. Because intact bullae are rare, small isolated foci of acantholysis may be all that are found. Parakeratosis is common, and the granular layer may be increased, especially in older lesions. A diffuse infiltrate of eosinophils and lymphocytes is present in the underlying dermis.

Differential Diagnosis

The pemphigus foliaceus pattern of transient acantholytic dermatosis may be virtually identical to pemphigus foliaceus. Direct immunofluorescence is required for accurate separation. A few acantholytic cells are common in bullous impetigo. Neutrophils are numerous and form a subcorneal pustule.

Pemphigus Erythematosus

Clinical Features

Pemphigus erythematosus combines the clinical findings of pemphigus foliaceus and lupus erythematosus. The typical presentation includes scaly, crusted plaques on the nose, cheeks, scalp, and upper trunk.[31–34] Individual lesions closely resemble those of pemphigus foliaceus. Bullae are rare. Serologic tests for lupus erythematosus, such as the antinuclear factor and the lupus band assay, may be positive, but patients rarely have other cutaneous or systemic findings of lupus.[1]

Histopathologic Features and Differential Diagnosis

The microscopic appearance of pemphigus erythematosus is indistinguishable from that of pemphigus foliaceus (Fig. 10-7). The two diseases cannot be reliably separated on the basis of histopathology alone; clinical and serologic data are needed.[31,32] No histologic features of lupus erythematosus, such as vacuolar interface change, are found.

Adjuncts to the Microscopic Diagnosis of Pemphigus

Fluid may be obtained from vesicles, bullae, or pustules and gently smeared onto a glass slide in the Tzanck preparation.[35,36] When stained with toluidine blue, methylene blue, or hematoxylin and eosin, groups of rounded, acantholytic cells are usually readily identified. The Tzanck preparation may be of value in differentiating the bullae of pemphigus vulgaris from bullous pemphigoid. However, cytologic evaluation alone does not help to define the level of acantholysis or to differentiate between the various intraepidermal acantholytic bullous diseases.

Direct and indirect immunofluorescence are essential in the assessment of lesions in which the histopathology suggests one of the above subtypes of pemphigus, because this group of acantholytic diseases is the only one with routinely positive intercellular staining.[37,38] Intercellular IgG deposits are invariably present in patients who have pemphigus. Nuclear or basement membrane staining may also be seen in pemphigus erythematosus.[39] Indirect immunofluorescence studies are essential to confirm the clinical and microscopic diagnosis of paraneoplastic pemphigus. Autoantibodies to desmoplakin I and desmoplakin II, bullous pemphigoid antigen, and, possibly, other antigens in the desmosomal complex are found in affected patients' sera.[18–20,40,41]

Figure 10-6. Pemphigus foliaceus. Acantholysis is confined to the upper levels of the epidermis leading to the formation of subcorneal bullae that are only rarely intact in histologic preparations. (× 200.)

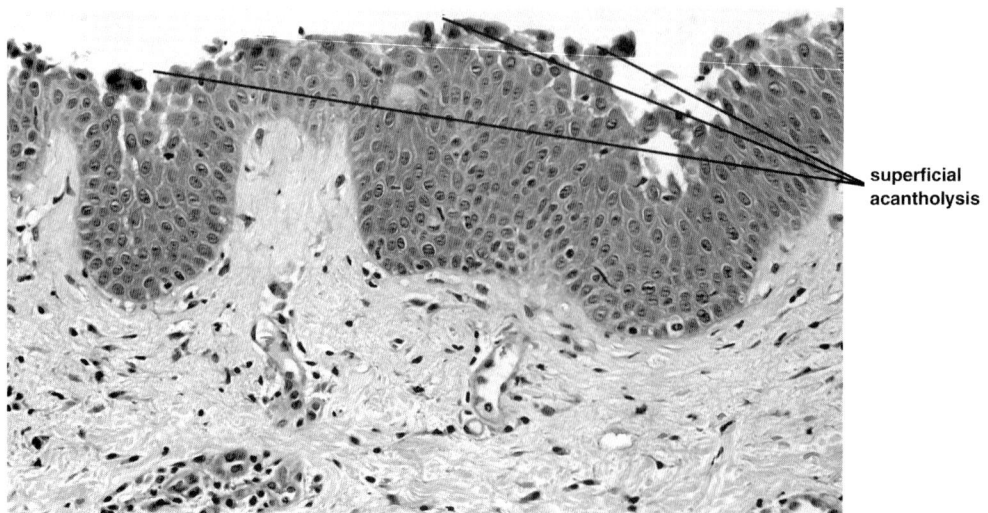

superficial
acantholysis

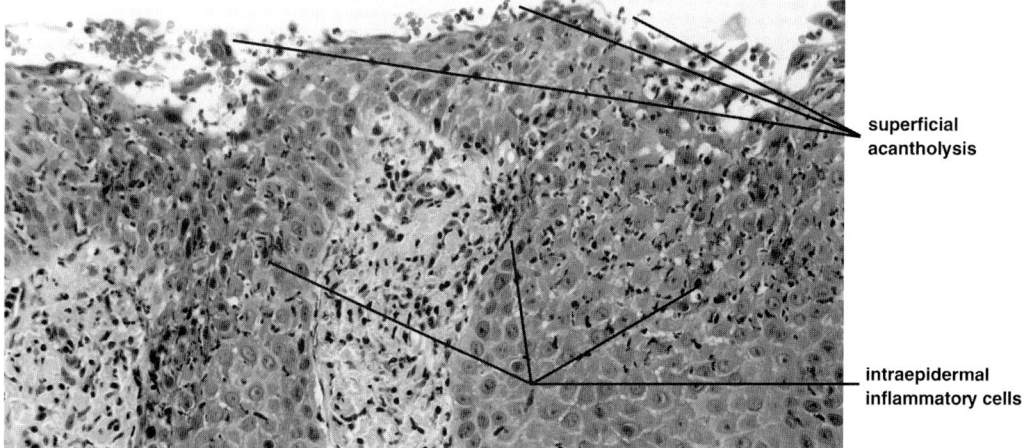

superficial
acantholysis

intraepidermal
inflammatory cells

Figure 10-7. Pemphigus erythematosus. The superficial acantholysis is indistinguishable from pemphigus foliaceus. (× 200.)

Transient Acantholytic Dermatosis (Grover's Disease)

Clinical Features

In most patients, transient acantholytic dermatosis is a relatively trivial eruption that occurs most commonly on the upper back and chest.[42,43] A zosteriform pattern has been reported.[44] The pinhead-sized, skin-colored or erythematous papules are slightly pruritic. In extensive cases, the papules are larger and the pruritus severe. The eruption is not invariably "transient." It may be persistent.[45] All five types of transient acantholytic dermatosis appear the same clinically.[43]

Histopathologic Features

Grover's disease has been divided into five histopathologic subtypes: (1) pemphigus vulgaris pattern (Fig. 10-8), (2) pemphigus foliaceus pattern (Fig. 10-9), (3) Hailey-Hailey pattern (Fig. 10-10), (4) Darier's pattern (Fig. 10-11) and (5) spongiotic pattern[46] (Fig. 10-12). The changes within the epidermis in each of these subtypes mimic the disease for which each is named. In most cases, the acantholysis is focal and limited. Inflammation ranges from minimal to dense diffuse lymphocytic infiltrates in the papillary and upper reticular dermis. Considerable overlap among the five subtypes is common.

Figure 10-8. Transient acantholytic dermatosis, pemphigus vulgaris subtype. Limited areas of basal and suprabasal acantholysis are present. (× 200.)

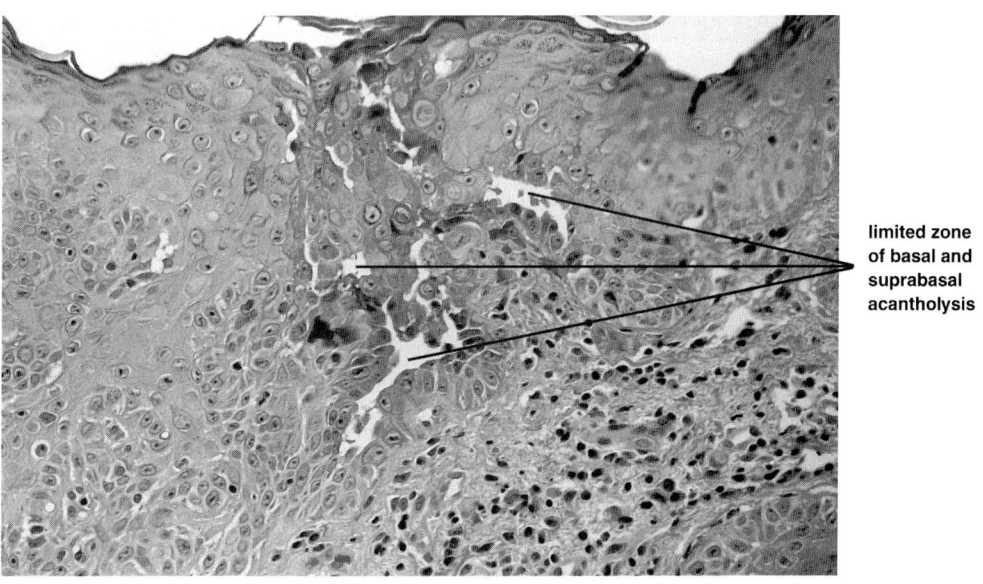

limited zone
of basal and
suprabasal
acantholysis

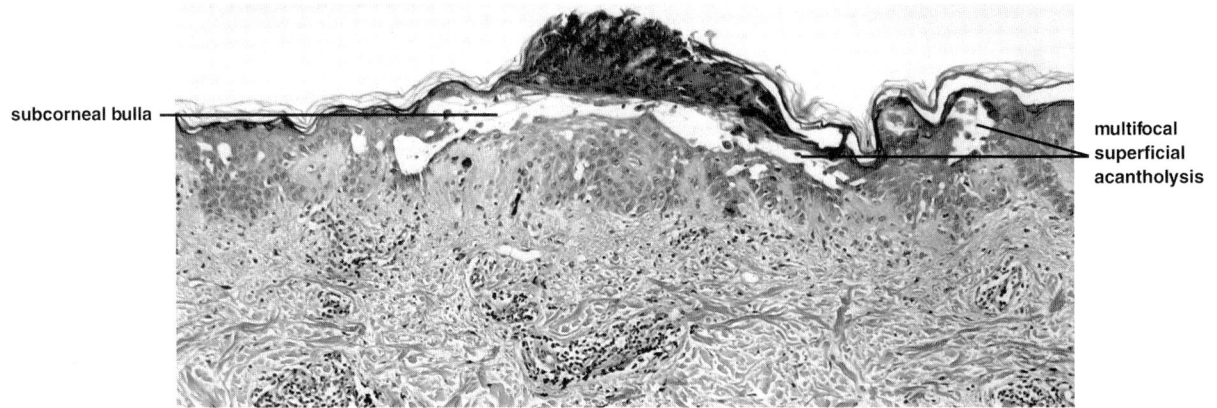

subcorneal bulla

multifocal superficial acantholysis

Figure 10-9. Transient acantholytic dermatosis, pemphigus foliaceus subtype. The acantholysis is limited and superficial. (× 80.)

Differential Diagnosis

Each subtype must be distinguished from the entity it is named for. In most instances transient acantholytic dermatosis tends to be limited in extent, whereas the other diseases are not. Clinical correlation can be helpful and is essential in some cases in which the changes are extensive. Pemphigus vulgaris and pemphigus foliaceus can be separated from transient acantholytic dermatosis by direct immunofluorescence examination, because the pemphigus pattern of immunoreactants (intercellular IgG) is not present in transient acantholytic dermatosis.[47] True benign familial pemphigus will have more extensive acantholy-

sis and keratosis follicularis will have more extensive dyskeratosis than their transient acantholytic dermatosis counterparts.

Benign Familial Pemphigus (Hailey-Hailey Disease)

Clinical Features

In contrast to transient acantholytic dermatosis, benign familial pemphigus is a potentially disabling dermatosis because of the presence of pruritic, oozing, foul-smelling, crusted, circinate plaques primarily localized to flexural surfaces such as the ax-

Figure 10-10. Transient acantholytic dermatosis, Hailey-Hailey subtype. Acantholysis is most prominent in the midepidermis, but is also present in the basal and suprabasal zones. (× 80.)

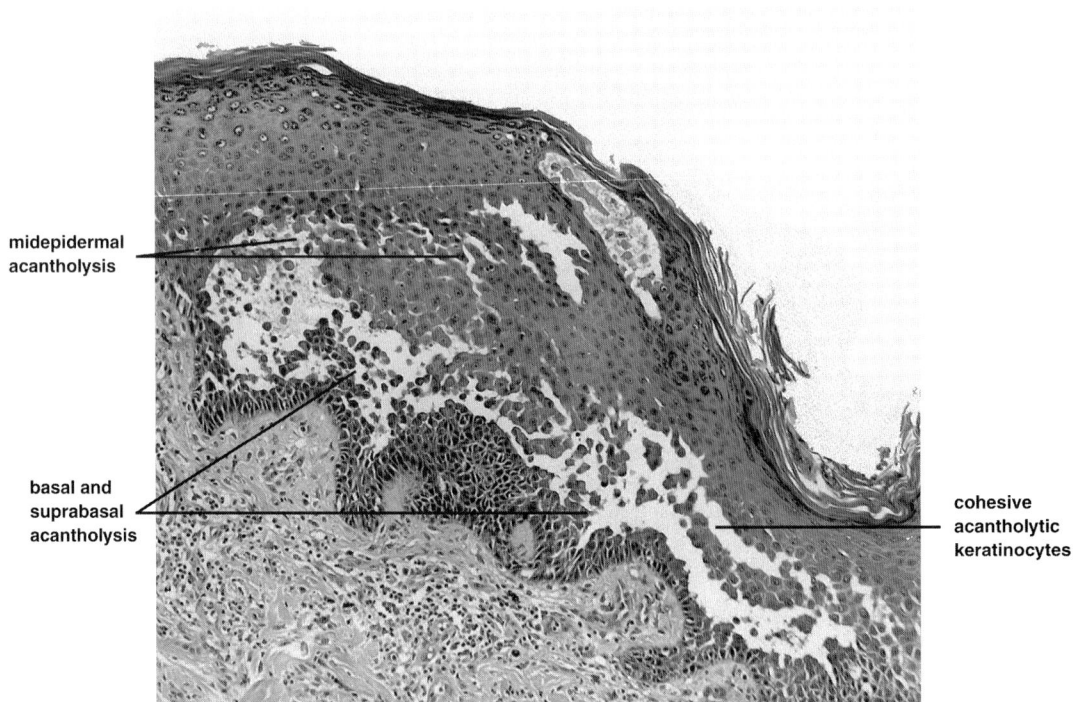

midepidermal acantholysis

basal and suprabasal acantholysis

cohesive acantholytic keratinocytes

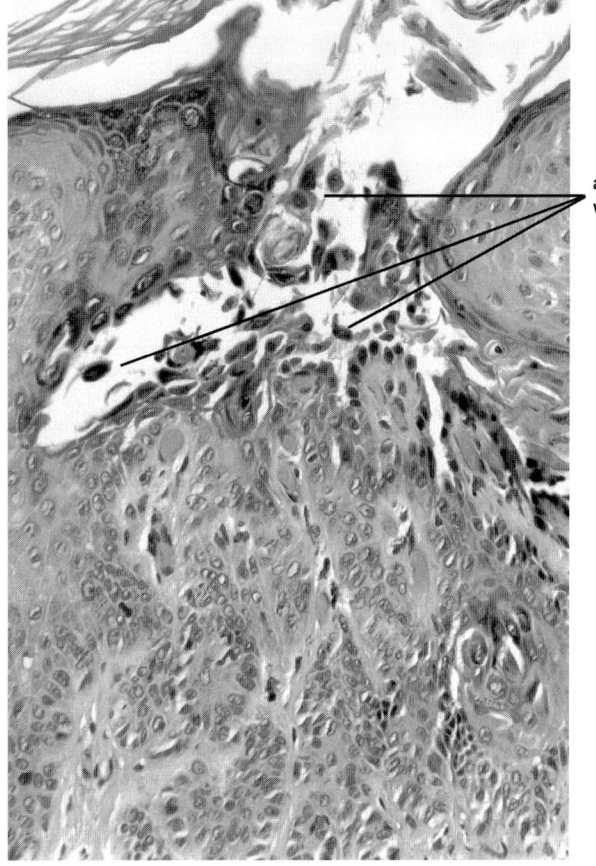

acantholytic keratinocytes
with prominent dyskeratosis

Figure 10-11. Transient acantholytic dermatosis, Darier's subtype. Dyskeratotic keratinocytes are present in addition to acantholytic cells. (× 80.)

illa and groin.[48] Vesicles may be discernible on the erythematous edges of the plaques. Although usually inherited as an autosomal dominant trait, some patients with benign mucosal pemphigus have no family history of the disease. Bacterial or mycotic superinfection (or both) are common. Trauma is suspected to play a role in the localization to flexural areas.

Histopathologic Features

Acantholytic cells extend through the full thickness of the epidermis from the basal cells to the granular layer to form an intraepidermal bulla[49,50] (Fig. 10-13). Observers have likened this change to a "dilapidated brick wall." The acantholytic cells fre-

Figure 10-12. Transient acantholytic dermatosis, spongiotic subtype. Acantholytic keratinocytes may be difficult to find. Spongiosis is multifocal. (× 200.)

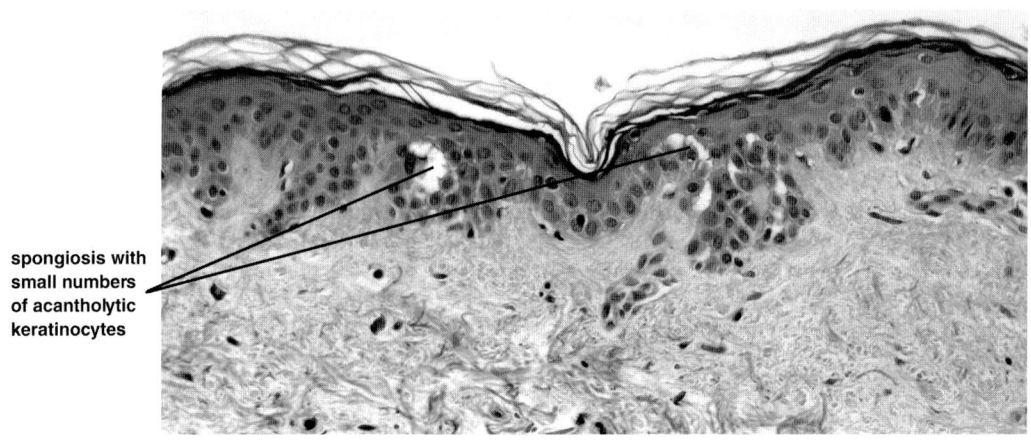

spongiosis with
small numbers
of acantholytic
keratinocytes

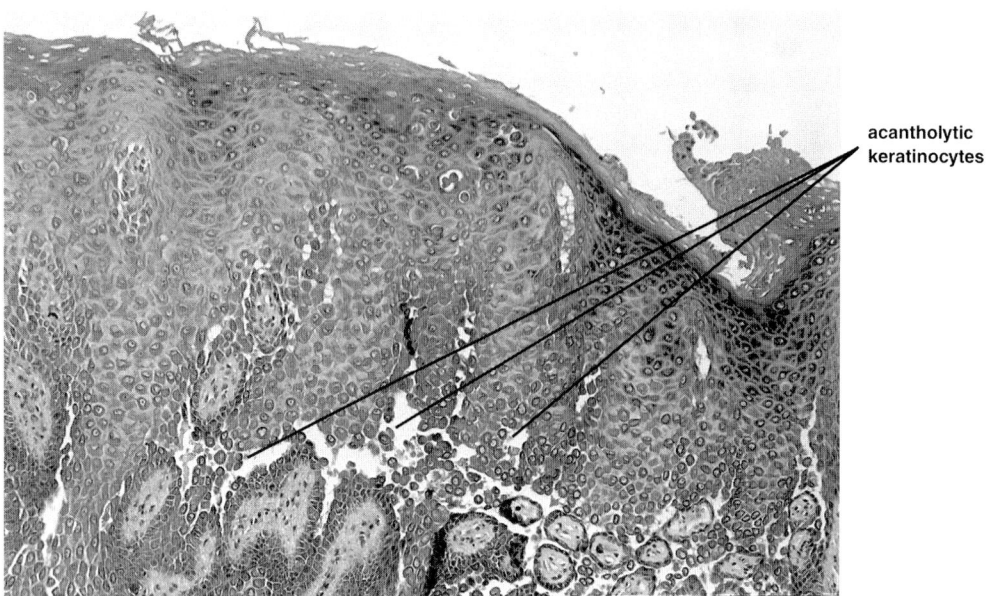

acantholytic
keratinocytes

Figure 10-15.   Papular acantholytic dyskeratosis of the genitalia. A dispersed zone of acantholysis is present in the lower to midepidermis. (× 80.)

Figure 10-16.   Herpesvirus infection. Giant, multinucleate keratinocytes with nuclei that have a ground-glass appearance and are molded together are characteristic of both herpes simplex and varicella-zoster infections. Numerous neutrophils are usually present. (× 200.)

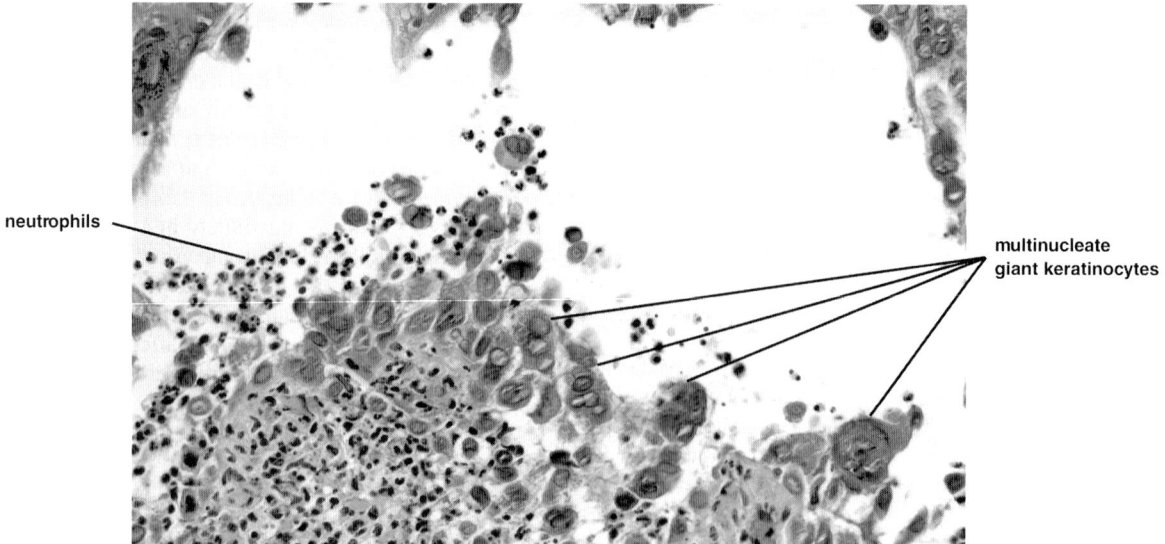

neutrophils

multinucleate
giant keratinocytes

When multinucleate, the nuclei appear to be molded together and have sharply faceted contours. Intranuclear eosinophilic inclusions may be present in some lesions, but are not required for diagnosis. The prominent acantholysis results in an intraepidermal bulla that eventually becomes filled with infected keratinocytes in various stages of degeneration.

Herpesvirus infection provokes an intense inflammatory response in immunocompetent persons within both the epidermis and the dermis. Leukocytoclastic vasculitis with subsequent epidermal and dermal necrosis may be present.[62,63] A destructive pustular folliculitis is common, especially in the beard area.[64] In immunosuppressed patients there may be minimal inflammation.[65]

Differential Diagnosis

Failure to recognize the diagnostic nuclear changes of herpesvirus infection can result in confusion with other intraepidermal acantholytic diseases, especially Darier's disease. In the latter disease prominent dyskeratosis may resemble herpesvirus-infected keratinocytes. The large viral inclusions of molluscum contagiosum, inclusion (myrmecial) warts, and orf/milkers' nodule can be confused with herpesvirus infection. The viral inclusions in all these infections are intracytoplasmic, not intranuclear. Multinucleation, so common in herpesvirus infection, is not present.

Adjuncts to the Diagnosis of Herpesvirus Infection

Cytologic evaluation of touch preparations (Tzanck smears) obtained from the blister fluid of either HSV or VZV lesions can be a useful adjunct in the rapid diagnosis of herpesvirus infection.[36,66–70] The best preparations are made from vesicles and pustules; crusts are rarely adequate. The blister fluid is allowed to dry on a glass slide and is then stained with any of a variety of quick-staining dyes such as toluidine blue, methylene blue, Giemsa, or Wright's. Keratinocytes infected with either virus demonstrate distinctive changes consisting of nuclear enlargement, homogenization of nucleoplasm, and multinucleation with molding of nuclear contours. The Tzanck smear is an economical, rapid, sensitive, and specific diagnostic test that can be a useful aid in the diagnosis of herpesvirus infection with only minimal interpretive experience.[67] Definitive diagnostic methods include viral culture and the polymerase chain reaction technique.[68,71,72]

Molluscum Contagiosum

Clinical Features

Molluscum contagiosum is a common poxvirus infection that presents as solitary or multiple waxy, skin-colored papules several millimeters in diameter. Common in childhood, they are also found in adults. Giant molluscum contagiosum up to several centimeters in diameter have been reported in patients with acquired immunodeficiency syndrome.[59,73,74]

Histopathologic Features

Cystic invaginations of the epidermis or follicular infundibulum are filled with acantholytic keratinocytes containing large basophilic and eosinophilic cytoplasmic viral inclusions[75,76] (Fig. 10-17). The easily recognized diagnostic inclusions eventually encompass the entire cell. Myriad molluscum bodies fill the epidermal invaginations in completely developed lesions. The adjacent granular layer is increased in thickness.

If the cystic epidermal invaginations or dilated infundibula rupture into the dermis, an intense inflammatory response ensues.[77] Antigenic stimulation can result in an infiltrate of large lymphocytes with prominent nuclei and even mitoses.

Figure 10-17. Molluscum contagiosum. Large basophilic and eosinophilic inclusion bodies are present within the cytoplasm of keratinocytes. Molluscum bodies are usually invaginated or cystic. (× 40.)

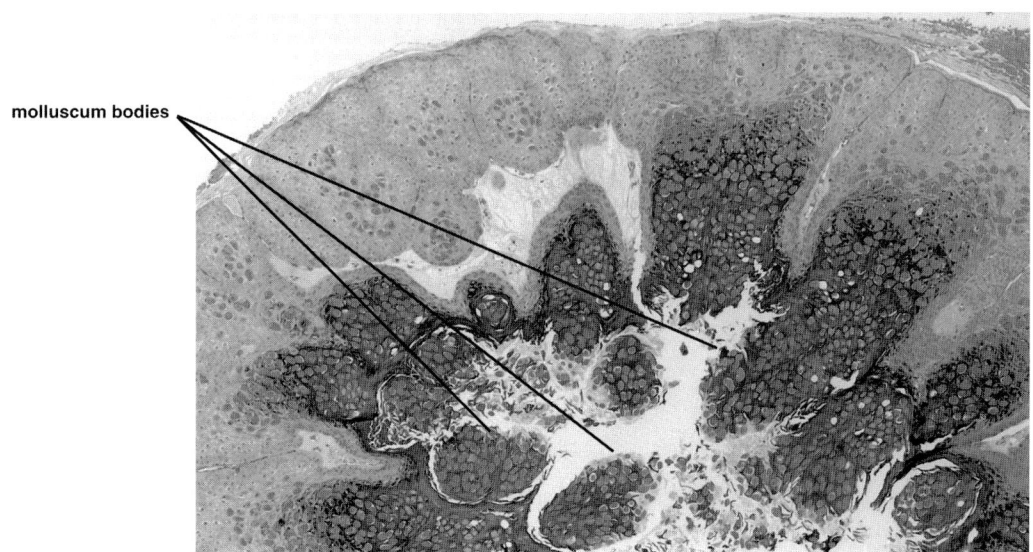

molluscum bodies

Differential Diagnosis

Myrmecial (inclusion) warts have similar large basophilic intracytoplasmic inclusions, but exophytic verrucous acanthosis is present rather than the cystic invaginations of molluscum contagiosum.[78] The viral changes of herpesvirus infection are intranuclear and rarely as prominent. If the molluscum bodies are inconspicuous, the dense lymphocytic infiltrate may simulate lymphoma, especially when many of these cells have large open nuclei and mitoses are numerous.[77]

Hand, Foot, and Mouth Disease

Clinical Features

A transient eruption of small discrete vesicles develops on the oral mucosa, palms, and soles in this Coxsackie virus infection.

Histopathologic Features

The early lesions are multilocular intraepidermal vesicles bounded by elongated keratinocytes with brightly eosinophilic cytoplasm (reticular degeneration)[79,80] (Fig. 10-18). No inclusions are found. In older lesions, the vesicles become subepidermal. Lymphocytic infiltrates are present in the superficial dermis beneath the vesicles.

Differential Diagnosis

Since the multilocular spongiotic vesicles of dyshidrotic eczema can closely mimic hand, foot, and mouth disease, the diagnostic reticular degeneration of keratinocytes must be differentiated from spongiosis.

Orf (Ecthyma Contagiosum) and Milkers' Nodule

Clinical Features

These parapoxvirus infections result in polymorphic lesions that are typically found on the fingers or hands of persons who have had contact with sheep (orf) or cows (milkers' nodule).[81–84] Early lesions are solitary vesicles; late ones are firm nodules.

Histopathologic Features

Multilocular, intraepidermal vesicles associated with eosinophilic cytoplasmic inclusions in keratinocytes are present in early lesions.[81–84] With time, the infected keratinocytes completely disintegrate. In the later stages, rete ridges proliferate downward where they are surrounded by a dense lymphocytic infiltrate.

Differential Diagnosis

In addition to the viral diseases discussed above, erythema multiforme can simulate orf or milkers' nodule. Extensive destruction of keratinocytes is common to both diseases, and the eosinophilic viral inclusions can be confused with the dyskeratotic keratinocytes of erythema multiforme.

Bullous Impetigo and Staphylococcal Scalded Skin Syndrome

Clinical Features

Golden- or honey-colored crusts with surrounding erythema occurring in combination with scattered pustules are characteristic of bullous impetigo. Staphylococci are the most common bacterial etiology of bullous impetigo, although streptococci are occasionally isolated. Bullous impetigo is most common in infants and children, but may also develop in adults, especially in persons with atopic dermatitis.[85] The staphylococcal scalded skin syndrome (Ritter's disease) is also more common in infants and children.[86] Infection with certain strains of staphylococci leads to the formation of large flaccid bullae that coalesce and quickly exfoliate as large sheets. The blisters and exfoliation are accompanied by fever.

Histopathologic Features

In both bullous impetigo and staphylococcal scalded skin syndrome the bullae are either subcorneal or intragranular. Numerous neutrophils are present along with few or many acantholytic keratinocytes.[85] Spongiosis and parakeratotic scale crust are also found in the adjacent epidermis (Fig. 10-19). In the staphylococcal scalded skin syndrome, a relative paucity of neutrophils are present within the epidermis.[86] The keratinocytes of the upper granular layer are usually completely necrotic, leading to a well-defined split in the epidermis in the middle of the granular layer.

Differential Diagnosis

Bullous impetigo can readily be confused with *Candida* infections; thus special stains may be of value in identifying the pseudohyphae and yeasts. Acantholysis is more pronounced in pemphigus foliaceus and fewer neutrophils are typically present.[87] The pustules of subcorneal pustular dermatosis are limited to the subcorneal epidermis alone and are usually much larger. Acantholytic keratinocytes are rare. The most important processes to differentiate from the staphylococcal scalded skin syndrome are toxic epidermal necrolysis and severe forms of erythema multiforme.[88] In the latter, the full thickness of the epidermis is completely or partially necrotic, whereas in the staphylococcal scalded skin syndrome the necrotic component is limited to the granular layer or higher. The subjacent keratinocytes are preserved.

NONACANTHOLYTIC INTRAEPIDERMAL PUSTULAR AND BULLOUS DISEASES

Necrolytic Migratory Erythema (Glucagonoma Syndrome)

Clinical Features

Patients with a glucagonoma may develop perioral, perineal, and acral vesicles and pustules that rupture to form weeping, scaling, circinate erythematous plaques and erosions.[89–95] Cyclical clearing and new vesicle formation results in rapid fluctuations in individual lesions. Cheilitis, stomatitis, and glossitis are common.

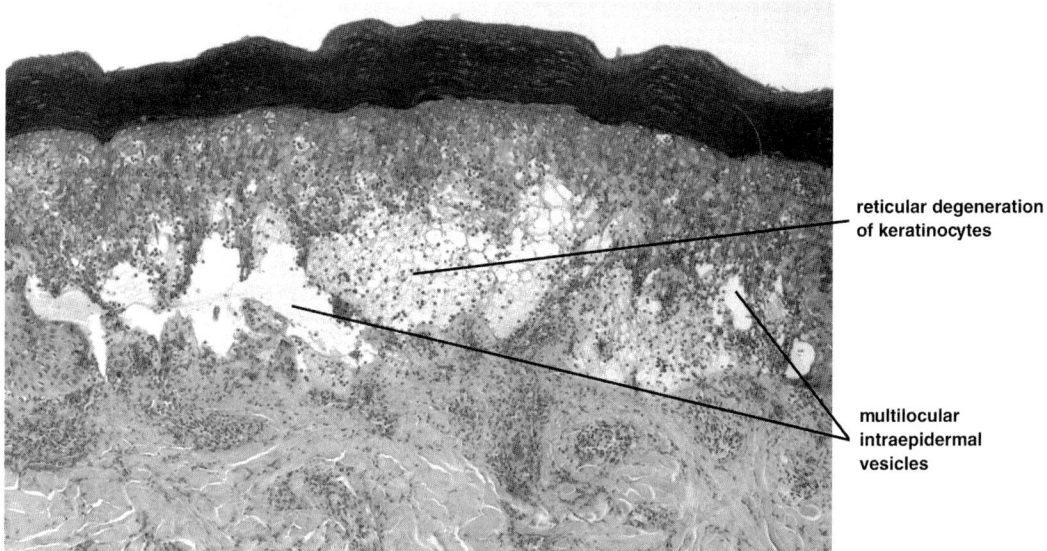

Figure 10-18. Hand, foot, and mouth disease. Reticular (net-like) degeneration of keratinocytes results in formation of multilocular intraepidermal vesicles. (× 40.)

Histopathologic Features

Zonal necrosis of the upper one-half or one-third of the epidermis is the characteristic feature of necrolytic migratory erythema.[89-93] The lower epidermis remains nearly normal. This peculiar change is best found in specimens taken from the periphery of a plaque. Intact bullae, when present, are subcorneal. *Necrolysis* refers to pale cytoplasmic staining, pyknotic nuclei, and loss of sharply defined cell outlines. Spongiosis surrounds the bulla and necrolytic areas. An influx

of neutrophils, sometimes massive, occurs in older plaques after the bullae rupture.

Differential Diagnosis

The superficial necrosis of the epidermis suggests an exogenous etiology such as freeze artifact or excoriation. Rarely, however, are the effects of physical trauma limited to the upper epidermis alone. The subcorneal bullae in pemphigus foliaceus and erythematosus are formed from acantholytic, not necrolytic, cells.

Figure 10-19. Bullous impetigo. Colonies of bacteria are embedded within parakeratotic stratum corneum and extravasated plasma. Karyorrhectic neutrophils are also present. The epidermis is spongiotic. (× 200.)

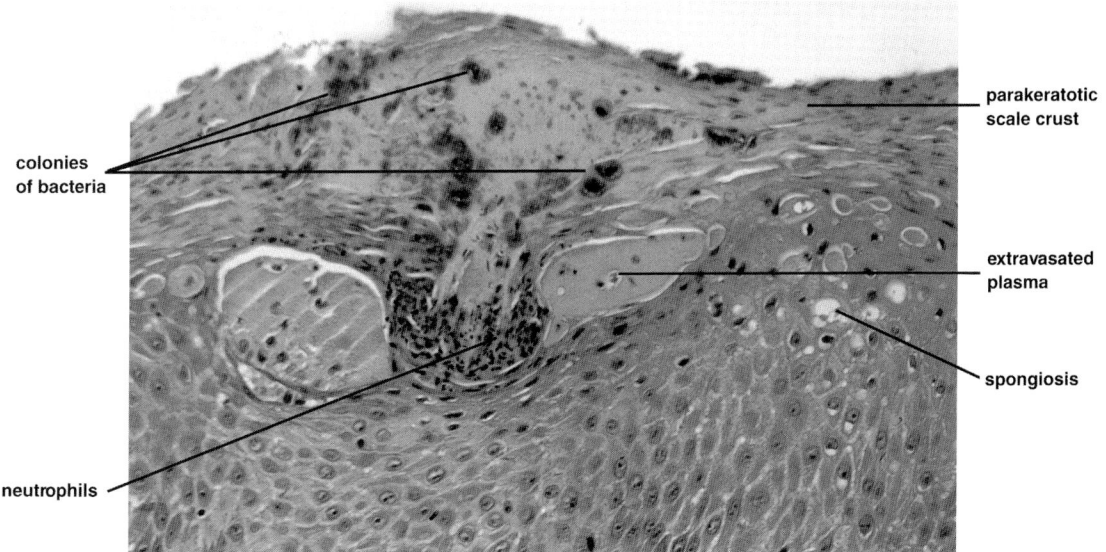

Subcorneal Pustular Dermatosis (Sneddon-Wilkinson Disease)

Clinical Features

The flaccid pustules of subcorneal pustular dermatosis typically occur in the groin or other body folds of middle-aged women.[96–98] The pustules range from several millimeters to several centimeters in diameter. A peculiar and distinctive finding is the tendency for pus to accumulate in the lower half of the pustule. The pustules easily rupture and leave behind coalescent, serpiginous erosions with a scaly edge and hyperpigmentation. The lesions are not pruritic. Similarities with pustular psoriasis exist, but subcorneal pustular dermatosis appears to be a separate, unrelated disease.[99] Subcorneal pustular dermatosis has been associated with a monoclonal gammopathy, most commonly an IgA paraprotein, and IgA-secreting myeloma.[100–102] Intercellular IgA may be present with direct immunofluorescence examination.[103] Subcorneal pustular dermatosis has also been reported to occur in association with Crohn's disease and Graves' disease.[104,105]

Histopathologic Features

A unilocular subcorneal pustule filled with neutrophils and rare eosinophils is the primary lesion of subcorneal pustular dermatosis (Fig. 10-20). Acantholytic cells are rare within the pustules. The granular layer beneath the pustule is at least partly intact, and the remainder of the epidermis is altered only by spongiosis and occasional neutrophils permeating through it. Sparse perivascular mixed neutrophilic and lymphocytic infiltrates are found in the papillary dermis.

Differential Diagnosis

Subcorneal pustular dermatosis may be confused with pustular psoriasis. In the latter, discrete collections of neutrophils, the so-called neutrophilic microabscesses of Kogoj and Monro, are small and scattered irregularly throughout the upper epidermis and the stratum corneum, respectively. The pustules of subcorneal pustular dermatosis are limited to the subcorneal epidermis alone and are usually much larger than the neutrophilic microabscesses of psoriasis.[96,97] The other characteristic findings of psoriasis, such as regular epidermal hyperplasia, apparent suprapapillary thinning of the epidermis, and uniform loss of the granular layer, are not present in subcorneal pustular dermatosis. The pustule of impetigo is found in a virtually identical location. Acantholytic keratinocytes are more abundant in impetigo. Although neutrophils are frequently present in the bullae of pemphigus foliaceus and pemphigus erythematosus, acantholytic keratinocytes are found in greater numbers. Neutrophils are less prominent and eosinophils are more conspicuous in these two types of pemphigus. Diagnostic yeast forms and nuclear changes are found in candidiasis and herpesvirus infection, respectively.

Erythema Toxicum Neonatorum

Clinical Features

Erythema toxicum neonatorum is a benign, but frequently alarming, pustular eruption in an otherwise healthy neonate. The pustules are usually not present at birth, but typically appear during the first week of life.[106–108] Individual pustules are 1 to 3 mm in diameter on a blotchy, erythematous base. Few or many pustules erupt in crops on the trunk, face, and limbs.

Figure 10-20. Subcorneal pustular dermatosis. The subcorneal neutrophilic pustule is characteristic. (× 80.)

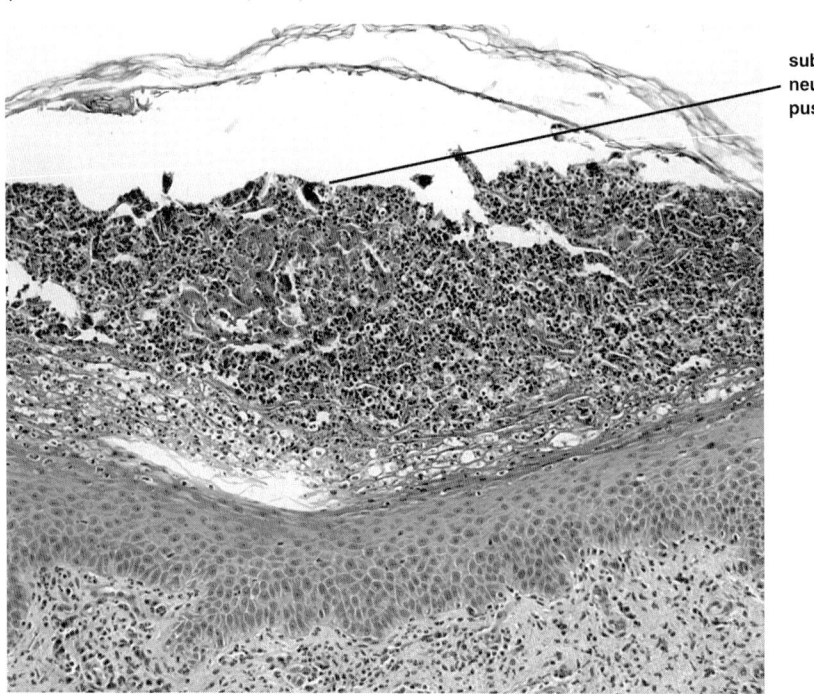

subcorneal
neutrophilic
pustule

Table 10-2. Infantile Vesiculobullous and Pustular Diseases

Name	Main Inflammatory Cell	Location of Vesicle/Pustule	Comment
Erythema toxicum neonatorum	Eosinophils	Early lesion in lower epidermis; late lesion is subcorneal	Adjacent to acrotrichium
Transient neonatal pustular melanosis	Neutrophils	Upper epidermis or subcorneal	Increased melanin pigment in basal keratinocytes in older lesions
Infantile acropustulosis	Neutrophils	Throughout the epidermis	Eosinophils may be present in the pustule
Miliaria crystallina	Rare neutrophils and lymphocytes	Intra- or subcorneal	Adjacent to acrosyringium
Candidiasis	Neutrophils	Any level of the epidermis	Yeasts and/or pseudohyphae present
Impetigo/bacterial sepsis	Neutrophils	Any level of the epidermis	Bacteria present
Herpesvirus infection	Neutrophils	Any location within the epidermis; frequently perifollicular	Homogenization and molding of nuclei; extensive necrosis of keratinocytes
Epidermolysis bullosa	None	Subepidermal	Ultrastructural examination or immunofluorescence required for definitive diagnosis

Histopathologic Features

The pustules are filled with eosinophils. The early lesions are found adjacent to the acrotrichium (the intraepidermal portion of the hair follicle) in the lower epidermis.[106] As the pustules age, they increase in size and move progressively higher within the epidermis so that the mature lesions are subcorneal. Eosinophils are present in the underlying papillary dermis in both a perivascular and a diffuse distribution. Table 10-2 summarizes the histopathologic features.

Differential Diagnosis

Erythema toxicum neonatorum must be differentiated from the first phase of incontinentia pigmenti, which also is characterized by numerous eosinophils within spongiotic epidermis. In incontinentia pigmenti, dyskeratotic keratinocytes are present, and the eosinophils are distributed throughout the epidermis, rather than being localized to discrete, perifollicular pustules as in erythema toxicum neonatorum. Disseminated candidiasis, bacterial sepsis, impetigo, and herpesvirus infection must always be considered in a pustular eruption in a neonate. Neutrophils, not eosinophils, predominate in these potentially serious diseases.

Transient Neonatal Pustular Melanosis

Clinical Features

In contrast to erythema toxicum neonatorum, the pustules of transient neonatal pustular melanosis are present at birth.[107–110] The pustules are the same size in both, but in transient neonatal pustular melanosis they do not occur on an erythematous base. As can be assumed by the name of the disorder, the asymptomatic pustules are transient. They erupt in crops, rupture in about 1 week, and leave residual fine scale and hyperpigmenta-

tion. Pustules are most common on the head, neck, trunk, palms, and soles. Transient neonatal pustular melanosis is more common in black infants.

Histopathologic Features

Numerous neutrophils are present both within the spongiotic epidermis and in discrete high epidermal or subcorneal pustules.[109] A rare eosinophil may be found in the pustules. Sparse infiltrates of neutrophils are evident in the papillary dermis. In older lesions, melanin pigment is increased in the cytoplasm of the basal keratinocytes. Table 10-2 summarizes the histopathologic features.

Differential Diagnosis

As in erythema toxicum neonatorum, candidal and bacterial sepsis and herpesvirus viremia must be in the differential diagnosis of transient neonatal pustular melanosis. Pustules secondary to bacterial sepsis or localized impetigo may be virtually identical to transient neonatal pustular melanosis. If present, acantholytic keratinocytes can help to separate these two diseases. If not, bacterial culture is necessary. Diagnostic yeast forms and nuclear changes are found in candidiasis and herpesvirus infection, respectively. Neutrophils are found in the pustules of transient neonatal pustular melanosis instead of the eosinophils of erythema toxicum neonatorum, but the composition of the pustules may change with the duration of the lesions.[111]

Infantile Acropustulosis

Clinical Features

The pustules of infantile acropustulosis resemble erythema toxicum neonatorum and transient neonatal pustular melanosis,

pustules and plaques: pemphigus vegetans, Hallopeau type. Arch Dermatol 123:393, 1987

16. Nelson CG, Apisarnthanarax P, Bean SF, Smith Y: Pemphigus vegetans of Hallopeau. Arch Dermatol 113:942–945, 1977

17. Anhalt GJ, Kim SC, Stanley JR et al: Paraneoplastic pemphigus: an autoimmune mucocutaneous disease associated with neoplasia. N Engl J Med 323:1729–1735, 1990

18. Horn TD, Anhalt GJ: Histologic features of paraneoplastic pemphigus. Arch Dermatol 128:1091–1095, 1992

19. Camisa C, Helm TN, Liu YC et al: Paraneoplastic pemphigus: a report of three cases including one long-term survivor. J Am Acad Dermatol 27:547–553, 1992

20. Mutasim DF, Pelc NJ, Anhalt GJ: Paraneoplastic pemphigus, pemphigus vulgaris, and pemphigus foliaceus. Clin Dermatol 11:113–117, 1993

21. Jansen T, Plewig G, Anhalt GJ: Paraneoplastic pemphigus with clinical features of erosive lichen planus associated with Castleman's tumor. Dermatology 190:245–250, 1995

22. Meyers SJ, Varley GA, Meisler DM et al: Conjunctival involvement in paraneoplastic pemphigus. Am J Ophthalmol 114:621–624, 1992

23. Stevens SR, Griffiths CE, Anhalt GJ, Cooper KD: Paraneoplastic pemphigus presenting as a lichen planus pemphigoides-like eruption [see comments]. Arch Dermatol 129:866–869, 1993

24. Perry HO, Brunsting LA: Pemphigus foliaceus. Arch Dermatol 91:10–23, 1965

25. Castro RM, Roscoe JT, Sampaio SA: Brazilian pemphigus foliaceus. Clin Dermatol 1:22–41, 1983

26. Diaz LA, Sampaio SA, Rivitti EA et al: Endemic pemphigus foliaceus (fogo selvagem). I. Clinical features and immunopathology. J Am Acad Dermatol 20:657–669, 1989

27. Goodyear HM, Abrahamson EL, Harper JI: Childhood pemphigus foliaceus. Clin Exp Dermatol 16:229–230, 1991

28. Iwatsuki K, Takigawa M, Hashimoto T et al: Can pemphigus vulgaris become pemphigus foliaceus? J Am Acad Dermatol 25:797–800, 1991

29. Kawana S, Hashimoto T, Nishikawa T, Nishiyama S: Changes in clinical features, histologic findings, and antigen profiles with development of pemphigus foliaceus from pemphigus vulgaris. Arch Dermatol 130:1534–1538, 1994

30. Furtado TA: Histopathology of pemphigus foliaceus. Arch Dermatol 80:66–71, 1959

31. Freiburger D: Pemphigus erythematosus. Arch Dermatol 104:449–450, 1971

32. Amerian ML, Ahmed AR: Pemphigus erythematosus: Senear-Usher syndrome. Int J Dermatol 24:16–25, 1985

33. Wieselthier JS, Treloar V, Koh HK et al: Multiple crusted plaques in a woman with systemic lupus erythematosus: pemphigus erythematosus (PE). Arch Dermatol 127:1572–1573, 1575–1576, 1991

34. Deloach-Banta LJ, Tenaro LJ: Superficial erosions with some oozing and marked crusting: pemphigus erythematosus (PE). Arch Dermatol 129:633, 636–637, 1993

35. Graham JH, Bingul O, Burgoon CB: Cytodiagnosis of inflammatory dermatoses. Arch Dermatol 87:118–127, 1963

36. Solomon AR: The Tzanck smear: viable and valuable in the diagnosis of herpes simplex, zoster, and varicella. Int J Dermatol 25:169–170, 1986

37. Izuno GT: Cutaneous immunofluorescence. Clin Lab Med 6:85–102, 1986

38. Fitzmaurice M: The immunopathology of pemphigus vulgaris: recent advances. Cleve Clin Q 53:283–289, 1986

39. Jablonska S, Chorzelski T, Blaszcyk M: Pathogenesis of pemphigus erythematosus. Arch Dermatol Res 258:135–140, 1977

40. Kanitakis J, Wang YZ, Roche P et al: Immunohistopathological study of autoimmune pemphigus: lack of strictly specific histological and indirect immunofluorescence criteria for paraneoplastic pemphigus. Dermatology 188:282–285, 1994

41. Helou J, Allbritton J, Anhalt GJ: Accuracy of indirect immunofluorescence testing in the diagnosis of paraneoplastic pemphigus. J Am Acad Dermatol 32:441–447, 1995

42. Grover RW, Duffy JL: Transient acantholytic dermatosis. J Cutan Pathol 2:111–127, 1975

43. Chalet M, Grover R, Ackerman AB: Transient acantholytic dermatosis. Arch Dermatol 113:431–435, 1977

44. Liss WA, Norins AL: Zosteriform transient acantholytic dermatosis. J Am Acad Dermatol 29:797–798, 1993

45. Mokni M, Aractingi S, Grossman R et al: Persistent acantholytic dermatosis: sex-related differences in clinical presentation? Acta Derm Venereol 73:69–71, 1993

46. Ackerman AB: Histologic Diagnosis of Inflammatory Skin Diseases. Lea & Febiger, Philadelphia, 1978

47. Bystryn JC: Immunofluorescence studies in transient acantholytic dermatosis (Grover's disease). Am J Dermatopathol 1:325–327, 1979

48. Winer LH, Leeb AJ: Benign familial pemphigus. Arch Dermatol 67:77–83, 1953

49. Wilkin JK: Chronic benign familial pemphigus. Arch Dermatol 114:136–138, 1978

50. Galimberti RL, Kowalczuk AM, Bianchi O et al: Chronic benign familial pemphigus. Int J Dermatol 27:495–500, 1988

51. Gottlieb SK, Lutzner MA: Darier's disease. Arch Dermatol 107:225–230, 1973

52. Deroo H, Van HE, Cuelenaere C, Kudsi S: Darier's disease—dyskeratosis follicularis. Dermatologica 180:191, 1990

53. Heymann WR: Warty dyskeratoma appearing in a patient with Darier's disease. Int J Dermatol 27:521–522, 1988

54. Duray PH, Merino MJ, Axiotis C: Warty dyskeratoma of the vulva. Int J Gynecol Pathol 2:286–293, 1983

55. Barrett JF, Murray LA, MacDonald HN: Darier's disease localized to the vulva: case report. Br J Obstet Gynaecol 96:997–999, 1989

56. Wong TY, Mihm MC, Jr: Acantholytic dermatosis localized to genitalia and crural areas of male patients: a report of three cases. J Cutan Pathol 21:27–32, 1994

57. Wong KT, Wong KK: A case of acantholytic dermatosis of the vulva with features of pemphigus vegetans. J Cutan Pathol 21:453–456, 1994

58. Siegal FP, Lopez C, Hammer GS: Severe acquired immunodeficiency in male homosexuals, manifested by chronic perianal ulcerative herpes simplex lesions. N Engl J Med 305:1439–1444, 1981

59. Berger TG, Obuch ML, Goldschmidt RH: Dermatologic manifestations of HIV infection. Am Fam Physician 41:1729–1742, 1990

60. Solomon AR, Rasmussen JE, Weiss JS: A comparison of the

Tzanck smear and viral isolation in varicella and herpes zoster. Arch Dermatol 122:282–285, 1986

61. McSorley J, Shapiro L, Brownstein MH: Herpes simplex and varicella-zoster: comparative histopathology of 77 cases. Int J Dermatol 13:69–75, 1974

62. Cohen C, Trapuckd S: Leukocytoclastic vasculitis associated with cutaneous infections by herpesvirus. Am J Dermatopathol 6:561–565, 1984

63. Langenberg A, Yen TS, LeBoit PE: Granulomatous vasculitis occurring after cutaneous herpes zoster despite absence of viral genome. J Am Acad Dermatol 24:429–433, 1991

64. Izumi AK, Kim R, Arnold H: Herpes sycosis. Arch Dermatol 106:372–374, 1972

65. Kaplan MH, Sadick N, McNutt NS: Dermatologic findings and manifestations of AIDS. J Am Acad Dermatol 16:485–506, 1987

66. Solomon AR, Rasmussen JE, Varani J, Pierson CL: The Tzanck smear in the diagnosis of cutaneous herpes simplex. JAMA 251:633–635, 1984

67. Grossman MC, Silvers DN: The Tzanck smear: can dermatologists accurately interpret it? J Am Acad Dermatol 27:403–405, 1992

68. Nahass GT, Goldstein BA, Zhu WY et al: Comparison of Tzanck smear, viral culture, and DNA diagnostic methods in detection of herpes simplex and varicella-zoster infection. JAMA 268:2541–2544, 1992

69. Tyring SK: Natural history of varicella zoster virus. Semin Dermatol 11:211–217, 1992

70. Cohen PR: Tests for detecting herpes simplex virus and varicella-zoster virus infections. Dermatol Clin 12:51–68, 1994

71. Nahass GT, Penneys NS, Leonardi CL: Analysis of the polymerase chain reaction in the detection of herpesvirus DNA from fixed and stained tissue sections. Arch Dermatol 131:805–808, 1995

72. Nahass GT, Mandel MJ, Cook S et al: Detection of herpes simplex and varicella-zoster infection from cutaneous lesions in different clinical stages with the polymerase chain reaction. J Am Acad Dermatol 32:730–733, 1995

73. Hughes WT, Parham DM: Molluscum contagiosum in children with cancer or acquired immunodeficiency syndrome. Pediatr Infect Dis J 10:152–156, 1991

74. Izu R, Manzano D, Gardeazabal J, Diaz-Perez JL: Giant molluscum contagiosum presenting as a tumor in an HIV-infected patient. Int J Dermatol 33:266–267, 1994

75. Ive FA: Follicular molluscum contagiosum. Br J Dermatol 113:493–495, 1985

76. Park SK, Lee JY, Kim YH et al: Molluscum contagiosum occurring in an epidermal cyst—report of 3 cases. J Dermatol 19:119–121, 1992

77. Henao M, Freeman RG: Inflammatory molluscum contagiosum. Arch Dermatol 90:479–482, 1964

78. Lyell A, Miles JAR: The myrmecia: a study of inclusion bodies in warts. BMJ 1:912–915, 1951

79. Fields JP, Mihm MC, Hellreich PD: Hand, foot, and mouth disease. Arch Dermatol 99:243–246, 1969

80. Thomas I, Janniger CK: Hand, foot, and mouth disease. Cutis 52:265–266, 1993

81. Johannessen JV, Krogh KH, Solberg J: Human orf. J Cutan Pathol 2:265–283, 1975

82. Leavell UW, Phillips JA: Milker's nodules. Arch Dermatol 111:1307–1311, 1975

83. Bassioukas K, Orfanidou A, Stergiopoulou CH, Hatzis J: Orf: clinical and epidemiological study. Australas J Dermatol 34:119–123, 1993

84. Amichai B, Grunwald MH, Abraham A, Halevy S: Tense bullous lesions on fingers: orf. Arch Dermatol 129:1043,1046, 1993

85. Elias PM, Levy SW: Bullous impetigo: occurrence of localized scalded skin syndrome in an adult. Arch Dermatol 112:856–858, 1976

86. Elias PM, Fritsch P, Epstein EH: Staphylococcal scalded skin syndrome. Arch Dermatol 113:207–219, 1977

87. Kouskoukis CE, Ackerman AB: What histologic finding distinguishes superficial pemphigus and bullous impetigo? Am J Dermatopathol 6:179–181, 1984

88. Amon RB, Dimond RL: Toxic epidermal necrolysis: rapid differentiation between staphylococcal and drug induced disease. Arch Dermatol 111:1433–1437, 1975

89. Myatt AE, Hargreaves GK: Necrolytic migratory erythema (glucagonoma syndrome). J R Soc Med 4:31–32, 1984

90. Parker CM, Hanke CW, Madura JA, Liss EC: Glucagonoma syndrome: case report and literature review. J Dermatol Surg Oncol 10:884–889, 1984

91. Skouge JW, Farmer ER: Papulosquamous eruption with weight loss: necrolytic migratory erythema (glucagonoma syndrome). Arch Dermatol 121:400, 1985

92. Vandersteen PR, Scheithauer BW: Glucagonoma syndrome: a clinicopathologic, immunocytochemical, and ultrastructural study. J Am Acad Dermatol 12:1032–1039, 1985

93. Rappersberger K, Wolff SE, Konrad K, Wolff K: [The glucagonoma syndrome.] Hautarzt 38:589–598, 1987

94. Chong LY, Lai CF, Woo CH et al: Necrolytic migratory erythema in glucagonoma syndrome. J Dermatol 19:369–374, 1992

95. Wynick D, Hammond PJ, Bloom SR: The glucagonoma syndrome. Clin Dermatol 11:93–97, 1993

96. Sneddon IB, Wilkinson DS: Subcorneal pustular dermatosis. Br J Dermatol 100:61–68, 1979

97. Murphy GM, Griffiths WA: Subcorneal pustular dermatosis. Clin Exp Dermatol 14:165–167, 1989

98. Boyd AS, Stroud MB: Vesiculopustules of the thighs and abdomen: subcorneal pustular dermatosis (Sneddon-Wilkinson disease). Arch Dermatol 127:1571, 1574, 1991

99. Sanchez NP, Perry HO, Muller SA, Winkelmann RK: Subcorneal pustular dermatosis and pustular psoriasis: a clinicopathologic correlation. Arch Dermatol 119:715–721, 1983

100. Dal TR, Di VF, Salvi F: Subcorneal pustular dermatosis and IgA myeloma. Dermatologica 170:240–243, 1985

101. Kasha EEJ, Epinette WW: Subcorneal pustular dermatosis (Sneddon-Wilkinson disease) in association with a monoclonal IgA gammopathy: a report and review of the literature. J Am Acad Dermatol 19:854–858, 1988

102. Bolcskei L, Husz S, Hunyadi J et al: Subcorneal pustular dermatosis and IgA multiple myeloma. J Dermatol 19:626–628, 1992

103. Wallach D: Intraepidermal IgA pustulosis. J Am Acad Dermatol 27:993–1000, 1992

104. Delaporte E, Colombel JF, Nguyen-Mailfer C et al: Subcorneal pustular dermatosis in a patient with Crohn's disease. Acta Derm Venereol 72:301–302, 1992

105. Taniguchi S, Tsuruta D, Kutsuna H, Hamada T: Subcorneal pustular dermatosis in a patient with hyperthyroidism. Dermatology 190:64–66, 1995

106. Freeman RG, Spiller R, Knox JM: Histopathology of erythema toxicum neonatorum. Arch Dermatol 82:586–589, 1960

107. Hansen LP, Brandrup F, Zori R: [Erythema toxicum neonatorum with pustulation versus transient neonatal pustular melanosis.] Hautarzt 36:475–477, 1985

108. Leung AK: Erythema toxicum neonatorum present at birth. J Singapore Paediatr Soc 28:163–166, 1986

109. Barr RJ, Globerman LM, Werber FA: Transient neonatal pustular melanosis. Int J Dermatol 18:636–638, 1979

110. Laude TA: Approach to dermatologic disorders in black children. Semin Dermatol 14:15–20, 1995

111. Ferrandiz C, Coroleu W, Ribera M et al: Sterile transient neonatal pustulosis is a precocious form of erythema toxicum neonatorum. Dermatology 185:18–22, 1992

112. Newton JA, Salisbury J, Marsden A, McGibbon DH: Acropustulosis of infancy. Br J Dermatol 115:735–739, 1986

113. Kahana M, Schewach MM, Feinstein A: Infantile acropustulosis—report of a case. Clin Exp Dermatol 12:291–292, 1987

114. Klein CE, Weber L, Kaufmann R: [Infantile acropustulosis.] Hautarzt 40:501–503, 1989

115. Dromy R, Raz A, Metzker A: Infantile acropustulosis. Pediatr Dermatol 8:284–287, 1991

116. Vignon PMD, Wallach D: Infantile acropustulosis: clinicopathologic study of six cases. Arch Dermatol 122:1155–1160, 1986

117. Straka BF, Cooper PH, Greer KE: Congenital miliaria crystallina. Cutis 47:103–106, 1991

118. Arpey CJ, Nagashima-Whalen LS, Chren MM, Zaim MT: Congenital miliaria crystallina: case report and literature review. Pediatr Dermatol 9:283–287, 1992

119. Feng E, Janniger CK: Miliaria. Cutis 55:213–216, 1995

120. Sulzberger MB, Cortese TA, Fishman L, Smith A: Studies on blisters produced by friction. J Invest Dermatol 47:456–465, 1966

121. Foley FD: Pathology of cutaneous burns. Surg Clin North Am 50:1200–1210, 1970

122. Winer LH, Levin GH: Changes in the skin as a result of electric current. Arch Dermatol 78:386–390, 1958

123. Burge SM, Bristol M, Millard PR, Dawber RP: Pigment changes in human skin after cryotherapy. Cryobiology 23:422–432, 1986

11

SUBEPIDERMAL VESICULOBULLOUS DISEASES

Walter H.C. Burgdorf

The evaluation of subepidermal blisters is based on an understanding of the dermoepidermal junction or epidermal basement membrane zone (BMZ) (Fig. 11-1). Figure 11-1 only includes an arbitrarily selected portion of the many antigens identified in the BMZ. The structure of the BMZ has been reviewed extensively[1–5] and we do not attempt to document the many individual contributions.

In simplest terms, the keratin intermediate filaments, primarily those of keratins 5 and 14, attach to the hemidesmosomes, which contain plectin, bullous pemphigoid antigen 1 (BPAG 1), bullous pemphigoid antigen 2 (BPAG 2), and integrin $\alpha6\beta4$. Extending from the hemidesmosomes through the lamina lucida to the lamina densa are the anchoring filaments; antigens associated with them include laminin 1, laminin 5, laminin 6, and uncein. Nidogen helps to attach laminin 1 to the lamina densa, which is comprised primarily of type IV collagen and perlecan. The anchoring fibrils composed of type VII collagen anchor the lamina densa to the dermis. Table 11-1 gives some of the alternate names for these structural elements.

Study of this region has undergone a number of changes as new techniques have become available. Light microscopy alone seldom allows a specific diagnosis; even when a blister is identified, its exact level and associated disease are difficult to determine. Both Achilles Civatte during World War II and Walter Lever a decade later employed light microscopy to separate pemphigus from dermatitis herpetiformis and bullous pemphigoid based primarily on the presence of acantholysis in the former. In the mid-1960s, Jordon, Beutner and colleagues introduced immunofluorescent examination, both direct and indirect, to more accurately define diseases such as pemphigus vulgaris and bullous pemphigoid. Electron microscopy was used to identify the major divisions of the BMZ—the lamina lucida, lamina densa, and sublamina densa zones. Many forms of epidermolysis bullosa are still defined at least in part by electron microscopic findings. Immunoelectron microscopy made it possible to more accurately identify the site of deposition of immunoreactants.

Several modifications of the above techniques have proven highly useful. When normal human epidermis is exposed to a 1 M NaCl solution, separation occurs in the lamina lucida and various antigens are made more accessible. Thus, indirect immunofluorescent examination using salt split skin allows one to map the epidermolysis bullosa acquista antigen (type VII collagen) to the base of the separation and the bullous pemphigoid antigens to the top. Some laboratories now routinely use salt split skin for indirect immunofluorescent examination.[6] The same technique can be used for direct immunofluorescent testing, as the patient's tissue is incubated in the salt solution.

Immunomapping is another valuable tool. If a panel of antibodies is used, such as antibodies to a bullous pemphigoid antigen, laminins, and type IV collagen, the level of separation can be mapped as discussed under epidermolysis bullosa. In the past few years, the use of a wide variety of molecular genetic techniques, including immunoblotting, gene sequencing, protein analysis, and creation of partial antigenic epitopes, have allowed an even more accurate understanding of the dermoepidermal junction and its associated diseases. Structures that are damaged in acquired blistering diseases have also been shown to be the site of mutations in inherited blistering disorders such as epidermolysis bullosa. For example, patients with one type of cicatricial pemphigoid have antibodies against laminin 5, while mutations in the same molecule cause the Herlitz or letalis form of junctional epidermolysis bullosa. Table 11-2 shows some of these associations.

The pathogenesis of the blistering diseases has remained harder to elucidate. Even though intuitively one assumes that the autoantibodies are causing disease, they could just as easily reflect another process; for example, inflammation or trauma, such as a burn, could expose or alter normal proteins, making them more antigenic and resulting in autoantibodies. Since in most instances simply injecting the autoantibodies into an experimental animal does not reproduce disease, a wide variety of tricks have been employed to create disease models, such as producing antibodies in one species of laboratory animal and transferring them to another or immunizing an animal with an epitope of a suspected antigen.

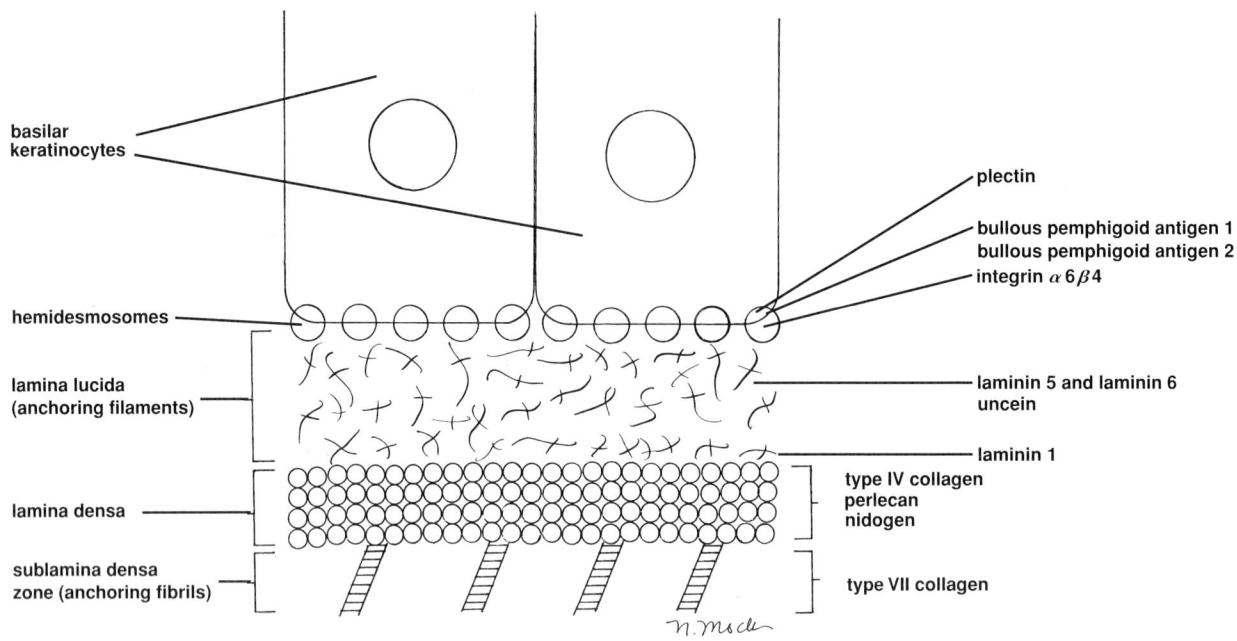

Figure 11-1. Chemical constituents of the epidermal basement membrane zone. (Courtesy of Stephen I. Katz, M.D, Ph.D., and Kim B. Yancey, M.D., Bethesda, MD.)

Table 11-1. Alternative Terms for Components of the Epidermal Basement Membrane Zone

Accepted Name	Synonyms
Plectin	HD 1
Bullous pemphigoid antigen 2 (BPAG 2)	Type XVII collagen
Uncein	19-DEJ-1
Laminin 5	Nicein, kalinin, GB3, epiligrin
Laminin 6	K-laminin
Nidogen	Entactin
Perlecan	Heparan sulfate proteoglycan
Type VII collagen	Epidermolysis bullosa acquisita antigen

Table 11-2. Acquired and Inherited Diseases Associated with Various Components of the Epidermal Basement Membrane Zone

Antigen	Autoantibodies	Inherited Defects
Keratins 5, 14		EB simplex
Plectin		EB with neuromuscular disorder
BPAG 1	Bullous pemphigoid, herpes gestationis	
BPAG 2	Bullous pemphigoid, herpes gestationis, cicatricial pemphigoid	Generalized atrophic benign (junctional) EB
Integrin $\alpha6\beta4$		Junctional EB with pyloric atresia
Laminin 5	Cicatricial pemphigoid	Junctional EB Herlitz type
Type VII collagen	EB acquisita, porphyria cutanea tarda, bullous eruption of systemic lupus erythematosus	Dystrophic EB

Abbreviation: EB, epidermolysis bullosa.

Most patients with blistering disorders are initially evaluated with traditional tools: clinical examination, routine light microscopy and direct and indirect immunofluorescent examinations. However, when cases are clinically atypical, reveal conflicting histologic or immunofluorescent results, or fail to respond to therapy, advanced techniques should be employed, most often at specialized centers.

The field of subepidermal blistering diseases is changing so fast that what we write (in 1997) will be out of date by the time it is read. The reader must thus depend on the current literature for guidance. We attempt to address the light microscopy and suggest how direct and indirect immunofluorescent techniques are employed, as well as briefly discuss the current understanding of the molecular aspects of the disease. While most readers will have access to electron microscopy, we have not emphasized this approach because often one is dealing with an extremely rare disorder where considerable experience is required to interpret even technically perfect images. Finally, new antigens and thus new diseases are continuously being reported[7]; we have restricted ourselves to the clinically established disorders. From a clinical perspective, five major types of subepidermal blistering disorders occur:

1. Large blisters often on an urticarial base
   Bullous pemphigoid
   Epidermolysis bullosa acquisita
   Chronic bullous disease of childhood
   Linear IgA disease
   Herpes gestationis
   Erythema multiforme

2. Multiple small pruritic blisters, often grouped
   Dermatitis herpetiformis
   Vesicular bullous pemphigoid
   Linear IgA disease
   Bullous eruption of systemic lupus erythematosus

3. Large relatively uninflamed blisters
   Epidermolysis bullosa
   Epidermolysis bullosa acquisita
   Bullous pemphigoid
   Bullous disease of diabetes
   Porphyria cutanea tarda
   Traumatic blisters (burns, suction, hypoxia, gangrene, autolysis)

4. Fragile sun-exposed skin, uninflamed blisters, milia
   Porphyria cutanea tarda
   Epidermolysis bullosa acquisita
   Bullous disease of dialysis
   Drug-induced pseudoporphyria

5. Mucosal blisters
   Cicatricial pemphigoid
   Bullous pemphigoid
   Linear IgA disease
   Epidermolysis bullosa acquisita
   Lupus erythematosus

The histopathologic diagnostic approach may be difficult. Farmer[8] has suggested an approach incorporating the type of inflammatory cell and the presence or absence of epidermal necrosis. Unfortunately, as blisters evolve, the predominant inflammatory cell may change. Similarly, older blisters often show necrosis. We recommend combining the clinical history and light microscopic appearance to suggest a working diagnosis, which usually should be confirmed by direct immunofluorescent examination.[9] That experienced dermatologists for generations were unable to accurately separate the various subepidermal blistering diseases without immunofluorescent studies supports this approach. Figure 11-2 shows an algorithmic plan.

A further complication is that several disorders considered elsewhere in the text can present clinically or histologically as subepidermal blisters because of inflammation, edema, or deposition in the BMZ. Included in this group are

Lichen planus
Urticaria
Erysipelas
Mast cell disease
Insect bite reactions
Polymorphic light eruption
Lichen sclerosus et atrophicus
Bullous amyloidosus

With these complexities in mind, we can now consider the individual subepidermal blistering diseases.

BULLOUS PEMPHIGOID

Bullous pemphigoid is a subepidermal blistering disorder characterized by large tense blisters with deposition of immunoreactants at the BMZ.[10,11]

Clinical Features

Bullous pemphigoid is most commonly a disease of the elderly; nonetheless, a number of cases in children have been documented.[12] It typically begins as an urticarial eruption that evolves into large blisters. Cases may be misdiagnosed as bullous impetigo early in their course. The bullae are most often generalized. Mucosal involvement is far less common than in pemphigus vulgaris and is rarely a presenting sign or major complaint. The individual lesion of bullous pemphigoid is usually a large tense blister that arises on an erythematous urticarial base or on normal skin. To some extent, the former lesions correspond to cell-rich bullous pemphigoid and the latter to cell-poor bullous pemphigoid. The blisters usually heal without scarring. Most patients have some itching; rarely, bullous pemphigoid patients may present with pruritus. Some reports suggest that bullous pemphigoid can be associated with internal malignancies; however, most studies in which the disease was defined immunologically and appropriate age-matched controls were included do not show bullous pemphigoid as a tumor marker.[13]

There are several clinical variants of bullous pemphigoid.[14]

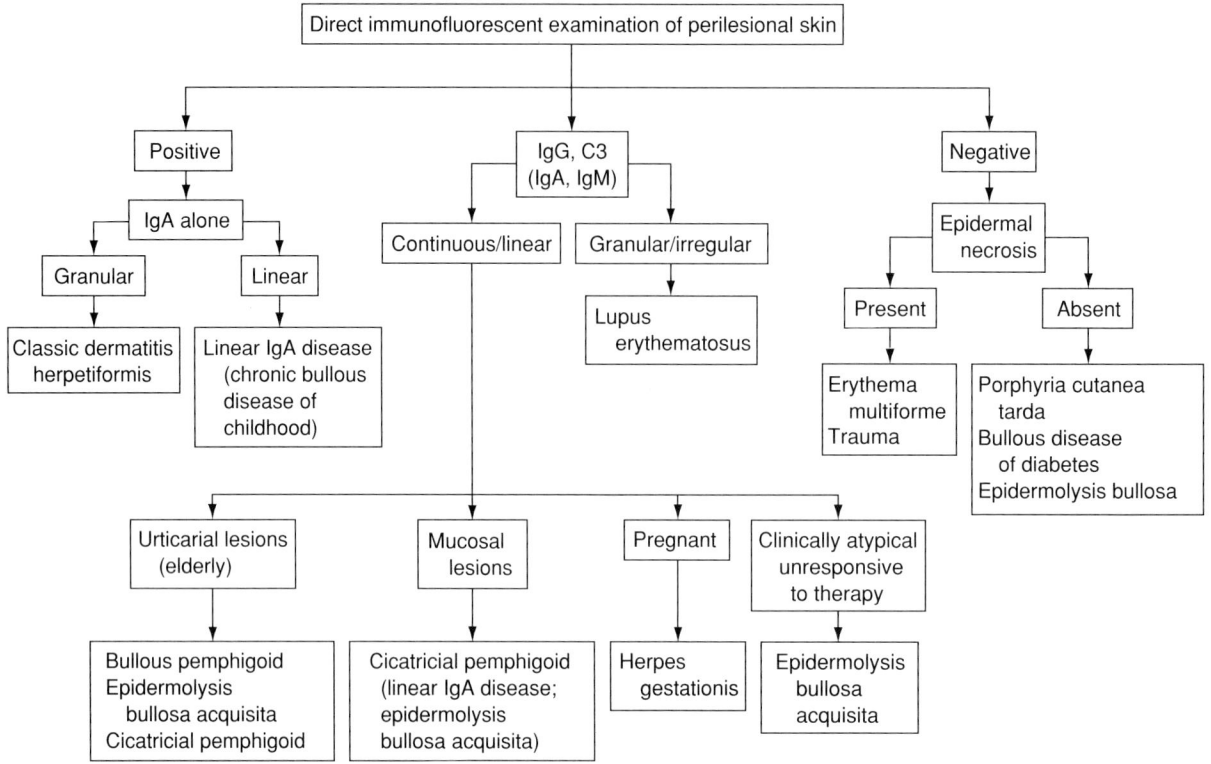

Figure 11-2. Evaluation of subepidermal blisters.

They include

1. *Urticarial bullous pemphigoid*: most bullous pemphigoid patients have urticarial lesions. Sometimes, most often early in the disease, only urticarial lesions are present.
2. *Vesicular bullous pemphigoid or polymorphic bullous pemphigoid*: these patients with tiny grouped vesicles resemble patients with dermatitis herpetiformis but differ histologically and immunopathologically from the latter.
3. *Localized bullous pemphigoid*: blisters are confined to one area of the body, usually the legs. They are nonscarring in contrast to localized cicatricial pemphigoid (Brunsting-Perry pemphigoid), which is usually on the head and neck. Localized bullous pemphigoid may remain so or progress to more generalized involvement.
4. *Vegetating bullous pemphigoid*: rarely pemphigoid may evolve into vegetating lesions in the groin and axillae, analogous to pemphigus vegetans.
5. *Prurigo nodularis bullous pemphigoid*: patients present with prurigo nodularis, but may have associated bullae.[15]
6. *Lichen planus pemphigoides*: some patients with lichen planus develop large blisters on clinically normal skin. This phenomenon, lichen planus pemphigoides, is considered an overlap between bullous pemphigoid and lichen planus. Its exact nature remains unclear.[16]

All these variants are identified by immunofluorescent examination as bullous pemphigoid; they are difficult to diagnose on clinical grounds alone. Thus the dermatopathologist must be alert to possible signs of subepidermal separation even when the submitting diagnosis does not mention the possibility of a blistering disorder.

Histopathologic Features

The typical bullous pemphigoid lesion is a subepidermal blister with little epidermal damage and a relatively cell-rich dermal inflammatory infiltrate dominated by eosinophils with few neutrophils (Fig. 11-3). The blister cavity contains fibrin and inflammatory cells, usually eosinophils. Adjacent skin or early lesions may show exocytosis of eosinophils (eosinophilic spongiosis) or basal cell vacuolization. The nature of the infiltrate varies between patients and in a given patient over time. Sometimes the infiltrate is dominated by neutrophils but usually without microabscesses in the adjacent papillae. In other cases, mononuclear cells are prominent. The dermal papillae are often edematous but usually well preserved (Figs. 11-4 and 11-5). Perivascular inflammation is common, but vasculitis is not. Epidermal necrosis is uncommon except in older lesions. Occasionally these older lesions can mimic intraepidermal separation as the blister base regenerates. Thus it is best to sample the edge of an early blister. Sometimes an urticarial lesion will not show a blister but instead have intense eosinophilic inflammation and high dermal edema that mimic urticaria.[17]

Direct immunofluorescent examination remains the standard way to confirm the diagnosis of bullous pemphigoid. Perilesional skin should be biopsied; there is a higher yield if a specimen from the legs is not used.[18] If a blistered area is biopsied,

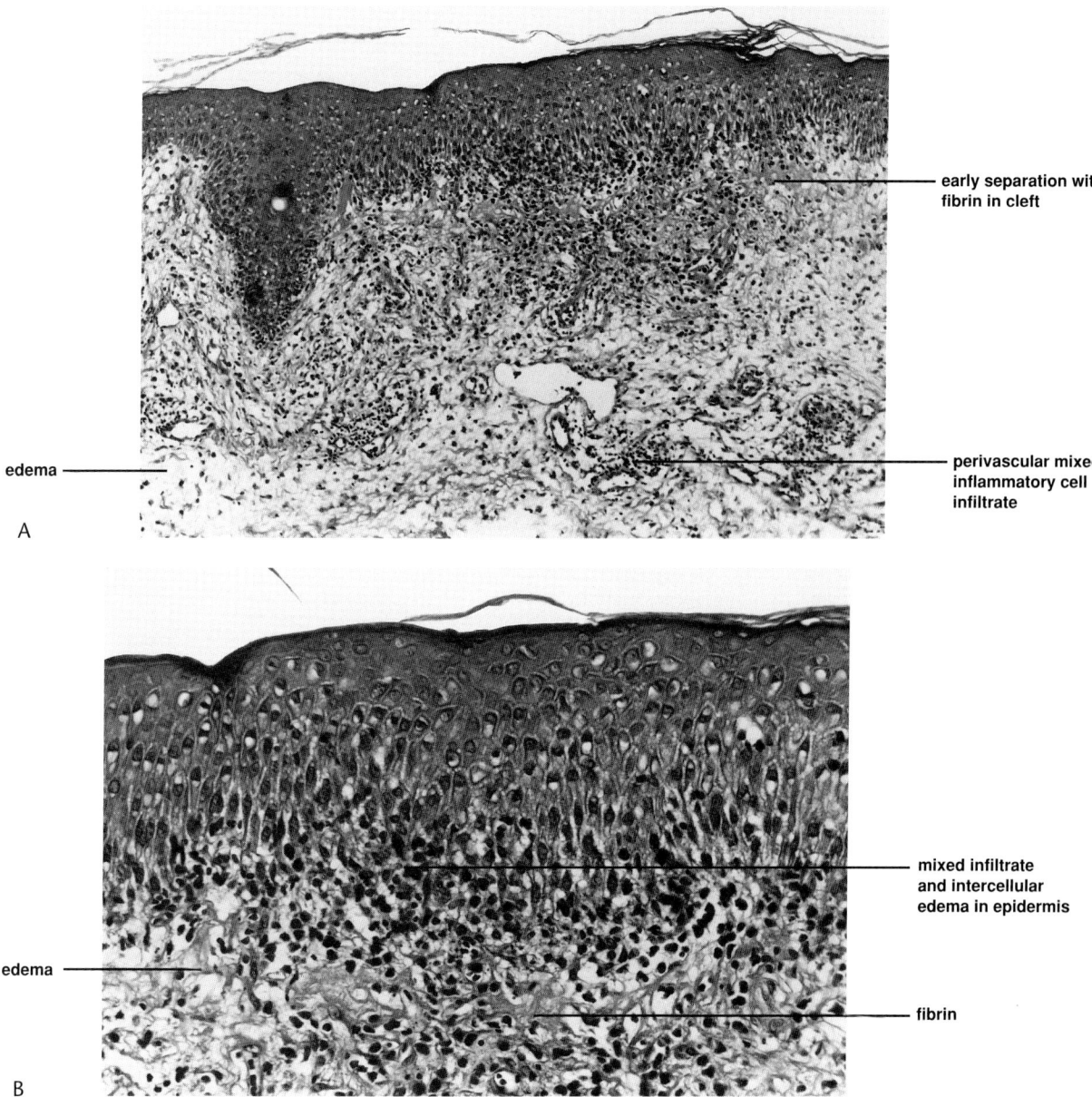

edema ——

A

early separation with
fibrin in cleft

perivascular mixed
inflammatory cell
infiltrate

edema ——

B

mixed infiltrate
and intercellular
edema in epidermis

fibrin

Figure 11-3. Bullous pemphigoid. (**A**) This early inflammatory lesion shows minimal separation at the dermoepidermal junction, but an intense mixed infiltrate is present in the papillary and upper reticular dermis. (**B**) Higher power view showing a mixed inflammatory infiltrate at the dermoepidermal junction.

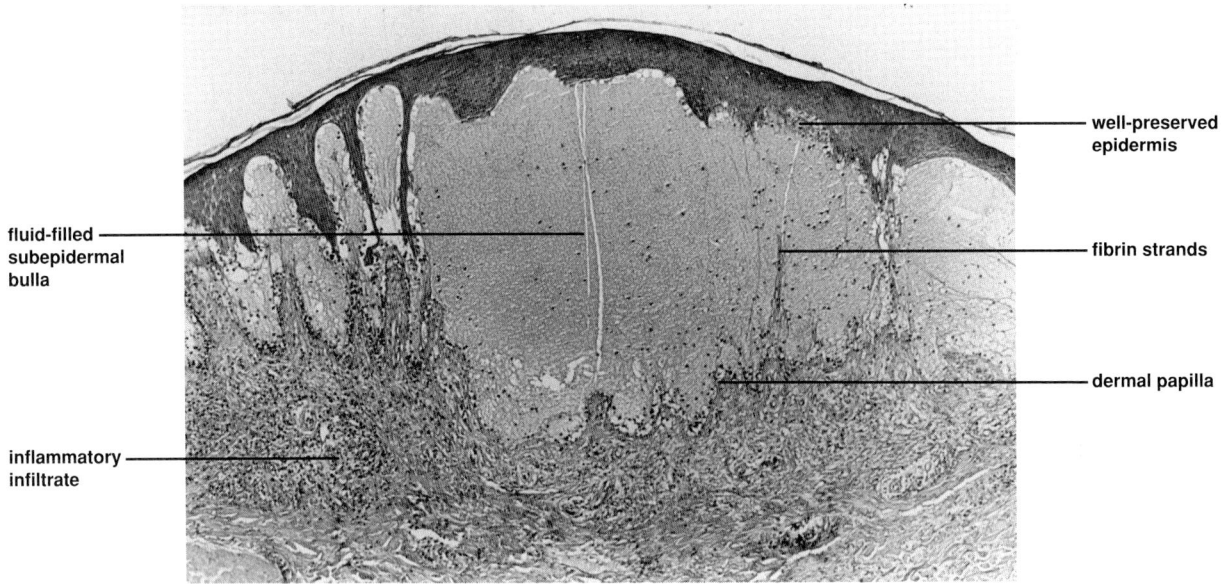

well-preserved
epidermis

fluid-filled
subepidermal
bulla

fibrin strands

dermal papilla

inflammatory
infiltrate

Figure 11-4. Bullous pemphigoid. Large subepidermal blister showing a moderately dense mixed inflammatory cell infiltrate and preservation of the architecture of the dermal papillae and the rete ridges.

the immunofluorescent examination may be unreliable. More than 80% of patients have deposition of IgG and C3, the third component of complement, in a continuous band along the BMZ. The frequency of C3 deposition in appropriate biopsy specimens approaches 100%. The main subclass of immunoglobulin is IgG4, which, paradoxically, is not a potent activator of complement.

About 70% of bullous pemphigoid patients have circulating antibodies against the epidermal BMZ as detected by indirect immunofluorescent examination. When 1 M NaCl split normal human skin is used as an indirect immunofluorescent test substrate, IgG autoantibodies from patients with bullous pemphigoid typically bind the epidermal side. When bullous pemphigoid autoantibodies react with both sides of this split substrate, their titer against the epidermal side is typically greatest. Circulating antiepidermal BMZ IgG may also occur in other conditions, such as herpes gestationis, cicatricial pemphigoid, and epidermolysis bullosa acquisita.

Figure 11-5. Bullous pemphigoid. Inflammation at the periphery with serum and inflammatory cells in the bulla and well-preserved dermal papillae. Sometimes the bullae are even more cell poor.

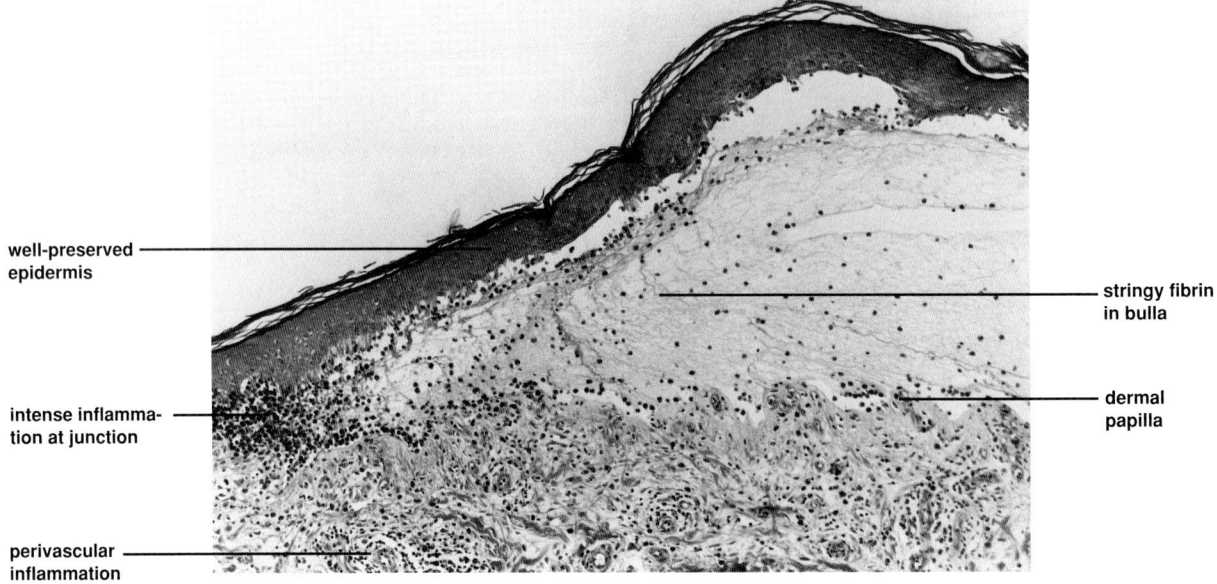

well-preserved
epidermis

stringy fibrin
in bulla

intense inflamma-
tion at junction

dermal
papilla

perivascular
inflammation

Clinicopathologic Correlation

The study of bullous pemphigoid has helped to define the structure of the epidermal BMZ. IgG autoantibodies in the sera of bullous pemphigoid patients have been used to isolate and identify BPAG 1 and BPAG 2. These two separate gene products are 230 and 180 kd proteins, respectively, which comprise part of the hemidesmosomes, ultrastructural elements in basal keratinocytes that promote these cells' adhesions to the epidermal BMZ. BPAG 1 is associated with inner plaques of hemidesmosomes; it is thought to interface with the keratin intermediate filament cytoskeleton of basal keratinocytes. BPAG 2 (also known as type XVII collagen) is a transmembrane component of hemidesmosomes that extends well into the lamina lucida. BPAG 1 is recognized by IgG from most patients with bullous pemphigoid, while BPAG 2 is recognized by about half these patients' sera. In addition to their role in cell adhesion, BPAG 1 and BPAG 2 may be important in early epidermal migration and wound healing.

The pathogenicity of BPAG 1 and BPAG 2 has been difficult to show in animal models. Mast cells and complement activation both are important in the cascade of inflammation in bullous pemphigoid. However, using a variety of elegant manipulations such as immunizing animals against epitopes of the antigens, autoimmunity against these hemidesmosome components has been shown to be sufficient to cause disease.

Differential Diagnosis

A relatively cell-free subepidermal blister can be seen in herpes gestationis, cicatricial pemphigoid, epidermolysis bullosa acquisita, linear IgA disease, chronic bullous disease of childhood, and erythema multiforme. The latter usually has more epidermal necrosis. The others are best separated by clinical findings and immunofluorescent examination. More inflammatory lesions overlap with urticaria and other inflammatory dermatoses, as well as dermatitis herpetiformis.

HERPES GESTATIONIS

Herpes gestationis (pemphigoid gestationis) is an uncommon subepidermal blistering disease of pregnancy and the immediate postpartum period.[19,20]

Clinical Features

Herpes gestationis usually starts on the gravid abdomen as urticarial plaques that progress to blisters. The intensely pruritic lesions may spread to cover most of the body but rarely involve the oral mucosa. Most patients develop the disease during the last trimester, often flare at delivery, and clear within a few weeks to months thereafter. In some patients the disease persists; in others, flares occur with the use of oral contraceptives or during menses. The disease usually recurs with subsequent pregnancies. Children born to mothers with herpes gestationis may experience a transient urticarial or blistering eruption during the first days or weeks of life. There is a strong predilection for HLA-DR3 and/or HLA-DR4.

Histopathologic Features

Herpes gestationis closely resembles bullous pemphigoid when studied by routine light microscopy. There may be slightly more epidermal damage. Necrotic keratinocytes can be seen at the base of the epidermis especially over the edematous dermal papillae. The "tear drop sign" refers to these edematous papillae that then coalesce to form a blister. Eosinophils appear in about the same numbers and pattern as in bullous pemphigoid; they may be aligned along the dermoepidermal junction in early cases. In addition, eosinophils may be found within in the epidermis, sometimes with spongiosis.

Immunofluorescent findings in bullous pemphigoid and herpes gestationis are also similar. Direct immunofluorescent examination of herpes gestationis perilesional skin shows a continuous band of C3 and occasionally IgG at the BMZ. Circulating IgG antibodies are rarely demonstrated by indirect immunofluorescent examination; the herpes gestationis factor, an IgG1 that avidly fixes C3, can usually be identified when complement is added to the indirect examination.

Clinicopathologic Features

IgG anti-BMZ autoantibodies from patients with herpes gestationis typically bind BPAG 2 but may also target BPAG 1—immunopathologic findings that (like clinical and histological findings) represent a common denominator between these subepidermal blistering diseases.

Differential Diagnosis

The lesions are identical to those of bullous pemphigoid and have the same differential diagnosis. A history of pregnancy is usually the deciding factor.

CICATRICIAL PEMPHIGOID

Cicatricial pemphigoid is a scarring erosive disease primarily of the ocular and oral mucosa.

Clinical Features

Cicatricial pemphigoid most commonly involves the conjunctival or oral mucosa of elderly patients. Although the primary lesion is a blister, often only erosions or scarring can be identified. In the oral cavity, cicatricial pemphigoid often presents as desquamative gingivitis with smooth-bordered erosions along the gingiva. Intact oral blisters are rarely seen. Mucosal peeling is a useful clinical sign. On the conjunctiva, erosions are rare and patients are more likely to have inflammation, symblepharon, and eventually entropion. The larynx, esophagus, and genital mucosa may also be affected.[21] The skin is involved infrequently (less than 20%); small transient blisters and erosions may occur on the head and neck. The blisters usually scar. The Brunsting-Perry variant of cicatricial pemphigoid refers to patients who have blisters of the head and neck without mucosal involvement.[22]

Histopathologic Features

Cicatricial pemphigoid shows a subepidermal blister often with inflammation. The predominant inflammatory cell is usually the neutrophil. Many biopsy specimens will be from mucosa, which serves as a clue in itself (Fig. 11-6). Often, routine sections have considerable artifact, either because erosions and fragility are present or because of damage during the biopsy.

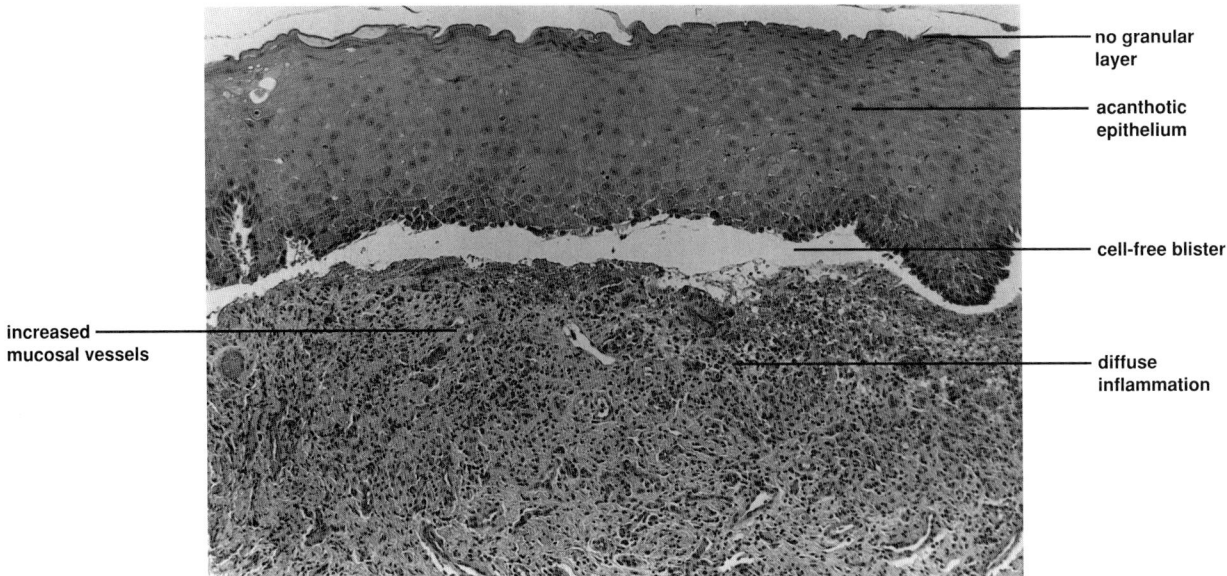

Figure 11-6. Cicatricial pemphigoid. There is a subepidermal blister that is relatively cell free. Two clues to the diagnosis are the overlying mucosal epithelium and the intense vascularity and inflammation of the underlying lamina propria.

Direct immunofluorescent examination of perilesional skin or mucosa is the most satisfactory way to diagnose cicatricial pemphigoid. IgG, IgA, and C3 are deposited in the BMZ. Occasionally only IgA is present. Indirect immunofluorescent examination is often negative.

Clinicopathologic Correlation

Recent studies suggest that cicatricial pemphigoid is a heterogeneous disease in that different subregions and antigens within the epidermal BMZ are targets for these patients' autoantibodies. For example, some patients with cicatricial pemphigoid have IgG autoantibodies directed against BPAG 2 on the epidermal side of 1 M salt split skin. Others have IgG autoantibodies directed against laminin 5, an adhesion molecule located at the interface of the lamina lucida and lamina densa, on the dermal side of 1 M salt split skin.[23]

Differential Diagnosis

A number of diseases can mimic cicatricial pemphigoid. In the oral mucosa, lichen planus and lupus erythematosus may appear clinically similar but have different findings on direct immunofluorescent examination. In addition, both linear IgA dermatosis and epidermolysis bullosa acquisita may present as desquamative gingivitis; they are distinguished by immunopathologic and electron microscopic techniques. On the ocular mucosa, mechanical scars, pressure blebs, erythema multiforme, and drug reactions (including reactions to the chronic use of ocular medications) are the main diseases to be differentiated from cicatricial pemphigoid. The cutaneous lesions that rarely occur in cicatricial pemphigoid are indistinguishable from those of bullous pemphigoid, herpes gestationis, or epidermolysis bullosa acquisita.

DERMATITIS HERPETIFORMIS

Dermatitis herpetiformis is a pruritic vesicular dermatitis associated with a specific HLA pattern.[24,25]

Clinical Features

Dermatitis herpetiformis presents either as a pruritic eruption with excoriations or, less often, as tiny grouped blisters that are soon excoriated. Areas of predilection include the knees, elbows, sacrum, and scalp. Occasionally larger blisters can be present. Oral involvement is rare. Pruritus in this disorder often has a distinctive stinging quality initially; patients can often predict the development of lesions on the basis of localized pruritus.

Most patients with "classic" dermatitis herpetiformis have other features. They are likely to have the HLA patterns HLA-A1 (75%), -B8 (88%), -DR3 (95%), and -DQw2 (>95%). A small bowel biopsy specimen reveals villous atrophy and a lymphocytic infiltrate similar to celiac sprue. Patients with dermatitis herpetiformis are also at risk to develop an intestinal lymphoma and often respond to a gluten-free diet.

Histopathologic Features

Dermatitis herpetiformis usually presents as small vesicles with subepidermal separation. In a low-power field, several tiny microvesicles can be seen (Fig. 11-7). Both in the vesicle and at the tips of the dermal papillae the characteristic inflammatory cell is the neutrophil (Fig. 11-8). Nuclear dust or debris may be present. If eosinophils are present, they usually appear late and in small numbers. Epidermal necrosis is relatively common in dermatitis herpetiformis. Another typical feature is the presence of neutrophilic abscesses in the papillae adjacent to the vesicle. Even when a large blister similar to bullous pemphigoid is found, papillary accumulations of neutrophils at its periphery can usually be identified.[26]

Direct immunofluorescent examination is the most accurate method to diagnose dermatitis herpetiformis. Over 90% of patients diagnosed with dermatitis herpetiformis have granular deposits of IgA in the dermal papillae. These deposits are present throughout the skin and are relatively permanent independent of the course of the disease or its response to medical therapy. However, in patients maintained on a gluten-free diet for long periods of time, the granular deposits of IgA may disappear from their skin. Those patients with granular deposits of IgA have classic dermatitis herpetiformis with HLA predilection and gut changes. The remainder have linear deposition of IgA, and this is discussed separately. Patients with classic or "granular" dermatitis herpetiformis rarely have circulating IgA anti-BMZ autoantibodies; hence, one should not rely on indirect immunofluorescent microscopy to assist in the diagnosis of this disease. Patients may have circulating antibodies against other structures such as gliadin, reticulin, and smooth muscle endomysium.

Clinicopathologic Correlation

The granular deposits of IgA in classic dermatitis herpetiformis are in the upper papillary dermis, just beneath the lamina densa about the elastin microfibrils. Despite this deposition, blisters develop in the lamina lucida perhaps because it is a mechanical point of least resistance.[27] No target antigen for dermatitis herpetiformis has been identified. Most suggest that the deposits are circulating IgA immune complexes, perhaps with dietary proteins, that wind up in the skin. There is conflicting information regarding how many dermatitis herpetiformis patients have circulating IgA immune complexes and the role of dietary challenge in inducing such complexes.

Differential Diagnosis

Small subepidermal blisters and intense papillary inflammation may also be seen in linear IgA disease, bullous lupus erythematosus, and epidermolysis bullosa acquisita. Larger blisters may

mimic bullous pemphigoid and related disorders, but usually demonstrate neutrophil microabscesses in the adjacent papillae, which are not a histopathologic feature of bullous pemphigoid.

LINEAR IGA DERMATOSIS

Linear IgA disease is an acquired disease of adults that resembles either dermatitis herpetiformis or bullous pemphigoid.[28]

Clinical Features

As mentioned above, about 10% of patients with clinically typical dermatitis herpetiformis actually have linear IgA disease. They lack the HLA association, gluten sensitivity, bowel abnormalities, and exquisite sulfone responsiveness of dermatitis herpetiformis. In addition, there are patients with large blisters on an erythematous base (typical for bullous pemphigoid) who actually have linear IgA disease. Yet others may present with mucosal lesions. Linear IgA dermatosis has been induced by a variety of medications, especially vancomycin and cytokines.[29]

Histopathologic Features

The histologic features of linear IgA disease resemble those of whichever bullous disease is clinically mimicked.[30] On direct immunofluorescent examination there is a linear band of IgA at the BMZ. Occasional individuals may also have IgG.[31] Indirect immunofluorescent examination is positive in over half the patients. The majority of IgA deposition occurs in the lamina lucida, although some may be seen about the anchoring fibrils in the sublamina densa region.

Clinicopathologic Correlation

The best identified target antigen appears to be a 97 kd molecule in the upper lamina lucida,[32] but another candidate is a 285 kd molecule that appears to be located lower in the epidermal BMZ.[33]

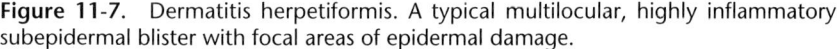

Figure 11-7. Dermatitis herpetiformis. A typical multilocular, highly inflammatory subepidermal blister with focal areas of epidermal damage.

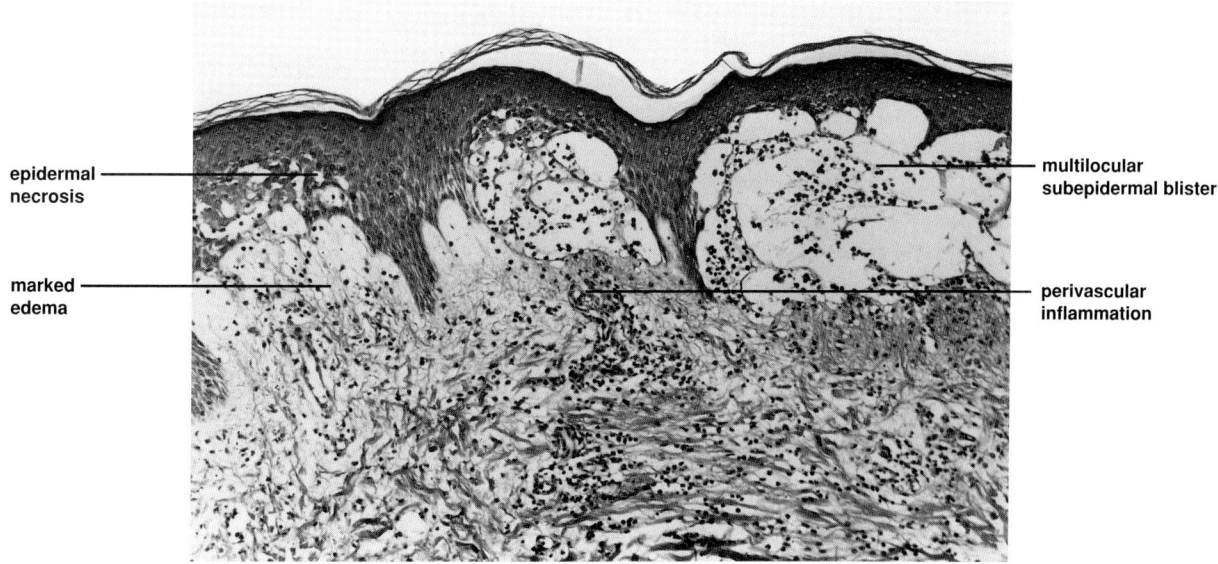

epidermal necrosis

marked edema

multilocular subepidermal blister

perivascular inflammation

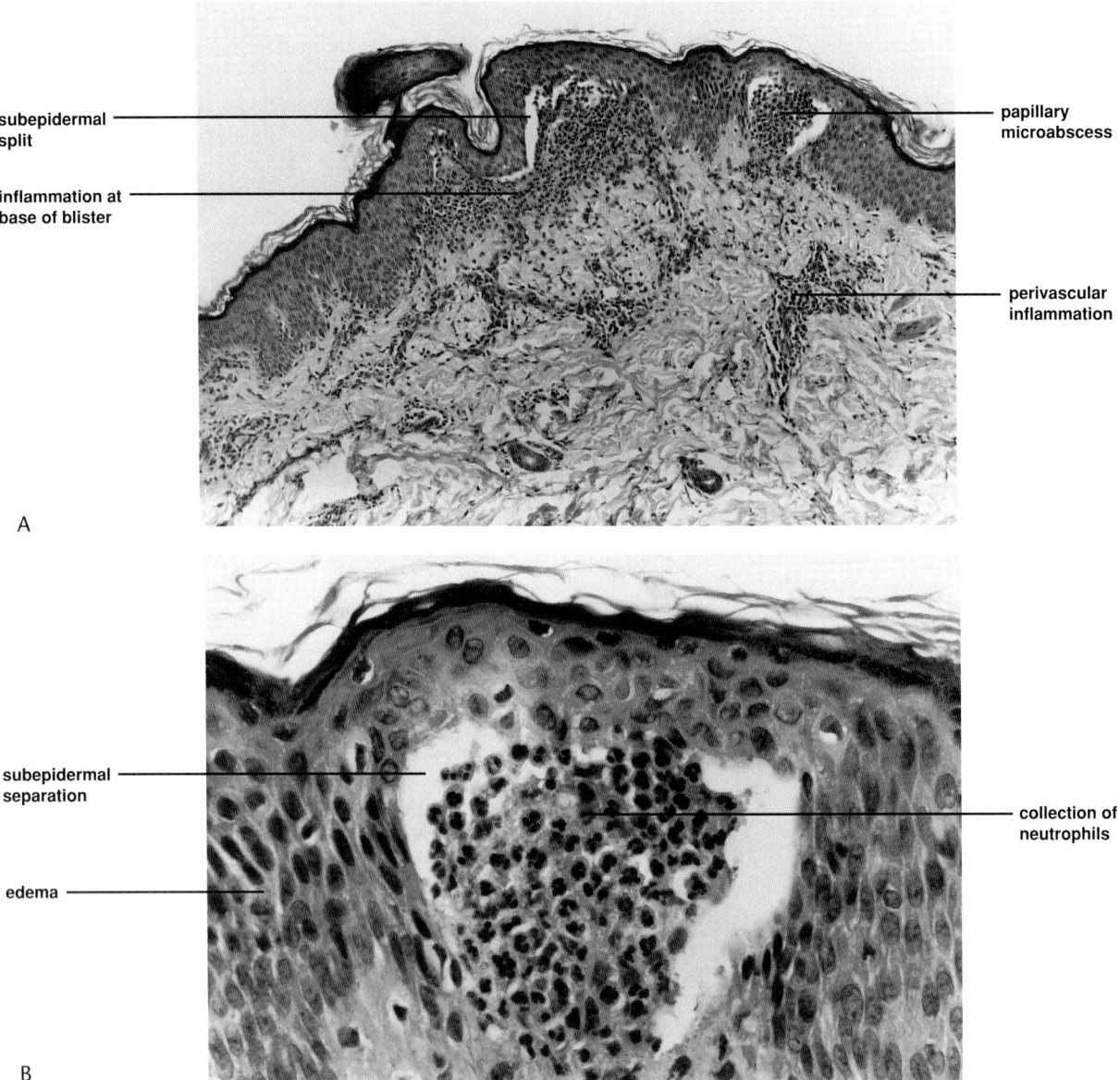

Figure 11-8. Dermatitis herpetiformis. (**A**) This is an early vesicle showing accumulation of neutrophils and beginning subepidermal separation. (**B**) A higher power view of intense inflammation in a single papilla. The predominant cell is a neutrophil.

Differential Diagnosis

Linear IgA disease can be suggested when either cell-poor or cell-rich subepidermal blisters are seen. However, it is a rare disorder that is diagnosed only by direct immunofluorescent examination.

CHRONIC BULLOUS DISEASE OF CHILDHOOD

Chronic bullous disease of childhood is a blistering disease that occurs only in children.[34] It was defined clinically and included patients with childhood bullous pemphigoid, epidermolysis bullosa acquisita, and dermatitis herpetiformis. Now it is synonymous with linear IgA disease in childhood.

Clinical Features

Patients with chronic bullous disease of childhood have a persistent eruption that usually consists of large blisters in a rosette pattern. The flexural areas are the most common site. These blisters are frequently mistaken for bullous impetigo initially.

Histopathologic Features

Most often large subepidermal blisters are seen, usually with a prominent inflammatory infiltrate rich in eosinophils. Thus, the routine picture is that of bullous pemphigoid. However, most patients have deposition of IgA in a linear fashion along the BMZ. Direct immunofluorescent examination is most likely to be helpful; often several biopsy specimens are required. Indirect immunofluorescent examination may be positive. The target antigen is identical to that of linear IgA disease.[35]

Differential Diagnosis

Most large subepidermal blisters in biopsy specimens from children represent chronic bullous disease of childhood and show linear IgA deposition on direct immunofluorescent examination. Bullous pemphigoid is not as uncommon in childhood as previously thought and must be excluded. Patients have been described with the immunologic profiles of both linear IgA disease and bullous pemphigoid.[36]

ERYTHEMA MULTIFORME

Erythema multiforme is a cutaneous reaction pattern characterized by a variety of skin and mucosal lesions.[37,38]

Clinical Features

Erythema multiforme takes many forms. The classic clinical manifestation is target or iris lesions often on the palms and soles, usually associated with a recent oral herpes simplex lesion. On the rest of the skin, a variety of changes may be seen. These include erythematous patches and plaques, urticaria, and bullae. The classification of the more severe forms of erythema multiforme, especially with significant mucosal involvement, are confusing. Assier and co-workers[39] have suggested the following categories:

1. *Erythema multiforme major*: acral target lesions and oral or mucosal involvement with blisters and erosions involving less than 10% of the body surface. Almost all cases are caused by herpes simplex virus I infections, especially if recurrent.
2. *Stevens-Johnson syndrome:* macular or purpuric, often atypical, target lesions on the trunk with oral or mucosal involvement, once again with less than 10% of the body surface involved with erosions.
3. *Stevens-Johnson/toxic epidermal necrolysis overlap*: oral or mucosal lesions and 10% to 30% of the body surface involved with blisters and erosions.
4. *Toxic epidermal necrolysis*: greater than 30% body surface involved, with blisters arising from both maculae and large erythematous patches; most patients also have mucosal involvement.

Stevens-Johnson syndrome and toxic epidermal necrolysis are most often caused by a medication reaction, although occasionally *Mycoplasma* or other infectious agents may be responsible.

A final confusing clinical variant is oral erythema multiforme, which is typically ulcerated, as the vesicles are short lived and rarely seen. Patients often have oral erythema multiforme without skin involvement.[40]

Histopathologic Features

Despite the confusion in clinical nomenclature, the histologic features of all the above disorders represent part of a spectrum, with frequent overlapping. As expected, erythema multiforme

has multiple microscopic patterns.[41,42] It is included in this chapter because one relatively characteristic lesion is a subepidermal blister that is usually a secondary or later change, following the prototypic vacuolar interface dermatitis (see Ch. 5) (Fig 11-9). Epidermal necrosis most often involves the basal cells but may include the entire epidermis (Figs. 11-10 and 11-11). In the dermis, there is usually a perivascular infiltrate with exocytosis of both lymphocytes and red blood cells. Edema is often prominent, and the blisters may arise from the combination of basal cell damage and pressure from the extradermal fluid. The blister roof may be spongiotic or even necrotic, but the damage occurs so rapidly that the stratum corneum usually retains its normal pattern. Leukocytoclastic vasculitis is not seen in erythema multiforme. In infants, vasculitis may be associated with target lesions and bullae that superficially resemble erythema multiforme; this unusual pattern is known as *acute hemorrhagic edema of infancy*.

When widespread erythema with loss of sheets of skin is the presenting sign, the two major diagnostic considerations are staphylococcal scalded skin syndrome and toxic epidermal necrolysis.[43] Although these diseases can appear similar clinically, they can be differentiated histologically. The quickest distinction is made by frozen section. Some have tried to take the shed skin from the patient and section it, but we have found this to be unreliable. We prefer a biopsy specimen. Staphylococcal scalded skin syndrome is usually a disease of children, but can occur in immunocompromised adults. It is caused by secretion of a toxin that damages the upper epidermis. The split occurs in the granular layer (Fig. 11-12). By contrast, toxic epidermal necrolysis shows full-thickness epidermal damage and may have subepidermal separation (Fig. 11-13). In the appropriate clinical settings, both acute graft-versus-host reaction and cutaneous damage from pretransplant radiation and chemotherapy can cause a similar loss of skin, as can desquamative drug eruptions that do not have the full-thickness epidermal damage of toxic epidermal necrolysis.

Clinicopathologic Correlation

The herpes simplex virus can be identified in most lesions of recurrent erythema multiforme. Antibodies against desmoplakins, key components of the desmosomes and related to BPAG 1 in the hemidesmosomes, have been found in erythema multiforme, but their role in epidermal necrosis remains to be demonstrated.[44]

Differential Diagnosis

Epidermal damage and dermal edema are the most useful clues to distinguish erythema multiforme from bullous pemphigoid and related diseases. Full-thickness epidermal necrosis separates toxic epidermal necrolysis from staphylococcal scalded skin syndrome, but similar damage may be seen in traumatic blisters.

PORPHYRIA CUTANEA TARDA

The porphyrias are a family of disorders characterized by enzymatic defects in hemoglobin synthesis. Most have cutaneous involvement: despite clinical differences, the cutaneous histo-

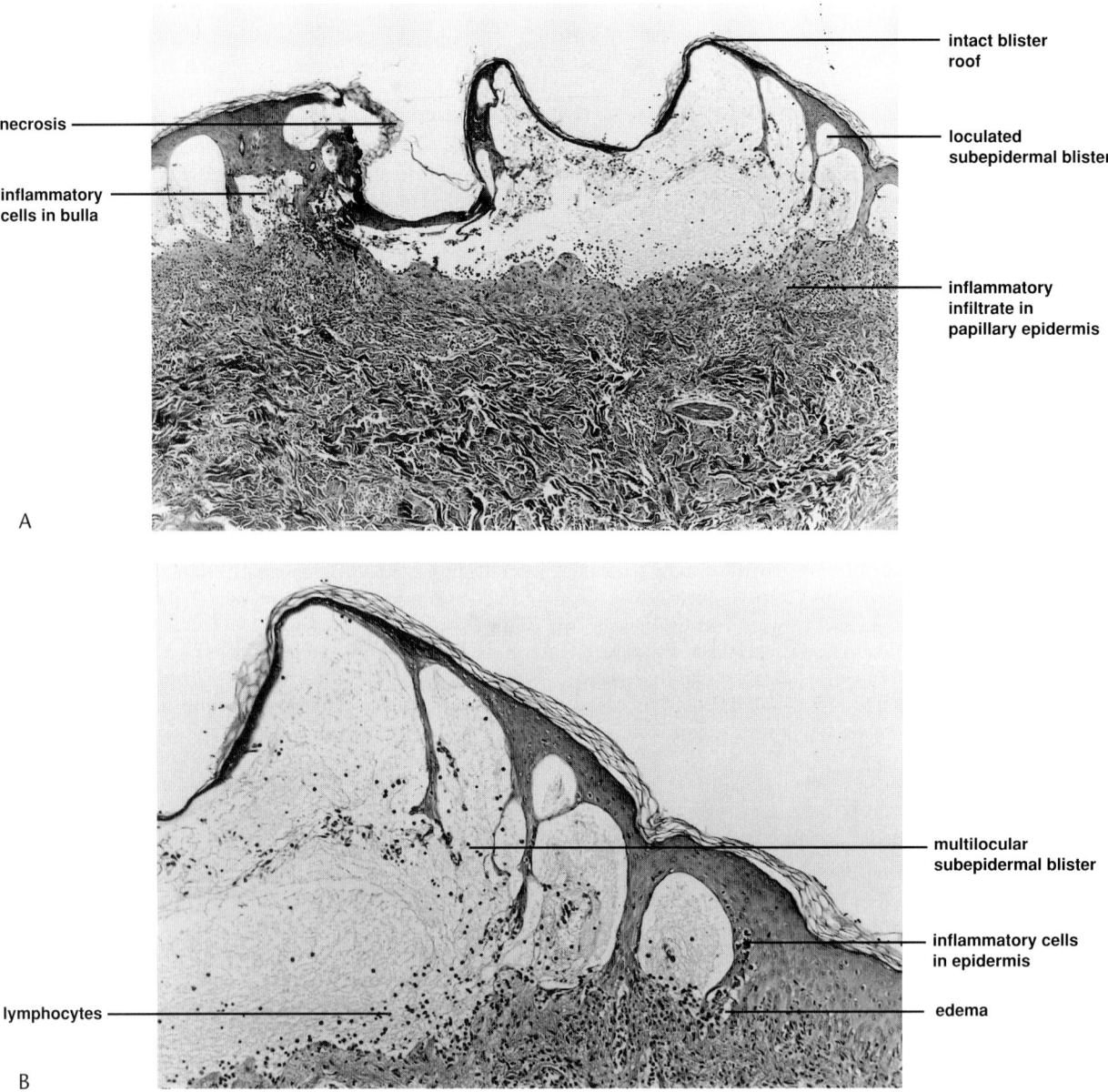

necrosis

inflammatory
cells in bulla

intact blister
roof

loculated
subepidermal blister

inflammatory
infiltrate in
papillary epidermis

A

multilocular
subepidermal blister

inflammatory cells
in epidermis

lymphocytes

edema

B

Figure 11-9.   Erythema multiforme. (**A**) Large multiloculated subepidermal bulla. (**B**) The edge of the bulla with considerable architectural similarities to bullous pemphigoid but with epidermal necrosis.

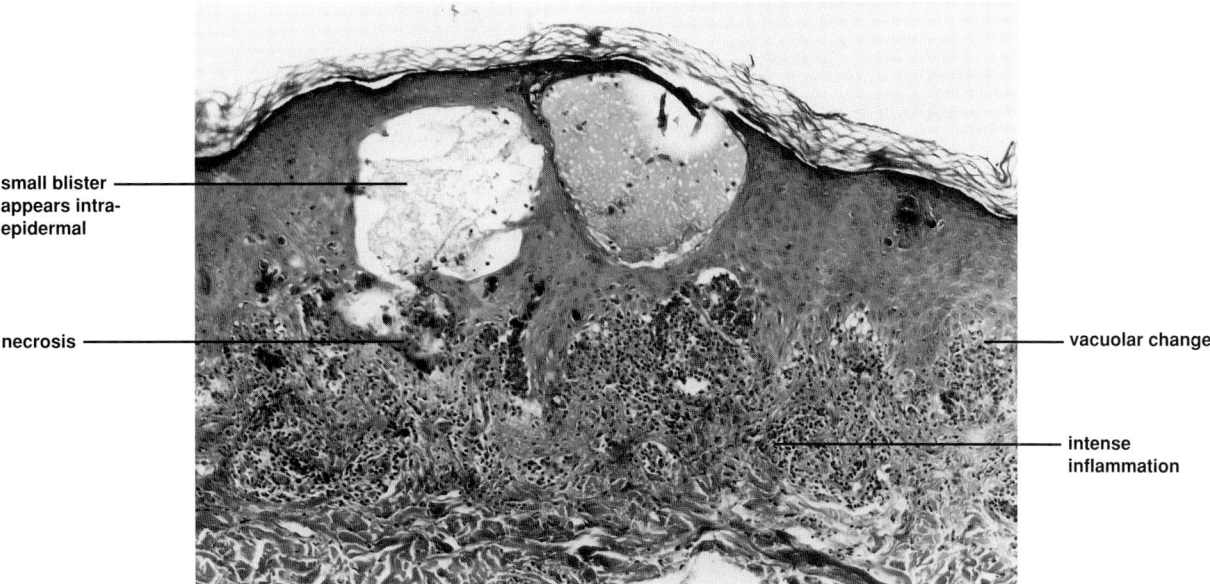

small blister appears intra-epidermal

necrosis

vacuolar change

intense inflammation

Figure 11-10. Erythema multiforme. There are smaller blisters here with more exocytosis of inflammatory cells at the dermoepidermal junction, a more intense dermal infiltrate, and more epidermal necrosis than in Fig. 11-9.

Figure 11-11. Erythema multiforme. There is frank interface dermatitis with necrotic keratinocytes. There is also a perivascular infiltrate of mononuclear cells.

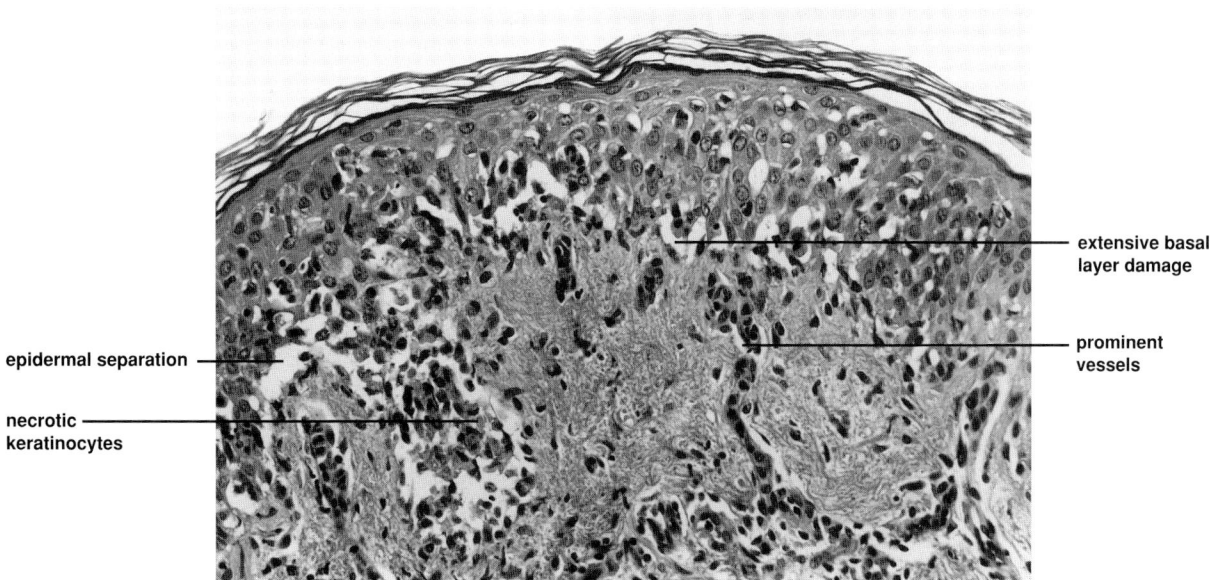

extensive basal layer damage

prominent vessels

epidermal separation

necrotic keratinocytes

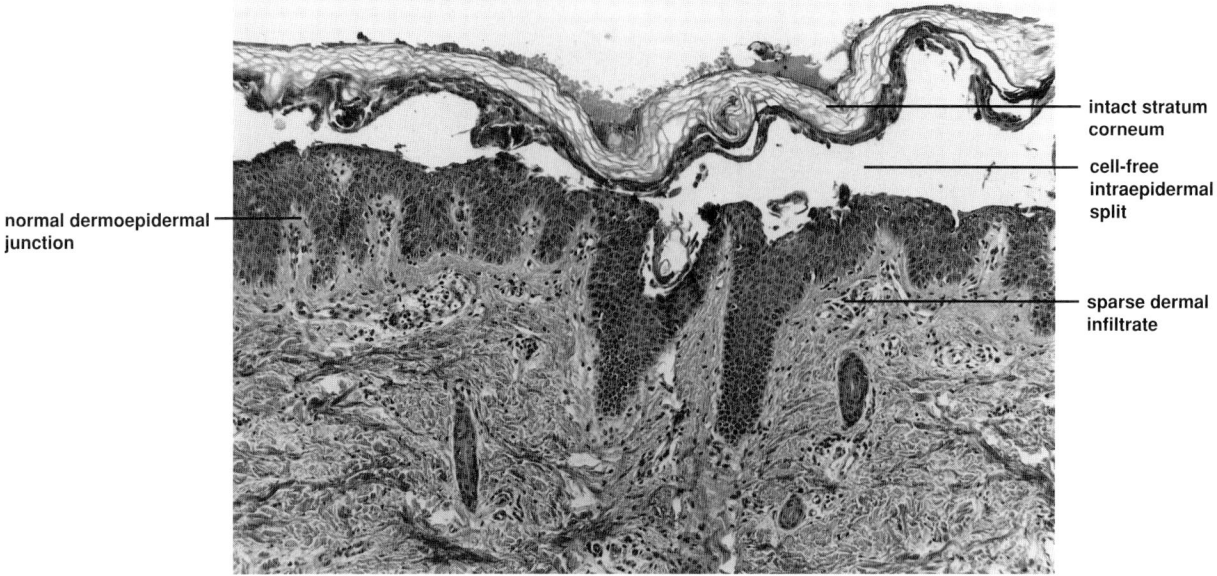

intact stratum
corneum

cell-free
intraepidermal
split

normal dermoepidermal
junction

sparse dermal
infiltrate

Figure 11-12. Staphylococcal scalded skin syndrome. There is high epidermal separation with minimal acantholysis. The rest of the epidermis is normal.

pathology is similar. Table 11-3 reviews the major porphyrias; there are other types that are discussed in specialized sources.[45–47] The most common type of porphyria encountered by dermatopathologists is porphyria cutanea tarda. Porphyria cutanea tarda patients usually present with skin fragility, but on examination may be found to have blisters, scars, and milia on the backs of their hands and on their face. Facial hypertrichosis may occur. Some have dermal sclerosis (see Ch. 16). Although the skin manifestations of porphyria cutanea tarda are most common in sun-exposed skin, patients are rarely clinically pho-

tosensitive. The hepatitis C virus appears to be a trigger for porphyria cutanea tarda, especially in human immunodeficiency virus-infected patients. In most patients, the disease is acquired, although familial patterns are also seen. Variegate porphyria patients have skin changes identical to those of porphyria cutanea tarda, but also have neurologic disease similar to acute intermittent porphyria. The latter has no skin findings.

By contrast, patients with erythropoietic porphyria and erythropoietic protoporphyria present with photosensitivity that usually begins in childhood. Patients with erythropoietic proto-

Figure 11-13. Toxic epidermal necrolysis. The entire epidermis is necrotic with subepidermal separation in several areas. There is only a sparse superficial perivascular mononuclear cell inflammatory infiltrate.

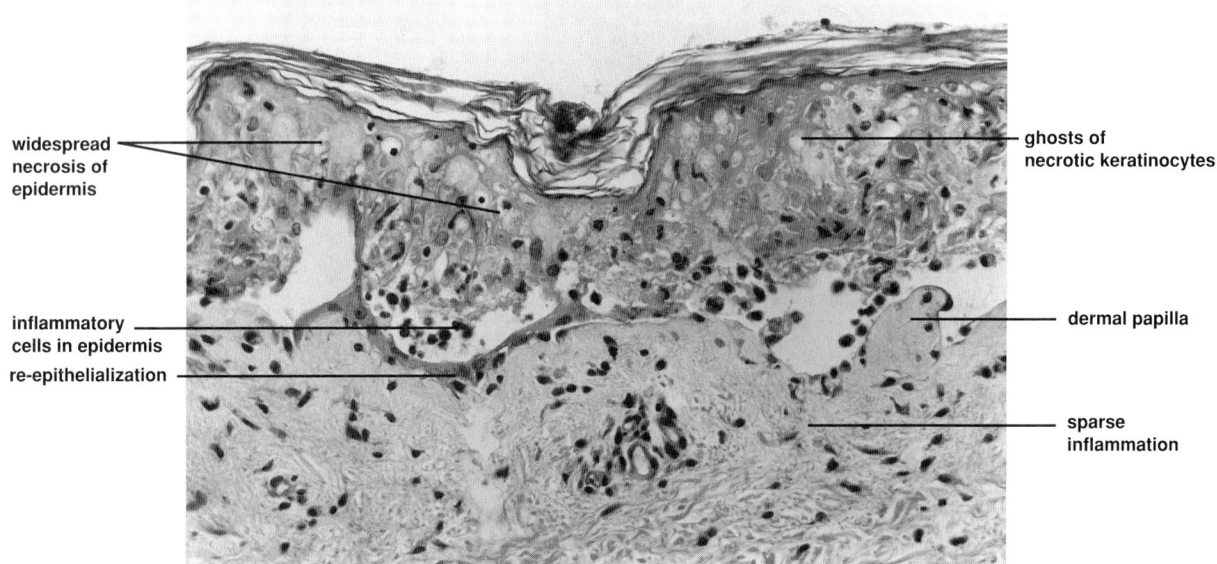

widespread
necrosis of
epidermis

ghosts of
necrotic keratinocytes

inflammatory
cells in epidermis
re-epithelialization

dermal papilla

sparse
inflammation

Table 11-3. The Major Porphyrias

Disease	Inheritance	Skin Findings
Porphyria cutanea tarda	Sporadic AD	Fragile skin, blisters, milia, hypertrichosis, pseudoscleroderma
Erythropoietic porphyria	AR	Extreme photosensitivity with hypertrichosis, scarring, mutilation
Erythropoietic protoporphyria	AD	Photosensitivity with scarring, waxy plaques, leathery skin
Variegate porphyria	AD	Identical to porphyria cutanea tarda
Acute intermittent porphyria	AD	None

Abbreviations: AD, autosomal dominant; AR, autosomal recessive.

porphyria have a mild photosensitivity accompanied by edema, scaling, crusting, and flat scars, especially on the nose. Their skin may also be thickened. Erythropoietic porphyria patients were probably the "werewolves" of old with the early development of extreme photosensitivity and the onset of mutilating scarring, pigmentary changes, alopecia, ectropion, and eventually cutaneous malignancies.

Histopathologic Features

Despite their varying clinical appearances, all porphyrias with skin involvement have varying degrees of damage around dermal vessels and at the epidermal BMZ.[48,49] The epidermal and perivascular BMZ are thickened; the exact molecular explanation for this abnormality is unclear. Proteoglycans and type IV collagen, two constituents of the lamina densa, have been identified, but so have many other substances. In porphyria cutanea tarda, the changes at the dermoepidermal junction predominate, while in the other forms the perivascular lesions are most prominent.

The dermatopathologist is most likely to encounter blisters on a patient with porphyria cutanea tarda. These lesions are characterized by lack of an inflammatory cell infiltrate, preserved or naked papillae that push into the blister cavity, and an acral location (Fig. 11-14). One distinctive clue to the diagnosis is the presence of amorphous globules known as *caterpillar bodies* in the blister roof. These eosinophilic caterpillar bodies contain degenerating keratinocytes, colloid bodies, and basement membrane structures.[50,51] The level of separation is not as clearly defined for porphyria cutanea tarda as for other blistering disorders. Sometimes the periodic acid-Schiff (PAS)-positive thickened basement membrane is on top of the blister; at other times it is beneath it (Fig. 11-15). Electron microscopic studies indicate that separation occurs mainly in the lamina lucida. Direct immunofluorescent examination shows deposition of broad linear deposits of IgG, other immunoglobulins, and complement components in the BMZ both of the vessel walls and the epidermis. The immune reactants are presumably passively trapped in the thickened structures. Indirect immunofluorescent examination is negative.

In erythropoietic protoporphyria and erythropoietic porphyria, the perivascular changes predominate. The acute photosensitivity reaction is perivascular, presumably as the photoreactive porphyrins leak from vessels and are exposed to light. Lymphocytes and edema are seen, but there are no good diagnostic clues. Later vessel wall BMZ changes are more striking; they can usually be appreciated on routine sections or enhanced with a PAS stain. Sometimes large amorphous deposits are

Figure 11-14. Porphyria cutanea tarda. The typical naked papillae of porphyria cutanea tarda project into a subepidermal blister in acral skin. There is relatively little inflammation.

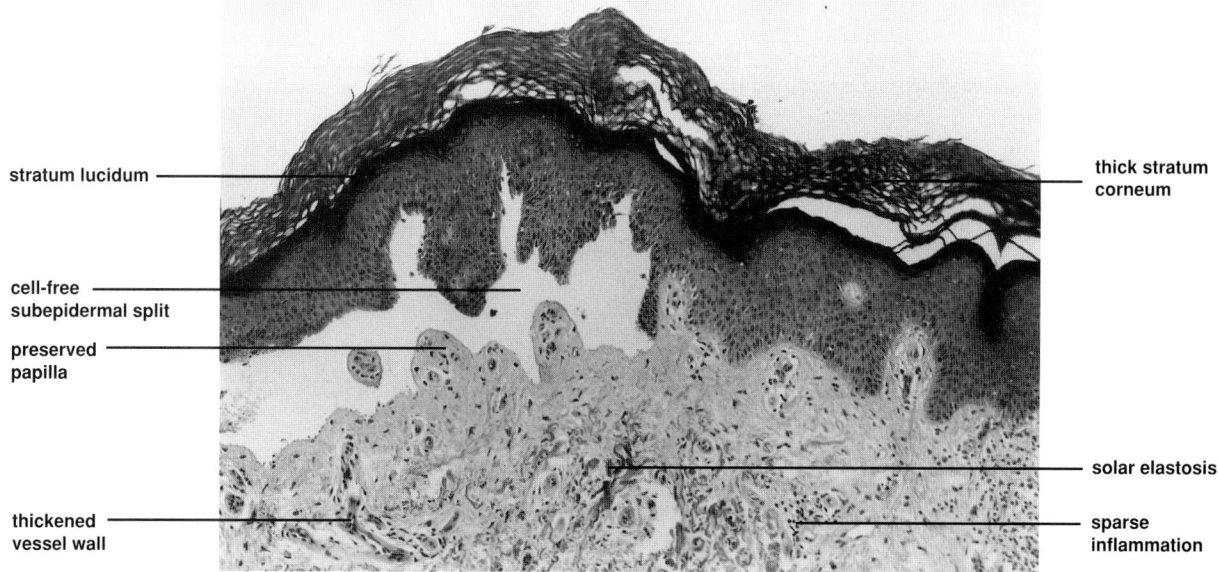

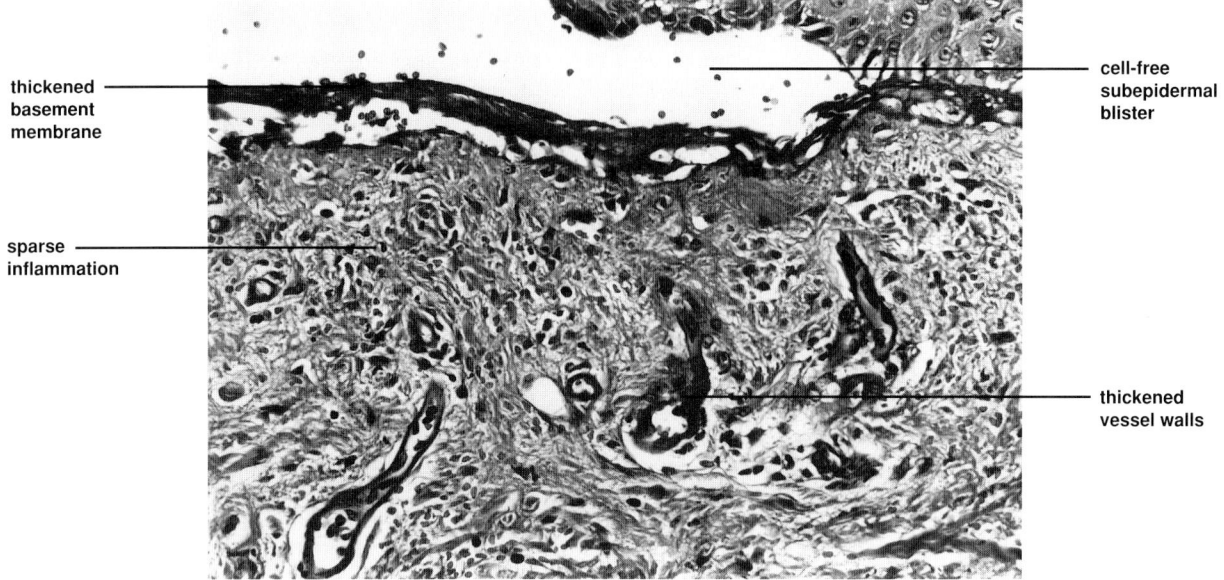

thickened basement membrane

cell-free subepidermal blister

sparse inflammation

thickened vessel walls

Figure 11-15. Porphyria cutanea tarda. The PAS-positive basement membrane is thickened around blood vessels and beneath the dermoepidermal junction.

formed, similar to lipid proteinosis (see Ch. 16); the source is the peculiar proliferation of the BMZ structures.

Pseudoporphyria

Clinical Features

Some patients have skin findings that mimic porphyria cutanea tarda but do not have measurable porphyrin abnormalities. Included among the pseudoporphyrias are

1. *Epidermolysis bullosa acquisita.*
2. *Drug-induced pseudoporphyria*: nonsteroidal anti-inflammatory agents, nalidixic acid, tetracycline, and furosemide have been reported to cause an eruption similar to porphyria cutanea tarda.[52]
3. *Bullous disease of renal dialysis*: patients in renal failure or on dialysis also may develop blisters in sun-exposed skin; some have elevated serum porphyrin levels, but the mechanism is unclear.[53]
4. *Light*: over-use of tanning devices can produce blisters and skin fragility.[54]

Histopathologic Features

The lesions are virtually indistinguishable on a light microscopic level from porphyria cutanea tarda. In all forms of pseudoporphyria, the vessel wall and epidermal BMZ thickening is minimal or absent. Immunofluorescent examination is also usually negative. In epidermolysis bullosa acquisita, the perivascular changes are not seen.

Differential Diagnosis

When a cell-poor subepidermal blister with well-preserved papillae is identified, the correct diagnosis must be confirmed by other means. Porphyria cutanea tarda is proven by elevated urine porphyrin levels. Pseudoporphyria is usually diagnosed on the basis of history (drug exposure, renal disease), the absence of abnormal porphyrins in the blood, urine, or stool, and the lack of circulating and/or tissue-bound anti-BMZ autoantibodies. Because epidermolysis bullosa acquisita presents with porphyria-like lesions in some cases, studies to exclude epidermolysis bullosa acquisita should be performed if the above tests are negative, especially if lesions are present in unexposed sites.

EPIDERMOLYSIS BULLOSA

Epidermolysis bullosa refers to a group of inherited diseases characterized by fragile skin. This group is also referred to as *mechanobullous disorders*.[5,55,56]

Clinical Features

The various types of epidermolysis bullosa traditionally have been identified partly on clinical features, partly on histologic features, and partly on pattern of inheritance. Epidermolysis bullosa is subdivided into three major groups based on the level of separation between the epidermis and dermis:

1. Epidermolysis bullosa simplex (keratinocytolytic epidermolysis bullosa)
2. Junctional epidermolysis bullosa
3. Dystrophic epidermolysis bullosa

Today, all are best explained in molecular biologic terms. Epidermolysis bullosa simplex is a disease of keratins, primarily 5 and 14, which are expressed in the basal layer. The type of mutation and the nature of the subsequent abnormal protein determine the clinical features. Thus epidermolysis simplex is usually inherited in an autosomal dominant pattern. A rare variant, epidermolysis bullosa simplex associated with neuromuscular disease, appears to involve a plectin mutation. Junctional epidermolysis bullosa is caused by mutations in a wide variety of components of the epidermal BMZ, such as BPAG 2 (type XVII collagen) in generalized atrophic benign epidermolysis bullosa, several components of laminin 5 in the Herlitz or lethal form, and integrin $\alpha6\beta4$ in junctional epidermolysis bullosa with pyloric atresia. Dystrophic epidermolysis bullosa is caused by mutations in type VII collagen. The autosomal dominant forms are caused by missense mutations that alter function, while the recessive forms are secondary to more damaging mutations that produce nonfunctional proteins.

There are some clinical correlations to the level of damage—most notably the tendency to scar. Epidermolysis bullosa simplex generally heals without scarring. Junctional epidermolysis bullosa may scar, but usually not severely, while dystrophic epidermolysis bullosa is characterized by dramatic scarring, producing the classic mitten changes of the hands. In addition, patients with dystrophic epidermolysis bullosa are at risk for cutaneous malignancies, many of which behave aggressively.

Pitfalls: It is wise to consider the pitfalls in diagnosing epidermolysis bullosa before considering the histologic features. How the biopsy specimen is obtained is crucial. The ideal blister for study is one that is fresh and minimal. When skin fragility is marked, as in some forms of dystrophic epidermolysis bullosa, the trauma of the biopsy will produce separation. Blisters produced by mild trauma such as rubbing with a pencil eraser can also be used, but too vigorous rubbing can produce false results. Study of the blister roof or eroded base is not helpful. Finally, the age of the lesion is crucial because healing can change the pattern. Because routine light microscopy rarely, if ever, is sufficient to diagnose any epidermolysis bullosa correctly, it may be wise to simultaneously obtain specimens for immunofluorescent mapping and electron microscopic studies.

Histopathologic Features

Two histologic patterns may be seen. Both are characterized by little or no inflammatory infiltrate.

1. *Basal layer separation*: almost all forms of epidermolysis bullosa simplex appear similar with light microscopy. In very early lesions, vacuolar change in the basal layer may be hinted at. Fragments of epidermal basal cells can often be seen on the dermal side of the blister. Blisters are often multiloculated (Fig 11-16). Eosinophils may be present, mimicking bullous pemphigoid.[57]

Dowling-Meara epidermolysis bullosa simplex may have more dyskeratosis and because of severe degeneration of the basal cells frequently appears to be subepidermal on routine sections. In Weber-Cockayne epidermolysis bullosa, the biopsy will usually be from acral skin, which provides a clue. Superficial epidermolysis bullosa simplex is characterized by a higher level split near or in the granular layer.

2. *Sharp epidermal-dermal separation*: most junctional and dermolytic epidermolysis bullosa cases look the same histologically with a relatively noninflamed subepidermal blister (Fig 11-17). In addition, biopsy specimens from patients with epidermolysis bullosa simplex may also show a subepidermal blister; thus routine light microscopy does not allow a reliable diagnosis of epidermolysis bullosa.

Electron microscopic evaluation has long provided the gold standard, although today genetic techniques are providing the definitive answer in more and more situations. Examples of the utility of electron microscopic studies include clumped tonofilaments in Dowling-Meara epidermolysis bullosa simplex, reduced or absent hemidesmosomes in Herlitz or lethal junctional epidermolysis bullosa, and absent or reduced anchoring fibrils in various types of dystrophic epidermolysis bullosa.[58]

Figure 11-16. Epidermolytic epidermolysis bullosa. There is intraepidermal separation with minimal inflammation. In several areas the split appears to be subepidermal, but in other sites there are clearly adherent basal cells.

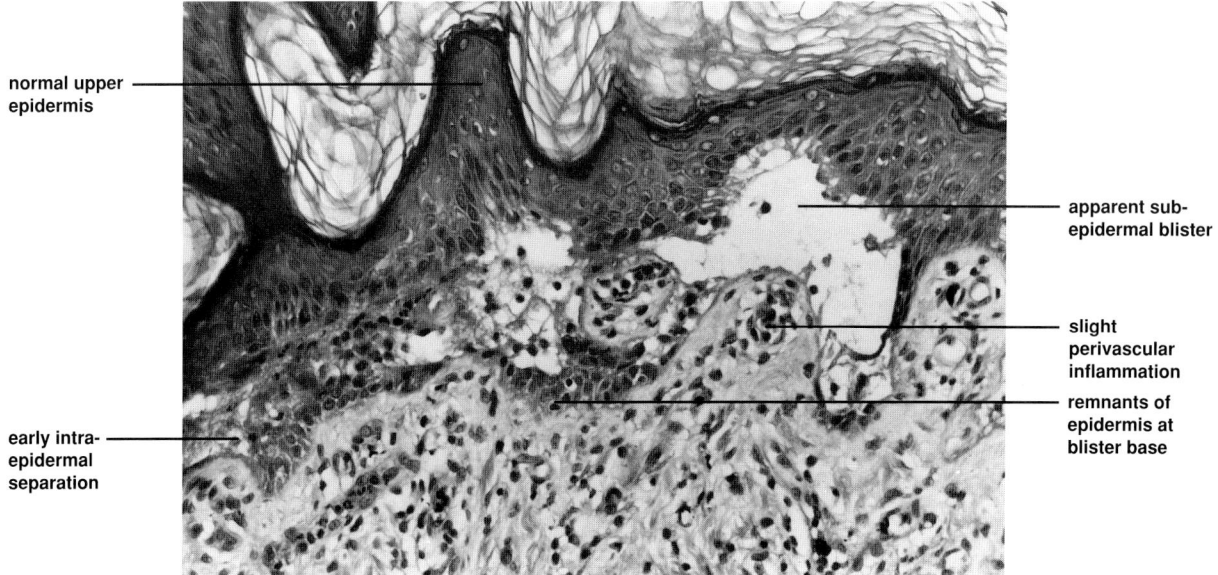

normal upper epidermis

apparent sub-epidermal blister

slight perivascular inflammation

remnants of epidermis at blister base

early intra-epidermal separation

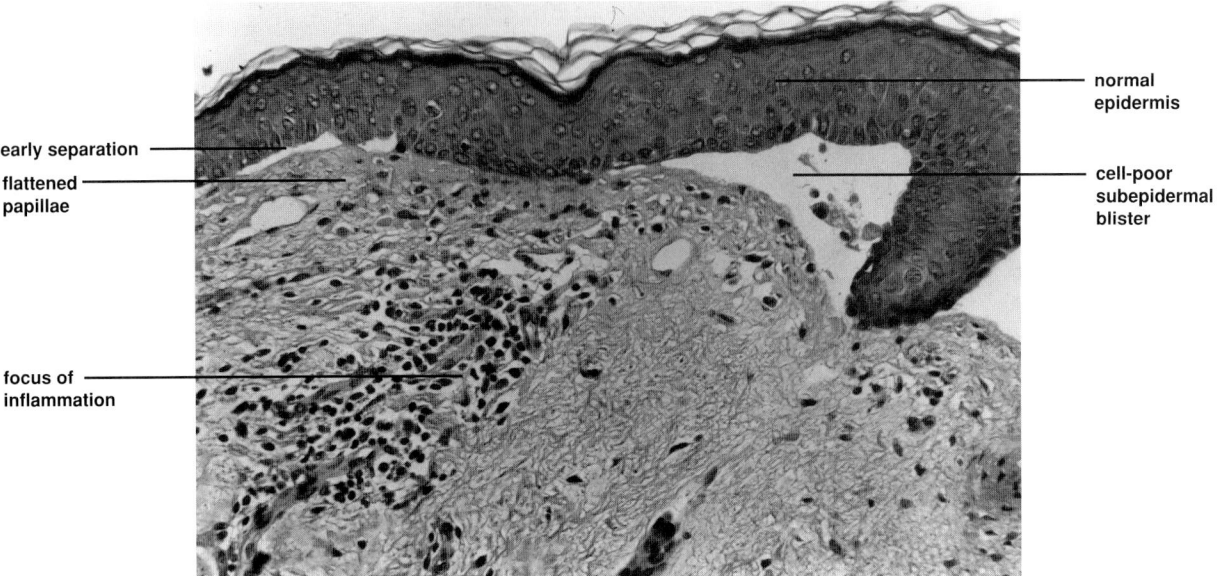

Figure 11-17. Dermolytic epidermolysis bullosa. Separation is subepidermal. There is a generous separation at one side and early separation at the other. Inflammation is minimal.

Immunofluorescent mapping can confirm the location of the split in the lamina lucida with bullous pemphigoid antigen on top and laminin and type IV collagen below, as Table 11-4 shows.[55] Specific antibodies can also be used to search for particular problems. For example, uncein, part of the anchoring filaments, is absent in most cases of junctional epidermolysis bullosa.[59] Antibodies against laminin 5 also typically fail to stain specimens from the Herlitz form of junctional epidermolysis bullosa. In generalized atrophic benign (junctional) epidermolysis bullosa, BPAG 2 is reduced or absent. Recessive and dominant dystrophic epidermolysis bullosa can be separated with antibodies against type VII collagen, since it does not stain in the recessive form, while in the dominant form it is present but dysfunctional.

Differential Diagnosis

The challenge is twofold: to diagnose epidermolysis bullosa and then to help identify the subtype. In the neonatal period, herpes simplex infections, impetigo and more severe bacterial infections, and congenital syphilis should all be considered. Occasionally, incontinentia pigmenti and some of the ichthyoses, especially epidermolytic hyperkeratosis, may appear similar. Often a specific diagnosis is not possible at birth, although im-

Table 11-4. Immunofluorescent Mapping of Epidermolysis Bullosa Blisters

Type of Blister	BPAGs	Laminins	Type IV Collagen
Epidermal (simplex)	Base	Base	Base
Junctional	Roof	Base	Base
Dermal (dystrophic)	Roof	Roof	Roof

munofluorescent mapping has made rapid working diagnoses possible. In older infants, the history of congenital onset and mechanical fragility usually points one in the right direction, but linear IgA disease, bullous pemphigoid, and even epidermolysis bullosa acquisita can appear in the first year of life.

EPIDERMOLYSIS BULLOSA ACQUISITA

Epidermolysis bullosa acquisita is an acquired subepidermal blistering disease characterized by antibodies to type VII collagen.[60,61]

Clinical Features

Epidermolysis bullosa acquisita takes multiple clinical patterns. About half the patients resemble porphyria cutanea tarda with fragile skin and blisters on sun-exposed areas. In contrast to porphyria cutanea tarda patients, these individuals usually if not always have blisters on nonexposed areas. Others more closely resemble bullous pemphigoid with more extensive blistering on an inflamed urticarial base. The latter subgroup was identified as more advanced methods were used to study atypical bullous pemphigoid patients who often had not responded to standard therapy. Furthermore, some patients have mucosal lesions and resemble cicatricial pemphigoid. Yet other patients may have mutilating acral changes.[62] The disease pattern may shift during its course. Patients with epidermolysis bullosa acquisita may have Crohn's disease or more often lupus erythematosus, but most have no associated disorder; they are more likely to have HLA-DR2.

Histopathologic Features

In the porphyria cutanea tarda variant, noninflamed subepidermal blisters are found. Older healed lesions may show scarring and thickened dermal collagen as in porphyria cutanea tarda, but thickening of the epidermal and vascular basement membranes is not seen. No epidermal damage is present. In the inflammatory variant, the histology closely mimics bullous pemphigoid, herpes gestationis, and cicatricial pemphigoid. Eosinophils are uncommon, as neutrophils usually predominate.

Routine direct and indirect immunofluorescent examinations may be identical to bullous pemphigoid, although the likelihood of a positive reaction is somewhat less. When indirect immunofluorescent examination is done using a patient's serum and 1 M salt split skin, epidermolysis bullosa acquisita serum will stain the dermal side exclusively in contrast to bullous pemphigoid serum, which stains the epidermal side. Less than 50% of epidermolysis bullosa acquisita patients have circulating IgG anti-BMZ autoantibodies, which is the main limitation of the above technique. In such cases direct immunofluorescent examination can be done on perilesional salt split skin to distinguish between epidermolysis bullosa acquisita and bullous pemphigoid.[63] Immunoelectron microscopy shows the deposits in the sublamina densa zone and offers final confirmation.

Ultrastructural and immunohistochemical studies have also helped to define epidermolysis bullosa acquisita. When protein is extracted from the lamina lucida and lamina densa of human epidermal basement membrance and studied by immunoblotting with epidermolysis bullosa acquisita antiserum, two proteins are identified with molecular weights of 290 and 145 kd. These proteins correspond to intact type VII collagen (290 kd) and its components: a rod-like 145 kd collagenous domain that extends into the sublamina densa and a globular 145 kd noncollagenous domain (NC 1) that attaches to the lamina densa.

Differential Diagnosis

In a series of 100 sequential patients whose sera contained BMZ antibodies, about 5% had epidermolysis bullosa acquisita instead of the clinically suspected bullous pemphigoid.[64] Patients with epidermolysis bullosa acquisita are unlikely to have deposition of C3.[65] Table 11-5 shows the various methods of separating epidermolysis bullosa acquisita from bullous pemphigoid. Both porphyria cutanea tarda and the bullous eruption of systemic lupus erythematosus also show separation in the sublamina densa zone; fortunately, both can be excluded by other laboratory tests (urine porphyrins and ANA, respectively).

BULLOUS ERUPTION OF SYSTEMIC LUPUS ERYTHEMATOSUS

The bullous eruption of systemic lupus erythematosus is a rare blistering eruption.[66,67] It should not be confused with either the oral erosions or occasional bullae that arise secondary to destruction of the basal layer keratinocytes in severe acute cutaneous reactions in systemic lupus erythematosus.

Clinical Features

The typical patient is a young black who meets the criteria for systemic lupus erythematosus and develops inflamed grouped blisters often on the face. The blisters most often resemble dermatitis herpetiformis, but occasionally may be larger and then mimic bullous pemphigoid. The blisters do not correlate with the course of the systemic lupus erythematosus and often respond dramatically to dapsone.

Histopathologic Features

The blisters most closely resemble dermatitis herpetiformis with an intense neutrophilic infiltrate (Fig. 11-18). Even more extensive lesions clinically thought to be bullous pemphigoid have an intense neutrophilic infiltrate. Direct immunofluorescent examination usually shows linear or granular deposits of IgG, IgM, IgA, and C3 along the BMZ, while indirect immunofluorescent examination usually is negative.[68]

The diagnosis can best be made by showing that the immunoreactants are deposited in the sublamina densa zone as in epidermolysis bullosa acquisita and porphyria cutanea tarda. Sera from some patients with the bullous eruption of systemic lupus erythematosus contains IgG anti-BMZ autoantibodies that bind to salt split skin on the dermal side and to the epidermolysis bullosa acquisita antigen on immunoblotting. Therefore, at least some patients with the bullous eruption of systemic lupus erythematosus have an autoimmune profile and immunopathologic findings that are similar to those documented in epidermolysis bullosa acquisita patients. Classic epidermolysis bullosa acquisita may be associated with systemic lupus erythematosus, which further confuses the issue.[69]

Table 11-5. Separation of Bullous Pemphigoid from Epidermolysis Bullosa Acquisita

Technique	Bullous Pemphigoid	Epidermolysis Bullosa Acquista
Direct immunofluorescence of patient's 1 M salt split skin	In situ IgG (at least partially) on the epidermal side	In situ IgG strictly on the dermal side
Indirect immunofluorescence of 1 M salt split normal human skin	IgG autoantibodies stain epidermal side of test substrate; if both sides stain, titer highest against epidermal side	IgG autoantibodies stain dermal side of test substrate
Immunoelectronmicroscopy	In situ immunoreactants in lamina lucida adjacent to plasma membrane of basal keratinocytes	In situ immunoreactants on anchoring fibrils in the sublamina densa region
Immunoblotting or immunoprecipitation	BPAG 1, BPAG 2	Type VII collagen

(Data courtesy of Kim B. Yancey, M.D., Bethesda, MD.)

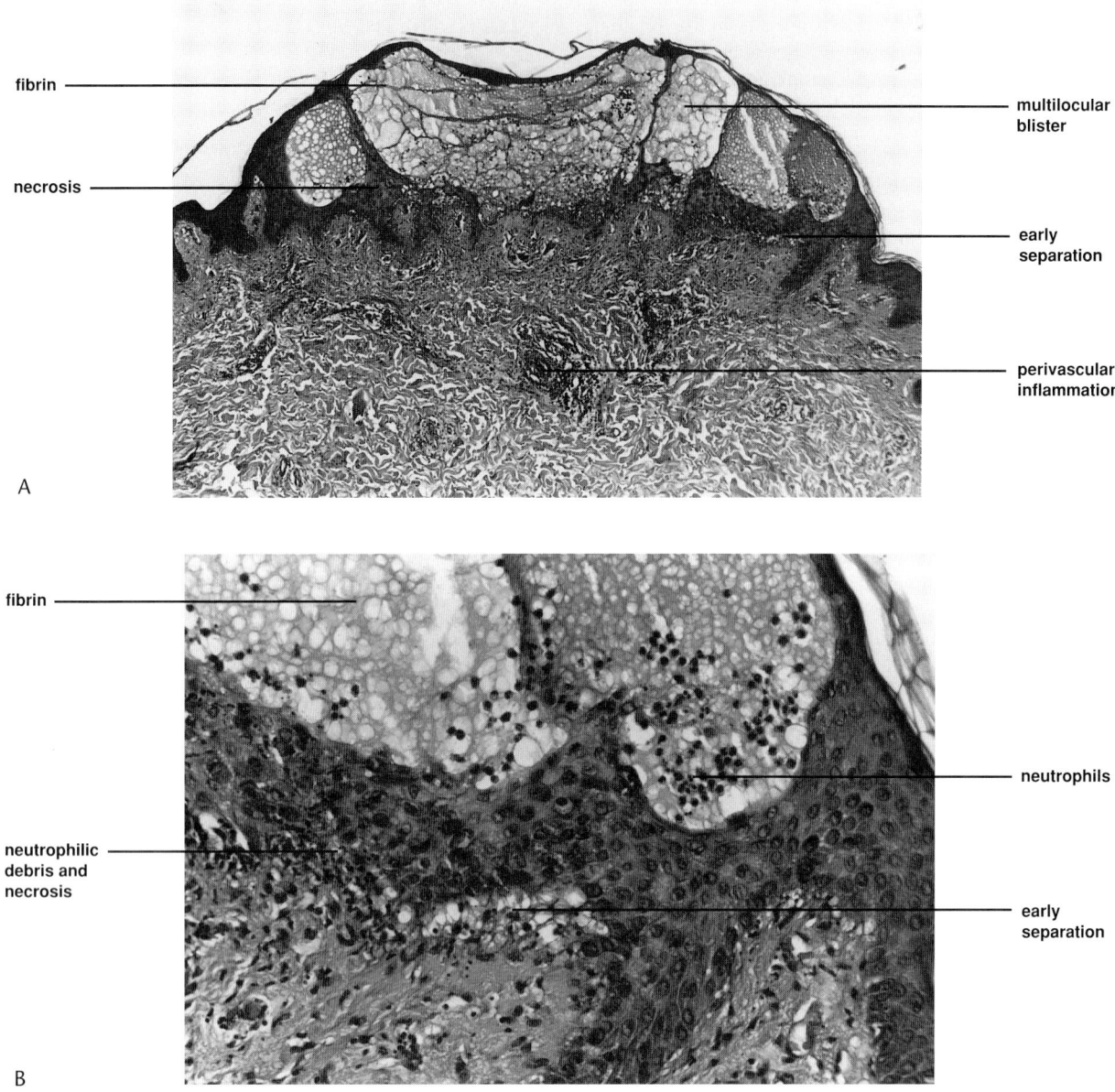

fibrin

necrosis

multilocular
blister

early
separation

perivascular
inflammation

A

fibrin

neutrophilic
debris and
necrosis

neutrophils

early
separation

B

Figure 11-18. Bullous eruption of systemic lupus erythematosus. (**A**) This multilocu-lated blister resembles dermatitis herpetiformis. There is a mixed inflammatory infiltrate and some separation at the dermoepidermal junction. (**B**) At higher power, the der-moepidermal separation, as well as the large number of neutrophils that characterize this disease, is more easily visible

Differential Diagnosis

When subepidermal blisters rich in neutrophils are seen in a sys-temic lupus erythematosus patient, of course one should think of the bullous eruption associated with the disorder. Direct im-munofluorescent examination and a trial of dapsone will usually clarify the diagnosis.

BULLOUS DISEASE OF DIABETES

Bullous disease of diabetes (bullosis diabeticorum) is a rare complication of diabetes mellitus in which patients develop large blisters usually on the legs or pressure sites.[70,71]

Clinical Features

Bullous disease of diabetes is rare, especially considering how common diabetes mellitus is. Less than 50 cases have been re-ported. Patients tend to develop large relatively painless and unin-flamed blisters on the lower extremities. Rarely involvement of other areas may occur. Possible cofactors are trauma and ischemia.

Histopathologic Features

In contrast to other subepidermal blistering diseases, the histopathology of bullous disease of diabetes has not been pre-cisely defined. Both subepidermal and intraepidermal blisters have been identified, but most studies indicate a subepidermal location. If a typical case exists, it has large subepidermal blisters without dermal changes and without immunofluorescent findings. In the few cases in which special examinations have been done, findings are confusing. In sum, bullous disease of diabetes has not been unraveled.

Differential Diagnosis

If a large cell-free subepidermal blister is identified in a diabetic, it is either bullous pemphigoid or bullous disease of diabetes. A single negative direct immunofluorescent examination does not entirely exclude bullous pemphigoid, because many specimens taken from the legs of patients with well-proven bullous pemphigoid lack immunoreactants.[18]

TRAUMATIC BLISTERS

Many types of cutaneous trauma can produce relatively cell-free subepidermal blisters often associated with accompanying epidermal damage:

Thermal burns: the traditional clinical classification of burns can be extended to histology. A first-degree burn shows only epidermal damage with necrotic keratinocytes, while a second-degree burn will show the same epidermal changes with separation at the BMZ with edema. A third-degree burn will show deeper dermal damage, including destruction of appendages. Chemical and thermal burns look identical. Phototoxic reactions, sunburn, and liquid nitrogen blistering are also similar, but usually more superficial. Electrodesiccation or electrical burns cause rearrangement of the cells of the epidermis that overlie the blister.[72] The keratinocytes are elongated perpendicular to the BMZ with a tufted or fringed appearance at the separation. This is often seen as a side effect in tissue that has been electrodesiccated before surgical excision.

Suction blister: suction produces a naked blister with preservation of the normal epidermis and dermal papilla. Separation usually occurs at the lamina lucida. Occasionally, if suction is severe enough, there can be hemorrhage or epidermal damage.[73]

Friction blisters: when acral surfaces are subjected to excessive trauma, such as by prolonged walking, blisters may develop. They are almost always intraepidermal and usually arise in the stratum malpighii,[74] so that in theory at least they are higher in the epidermis than those of epidermolysis bullosa simplex.

Hypoxia and pressure blisters: patients who have been unconscious and have been lying for some time without moving may develop blisters. The epidermis may show necrosis and inflammation. The separation is usually intraepidermal. A histologic clue to this process is damage to the eccrine sweat glands that results in a homogenization of their cytoplasm. The combination of pressure and perhaps toxic ingredients that accumulate in the glands may be responsible for the epithelial necrosis.[75,76]

Other traumatic blisters: nonimmune blisters may develop secondary to edema in stasis dermatitis and fracture patients,[77] as well as in reflex sympathetic dystrophy.[78] In the oral cavity, superficial blood-filled blisters, known as *angina bullosa hemorrhagica*, may arise on the buccal surfaces secondary to superficial trauma.[79]

Differential Diagnosis

Traumatic blisters have little inflammation and varying types of epidermal damage. Sometimes they can be distinguished on the basis of these unique changes. Erythema multiforme, epidermolysis bullosa, and bullous disease of diabetes may cause histopathologic confusion.

REFERENCES

1. Briggaman RA, Yoshike T, Cronce DJ: The epidermal-dermal junction and genetic disorders of this area. p. 1243. In Goldsmith LA (ed): Physiology, Biochemistry and Molecular Biology of the Skin. 2nd Ed. Oxford University Press, New York, 1991
2. Marinkovich MP: The molecular genetics of basement membrane diseases. Arch Dermatol 129:1557, 1993
3. Yancey KB: From bedside to bench and back; the diagnosis and biology of bullous diseases. Arch Dermatol 130:983, 1994
4. Yancey KB: Adhesion molecules. II. Interactions of keratinocytes with epidermal basement membrane. J Invest Dermatol 104:1008, 1995
5. Christiano AM, Uitto J: Molecular complexity of the cutaneous basement membrane zone. Revelations from the paradigms of epidermolysis bullosa. Exp Dermatol 5:1, 1996
6. Gammon WR, Fine J-D, Forbes M, Briggaman RA: Immunofluorescence on split skin for the detection and differentiation of basement membrane zone autoantibodies. J Am Acad Dermatol 27:79, 1992
7. Chan LS, Cooper KD: A novel immune-mediated subepidermal bullous dermatosis characterized by IgG autoantibodies to a lower lamina lucida component. Arch Dermatol 130:344, 1994
8. Farmer ER: Subepidermal bullous disease. J Cutan Pathol 12:316, 1985
9. Mutasim DF, Diaz LA: The relevance of immunohistochemical techniques in the differentiation of subepidermal bullous disease. Am J Dermatopathol 13:77, 1991
10. Korman N: Bullous pemphigoid. J Am Acad Dermatol 16:907, 1987
11. Anhalt GJ, Morrison LH: Pemphigoid: bullous, gestational, and cicatricial. Curr Prob Dermatol 1:125, 1989
12. Nemeth AJ, Klein AD, Gould EW, Schachner LA: Childhood bullous pemphigoid. Clinical and immunologic features, treatment and prognosis. Arch Dermatol 127, 378, 1991
13. Stone SP, Schroeter AL: Bullous pemphigoid and associated malignant neoplasms. Arch Dermatol 111:991, 1985
14. Liu H-NH, Su WPD, Rogers RS III: Clinical variants of pemphigoid. Int J Dermatol 25:17, 1986

12

FOLLICULITIS AND ALOPECIA

This chapter is divided into four parts: infundibulofolliculitis, acneiform folliculitis, follicular mucinosis, and alopecia. The classification of folliculitis is presented as an algorithm in Figure 12-1.

INFUNDIBULOFOLLICULITIS

The follicular infundibulum, the part of the hair follicle that extends from the opening of the sebaceous duct to the epidermis, is a frequent site of microscopic alterations. Irritants, allergens, and infectious agents first encounter the follicle here because of its proximity to and continuity with the epidermis.

Spongiotic Infundibulofolliculitis

Clinical Features

Atopic dermatitis frequently involves the hair follicle, which is observed clinically as follicular prominence.[1] Irritant or allergic contact dermatitis may also involve the follicle.[2] Disseminate and recurrent infundibulofolliculitis is a mildly pruritic, recurrent eruption in black patients that resembles follicular atopic dermatitis.[3,4] It tends to be widespread and resistant to topical corticosteroid therapy.

Histopathologic Features

In early lesions, spongiosis produces increased thickness of the infundibular epithelium. A variably dense lymphocytic infiltrate is present within both the epidermis and the dermis. The dermal lymphocytic infiltrate is peri-infundibular and perivascular (Fig. 12-2). Spongiosis is also usually present in the overlying and adjacent epidermis. Eosinophils are more prominent in allergic contact and atopic dermatitis than in irritant dermatitis. In chronic lesions, orthokeratosis and parakeratosis are present in the infundibulum in a pattern similar to subacute and chronic spongiotic dermatitis.[5] The microscopic changes of disseminate and recurrent infundibulofolliculitis are similar.[3,4] In contrast to atopic infundibulofolliculitis, eosinophils are not present.

Infectious Infundibulofolliculitis

Bacterial (Staphylococcal) Folliculitis

Clinical Features

Staphylococci are the most common cause of bacterial folliculitis. The folliculitis may be part of a larger pyoderma. Bacterial folliculitis tends to occur on the extremities and trunk.

Histopathologic Features

Because staphylococci are normal occupants of the follicular canal, the presence of these organisms per se does not imply infection. In bacterial folliculitis neutrophils permeate the spongiotic infundibular epithelium.[5,6] Acantholytic keratinocytes are also frequently present in the infundibulum. Colonies of bacteria may be found in large clumps in routine sections and in those stained with tissue Gram stains such as the Brown-Brenn stain. If inflammation is marked, the infundibulum may eccentrically rupture and deposit its finely granular, deeply basophilic follicular contents into the adjacent dermis (Fig. 12-3). A dense mixed inflammatory cell infiltrate composed primarily of neutrophils and lymphocytes admixed with varying numbers of macrophages, both mono- and multinucleate, surrounds the point of perforation. Bacteria, however, are rarely found in the dermis. This pattern of microscopic "perforating folliculitis" is common to all forms of infundibulofolliculitis in which the degree of inflammation is extensive.

Fungal Folliculitis (Dermatophytosis, Majocchi's Granuloma) and Pityrosporon Folliculitis

Clinical Features

Dermatophytes frequently involve the follicular infundibulum in both glabrous skin (tinea corporis) and the scalp (tinea capitis). Follicular pustules are often present in the annular plaques of tinea corporis. Dermatophytes invade (endothrix) or sur-

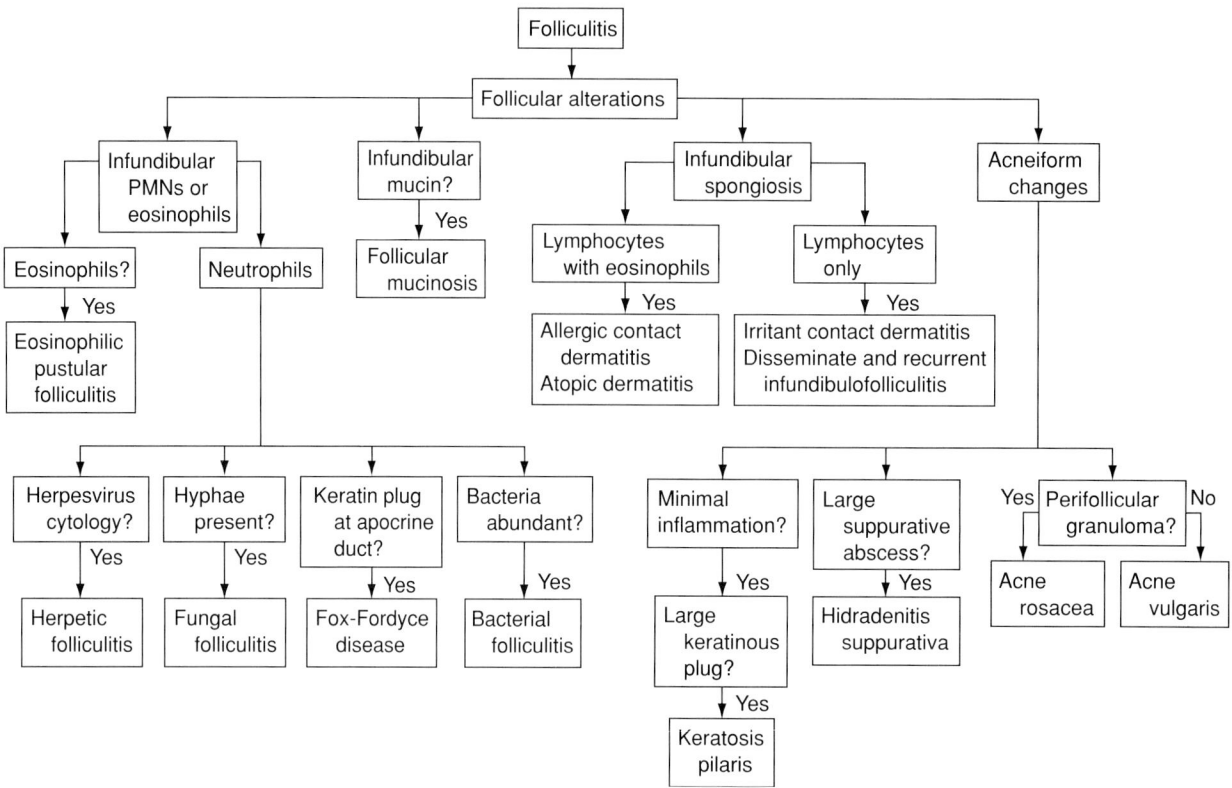

Figure 12-1. Algorithmic classification of folliculitis. PMNs, polymorphonuclear neutrophils.

Figure 12-2. Spongiotic infundibulofolliculitis. Spongiosis is present within the follicular infundibular epithelium. Parakeratosis is variable. The infundibulum is encompassed by lymphocytes with focal exocytosis into the infundibular epithelium. (× 80.)

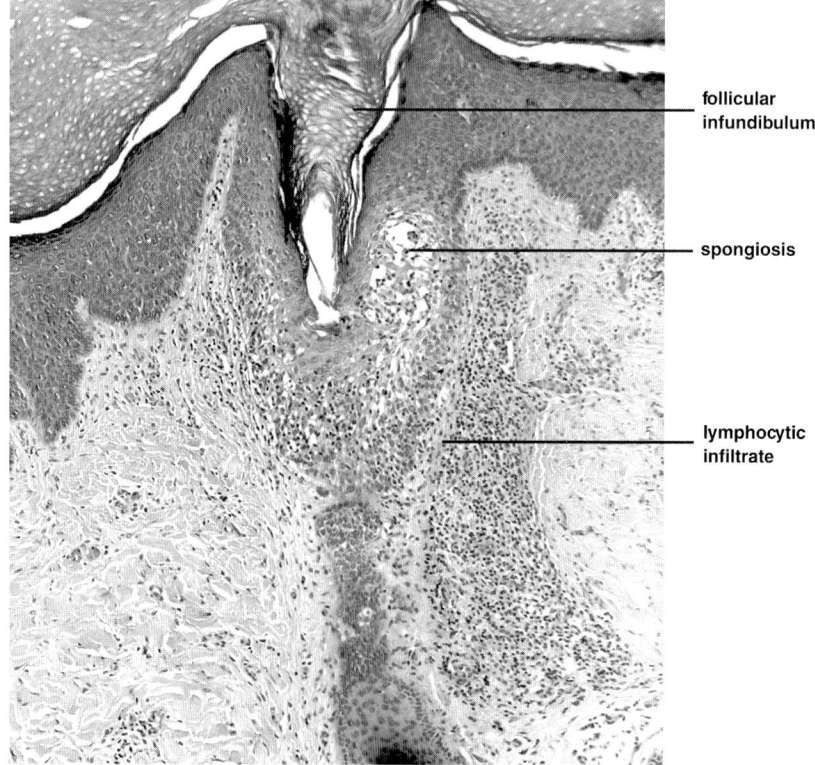

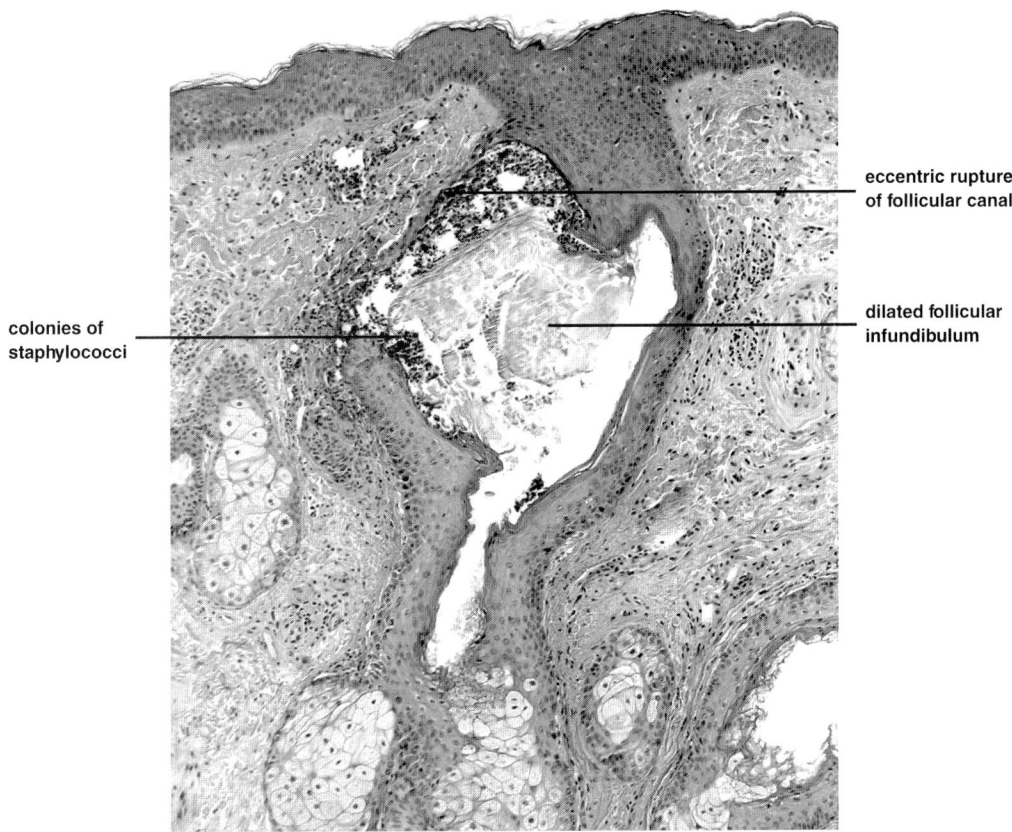

Figure 12-3. Bacterial folliculitis. Eccentric perforation of the follicular canal is common. Colonies of staphylococci are present within the dilated follicular canal. (× 80.)

colonies of
staphylococci

eccentric rupture
of follicular canal

dilated follicular
infundibulum

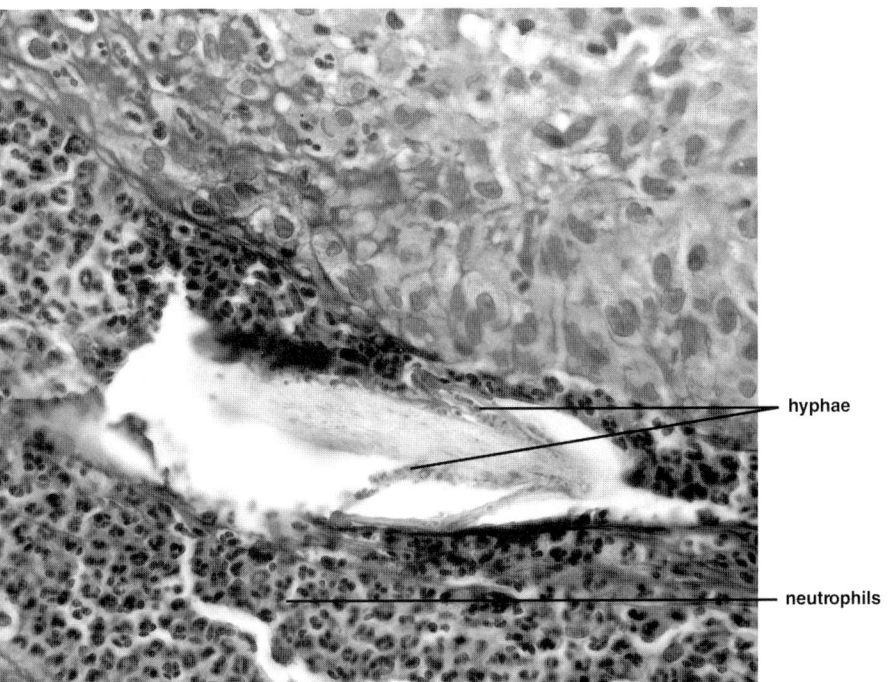

Figure 12-4. Fungal (dermatophyte) folliculitis. Hyphae surround a hair shaft. Numerous neutrophils are present adjacent to the hair shaft. (× 100.)

hyphae

neutrophils

Figure 12-5. Fungal (dermatophyte) folliculitis, Majocchi's granuloma. Neutrophilic and granulomatous inflammation is present around a ruptured follicle. ($\times$ 20.)

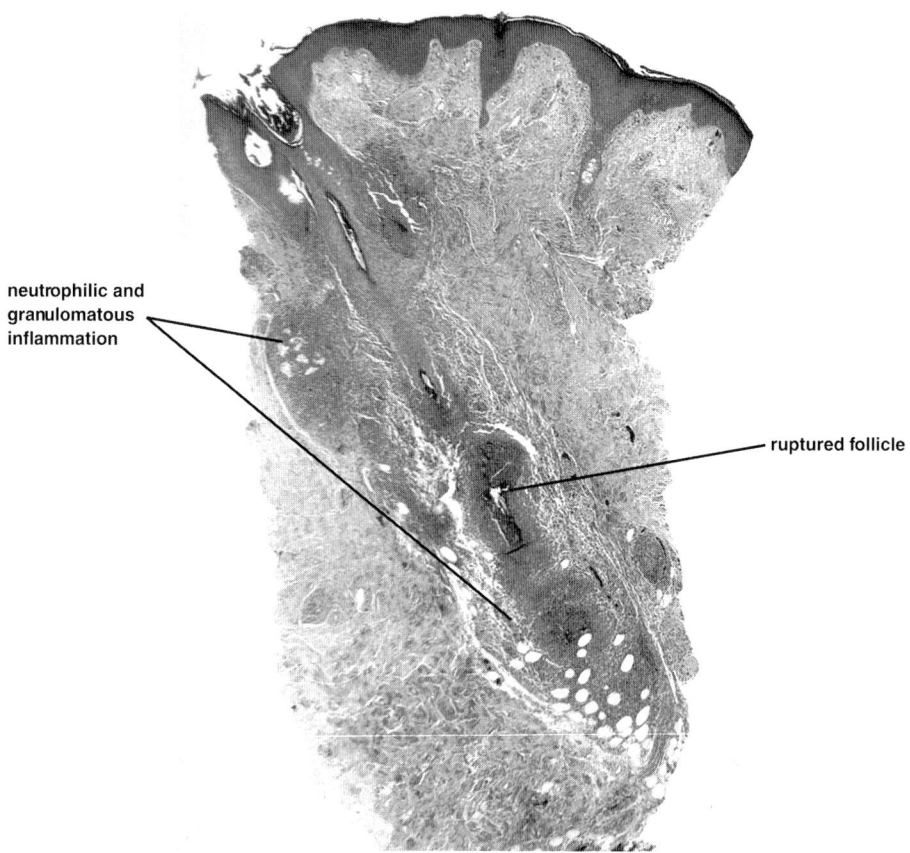

neutrophilic and granulomatous inflammation

ruptured follicle

round (ectothrix) hair shafts in tinea capitis. *Majocchi's granuloma* is the term applied to the chronic erythematous and indurated plaques that result from rupture of a dermatophyte-infected infundibulum.[7] It is frequently found on the anterior legs of women. Although the pityrosporon yeast is a normal inhabi-

tant of the epidermis and the follicular infundibulum, it can cause tinea versicolor and pityrosporon folliculitis.[8] The latter disease is characterized by small, pruritic, follicular pustules most commonly located on the face, neck, upper back, shoulders, or chest.

Figure 12-6. Pityrosporon folliculitis. Clumps of pityrosporon yeasts are present within the follicular canal near sebaceous lobules. ($\times$ 400.)

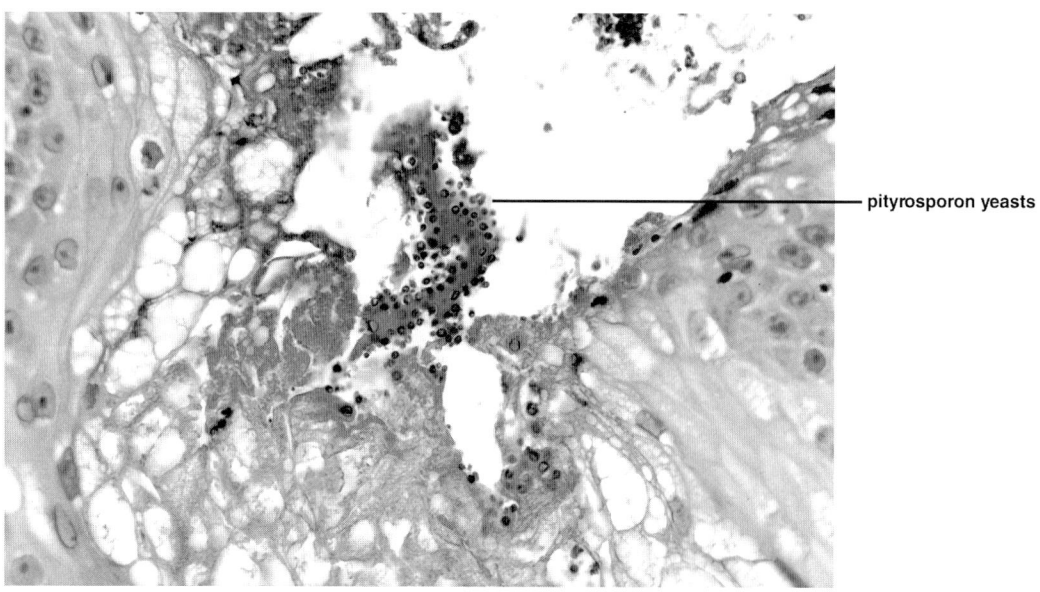

pityrosporon yeasts

Histopathologic Features

Neutrophils are present within the spongiotic infundibulum in dermatophyte infections.[5] Hyphae within or around hair shafts are usually easily visible in hematoxylin and eosin (H&E)–stained sections; they stand out vividly in periodic acid–Schiff (PAS) or silver-impregnated sections[6] (Fig. 12-4). Hyphae are also usually present in the adjacent epidermis. The inflammation in Majocchi's granuloma is more extensive due to rupture of the follicle with spillage of its contents into the dermis. A mixed neutrophilic and lymphocytic infiltrate at the site of the perforation precedes necrotizing, granulomatous inflammation (Fig. 12-5). Neutrophils usually surround the necrotic areas, but eosinophils may be prominent.[9] Hyphae are difficult to identify in the dermal inflammatory cell infiltrate and are usually best seen in the stratum corneum adjacent to the ruptured follicle. The inflammation eventually subsides, resulting in a perifollicular scar.

The intensity of the inflammatory response in pityrosporon folliculitis is variable.[5] Lymphocytes predominate, but a few neutrophils are also usually present in the peri-infundibular infiltrates.[8] Numerous pityrosporon yeasts are present and are easily visible within the follicle in routinely stained sections (Fig. 12-6). Special stains are rarely required to visualize the yeasts.

Herpetic Folliculitis (Herpes Simplex and Zoster)

Clinical Features

The vesicles and pustules of both herpes simplex and zoster often form around hair follicles.[10]

Histopathologic Features

The characteristic nuclear changes of herpesvirus infection (i.e., "ground-glass" homogeneous chromatin, multinucleation, fused, molded nuclear contours, and rare eosinophilic intranuclear inclusions) are found in the keratinocytes of the infundibulum[11] (Fig. 12-7). Acantholysis and dyskeratosis are prominent. A mixed dense inflammatory cell infiltrate that includes numerous neutrophils is found both within the follicle and adjacent to it. Leukocytoclastic vasculitis may occur around the affected follicle. Keratinocyte necrosis is extensive and leads to eventual destruction of the hair follicle.

Special Variants of Infundibulofolliculitis

Fox-Fordyce Disease

Clinical Features

Fox-Fordyce disease affects the axillae and less commonly the areolae and anogenital areas of women, anatomic sites with apocrine glands.[12] Multiple discrete pruritic papules form around hair follicles. The course is characterized by intermittent exacerbations and remissions. Follicular occlusion in the affected sites leads to obstruction of apocrine secretion.

Histopathologic Features

Spongiosis is limited to an area adjacent to the opening of the apocrine sweat duct into the follicular infundibulum.[12] A keratotic plug occludes the dilated infundibulum. Exocytotic lymphocytes are present in the spongiotic areas. Eventually, the up-

Figure 12-7. Herpetic folliculitis. Multinucleate giant keratinocytes with homogenization of the nuclear chromatin are found within follicular epithelium. (× 200.)

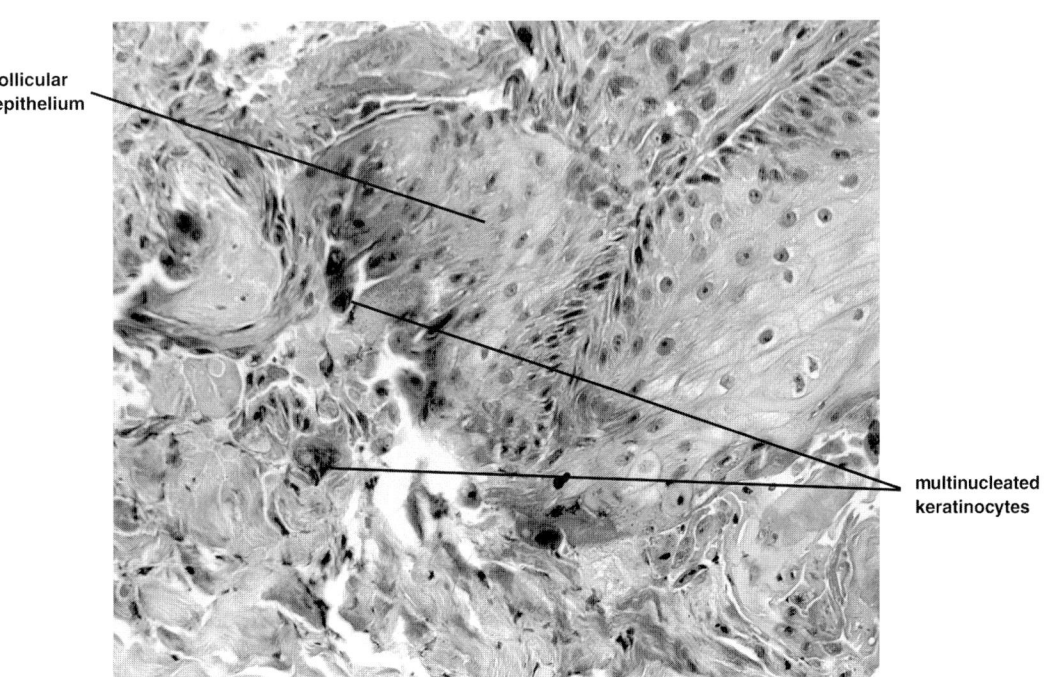

follicular epithelium

multinucleated keratinocytes

per part of the apocrine duct becomes cystically dilated, and the apocrine secretory apparatus degenerates. Serial sections may be needed to demonstrate the periductal spongiosis and the dilated apocrine duct.

Eosinophilic Pustular Folliculitis (Ofuji Syndrome)

Clinical Features

Originally described in Japanese men, eosinophilic pustular folliculitis (EPF) was first thought to be rare in the United States.[13–16] However, EPF in patients with acquired immunodeficiency syndrome is now being diagnosed with relative frequency in this country.[17–21] EPF is more common in men. Intensely pruritic papules and pustules are typically found on the face, trunk, and extremities. The individual lesions may coalesce to form erythematous plaques with irregular borders and a tendency toward central clearing. EPF remits spontaneously but frequently recurs. Patients with EPF may have leukocytosis and eosinophilia. Eosinophilic pustular folliculitis may occur in infants and children[22–24] and has also been reported in association with hematologic malignancies.[16,21,25,26]

Histopathologic Features

Early vesicles are characterized by a spongiotic follicular infundibulum laced with eosinophils.[13–15,21] Similar changes may be present in the epidermis adjacent to the follicles. The spongiotic vesicles rapidly progress to an eosinophil-filled pustule that distends and distorts the infundibulum, ultimately resulting in follicular rupture (Fig. 12-8). Eosinophils may also extend proximally within the follicle to the outer root sheath and along the sebaceous duct into the sebaceous gland lobules. Eosinophils, along with lymphocytes and neutrophils, are also found in the dermis adjacent to the follicle. They may be present in sufficient numbers to form a dermal abscess. Mucin production within follicles has been reported.[13–15,21]

Differential Diagnosis

Each of the different types of infundibulofolliculitis is characterized by the same basic inflammatory pattern (i.e., infundibular spongiosis and inflammatory cell infiltrates). Each has distinguishing features (Table 12-1).

In routinely stained sections, the mucin deposits of follicular mucinosis may appear as clear spaces that separate stretched infundibular keratinocytes and can be easily mistaken for spongiosis. Special stains for mucin, such as the Alcian blue or colloidal iron stains, allow differentiation of the two processes.

ACNEIFORM FOLLICULITIS

Acneiform folliculitis is a group of related diseases characterized by cystic dilation of the follicular infundibulum. The initial

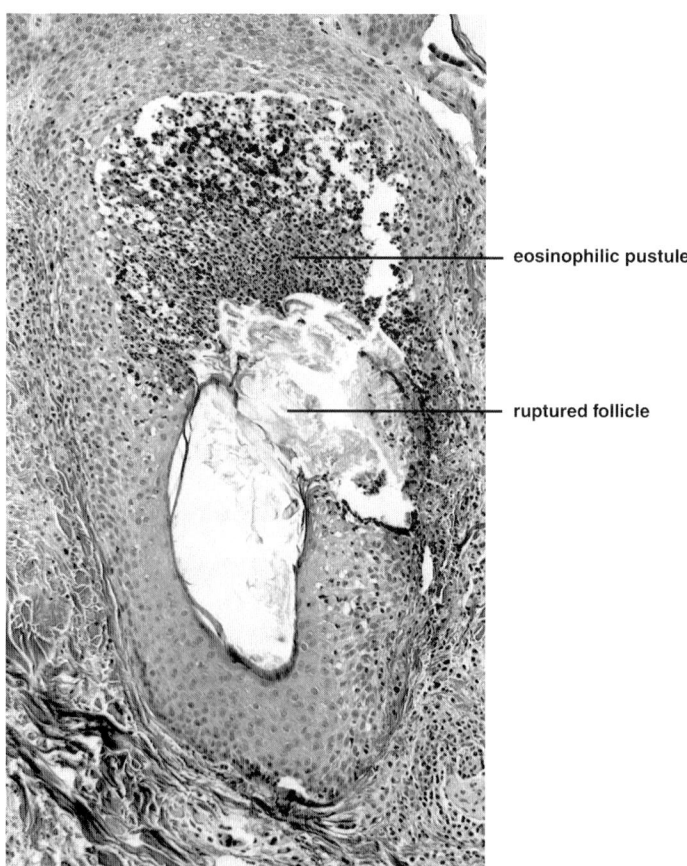

Figure 12-8. Eosinophilic folliculitis. An abscess formed from eosinophils is present near the site of follicular rupture. (× 100.)

eosinophilic pustule

ruptured follicle

Table 12-1. Differential Features of Infundibulofolliculitis

Diagnosis	Infundibular Change
Spongiotic	Intra- and perifollicular lymphocytic infiltrates; ± eosinophils
Staphylococcal	Clumps of cocci; neutrophils
Fungal	Hyphae or yeasts; neutrophils
Herpetic	Multinucleate keratinocytes with glassy, molded, and fused nuclei; necrosis
Fox-Fordyce	Keratinous plug at entrance of apocrine duct
Eosinophilic pustular folliculitis	Large numbers of eosinophils

pathogenic event in each of these diseases is obstruction of the infundibular orifice with subsequent distention of this part of the follicle.[27] Cystically dilated follicles are the microscopic equivalent of the clinical comedo. Continued distortion of the cystically dilated infundibulum results in necrosis of the keratinocytes and loss of integrity of the investing basement membrane. If the obstruction is not alleviated, the follicle will eventually rupture and spew its contents into the adjacent dermis. An exuberant, primarily neutrophilic, inflammatory response initially develops. A frank intra- and perifollicular abscess may follow. The neutrophilic inflammatory infiltrate is eventually replaced by lymphocytes and macrophages. Finally, the infiltrate becomes more or less granulomatous. Resolution results in varying degrees of perifollicular fibrosis. The follicle may be destroyed.

This sequence takes place to a greater or lesser degree depending on the particular disease. In mild to moderate acne vulgaris and folliculitis decalvans inflammation is limited to the cystically dilated infundibulum and adjacent dermis.[27,28] Even this limited inflammation may lead to follicular destruction, especially in folliculitis decalvans. The extent of dermal abscess formation is much greater in cystic acne, hidradenitis suppurativa, and dissecting cellulitis of the scalp.[27–30] Follicular destruction is the rule here. The perifollicular inflammation is frequently granulomatous in rosacea.[31] Inflammation is limited in keratosis pilaris. Prominent perifollicular scarring characterizes acne keloidalis.

Acne Vulgaris

Clinical Features

Acne vulgaris of some extent is present in most adolescents.[27] Involvement is remarkably variable and ranges from a few intermittent papules of only cosmetic significance to severe, disfiguring disease. The face, upper back, shoulders, and upper chest are most frequently involved. Men and women are equally affected. Hormonal stimulation of sebaceous glands to form excessive amounts of sebum is thought to incite a cascade of events, including overgrowth of *Propionibacterium acnes*. The infundibular keratinocytes then proliferate, and the intrainfundibular stratum corneum increases in thickness. The dilated infundibulum (comedo) either remains closed (whitehead) or open (blackhead). Continued dilation of the follicle results in an erythematous papule (papular acne). After it ruptures, a perifollicular abscess may form and eventually connect with other follicles (acne conglobata). Several clinical variants have been described (e.g., acne mechanica from chronic irritation, acne cosmetica from occlusive cosmetics, and corticosteroid-induced acne).

Histopathologic Features

A comedo is a cystically dilated follicular infundibulum with keratotic debris filling its lumen[27] (Fig. 12-9). Inflammatory cells, primarily neutrophils and lymphocytes, are initially sparse inside the follicle.[32] Perifollicular inflammation is greater and is composed primarily of lymphocytes and neutrophils. With rupture of the dilated infundibulum, abscess formation and liquefaction necrosis develop in the perifollicular dermis. Macrophages and multinucleate giant cells surround the abscess. Eventually fibrous scar replaces the inflammation. If the follicle is destroyed in this process, "naked" hair shafts may be found either within the inflammatory cell infiltrate or entrapped in the fibrotic scar.

Differential Diagnosis

Majocchi's granuloma (see above) develops after a dermatophyte infection of the hair shaft.[7] Rupture of the infected follicle leads to perifollicular granulomatous inflammation similar to that in acne. Special stains such as the PAS stain may facilitate recognition of the hyphae. Other forms of infundibulofolliculitis may resemble acne (Table 12-1). Acne vulgaris and its variants are virtually limited to the face, neck, chest, shoulders, and upper back. The epidermis adjacent to the affected follicle in perforating folliculitis, a disease most often found in patients with diabetes, is markedly acanthotic.[33] The perifollicular inflammation in acne rosacea is frequently granulomatous.

Hidradenitis Suppurativa

Clinical Features

Hidradenitis suppurativa is limited to areas with apocrine glands.[29,30] It is usually most severe in the axillary, groin, and perianal areas. The inframammary skin may also be involved. The disease begins at puberty or during adolescence. Both men and women are affected. Initially the fluctuant abscesses are solitary, but they eventually become linked by deep purulent channels. Both the nodular abscesses and the connecting channels frequently rupture to the skin surface so that abundant foul-smelling pus is extruded. Eventually the entire affected area becomes a network of draining abscesses, fluctuant sinus tracts, and firm linear scars.

Histopathologic Features

The earliest changes in hidradenitis suppurativa consist of spongiosis of the apocrine duct and follicular infundibulum near the entrance of the duct into the follicle.[29,30,34] The infundibulum

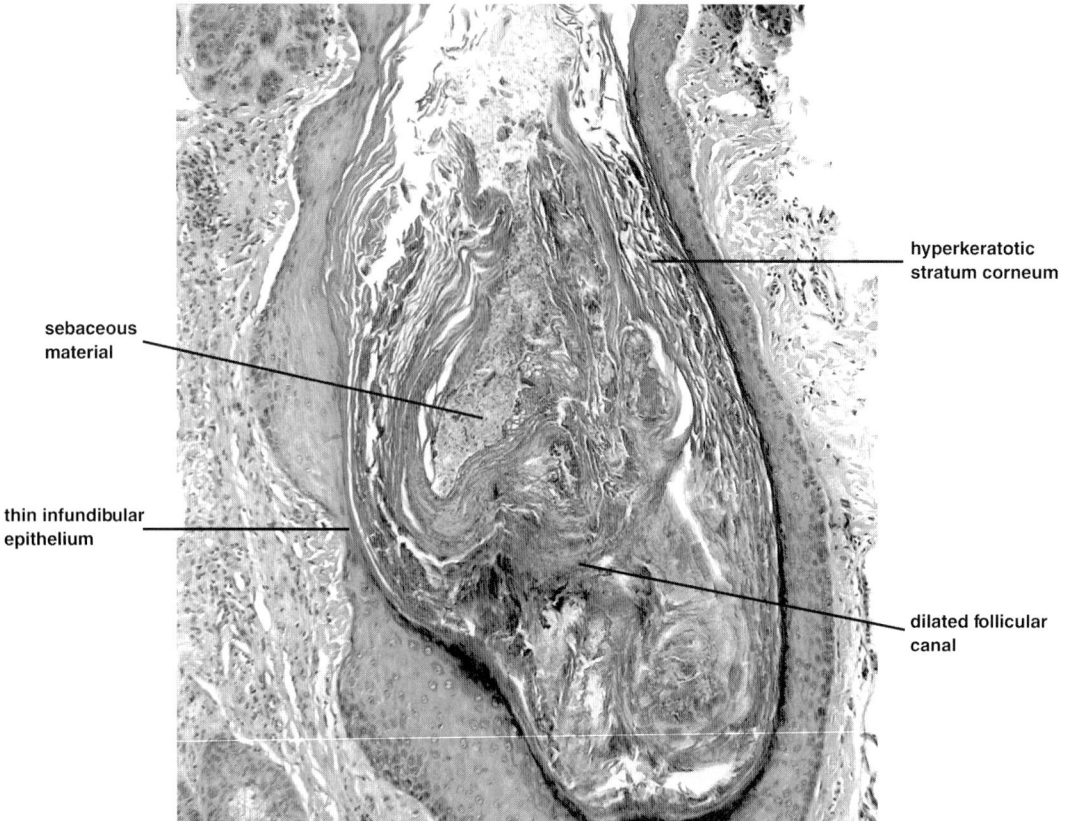

Figure 12-9. Acne comedo (acneiform folliculitis). The cystically dilated follicular canal is filled with hyperkeratotic stratum corneum and sebaceous material. The infundibular epithelium is focally thinned. (× 80.)

labels: hyperkeratotic stratum corneum; sebaceous material; thin infundibular epithelium; dilated follicular canal

then fills with keratinous debris, resulting in comedo-like infundibular distention. These follicles then rupture, leading to the formation of perifollicular and periapocrine abscesses that are connected by dermal and subcutaneous sinus tracts filled with neutrophils and necrotic debris (Fig. 12-10). Granulomatous inflammation, including foreign body-type giant cells, is present at the periphery of the purulent inflammation. Pseudoepitheliomatous hyperplasia is evident where the sinus tracts open to the epidermis. Lobules of reactive, proliferated epidermis may extend into the deep dermis and even subcutis. The inflammatory and proliferative changes are adjacent to dermal scars that increase in thickness as the inflammatory component decreases in extent. In quiescent areas, nodular foci of mixed inflammatory cell infiltrates and varying degrees of pseudoepitheliomatous hyperplasia are found in addition to dermal and subcutaneous scarring.

Differential Diagnosis

The purulent abscesses of hidradenitis suppurativa must be differentiated from infectious diseases such as deep fungal and atypical mycobacterial infections by special stains and inoculation of the appropriate culture media. Foreign body–type granulomatous inflammation with flakes of stratum corneum and possibly rem-

nants of the squamous epithelium are found in ruptured epidermoid cysts, but interconnecting sinus tracts are not present.

Acne Rosacea and Perioral Dermatitis

Clinical Features

Acne rosacea is a multiphasic eruption of adults that is essentially limited to the face.[35] Initially, only erythema and blushing are present. Telangiectasia becomes prominent as the disease progresses. The skin is oily. Eventually scattered papules, pustules, and small cysts form within the telangiectatic, erythematous areas. The latter are more prominent in some patients than others and may extend onto the eyelids and forehead. Furrowed, lobulated thickening of the skin of the nose (rhinophyma) may occur alone, but usually is present in conjunction with the other components.

Granulomatous rosacea (lupus miliaris disseminatus faciei) most commonly occurs on the cheeks without a background of erythema and telangiectasia.[36–38]

Perioral dermatitis is limited to the skin around the lips and chin. The combination of papules and erythema resembles rosacea, but the papules tend to be smaller and the skin is dry and scaly rather than oily.[39] Perioral dermatitis is commonly associated with prolonged use of fluorinated topical corticosteroids.

Histopathologic Features

Specimens from the erythematous and telangiectatic areas show only minimal perivascular and perifollicular neutrophilic and lymphocytic infiltrates along with ectasia of the capillaries of the superficial dermis.[31] The follicular changes in the papules and cysts are virtually identical to those in acne vulgaris. Perifollicular granulomas composed of epithelioid macrophages, multinucleate giant cells, and lymphocytes are characteristic of papular and granulomatous rosacea. The granulomas may be large and conspicuous or small and subtle.[36,38] They resemble the granulomas of sarcoidosis in that they tend to be well circumscribed. Small, focal areas of necrosis are common within the granulomas, but necrosis may be extensive in the purely granulomatous variant.[38] Special stains for organisms, including acid-fast bacilli, are negative. Rarely the granulomas may be found in the subcutis or dermis with no demonstrable spatial relationship to the hair follicles.

Follicular alterations similar to rosacea, but less extensive, are found in perioral dermatitis.[39] Spongiosis, parakeratosis, and acanthosis are common features in both the acrotrichia and interfollicular epidermis.

Differential Diagnosis

Discrete perifollicular granulomas distinguish rosacea and its variants from acne vulgaris. Although perifollicular granuloma-tous inflammation may occasionally occur in acne, the granulomas are not as well demarcated as in rosacea. Infections, especially deep fungal and mycobacterial, must be differentiated from rosacea with special stains and appropriate cultures.[40] Cutaneous sarcoidosis, especially lupus pernio, may be impossible to differentiate from rosacea by microscopy alone. Clinical correlation is essential.

Keratosis Pilaris

Clinical Features

Pinhead-sized erythematous or skin-colored acneiform papules occur on the dorsal surface of the upper arms, thighs, and buttocks.[41] The keratinous plugs that protrude from the papules impart a sandpaper-like feel to the skin surface. Keratosis pilaris is usually asymptomatic. It is most common in adolescents and in atopic persons with xerosis. Keratosis pilaris may rarely be associated with scarring alopecia.[42]

Histopathologic Features

The papules of keratosis pilaris are formed from individual follicular infundibula expanded by a dense orthokeratotic plug that surrounds the hair shaft[41] (Fig. 12-11). The infundibular epithelium is spongiotic. A minimal lymphocytic infiltrate surrounds the infundibulum.

Figure 12-10. Hidradenitis suppurativa. Remnants of a hair follicle are surrounded by a large dermal and subcutaneous abscess. (× 20.)

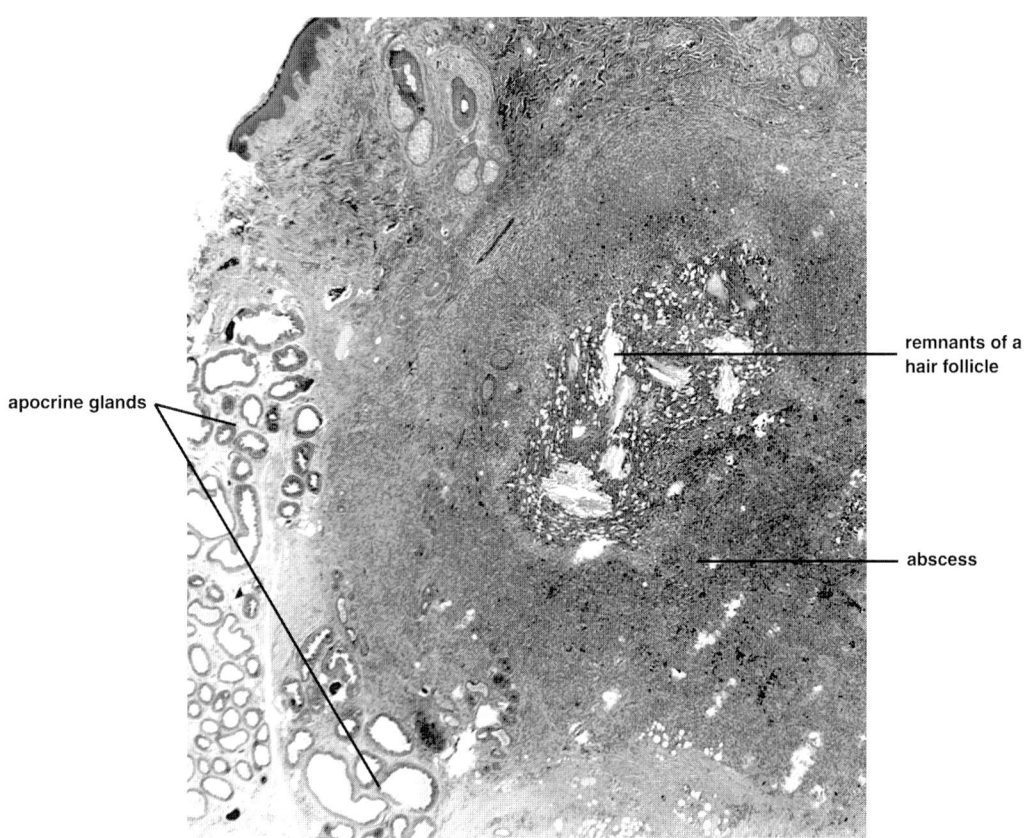

apocrine glands

remnants of a hair follicle

abscess

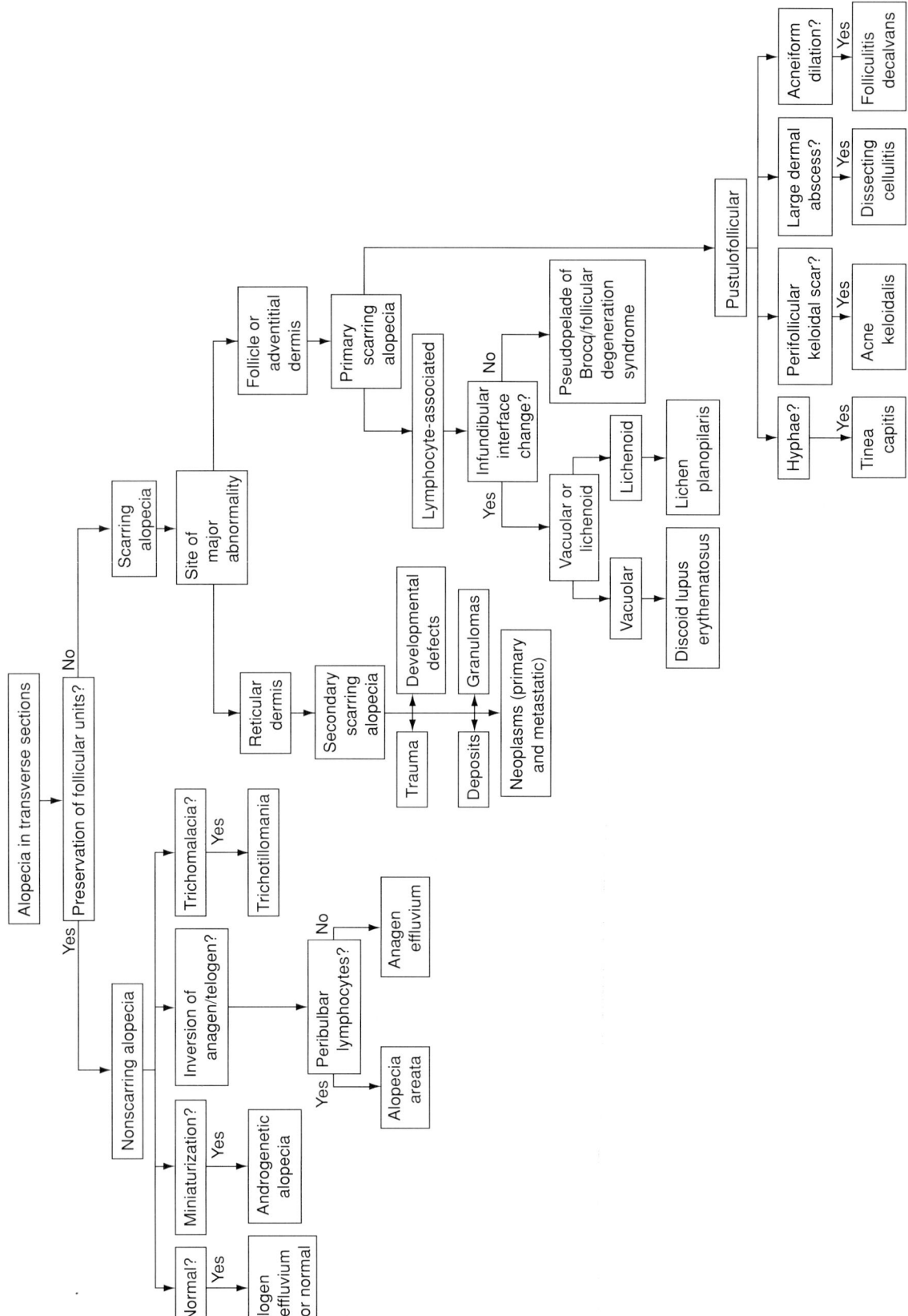

Figure 12-13.   Algorithm describing the classification of alopecia by transverse section evaluation.

tions are taken perpendicular to the follicle, a partial rim of epidermis is usually present in the most superficial sections from a properly prepared specimen (see below). Therefore, evaluation of epidermal or interface changes can be done on transverse sections as well. Interpretation of transversely sectioned scalp biopsy specimens are emphasized in the following discussions, especially in the evaluation of nonscarring alopecias.

Transverse Section Scalp Biopsy Technique

The only change required in the gross processing of punch biopsy specimens from the scalp is that instead of the traditional longitudinal bisection, the specimen is cut transversely, perpendicular to the plane of the hair shafts protruding from the epidermal surface (not perpendicular to the plane of the epidermis).[52] If no hair shafts are present, the cut should be made at a slight (10 to 15 degree) angle to the epidermis. This cut is best made through the dermis approximately 1 mm above its junction with the subcutis. To aid in orientation of the tissue blocks for microtome sectioning, a drop of India ink can be placed on the cut edge of each half of the specimen.

Each half of the transected specimen should be put in a separate cassette for sectioning, because multiple blocks in the same cassette are more difficult to orient to the microtome blade and may result in tangential sections. As the microtome blade cuts into the specimen, the sections from the superficial block will be of dermis, and each section will be closer to the epidermis. The sections from the deeper block will be progressively deeper moving toward the subcutis.

Examination of several levels of sections from each block is usually sufficient. Additional levels or serial sections can be obtained when necessary.

Clinical Considerations

Because the bulbs of terminal follicles extend into the subcutis, the punch biopsy specimen should include as much subcutis as possible. A sharp biopsy tool is essential, and long, curved scissors are helpful because straight scissor blades result in a diagonal rather than a horizontal deep excision margin. A 4-mm punch biopsy specimen is usually adequate, but a 6-mm specimen is optimal.

Scalp Microanatomy in Transverse Section

Features of scalp microanatomy seen in transverse section have been described by several authors.[52–62] *Terminal follicles* are the largest hair follicles in the scalp (Figs. 12-14 to 12-16). An arrector pili muscle is attached to each follicle. The hair bulb is located in the subcutis. The hair shaft is relatively large in diameter, and both a cortex and a medulla are present. In darkly pigmented hair shafts abundant melanin granules are readily apparent in the effete keratinocytes of the shaft. *Vellus follicles* are smaller in diameter and shorter in length (Figs. 12-14 to 12-16). The bulb is located in the dermis rather than the subcutis. These follicles do not have an arrector pili muscle attached. The keratinocytes in the shaft rarely contain melanin granules, and the shaft is not medullated.

Figure 12-14. Normal scalp in transverse section. Numerous follicular units are separated by reticular dermal collagen. This section is taken through a plane immediately below the opening of the sebaceous duct, since both the inner and outer root sheaths are seen in most of the terminal follicles. Most of the follicles are in the anagen growth phase. (× 20.)

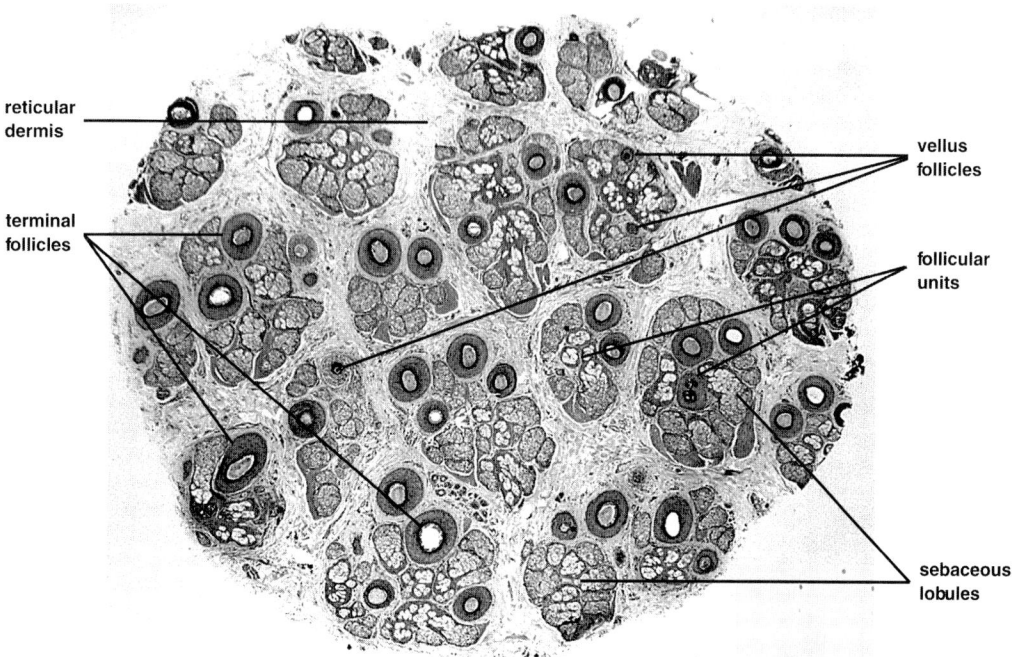

reticular dermis

terminal follicles

vellus follicles

follicular units

sebaceous lobules

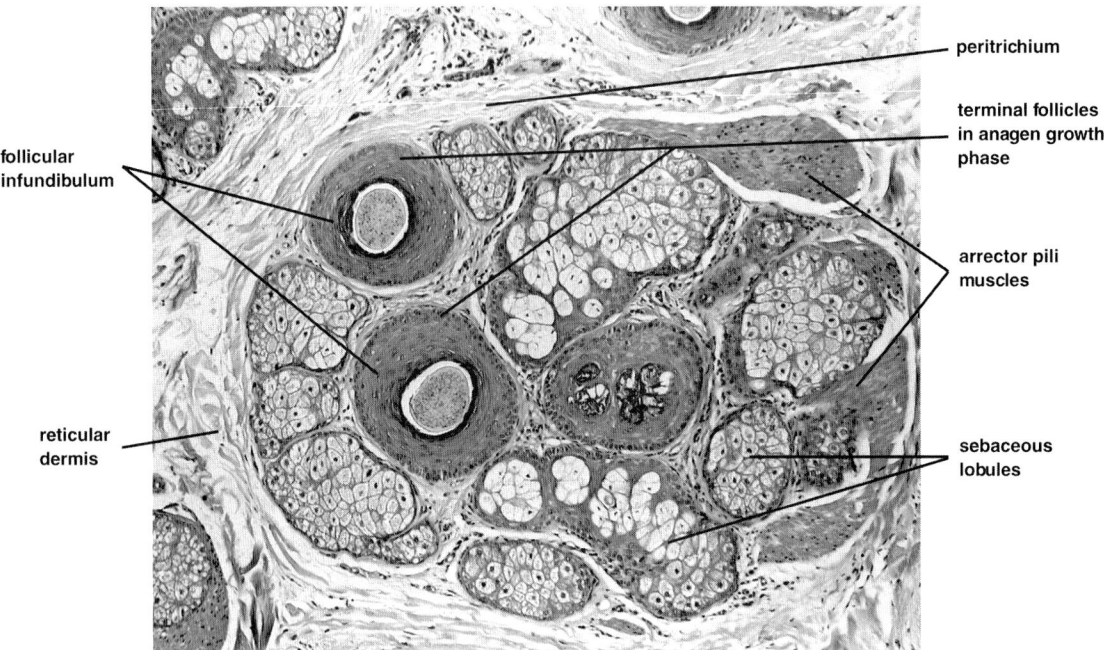

peritrichium

terminal follicles
in anagen growth
phase

follicular
infundibulum

arrector pili
muscles

reticular
dermis

sebaceous
lobules

Figure 12-15. Normal follicular unit in transverse section. This section was taken through a plane above the opening of the sebaceous duct because the follicular epithelium is keratinizing in an epidermal mode and neither the inner nor outer root sheath is present. This is the follicular infundibulum. No vellus follicles are seen in this follicular unit. ($\times$ 80.)

Figure 12-16. Normal follicular unit in transverse section. This section was taken through a plane below the opening of the sebaceous duct. Both the inner and outer root sheaths are visible; hence the follicles are in the anagen growth phase. ($\times$ 80.)

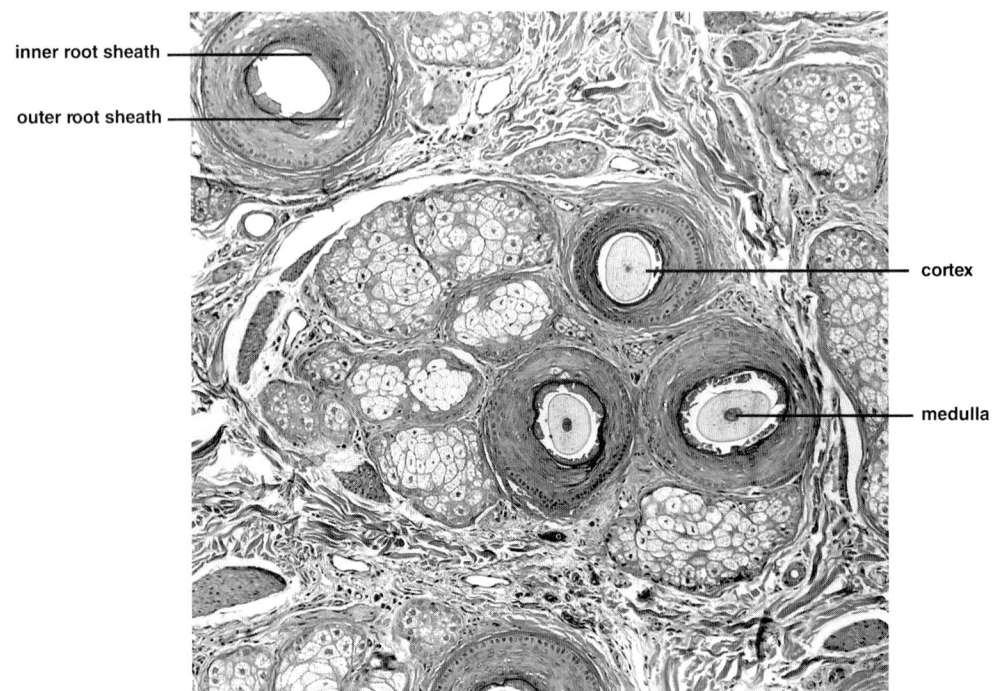

inner root sheath

outer root sheath

cortex

medulla

The Follicular Unit

In normal scalp, two to four terminal follicles and one or two vellus follicles are grouped together to form a *follicular unit* when viewed in transverse sections (Figs. 12-14 to 12-16). Two or more hair shafts may emerge from the same infundibulum within a follicular unit. The follicular units are normally oriented in geometric arrays (Fig. 12-14). Recognition of the normal grouping of human scalp follicles into follicular units is important, because abnormalities of the normal pattern are readily discernible at low magnification and usually indicate a loss of follicles. A 4-mm punch biopsy specimen from normal scalp contains 10 to 12 follicular units and, therefore, 20 to 48 terminal follicles.

Follicular Dynamics

Follicular dynamics have been described by several authors.[52–54,60,63]

The Anagen Follicle. Approximately 90% of terminal hair follicles on the normal scalp are in the anagen growth phase at any given time. All parts of the hair follicle are present in the anagen growth phase. Five different patterns of keratinization are evident. Each type of keratinization defines a different part of the anagen follicle and is of value in locating the plane of sectioning in transverse sections (Table 12-2).

Vellus follicles have a similar appearance in transverse sections, but the follicular diameters are smaller than terminal follicles and the bulbs are located in the dermis rather than the subcutis.

The *follicular infundibulum* is the most superficial part of the follicle and extends from the intraepidermal follicular orifice *(acrotrichium)* to the opening of the sebaceous duct into the follicular canal. It is formed from progressively flattened keratinocytes that keratinize like the epidermis (i.e., with basophilic [*keratohyaline*] granules in the keratinocytes adjacent

Table 12-2. Follicular Keratinization in Transverse Section

Level Within Follicle	Keratinization Type
Infundibulum	Epidermal: keratohyaline (basophilic) granule formation
Ostium of the sebaceous duct	Cuticular: thin, wavy, eosinophilic keratin layer; no granule formation
Outer root sheath	Trichilemmal: no granule formation
Inner root sheath	Trichohyaline: brightly eosinophilic granule in zone of keratinization
Hair bulb	Hair shaft formation: hair shaft keratins form without granule formation, dendritic melanocytes mixed between basophilic, basaloid keratinocytes of the hair matrix; dermal papilla formed from collagen, blood vessels, small nerves

to the lumen) (Fig. 12-15). These large basophilic granules allow easy recognition of the infundibulum in transverse sections.

The *sebaceous duct* is a short canal that connects the sebaceous lobules with the hair follicle. The luminal surface is lined by a distinctive brightly eosinophilic, wavy "cuticle" that extends a short distance into the infundibulum.

The *outer root sheath* (trichilemma) extends from the opening of the sebaceous duct distally to the hair bulb proximally (Figs. 12-14, 12-16, and 12-17). The keratinocytes of this layer are large and cuboidal. The cytoplasm of these cells contains abundant glycogen, imparting a pale or clear cytoplasm in H&E-stained sections. The keratinocyte cytoplasm is magenta in PAS-stained sections. The outer root sheath completely disintegrates immediately below the entrance of the sebaceous duct.

The *inner root sheath* closely invests the hair shaft. It begins proximally at the hair bulb and becomes fully keratinized below the opening of the sebaceous duct where it completely disintegrates along with the outer root sheath (Figs. 12-14, 12-16, and 12-17). Brightly eosinophilic granules (*trichohyaline*) are a unique marker for inner root sheath keratinization. The outer layer of the inner root sheath (Henle) interlocks with the outer root sheath, whereas the inner layer (Huxley) forms a cuticle that interlocks with the cuticle of the cortex of the hair shaft. Both cuticles are only one cell thick.

The *hair bulb* is the germinative part of the hair follicle (Fig. 12-17). From this structure arise all of the above follicular components except the infundibulum and the sebaceous duct. It is formed from both epithelial *(hair matrix)* and mesenchymal *(dermal papilla)* components (Fig. 12-17). The dermal papilla invests the epithelial cells of the hair matrix. The keratinocytes of the hair matrix are small, basaloid, basophilic cells. In persons with dark terminal hairs, numerous dendritic melanocytes are located among the keratinocytes of the hair matrix. Melanin pigment granules are prominent within the cytoplasm of both bulbar melanocytes and keratinocytes. The keratinocytes keratinize without granule formation in the center of the bulb to form the hair shaft. The hair shaft has a central *medulla* surrounded by the peripheral *cortex* in terminal follicles (Fig. 12-16). No medulla is present in the shafts of vellus follicles. The cuticle of the hair shaft is the outermost layer of the cortex. The peripheral keratinocytes of the hair matrix form the inner and outer root sheaths described above.

The dermal papilla is composed of collagen, elastic fibers, fibroblasts, small blood vessels, and nerves. It is continuous with a thin layer of collagen and capillaries, the *peritrichium* that invests the basement membrane of the entire follicle (Fig. 12-15).

Catagen-Telogen Follicle. When hair follicles cease to produce a hair shaft, they enter into the *catagen*, or initial phase of the resting follicle.[64] One of the first morphologic changes of catagen is scattered dyskeratotic *(apoptotic)* keratinocytes in the hair matrix. Next the basement membrane of the hair bulb and lower follicle becomes greatly thickened and undulated. Finally, the inner and outer root sheaths condense around the hair shaft to form a solid, eosinophilic keratinous ball at the proximal end (Fig. 12-18). Catagen is an irreversible process always followed by the *telogen* or resting phase of the growth cycle.

At the termination of the catagen phase, the inner and outer root sheaths completely disintegrate. The few remaining epithelial cells condense to form a cord of small basaloid cells termed the *telogen germinal unit*. As the telogen germinal unit forms, the epithelial cells regress to a point immediately below the sebaceous duct, where they remain until the anagen phase begins anew. Melanocytes become inconspicuous. A narrow tract of delicate collagen, elastic fibers, fibroblasts, and small blood vessels trails the regressing epithelial cells. Headington[53] termed this residual fibrous tract the follicular *stele* (Fig. 12-19; see also Fig. 12-42). This collagenous column is thought to be important in inducing and directing regrowth of the follicle when the anagen phase resumes. The telogen germinal unit and the stele form the *telogen phase follicle*. Normally, follicles remain in the telogen phase several months before anagen growth begins and the growth cycle continues.

Types of Alopecia

The traditional classification of alopecia into either scarring or nonscarring types is based on whether the alopecia results from destruction or atrophy (drop-out) of terminal follicles or alteration in the growth cycle dynamics alone.

Nonscarring Alopecias

Androgenetic Alopecia (Male Pattern Alopecia, Female Pattern Alopecia)

Clinical Features. Male and female patterns of alopecia are the most common forms of alopecia.[65–71] Men may become completely bald, whereas women rarely lose all of their hair. Androgenetic alopecia selectively affects certain areas of the scalp more than others so that the alopecia is "patterned" rather than random or diffuse. Men tend to lose hair from the frontoparietal areas bilaterally and from the occiput. By contrast, androgenetic alopecia results in diffuse thinning over the centrofrontal crown of the scalp in women. The frontal hairline is preserved. Androgenetic alopecia is usually slowly but relentlessly progressive, asymptomatic, and irreversible without treatment. It is inherited but not in a strict mendelian pattern. The onset of androgenetic alopecia is heralded by an increased shedding of normal telogen hairs and a gradual reduction in the diameter of the hair shafts in the affected areas. Loss of pigment in the remaining smaller shafts is common.

Androgenetic alopecia may be the result of androgen excess in some women. In such instances, other signs of virilism are usually present.

Histopathologic Features. The earliest finding in androgenetic alopecia is a decreased anagen/telogen ratio.[52,62] The in-

Figure 12-17. Anagen growth phase in longitudinal section. The hair matrix epithelium is continuous with the epithelium of the inner and outer root sheaths. The brightly eosinophilic trichohyaline granules are limited to the inner root sheath. (× 80.)

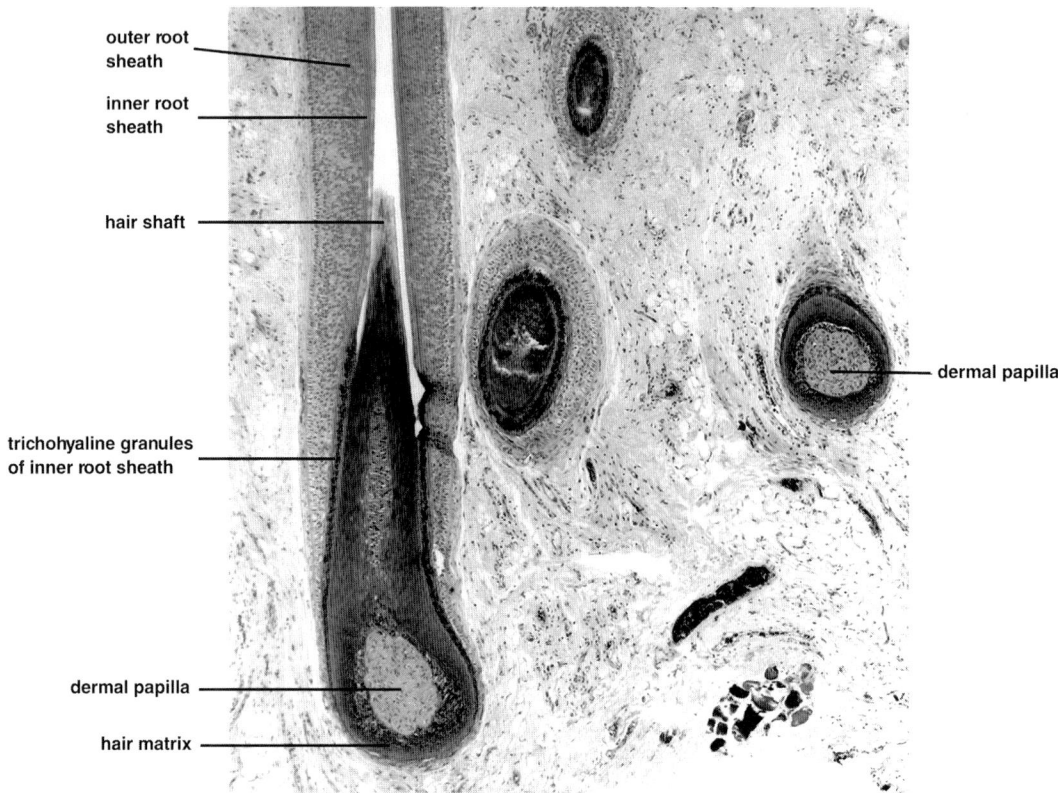

outer root sheath

inner root sheath

hair shaft

trichohyaline granules of inner root sheath

dermal papilla

hair matrix

dermal papilla

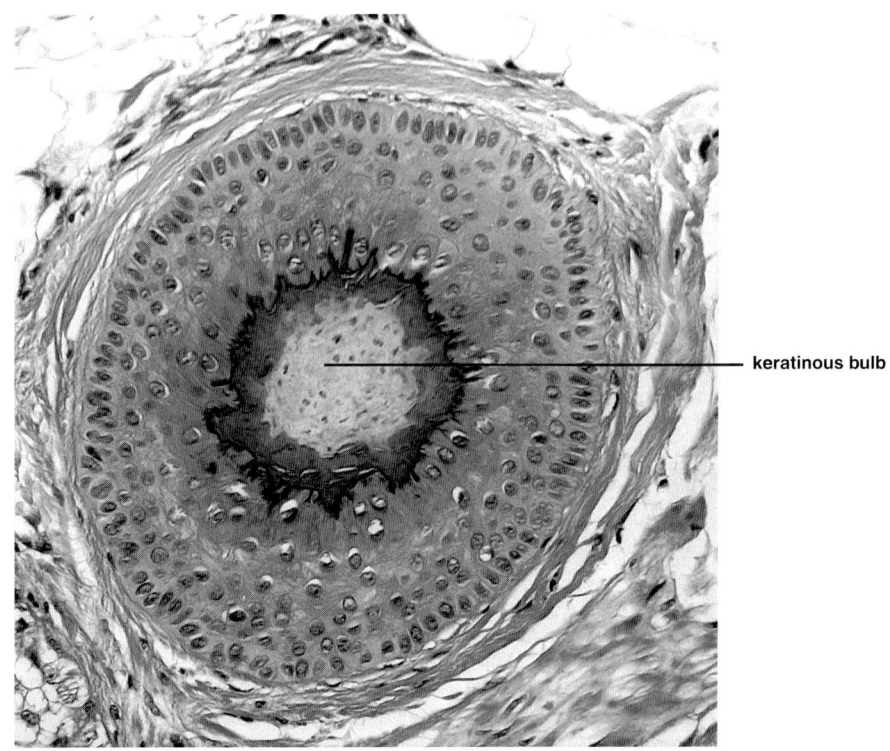

Figure 12-18. Catagen follicle. The early involuting phase is termed *catagen*. At the end of catagen the proximal end of the hair shaft becomes bulbous. This process is irreversible. Eventually the inner and outer root sheath epithelium collapses around the bulbous keratinous material. (× 200.)

keratinous bulb

creased telogen bulbs are evenly and randomly distributed throughout the biopsy specimen. Both terminal and vellus follicles are affected.

With time, the diagnostic microscopic changes of androgenetic alopecia emerge.[52,60,62,67–73] Progressive, random diminution in follicular diameters results in the formation of follicles with a hair shaft of intermediate diameter between a normal terminal and vellus follicle *(miniaturization)* (Fig. 12-20). As the severity of the alopecia progresses, these intermediate follicles increase in number while the normal-diameter follicles decrease proportionately. In addition to decreased follicle and shaft diameters, the intermediate follicles contain less melanin pigment in the keratinocytes of the shafts and bulbs.

Eventually even the intermediate follicles are reduced to the

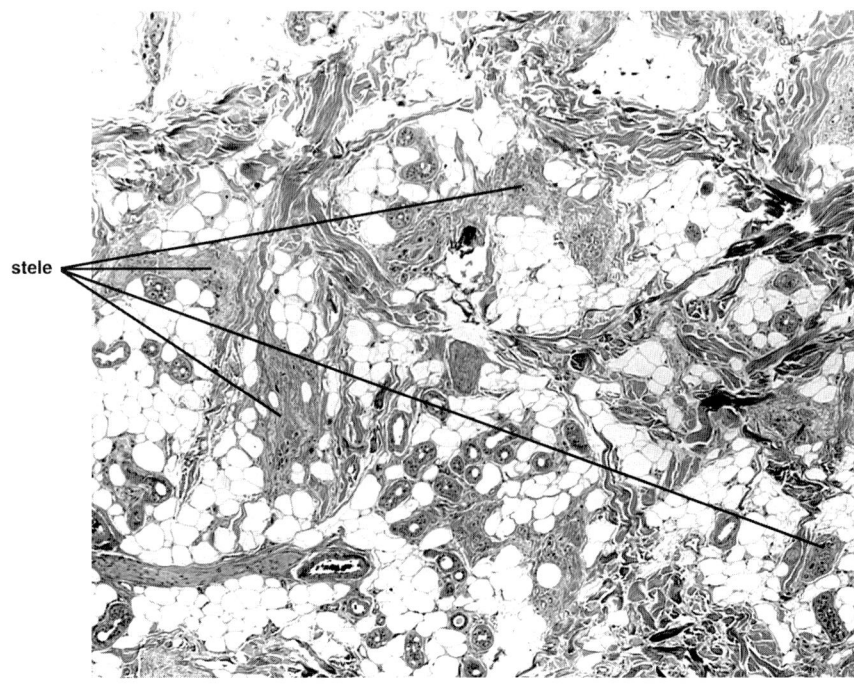

Figure 12-19. Follicular stele. Fine fibrillar collagen and small blood vessels form the residual fibrous tract of the telogen phase follicle. (× 40.)

stele

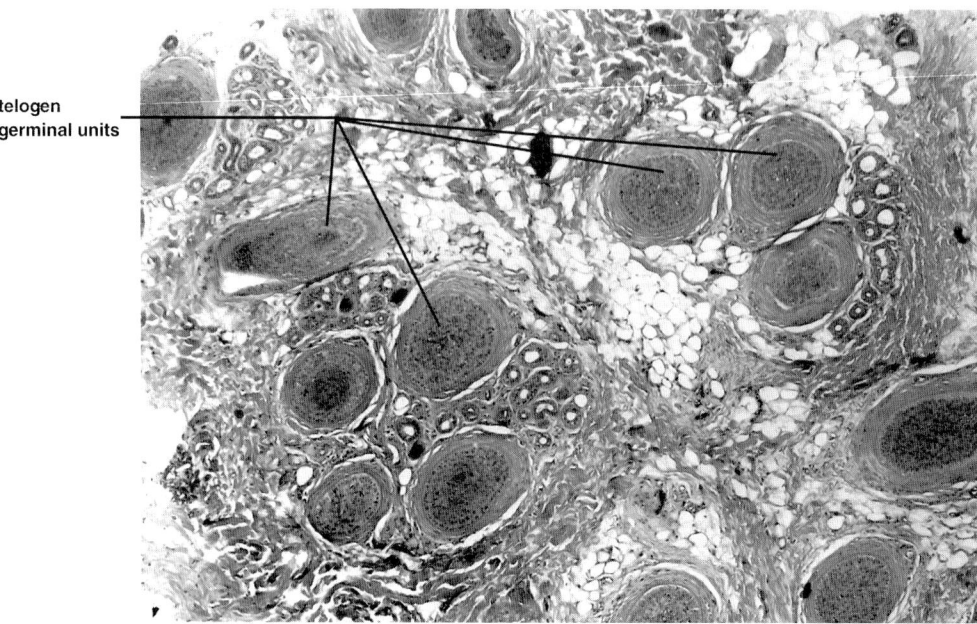

telogen
germinal units

Figure 12-22. Anagen effluvium in transverse section. Virtually all of the terminal follicles are in telogen. No inflammation is present. (× 40.)

morphic catagen bulb. Eventually these follicles regress to form telogen germinal units that are morphologically identical to normal telogen bulbs. This entire process occurs in the absence of inflammation (Fig. 12-22).

Differential Diagnosis. Transverse sections are of great value in making the diagnosis of anagen effluvium. Dysmorphic catagen bulbs are easily identified in transverse section by the presence of numerous dyskeratotic matrical keratinocytes, irregular, seemingly random keratinization, and reverse taper hair shafts in the absence of inflammation. These epithelial changes closely resemble the dysmorphic follicles of alopecia areata. The hair bulbs in the latter are typically, but not invariably, surrounded by sparse, peribulbar lymphocytic infiltrates. Fewer telogen-phase follicles are present in early, evolving telogen effluvium.

Alopecia Areata

Clinical Features. Alopecia areata is a common form of alopecia.[77–80] It is frequently classified as an "autoimmune" disorder because it may coexist with vitiligo and Hashimoto's thyroiditis. Patients with alopecia areata are frequently atopic. The lymphocytic infiltrate of alopecia areata is composed of helper T cells, which presumably induce the characteristic morphologic changes in the affected follicles.[79–82]

Alopecia areata may occur at any age and in all races and affects men and women equally.[78,79] Although autoantibodies directed against organs such as the thyroid gland are common in alopecia areata, these rarely result in symptoms or signs of disease. No other cutaneous changes accompany the alopecia other than nail pitting (common) and nevus flammeus of the scalp (rare).

Rapid shedding of hair shafts to form small, well circumscribed, round or oval patches is the most common presentation of alopecia areata. The hairless scalp is usually asymptomatic and appears normal. Only rarely does the patient notice a tingling sensation or a slight degree of erythema. The patches of alopecia are typically 3 to 5 cm in diameter. The hair shafts at the periphery of the patches can be dislodged from their follicle with minimal force in active disease (positive pull test). Patches may enlarge peripherally to form more irregular patches and may coalesce to cover large expanses of scalp. In addition to this classic presentation, alopecia areata may present as bilateral bands of alopecia that begin at the sideburns and extend posteriorly over the ears to the nape of the neck (*ophiasis* pattern).

Severe forms of alopecia areata include *alopecia totalis*, when the scalp alopecia is total or nearly total, and *alopecia universalis*, when there is complete loss of scalp and body hair. Although the latter is uncommon, small patches of alopecia in the beard and eyebrow areas frequently accompany the common patch-type alopecia areata of the scalp.

In most patients with one or a few small patches of alopecia areata on the scalp, hair loss is temporary and regrowth is spontaneous. New patches may form while older ones regrow hair. In general, the greater the extent of hair loss, the worse the prognosis for spontaneous regrowth.[78,79]

Histopathologic Features. The earliest diagnostic changes in alopecia areata are virtually indistinguishable from those of anagen effluvium: apoptosis of matrical keratinocytes, errant and random keratinization, and abrupt cessation of hair shaft formation such that no bulbous keratinous proximal end is formed[52,60,62,77,83] (Figs. 12-23 and 12-24). Unlike anagen effluvium, and helpful in differentiating the two, are a decrease in the number of bulbar melanocytes and the presence of a peribulbar lymphocytic infiltrate.[52,60,62,77–80,82,84] The infiltrate is usually sparse with only a few lymphocytes actually in the hair bulbs[52,62,85] (Fig. 12-25). No interface change is present. As in anagen effluvium, rapid cycling out of anagen soon results in an inversion of the anagen/telogen ratio.[52,61,62,86] The telogen bulbs are found in the lower and middle reticular dermis.

In persistent alopecia areata, the follicles remain fixed in the telogen phase.[52,61,62] Variable numbers of lymphocytes remain around the bulbs, but the lymphocytes continue to diminish in number as the chronicity sets in. In long-standing alopecia areata only rare lymphocytes are found around the telogen bulbs.[52,61,62]

The number of anagen follicles is variable in the regrowth phase.[52,61,62,77] In the early regrowth phase the new anagen follicles are smaller than normal. Their hair shafts are reduced in diameter with less than normal amounts of melanin pigment. There is a corresponding decrease in the number of dendritic melanocytes within the matrix of the hair bulb.[82,87] Eccrine glands may be reduced in number.[84]

If the patient's recovery is complete, the follicles return to normal size and morphology. If the alopecia is prolonged, a gradual but progressive loss of follicles occurs.

Differential Diagnosis. Transverse sections facilitate the microscopic diagnosis of alopecia areata. As discussed above,

anagen effluvium can usually be differentiated from alopecia areata by the lack of peribulbar lymphocytic infiltrates in the former, but in prolonged alopecia areata inflammation may be minimal or absent. Dysmorphic catagen follicles are not features of telogen effluvium, and telogen germinal units are found to be increased in number only when biopsy specimens are obtained early in the course of the alopecia. An increased number of catagen- and telogen-phase follicles and peribulbar lymphocytic infiltrates may be present in the patchy or generalized alopecia of secondary syphilis. An admixture of plasma cells in the infiltrate is suggestive of secondary syphilis, but plasma cells may be few in number or even absent.[88,89]

Trichotillomania and Traction Alopecia

Clinical Features. *Trichotillomania*, the compulsive, irresistible urge to twist or pluck one's hair, is classified as a disturbance of impulse control.[90–94] This disorder is more common in children but is not limited to this age group. Although patients with trichotillomania usually fixate on plucking scalp hair, eyebrows and even eyelashes may be extracted. Patients may either be fully aware of their compulsion or deny it completely.

The characteristic clinical finding in trichotillomania is irregular patches of partial alopecia with many broken shafts. The scalp surface may be excoriated. The crown of the scalp is a common site of alopecia in trichotillomania, but any area may be involved.

In *traction alopecia* the damage to hair follicles is not the re-

Figure 12-23. Alopecia areata in transverse section. The majority of terminal follicles are in telogen (inverted anagen/telogen ratio). (× 40.)

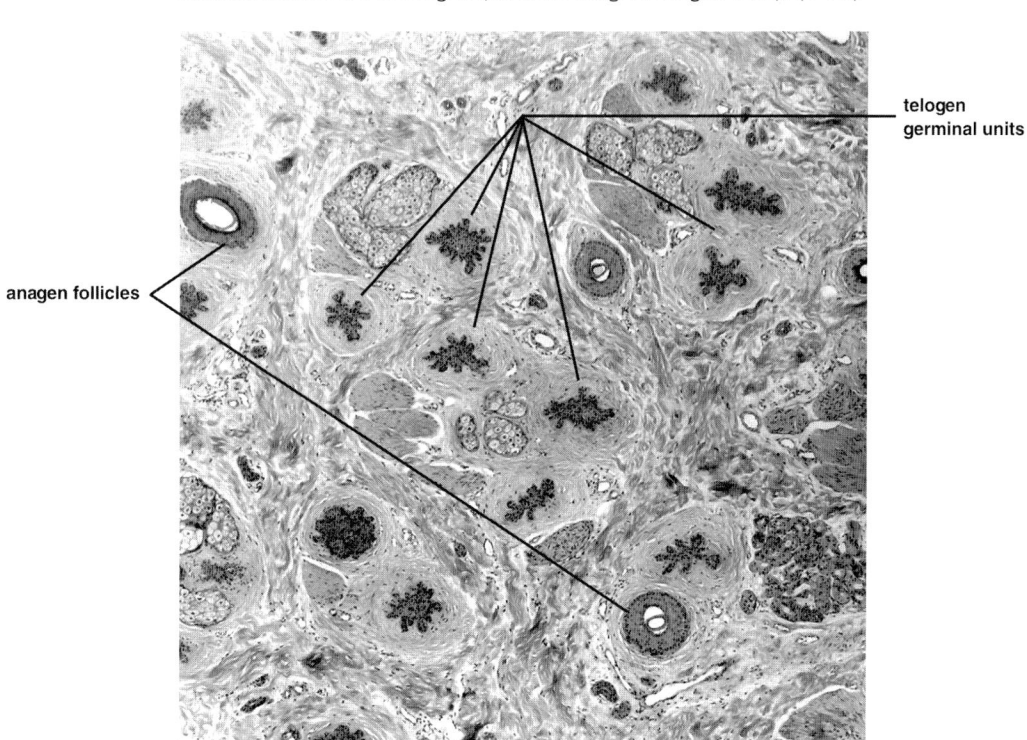

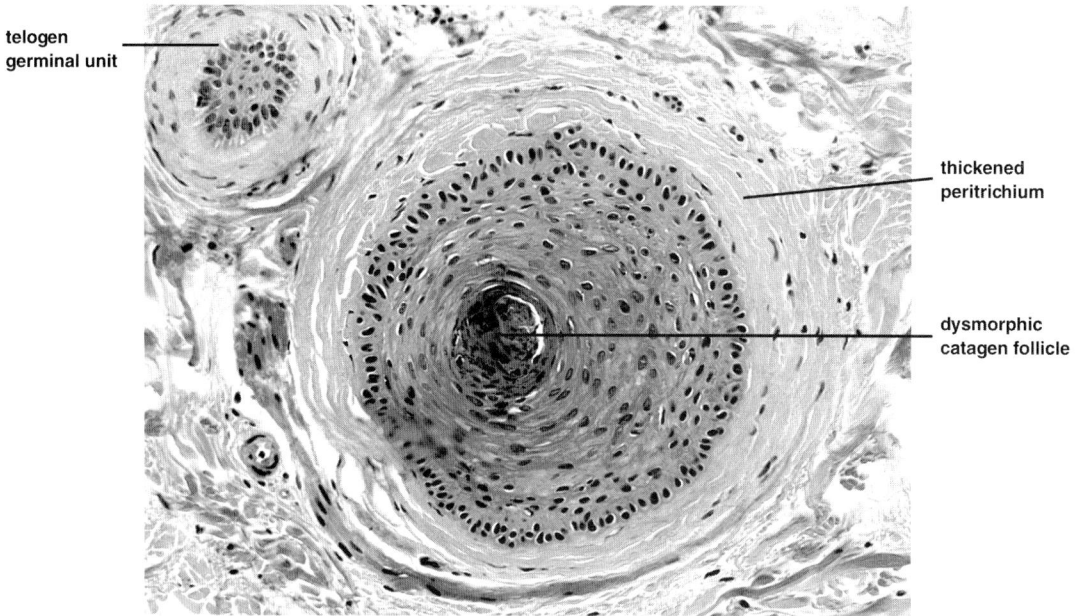

telogen
germinal unit

thickened
peritrichium

dysmorphic
catagen follicle

Figure 12-24. Alopecia areata in transverse section, dysmorphic follicle. Only irregular keratinous remnants of the hair shaft are present in this dysmorphic catagen follicle, in contrast to the bulbous keratinous material seen in the normal catagen phase. (× 200.)

sult of plucking but rather the result of prolonged tension on the hair shaft that is transmitted to the hair bulb.[95,96] Tightly rolled or braided hair styles are common causes.[97,98] The alopecia is typically greatest in the frontal and parietal scalp.

Neither trichotillomania nor traction alopecia results in destruction of follicles in the early stages, but, with prolonged and repeated insults, the follicles may atrophy.[52,60,62]

Histopathologic Features. The initial change in trichotillomania is an increase in the number of catagen and telogen follicles that is easily observed in transverse sections[52,60,62] (Fig. 12-26). In addition, distorted, fractured hair shafts or bulbs are found within follicles (*trichomalacia*) along with amorphous intrafollicular deposits of melanin pigment (*melanin casts*)[90–94] (Fig. 12-27). The melanin is embedded in inner root sheath ker-

Figure 12-25. Alopecia areata in transverse section, peribulbar lymphocytic infiltrates. Sparse peribulbar lymphocytic infiltrates are variably present around the telogen germinal units. The peribulbar infiltrates becomes less prominent in long-standing alopecia and are not infrequently absent. The low density of lymphocytes and their peribulbar location has been stated to resemble a "swarm of bees." (× 80.)

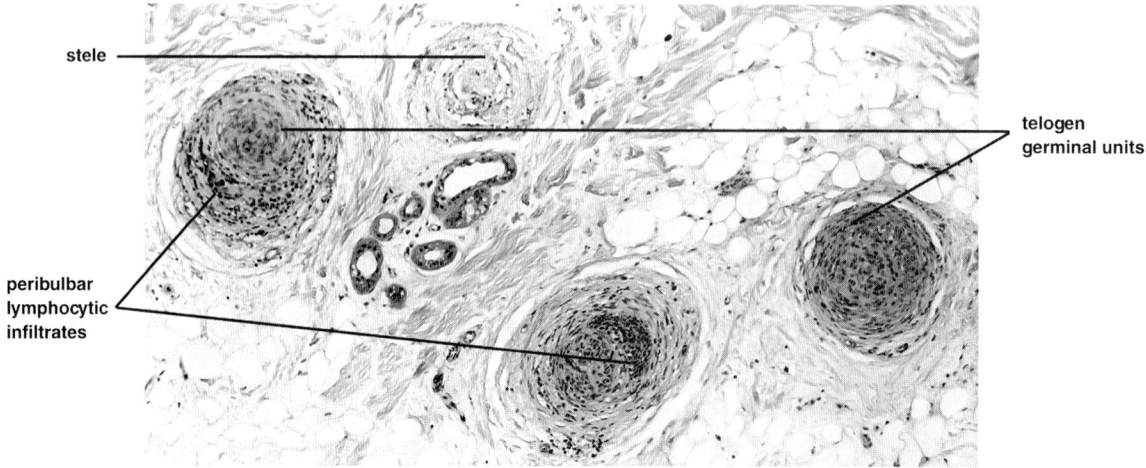

stele

telogen
germinal units

peribulbar
lymphocytic
infiltrates

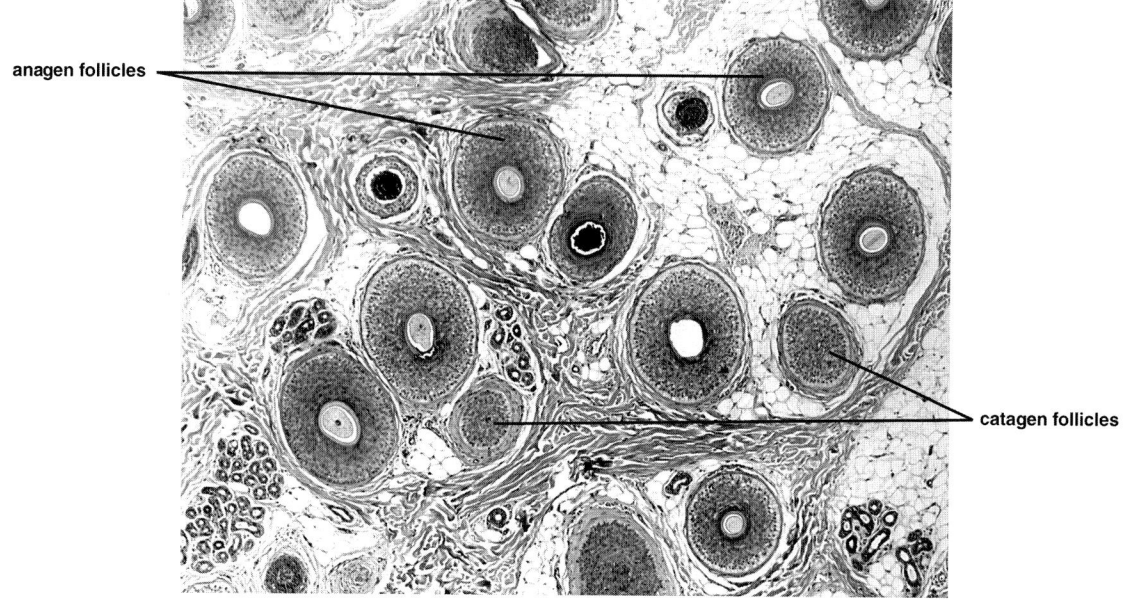

anagen follicles

catagen follicles

Figure 12-26. Trichotillomania/traction alopecia, early phase, a transverse section. Catagen follicles are increased in number. Inflammation is absent. (× 80.)

atin and not associated with a hair shaft[90,99] (Fig. 12-28). Melanin casts are absent or less prominent in blond or red hair because of the smaller amounts of melanin normally present in the hair shafts. Disrupted follicles with peri- or intrafollicular hemorrhage or hemosiderin deposits are uncommon, but diagnostic of trichotillomania.

Evidence of external epidermal trauma (e.g., superficial well-demarcated erosions, scale-crust, and spongiosis) adds additional evidence for the diagnosis of trichotillomania, but is rarely present. Continued, prolonged plucking eventually results in follicular atrophy (Fig. 12-29).

Shaft fragmentation and disruption of the hair follicles are

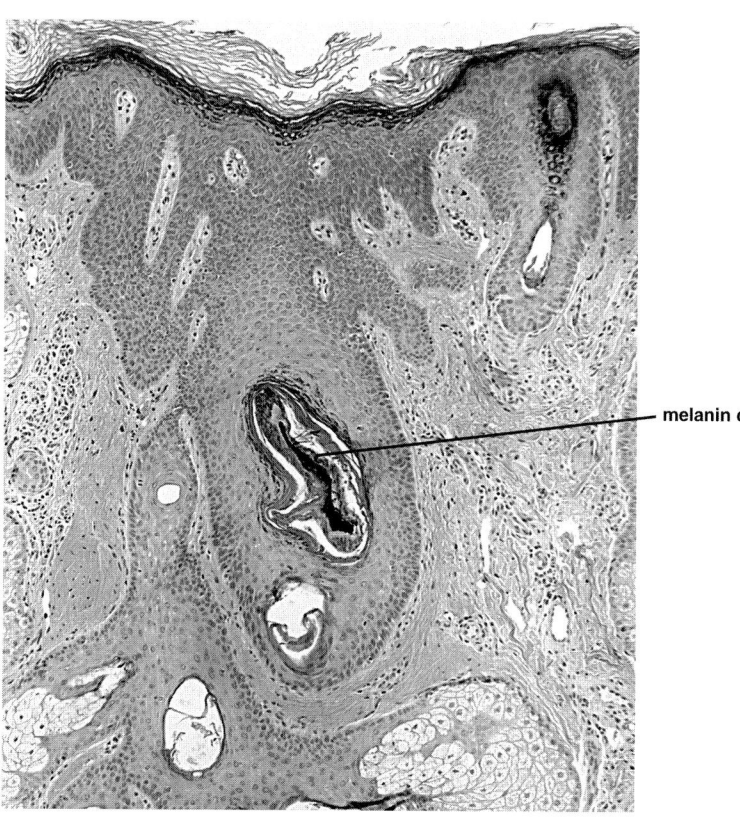

melanin cast

Figure 12-27 Trichotillomania/traction alopecia in longitudinal section. A melanin cast is visible in the follicular canal at the level of the infundibulum. (× 80.)

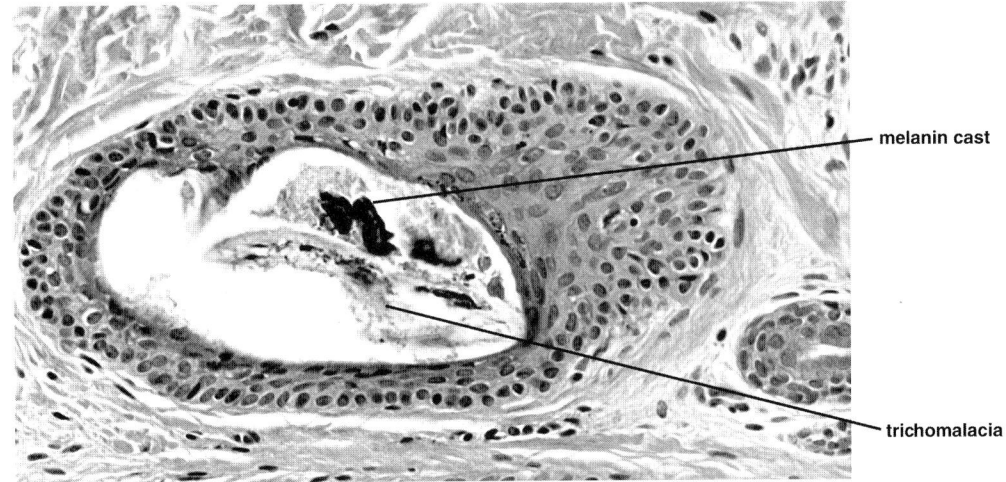

melanin cast

trichomalacia

Figure 12-28. Trichotillomania/traction alopecia in transverse section. A melanin cast is enmeshed with hair shaft fragments (trichomalacia). (× 200.)

unusual in traction alopecia. In general, the only finding is a decreased anagen/telogen ratio. As with trichotillomania, long-standing traction alopecia leads to telogen arrest and loss of follicles.

Differential Diagnosis. Distorted hair shafts in trichotillomania may easily be confused with the dysmorphic follicles of alopecia areata or anagen effluvium, especially if the traumatized follicle has cycled into the catagen or telogen phase. In trichotillomania, the increased numbers of catagen and telogen follicles are distributed more or less randomly, whereas in alopecia areata and anagen effluvium virtually all of the follicles are affected. Peribulbar lymphocytic infiltrates, when present, help in the recognition of alopecia areata. Small clumps of melanin pigment that resemble the pigment casts of trichotillomania may be found in the follicles of alopecia areata or

anagen effluvium that are undergoing rapid involution. This adds futher difficulty to the differential diagnosis.

Scarring (Cicatricial) Alopecias

In contrast to the nonscarring alopecias, hair follicles are destroyed in scarring alopecias. One approach to the microscopic classification of scarring alopecias is to divide them into two broad categories based on whether the hair follicle and its associated structures are the primary or secondary target (i.e., primary or secondary scarring alopecias).[28,52,58,62] The follicle and the peritrichium are the principal site of the abnormality in primary scarring alopecia, whereas the reticular dermis is the main location in secondary scarring alopecia. The distinction is not perfect; mixed patterns exist. Scarring alopecias are classified as primary or secondary on the basis of where the most diag-

Figure 12-29. Trichotillomania/traction alopecia, late phase, in transverse section. Stele have replaced all of the terminal follicles within a single follicular unit (drop-out of terminal follicles). This is a permanent process that eventuates in decreased follicle density. (× 80.)

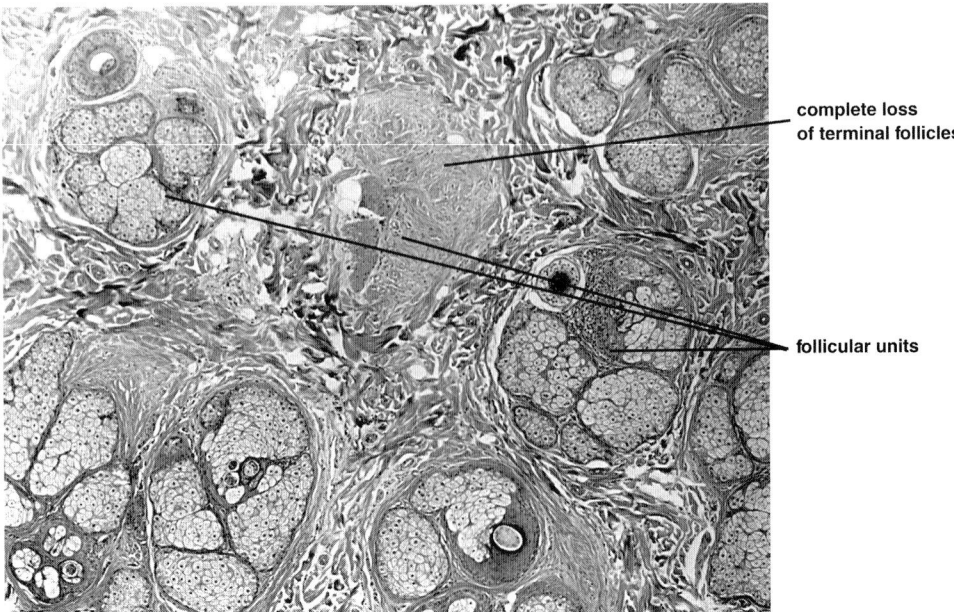

complete loss of terminal follicles

follicular units

nostic feature is located. Primary scarring alopecia can be further subclassified into lymphocytic- or neutrophilic-associated subtypes based on the predominate inflammatory cell present around or within the affected follicles.

Primary Scarring Alopecias

Lymphocyte-Associated Primary Scarring Alopecia.
Clinical Features. Discoid lupus erythematosus, lichen planopilaris, and pseudopelade of Brocq are discussed together. These three types of scarring alopecia have the following in common: perifollicular lymphocytic infiltrates and eventual destruction of hair follicles resulting in scar formation.[28,52,58,62] Although there is much overlap among these diseases, especially in the advanced stages of follicle destruction (end-stage alopecia), certain differences aid in separating them microscopically.[100,101]

The scalp is involved in approximately half the patients with discoid lupus erythematosus.[28,102] Ten percent of patients with discoid lupus erythematosus have scalp involvement only. The characteristic lesions are erythematous, scaly plaques within which there is a variable degree of hair loss. Although not invariably present, keratotic plugs adherent to patulous, dilated follicles are helpful in the clinical diagnosis. These plugs resemble an inverted, cone-shaped flask. Older plaques are frequently hypopigmented. The end stage is an atrophic scar with little or no remaining hair follicles. Hypertrophic plaques are less common on the scalp. Discoid plaques of lupus erythematosus may occur in patients with systemic lupus erythematosus. This is not the patchy, nonscarring telogen effluvium of systemic lupus erythematosus.

Lichen planopilaris may present as either large, violaceous to erythematous plaques that closely resemble discoid lupus erythematosus or as smaller spinous or acuminate papules.[28,103–105] The papules may be closely grouped and can coalesce. Both forms are characterized by follicular spines that tend to be smaller and more numerous than those of discoid lupus erythematosus. Progressive disease leads to small, irregular, angular atrophic patches of alopecia with total or nearly total loss of follicular orifices. Typical lesions of lichen planus on other anatomic sites may coexist with scalp lesions. Pruritus is frequently minimal or absent on the scalp in contrast to lichen planus elsewhere.

Some confusion exists as to whether pseudopelade of Brocq is a single clinicopathologic entity. In this chapter, the term is used to describe a form of scarring alopecia characterized by multiple, round to oval, minimally pruritic patches of alopecia that may coalesce into larger, irregular areas.[28,101,106,107] No induration, pustule formation, or follicular plugging is apparent. Erythema, if present, is limited to perifollicular skin and is mild. With progression of the disease, follicles are lost so that the scalp becomes smooth and shiny. Sperling and Sau[55] have proposed the term *follicular degeneration syndrome* for a similar, if not identical, form of scarring alopecia that is typically, but not exclusively, found on the centrofrontal scalp of black American women.[57,108]

Histopathologic Features. Vacuolar interface change in basal keratinocytes is the histologic hallmark of discoid lupus erythematosus[28,52,58,62] (Fig. 12-30). Clear vacuoles form in the cytoplasm of basal keratinocytes, eventually leading to necrosis of these cells. In the scalp lesions of discoid lupus erythematosus, the vacuolar interface change is usually greater at the level of the follicular infundibulum than along the basement membrane of the epidermis. Accompanying the interface change is a dense lymphocytic infiltrate around both superficial and deep dermal

Figure 12-30. Discoid lupus erythematosus in transverse section. Dense perifollicular lymphocytic infiltrates are present adjacent to a follicular infundibulum. Prominent vacuolar interface change is present. (× 200.)

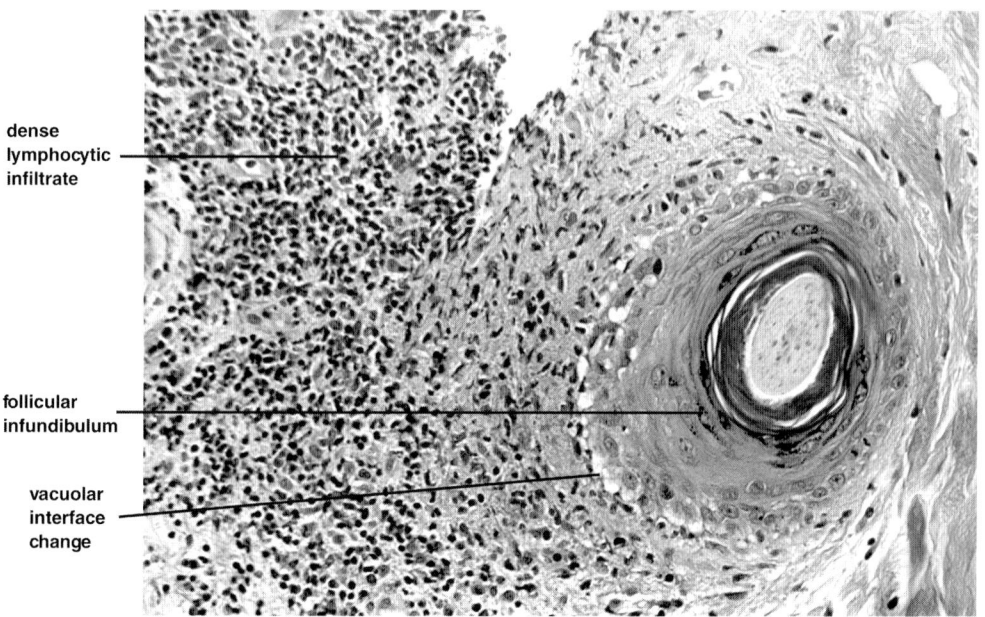

dense lymphocytic infiltrate

follicular infundibulum

vacuolar interface change

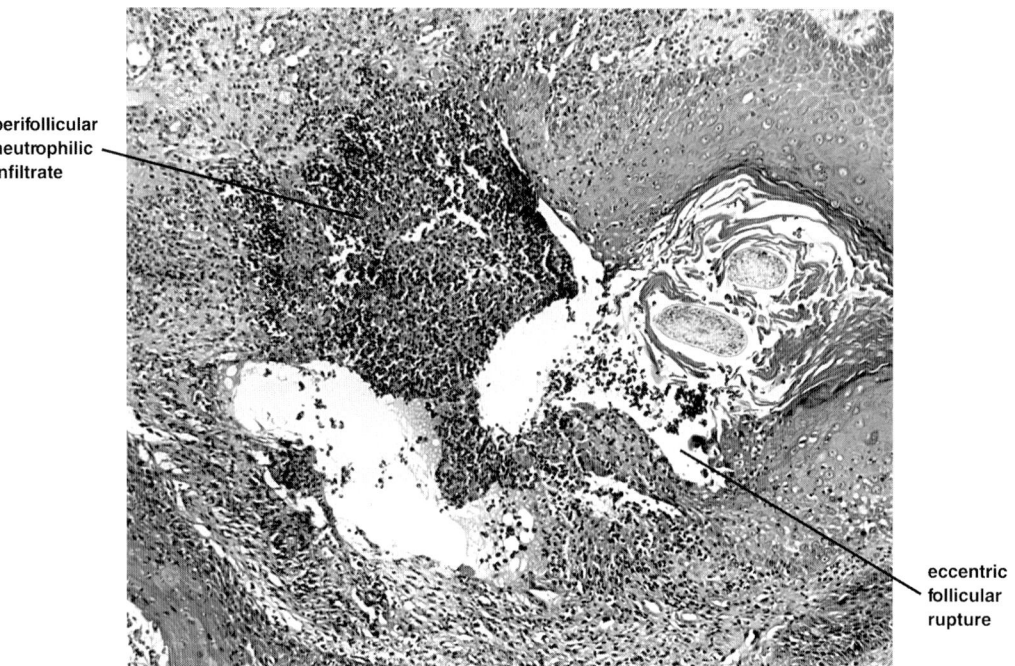

perifollicular
neutrophilic
infiltrate

eccentric
follicular
rupture

Figure 12-38. Folliculitis decalvans. A small neutrophilic abscess is present at the site of eccentric follicular rupture. (× 80.)

lesce to form sinus tracts that perforate the epidermis at multiple sites (Fig. 12-37). Pseudoepitheliomatous hyperplasia then develops around the purulent infiltrates. With time, a complex network of partially squamous epithelium-lined channels and dilated follicular infundibula is formed that may extend into the subcutis. Dense fibrotic scar eventually surrounds the sinus tracts. The affected follicles are destroyed by the fibroinflammatory process.

The neutrophilic infiltrate is limited to the perifollicular dermis in folliculitis decalvans[28,52,58,62,113] (Fig. 12-38). The affected follicles soon cycle into the telogen phase and ultimately are destroyed. Plasma cells may be present in the neutrophilic infiltrate.

The suppurative inflammation in acne keloidalis is variable in extent, but is usually less extensive than the infiltrate of dissecting cellulitis of the scalp. Perifollicular keloidal scars develop with a concomitant loss of follicles[28,52,58,62,114–116] (Fig. 12-39).

Ruptured neutrophil-laden infundibula that result in perifollicular abscesses, granulomatous inflammation, and eventually scar formation with destruction of follicles combine to form a kerion. Hyphae are found either within (endothrix) or surrounding (ectothrix) hair shafts[28,52,58,62,117] (Fig. 12-40).

Secondary Scarring Alopecia

The causes of secondary scarring alopecia are many and varied. Some of the more common ones include trauma (thermal or chemical burns, prolonged pressure, laceration), connective tissue diseases (morphea/scleroderma), developmental anomalies (aplasia cutis congenita), deposits (amyloid), granulomatous diseases (sarcoidosis), and neoplasms (adnexal neoplasms, dermatofibrosarcoma protuberans, metastatic neoplasms)[28,52,58,62] (Fig. 12-41).

In secondary scarring alopecia the hair follicles are not the primary site of pathologic change. They are only secondarily involved in the destructive process. The diagnostic microscopic features are those of the causative disease process.[28,52,58,62] These diseases are not limited to the scalp.

Combined Alopecias

Two or more types of alopecia may exist concurrently, resulting in confusing clinical and microscopic findings. A particularly common combined alopecia occurs when superimposed telogen effluvium, secondary to a drug or to stress, accentuates pre-existing androgenetic alopecia.[52,58,62]

Differential Diagnosis of Scarring Alopecia

Evaluation of specimens from relatively early in the course of the disease is essential in differentiating one scarring alopecia from another (Table 12-3). Each of these alopecias eventually

Table 12-3. Differential Microscopic Features of Scarring Alopecia

Alopecia	Microscopic Findings
Discoid lupus erythematosus	Lymphocytic; vacuolar interface change at the infundibulum; ± dermal mucin
Lichen planopilaris	Lymphocytic; lichenoid interface change at the infundibulum; colloid bodies; no dermal mucin
Pseudopelade of Brocq	Lymphocytic; minimal or no interface change at the infundibulum (clefts may be present); no dermal mucin
Dissecting cellulitis	Neutrophilic; large perifollicular interconnecting abscesses
Folliculitis decalvans	Neutrophilic; smaller perifollicular abscesses
Acne keloidalis	Neutrophilic; variable perifollicular abscesses; extensive perifollicular scar
Tinea capitis	Neutrophilic; perifollicular abscess; hyphae in or around hair shaft

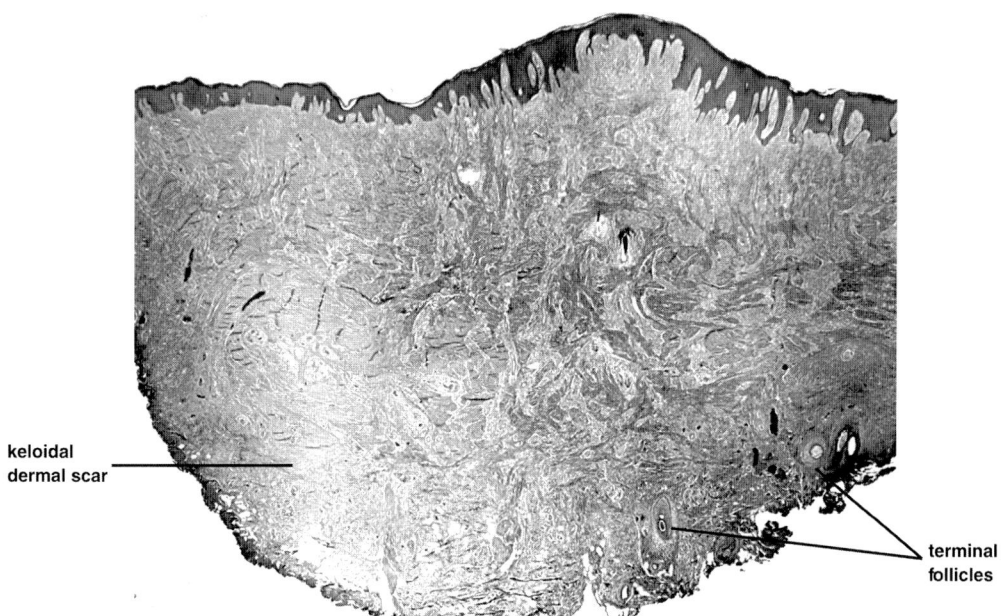

keloidal
dermal scar

terminal
follicles

Figure 12-39. Acne keloidalis in longitudinal section. Keloidal dermal scar replaces the normal reticular dermis. Only a small number of terminal follicles remain at the periphery of the scar. (× 10.)

Figure 12-40. Tinea capitis. Numerous fungal hyphae and spores are present within a hair shaft (endothrix). The affected follicle is surrounded by a neutrophilic abscess. (× 200.)

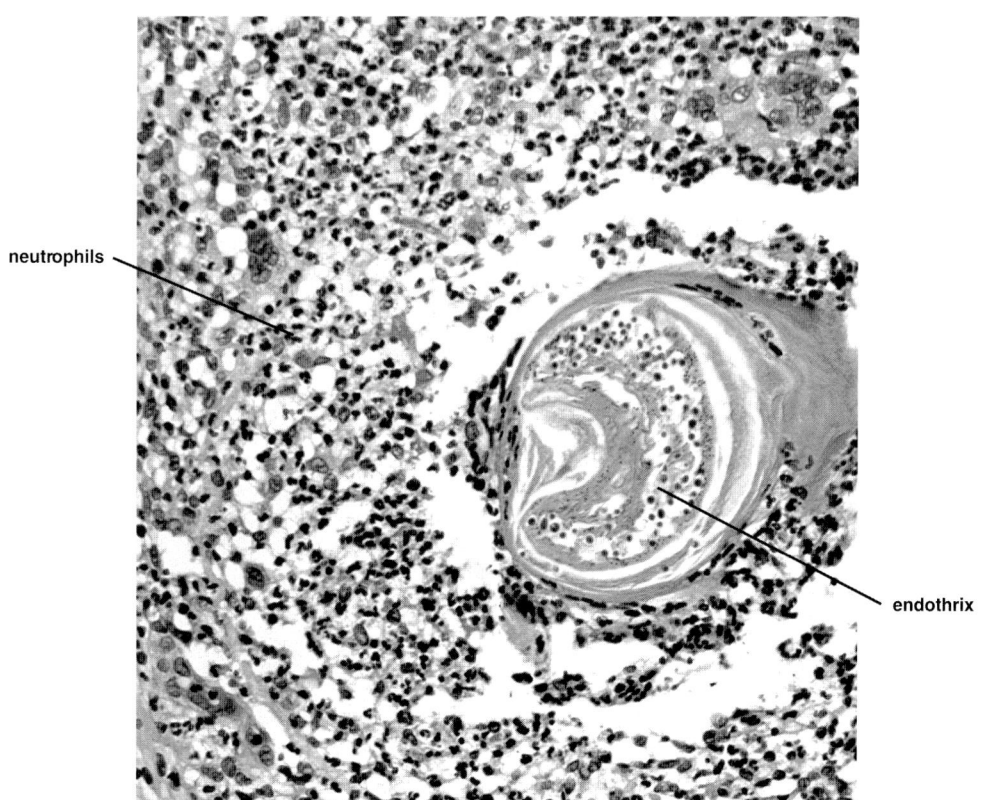

neutrophils

endothrix

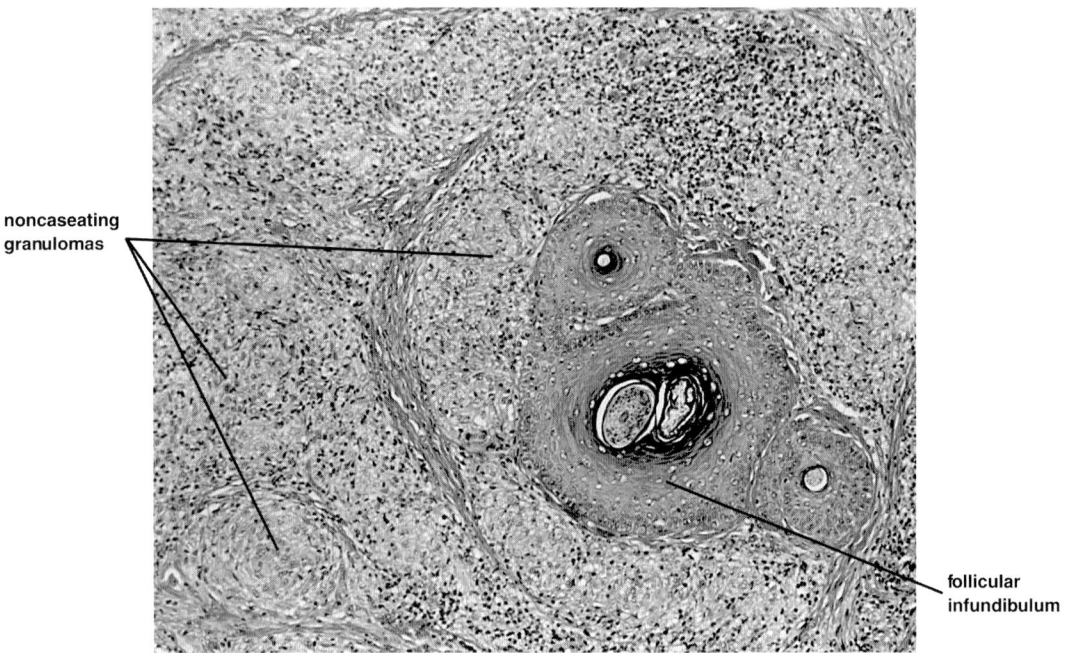

noncaseating granulomas

follicular infundibulum

Figure 12-41. Cutaneous sarcoidosis. Confluent noncaseating granulomas surround a follicular infundibulum. (× 80.)

progresses to an alopecia characterized by the residual follicle stele, remnants of hair shafts surrounded by foreign body-type granulomatous inflammation, and variably dense primarily lymphocytic inflammatory cell infiltrates. The lack of characteristic findings in this advanced stage of alopecia usually precludes accurate differentiation between the various types of scarring alopecia and nonscarring alopecia with extensive follicular atrophy. I apply the term *end-stage alopecia* to emphasize the poor prognosis for cosmetically significant regrowth resulting from the extensive destruction of the follicles (Fig. 12-42).

Figure 12-42. End-stage alopecia. In end-stage alopecia only follicular stele remain to mark the previous location of terminal follicles. (× 40.)

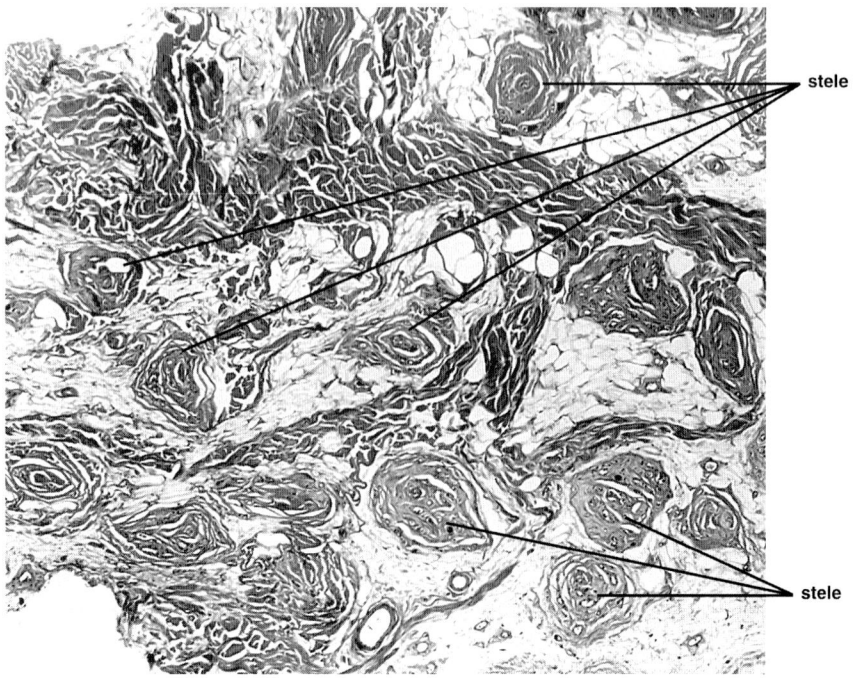

stele

stele

REFERENCES

1. Uehara M, Ofuji S: Primary eruption of prurigo simplex subacuta. Dermatologica 153:49–56, 1976
2. Miyauchi H, Uehara M: Follicular occurrence of prurigo nodularis. J Cutan Pathol 15:208–211, 1988
3. Hitch JM, Lund HZ: Disseminate and recurrent infundibulofolliculitis. Arch Dermatol 105:580–583, 1972
4. Owen WR, Wood C: Disseminate and recurrent infundibulofolliculitis. Arch Dermatol 115:174–175, 1979
5. Herman LE, Harawi SJ, Ghossein RA, Kurban AK: Folliculitis: a clinicopathologic review. Pathol Annu 26:201–246, 1991
6. Pinkus H: Furuncle. J Cutan Pathol 6:517–518, 1979
7. Mikhail GR: Trichophyton rubrum granuloma. Int J Dermatol 9:41–46, 1970
8. Back O, Faergemann J, Hornqvist R: Pityrosporon folliculitis: a common disease of the young and middle-aged. J Am Acad Dermatol 12:56, 1985
9. Dyall-Smith D, Mason G: Fungal eosinophilic pustular folliculitis. Australas J Dermatol 36:37–38, 1995
10. Sexton M: Occult herpesvirus folliculitis clinically simulating pseudolymphoma. Am J Dermatopathol 13:234–240, 1991
11. Solomon AR: The Tzanck smear—viable and valuable. Int J Dermatol 25:169–170, 1986
12. Macmillan DC, Vickers HR: Fox-Fordyce disease. Br J Dermatol 84:181, 1971
13. Ofuji S, Ogino A, Horio T et al: Eosinophilic pustular folliculitis. Acta Derm Venereol (Stockh) 50:195–203, 1970
14. Dinehart SM, Noppakun N, Solomon AR, Smith EB: Eosinophilic pustular folliculitis. J Am Acad Dermatol 14:475–479, 1986
15. Teraki Y, Konohana I, Shiohara T et al: Eosinophilic pustular folliculitis (Ofuji's disease): immunohistochemical analysis. Arch Dermatol 129:1015–1019, 1993
16. Brenner S, Wolf R, Ophir J: Eosinophilic pustular folliculitis: a sterile folliculitis of unknown cause? J Am Acad Dermatol 31:210–212, 1994
17. Buchness MR, Lim HW, Hatcher VA et al: Eosinophilic pustular folliculitis in the acquired immunodeficiency syndrome: treatment with ultraviolet B phototherapy. N Engl J Med 318:1183–1186, 1988
18. Jenkins DJ, Fisher BK, Chalvardjian A, Adam P: Eosinophilic pustular folliculitis in a patient with AIDS. Int J Dermatol 27:34–35, 1988
19. Darmstadt GL, Tunnessen WW, Jr, Swerer RJ: Eosinophilic pustular folliculitis. Pediatrics 89:1095–1098, 1992
20. Ferrandiz C, Ribera M, Barranco JC et al: Eosinophilic pustular folliculitis in patients with acquired immunodeficiency syndrome. Int J Dermatol 31:193–195, 1992
21. Magro CM, Crowson AN: Eosinophilic pustular follicular reaction: a paradigm of immune dysregulation. Int J Dermatol 33:172–178, 1994
22. Duarte AM, Kramer J, Yusk JW et al: Eosinophilic pustular folliculitis in infancy and childhood. Am J Dis Child 147:197–200, 1993
23. Garcia-Patos V, Pujol RM, de Moragas JM: Infantile eosinophilic pustular folliculitis. Dermatology 189:133–138, 1994
24. Dupond AS, Aubin F, Bourezane Y et al: Eosinophilic pustular folliculitis in infancy: report of two affected brothers. Br J Dermatol 132:296–299, 1995
25. Patrizi A, Di Lernia V, Neri I, Gherlinzoni F: Eosinophilic pustular folliculitis (Ofuji's disease) and non-Hodgkin lymphoma. Acta Derm Venereol 72:146–147, 1992
26. Lambert J, Berneman Z, Dockx P et al: Eosinophilic pustular folliculitis and B-cell chronic lymphatic leukaemia. Dermatology 189:58–59, 1994
27. Webster G: Inflammatory acne. Int J Dermatol 29:34–35, 1990
28. Newton RC, Hebert AA, Freese TW, Solomon AR: Scarring alopecia. Dermatol Clin 5:603–618, 1987
29. Yu CC, Cook MG: Hidradenitis suppurativa: a disease of follicular epithelium, rather than apocrine glands. Br J Dermatol 122:763–769, 1990
30. Attanoos RL, Appleton MA, Douglas-Jones AG: The pathogenesis of hidradenitis suppurativa: a closer look at apocrine and apoeccrine glands. Br J Dermatol 133:254–258, 1995
31. Marks R, Harcourt-Webster JN: Histopathology of rosacea. Arch Dermatol 100:683–691, 1969
32. Strauss JS, Kligman AM: The pathologic dynamics of acne vulgaris. Arch Dermatol 82:779–790, 1960
33. Golitz L: Follicular and perforating disorders. J Cutan Pathol 12:282–288, 1985
34. Attanoos RL, Appleton MA, Hughes LE et al: Granulomatous hidradenitis suppurativa and cutaneous Crohn's disease. Histopathology 23:111–115, 1993
35. Wilkin JK: Rosacea. Int J Dermatol 22:393–400, 1983
36. Mullanax MG, Kierland RR: Granulomatous rosacea. Arch Dermatol 101:206–211, 1970
37. Shitara A: Lupus miliaris disseminatus faciei. Int J Dermatol 23: 542–544, 1984
38. Helm KF, Menz J, Gibson LE, Dicken CH: A clinical and histopathologic study of granulomatous rosacea. J Am Acad Dermatol 25:1038–1043, 1991
39. Wilkinson DS, Kirton V, Wilkinson JD: Perioral dermatitis: a 12-year review. Br J Dermatol 101:245–257, 1979
40. Hruza GJ, Posnick RB, Weltman RE: Disseminated lupus vulgaris presenting as granulomatous folliculitis. Int J Dermatol 28:388–392, 1989
41. Sallakachart P, Nakjang Y: Keratosis pilaris: a clinico-histopathologic study. J Med Assoc Thai 70:386–389, 1987
42. Maroon M, Tyler WB, Marks VJ: Keratosis pilaris and scarring alopecia. Keratosis follicularis spinulosa decalvans. Arch Dermatol 128:397–400, 1992
43. Emmerson RW: Follicular mucinosis: a study of 47 patients. Br J Dermatol 81:395–413, 1969
44. Sentis HJ, Willemze R, Scheffer E: Alopecia mucinosa progressing into mycosis fungoides: a long-term follow-up study of two patients. Am J Dermatopathol 10:478–486, 1988
45. Mehregan DA, Gibson LE, Muller SA: Follicular muci-

nosis: histopathologic review of 33 cases. Mayo Clin Proc 66:387–390, 1991

46. Buchner SA, Meier M, Rufli T: Follicular mucinosis associated with mycosis fungoides. Dermatologica 183:66–67, 1991

47. Ramon D, Jorda E, Molina I et al: Follicular mucinosis and Hodgkin's disease. Int J Dermatol 31:791–792, 1992

48. Roth DE, Owen LG, Hodge SJ, Callen JP: Follicular mucinosis associated with pregnancy. Int J Dermatol 31:441–442, 1992

49. Hempstead RW, Ackerman AB: Follicular mucinosis: a reaction pattern in follicular epithelium. Am J Dermatopathol 7:245–257, 1985

50. Fanti PA, Tosti A, Morelli R et al: Follicular mucinosis in alopecia areata. Am J Dermatopathol 14:542–545, 1992

51. Nickoloff BJ: Epidermal mucinosis in mycosis fungoides. J Am Acad Dermatol 15:83–86, 1986

52. Solomon AR: The transversely sectioned scalp biopsy specimen: the technique and an algorithm for its use in the diagnosis of alopecia. Adv Dermatol 9:127–157, 1994

53. Headington JT: Transverse microscopic anatomy of the human scalp. Arch Dermatol 120:449–456, 1984

54. Sperling LC: Hair anatomy for the clinician. J Am Acad Dermatol 25:1–17, 1991

55. Sperling LC, Sau P: The follicular degeneration syndrome in black patients: "hot comb alopecia" revisited and revised. Arch Dermatol 128:68–74, 1992

56. Whiting DA: Diagnostic and predictive value of horizontal sections of scalp biopsy specimens in male pattern androgenetic alopecia [published erratum appears in J Am Acad Dermatol 29:554, 1993]. J Am Acad Dermatol 28:755–763, 1993

57. Sperling LC, Skelton HGR, Smith KJ et al: Follicular degeneration syndrome in men. Arch Dermatol 130:763–769, 1994

58. Templeton SF, Solomon AR: Scarring alopecia: a classification based on microscopic criteria. J Cutan Pathol 21:97–109, 1994

59. Elston DM, McCollough ML, Angeloni VL: Vertical and transverse sections of alopecia biopsy specimens: combining the two to maximize diagnostic yield. J Am Acad Dermatol 32:454–457, 1995

60. Sperling LC, Lupton GP: Histopathology of non-scarring alopecia. J Cutan Pathol 22:97–114, 1995

61. Whiting DA: Histopathology of alopecia areata in horizontal sections of scalp biopsies. J Invest Dermatol 104:26S–27S, 1995

62. Templeton SF, Santa Cruz DJ, Solomon AR: Alopecia: histologic diagnosis by transverse sections. Semin Diagn Pathol 13:2–18, 1996

63. Headington JT: Telogen effluvium. Arch Dermatol 129:356–363, 1993

64. Weedon D, Strutton G: The recognition of early stages of catagen. Am J Dermatopathol 6:553–555, 1984

65. Hamilton JB: Patterned long hair in man: types and incidence. Ann NY Acad Sci 53:708, 1951

66. Bergfeld WF, Redmond GP: Androgenic alopecia. Dermatol Clin 5:491–500, 1987

67. Brodland DG, Muller SA: Androgenetic alopecia (common baldness). Cutis 47:173–176, 1991

68. Rushton DH, Ramsay ID, Norris MJ, Gilkes JJ: Natural progression of male pattern baldness in young men. Clin Exp Dermatol 16:188–192, 1991

69. Alcaraz MV, Villena A, Perez de Vargas I: Quantitative study of the human hair follicle in normal scalp and androgenetic alopecia. J Cutan Pathol 20:344–349, 1993

70. Bergfeld WF: Androgenetic alopecia: an autosomal dominant disorder. Am J Med 98:95S–98S, 1995

71. Callan AW, Montalto J: Female androgenetic alopecia: an update. Australas J Dermatol 36:51–55, 1995

72. Abell E: Pathology of male-pattern alopecia. Arch Dermatol 120:1607–1608, 1984

73. Sperling LC, Winton GB: The transverse anatomy of androgenic alopecia. J Dermatol Surg Oncol 16:1127–1133, 1990

74. Ebling FJG: The biology of hair. Dermatol Clin 5:467–481, 1987

75. Rebora A: Telogen effluvium: an etiopathogenetic theory. Int J Dermatol 32:339–340, 1993

76. Tosi A, Misciali C, Piraccini BM et al: Drug-induced hair loss and hair growth: incidence, management and avoidance. Drug Saf 10:310–317, 1994

77. Headington JT, Mitchell AJ, Swanson N: New histopathological findings in alopecia areata studied in transverse sections. J Invest Dermatol 76:325, 1981

78. Mitchell AJ, Balle MR: Alopecia areata. Dermatol Clin 5:553–564, 1987

79. Sawaya ME, Hordinsky MK: Advances in alopecia areata and androgenetic alopecia. Adv Dermatol 7:211–226, 1992

80. Fanti PA, Tosti A, Bardazzi F et al: Alopecia areata: a pathological study of nonresponder patients. Am J Dermatopathol 16:167–170, 1994

81. Perret C, Wiesner-Menzel L, Happle R: Immunohistochemical analysis of T-cell subsets in the peribulbar and intrabulbar infiltrates of alopecia areata. Acta Derm Venereol (Stockh) 64:26–30, 1984

82. Randall VA, Hull SP, Nutbrown M et al: Is the dermal papilla a primary target in alopecia areata? J Invest Dermatol 104:7S–8S, 1995

83. Tobin DJ, Fenton DA, Kendall MD: Cell degeneration in alopecia areata: an ultrastructural study. Am J Dermatopathol 13:248–256, 1991

84. Elieff D, Sundby S, Kennedy W, Hordinsky M: Decreased sweat-gland number and function in patients with alopecia areata. Br J Dermatol 125:130–135, 1991

85. Tobin DJ, Fenton DA, Kendall MD: Ultrastructural observations on the hair bulb melanocytes and melanosomes in acute alopecia areata. J Invest Dermatol 94:803–807, 1990

86. Messenger AG, Slater DN, Bleehen SS: Alopecia areata: alterations in the hair growth cycle and correlation with the follicular pathology. Br J Dermatol 114:337–347, 1986

87. Hordinsky MK, Kennedy W, Wendelschafer-Crabb G, Lewis S: Structure and function of cutaneous nerves in alopecia areata. J Invest Dermatol 104:28S–29S, 1995

88. Lee JY, Hsu ML: Alopecia syphilitica, a simulator of alopecia areata: histopathology and differential diagnosis. J Cutan Pathol 18:87–92, 1991

89. Cuozzo DW, Benson PM, Sperling LC, Skelton HG III: Essential syphilitic alopecia revisited. J Am Acad Dermatol 32:840–843, 1995

90. Muller SA: Trichotillomania: a histopathologic study in sixty-six patients. J Am Acad Dermatol 23:56–62, 1990

91. Graber J, Arndt WB: Trichotillomania. Compr Psychiatry 34:340–346, 1993

92. Rothbaum BO, Ninan PT: The assessment of trichotillomania. Behav Res Ther 32:651–662, 1994

93. Schneider D, Janniger CK: Trichotillomania. Cutis 53:289–290, 294, 1994

94. Clark J, Jr, Helm TN, Bergfeld WF: Chronic alopecia: trichotillomania. Arch Dermatol 131:720–721, 723–724, 1995

95. Aaronson CM: Etiologic factors in traction alopecia. South Med J 62:185–186, 1969

96. Halder RM: Hair and scalp disorders in blacks. Cutis 32:378–380, 1983

97. Nicholson AG, Harland CC, Bull RH et al: Chemically induced cosmetic alopecia. Br J Dermatol 128:537–541, 1993

98. Trueb RM: "Chignon alopecia": a distinctive type of non-marginal traction alopecia. Cutis 55:178–179, 1995

99. LaChapelle JM, Pierard SE: Traumatic alopecia in trichotillomania: a pathogenic interpretation of histologic lesions in the pilosebaceous unit. J Cutan Pathol 4:51, 1977

100. Nayar M, Schomberg K, Dawber RP, Millard PR: A clinicopathological study of scarring alopecia. Br J Dermatol 128:533–536, 1993

101. Silvers DN, Katz BE, Young AW: Pseudopelade of Brocq is lichen planopilaris: report of four cases that support this nosology. Cutis 51:99–105, 1993

102. Laman SD, Provost TT: Cutaneous manifestations of lupus erythematosus. Rheum Dis Clin North Am 20:195–212, 1994

103. Silver H, Chargin L, Sachs PM: Follicular lichen planus (lichen planopilaris). Arch Dermatol Syph 67:346–354, 1953

104. Kubba R, Rook A: The Graham-Little syndrome: follicular keratosis with scarring alopecia. Br J Dermatol 93:53–55, 1975

105. Mehregan DA, Van Hale HM, Muller SA: Lichen planopilaris: clinical and pathologic study of forty-five patients. J Am Acad Dermatol 27:935–942, 1992

106. Braun-Falco O, Imai S, Schmoeckel C et al: Pseudopelade of Brocq. Dermatologica 172:18–23, 1986

107. Collier PM, James MP: Pseudopelade of Brocq occurring in two brothers in childhood. Clin Exp Dermatol 19:61–64, 1994

108. Solomon AR: Alopecia by a different name: a matter of splitting hairs. Arch Dermatol 128:102–103, 1992

109. Matta M, Kibbi AG, Khattar J et al: Lichen planopilaris: a clinicopathologic study. J Am Acad Dermatol 22:594–598, 1990

110. Moschella SL, Klein MH, Miller RJ: Perifolliculitis capitis abscedens et suffodiens. Arch Dermatol 69:195–197, 1967

111. Benvenuto ME, Rebora A: Fluctuant nodules and alopecia of the scalp: perifolliculitis capitis abscedens et suffodiens. Arch Dermatol 128:1115–1119, 1992

112. Dyall-Smith D: Signs, syndromes and diagnoses in dermatology: dissecting cellulitis of the scalp. Australas J Dermatol 34:81–82, 1993

113. Boggs A: Folliculitis decalvans. Acta Dermatol Venereol 43:14–24, 1963

114. Dinehart SM, Herzberg AJ, Kerns BJ, Pollack SV: Acne keloidalis: a review. J Dermatol Surg Oncol 15:642–647, 1989

115. Dinehart SM, Tanner L, Mallory SB, Herzberg AJ: Acne keloidalis in women. Cutis 44:250–252, 1989

116. George AO, Akanji AO, Nduka EU et al: Clinical, biochemical and morphologic features of acne keloidalis in a black population. Int J Dermatol 32:714–716, 1993

117. Sperling LC: Inflammatory tinea capitis (kerion) mimicking dissecting cellulitis: occurrence in two adolescents. Int J Dermatol 30:190–192, 1991

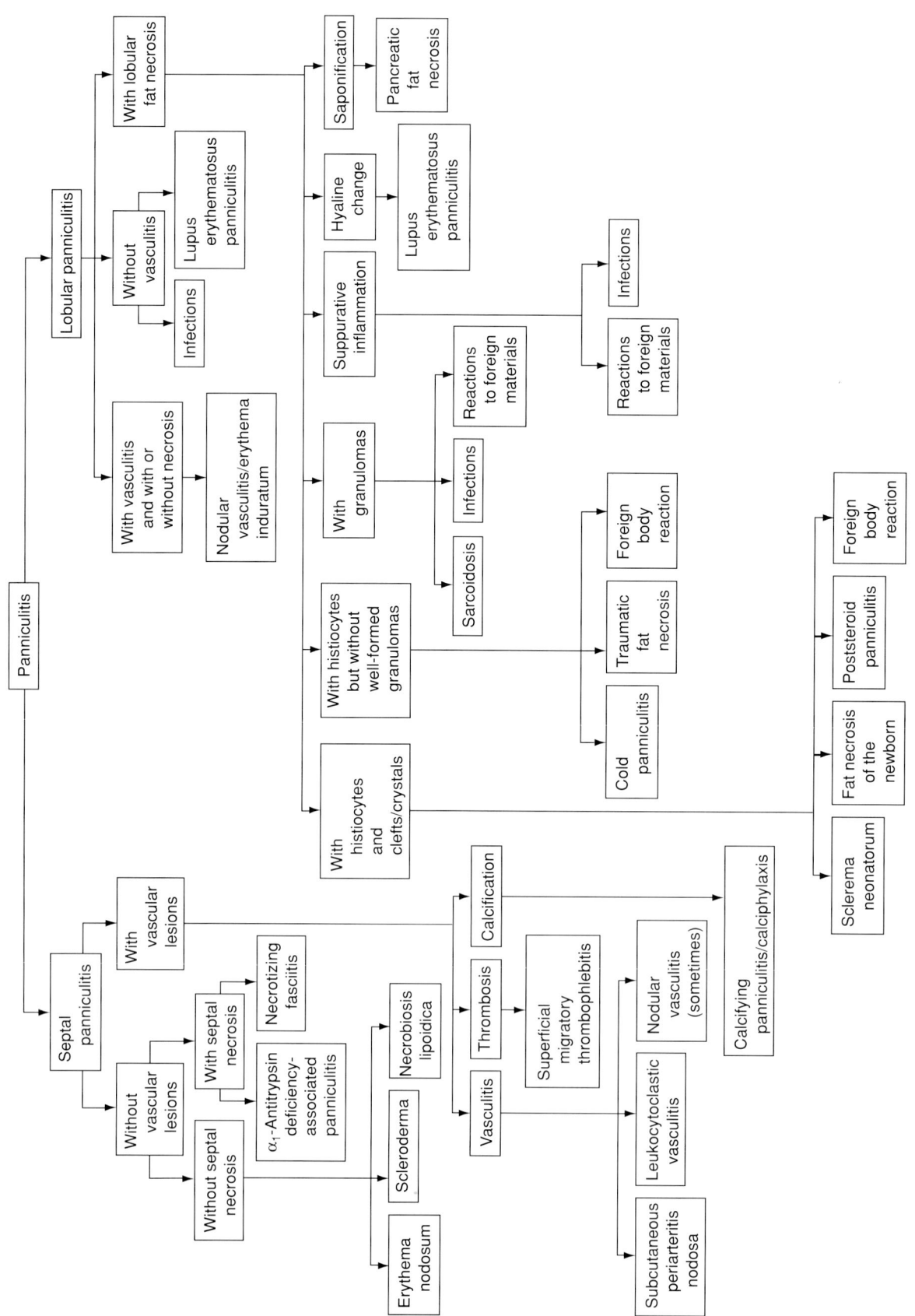

Figure 13-1. Algorithmic classification of panniculitis.

Table 13-1. Classification Based on Etiology

Immunologic or autoimmune
  Erythema nodosum
  Nodular vasculitis
  Lupus erythematosus panniculitis
  Scleroderma
Metabolic disorders
  Sclerema neonatorum
  Fat necrosis of the newborn?
  α_1-Antitrypsin deficiency panniculitis
  Pancreatic fat necrosis
Physical panniculitis
  Traumatic panniculitis
  Cold panniculitis (possible metabolic predisposition?)
  Reaction to foreign substances
Infectious panniculitis
Neoplastic panniculitis
  Histiocytic cytophagic panniculitis

contraceptives), and various diseases of unknown cause (sarcoidosis, ulcerative colitis, and Behçet syndrome).[2,3]

Histopathologic Features

The microscopic changes in erythema nodosum are concentrated in the interlobular septa. Early findings include infiltration of the fibrous tissue around septal vessels by neutrophils and lymphocytes (Fig. 13-2). Later, septal fibrosis becomes prominent (Fig. 13-3). At this stage, macrophages may be numerous. Sometimes they cluster in the septa and form non-necrotizing granulomas complete with multinucleate giant cells (Fig. 13-4). With time, the infiltrate diminishes and the fibrosis becomes more collagenized. Nodular aggregates of small monocyte/macrophages frequently surround a central cleft with a well-defined border. These have been called *Miescher's radial granulomas* and are thought to be specific for erythema nodosum.[4] Although the inflammatory changes are concentrated in the septa, the periphery of the fat lobules is usually involved to some degree by the infiltrate and the fibrosis.

Vasculitic changes have been described in erythema nodosum.[1] Although lymphocytic infiltration of vein walls is seen, the picture is not that of a leukocytoclastic vasculitis.

Pathophysiology

The mechanisms that produce erythema nodosum are poorly understood. Although the disease was linked to tuberculosis by early observers, many infections can precipitate the process. Whatever the stimulus, there is no evidence of an immune complex-related vasculitis. The microscopic findings are more consistent with a cell-mediated, delayed-hypersensitivity reaction that chiefly affects the septal vessels.

Differential Diagnosis

Histologically, early scleroderma with its infiltrate of lymphocytes and plasma cells around the vessels of the dermis that ex-

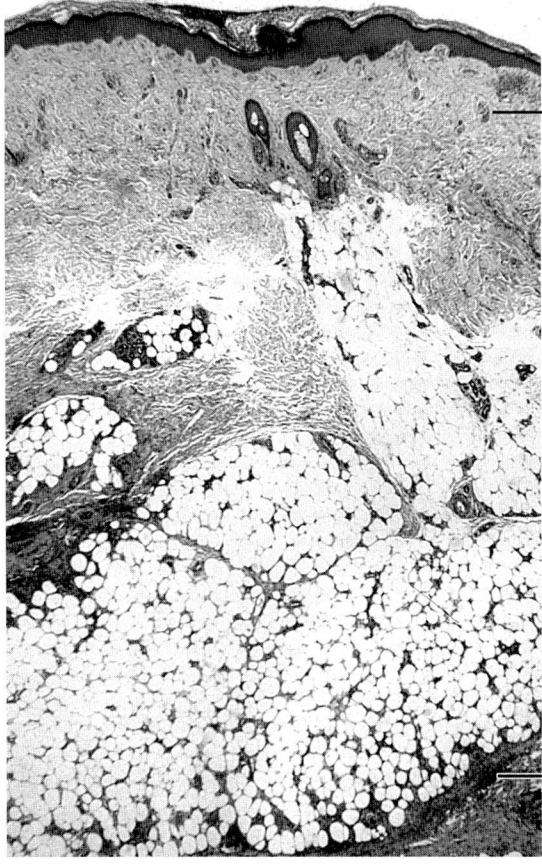

sparse dermal perivascular infiltrate

septal inflammatory infiltrate

Figure 13-2. Erythema nodosum. At scanning magnification there is a sparse perivascular dermal infiltrate with the chief changes centered in the subcutis where the septa contain an inflammatory infiltrate.

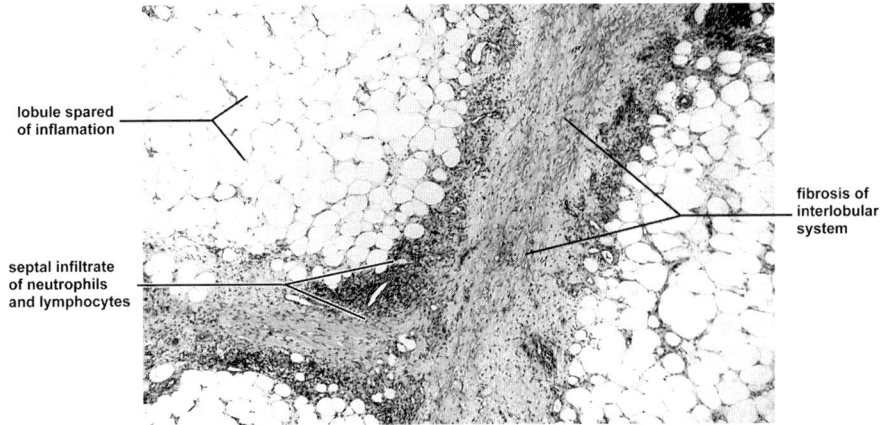

Figure 13-3. Erythema nodosum. The interlobular septa are thickened, and the lobules are relatively spared. The septal infiltrate consists of neutrophils and lymphocytes, and there is early septal fibrosis.

tends into the septa of the pannus is somewhat similar to erythema nodosum. However, dermal involvement tends to be more pronounced, and, in its later stages, scleroderma lacks the giant cells and granulomatous nodules frequently seen in erythema nodosum. The clinical appearance is also helpful in distinguishing these diseases.

Infectious granulomas can result in septal inflammation and a microscopic picture virtually identical to erythema nodosum. However, the clinical appearance is usually dissimilar, and there is frequently necrosis microscopically.

Noninfectious granulomatous diseases can also mimic erythema nodosum clinically. Sarcoidosis, cited as a cause of some cases of erythema nodosum, seldom involves the subcutis; when it does, it can simultaneously involve the dermis. Sarcoid should be considered in the differential diagnosis of

septal granulomatous inflammation particularly when the clinical presentation of the panniculitis is not typical of erythema nodosum and when there is involvement of other organs. Crohn's disease also can result in a septal panniculitis with microscopic features virtually identical to erythema nodosum. Clinical data are essential to resolve the differential diagnosis.

Necrobiosis lipoidica, a palisading granulomatous panniculitis, can show septal inflammation. Clues to diagnosis rest in the extensive changes in the dermis, with areas of collagen degeneration, fibroblastic proliferation, and associated mononuclear cell infiltrate sometimes accompanied by epithelioid granulomas with giant cells. Subcutaneous granuloma annulare is usually more localized than erythema nodosum and results in a well-formed palisaded granuloma.

Figure 13-4. Erythema nodosum (late stage). Fibrotic septa contain non-necrotizing granulomas and a few scattered lymphocytes.

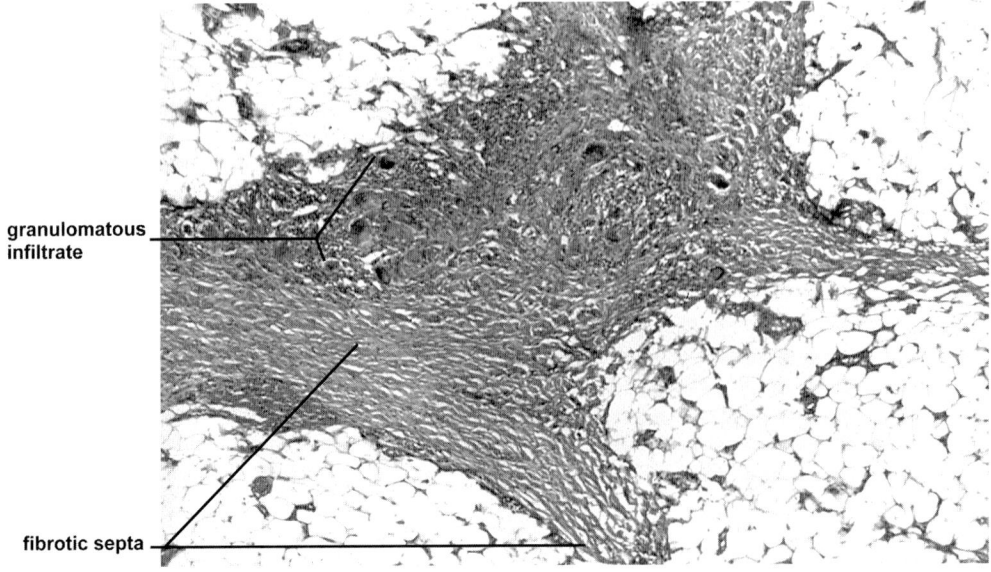

α_1-*Antitrypsin Deficiency-Associated Panniculitis*

Clinical Presentation

Erythematous nodules and plaques on the trunk and/or proximal extremities characterize the panniculitis associated with α_1-antitrypsin deficiency. In many patients there is breakdown of nodules with drainage of serous or serosanguineous fluid.[5] The disease affects all ages and is distributed about equally between the sexes.

Histopathology

Early in its course the septa and peripheral lobules are infiltrated by numerous neutrophils, and there is interstitial hemorrhage. Later, monocytes participate in the inflammatory response. There is necrosis of the septa, and often the necrosis and neutrophilic infiltrate involve the dermis and result in ulceration (Fig. 13-5). As monocytes become more numerous they spread from the septa to the lobules, and sometimes cluster to form granulomas. Lipid-filled monocytes are seen in areas of fat necrosis, and, late in the course of the disease, large numbers of lipophages and some giant cells can be found in the panniculus.[6]

Pathogenesis

α_1-Antitrypsin is a polypeptide glycoprotein that is made in the liver and regulates trypsin and some other proteolytic enzymes. Of the more than 26 alleles that affect α_1-antitrypsin production, the most common is designated M. Several alleles such as S and Z types result in deficient α_1-antitrypsin production. Severe deficiencies result from homozygous pairing of deficiency-related alleles such as SS and ZZ.[6]

α_1-Antitrypsin deficiency affects many organs, including the lungs (severe and progressive emphysema) and the liver (hepatitis and cirrhosis). When there are insufficient amounts of α_1-antitrypsin (or presumably other protease inhibitors) to regulate normally protective inflammatory reactions, protease activation can lead to severe tissue damage. This is postulated to be the mechanism that underlies α_1-antitrypsin-associated panniculitis.[7]

Differential Diagnosis

The histopathologic changes are similar to those of Weber-Christian disease, and it is likely that α_1-antitrypsin deficiency is the underlying mechanism of the panniculitis in many patients assigned this diagnosis. Factitial panniculitis and necrotizing fasciitis can also have a similar histopathologic appearance. Determination of blood levels of α_1-antitrypsin is important. The results of this test, when considered with the clinical presentation and microscopic morphology, often enable a specific diagnosis to be made.

With Vasculitis

Cutaneous Periarteritis Nodosa

Clinical Features

Cutaneous periarteritis nodosa presents as painful erythematous nodules usually located on the extremities, head, or neck. They range in size from 0.5 to 2.0 cm and may erupt in clusters. Ulceration sometimes occurs. Livedo reticularis may develop after the formation of the nodules. With time, the erythema fades and the nodules heal; the livedo pattern can persist.

In contrast to systemic periarteritis nodosa, patients with these lesions have a benign but chronic course. Systemic symptoms other than arthralgias and fever (during acute episodes) are uncommon.

Cutaneous periarteritis nodosa has been found in association with Crohn's disease.[8] It can be preceded by pharyngitis or an upper respiratory tract infection.[9]

Figure 13-5. α_1-Antitrypsin deficiency-associated panniculitis. There is necrosis of interlobular septa with an associated neutrophilic infiltrate. (Pathologic material courtesy of W.P.D. Su, M.D.)

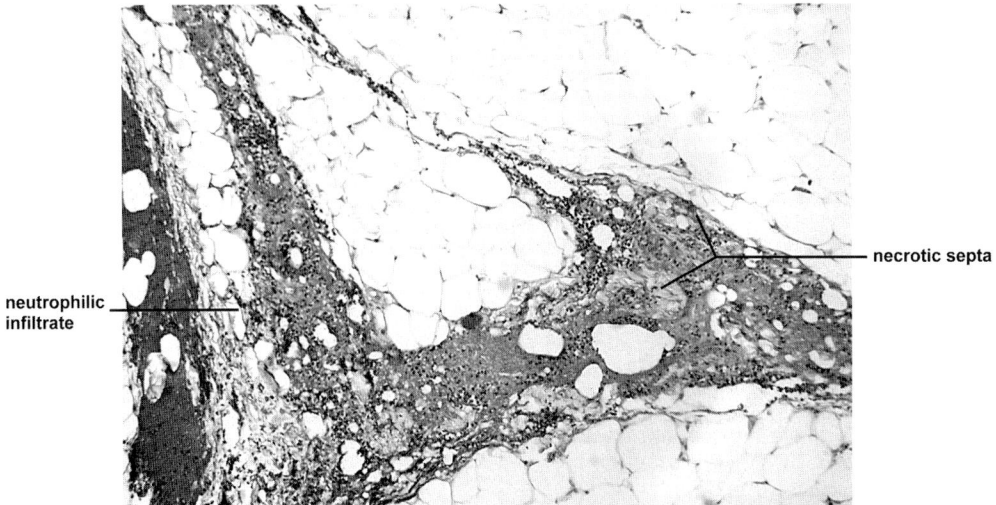

neutrophilic infiltrate

necrotic septa

Histopathologic Features

An excised nodule shows a necrotizing vasculitis of small and medium-sized arteries in the septa of the panniculus and in the lower dermis. Small vessels of the more superficial reticular dermis and papillary dermis are often surrounded by an infiltrate of lymphocytes. Walls of muscular arteries are diffusely infiltrated by neutrophils and show varying degrees of leukocytoclasis (Fig. 13-6). Frequently, scattered eosinophils can be identified in the infiltrate. There is fibrinoid necrosis of the vessel walls. As a result of vascular thrombosis, there is sometimes ischemic necrosis of the overlying skin that results in ulceration.

In contrast to other forms of panniculitis, the septal infiltrate remains fairly localized to the region around the involved vessels.[10]

Pathophysiology

The mechanisms that produce cutaneous periarteritis nodosa are poorly understood. In some cases, the finding of IgM deposits in the walls of uninvolved dermal vessels and vessels undergoing destruction by the panarteritis suggests that circulating immune complexes play a role. Their presence has been observed in a case associated with Crohn's disease.[8,11]

Differential Diagnosis

The differential diagnosis includes other forms of necrotizing arteritis that involve the subcutaneous fat such as nodular vasculitis (erythema induratum) and those that involve both the subcutaneous vessels and the small vessels of the dermis (leukocytoclastic vasculitis). Unlike erythema induratum, cutaneous periarteritis nodosa is not associated with caseous necrosis or a prominent granulomatous reaction, and the fat lobules are relatively spared. Although leukocytoclasis is present in the vascular lesions, it does not involve the small vessels of the superficial dermis as is the hallmark of leukocytoclastic vasculitis. The presence of systemic involvement distinguishes systemic periarteritis nodosa from subcutaneous periarteritis.

With Vascular Thrombosis

Superficial Migratory Thrombophlebitis

Clinical Features

Superficial migratory thrombophlebitis presents as crops of erythematous nodules that usually occur on the legs but may affect other parts of the body. As the process evolves, the nodules may become linear or cord-like.

Superficial migratory thrombophlebitis is frequently a sign of advanced visceral adenocarcinoma, usually of pancreatic origin. Similar lesions have been described in patients with Behçet's disease and systemic lupus erythematosus with lupus "anticoagulant."[12,13]

Histopathologic Features

There is thrombosis of superficial veins and virtually no associated inflammatory infiltrate or fat necrosis. Therefore, in the strict sense, this disease is not a true panniculitis.

Differential Diagnosis

The differential diagnosis includes septic vasculitis and erythema induratum from which superficial migratory thrombophlebitis can be distinguished by the relative absence of an inflammatory infiltrate and the lack of either vascular or fat necrosis. The histologic picture is similar to that seen in other forms of venous thrombosis.

Figure 13-6. Cutaneous periarteritis nodosa. Walls of muscular arteries of the subcutis are infiltrated by neutrophils and a few eosinophils. There is a variable amount of nuclear dust and often fibrinoid necrosis.

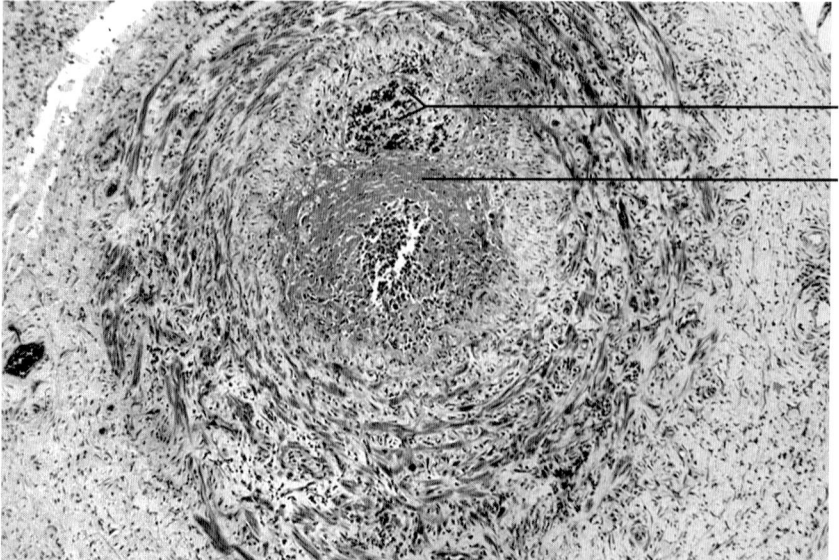

mixed infiltrate of eosinophils and neutrophils

fibrinoid necrosis

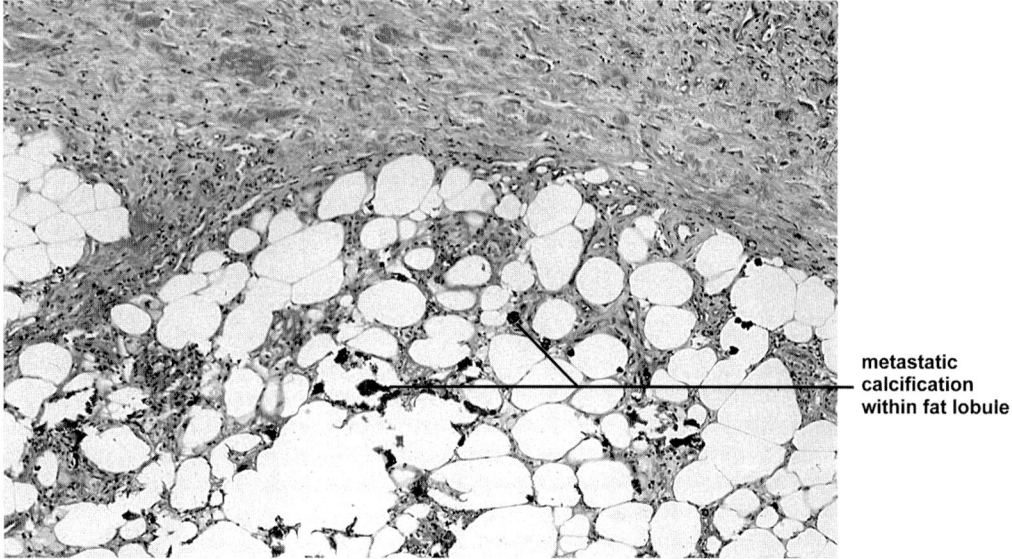

metastatic
calcification
within fat lobule

Figure 13-7. Calcifying panniculitis. Deposits of metastatic calcification are sometimes seen within fat lobules.

With Vascular Calcification

Calcifying Panniculitis

Clinical Features

Calcifying panniculitis is rare and occurs in patients with hypercalcemia or in whom calciphylaxis is operative. It is characterized by tender induration, erythema, and necrosis. The lower abdomen and thighs are the most frequent sites of involvement.[14–17]

Histopathologic Features

The most important feature is calcification of vessels[14,17] or fat lobules[15] (Fig. 13-7). Vascular occlusion that sometimes resulted in infarction was reported by Winkelmann and Keating[14] (Fig. 13-8). Inflammation, except as a response to necrosis or ulceration, is not characteristic.

Pathophysiology

Calcifying panniculitis is a sign of defective calcium metabolism. In some instances the changes can be brought about by metastatic

Figure 13-8. Calcifying panniculitis. Metastatic calcification of vessels can lead to thrombosis. Infarction sometimes results.

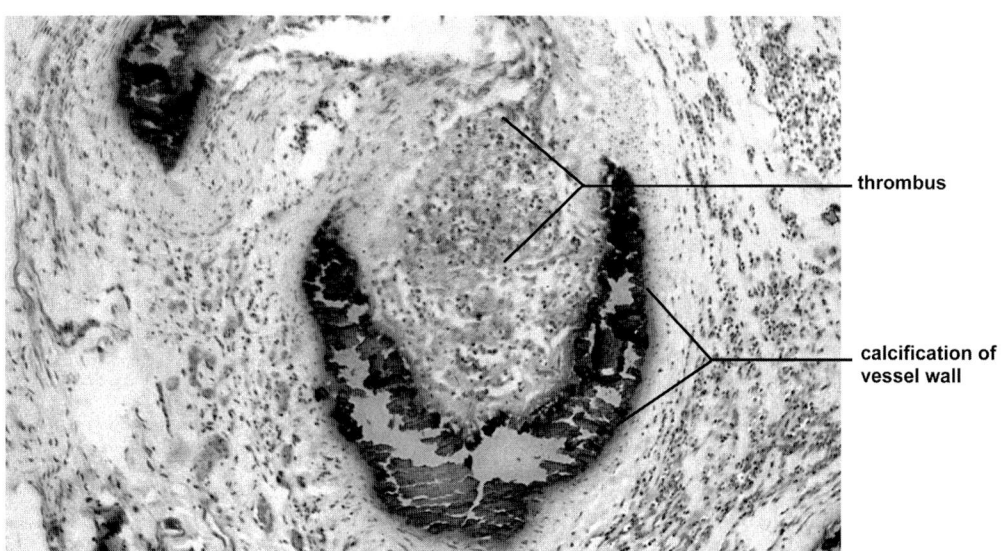

thrombus

calcification of
vessel wall

Figure 13-9.   (**A & B**) Nodular vasculitis. There is severe inflammation and necrosis of the fat lobules.

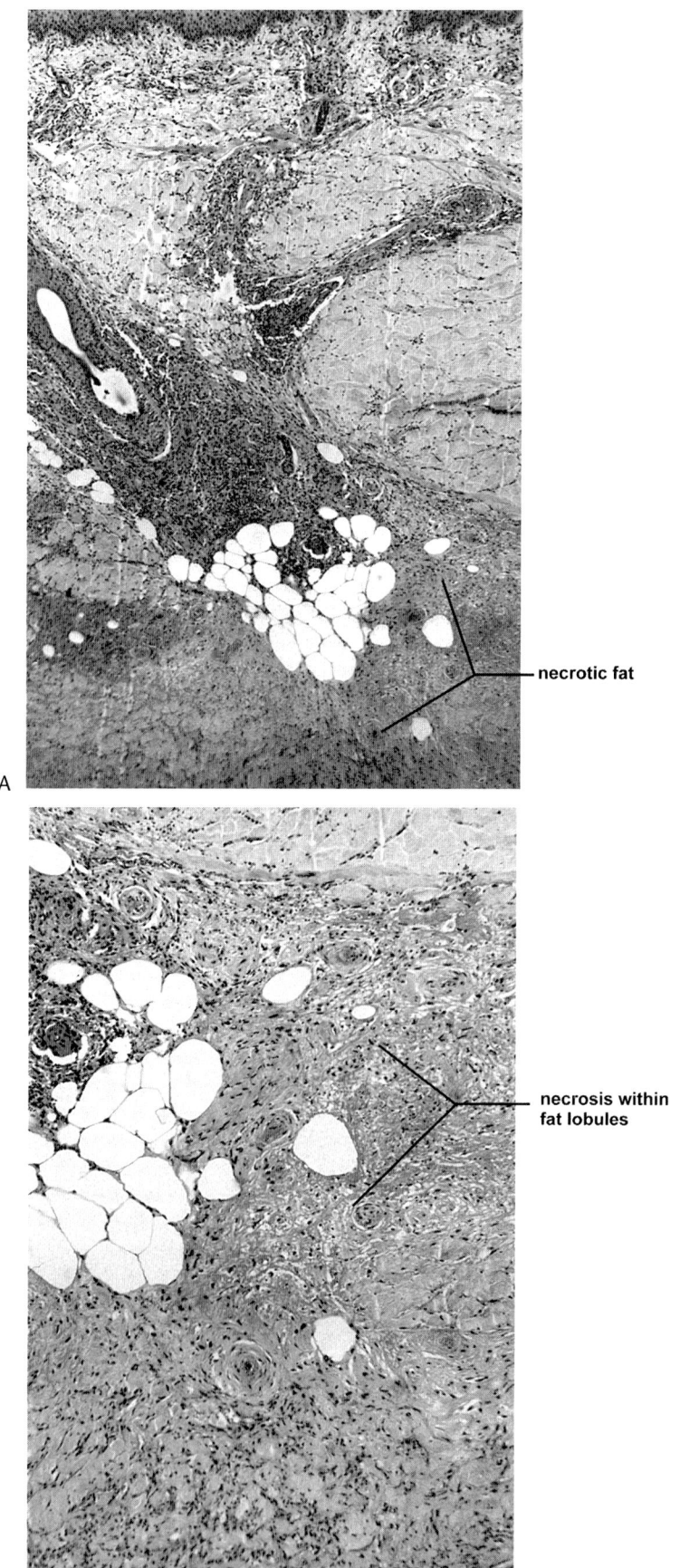

necrotic fat

A

necrosis within
fat lobules

B

calcification. At other times, the serum calcium level is insufficient to invoke this mechanism. Seyle,[18] in 1962, described "calciphylaxis," in which soft tissue calcification and necrosis in rats resulted from sensitization by parathyroid hormone or other systemic agents followed by challenge with a precipitating agent such as egg albumin, metallic salts, or local trauma.

Differential Diagnosis

The distinction between calcifying panniculitis and pancreatic panniculitis is the nature of the necrosis and the site of calcification. In pancreatic panniculitis the adipocytes are the primary target of circulating pancreatic enzymes and undergo saponification. In calcifying panniculitis the necrosis, if present, appears to result from ischemia and takes the form of an infarct.

LOBULAR PANNICULITIS

With Coagulative or Caseous Necrosis

With Vasculitis: Nodular Vasculitis and Erythema Induratum

In those instances in which there is vasculitis accompanying marked lobular damage, there is almost always a septal component as well (because of the location of the larger vessels). Nodular vasculitis (erythema induratum) is the prototype for this group.

Clinical Features

Nodular vasculitis can be a manifestation of an infection or a primary vascular abnormality. Although the term *erythema induratum (Bazin)* has been used synonymously with *nodular vasculitis* by several authors, others have found it useful to reserve the former for lesions related to a tuberculous infection.[19–21]

Nodular vasculitis presents as painful red to blue nodules that are located typically on the posterior legs. They sometimes ulcerate and occur most frequently in middle-aged women. There is a tendency toward chronicity and recurrence. In those instances in which there is a concurrent tuberculosis infection the lesions can affect a broader age range, from adolescence to old age, and can involve other body sites.

Histopathologic Features

The characteristic feature of nodular vasculitis is severe inflammation of muscular arteries and sometimes veins in the interlobular septa of the panniculus (Fig. 13-9). This is associated with severe inflammation and necrosis of the fat lobules. The necrosis has often been described as "caseous." However, in our experience, coagulation necrosis is far more frequent. There is infiltration of muscular arteries and sometimes veins by neutrophils, lymphocytes, and monocytes, associated with intimal swelling and sometimes thrombosis (Fig. 13-10). There is edema within the media and fragmentation of internal and external elastic lamina. The lobular infiltrate is initially neutrophil rich, but with progressive fat necrosis foamy macrophages and some giant cells appear that sometimes cluster to form granulomas.

Differential Diagnosis

The vasculitis in the septa and the lobular panniculitis are both necessary for the diagnosis of nodular vasculitis. Clinical evidence of tuberculosis is required for the more specific diagnosis of erythema induratum, although acid-fast bacilli are not characteristically found in the subcutaneous lesions. Special stains for elastic fibers are potentially useful in the identification of vessel remnants. In the absence of identifiable vasculitis, the presence of which often requires an incisional biopsy specimen, it is important to rule out an infectious etiology by special stains. Unlike subcutaneous periarteritis nodosa, there is characteristically intense lobular inflammation and often necrosis. When

Figure 13-10. Nodular vasculitis. The panniculitis is associated with a vasculitis of muscular arteries.

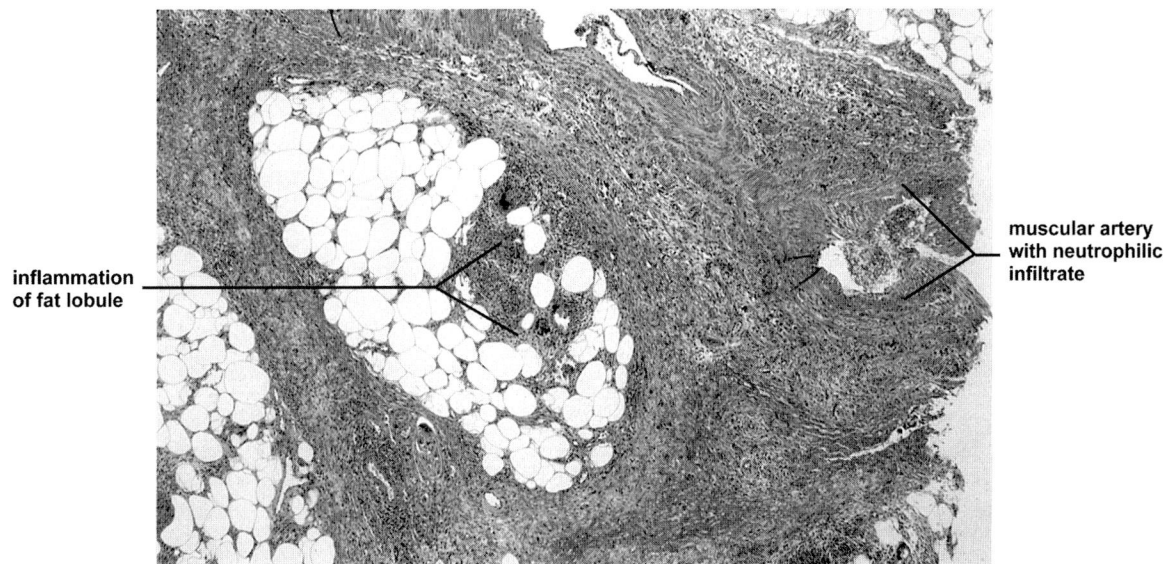

inflammation of fat lobule

muscular artery with neutrophilic infiltrate

caseous necrosis is present it is important that infectious panniculitis be ruled out by culture and special stains.

Without Vasculitis: Infectious Panniculitis
Clinical Features

Infectious panniculitis presents clinically as inflammatory subcutaneous nodules or plaques that can closely mimic erythema nodosum or nodular vasculitis in both appearance and location. Sometimes the nodules become fluctuant and can ulcerate. In some cases, lesions are located on the trunk, buttocks, or upper extremities. Cultures obtained at the time of biopsy can be useful to identify causative organisms. Although many patients with infectious panniculitis are predisposed to infection, in some there is no known immunosuppression or prior infection.

Histopathologic Features

Subcutaneous infections can result in a lobular, septal, or mixed pattern of inflammation (Fig. 13-11). Neutrophils are usually prominent in the infiltrate. Granulomas are uncommon in bacterial infections but are prominent in mycobacterial and fungal infections. There is often focal necrosis, abscess formation, and

Figure 13-11. Infectious panniculitis. (**A**) In this example of primary inoculation tuberculosis (*Mycobacterium tuberculosis*) there is a lobular panniculitis with a prominent granulomatous component. (**B**) The acid-fast stain (Kinyoun's method) demonstrates rare acid-fast rods.

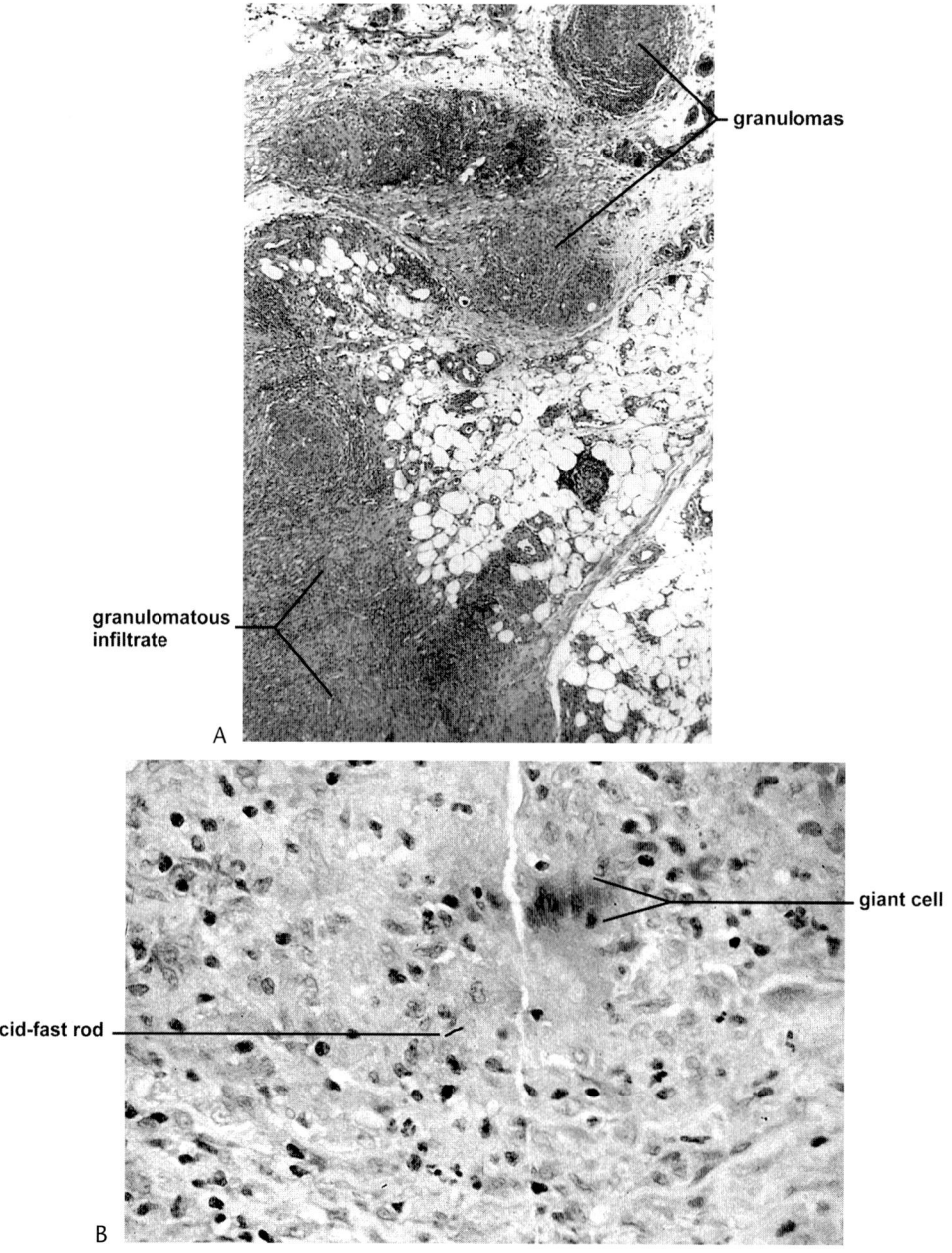

hemorrhage. Vasculitis may accompany panniculitis associated with septicemia.[22]

Differential Diagnosis

In some instances with predominantly septal involvement and little necrosis, the histologic picture mimics that of erythema nodosum, and in these instances the clues to proper diagnosis may lie in location and history. Confirmation is made by special stains and cultures. When there is prominent granulomatous inflammation and necrosis of fat lobules, infectious panniculitis is distinguished from nodular vasculitis by the absence of vasculitis and the identification of organisms.

With Needle-Like Clefts in Histiocytes or Lipocytes (or Both)

Sclerema Neonatorum

Much of the literature on sclerema neonatorum is confusing, as there has been a tendency to include discussions of subcutaneous fat necrosis of the newborn under this heading.

Clinical Features

In its restrictive sense, sclerema neonatorum refers to a peculiar, rapidly evolving, and widespread solidification of the subcutaneous fat of a newborn infant who almost always has another concurrent or antecedent major debilitating illness. Difficulties in temperature regulation are common.[23] The vast majority die within days of onset. In many instances, there is evidence of maternal illness before delivery.

The condition results in skin that cannot move over the underlying structures because the subcutis has lost its mobility. This change is widespread but spares the palms, soles, and genitalia.[24]

Histopathologic Features

Epidermis and dermis are unaltered histologically. The pannus appears thickened. Interlobular septa are thickened, but contain no inflammatory infiltrate. Adipocytes of the lobules are filled with cytoplasmic crystalline structures.[23]

Pathophysiology

The clinical and microscopic features are thought to reflect either an alteration in chemical composition of the intracellular lipids or a defect in the metabolism or transport of them. An abnormally high ratio of saturated to unsaturated fatty acids has been postulated to result in their solidification at temperatures at which normal fat would remain in its liquid state.

Fat Necrosis of the Newborn

The distinction between this disease and sclerema neonatorum has not always been made clearly in the literature. However, their clinical presentations, histologic appearances, and clinical courses are substantially different. Therefore, their separation is warranted.

Clinical Features

Unlike infants with sclerema neonatorum, infants with subcutaneous fat necrosis of the newborn usually have no other significant disease, although hypercalcemia is present in some.[25] The disease usually presents as one or several erythematous nodules or plaques that are freely movable. Although commonly located on the shoulders or back, the lesions may be located anywhere. Some may become fluctuant or drain (or both). Affected infants usually continue to thrive, and the lesions resolve in several months, sometimes with residual atrophy.[26]

Histopathologic Features

The inflammatory infiltrate is conspicuous with numerous lymphocytes and macrophages along with multinucleate giant cells, usually of the foreign body type (Fig. 13-12). There is associ-

Figure 13-12. Fat necrosis of the newborn. There is a lobular infiltrate of lymphocytes and foamy histiocytes. Some of the latter contain arrays of needle-like clefts. Multinucleate giant cells are also present.

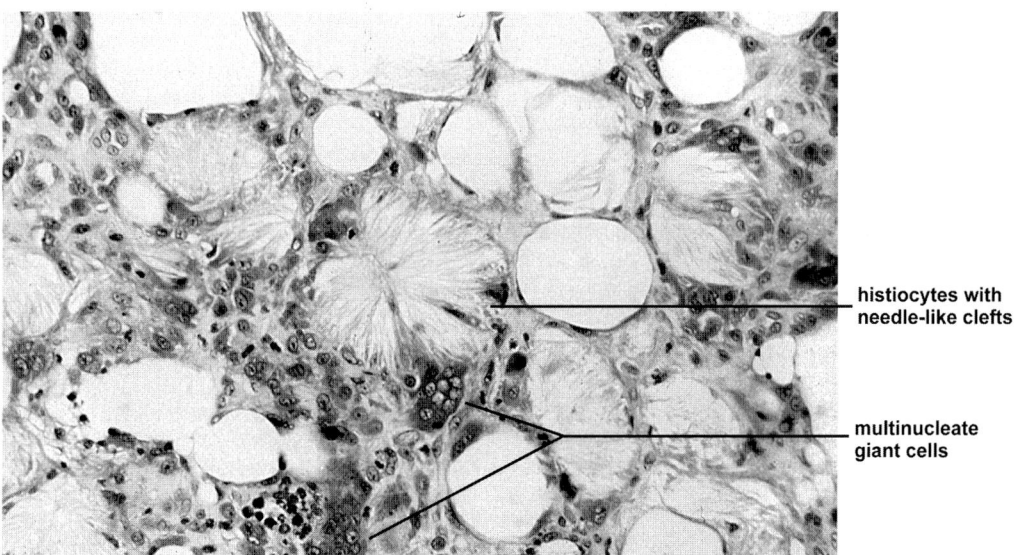

histiocytes with needle-like clefts

multinucleate giant cells

ated fibroplasia. The morphology of this condition is similar to that of fat necrosis induced by trauma except that needle-like clefts can be identified in lipocytes, multinucleate giant cells, and areas of necrosis.

Pathophysiology

The pathogenesis is poorly understood, but abnormal crystallization of fat, as in sclerema neonatorum, is thought to play a role. However, in this instance, the abnormality results in destruction of many lipocytes with resulting granulomatous inflammation.[27]

Differential Diagnosis

Subcutaneous fat necrosis of the newborn is similar in some respects to sclerema neonatorum, but there are major differences in both clinical presentation and histology. In subcutaneous fat necrosis, there is a panniculitis that manifests as nonfixed nodules or erythematous plaques. There is spontaneous resolution. In contrast to sclerema neonatorum, there is microscopic evidence of inflammation with lymphocytes, monocytes, and multinucleate giant cells. Sclerema neonatorum represents a physical alteration of the lipocytes and is not truly an inflammatory process and lacks an inflammatory infiltrate. Subcutaneous fat necrosis is virtually identical morphologically to poststeroid panniculitis and must be distinguished from it by history.

Poststeroid Panniculitis

Clinical Features

This disease apparently occurs only in infants and children upon cessation of high-dose corticosteroid therapy. Several tender subcutaneous nodules, sometimes with overlying erythema, form in the cheeks or in the skin of the trunk or extremities. The process is self-limited, with resolution in weeks to months.

Histopathologic Features

There is a lobular panniculitis with fat necrosis and infiltration by monocytes, multinucleate giant cells, foam cells, and lymphocytes. Interlobular septa are largely spared. Needle-like clefts can be seen within lipocytes[28,29] or macrophages.[30]

Differential Diagnosis

There are marked morphologic similarities between this disease and fat necrosis of the newborn. A history of steroid therapy is required for the diagnosis. Distinction from other lobular panniculitides is made by the identification of granulomatous inflammation that mostly spares the septa and needle-like clefts in lipocytes or macrophages (or both).

With Hyaline Sclerosis of Fat

Lupus Panniculitis

Clinical Features

The tender subcutaneous nodules and plaques of lupus panniculitis can form before, during, or after other manifestations of lupus erythematosus and in some patients is the sole clinical manifestation of the disease. The lesions can be associated with characteristic epidermal changes of lupus erythematosus and usually involve the head and neck, trunk, or proximal extremities. Ulceration sometimes occurs. The course is chronic with a tendency for relapses to occur. Loss of adipose tissue occurs with resolution of the inflammatory stage and results in a clinical picture similar to that of localized lipodystrophy.[31]

Histopathologic Features

Lupus panniculitis often has a characteristic appearance. There is an infiltrate of chiefly lymphocytes in the fat lobules (Fig. 13-13A & B). These may aggregate to form follicles, sometimes with germinal centers. A few plasma cells are often present.

A peculiar and characteristic form of fat necrosis is seen in fully developed lesions in which the lipocytes are surrounded by an eosinophilic "hyaline" material. Septa are thickened with thickened vessels surrounded by the hyaline material (Fig. 13-13C). Granulomas are sometimes present in the septa, and focal aggregates of neutrophils may be associated with areas of fat necrosis.

The overlying epidermis and dermis often show the changes of lupus erythematosus with a vacuolar interface dermatitis that progresses to epidermal thinning, follicular plugging, and epidermal basement membrane thickening. Perivascular and periadnexal infiltrates of lymphocytes and some plasma cells can be seen throughout the dermis. Sometimes connective tissue mucin accumulates in the reticular dermis and the involved subcutaneous tissues.[32]

Differential Diagnosis

The peculiar hyaline necrosis of the fat lobules is characteristic of this disease, and epidermal and dermal changes are often of great help in making the diagnosis. In the absence of these changes a lupus band test is helpful in confirming the diagnosis in many cases as are serologic tests for the diagnosis of lupus erythematosus. The distribution of these lesions is unlike that of either erythema nodosum or nodular vasculitis, as lupus panniculitis usually spares the legs.

With Saponification

Pancreatic Panniculitis

Pancreatic disease, either inflammatory or neoplastic, can present with or be complicated by fat necrosis. Although this is frequently limited to the peritoneum, it can take the form of a panniculitis that can clinically mimic erythema nodosum.

Clinical Features

Pancreatic (enzymatic) fat necrosis of the subcutaneous fat is characterized by erythematous nodules that usually occur first on the legs and later may involve the trunk, arms, and even scalp. They may resemble lesions of erythema nodosum or allergic vasculitis.[33] As in erythema nodosum, some patients have concurrent arthritis most commonly of the ankles.[34]

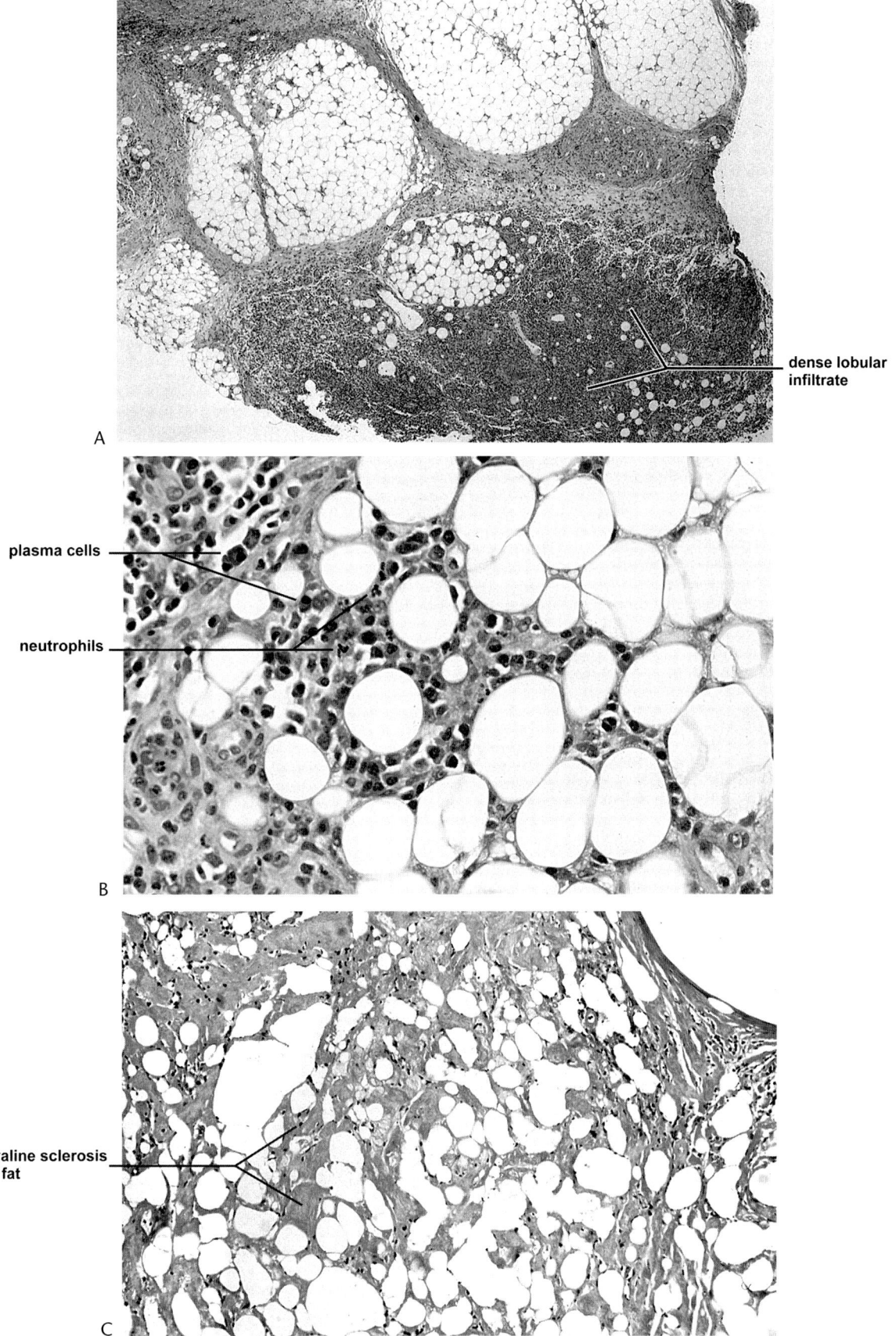

Figure 13-13. Lupus erythematosus panniculitis. (**A & B**) There is a dense lobular infiltrate of lymphocytes, plasma cells, and a few neutrophils. (**C**) With resolution of the inflammatory infiltrate there is frequently a characteristic hyaline sclerosis of the fat lobules.

Histopathologic Features

Microscopically, the changes in the subcutaneous fat are pathognomonic and are identical to those seen in the peritoneal fat in patients with acute pancreatitis. There is necrosis of lipocytes with loss of nuclei. Cytoplasmic membranes appear thickened and poorly defined. In some areas there is deposition of granular basophilic material, probably calcium, both between cells and within them (Fig. 13-14).

Pathophysiology

The changes are thought to result from the action of lipases on intracytoplasmic lipid. Elevated serum trypsin levels may facilitate the escape of these lipases from the vasculature.

Differential Diagnosis

No other panniculitis exhibits similar changes within necrotic fat.

Lipodystrophy (Lipoatrophy)

Clinical Features

Total, partial, and localized lipodystrophy are conditions in which subcutaneous fat is lost. Total lipodystrophy may be either congenital or acquired and refers to the complete loss of the subcutaneous fat. It is often associated with hepatic enlargement, hyperlipemia, hyperglycemia, and an increased metabolic rate.[35] Other endocrine and developmental disorders have also been reported in these patients.[36–38]

Partial lipodystrophy refers to regional loss of adipose tissue. Symmetric involvement of the face, thorax, and arms is the most common and, like total lipodystrophy, has been associated with renal disease, hirsutism, hyperpigmentation, hepatomegaly, hyperlipemia, and diabetes. Hemilipodystrophy, which involves half of the face or body, is an infrequent pattern of involvement.

Localized lipodystrophy refers to fat loss in one or several localized circumscribed areas. There is sometimes associated morphea, lichen sclerosus, or lupus erythematosus.

Histopathologic Features

Lipodystrophy in its fully developed form is characterized by an absence or reduction in the amount of subcutaneous fat. An early inflammatory stage in which there is a lymphocytic infiltrate of the subcutis has been described in several cases of localized lipodystrophy.[39] A second form or localized lipodystrophy has been described in which there is no inflammatory infiltrate, but an "involutional" appearance of the fat with lobules that contain small lipocytes in a background of hyaline material and numerous capillaries.[40] Whether the inflammatory pattern represents a precursor to the involutional pattern is unclear.

Pathophysiology

The pathogenesis of these diseases is poorly understood. Although an inflammatory process has been implicated in some instances of localized lipodystrophy, there is currently little histologic evidence to support an inflammatory process in total or partial lipodystrophy.

Differential Diagnosis

The absence of subcutaneous adipose tissue is pathognomonic of lipodystrophy. The distribution of the atrophy, its clinical history, and associated conditions are clues to its etiology.

Physical Panniculitis

Cold Panniculitis

Clinical Features

Cold panniculitis has been most frequently reported in children less than 10 years of age. It has been infrequently identified in older patients, usually women.

Characterized by tender red plaques that form shortly after exposure to cold and resolve in several weeks, these lesions usually are located on the face but have been described on the legs and thighs.

Histopathologic Features

The inflammatory reaction is similar to that seen in traumatic fat necrosis but tends to involve the superficial subcutis preferentially. Early in its course (24 hours after cold exposure) a perivascular infiltrate of lymphocytes and monocytes is noted. Later in its course, there is rupture of lipocytes with cyst formation and a mixed infiltrate of lymphocytes, monocytes, and a few neutrophils.[41]

Pathophysiology

The pathogenesis of this condition is unknown, but two mechanisms have been postulated: (1) an abnormal ratio of saturated to unsaturated fats results in solidification at higher than normal temperatures[42] and (2) cellular hypersensitivity produces the lymphomonocytic infiltrate seen in the first stages of the disease.[41] The former mechanism, which is similar to that postulated for sclerema neonatorum, might explain the susceptibility of young children to this panniculitis and the relative resistance of adults. The latter mechanism is suggested by the morphologic changes early in the course of the disease when the inflammatory infiltrate precedes morphologic evidence of dissolution of lipocytes.

Differential Diagnosis

The histopathologic findings are similar to those found in traumatic fat necrosis. The location of the lesions, the history of cold exposure, and the tendency for the disease to occur in young children enables the distinction to be made. Unlike sclerema neonatorum and neonatal fat necrosis, intracytoplasmic crystalline structures are not generally seen in either monocytes or lipocytes.

Traumatic Panniculitis

Clinical Features

Traumatic fat necrosis of the breast is the most common manifestation of traumatic panniculitis. This reaction can also be seen in other subcutaneous tissues exposed to physical trauma.

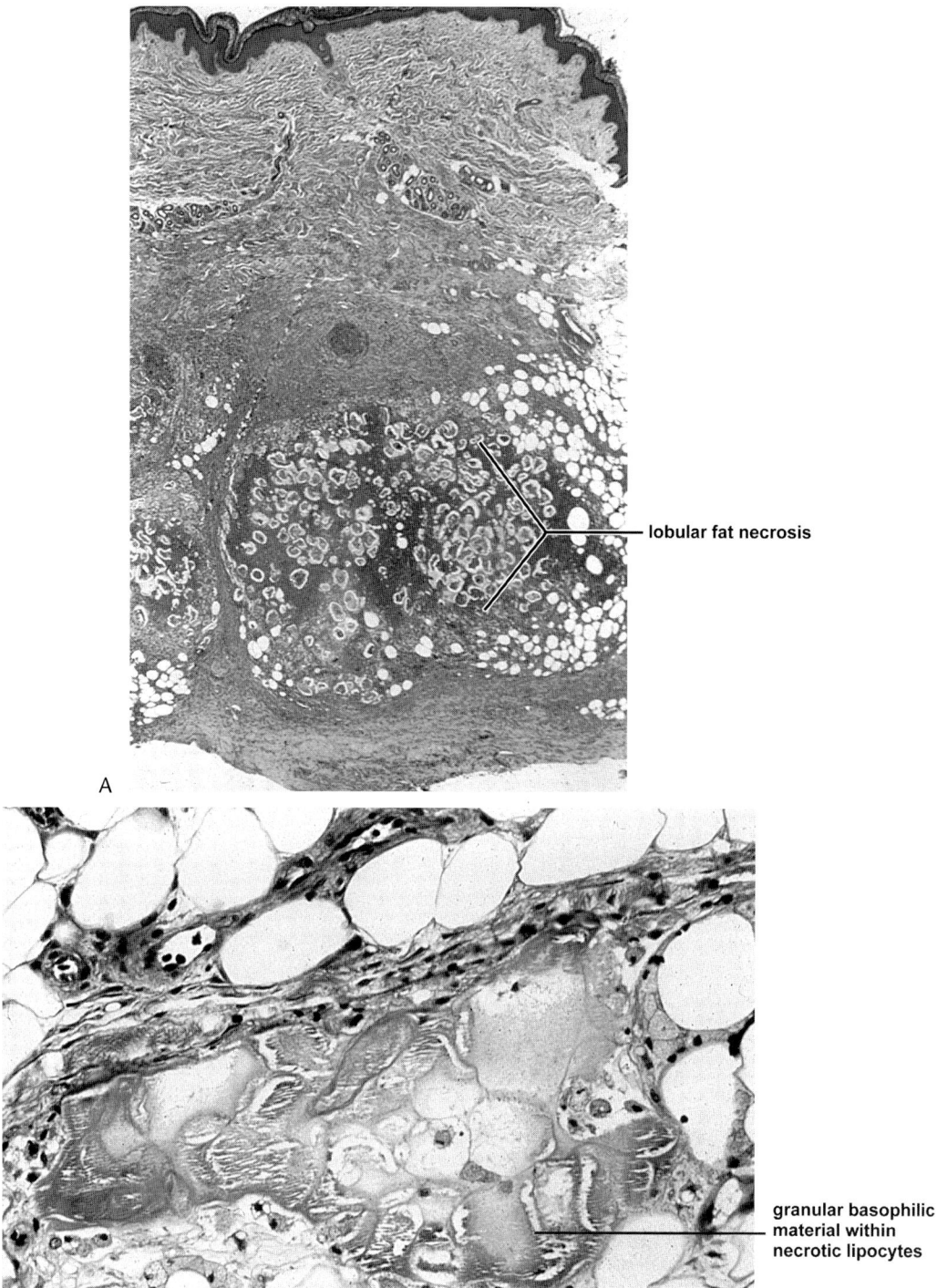

lobular fat necrosis

granular basophilic
material within
necrotic lipocytes

Figure 13-14. **(A & B)** Pancreatic panniculitis (enzymatic fat necrosis). There is lobular fat necrosis with deposition of granular basophilic material within lipocytes.

Although blunt trauma is the usual cause, a similar reaction can occur adjacent to a cutaneous surgical site. In some patients no history of trauma can be elicited.

In its early stages there is redness and swelling and sometimes ecchymosis, pain, and tenderness. Later there may be skin retraction.

Histopathologic Features

The early changes occur primarily within the fat lobule with rupture and dissolution of adipocytes to form lipid-filled cysts. Sometimes these cysts are lined by distinct eosinophilic membranes that may have a scalloped contour and the staining pattern of ceroid.[43] There may be interstitial hemorrhage or even the formation of a hematoma. Lymphocytes and monocytes migrate into the site of injury, and the latter engulf liberated lipids and develop abundant foamy cytoplasm. There is often formation of multinucleate giant cells.

Fibroplasia surrounds areas of necrosis and may involve the interlobular septa. Fibrosis eventually replaces the necrotic fat and results in a dense scar.

Pathophysiology

Lipocytes may be injured directly through mechanical injury (crushing) or as the result of ischemia caused by vascular damage. The inflammatory reaction is a response to released lipid and components of necrotic cells.

Differential Diagnosis

The differential diagnosis includes panniculitis caused by injection of foreign substances. Demonstration of birefringent foreign debris by polarized light is helpful in this regard. Clinical history is also of great importance.

Panniculitis Caused by Foreign Substances

Clinical Features

The clinical presentation of these factitial panniculitides is extremely variable and depends on the nature of the foreign material, the manner by which it was introduced, and its location. Substances that are relatively inert biologically do not often produce the clinical signs of acute inflammation but result in indurated masses. Injection of paraffins (usually for penile or scrotal enlargement)[44] or the introduction of silicone, either injected or released from prosthetic implants, results in this reaction.

Reactions to the injection of various drugs depend on the nature of the compound. Some, such as povidone and meperidine hydrochloride, produce the signs and symptoms of acute inflammation at the site of injection.[45,46] Others, such as pentazocine, can produce cutaneous ulcerations.[47] A reaction that simulates Weber-Christian syndrome resulted from the injection of milk into the subcutis.[48] Other organic substances, when injected, can produce severe inflammation of the pannus.

Histopathologic Features

Reactions to paraffins and silicone produce lipophagic granulomas with areas of fat necrosis and fibrosis. Lymphocytes and monocytes are the reacting cells, but other cells may be admixed depending on the nature of the substance and its location.

Toxic drugs can cause direct injury to the subcutaneous tissues. Some therapeutic agents are vasoactive or can cause vascular thrombosis and thus can lead to infarction and subsequent necrosis of the subcutis and skin.[47] Still others are thought to result in panniculitis through immunologic mechanisms.

The injection of organic materials can result in various inflammatory reactions. The injection of milk has been reported to result in a panniculitis that simulates the early stages of Weber-Christian disease.[48] The injection of feces results in subcutaneous abscess formation.[49]

Miscellaneous

Weber-Christian Disease (Syndrome)

Clinical Features

This disease has been described as a recurring febrile illness associated with nodules within the subcutaneous fat that resolve with atrophy.[50]

Histopathologic Features

The histology is that of a lobular or lobular and septal panniculitis. Destruction of lipocytes and infiltration of the affected area by neutrophils, lymphocytes, and lipophagic histiocytes have been described along with scarring upon resolution.[51]

Pathophysiology

With increasing understanding of the pathogenesis of the panniculitides, the clinical and histologic features once thought diagnostic of Weber-Christian disease are now known to be caused by a variety of mechanisms. Lupus panniculitis, α_1-antitrypsin deficiency-related panniculitis, and histiocytic cytophagic panniculitis are recognized as distinct entities. These diseases and others were probably grouped under the heading of Weber-Christian disease in the past. It is, therefore, useful to consider Weber-Christian disease as a reaction pattern that can result from diverse mechanisms, some of which are beginning to be recognized and some of which are yet to be elucidated.[52]

Histiocytic Cytophagic Panniculitis

Whether this peculiar and rare process that results in subcutaneous nodules should be classified as a true panniculitis or is better regarded as a manifestation of a neoplastic proliferation of monocyte macrophages is debatable. It is included here because of its morphologic appearance, which closely resembles inflammatory processes that involve the pannus. It is likely that it was known under the term "Weber-Christian" disease before the recognition of its progressive and fatal clinical course by Winkelmann and Bowie,[53] who also defined the microscopic features that characterize it as a morphologic entity.

Clinical Features

The patients, often young women, present with tender subcutaneous nodules of variable size that are sometimes erythematous. These are distributed widely and are associated with febrile episodes. Biopsy sites heal poorly. Associated signs include hepatosplenomegaly, mucosal ulcers, and pleural effusion. The course is characterized by progressive deterioration with increasing hepatic dysfunction. Ecchymoses or bleeding from the gastrointestinal, respiratory, or urinary tract usually occurs preterminally.

Histopathologic Features

Microscopic examination of an excised subcutaneous nodule shows necrosis of fat lobules. There is an associated dense infiltrate of cytologically benign monocytes admixed with lymphocytes and plasma cells. The macrophages have foamy cytoplasm, and many contain remnants of neutrophils and erythrocytes to produce a "bean-bag" appearance. Infiltrates of similar cells can be seen replacing lymph nodes and in the spleen and bone marrow.

Pathophysiology

Histiocytic cytophagic panniculitis is probably a malignant infiltrative process despite the absence of cytologic atypia. Its aggressive clinical course and its pattern of systemic involvement suggest a neoplastic process. A case in which remission was induced with combination chemotherapy has been reported.[54]

Differential Diagnosis

The differential diagnosis includes other forms of lobular panniculitis from which cytophagic histiocytic panniculitis can be usually distinguished by the presence of numerous "bean-bag" cells and subsequent clinical course.

SUMMARY

Panniculitis can be classified according to the anatomic site of involvement. Figure 13-1 includes such a classification.

Diseases in which the inflammatory infiltrate is located chiefly in the interlobular septa are called *septal panniculitides*. The differential diagnosis of this group rests on the presence or absence of vascular lesions, the nature of the vascular lesions, if present, the nature of the inflammatory infiltrate, and the presence or absence of septal necrosis if vascular lesions are not identified.

Diseases in which the fat lobule is primarily affected are called *lobular panniculitides*. They are classified here according to the histologic characteristics of the fat necrosis, if present. Physical panniculitis is included as a major category because its clinical presentation and history are often more important than its microscopic features.

Finally, Weber-Christian disease is becoming recognized as a clinical reaction pattern that results from a variety of diseases of differing pathogenesis. As such, it cannot be logically included in this (chiefly morphologic) schema.

REFERENCES

1. Winkelmann RK, Forstrom L: New observations in the histopathology of erythema nodosum. J Invest Dermatol 65:441–446, 1975
2. Favour CV, Sosman MC: Erythema nodosum. Arch Intern Med 80:435–453, 1947
3. Chun SI, Su WPD: Erythema nodosum-like lesions in Behçet's syndrome: a histopathologic study of 30 cases. J Cutan Pathol 16:259–265, 1989
4. Yus ES, Vico MDS, Diego VD: Miescher's radial granuloma: a characteristic marker of erythema nodosum. Am J Dermatopathol 11:434–442, 1989
5. Smith KC, Pittelkow MR, Su WPD: Panniculitis associated with severe alpha-1 antitrypsin deficiency. Arch Dermatol 123:1655–1661, 1987
6. Su WPD, Smith KC, Pittelkow MR, Winkelmann RK: Alpha-1 antitrypsin deficiency panniculitis. Am J Dermatopathol 9:483–490, 1987
7. Hendrick SJ, Silverman AK, Solomon AR, Headington JT: Alpha-1 antitrypsin deficiency associated with panniculitis. J Am Acad Dermatol 18:684–692, 1988
8. Goslen JB, Graham W, Lazarus GS: Cutaneous polyarteritis nodosa. Arch Dermatol 119:326–329, 1983
9. Braverman IM: Skin Signs of Systemic Disease. 2nd Ed. WB Saunders, Philadelphia 1981
10. Diaz-Perez JL, Schroeter AL, Winkelmann RK: Cutaneous periarteritis nodosa. Arch Dermatol 110:407–414, 1974
11. Diaz-Perez JL, Schroeter AL, Winkelmann RK: Cutaneous periarteritis nodosa. Arch Dermatol 116:56–58, 1980
12. Durham RH: Thrombophlebitis migrans and visceral carcinoma. AMA Arch Intern Med 96:380–386, 1955
13. Blum F, Gilkeson G, Greenberg C, Murray J: Superficial migratory thrombophlebitis and the lupus anticoagulant. Int J Dermatol 29:190–192, 1990
14. Winkelmann RK, Keating FR Jr: Cutaneous vascular calcification, gangrene and hyperparathyroidism. Br J Dermatol 83:263–268, 1970
15. Richens G, Piepkorn MW, Krueger GG: Calcifying panniculitis associated with renal failure. J Am Acad Dermatol 6:537–539, 1982
16. Rees JKH, Coles GA: Calciphylaxis in man. BMJ 2:670–672, 1969
17. Richardson JA, Herron G, Reitz R, Layzer R: Ischemic ulcerations of skin and necrosis of muscle in azotemic hyperparathyroidism. Ann Intern Med 71:129–138, 1969
18. Seyle H: Calciphylaxis. University of Chicago Press, Chicago, 1962
19. Kuramoto Y, Aiba S, Tagami H: Erythema induratum of Bazin as a type of tuberculid. J Am Acad Dermatol 22:612–616, 1990
20. Rademaker M, Lowe DG, Munro DD: Erythema induratum (Bazin's disease). J Am Acad Dermatol 21:740–745, 1989
21. Lebel M, Lassonde M: Erythema induratum of Bazin. J Am Acad Dermatol 14:738–742, 1986
22. Patterson JW, Brown PC, Broecker AH: Infection-induced panniculitis. J Cutan Pathol 16:183–193, 1989
23. Kellum RE, Ray TL, Brown GR: Sclerema neonatorum. Arch Dermatol 97:372–380, 1968
24. Hughes WE, Hammond ML: Sclerema neonatorum. J Pediatr 32:676–692, 1948
25. Holzel A: Subcutaneous fat necrosis of the newborn. Arch Dis Child 26:89–91, 1951
26. Fretzin DF, Arias AM: Sclerema neonatorum and subcutaneous fat necrosis of the newborn. Pediatr Dermatol 4:112–122, 1987
27. Proks C, Valvoda C: Fatty crystals in sclerema neonatorum. J Clin Pathol 19:193–195, 1966
28. Roenigk HH Jr, Haserick JR, Arundell FD: Poststeroid panniculitis: report of a case and review of the literature. Arch Dermatol 90:387–391, 1964
29. Saxena AK, Nigam PK: Panniculitis following steroid therapy. Cutis 42:156–157, 1988

30. Silverman RA, Newman AJ, LeVine MJ, Kaplan B: Post-steroid panniculitis: a case report. Pediatr Dermatol 5:92–93, 1988
31. Peters M, Su WPD: Lupus erythematosus panniculitis. Med Clin North Am 73:1113–1126, 1989
32. Sanchez NP, Peters MS, Winkelmann RK: The histopathology of lupus erythematosus panniculitis. J Am Acad Dermatol 5:673–680, 1981
33. Szymanshi FJ, Bluefarb SM: Nodular fat necrosis and pancreatic diseases. Arch Dermatol 83:224–229, 1961
34. Hughes PSH, Apisarnthanarax P, Mullins JF: Subcutaneous fat necrosis associated with pancreatic disease. Arch Dermatol 111:506–510, 1975
35. Senior B, Gellis SS: The syndromes of total lipodystrophy and of partial lipodystrophy. Pediatrics 33:593–612, 1964
36. Brubaker MM, Levan NE, Collipp PJ: Acanthosis nigricans and congenital total lipodystrophy. Arch Dermatol 91:320–325, 1965
37. Reed WB, Dexter R, Corley C, Fish C: Congenital lipodystrophic diabetes and acanthosis nigricans: the Seip-Lawrence syndrome. Arch Dermatol 91:326–334, 1965
38. Seip M: Lipodystrophy and gigantism with associated endocrine manifestations – a new diencephalic syndrome? Acta Paediatr 48:555–574, 1959
39. Peters MS, Winkelmann RK: Localized lipoatrophy (atrophic connective tissue disease panniculitis). Arch Dermatol 116:1363–1368, 1980
40. Peters MS, Winkelmann RK: The histopathology of localized lipoatrophy. Br J Dermatol 114:27–36, 1986
41. Duncan WC, Freeman RG, Heaton CL: Cold panniculitis. Arch Dermatol 94:722–724, 1966
42. Lowe LB Jr: Cold panniculitis in children. Am J Dis Child 115:709–713, 1968
43. Poppiti RJ, Margulies M, Cabello B, Rywlin AM: Membranous fat necrosis. Am J Surg Pathol 10:62–69, 1986
44. Oertel YC, Johnson FB: Sclerosing lipogranuloma of male genitalia. Arch Pathol Lab Med 101:321–326, 1977
45. Forstrom L, Winkelmann RK: Factitial panniculitis. Arch Dermatol 110:747–750, 1974
46. Kossard S, Ecker RI, Dicken CH: Povidone panniculitis. Arch Dermatol 116:704–706, 1980
47. Palestine RF, Millns JL, Spigel GT, Schroeter AL: Skin manifestations of pentazocine abuse. J Am Acad Dermatol 2:47–55, 1980
48. Ackerman AB, Mosher DT, Schwamm HA: Factitial Weber-Christian syndrome. JAMA 198:731–736, 1966
49. Sullivan M, Trosow A: Multiple subcutaneous abscesses produced by the hypodermic injection of feces. South Med J 42:402–404, 1949
50. Christian HA: Relapsing febrile nodular non-suppurative panniculitis. Arch Intern Med 42:338, 1928
51. MacDonald A, Feiwel M: A review of the concept of Weber-Christian panniculitis with a report of five cases. Br J Dermatol 80:355–361, 1968
52. Panush RS, Yonker RA, Dlesk A et al: Weber-Christian disease. Medicine (Baltimore) 64:181–191, 1985
53. Winkelmann RK, Bowie W: Hemorrhagic diatheses associated with benign histiocytic, cytophagic panniculitis and systemic histiocytosis. Arch Intern Med 140:1460–1463, 1980
54. Barron DR, Davis BR, Pomeranz JR et al: Cytophagic histiocytic panniculitis: a variant of malignant histiocytosis. Cancer 55:2538–2542, 1985

14

DISORDERS OF PIGMENTATION

Many processes can lead to discoloration of the skin. Of major concern to dermatopathologists are abnormalities in melanocytes. Excesses either in the number of melanocytes or in melanin production lead to hyperpigmentation, while corresponding decreases lead to hypopigmentation. In this chapter most types of hypopigmentation as well as hyperpigmentation caused by excess melanin and other factors are considered. Hyperpigmentation secondary to an increased number of melanocytes is discussed in Chapter 20.

Melanocytes in the basal layer usually have a small dark nucleus and a clear cytoplasm. They contain melanin that can be identified by silver stains such as the Fontana-Masson stain. Melanocytes can also be stained by the Bloch dopa reaction because they are capable of synthesizing melanin. An anti-S-100 stain will also identify melanocytes, as well as a variety of other cells. The definitive method for identifying melanocytes is ultrastructural examination, for only with this technique can melanosomes, their transfer, and their life history be studied. Identification of early melanosomes in a cell proves it is a melanocyte. More mature melanosomes occur in many types of cells after transfer. It is also difficult to assess melanocyte numbers by routine light microscopy. First, melanocytes may be hard to identify. Second, other epidermal clear cells, especially Langerhans cells, may be seen in the basal layer. Then, too, there are regional and age-related differences in the number of melanocytes. Reliable quantitative melanocyte counts are a research technique. Fortunately such detailed examinations are rarely ever needed to answer clinical questions.[1,2]

LEUKODERMA OR HYPOPIGMENTATION

It is perhaps better to use the term *leukoderma*, for it avoids the difficult distinction between hypopigmentation and depigmentation (or hypomelanosis and amelanosis). Leukoderma can be subdivided in melanocytopenic and melanopenic disorders, although the distinction is sometimes difficult, and overlapping occurs.

Melanocytopenic Disorders

In these diseases, the melanocytes are decreased in number or are absent. They may have been destroyed by immunologic or toxic means or may simply have failed to appear in the skin. In general, melanocytopenic disorders have more complete depigmentation.

Vitiligo

Vitiligo is the acquired patchy loss of pigment of skin and hair.

Clinical Features

Vitiligo may be subdivided into three groups based on pattern and degree of cutaneous involvement: localized (focal or segmental), generalized, and universal. The clinical diagnosis is usually obvious, as there are few other causes of sharply localized depigmentation without inflammation or epidermal change. Depigmentation in areas of trauma is a common occurrence. Only if leprosy is a serious differential diagnostic problem are biopsy specimens likely to be obtained. In addition, there are vitiligo-like lesions in progressive systemic sclerosis. Early lesions (trichrome vitiligo) may have areas of partial color loss, but well-developed lesions are without color. When either therapy-induced or spontaneous repigmentation occurs, it usually starts around hair follicles and produces a speckled appearance. Vitiligo is associated with a number of syndromes and associated disorders but the cutaneous pattern is independent of other organ involvement.[3]

Histopathologic Features

The skin appears relatively normal except for an absence of melanocytes (Fig. 14-1). Clear cells may be present in the basal layer, but they are Langerhans cells.[4] Before a definite diagnosis of vitiligo is made, the lack of melanocytes must be proven. A negative silver stain for melanin suffices; the dopa reaction

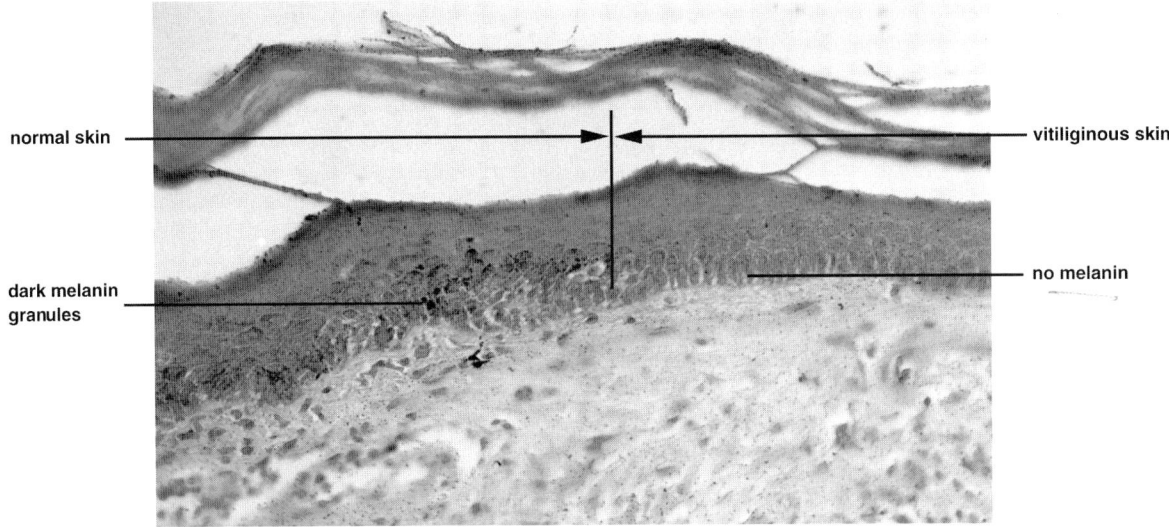

normal skin — — vitiliginous skin

dark melanin granules — — no melanin

Figure 14-1. Vitiligo. To the left of the epidermis at the basal layer is black-staining melanin; on the right this is absent. There are no other abnormalities. (Fontana-Masson stain.)

will also be negative. There may be lymphocytic inflammation especially underlying recent or erythematous lesions. The inflammation is usually lichenoid with little if any epidermal damage. However, vacuolated keratinocytes can be seen.[5] Melanophages may be found in the dermis. All forms of vitiligo, whether associated with a syndrome or not, and whether from a single patch or from almost total depigmentation, are identical microscopically.

Clinicopathologic Correlation

The mechanism of melanocyte destruction in vitiligo has been the subject of much research but is poorly understood. Centrally melanocytes are missing, while peripherally they may show degenerative changes. Most researchers have concentrated on autoantibodies against melanocytes that can be found in some vitiligo patients. Their toxicity has been shown in several in vitro systems, but the in vivo process remains unclear.

Piebaldism and Waardenberg Syndrome

Piebaldism is an autosomal dominantly inherited, permanent, stable leukoderma caused by a mutation in the *kit* gene, a proto-oncogene that codes for a tyrosinase kinase cell-surface receptor.[6] Piebaldism has a number of other names (e.g., partial albinism, albinoidism, and congenital vitiligo). Waardenberg syndrome is the association of piebaldism with congenital deafness, heterochromia irides, and other structural abnormalities of the face. It is also inherited in an autosomal dominant fashion, probably caused by several different genes.

Clinical Features

The leukodermic patches of piebaldism are present at birth. They are usually midline and most often involve the scalp (white forelock), chest, and abdomen. In contrast to vitiligo,

they frequently contain hyperpigmented macules within them; these darker areas are often brought out by sun exposure. In Waardenberg syndrome, the skin findings are identical.

Histopathologic Features

The skin has no or few melanocytes and is normal in all other aspects. The few remaining melanocytes may be the precursors of the hyperpigmented macules.[7,8]

Chemical Leukoderma

Chemical leukoderma is an acquired leukoderma most often caused by exposure to paraphenol compounds.

Clinical Features

A variety of chemicals that are for the most part para-substituted phenols that mimic tyrosine can cause complete depigmentation identical to vitiligo. Industrial cleaning agents are a common source of exposure. The hands are most often involved because they come in direct contact with the chemicals. Similar agents are used to bleach melasma (hydroquinone) or to complete depigmentation in universal vitiligo (monobenzyl ether of hydroquinone). When chemical exposure is stopped, some pigmentation may return.

Histopathologic Features

No melanocytes are found. The skin is otherwise normal. Thus, the histology is indistinguishable from that of vitiligo.[9]

Clinicopathologic Correlation

These compounds interfere with melanin production not only by competitive inhibition of tyrosine metabolism but also through toxicity to melanocytes.

Incontinentia Pigmenti Achromians (Ito Syndrome)

Incontinentia pigmenti achromians (IPA) is a congenital disorder characterized by swirls of hypopigmentation and a variety of systemic problems.

Clinical Features

IPA is usually congenital, but a variety of inheritance patterns have been discussed. Patients typically have diffuse swirls and streaks of hypopigmentation. In contrast to incontinentia pigmenti, the abnormal areas are the hypopigmented ones; thus, incontinentia pigmenti achromians has been referred to as a mirror image of incontinentia pigmenti.

Systemic problems include mainly musculoskeletal and neurologic defects. Mental retardation, seizures, and strabismus are most common.[10] IPA may well represent a group of disorders reflecting mosaicism for a variety of genes involved in pigment expression. Perhaps IPA, linear and whorled nevoid hypermelanosis, and nevus depigmentosus are all part of the same spectrum.[11]

Histopathologic Features

The histologic descriptions of IPA are somewhat confusing, perhaps reflecting the clinical difficulty in determining which skin is normal and which is abnormal. There appear to be fewer melanocytes that are also smaller, produce less melanin, and have fewer dendrites, suggesting impaired transfer. Pigment incontinence is not seen.

Melanopenic Disorders

In melanopenic disorders the lack of pigmentation is caused by absence or reduction in the amount of melanin. Thus, melanocytes are present, although not functioning properly. There may be a widespread disorder such as albinism in which enzymes essential to melanin production are missing or a localized disorder in which there is focal disruption in melanin synthesis or melanin transfer to keratinocytes.

Albinism

Albinism is the absence of melanin secondary to a variety of enzymatic defects that interfere with melanin synthesis.

Clinical Features

Albinism is not one disease but many. All have been extensively reviewed.[12] Depending on the biochemical defect, melanin may be lacking in the skin, eyes, or central nervous system to produce a variety of defects. In classic tyrosinase-negative albinism, any skin coloration is rare, but in other forms some degree of freckling may be seen. Melanocytic nevi occur but lack melanin. Albinos may develop cutaneous carcinomas at an early age because they lack natural photoprotection.

Histopathologic Features

The skin appears normal. X-linked ocular albinism patients, as well as female carriers, regularly have melanin macroglobules in their normal skin[13] (Fig. 14-2). Dopa incubation may or may not result in melanin production, depending on the nature of the enzyme defect. Ultrastructural examination reveals reduced to absent melanin in stages I to II melanosomes, while stages III to IV melanosomes are not seen and the silver stain is usually negative.

Figure 14-2.   X-linked ocular albinism. There are macromelanosomes in the cytoplasm of the melanocytes in the basal layer. No melanin pigment is detectable in the cytoplasm of the basal keratinocytes.

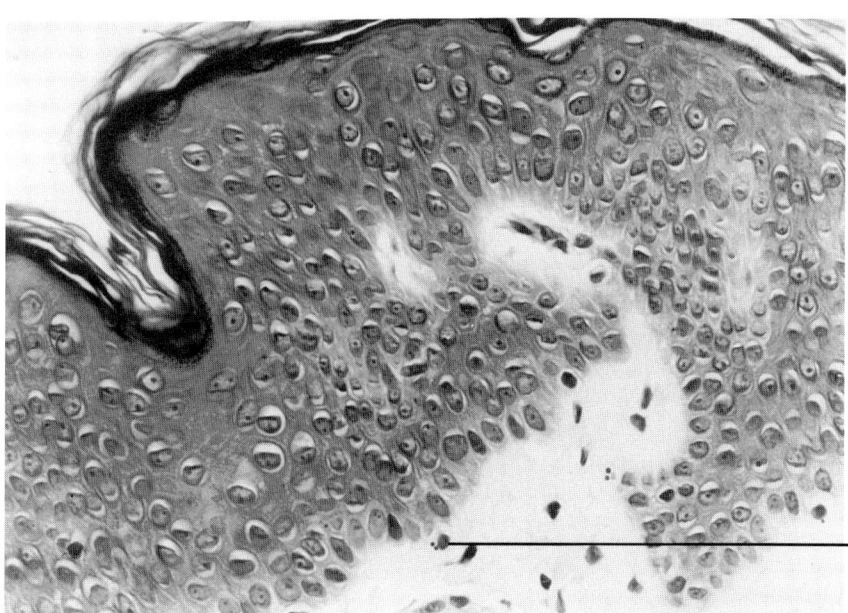

macromelanosomes
in cytoplasm of a
melanocyte

Clinicopathologic Correlation

The spectrum of albinism is beyond this text. Hair bulb incubation in dopa is a useful way of distinguishing tyrosinase-positive and -negative forms. Each form has a different mechanism of pigment failure.

Chédiak-Higashi Syndrome

Chédiak-Higashi syndrome is an autosomal recessive inherited disorder of pigmentation, immunity, and hematologic function.

Clinical Features

Patients are best described as having pigmentary dilution. Thus, white patients may appear almost totally white, like a tyrosinase-negative albino, while darker skinned patients may have a grayish tinge. The hair has a metallic color. More severe manifestations include failure to thrive, chronic recurrent infection, and, in the accelerated stage of the disease, a diffuse reactive lymphohistiocytic infiltrate.[14]

Histopathologic Features

Chédiak-Higashi syndrome is best diagnosed by examination of a peripheral blood smear, which will show large granules in granulocytes. A skin biopsy specimen appears entirely normal with normal melanocytes and perhaps sparse dermal melanin. However, ultrastructural examination reveals large abnormal melanosomes that are transferred to keratinocytes with difficulty and degraded more rapidly.[15]

Clinicopathologic Correlation

In Chédiak-Higashi syndrome, although patients have the diffuse color loss of an albino, they have a totally different mechanism of hypopigmentation—abnormal melanosomes that are transferred poorly and destroyed readily.

Ash-Leaf Macule of Tuberous Sclerosis

Tuberous sclerosis is an autosomal dominantly inherited genodermatosis with seizures, mental retardation, and a variety of systemic problems. Its cutaneous manifestations include connective tissue nevi, angiofibromas, and white macules.[16]

Clinical Features

The prototype leukodermic lesion in tuberous sclerosis is the elliptical ash-leaf macule. It usually occurs on the trunk and is often the first cutaneous sign of tuberous sclerosis. Wood's light examination is helpful in identifying these lesions. Other hypopigmented lesions can also occur. These include irregular macules, confetti-like spots, and segmental depigmentation. The lesions are often present at birth or in the early months of life and are stable.[17]

Histopathologic Features

On routine light microscopy an ash-leaf macule appears normal. However, when the skin is incubated in dopa a normal number of melanocytes with a markedly decreased melanin content are seen. One defect appears to be a reduced melanosome size with impaired transfer. Another may be immaturity of melanosomes with only types I and II present in hypopigmented areas.[18,19]

Nevus Depigmentosus

Nevus depigmentosus is a congenital stable patterned leukoderma.

Clinical Features

Nevus depigmentosus is usually apparent at birth or during the first few months of life. It is often segmental or patterned and may be related to other forms of pigmentary mosaicism involving Blaschko lines.[11]

Histopathologic Features

The skin is normal with normal melanocytes, but reduced melanin. There is some evidence that both increased destruction of melanosomes following complexing within melanocytes and abnormal transfer of melanin are responsible for the leukoderma.[18]

Idiopathic Guttate Hypomelanosis

Idiopathic guttate hypomelanosis is a widely distributed macular hypopigmentation, primarily of the extremities.

Clinical Features

Idiopathic guttate hypomelanosis is probably the most common leukoderma: some studies suggest as many as two-thirds of adults are affected. The incidence increases with advancing age. There are confetti-like hypopigmented macules on the arms and legs that are asymptomatic and usually not noticed by the patient.

Histopathologic Features

A subtle decrease in melanocytes is found with some loss of dendrites that suggests impaired melanosome transfer.[20] Melanin is also decreased.[21] Lesions are rarely biopsied.

Nevus Anemicus

Nevus anemicus is a pharmacologic nevus and represents an area of permanent vasoconstriction.

Clinical Features

Nevus anemicus is usually a large pale patch with sharp borders, but grouping of macules at the periphery may produce a jagged effect. The lesion disappears during Wood's light examination.

Histopathologic Features

The skin is entirely normal.

HYPERPIGMENTATION

Hyperpigmented lesions can be readily subdivided. The first step is to determine whether they are caused by melanin abnormalities or other changes. The Wood's light examination is helpful because it exaggerates hyperpigmentation caused by melanin and reduces or ablates hyperpigmentation from other causes. If melanin is determined to be responsible, the next question is, is there too much melanin or too many melanocytes? As mentioned previously, it is difficult to quantify either of these. Furthermore, pigmentation may not be related to melanin or melanocytes. For example, hyperkeratosis can cause darkening as in acanthosis nigricans. Foreign material, whether a tattoo or a fungus, may also mimic melanin pigmentation.

Finally, localized and diffuse hyperpigmentation should be distinguished. The former disorders are frequently biopsied to rule out a melanocytic proliferation. Most often, diffuse hyperpigmentation is diagnosed by other means. This is partially summarized in Table 14-1, which considers only those causes of diffuse hyperpigmentation in which a biopsy specimen may be useful in diagnosis.

Melanotic Disorders

Only disorders in which there is increased melanin without an obvious increase in the number of melanocytes are discussed in this chapter. There are several problems with this distinction. As Rhodes and co-workers[22] have repeatedly shown, melanocyte frequency must be assessed in a formal quantitative fashion to decide if one is dealing with a freckle or a lentigo. For many diseases, studies are conflicting or have not been performed in sufficient detail. We have tried to indicate the consensus opinion. In addition, lentigo is not a single lesion but is used to refer to early junctional melanocytic nevi, flat seborrheic keratoses, and both sunlight- and PUVA (psoralens plus longwave ultraviolet light)-induced pigmented macules. The following diseases have increased melanin and generally have a normal number of melanocytes.

Ephelis

An ephelis, or freckle, is a circumscribed hyperpigmented macule on sun-exposed skin.

Clinical Features

Ephelides are macules with irregular pigment and borders on sun-exposed skin, especially in fair-skinned persons. Ephelides are al-

most never biopsied unless they are large in size, have highly irregular pigmentation, or otherwise raise clinical concern.

Histopathologic Features

Ephelides traditionally have been described as having a normal number of melanocytes but an increased amount of melanin. In the only recent quantitative study, sun-induced freckles from children and young adults contained not only an increased number of melanocytes but also some atypical melanocytes.[22] Perhaps many sun-induced freckles are lentigines.

Clinicopathologic Correlation

The chief defect in ephelides appears to be an increase in the production and transfer of melanin in response to ultraviolet light. Freckles can be viewed as a partially successful attempt to create hyperpigmentation as photoprotection.

Café-au-Lait Macule

A café-au-lait macule is a stable patch of tan-colored skin.

Clinical Features

Café-au-lait macules are typically tan (hence the name "coffee with milk"). They may be present at birth or appear early in life. They are a diagnostic feature of neurofibromatosis type I, but they can also occur in normal persons and in other syndromes. There are clinical criteria based on age of patient as well as size and number of café-au-lait macules that help to determine whether neurofibromatosis type I is present.[23]

Histopathologic Features

A café-au-lait macule shows little under the microscope. The melanocytes are normal in number, but there may be an increased amount of melanin. Some café-au-lait macules have melanin macrogranules or giant melanosomes that are a type of autophagolysosome. They represent the fusion of autophagosomes that contain melanin with lysosomes.[24] Melanin macrogranules can be identified in routine biopsy specimens[25] (Fig. 14-3).

Table 14-1. Diffuse Hyperpigmentation

Disorder	Clinical Features	Cutaneous Pathology
Addison's disease	Weakness, hypotension	Increased basal layer melanin
Argyria	Blue-gray color	Pigment around sweat glands (see Ch. 16)
Chronic arsenic ingestion	Hyper- and hypopigmentation, keratoses, cutaneous and internal tumors	Incontinentia pigmenti
Cushing syndrome	Hypertension, obesity, striae, hirsutism	Increased basal layer melanin
Drug reactions		
Chlorpromazine	Slate-blue color in sun-exposed areas	Drug-melanin complexes in dermis
Minocycline	Several types of hyperpigmentation, blue-gray or brown, localized or diffuse	Increased dermal iron and/or melanin
Hemochromatosis	Diabetes, hepatomegaly, bronze color	Increased dermal iron and/or melanin (see Ch. 16)
Malignant melanoma with melanomatosis	Widespread metastases, melanuria, blue-gray skin	Melanin leaks into dermis from vessels
Ochronosis	Arthritis, patchy hyperpigmentation	Discolored, damaged collagen (see Ch. 16)

Differential Diagnosis

Histopathology cannot separate café-au-lait macules in neurofibromatosis patients from those that occur sporadically or in other syndromes. There is sufficient variation in the number of melanin macrogranules in café-au-lait macules based on the age and racial background of the patient that a search for these organelles is of little help in diagnosing neurofibromatosis in children.[26]

Melanotic Patches in McCune-Albright Syndrome

McCune-Albright syndrome is an autosomal dominantly inherited disease with fibrous dysplasia of bone, multiple endocrine abnormalities, and hyperpigmentation.

Clinical Features

Patients with McCune-Albright syndrome have large hyperpigmented patches, most commonly located on the sacral area and buttocks. They may present at birth but usually appear during the first few years of life. The patches may lie over the bony abnormalities and frequently follow Blaschko lines, reflecting somatic mosaicism.[27] The large size and pattern of distribution of the pigmented patches usually allow one to separate McCune-Albright syndrome from neurofibromatosis type I.

Histopathologic Features

There is an increase in melanin without other abnormalities. Giant melanosomes are less common than in café-au-lait macules in neurofibromatosis patients, but can be present.

Differential Diagnosis

It is more productive to obtain appropriate radiographic and endocrine studies to diagnose McCune-Albright syndrome than to perform a skin biopsy.

Mucocutaneous Melanoses

Several different mucosal lesions have increased melanin without other obvious abnormalities.

Clinical Features

There are many different clinical settings in which macules with increased melanin occur on mucosal surfaces:

1. Both Peutz-Jeghers syndrome and Carney syndrome may present with pigmented macules. In the latter, the lesions are more often lentigines.
2. Hyperpigmented macules in the mouth, whether of racial origin (physiologic variant), secondary to smoking, or a reflection of Addison's disease, usually contain excess melanin but no melanocytic abnormalities.
3. Labial melanotic macules are solitary or a few lesions on the lip, usually lower, perhaps just a lip freckle, but they can occur in patients with no other freckles.[28,29]
4. Both males and females may have hyperpigmented macules (genital melanosis) on the genital mucosa.[30]

Histopathologic Features

All these lesions contain increased melanin without overt proliferation of melanocytes. Each may have some subepithelial melanophages. The labial and genital lesions are often biopsied to rule out a malignant or premalignant melanocytic process, but the lack of melanocytic proliferation answers the question. The

Figure 14-3. Café-au-lait macule showing normal epidermis with a normal number of melanocytes, although there may be some that are increased in size. Some melanin macrogranules are present.

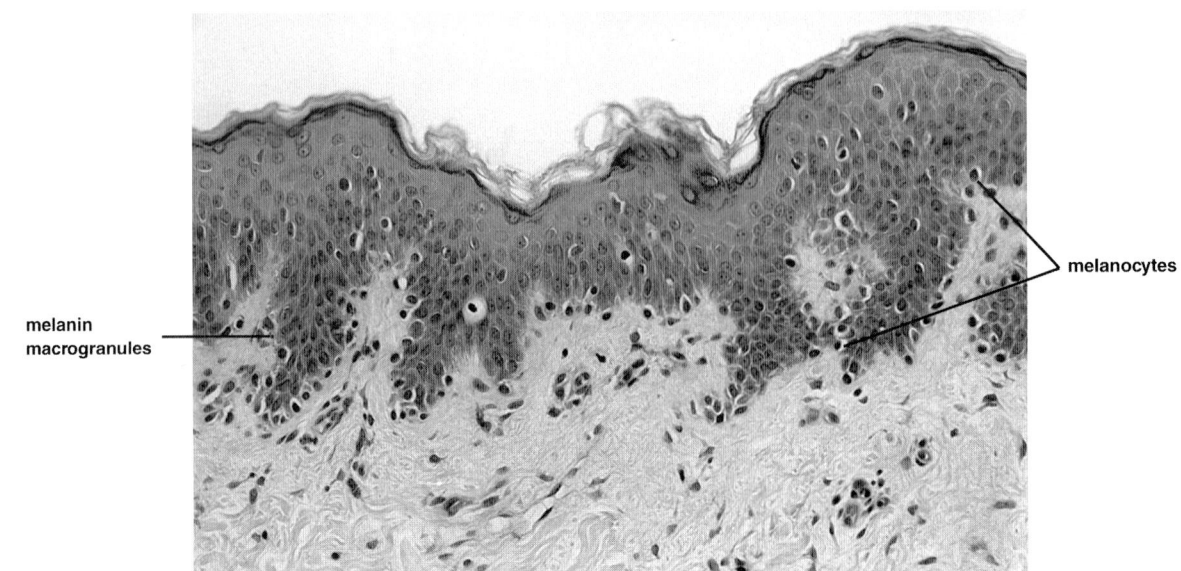

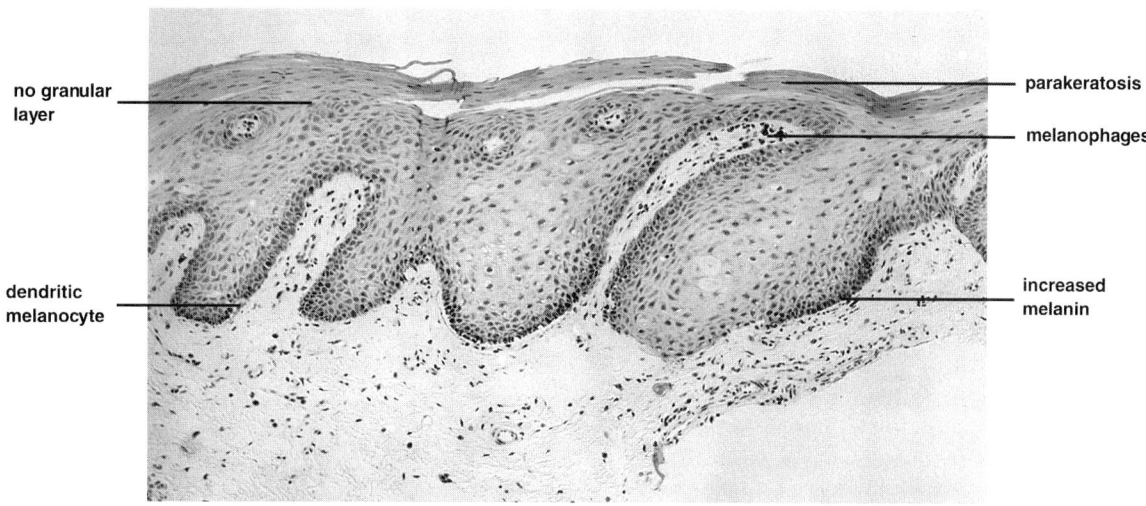

Figure 14-4. Labial melanotic macule. The epithelium shows slight hyperplasia and parakeratosis. There is increased pigment in the basal layer of the rete ridges without a detectable increase in melanocytes. A sparse mononuclear cell infiltrate that includes several melanophages is present in the lamina propria.

labial macule may show actinic damage as is typical for the lower lip, with slight epidermal hyperplasia and a sparse superficial mononuclear infiltrate (Fig. 14-4).

Melasma

Melasma (chloasma, mask of pregnancy) is an acquired patchy hyperpigmentation primarily of the face.

Clinical Features

Melasma is a blotchy hyperpigmentation of the face, especially the cheeks, forehead, and chin, which is caused by both hor-mones (pregnancy, oral contraceptives) and sunlight. It can occur in men, but is overwhelmingly more common in women, especially darker colored whites.[31]

Histopathologic Features

Melasma has an increased amount of basal layer pigment. Pigment incontinence and superficial dermal inflammation separate melasma from other disorders in this group. In some patients, most of the melanin may be in the superficial dermis[32,33] (Fig. 14-5).

Figure 14-5. Melasma. There is increased melanin in the basal layer as well as pigment incontinence and a sparse lymphocytic perivascular infiltrate. Chloasma represents a histologic overlap between increased basal layer melanin and postinflammatory hyperpigmentation.

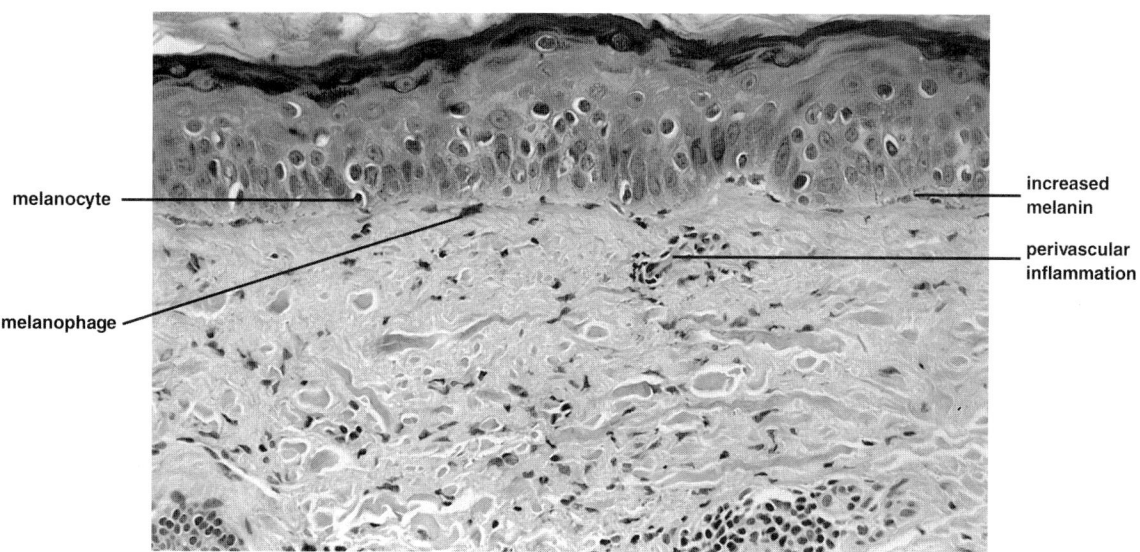

Clinicopathologic Correlation

Melasma is clinically similar to postinflammatory hyperpigmentation. However, the pigment is relatively superficial and therefore easier to treat with paraphenol bleaching compounds such as the hydroquinones.

Becker's nevus

Becker's nevus is an acquired hyperpigmented patch or plaque most often with hypertrichosis.

Clinical Features

Becker's nevus usually occurs on the shoulder or trunk. It is present at birth or in early childhood, but is often not apparent until puberty, when the hypertrichosis develops. Localized acneiform change may occur, and the nevus may become nodular. Becker's nevus is often mistaken for a congenital hairy nevus and thus biopsied.

Histopathologic Features

The pigmentary changes in Becker's nevus are due to increased melanin; a normal number of melanocytes is usually present. The melanocytes appear to be more active in pigment synthesis and in some cases may be increased in number.[34] There are other changes that help distinguish Becker's nevus from other hypermelanoses. There is usually epidermal hyperplasia sometimes with mild papillomatosis. The terminal hair follicles may have inflammation about them whether or not acneiform changes are present clinically. There may also be an increase in arrector pili smooth muscles; this perhaps represents an overlap between Becker's nevus and smooth muscle hamartoma (Fig. 14-6).

Dowling-Degos Disease

Dowling-Degos disease, or reticulated pigment anomaly of the flexures, is a macular reticulated hyperpigmentation especially of the axillae and other flexural areas.

Clinical Features

Dowling-Degos disease is an uncommon disorder perhaps more common in Orientals. There are numerous hyperpigmented macules in flexural areas that often blend together in a reticulated pattern. Some patients have pigmented pits of the perioral and acral areas. Many cases are familial, inherited in an autosomal dominant fashion. Basal cell carcinomas may develop in the pigmented areas.[35]

Histopathologic Features

There is increased basal layer melanin associated with an epidermal hyperplasia similar to an adenoid seborrheic keratosis. The rete ridges are elongated and form a lacy pattern, which may also be seen along follicle walls (in contrast to seborrheic keratoses). Horn pseudocysts are seen. The melanocytes are normal in size and number, but melanin may be increased (Fig. 14-7).

Differential Diagnosis

The nosology of Dowling-Degos is confusing. Two other syndromes are either similar or are perhaps variants.

Figure 14-6. Becker's nevus. The epidermis shows slight elongation of rete ridges and anastomosis. There is no increase of melanocytes and minimal increase in melanin. In the dermis there are numerous arrector pili smooth muscle bundles.

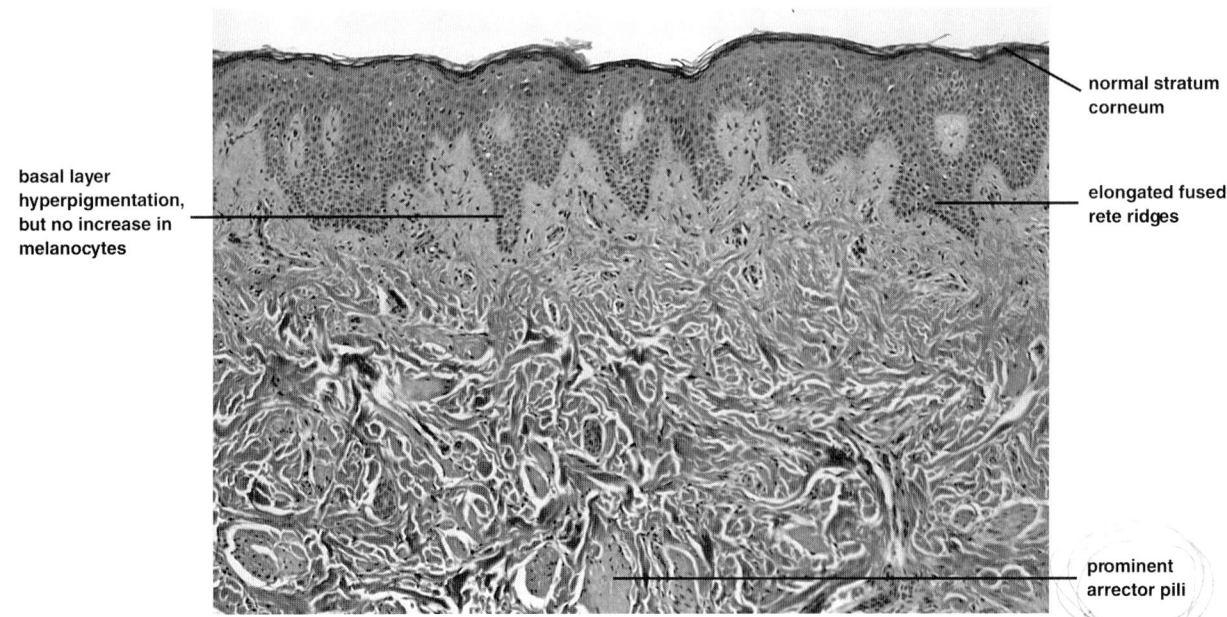

basal layer hyperpigmentation, but no increase in melanocytes

normal stratum corneum

elongated fused rete ridges

prominent arrector pili

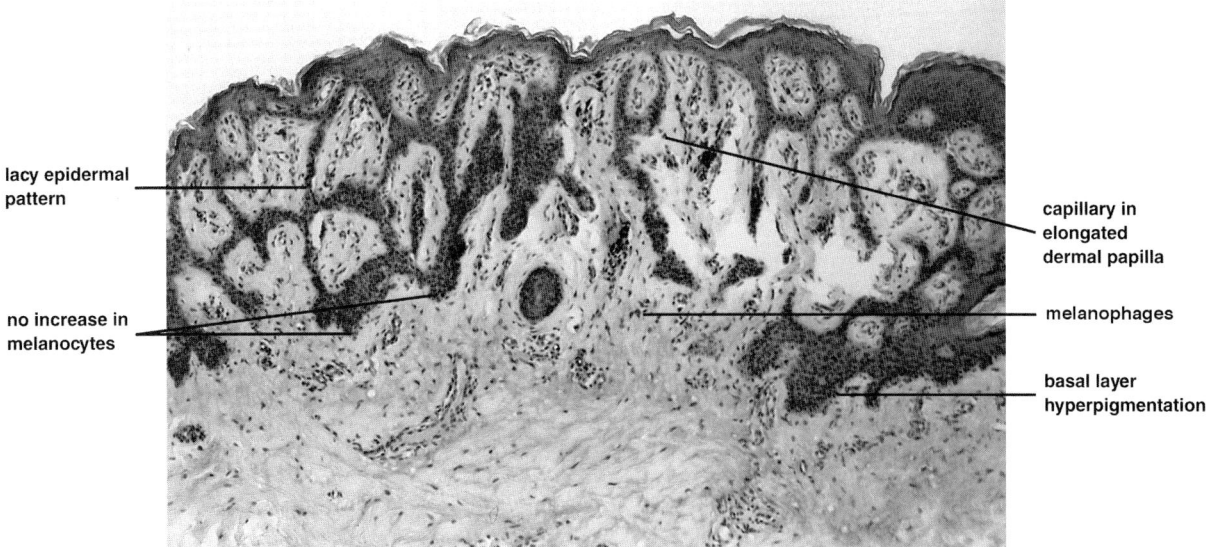

lacy epidermal pattern

no increase in melanocytes

capillary in elongated dermal papilla

melanophages

basal layer hyperpigmentation

Figure 14-7. Dowling-Degos disease. There is a lacy epidermal proliferation resembling a seborrheic keratosis. There is no proliferation of melanocytes. (Histologic material courtesy of Guenter Burg, M.D., Zurich, Switzerland.)

Haber syndrome is an autosomal dominant disorder with multiple pigmented seborrheic keratoses, facial erythema, and hyperpigmentation. It is also associated with basal cell carcinomas.[35]

Kitamura's reticulate acropigmentation consists of reticulate acral lesions, especially of the dorsal hands and feet, with palmoplantar pits.[36]

The hyperpigmentation in all three disorders is associated with the same lacy epithelial down growths associated with small plugged follicles. The clinical features may allow separation.

Nonmelanotic Disorders

A number of disorders may have hyperpigmentation totally unrelated to melanin or melanocytes. Included in this group are exogenous stains or deposits, many cutaneous tumors, and many hyperkeratotic disorders. All are included in the differential diagnostic section in which there are cross-references to other chapters where these entities are discussed. The following exogenous stains do not fit conveniently elsewhere and are covered briefly here.

Tinea Nigra

Tinea nigra is a fungal infection of the stratum corneum.

Clinical Features

Tinea nigra is caused by *Phaeoannellomyces wernickii* (formerly *Exophiala wernickii*), a dematiaceous soil fungus. Because its hyphae are brown and situated in the stratum corneum, they cause a dark spot that is occasionally biopsied to rule out a melanocytic lesion. Diagnosis can also be made by doing a KOH examination or culture.[37]

Histopathologic Features

The skin is normal except for thick brown hyphae in the stratum corneum. There is little if any inflammation (Fig. 14-8).

Dermal exogenous pigmentation is also a cause of hyperpigmentation. It tends to have a more bluish hue — whether it is a tattoo, argyria, or a foreign body. Several types of exogenous pigmentation are considered under dermal deposits. Those localized forms likely to be clinically diagnosed as a melanocytic lesion are considered here.

Black Heel

Black heel, or talon noir, is the deposition of blood in the epidermis secondary to trauma.

Clinical Features

Black heel occurs most commonly on the heels of participants in basketball and racquet sports. However, it may be seen anywhere on the foot as a result of trauma from a variety of activities. Black heel can be diagnosed by simply trimming the stratum corneum. It rarely needs to be biopsied.

Histopathologic Features

Brown pigment and red blood cells are seen in the stratum corneum. The skin is volar with a stratum lucidum. The dermis is usually poorly sampled but always normal (Fig. 14-9).

Tattoo

A tattoo is the result of the introduction of pigment into the skin.

Clinical Features

Tattoos may be intentionally produced by professional artists or amateurs or by accident. Most pigment has a blue-gray tint. The

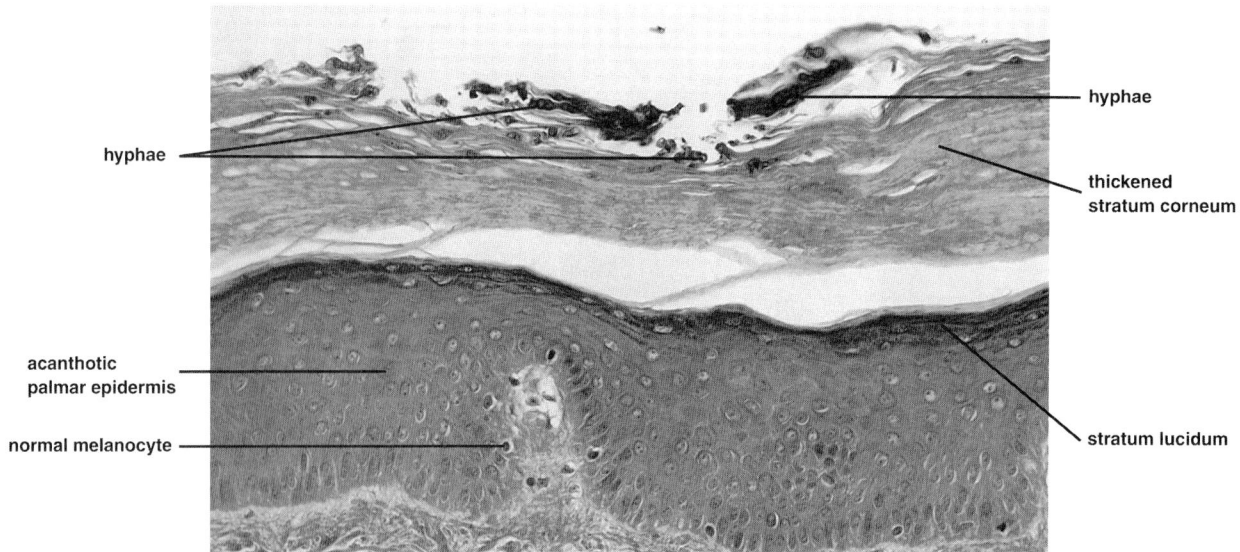

Figure 14-8. Tinea nigra. Thick dark hyphae are seen in the stratum corneum.

most common unintentional tattoo is the amalgam tattoo of the oral mucosa that occurs when inadvertent trauma introduces dental amalgam into the mucosa, usually adjacent to an amalgam repair.[38]

Histopathologic Features

Some tattoos are easy to identify, as large amounts of pigment are visible in the dermis. Occasionally, a foreign body or a sarcoidal granuloma will accompany the material and make the changes more obvious. However, only small amounts of pigment are sometimes present, and the diagnosis is difficult.[39] An amalgam tattoo shows black pigment in the highly vascular lamina propria of the oral cavity. The surrounding structures are the best clue to the diagnosis, as nonkeratinizing epithelium and occasionally minor salivary glands are seen (Fig. 14-10).

HYPO- AND HYPERPIGMENTATION

There are many disorders that can produce a mixture of hypo- and hyperpigmentation. The most common is tinea versicolor,

Figure 14-9. Black heel. There is a hemorrhage just above the granular layer in this shave biopsy from the heel. A layer of necrotic epithelium is evident between the collection of red blood cells and the overlying volar stratum corneum.

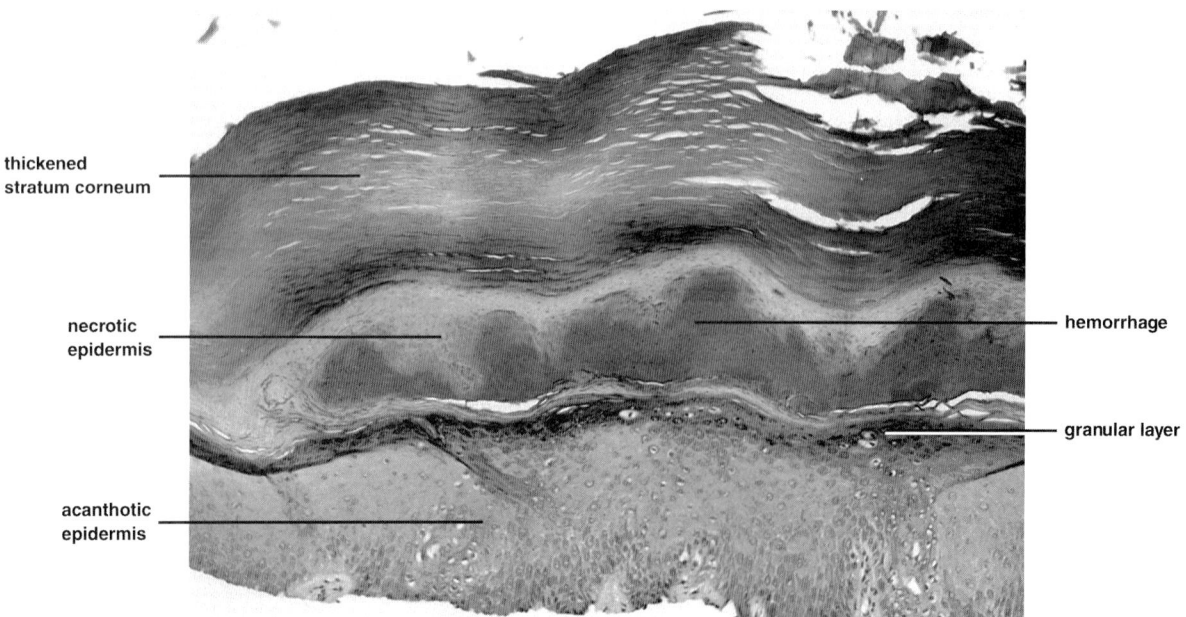

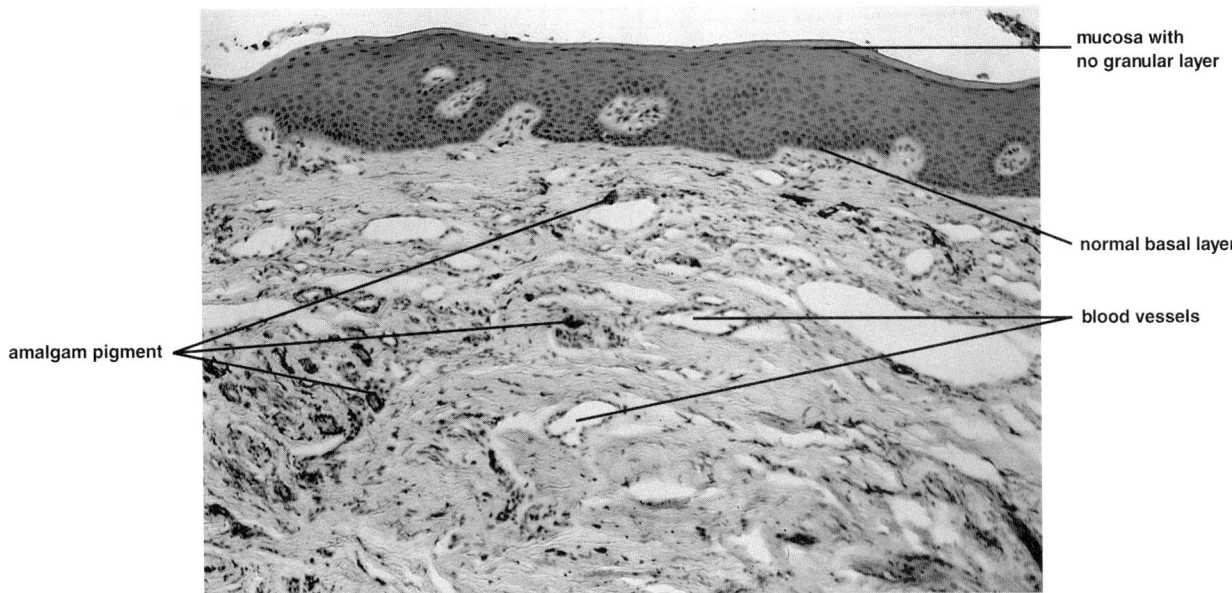

mucosa with
no granular layer

normal basal layer

blood vessels

amalgam pigment

Figure 14-10. Amalgam tattoo. The epithelium has normal parakeratosis, suggesting an intraoral location. The lamina propria is highly vascular, and there are scattered granules of black pigment.

although many presumably postinflammatory disorders also produce a variable appearance. Incontinentia pigmenti is a rare disorder that has several pigmentary changes.

Tinea Versicolor

Tinea versicolor is an infection of the epidermis by *Malassezia furfur*, a lipophilic yeast.

Clinical Features

M. furfur, formerly known as *Pityrosporum orbiculare* or *P. ovale*, in its spore form is part of the normal flora of the scalp and upper trunk. It may at times convert to a hyphal form and grow throughout the stratum corneum to produce scaly hypo- and hyperpigmented patches. The most common site of involvement is the upper trunk, but the abdomen, back, arms, and face can be involved. Usually the diagnosis is apparent and can be confirmed by KOH examination. Occasionally solitary or atypical lesions may be biopsied.

Histopathologic Features

Microscopically, tinea versicolor is an "invisible" dermatosis. The only clue usually is the presence of hyphae and spores ("spaghetti and meatballs") in the stratum corneum. Occasionally there is slight inflammation or follicular plugging. The hyphae can be distinguished from those of tinea nigra because they are smaller and not pigmented. Sometimes prominent basal layer melanin with incontinenti pigmenti is seen; on other occasions melanin appears to be reduced.[40,41] The hyphae and spores are limited to the stratum corneum and keratin-plugged follicles. Periodic acid–Schiff-stained sections allow better visualization of the fungal elements (Fig. 14-11).

Clinicopathologic Correlation

Tinea versicolor produces a variety of pigmentary changes. The organism produces azalaic acid that apparently inhibits melanin production and may damage melanocytes. Another cause of hypopigmentation may be the "umbrella effect," whereby the increased scale blocks tanning. Epidermal thickening and scaling can produce hyperpigmentation, as does stimulation of melanocytes. Despite this array of possible events, the histologic picture is bland.

Differential Diagnosis

The double-walled spores distinguish tinea versicolor from *Candida albicans* infection, which usually is associated with more inflammation, as well as single-walled spores and pseudohyphae. Tinea nigra has thick, dark hyphae.

Incontinentia Pigmenti (Bloch-Sulzberger Syndrome)

Incontinentia pigmenti is an X-linked dominantly inherited genodermatosis with multiple abnormalities of pigmentation and a variety of systemic problems.

Clinical Features

Incontinentia pigmenti goes through at least four cutaneous phases. The three classic stages are (1) blisters, (2) verrucous lesions, and (3) hyperpigmented macules. In addition, older patients often have scarred hypopigmentation. Neonates may present with a blistering linear eruption that can be initially mistaken for an infection until a smear reveals numerous eosinophils. These blisters resolve and heal with verrucous hy-

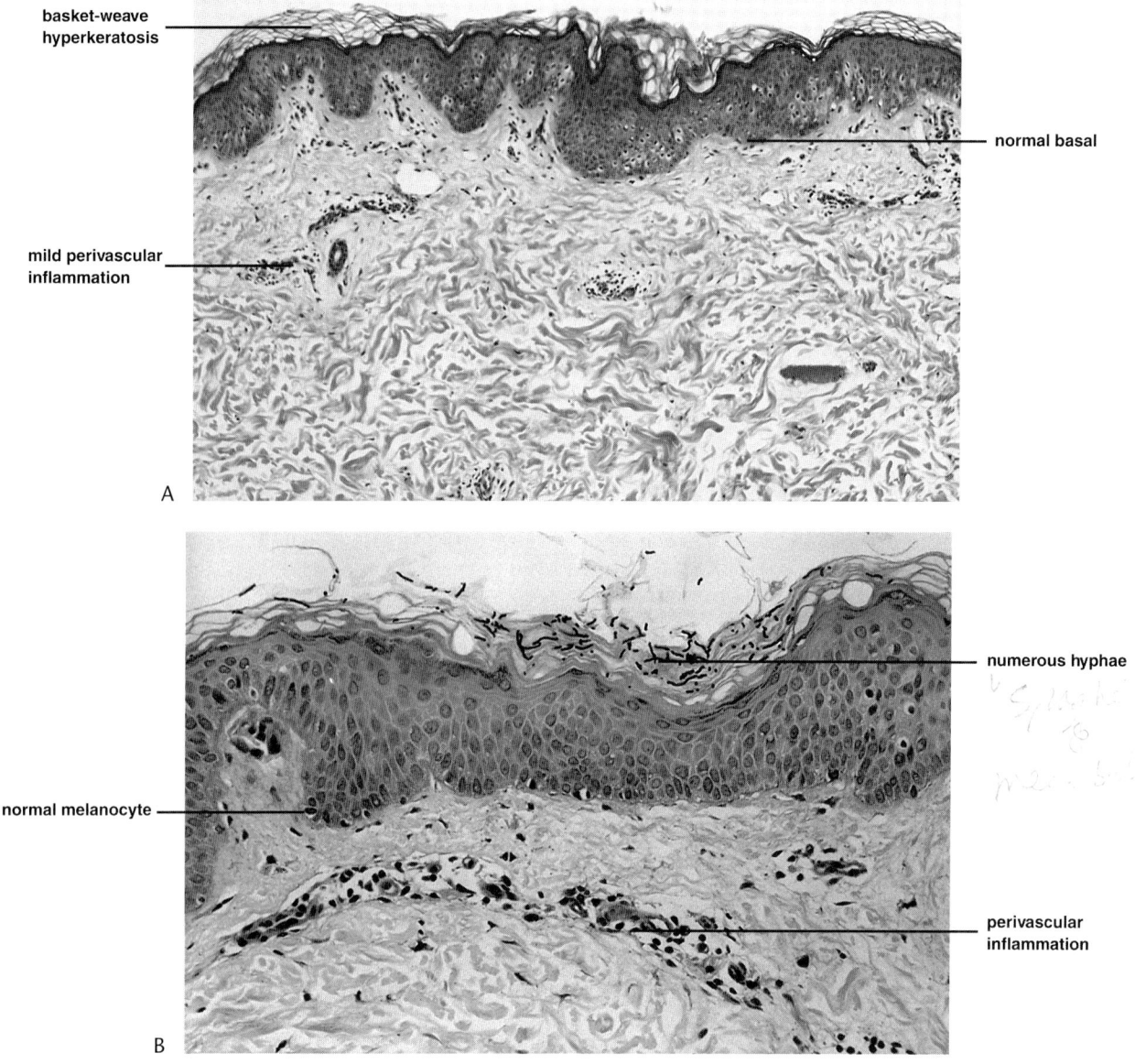

basket-weave
hyperkeratosis

normal basal

mild perivascular
inflammation

numerous hyphae

normal melanocyte

perivascular
inflammation

A

B

Figure 14-11. Tinea versicolor. (**A**) The lower power view shows a normal epidermis and dermis with a sparse lymphocytic perivascular infiltrate. (**B**) Higher power view with a PAS stain demonstrates smaller hyphae than in Fig. 14-7 easily visualized in the stratum corneum.

perplasia often in a linear fashion. The verrucous lesions also resolve during the first few years of life.

The main permanent stigma of incontinentia pigmenti is the so-called Chinese letter or marble cake hyperpigmentation that apparently results from dermal deposition of melanin. This pigment deposition is independent of the two previous stages and usually linear or segmental. Finally, most often on the legs, there can be atrophic white scars that are presumably sequelae of the initial blisters and verrucous lesions.

There are a number of systemic problems in incontinentia pigmenti. Additional ectodermal abnormalities include abnormal teeth and alopecia. The most serious changes involve the central nervous system, eyes, and skeletal system. Most patients

are females reflecting the X-linked dominant inheritance with decreased life expectancy in males.[42]

Histopathologic Features

The blisters often show only a large number of eosinophils. When epidermal changes are present, there is usually dyskeratosis. In the dermis there is a perivascular inflammation also dominated by eosinophils. The verrucous lesions show compact hyperkeratosis with large numbers of dyskeratotic cells. The "Chinese letter" hyperpigmentation shows slight, if any, basal layer vacuolar change and sparse to marked dermal melanin[43] (Fig. 14-12). Finally, the atrophic scars contain reduced or absent dermal appendages, fibrotic dermal collagen, and a normal to decreased number of melanocytes.[44] Just as the clinical appearance of incontinentia pigmenti can be diverse, so can its histologic pattern.

Differential Diagnosis

The pigmented lesions should be differentiated from linear and whorled nevoid hypermelanosis, which shows increased basal layer melanin but no significant incontinentia pigmenti.[45]

Postinflammatory Changes

Several disorders produce hypo- and hyperpigmentation secondary to damage at the dermoepidermal junction with either incontinentia pigmenti or destruction of melanocytes. This may be blended with scarring that destroys melanocytes by fibrosis and new vessel formation. Probably the most common cause of postinflammatory hyperpigmentation is the healing stage of an inflammatory dermatosis such as atopic dermatitis, pityriasis rosea, or lichen planus. The prototype of postinflammatory hypopigmentation is pityriasis alba in which patients develop white scaly patches, especially on the cheeks. In addition to these relatively nonspecific changes, there are several more specific postinflammatory disorders.

Fixed Drug Eruption

Fixed drug eruption is a recurrent localized cutaneous reaction to the ingestion of a drug.

Clinical Features

Patients who become sensitive to a drug, most often phenolphthalein, tetracycline, or barbiturates, develop one or more erythematous or dark plaques at the same cutaneous site on each re-

exposure to the drug. The most common sites are the face, genitalia, and extremities.[46]

Histopathologic Features

There is an acute dermatitis with spongiosis and ballooning of the epidermis. Vacuolar changes usually occur in the basal zone but are variable in severity. The inflammatory infiltrate is moderately dense, mixed, both superficial and deep, and interstitial. In the later phase melanophages can be identified, often deeper than in any other form of postinflammatory hyperpigmentation, presumably because of repeated insults[47,48] (Fig. 14-13).

Differential Diagnosis

Fixed drug eruption may be mimicked clinically and histologically by erythema multiforme. However, the latter has more vacuolar damage and a sparser, predominantly lymphocytic perivascular infiltrate.

Berloque Dermatitis

Berloque dermatitis is caused by application of a photosensitizing agent to the skin and subsequent sun exposure.

Clinical Features

A variety of furocoumarins in perfumes and plants are phototoxic when applied to the skin. Their application, followed by sun exposure, results in hyperpigmented areas often in an unusual pattern.

Histopathologic Features

The microscopic changes are minimal. There may be epidermal damage with occasional dyskeratotic cells. Sometimes vacuolar

Figure 14-12. Incontinentia pigmenti. This is the third stage of incontinentia pigmenti showing a normal epidermis with a large amount of melanin within melanophages in the superficial dermis. Note that neither of the typical changes of the first two stages, eosinophils or dyskeratosis, is still visible.

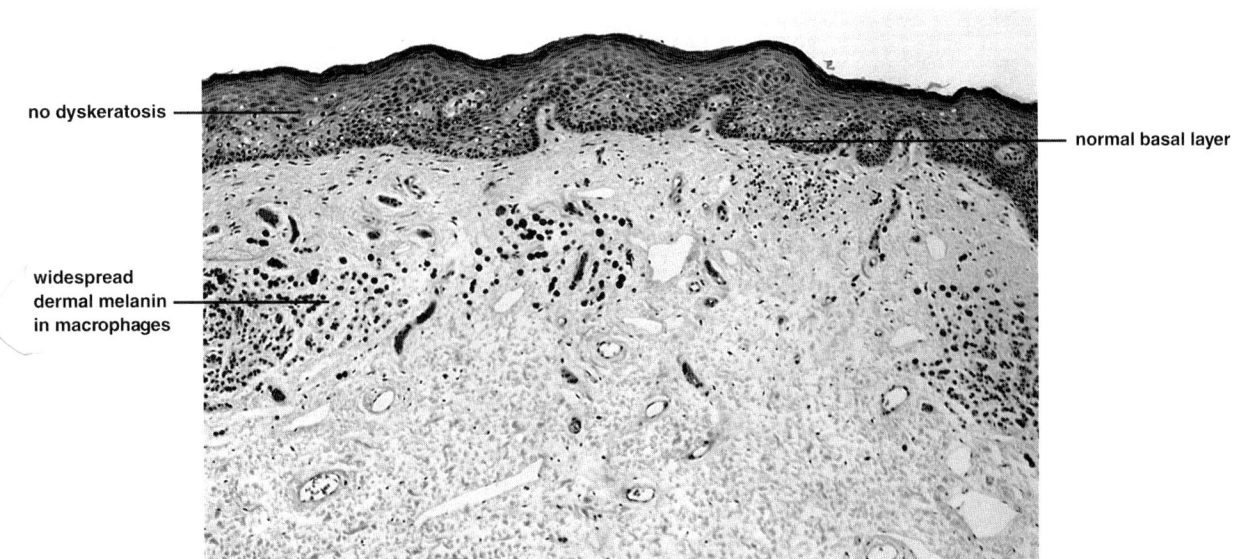

no dyskeratosis

normal basal layer

widespread
dermal melanin
in macrophages

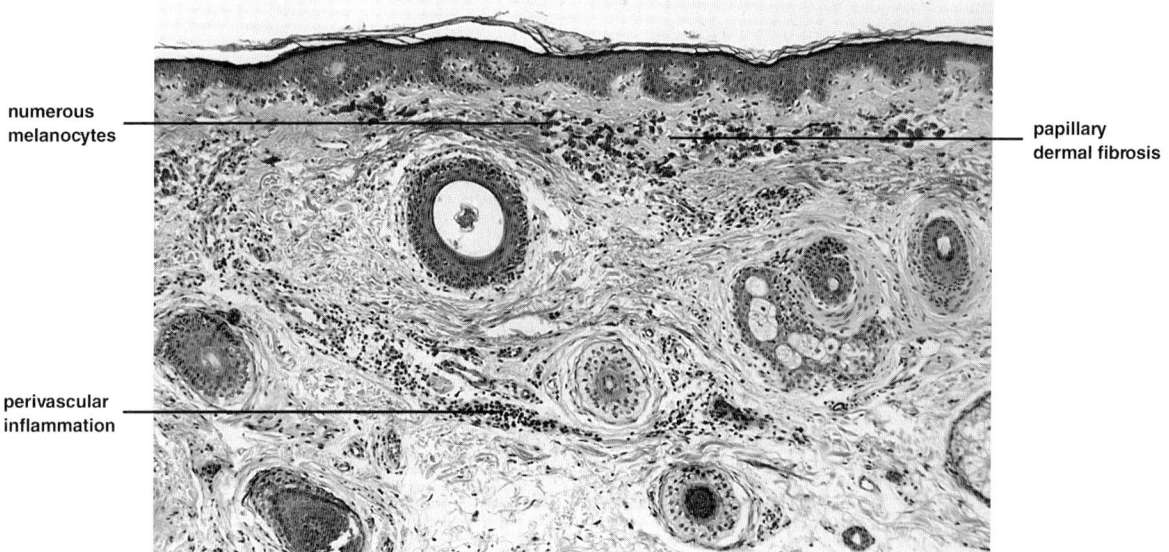

numerous melanocytes

papillary dermal fibrosis

perivascular inflammation

Figure 14-13. Fixed drug eruption. In this late phase lesion the inflammatory infiltrate is sparse around vessels at all levels of the dermis. There is little inflammation at the dermoepidermal junction. The chief pathologic feature is the presence of large accumulations of melanin in the superficial dermis.

changes are seen as well as incontinentia pigmenti. The main change is the presence of dermal melanophages. There may be mild dermal fibrosis and telangiectases.

Erythema Ab Igne

Erythema ab igne is a reticulated hyperpigmentation that results from chronic exposure to heat.

Clinical Features

Erythema ab igne is caused by long-term exposure to relatively low heat. A typical history is frequent sitting in front of an open fire or using a hot pad while sleeping. The skin shows both darkened areas and red patches presumably from vascular changes. Keratoses and even squamous cell carcinoma can arise in erythema ab igne.

Histopathologic Features

Microscopic examination shows dermal deposition of melanin without epidermal changes. There is usually a lichenoid infiltrate in most acute cases, while later the dermal blood vessels increase in number and develop thickened walls. The papillary dermis may become fibrotic.[49]

Erythema Dyschromicum Perstans

Erythema dyschromicum perstans is a mottled blue-gray hyperpigmentation that most often occurs on the trunk of darker skinned persons.

Clinical Features

Erythema dyschromicum perstans reflects the uncertainty of postinflammatory hyperpigmentation. It is most common in Latin Americans, who typically develop blue-gray patches on their backs often without clinically appreciated antecedent inflammation.

Histologic Features

There is striking dermal melanin, often quite deep, which explains the blue tinge. There may be vacuolar changes at the dermoepidermal junction; early lesions of erythema dyschromicum perstans exhibit a lichenoid tissue reaction.[50,51] Other patients who look clinically identical have little interface change.[52] In general, it is impossible to distinguish old erythema dyschromicum perstans from other types of postinflammatory hyperpigmentation.

Clinicopathologic Correlation

The major issue is whether erythema dyschromicum perstans is a disease sui generis or does it follow a variety of inflammatory dermatoses in a susceptible population? An answer to this question is not available.

DIFFERENTIAL DIAGNOSIS OF HYPO- AND HYPERPIGMENTED LESIONS

Figure 14-14 provides an approach to hypopigmented lesions. In a practical sense, most biopsy specimens from leukodermic patches will fall into the differential diagnosis of "nothing dermatoses" or "invisible dermatoses." The first step is to decide between melanocytopenic and melanopenic leukodermas. An S-100 stain is probably the simplest method to search for melanocytes. If no melanocytes are found, the answer is vitiligo, piebaldism, or chemical leukoderma. These three are histologically identical and must be sorted out by the clinician. When reduced melanocytes are found, the problem is cloudy, but incontinentia pigmenti achromians and idiopathic guttate hypomelanosis are the most likely candidates. When melanocytes are seen, a silver stain will confirm the lack of melanin. Then a clinical choice between albinism, tuberous sclerosis, and nevus depigmentosus must be made. Ultrastructural examination does show differences between these three disorders, but the differences are not distinct enough to be of practical use. Finally, subtle signs of scarring as might be seen in postinflammatory hypopigmentation and incontinentia pigmenti must be sought. A halo nevus will be suggested by the intense lymphocytic infiltrate, while in the appropriate clinical setting the stigmata of pinta or leprosy must be searched for, as a wide variety of lesions in these diseases are hypopigmented. When the skin is totally normal, perhaps nevus anemicus—a pharmacologic lesion with no structural changes—is the answer.

When considering hyperpigmented lesions, one must first ask, is the color change localized or diffuse? Diffuse hyperpigmentation is best evaluated by other clinical measures, as the skin biopsy is rarely helpful. Localized changes are of greatest concern when they involve an increased number of melanocytes. When no obvious increase is seen, the lesion can be approached as in Figure 14-15. First, one should examine the stratum corneum. If hyphae are present, the answer is either tinea versicolor or tinea nigra. The latter has pigmented larger hyphae. Hemorrhage into the stratum corneum is diagnostic of black heel or its variants. When the skin appears normal, with perhaps an increase in melanin, a freckle, café-au-lait macule, McCune-Albright syndrome, or melasma should be considered. In this setting, a search for melanin macrogranules may be helpful to support the diagnosis of café-au-lait macule. Incontinentia pigmenti plus increased basal layer melanin favors chloasma. When epidermal hyperplasia is present, Becker's nevus, Dowling-Degos syndrome, or an adenoid seborrheic keratosis should be suspected.

When the epidermis is normal, the source of color may be dermal. Incontinence of melanin suggests a postinflammatory change or incontinentia pigmenti. When this is coupled with dermal fibrosis or loss of appendages, a scar is likely. Exogenous pigment, such as a tattoo or foreign body, or dermal melanocytic hyperpigmentation as in a mongolian spot may also be present. Finally, dermal tumors such as blue nevi, mast cell tumors, dermatofibromas, vascular tumors, and many other neoplasms may appear as a hyperpigmented spot.

Figure 14-14. Algorithmic diagnosis of hypopigmentation.

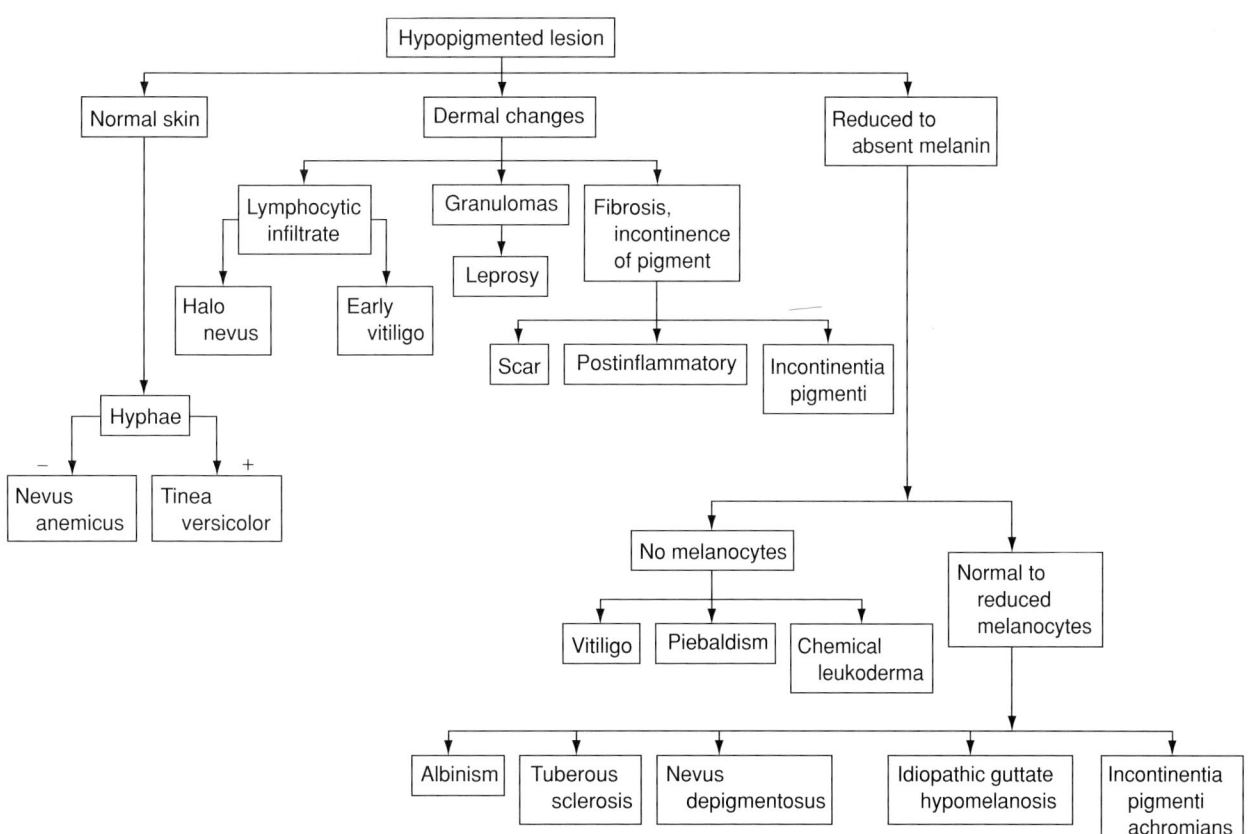

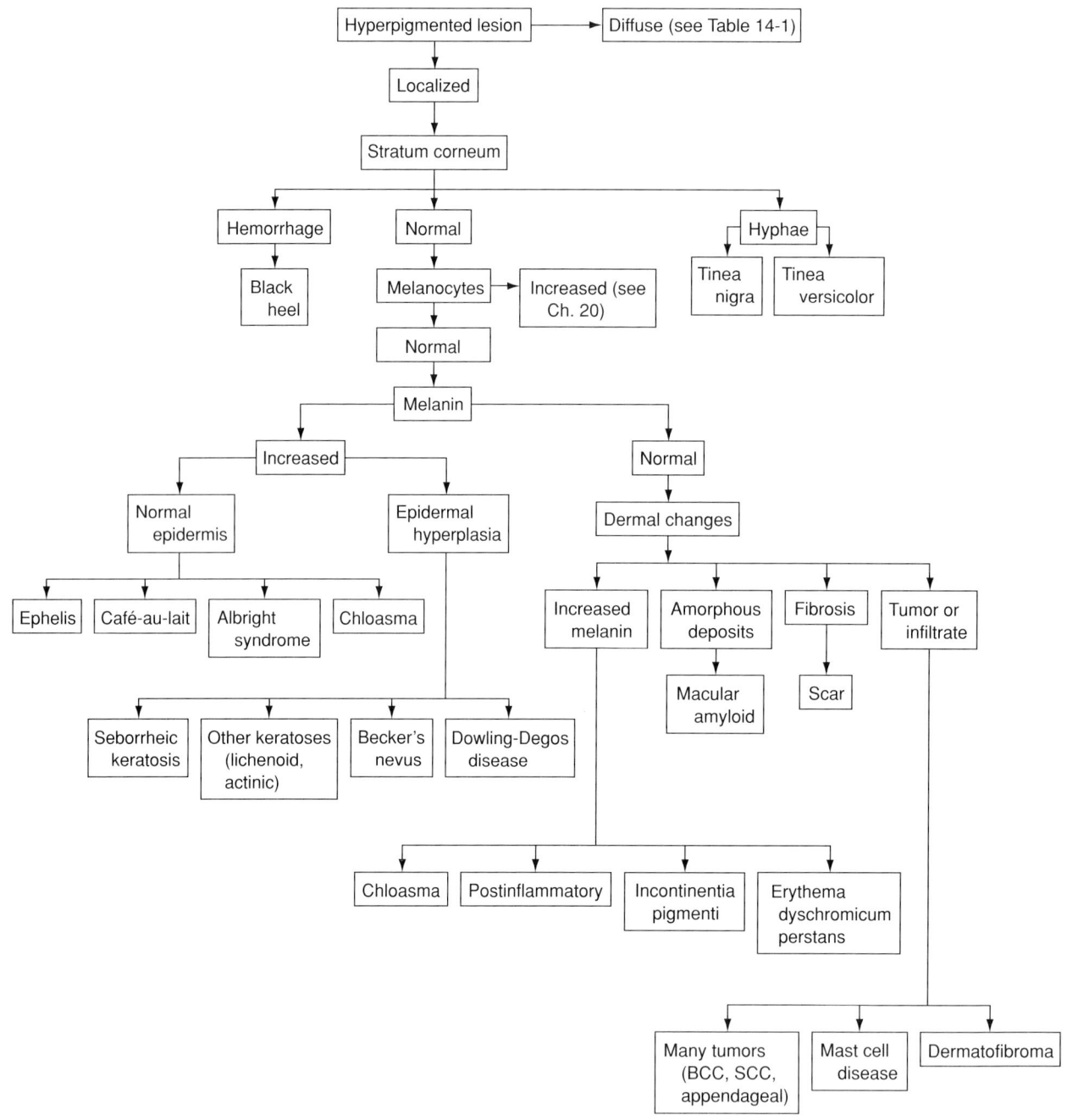

Figure 14-15. Algorithmic diagnosis of hyperpigmentation.

REFERENCES

1. Ortonne JP, Mosher DB, Fitzpatrick TB: Vitiligo and Other Hypomelanoses of Hair and Skin. Plenum, New York, 1983
2. Maize JC, Ackerman AB: Pigmented Lesions of the Skin. Lea & Febiger, Philadelphia, 1987
3. Nordlund JJ, Ortonne JP: Vitiligo and depigmentation. Curr Prob Dermatol 4:3, 1992
4. Claudy AL, Rouchouse B: Langerhans cells and vitiligo. Quantitative study of T6 and HLA-DR antigen-expressing cells. Acta Derm Venereol (Stockh) 64:334, 1984
5. Bhawan J, Bhutani LK: Keratinocyte damage in vitiligo. J Cutan Pathol 10:207, 1983
6. Ward KA, Moss C, Sanders DS: Human piebaldism: relationship between phenotype and site of *Kit* gene mutation. Br J Dermatol 132:929, 1995
7. Chang T, McGrae JD Jr, Hashimoto K: Ultrastructural study of two patients with both piebaldism and neurofibromatosis 1. Pediatr Dermatol 10:224, 1993
8. Dippel E, Haas N, Grabbe J et al: Expression of the c-*kit* re-

ceptor in hypomelanosis: a comparative study between piebaldism, naevus depigmentosus and vitiligo. Br J Dermatol 132:182, 1995

9. Nordlund JJ, Forget B, Kirkwood J, Lerner AB: Dermatitis produced by application of monobenzene in patients with active vitiligo. Arch Dermatol 121:1141, 1985

10. Ruiz-Maldonado R, Toussaint S, Tamayo L et al: Hypomelanosis of Ito: diagnostic criteria and report of 41 cases. Pediatr Dermatol 9:1, 1992

11. Nehal KS, PeBenito R, Orlow SJ: Analysis of 54 cases of hypopigmentation and hyperpigmentation along the lines of Blaschko. Arch Dermatol 132:1167, 1996

12. Witkop CJ Jr, Quevedo WC Jr, Fitzpatrick TB, King RA: Albinism. pp. 4353–4392. In Scriver CR, Beaudet AL, Sly WS, Valle D (eds): The Metabolic Basis of Inherited Disease. 7th Ed. McGraw-Hill, New York, 1995

13. Garner A, Jay BS: Macromelanosomes in X-linked ocular albinism. Histopathology 4:243, 1980

14. Anderson LL, Paller AS, Malpass D et al: Chédiak-Higashi syndrome in a black child. Pediatr Dermatol 9:31, 1992

15. Zelickson AS, Windhorst DB, White JG, Good RA: The Chédiak-Higashi syndrome: formation of giant melanosomes and the basis of hypopigmentation. J Invest Dermatol 49:575, 1980

16. Rogers RS III: Dermatologic manifestations. pp. 111–131. In Gomez MR (ed): Tuberous Sclerosis. 2nd Ed. Lippincott-Raven, Philadelphia, 1988

17. Fitzpatrick TB: History and significance of white macules, earliest visible sign of tuberous sclerosis. Ann NY Acad Sci 615:26, 1991

18. Jimbow K, Fitzpatrick TB, Szabo G et al: Congenital circumscribed hypomelanosis: characterization based on electron microscopic study of tuberous sclerosis, nevus depigmentosus, and piebaldism. J Invest Dermatol 64:50, 1975

19. Ruiter DJ, van Duinen SG, Peters ACB et al: Hypomelanotic macules in tuberous sclerosis: an ultrastructural and enzyme-histochemical study. Arch Dermatol Res 271:171, 1981

20. Wilson PD, Lavker RM, Kligman AM: On the nature of idiopathic guttate hypomelanosis. Acta Derm Venereol (Stockh) 62:301, 1982

21. Ploysangam T, Dee-Ananlap S, Suvanprakorn P: Treatment of idiopathic guttate hypomelanosis with liquid nitrogen: light and electron microscopic studies. J Am Acad Dermatol 23:681, 1990

22. Rhodes AR, Albert LS, Barnhill RL, Weinstock MA: Sun-induced freckles in children and young adults. Cancer 67:1990, 1991

23. Neurofibromatosis Conference Statement. National Institutes of Health Consensus Development Conference. Arch Neurol 45:575, 1988

24. Nakagawa H, Hori Y, Sato S et al: The nature and origin of the melanin macroglobule. J Invest Dermatol 83:134, 1984

25. Morris TJ, Johnson WG, Silvers DN: Giant pigment granules in biopsy specimens from café-au-lait spots in neurofibromatosis. Arch Dermatol 118:385, 1982

26. Silvers DN, Greenwood RS, Helwig EB: Café-au-lait spots without giant pigment granules. Arch Dermatol 110:87, 1974

27. Rieger E, Kofler R, Borkenstein M: Melanotic macules following Blaschko's lines in McCune-Albright syndrome. Br J Dermatol 130:215, 1994

28. Sexton FM, Maize JC: Melanotic macules and melanoacanthomas of the lip: a comparative study with a census of the basal melanocyte population. Am J Dermatopathol 9:438, 1987

29. Ho KK-L, Dervan P, O'Loughlin S, Powell FC: Labial melanotic macule: a clinical, histopathologic and ultrastructural study. J Am Acad Dermatol 28:33, 1993

30. Revuz J, Clerici T: Penile melanosis. J Am Acad Dermatol 20:567, 1989

31. Grimes PE: Melasma: etiologic and therapeutic considerations. Arch Dermatol 131:1453, 1995

32. Sanchez NP, Pathak MA, Sato S et al: Melasma: a clinical, light microscopic, ultrastructural, and immunofluorescence study. J Am Acad Dermatol 4:698, 1981

33. Vasquez M, Maldonado H, Benmaman C, Sanchez JL: Melasma in men: a clinical and histologic study. Int J Dermatol 27:25, 1988

34. Tate PR, Hodge SJ, Owen LG: A quantitative study of melanocytes in Becker's nevus. J Cutan Pathol 7:404, 1980

35. Kikuchi I, Inoue S, Narita H et al: The broad spectrum of Dowling-Degos disease, including Haber's syndrome. J Dermatol (Tokyo) 10:361, 1983

36. Crovato F, Desirello G, Rebora A: Is Dowling-Degos disease the same disease as Kitamura's reticulate acropigmentation? Br J Dermatol 109:105, 1983

37. Merwin CF: Tinea nigra palmaris: review of the literature and case report. Pediatrics 36:537, 1965

38. Buchner A, Hansen LS: Amalgam pigmentation (amalgam tattoo) of the oral mucosa: a clinicopathologic study of 268 cases. Oral Surg 49:139, 1980

39. Goldstein AP: Histologic reactions in tattoos. J Dermatol Surg Oncol 5:896, 1979

40. Dotz WI, Henrikson DM, Yu GSM, Galey CI: Tinea versicolor: a light and electron microscopic study of hyperpigmented skin. J Am Acad Dermatol 12:37, 1985

41. Galadari I, el Komy M, Mousa A et al: Tinea versicolor: histologic and ultrastructural investigation of pigmentary changes. Int J Dermatol 31:253, 1992

42. Landy SJ, Donnai D: Incontinentia pigmenti (Bloch-Sulzberger syndrome). J Med Genet 30:53, 1993

43. Schaumburg-Lever G, Lever WF: Electron microscopy of incontinentia pigmenti. J Invest Dermatol 61:151, 1973

44. Ashley JR, Burgdorf WH: Incontinentia pigmenti: pigmentary changes independent of incontinence. J Cutan Pathol 14:248, 1987

45. Kalter DC, Griffiths WA, Atherton DJ: Linear and whorled nevoid hypermelanosis. J Am Acad Dermatol 19:1037, 1988

46. Korkij W, Soltani K: Fixed drug eruption: a brief review. Arch Dermatol 120:520, 1984

47. Masu S, Seiji M: Pigmentary incontinence in fixed drug eruptions. J Am Acad Dermatol 8:525, 1983

48. Teraki Y, Moriya N, Shiohara T: Drug-induced expression of intercellular adhesion molecule-1 on lesional keratinocytes in fixed drug eruption. Am J Pathol 145:550, 1994

49. Finlayson GR, Sams WM Jr, Smith JG Jr: Erythema ab igne: a histopathological study. J Invest Dermatol 46:104, 1966

50. Pinkus H: Lichenoid tissue reactions: a speculative review of the clinical spectrum of epidermal basal cell damage with special reference to erythema dyschromicum perstans. Arch Dermatol 107:840, 1973

51. Miyagawa S, Komatsu M, Okuchi T et al: Erythema dyschromicum perstans. Immunopathologic studies. J Am Acad Dermatol 20:882, 1989

52. Tschen JA, Tschen EA, McGavran MH: Erythema dyschromicum perstans. J Am Acad Dermatol 2:295, 1980

15

EPIDERMAL MALFORMATIONS, DYSPLASIAS, AND HYPERPLASIAS

APPROACH TO EPIDERMAL DISORDERS

A variety of congenital and acquired disorders histologically present as perturbations of the normal epidermal architecture. The same changes may be found in a solitary lesion, a linear or segmental defect, palmar-plantar hyperkeratosis, and diffuse ichthyosis, so histopathologic findings rarely provide an unequivocal diagnosis. These patterns are also found in neoplasms of epidermal origin so that in some instances separation is arbitrary. The "brick and mortar" model of the epidermis has helped in understanding many of these disorders. The epidermal corneocytes are the "bricks," and the epidermal lipids and lamellar body membranes provide the "mortar" for the finished structure. Keratins are the intermediate filament proteins found in keratinocytes and are typically present in complementary acid-base pairs. These pairs are expressed in highly specific locations, such as keratins 5 and 14 in the basal layer and keratins 1 and 10 in differentiating keratinocytes. Different pairs are found in nails, hair, and other keratinizing epithelia. The genes for basic keratins are on chromosome 12q, while those for acidic keratins are on chromosome 17q.[1]

It is not correct to describe all the disorders discussed in this chapter as disorders of keratinization, as many other materials play a crucial role. Other important proteins include profilaggrin, which is found in keratohyaline granules; in the stratum corneum it is converted to filaggrin, where it plays a role in water retention and helps to bind the keratin filaments into bundles. The main proteins of the cornified envelope are involucrin and loricrin. The epidermal lipids are primarily delivered to the stratum corneum by the lamellar (membrane-coating or Odland) bodies.

The epidermis has two basic roles: (1) forming a protective barrier out of cornified keratinocytes, lamellar body membranes, and epidermal lipids to prevent water loss; and (2) shedding dead keratinocyte products. Abnormalities in this complex system have been described as disorders of cornification by Williams and Elias.[2] If the barrier function is abnormal, one response may be increased cell proliferation resulting in proliferative hyperkeratosis. If lipids are abnormal or filaggrin (keratohyaline granules) defective, the skin may be so dry that proteolytic enzymes do not function well and shedding is impaired, producing retention hyperkeratosis. These two processes are at play to varying degrees in the ichthyoses.

Disturbances in the keratin filaments may lead to distinct morphologic features. Mutations in the basal layer keratins 5 and 14 are found in epidermolysis bullosa simplex, while changes in keratins 1 and 10 are associated with the variants of epidermolytic hyperkeratosis. Some keratins such as 6 and 16 are expressed on palmar-plantar surfaces and mucosal surfaces and in the epithelial-producing hair and nails; their defects lead to disorders such as pachyonychia congenita and palmar-plantar keratoderma. Keratin 9 is only expressed in palmar-plantar skin and is defective in the form of palmar-plantar keratoderma with epidermolytic hyperkeratosis.

Because fixation removes all lipids, routine light microscopy is an unsatisfactory method to study the complexities of epidermal structure. Traditionally electron microscopy was the principal tool employed, for with it both proteins and lipids could be studied. Many of the ichthyoses and other disorders of cornification are defined and diagnosed based on ultrastructural features. Monoclonal antibodies allow one to type keratins, while genetic studies can identify abnormal keratin genes. A wide variety of elegant techniques are also available to study epidermal lipids.

The simplest approach to epidermal lesions is to compare their pattern to the normal picture:

1. Is the pattern of epidermal growth flat or papillomatous?
2. Is the type of hyperkeratosis compact or basket weave?
3. Is a granular layer present or absent?
4. Is there evidence for premature keratinization, dyskeratosis, acantholysis, or parakeratosis?

Table 15-1 lists several of the common abnormal epidermal patterns and the disorders in which they may be seen. All classifications of epidermal disorders, including ours, have overlaps, because some diseases are traditionally identified clinically (e.g., the ichthyoses) and others are identified by histologic features (e.g., porokeratosis must have cornoid lamellae).

ICHTHYOSES

The ichthyoses are a group of inherited diseases characterized by abnormalities of cornification. We concentrate on the histopathology of the various disorders; the reader should seek additional clinical and genetic information in the reviews. The subject has been reviewed extensively. Traupe's monograph[3] is the best source of both clinical information and detailed histopathologic material, but many other reviews[4,5] are available.

About the only matter on which "cutaneous ichthyologists" agree is that *ichthyosis* is a poor term. Not only do the clinical changes not at all resemble fish scales, but the pejorative nature of the name adds to the misery of an already uncomfortable patient. In their classic work, Frost and Van Scott[6] first divided the ichthyoses into two groups: proliferative hyperkeratosis with an increased number of mitoses and parakeratosis and retention hyperkeratosis with a compact thickened stratum corneum. Counting mitoses is not a practical way to study biopsy specimens from ichthyosis patients. Classification of the ichthyoses has changed as many new diseases have been identified but it still remains difficult. Williams and Elias[5] designated all ichthyoses as disorders of cornification (DOC) and assigned sequential numbers without any particular attention to pathophysiology or interrelationships. Traupe[3] suggested four categories: isolated vulgar ichthyoses, associated vulgar ichthyoses, isolated congenital ichthyoses, and associated congenital ichthyoses. Thus, by determining the presence or absence at birth and the involvement of other organs, the disorders can be quickly subdivided. Then, by using associated cutaneous and systemic findings, mode of inheritance, and histo-

logic patterns, the possibilities can be narrowed down. Cutaneous features that are often important in classification include presence of a collodion membrane at birth; involvement of the flexures, palms, or soles; ectropion; and alopecia. For several of the ichthyoses, other laboratory tests will produce a much more reliable diagnosis. In addition, molecular genetic studies have made some of the diagnoses even more secure.

Histopathologic Features

Microscopic evaluation is a disappointing method for subdividing the ichthyoses. Even when distinguishing between two relatively distinct and common forms, such as autosomal dominant ichthyosis vulgaris and X-linked recessive steroid sulfatase-deficient ichthyosis, the discriminatory value of the biopsy is limited.[7] The only situation in which the biopsy is essential to the diagnosis is in the forms of ichthyosis with epidermolytic hyperkeratosis. At least five epidermal patterns may be seen in ichthyoses. They are rarely specific, since a given patient may have variable features in different biopsy specimens due to location, age of lesion, age of patient, treatment, and many other factors. Electron microscopy is required for an exact diagnosis in many cases; most of the classic papers have been written by Anton-Lamprecht[8] and colleagues. Skin biopsies have been employed for prenatal diagnosis of ichthyosis[9]; bullous congenital ichthyosiform erythroderma was the first skin disorder to be diagnosed by prenatal biopsy. It may be possible in a fetus at risk to determine whether ichthyosis is present (i.e., whether the epidermis is normal). This should not be confused with the difficulties in diagnosing the type of ichthyosis with a biopsy.

Epidermolytic Hyperkeratosis

Epidermolytic hyperkeratosis is the most specific and readily recognizable histologic pattern in ichthyosis (Fig. 15-1). It is characterized by acanthokeratolysis. There is basket-weave or-

Table 15-1. Patterns of Epidermal Malformations

Pattern	Prototype	Other Lesions
Acanthokeratolysis (epidermolytic hyperkeratosis)	Bullous congenital ichthyosiform erythroderma	Other types of ichthyosis; epidermal nevus; Vörner-type keratoderma; isolated lesions; incidental finding
Acantholytic dyskeratosis	Darier's disease	Epidermal nevus; Grover's disease; warty dyskeratoma; isolated lesions
Papillomatosis ("church spiring")	Acanthosis nigricans	Epidermal nevus; seborrheic keratosis; acrokeratosis verruciformis; confluent and reticulated papillomatosis; some types of ichthyosis
Porokeratosis (cornoid lamella)	Porokeratosis of Mibelli	Epidermal nevus; disseminated superficial actinic porokeratosis; punctate porokeratosis; disseminated porokeratosis
Eosinophils and dyskeratosis	Incontinentia pigmenti	Epidermal nevus
Lichenoid infiltrate	Lichen planus	Epidermal nevus; lichenoid keratosis; Flege's disease; Lichen striatus; many others
Compact orthohyperkeratosis	Many types of ichthyosis (especially harlequin fetus)	Epidermal nevus; pachyonychia congenita; many others
"Psoriasiform" inflammation	Psoriasis	Epidermal nevus; ILVEN; CHILD nevus; some types of ichthyosis

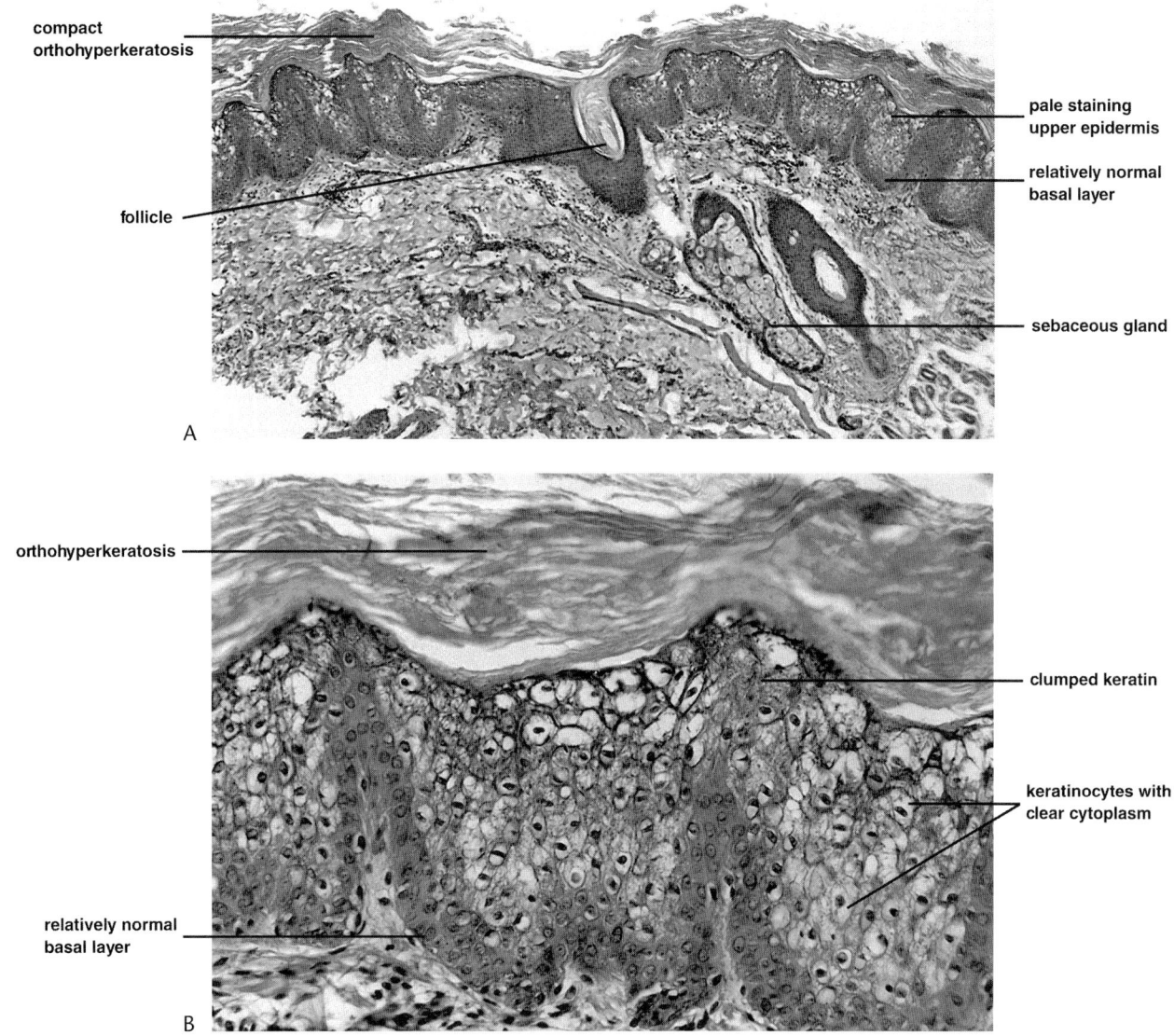

compact orthohyperkeratosis

pale staining upper epidermis

relatively normal basal layer

follicle

sebaceous gland

A

orthohyperkeratosis

clumped keratin

keratinocytes with clear cytoplasm

relatively normal basal layer

B

Figure 15-1. Epidermolytic hyperkeratosis. (**A**) There is compact orthohyperkeratosis overlying a hyperplastic epidermis. Even at low power one can see the degenerative changes with abnormal keratinization. (**B**) At higher power, the spaces around cells, the clumping of keratin, and the disruption of the epidermis are better appreciated.

thohyperkeratosis that overlies a granular layer with large clumps of keratohyaline, edema, and perinuclear vacuolar changes. Pink trichohyaline-like granules may also be seen in the granular layer. The basal and suprabasal keratinocytes are usually normal.[10] Ultrastructurally, thickened clumps and bundles of tonofilaments are seen in the cells of the upper layers of the epidermis. Widespread epidermolytic hyperkeratosis is caused by mutations in keratins 1 and 10; the same mutations have been shown in some epidermal nevi with the same histologic change, supporting the nature of the mosaicism. The Siemens variant may have a mutation in keratin 2e, while the epidermolytic hyperkeratosis seen in Vörner's palmar-plantar keratoderma is caused by mutations in keratin 9. Epidermolytic hyperkeratosis is seen in at least five ichthyotic disorders; all are inherited in an autosomal dominant pattern.

Epidermolytic hyperkeratosis (bullous congenital ichthyosiform erythroderma, bullous ichthyosis), a diffuse congenital erythroderma, is the prototype of epidermolytic hyperkeratosis. As patients get older, they become less erythrodermic but develop thickened scales.

Ichthyosis hystrix of Curth-Macklin is similar to epidermolytic hyperkeratosis, but patients do not blister. Ultrastructural examination shows shells of tonofilaments around the nucleus, and detailed light microscopic examination may show binucleated keratinocytes.[11] *Ichthyosis hystrix* is a very confusing term; it refers to all spiny ichthyoses. The Lambert family toured Europe over a century ago as the "porcupine men" and were diagnosed with ichthyosis hystrix. Unfortunately, today it is unclear what disorder they had. Probably the most common use of the term today is in describing an epidermal nevus that clinically is very verrucous or spiny and often shows epidermolytic hyperkeratosis microscopically, although several rare types of ichthyosis are also so labeled.

In *ichthyosis bullosa of Siemens*, there is more variability in the lesions, and a thick, well-developed plaque should be biopsied to increase the likelihood of finding epidermolytic hyperkeratosis.[12]

In *acral epidermolytic hyperkeratosis*, only the acral skin is involved. There is no erythema, but there is frequent blistering.[13]

In *annular epidermolytic ichthyosis*, there are annular and polycyclic, erythematous, hyperkeratotic plaques on the trunk and extremities. Blistering occurs in childhood, but ceases at puberty.[14]

Epidermolytic hyperkeratosis can also be seen in a variety of other clinical settings:

1. *Vörner palmar-plantar keratoderma*
2. *Linear epidermal nevi* patients with linear epidermal nevi that have epidermolytic hyperkeratotic changes are at risk of parenting children with bullous congenital ichthyosiform erythroderma through the mechanism of gonadal mosaicism. This same risk is not found in patients with other forms of epidermolytic hyperkeratosis.
3. *Epidermolytic acanthoma* patients may have single or multiple papules that on biopsy show epidermolytic hyperkeratosis.[15]
4. *Incidental finding:* epidermolytic hyperkeratosis is seen in a variety of lesions, including actinic keratosis, seborrheic keratosis, basal cell carcinoma, and trichilemmal cyst. Sometimes the epidermolytic hyperkeratosis may be very focal and limited to a single sweat duct or rete ridge.[16]

Compact Orthohyperkeratosis with Reduced to Absent Granular Layer

This is the prototypical pattern of ichthyosis vulgaris. There is compact hyperkeratosis over a reduced to absent granular layer.

In general, hyperkeratosis in associated with a prominent granular layer (Fig. 15-2). In addition, both epidermal atrophy and hyperplasia can be present, often in the same specimen. There may be flattening of the rete ridges. Frequently follicular orifices are blocked.[17] Ultrastructural examination shows reduced keratohyaline granules with a crumbly or spongy pattern, reflecting the abnormalities in profilaggrin and fitting with the autosomal dominant inheritance.[18]

These ultrastructural changes allow ichthyosis vulgaris to be distinguished from other diseases with a reduced granular layer. While there is a clinical overlap between the dry skin of atopic dermatitis and ichthyosis vulgaris, electron microscopy reveals that less than 5% of atopic dermatitis patients have ichthyosis vulgaris.[19]

Included in this group besides ichthyosis vulgaris are a number of rare disorders in which the granular layer may be diminished (all could just as easily be included in the next grouping, as they may also have a normal granular layer):

1. *X-linked recessive ichthyosis*: it is very difficult to discriminate between this disorder and ichthyosis vulgaris. Usually the granular layer is present, but it may be very sparse.
2. *Refsum syndrome* (phytanic acid storage disease): this rare autosomal recessive type may have a reduced granular layer; the keratinocytes and even melanocytes contain lipid droplets that can be seen with lipid stains or electron microscopy.[20]
3. *Trichothiodystrophy*: a number of interrelated autosomal recessively inherited syndromes have been grouped together; they may have a reduced granular layer. Examining the hair with polarized light will show banding.[21]
4. *X-linked dominant ichthyosis* (Conradi-Hünermann syndrome, chondrodysplasia punctata): epidermal calcification may be a distinguishing feature. In infants, the calcium can be seen with von Kossa stain on light microscopy, but later

Figure 15-2. Ichthyosis vulgaris. There is prominent orthohyperkeratosis with few if any other changes. The absence of a granular layer can be seen, as well as the relative normalcy of the epidermis and upper dermis.

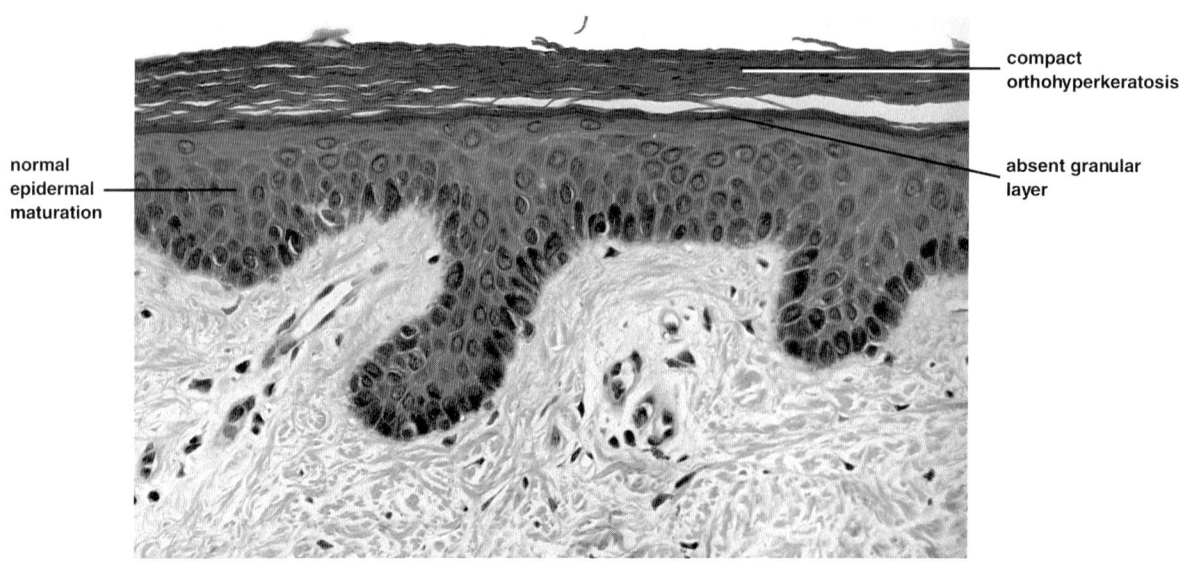

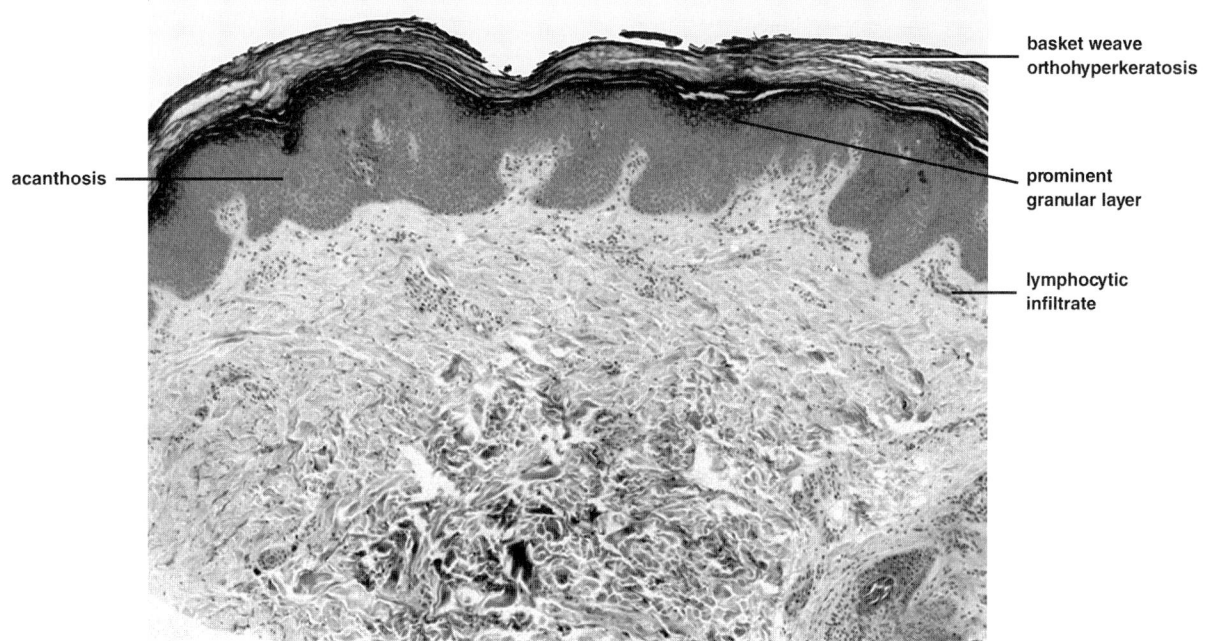

basket weave orthohyperkeratosis

acanthosis

prominent granular layer

lymphocytic infiltrate

Figure 15-3. Congenital ichthyosiform erythroderma. There is orthohyperkeratosis with a prominent granular layer coupled with epidermal hyperplasia and a sparse papillary dermal mononuclear cell infiltrate.

it is difficult to identify without electron microscopy.[22] Radiographic studies to search for stippled epiphyses is simpler.

Compact Hyperkeratosis with Normal or Prominent Granular Layer

Striking compact hyperkeratosis may develop, reflecting thick scales. Parakeratosis is present in the more rapidly proliferating variants, but often absent. The rete ridges may be broadened, resembling lichen simplex chronicus. Often there is papillomatosis, but it varies greatly from region to region.

Lamellar ichthyosis (nonerythrodermic lamellar ichthyosis) has laminated orthohyperkeratosis, little parakeratosis, and frequently papillomatosis.[23]

Congenital ichthyosiform erythroderma (nonbullous congenital ichthyosiform erythroderma; lamellar ichthyosis-erythrodermic type; erythrodermic lamellar ichthyosis) usually has some parakeratosis and psoriasiform changes (Fig. 15-3). It is impossible to separate accurately the "lamellar ichthyoses" histologically, but electron microscopy may be useful.[24,25]

Lamellar ichthyosis, dominant type, may have alternating areas of laminated orthohyperkeratosis and parakeratosis, both with a thickened granular layer pattern and papillomatosis. Electron microscopy may show a thickened transforming zone (transition from granular layer to stratum corneum).[26]

X-linked recessive ichthyosis has compact hyperkeratosis and a variable granular layer. Therefore, the presence of a granular layer cannot be used to distinguish ichthyosis vulgaris from X-linked ichthyosis with certainty.[7,17] Patients are most accurately diagnosed by documenting their steroid sulfatase deficiency.

Harlequin fetus is rarely diagnosed histologically, as it is so clinically dramatic. Patients present at birth with large plates of thickened skin separated by erythematous rhagades.[27] When biopsied, there is extraordinary hyperkeratosis so that the stratum corneum is often as thick as the rest of the epidermis and dermis.[28,29]

Neutral lipid storage disease (Chanarin-Dorfman syndrome) may have lipids in keratinocytes; electron microscopy shows abnormal lamellar bodies.[30]

Keratitis, ichthyosis, and deafness (KID) syndrome has ichthyosis-like hyperkeratosis with thickened leathery skin but no scales; the cutaneous involvement is localized especially on the face and extremities.[31]

Peeling skin syndrome A has orthohyperkeratosis but a stratum corneum split.[32] It is best distinguished from superficial epidermolysis bullosa simplex by its lack of mechanical fragility.

Acquired ichthyosis is usually secondary to lipid-altering medications or other lipid abnormalities; on rare occasions, it may be a paraneoplastic marker. Although accurate histologic reports are lacking, most cases seem to have compact hyperkeratosis without granular layer changes.

Papillomatosis

All the disorders discussed above may occasionally have papillomatosis. However, in some disorders it is frequently present and may be exaggerated.

Lamellar ichthyosis frequently has a pattern of epidermal undulations or "church spiring."

Sjögren-Larsson syndrome has prominent papillomatosis with compact hyperkeratosis[33] (Fig. 15-4). The lesions are clin-

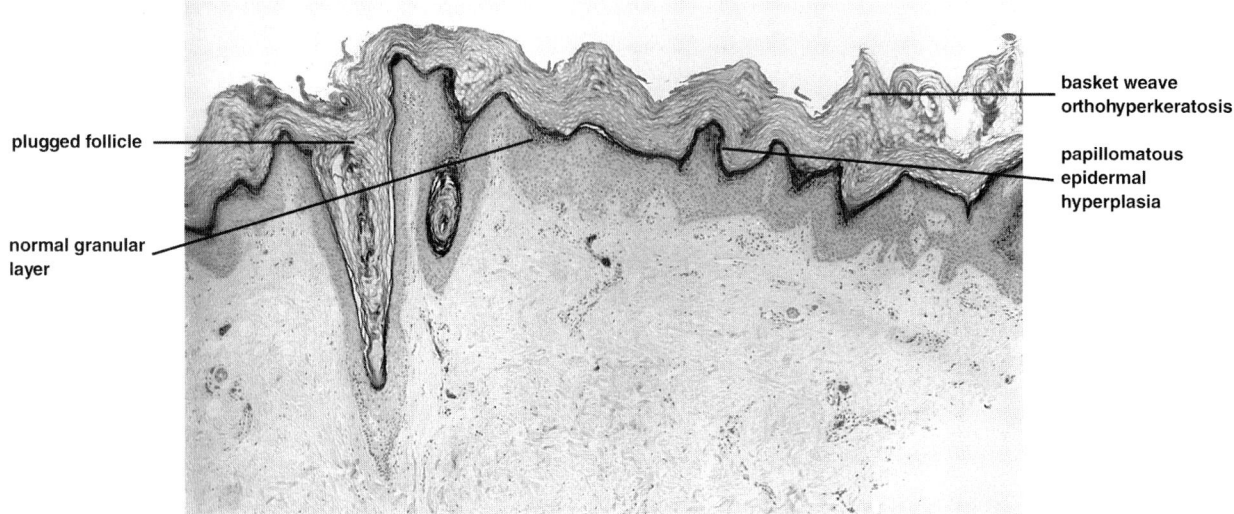

Figure 15-4. Sjögren-Larsson syndrome. There is prominent orthohyperkeratosis and papillomatosis with little if any inflammation.

ically often velvety, and histology may even resemble acanthosis nigricans or other extremely papillomatous lesions. The diagnosis is best confirmed biochemically.[34]

Erythrokeratodermia variabilis has wandering scaly patches that often show papillomatosis.[35]

Compact Hyperkeratosis with Inflammation

This group displays proliferative hyperkeratosis with acanthosis, normal to thickened granular layer, marked parakeratosis, and both dermal and epidermal inflammatory infiltrates. Neutrophils can be found in the stratum corneum. It is also designated *psoriasiform ichthyosis*, but rarely resembles true psoriasis histologically.

Congenital ichthyosiform erythroderma may have marked parakeratosis and some inflammation.

Netherton syndrome features ichthyosis linear circumflexa that has psoriasiform hyperplasia with parakeratosis. The characteristic double scale at the lesion's edge may also be seen histologically. The nonichthyosis linear circumflexa regions in Netherton patients are likely to show parakeratosis and periodic acid–Schiff staining of stratum corneum.[36] The simplest microscopic test is examining hairs for trichorrhexis invaginata and other structural abnormalities.[37]

Peeling skin syndrome A is characterized histologically by separation of the epidermis between the stratum corneum and the stratum granulosum.[38]

DARIER'S DISEASE

Darier's disease, or keratosis follicularis, is an autosomal dominant inherited genodermatosis with waxy verrucous papules and a characteristic histologic pattern of acantholytic dyskeratosis.

Clinical Features

Typically Darier's disease presents with waxy brown papules initially in a follicular distribution on the chest, back, or face that later may become widespread. Occasionally bullae may develop. The lesions are frequently intensely inflamed. Chemotactic defects have been identified in some cases. Patients are at risk to develop Kaposi's varicelliform eruption.[39,40]

Other areas involved include (1) palms and soles, which can be intensely hyperkeratotic and painful; (2) nails, with linear colored streaks, dystrophy, and distal notching; (3) oral mucosa which can have nodular hyperkeratotic papules (cobblestoning), especially on the hard palate; and (4) scalp, which may have marked scale or alopecia. Acrokeratosis verruciformis may be present. Cornifying Darier's disease is a variant with large cutaneous horns especially on the extremities.[41]

Histopathologic Features

The histologic features of Darier's disease are distinctive. In general, the disordered keratinization is characterized by corps ronds and/or grains (Fig. 15-5A). The corps ronds that arise in the upper epidermis are keratinocytes that contain a central pyknotic nucleus surrounded by a clear zone (halo) with a thick keratotic shell. The grains are large parakeratotic keratinocytes that are horizontally elongated and prematurely keratinized.

The epidermis is interrupted by frequent pits and clefts, in which both dyskeratosis and acantholysis are prominent. Clefting arises in the lower epidermis; the tiny suprabasal separations are called *lacunae*. Often dermal papillae are left covered by one layer of basal keratinocytes. Basal layer budding may be found beneath the clefts. While follicular involvement may occur (Fig. 15-5B), the older name of *keratosis follicularis* is misleading. Some inflammation may be seen histologically, but it is rarely as severe as clinically suggested.

Pathophysiology

The basic defect in Darier's disease remains unclear. While the gene has been localized to chromosome 12q, suggesting involvement of a keratin molecule, the responsible protein has not been identified. The main problems are acantholysis and dyskeratosis, but a unifying mechanism is absent. Acantholysis may reflect an intrinsic defect in the intercellular matrix or represent dissolution of one of the matrical constituents by enzymes released from keratinocytes.

The dyskeratotic changes reflect a variety of ultrastructural tonofilament abnormalities. The tonofilaments may clump with keratohyaline granules. The corps ronds are cells with a clear cytoplasm around pyknotic nuclei and a tonofilament shell. In the grains nuclear fragments and tonofilaments are aggregated.[42]

Other clinically distinct disorders may have identical histologic changes. They include

1. *Warty dyskeratoma* (solitary Darier's disease): usually a solitary facial or scalp nodule that resembles a large comedo or verruca. It is often excised to rule out an epithelial malignancy.[43,44]

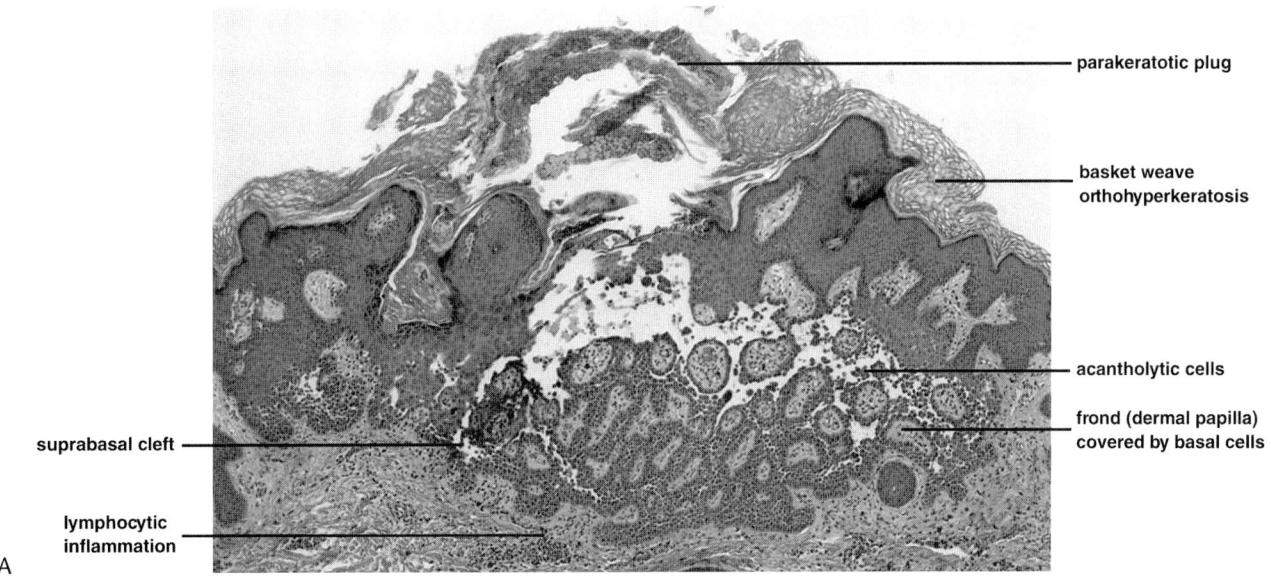

A

parakeratotic plug

basket weave orthohyperkeratosis

acantholytic cells

frond (dermal papilla) covered by basal cells

suprabasal cleft

lymphocytic inflammation

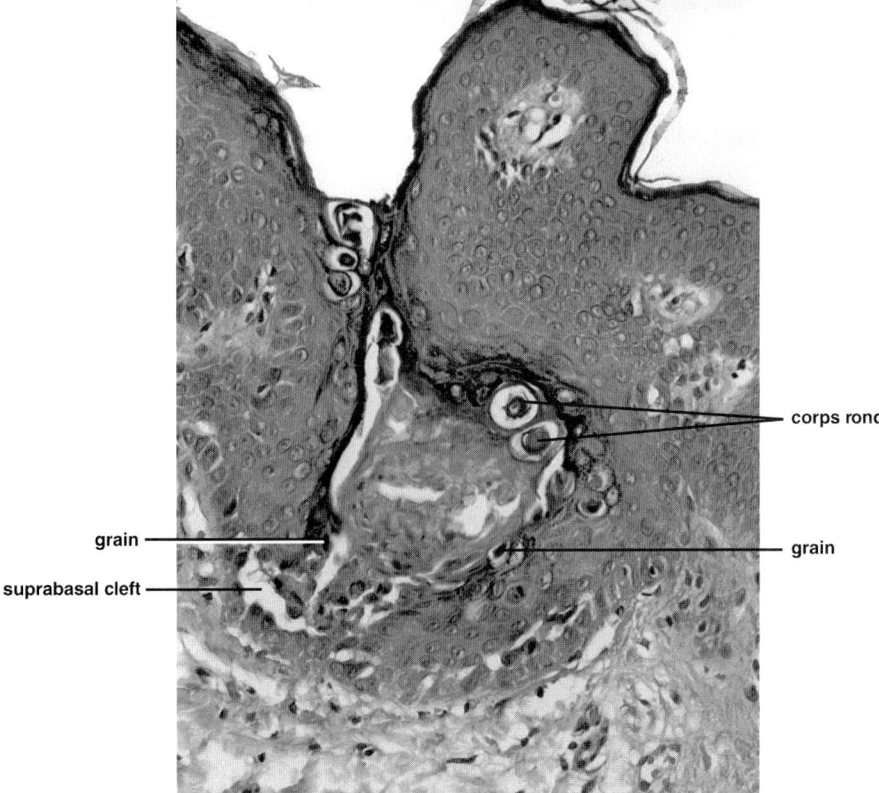

B

corps rond

grain

grain

suprabasal cleft

Figure 15-5. Darier's disease. (**A**) Sections show preserved dermal papillae or fronds covered by a layer of epithelial cells. There is also intraepidermal separation laterally and parakeratosis over the central cleft. (**B**) Higher magnification showing acantholysis as well as corps ronds and grains.

A central patulous follicle or dell is lined by an acanthotic epidermis rich in dyskeratotic cells. Suprabasilar acantholysis, corps ronds, and grains identical to those in Darier's disease are seen.

2. *Linear Darier's disease and linear epidermal nevus*: linear lesions otherwise clinically indistinguishable from linear epidermal nevi may have the histologic changes of Darier's disease.

3. *Familial dyskeratotic comedones:* may show focal acantholytic dyskeratotic changes in the follicular plugs.[45]

4. *Transient acantholytic dermatosis* (Grover's disease): patients have a highly pruritic papular eruption that is usually transient. It is more common in older men.[46] Many histologic patterns are seen that mimic several blistering disorders. One pattern is identical to Darier's disease with prominent dyskeratosis. When acantholysis dominates, the lesion may mimic Hailey-Hailey disease or even pemphigus, but can usually be distinguished by its focal nature.[47]

5. *Acantholytic acanthoma*[48]: patients have solitary or multiple papules dominated by acantholysis and/or dyskeratoses.[49] Multiple acantholytic acanthoma and papular acantholytic dyskeratosis differ from Grover's disease because they are nonpruritic, fewer in number, larger, and more likely to be permanent.[50] The differential diagnosis of Darier's disease has two parts:

A. Several disorders have identical histopathologic changes and can only be sorted out clinically.

B. Occasionally it can be impossible to distinguish between Hailey-Hailey disease (chronic benign familial pemphigus) and Darier's disease, either clinically or histologically. In general, Darier's disease has less intertriginous involvement, more scale, more dyskeratosis, and less acantholysis.

PALMAR-PLANTAR KERATODERMA

Permanent thickened plaques on the palms and soles characterize a variety of disorders, many of which represent inherited abnormalities in keratin.

Clinical Features

Many different types of palmar-plantar keratoderma have been described.[51,52] Stevens and colleagues[53] have proposed a new working classification incorporating the following clinical information as well as molecular genetic information when available. Useful data include

1. Family history—usually inherited in an autosomal dominant fashion
2. Age of onset
3. Nature of lesions—diffuse, focal (linear, striate), punctate
4. Associated lesions—skin or internal

Stevens et al[53] designate a long list of disorders as *palmoplantar ectodermal dysplasias* including pachyonychia congenita, Howel-Evans syndrome (tylosis-esophageal cancer), and Voh-

winkel syndrome (deafness and starfish-like keratoses on extensor surfaces, perhaps associated with a loricrin mutation). Defects may involve keratin 9, which is only expressed in the skin of the palms and soles, or keratins 6 and 16, which are typically paired and found not only on the palms and soles but also associated with hair, nails, and mucosae.

Histopathologic Features

The histologic pattern usually shows volar skin with an exaggeration of the compact orthohyperkeratosis (Fig. 15-6). The only unique finding on light microscopy is the presence of epidermolytic hyperkeratosis; this is found in Vörner or epidermolytic palmar-plantar hyperkeratosis, which may be the most common type and is caused by a defect in keratin 9. Many patients initially identified as Unna-Thost palmar-plantar hyperkeratosis have on restudy (including Thost's pedigree) been shown to have epidermolytic hyperkeratosis on biopsy and keratin 9 mutations.[54]

Hyperkeratosis of the palms and soles, whether reflecting an inherited disorder or a response to pressure and friction, has a limited histologic spectrum:

1. Diffuse hyperkeratosis: plaques with marked hyperkeratosis without a sharp border; when caused by chronic trauma, such a lesion is a callus
2. Localized hyperkeratosis[55]

A. Corn or clavus: punctate papule over a bony prominence with a central parakeratotic column

B. Punctate keratoderma: sharply defined area of acanthosis and extreme hyperkeratosis rising above adjacent skin

C. Keratotic pit: sharply demarcated invagination of epidermis, filled with keratin and most common in creases

D. Porokeratotic keratoderma (punctate plantar porokeratosis): when a volar keratotic pit has a column of parakeratosis, it is designated as porokeratosis. The granular layer may be poorly developed, as in classic nonvolar porokeratosis

PACHYONYCHIA CONGENITA

Pachyonychia congenita refers to at least three different autosomally dominant inherited genodermatoses, all characterized by nail changes and hyperkeratotic epithelial lesions.[53,56,57]

Clinical Features

The primary cutaneous lesion is a hyperkeratotic papule or plaque, often overlying an area of pressure or trauma. Other features are summarized in Table 15-2. In the past, there was controversy over how to best subdivide these disorders. Genetic studies have shown mutations in keratins 6 and 16 in the Jadassohn-Lewandowsky form and in keratin 17 in the Jackson-Lawler type, suggesting that some splitting is warranted.

Histopathologic Features

Microscopy is not a useful way to study pachyonychia congenita. Striking localized hyperkeratosis is found with little else

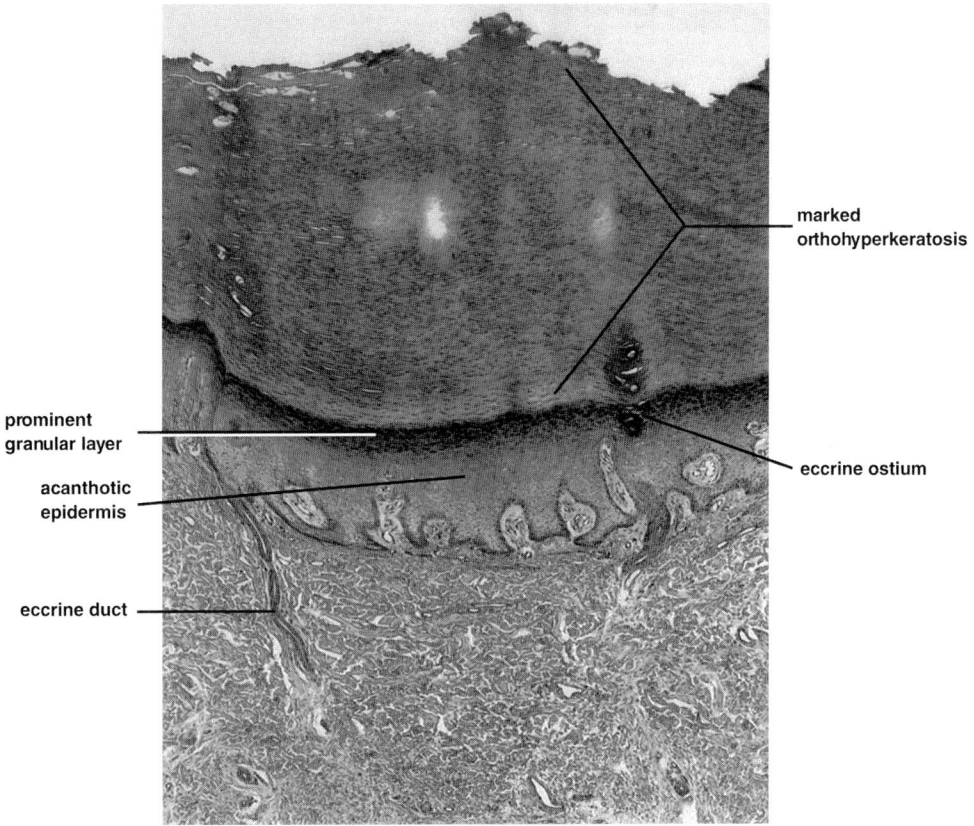

prominent granular layer

acanthotic epidermis

eccrine duct

marked orthohyperkeratosis

eccrine ostium

Figure 15-6. Keratoderma. Sections show volar skin with prominent eccrine glands and marked hyperkeratosis with a prominent granular layer. Clinically this was a punctate keratoderma.

(Fig. 15-7). The follicular nature of some hyperkeratotic plaques can be confirmed, but this is just as easily established clinically. Oral hyperkeratosis cannot be distinguished from white sponge nevus, hereditary benign intraepithelial dysplasia, and dyskeratosis congenita (unless the latter has progressed to have atypical changes). The amyloid changes in Tidman's variant are considered in Chapter 16.[58]

DYSKERATOSIS CONGENITA

Dyskeratosis congenita is an X-linked recessive genodermatosis with multisystem involvement.

Clinical Features

Patients have widespread poikiloderma or hyper- and hypopigmentation. Their nails are frequently dystrophic. They have leukokeratosis of their oral mucosa, which, in contrast to other congenital white oral hyperplasias, is premalignant and a significant cause of morbidity. Another major problem is pancytopenia, which occurs in about 50% of patients. This hematologic change produces a potential diagnostic problem.[59,60] In dyskeratosis congenita patients who have undergone a bone marrow transplant, the poikiloderma can mimic graft-versus-host disease both clinically and microscopically.[61]

Table 15-2. Pachyonychia Congenita

Disease	Inheritance	Thickened Nails	Keratoderma	Follicular Keratosis	Epidermoid Cyst	Natal Teeth	Leukoplakia	Hyperpigmentation	Amyloid
Jadassohn-Lewandowsky	AD	+	+	+	−	−	+	−	−
Jackson-Lawler	AD	+	+	+	+	+	±	−	−
Tidman-Wells-MacDonald	AD	+	+	−	−	−	−	±	+

Abbreviation: AD, autosomal dominant.

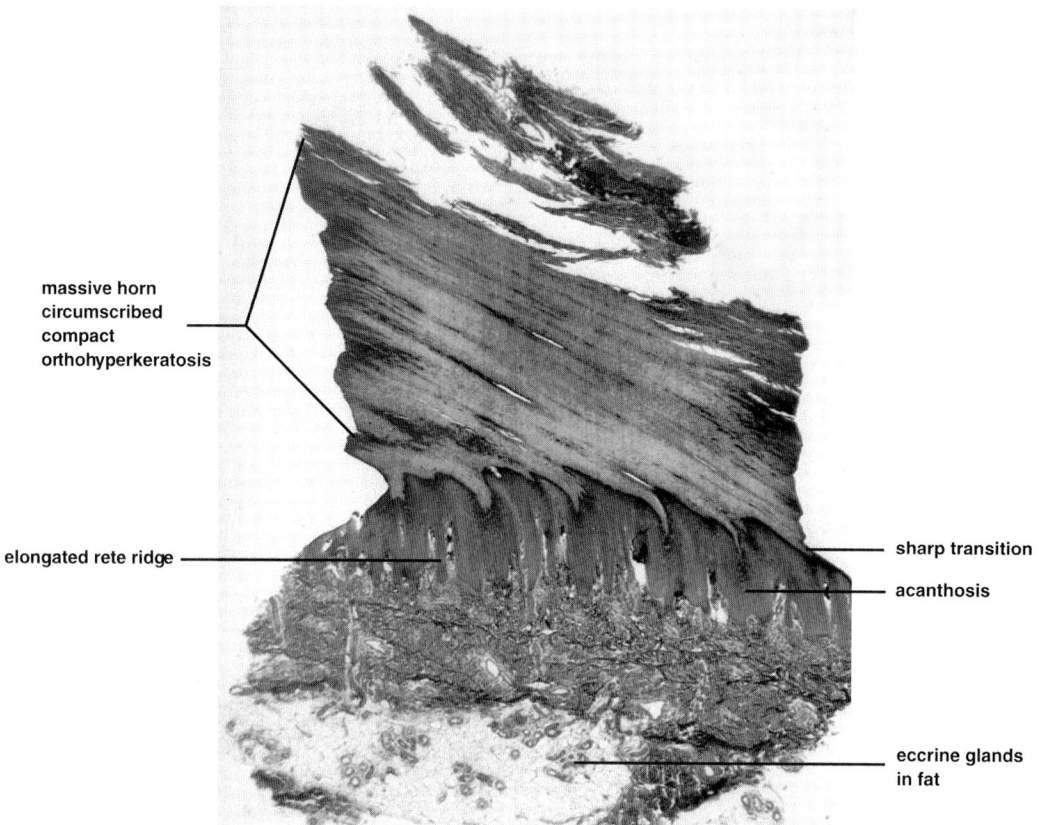

massive horn
circumscribed
compact
orthohyperkeratosis

elongated rete ridge

sharp transition

acanthosis

eccrine glands
in fat

Figure 15-7. Pachyonychia congenita. There is laminated compact orthohyperkeratosis and epidermal hyperplasia. This is indistinguishable from most forms of palmar-plantar keratoderma, except that it is not from acral skin. (Histologic material courtesy of W.P.D. Su, M.D., Rochester, MN.)

Histopathologic Features

The skin shows epidermal atrophy, incontinentia pigmenti, and telangiectasia; in short, it is the prototype of poikiloderma (Fig. 15-8). There may also be hyperkeratosis and minimal dyskeratosis. The oral mucosa has compact hyperkeratosis, which may eventually develop dyskeratotic changes and then squamous cell carcinoma.

ECTODERMAL DYSPLASIAS

Ectodermal dysplasia refers to several hundred genodermatoses summarized in an entire book.[62] These diseases are characterized by abnormalities of skin, hair, nails, and many other organs. Their nosologies are beyond the scope of this book, especially because their histologies are of little utility in classifying these disorders. We consider only the most classic form of ectodermal dysplasia.

Hypohidrotic (anhidrotic) ectodermal dysplasia is usually transmitted in an X-linked recessive fashion, so it is seen almost exclusively in males.[63] The physiognomy is so characteristic that all patients look enough alike to be siblings. There is frontal bossing with a saddle nose. Patients have hypodontia or anodontia; the few teeth are often conical. The lips tend to pro-

trude. The combination of lip and tooth abnormalities and laryngeal atrophy leads to a characteristic croaky voice. The skin is soft and dry, and sweating is reduced to absent, leading to heat intolerance. Some infants present with fever of unknown origin. The mothers have hypohidrosis in a segmental distribution, following the lines of Blaschko, as a vivid example of mosaicism. A skin biopsy specimen will show reduced to absent eccrine sweat glands,[64] but this finding can be more easily demonstrated with a sweat test. A palmar skin biopsy has also been recommended.[65]

EPIDERMAL NEVUS

An epidermal nevus is a circumscribed, long-lasting, congenital malformation of epidermis and epidermally derived structures, reflecting genetic mosaicism.[66]

Clinical Features

Epidermal nevi can have a variety of clinical patterns and also an array of histologic pictures. Happle[67] has pointed out that epidermal nevi represent somatic mosaicism. This is of great clinical importance, for if an individual has a localized nevus with a mutation in, for example, keratin 10, he has an epidermolytic epidermal nevus; if the same mutation has occurred in his testes, then he may father a child with bullous congenital ichthyosiform erythema (epidermolytic hyperkeratosis).[68,69]

The most common clinical patterns[70,71] are

1. *Linear epidermal nevus:* the typical patient has a linear verrucous epidermal proliferation. Lesions often extend down a limb. They may extend onto a mucosal surface. In infancy, the area may simply be hyperpigmented and confused with a congenital melanocytic nevus, café-au-lait macule, or Becker's nevus. With time, the lesions tend to thicken and darken. Small epidermal nevi may consist of grouped papules resembling papillomatous melanocytic nevi, verrucae, or seborrheic keratoses. The typical linear lesions usually follow the lines of Blaschko.

2. *Nevus sebaceus of Jadassohn:* an affected person is born with a patch of alopecia often on the temple or frontal hair line that usually remains stable until puberty and then becomes yellow and hyperkeratotic. While all epidermal nevi have the potential to give rise to adnexal neoplasms, the phenomenon is most common in nevus sebaceus where it can occasionally be recognized clinically when a papule or nodule develops.[72]

3. *Comedo nevus:* a single patch of skin is rich in comedones independent of acne vulgaris.[73,74] Some patients may have familial comedones but not in a nevoid pattern; often the plugged follicles show acantholytic dyskeratosis.[45] The lesions may also involve the palms or soles, where no follicles are present. Here eccrine ducts are involved; the term porokeratotic eccrine ostial and dermal duct nevus has been used. Overlaps between epidermal nevus and comedo nevus occur, supporting their close relationship.[75]

4. *Inflammatory linear verrucous epidermal nevus:* erythematous linear lesions look like a patch or streak of dermatitis, except that they are permanent.[76] They are often psoriasiform[77]; perhaps they represent a rather inapparent epidermal nevus that is susceptible to psoriasis, in contrast to the "resistant" adjacent normal skin.

5. *CHILD nevus:* CHILD (*c*ongenital *h*emidysplasia with *i*chthyosiform nevus and *l*imb *d*efects) is inherited in an X-linked dominant fashion. The epidermal nevus is erythematous, covered with waxy scales, displays an affinity for the body folds, and shows a strict midline demarcation.[78,79]

Patients with extensive linear epidermal nevi or extensive nevus sebaceus were originally described as having the epidermal nevus syndrome (Schimmelpenning-Feuerstein-Mims syndrome), with the likelihood of central nervous system, skeletal, and other internal involvement.[80] As Happle[81] has pointed out, there are many epidermal nevus *syndromes* rather than one entity. For example, the Proteus syndrome, with a range of skeletal, ocular, and central nervous system problems, as well as many skin changes (epidermal nevi, melanocytic nevi, connective tissue nevi, vascular malformations, and café-au-lait macules, among others) is also an epidermal nevus syndrome.[81]

Histopathologic Features

Under the microscope, epidermal nevi have an equally broad spectrum.[82] There is almost invariably epidermal hyperplasia, usually in a papillomatous or "church spire" pattern. Dyskeratosis is uncommon. When a pure pattern of papillomatous epidermal hyperplasia is seen, the term *nevus verrucous* may be appropriate. However, in our experience, this pure pattern is uncommon.

In nevus sebaceus, the same epidermal changes are seen (Fig. 15-9A). Nascent hair buds are frequently present at the base of the epidermis, but mature hair follicles are absent (Fig. 15-9B). In younger patients, there may be no striking increase in seba-

Figure 15-8.   Dyskeratosis congenita. There is epidermal vacuolar damage at the dermoepidermal junction with orthohyperkeratosis and minimal dyskeratosis. The rete ridges are effaced. In the superficial dermis there are telangiectases. This could be histologically mistaken for late graft-versus-host disease. (Histologic material courtesy of Neil Fenske, M.D., Tampa, FL.)

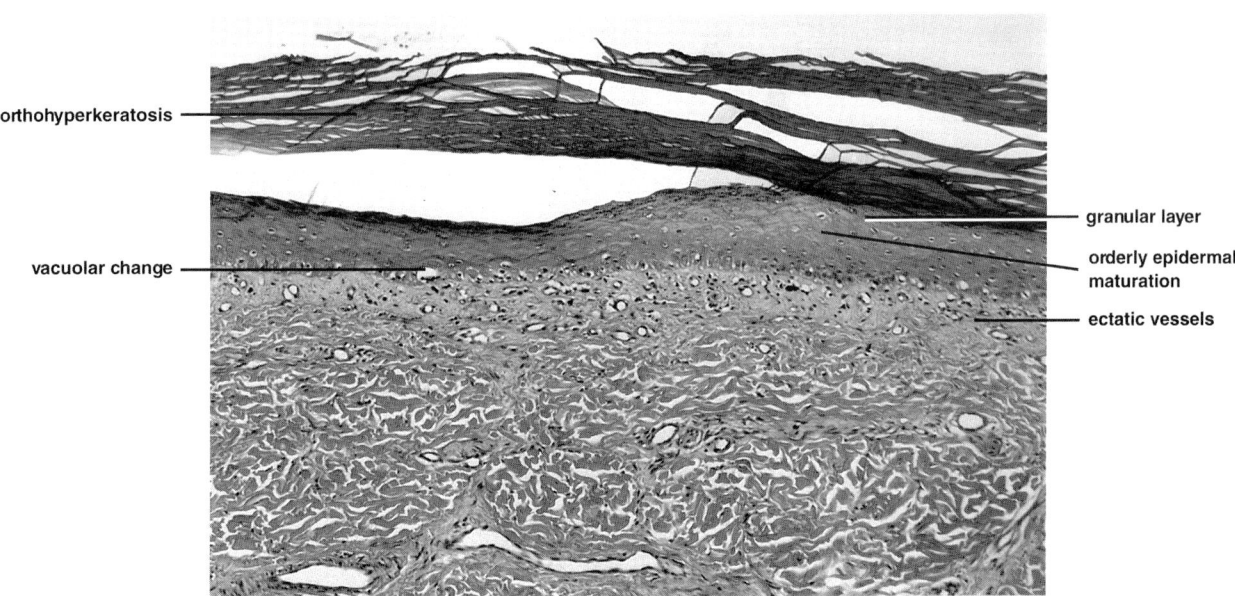

ceous glands, but in older patients varying degrees of adnexal hyperplasia are seen (Fig. 15-9C). Although sebaceous glands usually dominate, perhaps because of the scalp location, on careful search, evidence of eccrine or apocrine hyperplasia may also be found. The histologic diagnosis of the tumors that develop is usually trichoblastoma or syringocystadenoma papilliferum, although occasionally basal cell carcinoma, squamous cell carcinoma, or keratoacanthoma does occur.[72,83]

If a single adnexal element predominates, one may diagnose an eccrine nevus, for example. If multiple adnexal structures in-

terplay and the nevus clinically is not a nevus sebaceus, then organoid nevus seems the best diagnosis.[84]

Another unifying feature of epidermal nevi is that all the reaction patterns seen in other epidermal proliferations and tumors can be found within the nevi:

1. Acantholytic dyskeratosis resembling Darier's disease may occur. If a lesion is congenital and has focal dyskeratosis with corps ronds and grains, it is designated *linear epidermal nevus*; if it becomes apparent later in life, the term *linear*

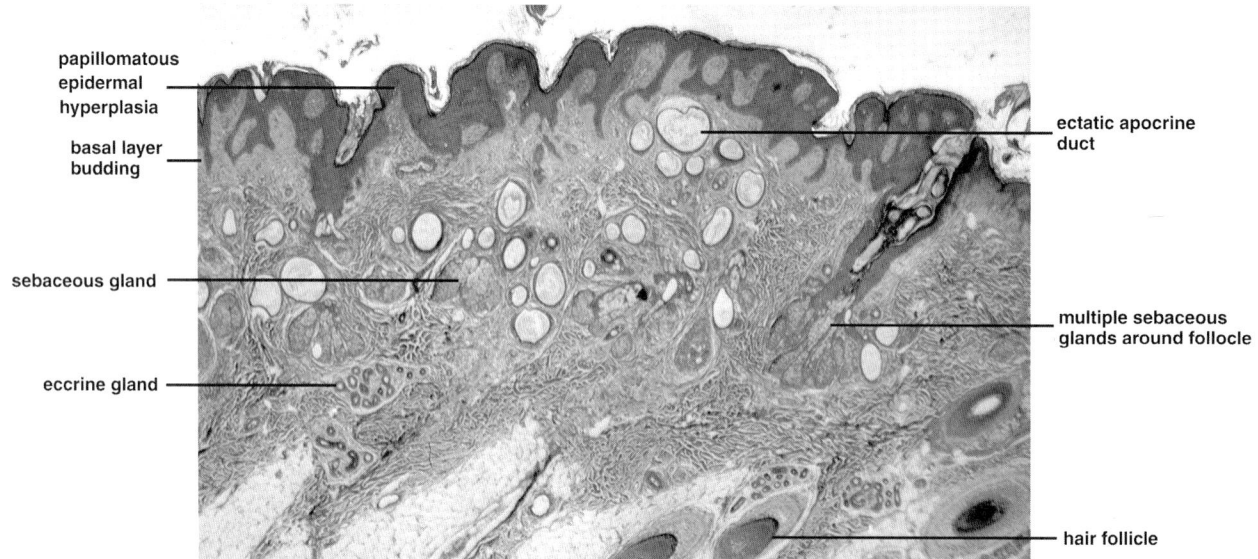

papillomatous epidermal hyperplasia — basal layer budding — sebaceous gland — eccrine gland — ectatic apocrine duct — multiple sebaceous glands around follocle — hair follicle

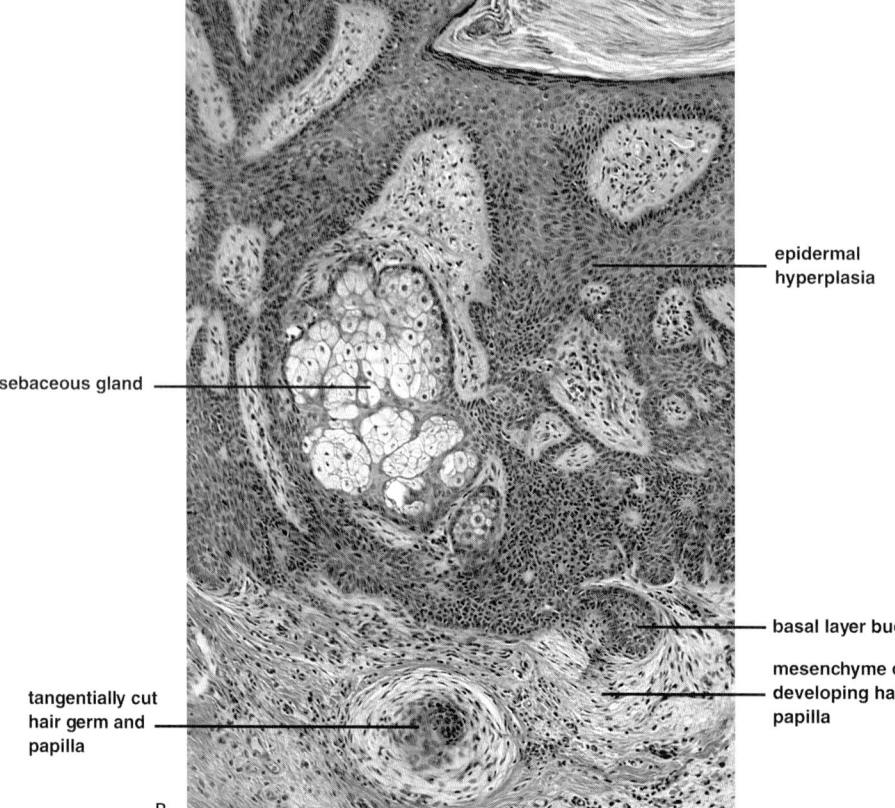

epidermal hyperplasia — sebaceous gland — basal layer bud — mesenchyme of developing hair papilla — tangentially cut hair germ and papilla — B

Figure 15-9. Epidermal nevus. (**A**) Many of the features of epidermal nevus are seen here, including a papillomatous epidermal pattern; eccrine, apocrine, and sebaceous glands; and some basal layer budding. Note the absence of terminal hair follicles compared with the perilesional follicles on the lower right. (**B**) These small follicular buds at the basal layer in this case around a sebaceous gland are typical in an epidermal nevus.

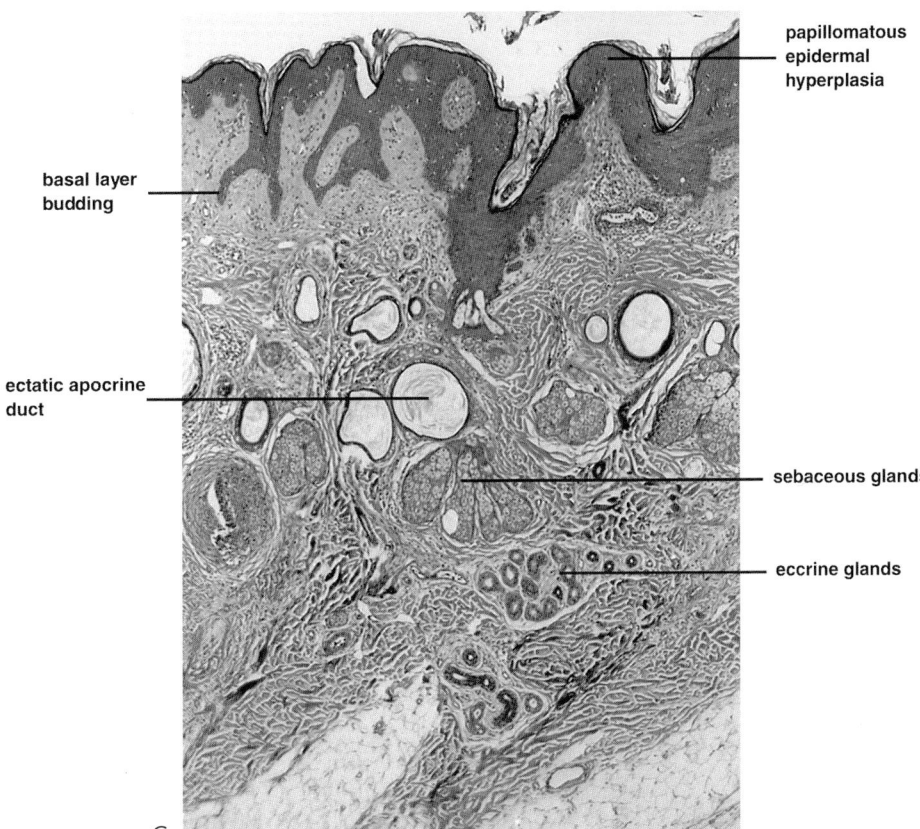

basal layer budding

ectatic apocrine duct

papillomatous epidermal hyperplasia

sebaceous glands

eccrine glands

C

Figure 15-9 *(continued).* **(C)** The abundant apocrine, eccrine, and sebaceous glands are seen in the dermis. Some apocrine ducts are markedly ectatic.

Darier's disease is used. The disorders are otherwise identical and probably represent the same mosaic process.[85,86]

2. Epidermolytic hyperkeratosis may be seen in a linear hyperkeratotic lesion without any clinical features of a congenital ichthyotic disorder. The old term of *ichthyosis hystrix* is sometimes applied to this lesion.

3. Acantholysis with only minimal dyskeratosis, as in Hailey-Hailey disease, may also be found.

4. Occasionally inflammation, dyskeratosis, and a predominance of eosinophils may be present, mimicking incontinentia pigmenti.

5. Porokeratosis with numerous cornoid lamellae may be seen. When other elements of an epidermal nevus are present, the cornoid lamellae are irrelevant. When they are found only in a linear lesion, either of two diagnoses may be applied: linear porokeratosis or porokeratotic epidermal nevus; we view them as the same process.[86]

6. Comedo nevi not surprisingly contain large dilated plugged hair follicles (Fig. 15-10). However, these changes are not identical to acne. The follicles are large, almost U shaped, with concentric hyperkeratosis and compact lamellate scale. There is little if any inflammation, and closed comedones as seen in acne are not present. On the palms and soles, the plugs involve eccrine ostia and ducts. Other features of linear epidermal nevus may also be seen.

7. Inflammatory linear verrucous epidermal nevus (ILVEN) has many features that are nonspecific: hyperkeratosis, parakeratosis, acanthosis, spongiosis, and a dermal mononuclear infil-

trate. One clue (Fig. 15-11) is an alternating epidermal pattern with parakeratotic caps over a missing granular layer admixed with compact hyperkeratosis over a normal granular layer. The papillary dermis also usually exhibits vertically oriented thickened collagen bundles as in lichen simplex chronicus because inflammatory linear verrucous epidermal nevus is frequently pruritic and rubbed. The histologic features of inflammatory linear verrucous epidermal nevus are psoriasiform, but the term *psoriasiform epidermal nevus* seems inappropriate.

8. The demarcated unilateral lesions in CHILD syndrome have been described as psoriasiform, as ichthyotic, or as ILVEN. None is correct, but psoriasiform comes closest. There is orthohyperkeratosis alternating with parakeratosis, and collections of neutrophils may be found in the stratum corneum, just as in psoriasis (Munro microabscesses). A unique feature is the accumulation of lipid-filled histiocytes in the dermal papillae; this change is known as verruciform xanthoma (see Ch. 16).

9. Lichenoid epidermal nevus: some epidermal nevi mimic lichen planus histologically.[88] The main differential diagnostic consideration is lichen striatus. Often one cannot make a confident diagnosis either clinically or histologically and must simply wait to see if the lesion is permanent (epidermal nevus) or resolves (lichen striatus).

POROKERATOSIS

Porokeratosis is a disorder of epidermal keratinization defined by a unique histologic feature, the cornoid lamella.[89]

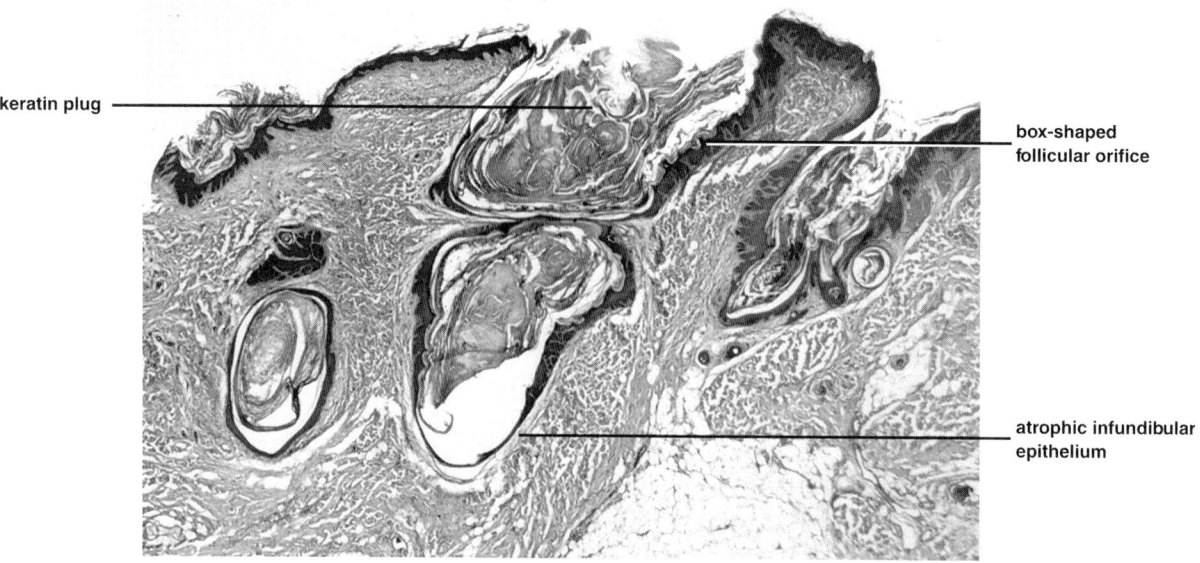

keratin plug

box-shaped
follicular orifice

atrophic infundibular
epithelium

Figure 15-10. Comedone nevus. The comedones have no inflammation around them and are more rectangular in shape than in acne.

Clinical Features

The two main types of porokeratosis are porokeratosis of Mibelli and disseminated superficial actinic porokeratosis. *Porokeratosis of Mibelli* consists of annular lesions with a sharp collarette scale. The disorder is usually sporadic and may develop in patients who are immunosuppressed. Especially in such hosts, porokeratosis of Mibelli may evolve into squamous cell carcinoma.[53]

In *disseminated superficial actinic porokeratosis*, patients have few to hundreds of annular well-defined scaly macules most often in sun-exposed regions, especially the arms and legs.[90] Lesions can be experimentally induced by light.[91] Not all lesions are in areas of sun exposure, and immunosuppression is another co-factor. Palmar-plantar lesions are not seen. The annular lesions start small, usually only a few millimeters in diameter, and gradually spread peripherally. They resemble ac-

Figure 15-11. Inflammatory linear verrucous epidermal nevus. There is a sharp transition from a granular layer and orthokeratosis to the absence of granular layer and parakeratosis.

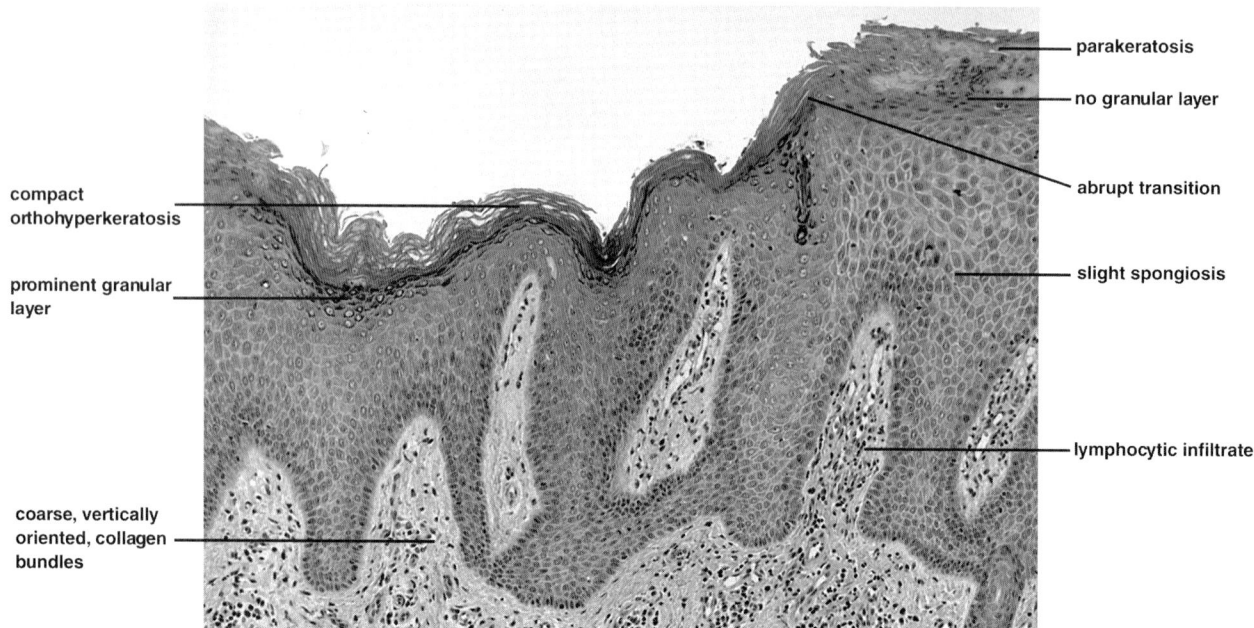

compact
orthohyperkeratosis

prominent granular
layer

coarse, vertically
oriented, collagen
bundles

parakeratosis

no granular layer

abrupt transition

slight spongiosis

lymphocytic infiltrate

tinic keratoses but are more uniform with raised borders and flat centers. Although they have the potential for malignant transformation, the risk is low.

Less common types of porokeratosis include the following:

1. Disseminated porokeratosis: patients have hundreds of lesions, not just in sun-exposed areas. Palmar-plantar involvement may be striking.[92]
2. Discrete palmar-plantar porokeratosis: similar to above, but localized.
3. Punctate plantar porokeratosis: these lesions look like corns, but have a parakeratotic column in their hyperkeratotic plug. The plug may originate in an acrosyringium.[53]
4. Linear porokeratosis: some linear epidermal nevi are dominated by porokeratosis.[87] Malignant transformation has also been reported in this setting.

Finally, there are situations in which a cornoid lamella is found, but porokeratosis is not present; for example, in many ordinary actinic keratoses, columns of parakeratosis are common and difficult to distinguish from cornoid lamellae.

Histopathologic Features

The hallmark of porokeratosis is the cornoid lamella, a focal area of granular layer change associated with a column of parakeratosis[93,94] (Fig. 15-12). The cornoid lamella corresponds to the clinically well-defined peripheral rim. It is important to obtain a specimen in which the orientation is clear so that the cornoid lamella is not lost. Usually a thin ellipse whose long axis is perpendicular to the rim is most ideal. The histopathology laboratory should be alerted to the suspected diagnosis so that sections will be cut along the long axis.

Other changes are less consistent. There may be varying degrees of inflammation. Disseminated superficial actinic porokeratosis lesions are usually less definite and have a less well-

Figure 15-12. Porokeratosis. (**A**) Both sides of the lesion are shown with two cornoid lamellae. The intervening epidermis is somewhat depressed, just as is seen clinically, but otherwise unaffected. (**B**) The left side of the above lesion at higher power shows two prominent cornoid lamellae or columns of parakeratosis with an absent granular layer at the base of each.

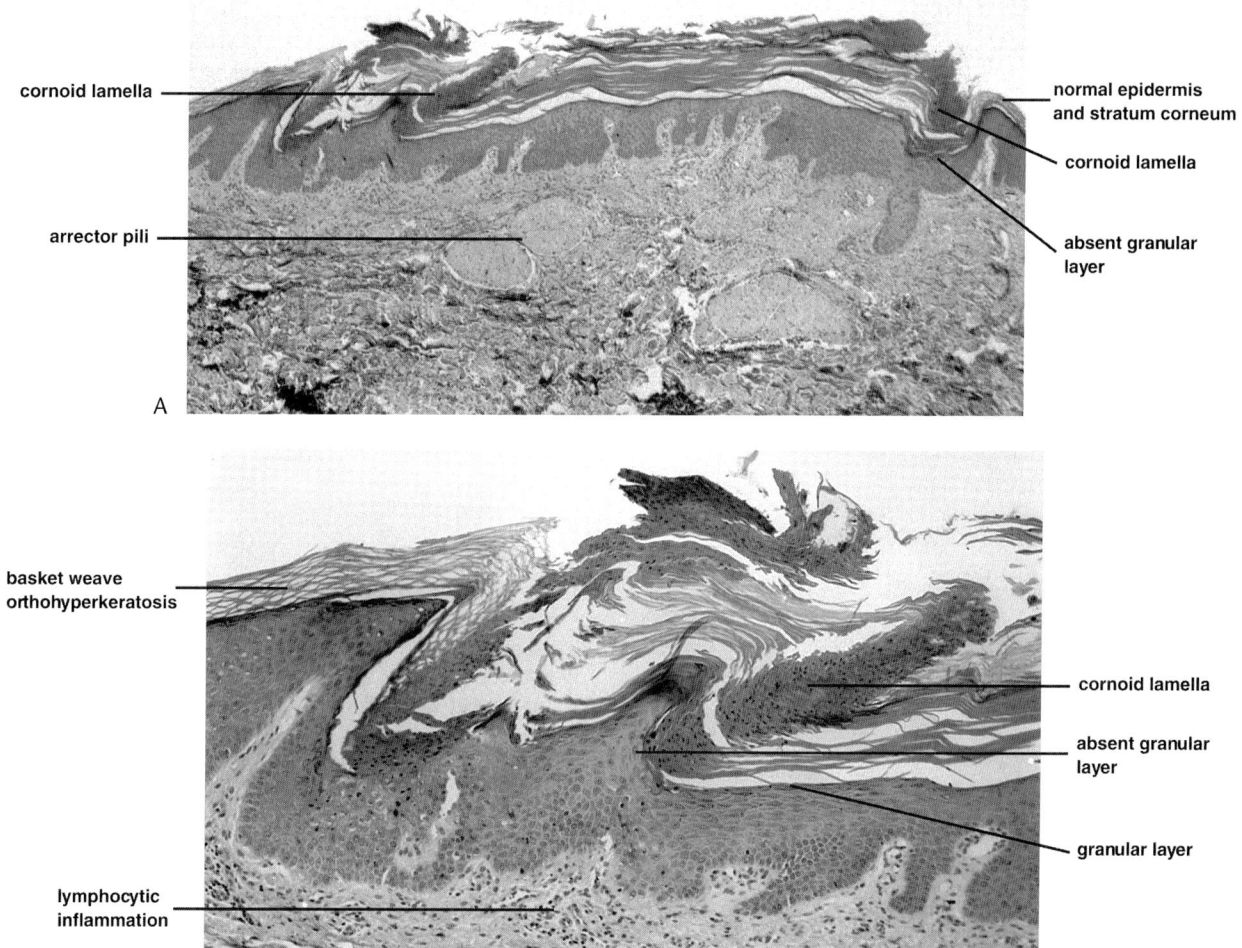

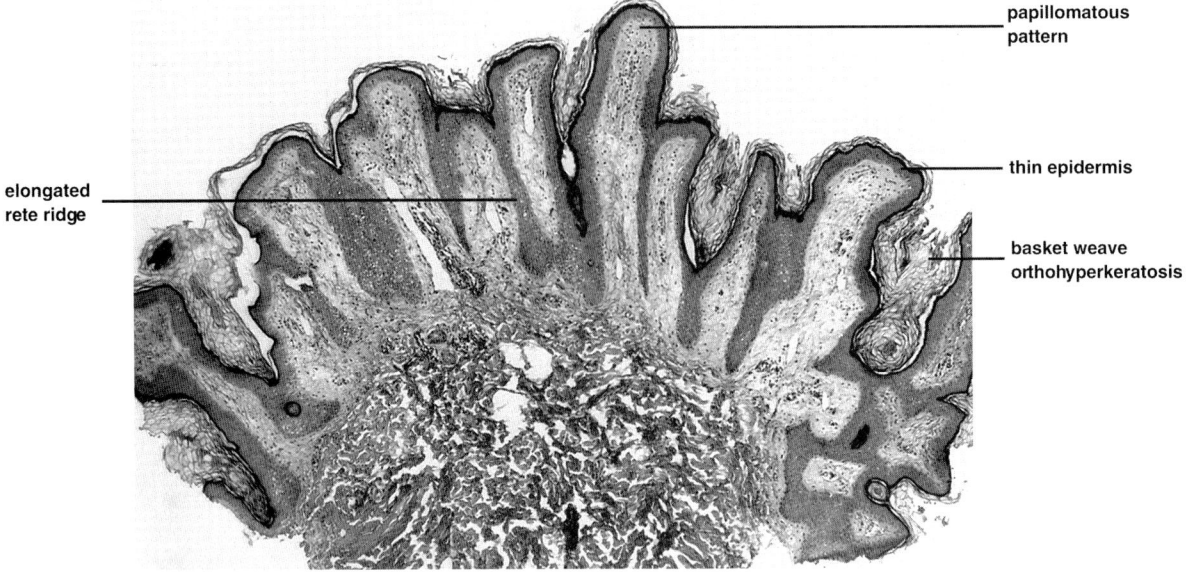

elongated
rete ridge

papillomatous
pattern

thin epidermis

basket weave
orthohyperkeratosis

Figure 15-13. Acanthosis nigricans. There is marked papillomatosis and focal basket-weave orthohyperkeratosis. In addition, the disease process extends to both edges of the specimen, for this was a punch biopsy from a large plaque. That is the best clue that this is not a focal lesion such as seborrheic keratosis or acrokeratosis verruciformis.

defined rim histologically. In their center disseminated superficial actinic porokeratosis lesions show effacement of rete ridges, vacuolar changes in the basal layer, a perivascular mononuclear infiltrate, and melanophages.[95]

Clinicopathologic Correlation

The origin of the cornoid lamella has remained an intriguing question for decades. Because many porokeratotic lesions are annular with the characteristic cornoid lamella occurring peripherally as central clearing appears, it has been suggested that porokeratosis represents a clone of atypical epithelial cells that spread peripherally.[96,97] Most other epithelial clones (such as warts) grow initially in a vertical fashion and do not have a centrifugal growth pattern. The relationship with immunosuppression has raised the question of a viral etiology, but no pathogenic organism has been found.

ACANTHOSIS NIGRICANS

Acanthosis nigricans is a papillomatous epidermal alteration most often in flexural areas.

Clinical Features

Acanthosis nigricans presents as velvety brown patches in the axilla, groin, and nape of the neck. It occurs in several different clinical settings[98–100]:

1. Familial: early onset, usually autosomal dominant, often associated with other abnormalities
2. Endocrine: overlaps with familial, as it is seen in familial insulin resistance, polycystic ovary syndrome, and many other disorders

3. Malignant: late onset, associated with internal malignancy, usually intestinal adenocarcinoma, but seen with lymphomas and sarcomas as well; may precede the signs or symptoms of the internal tumor
4. Idiopathic: tends to occur in obese patients, more commonly in blacks and Hispanics, who have no obvious endocrine basis for their weight problem

Histopathologic Features

All forms of acanthosis nigricans look identical under the microscope. The two cardinal features are papillomatosis and hyperkeratosis, which causes the darkening. There is no increase in the thickness of the epidermis above the elongated dermal papillae and little if any hyperpigmentation[101] (Fig. 15-13).

Differential Diagnosis

Acanthosis nigricans may be indistinguishable from many other papillomatous lesions, including old warts, seborrheic keratoses, epidermal nevi, acrokeratosis verruciformis, and confluent and reticulated papillomatosis.

Pathophysiology

Acanthosis nigricans may in some cases be modulated by epidermal growth factor or a related substance. Various patterns of keratin expression have been described.[102] One case report describes the waxing and waning of acanthosis nigricans as levels of mediator fluctuated in a patient with metastatic malignant melanoma.[103] There also appears to be an overlap between acanthosis nigricans, eruptive skin tags, and eruptive seborrheic keratoses (the sign of Leser-Trélat), as all are tumor markers.

CONFLUENT AND RETICULATED PAPILLOMATOSIS

Confluent and reticulated papillomatosis of Gougerot and Carteaud is a diffuse, minimally scaly truncal eruption.[104]

Clinical Features

Confluent and reticulated papillomatosis occurs most often on the chest and back of obese patients and is more common in dark-skinned persons. The lesions are tan or brown, scaly, and may coalesce into patches (confluent) or have a lacy pattern (reticulate). There may be clinical overlaps with acanthosis nigricans.[105]

Histopathologic Features

The pattern is similar to acanthosis nigricans, but generally the changes are less extreme[106] (Fig. 15-14).

Pathophysiology

Malassezia furfur has been suggested as a trigger for confluent and reticulated papillomatosis in some cases. Special stains for organisms, however, are usually negative.

ACROKERATOSIS VERRUCIFORMIS

Acrokeratosis verruciformis is a disorder with focal, usually acral, hyperkeratotic papules.

Clinical Features

There are many tiny, asymptomatic, flat-topped or warty papules on the dorsa of the hands and feet. They are usually white or light colored but often darken with sun exposure. They may occur alone or in association with Darier's disease, but in either event are inherited in an autosomal dominant pattern. They tend to be more persistent than the other cutaneous lesions of Darier's disease.[107,108]

Histopathologic Features

There are well-demarcated spikes of papillomatosis and ortho-hyperkeratosis—"church spiring" (Fig. 15-15). No granular layer abnormalities are seen. The dermis is normal. In cases associated with Darier's disease, dyskeratosis is seen in some lesions.

Differential Diagnosis

The clinical and histologic differential diagnoses differ. Clinically, stucco keratoses, verrucae vulgares, and seborrheic keratoses are usually considered. Warts should have granular layer changes, but small seborrheic keratoses or stucco keratoses are sometimes identical to acrokeratosis verruciformis histologically. The small size of acrokeratosis verruciformis usually suggests the diagnosis. However, if the size of the lesion cannot be determined, still other diseases also mimic acrokeratosis verruciformis. They include acanthosis nigricans, confluent and reticulated papillomatosis, and some forms of ichthyosis.

There are also a number of rarer disorders that present with acral papules. They remotely enter into the differential diagnosis:

1. *Acrokeratoelastoidosis*: patients have umbilicated papules. Most are concentrated at the junction of the dorsal and palmar skin (line of transgradience), but some may also occur on the dorsa of the hands. They are inherited in an autosomal dominant pattern. Trauma seems to induce the lesions.[109]

   There is compact orthohyperkeratosis over a hyperplastic acral epidermis. In the dermis, there are coarse fragmented elastic fibers, described as elastorrhexis.

2. *Keratoelastoidalis marginalis* (degenerative collagenous plaques, digital papular calcific elastosis): a type of solar elastosis that typically occurs along the line of transgradience in the notch between the thumb and index finger. The lesions are large plaques and are only confusing because of their name, not their clinical or histologic features.

Figure 15-14. Confluent and reticulated papillomatosis. There is hyperkeratosis and some papillomatosis, but not as extreme as in the example of acanthosis nigricans in Figure 15-13. This is histologically compatible with a relatively flat seborrheic keratosis, but it was from a widespread eruption on the back of a young adult.

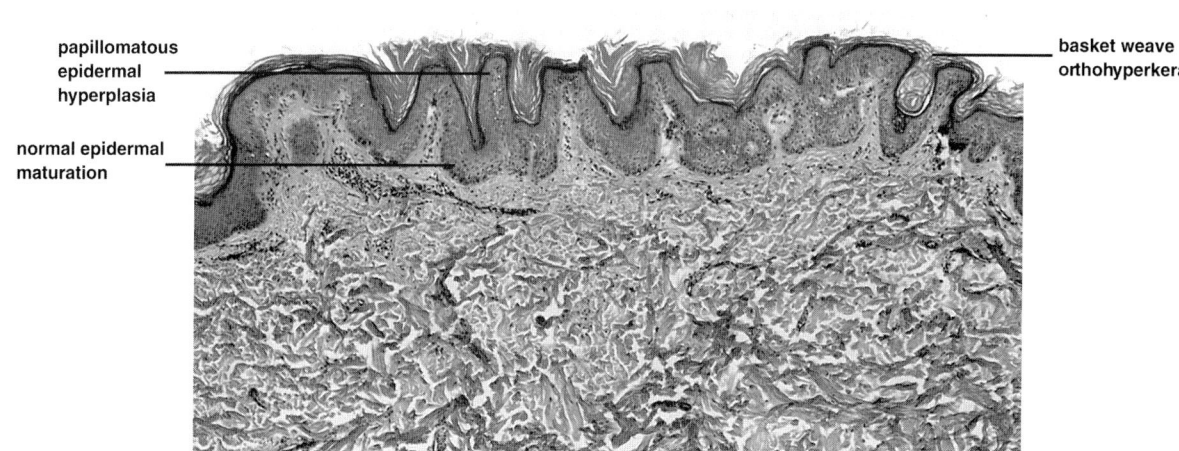

papillomatous epidermal hyperplasia

normal epidermal maturation

basket weave orthohyperkeratosis

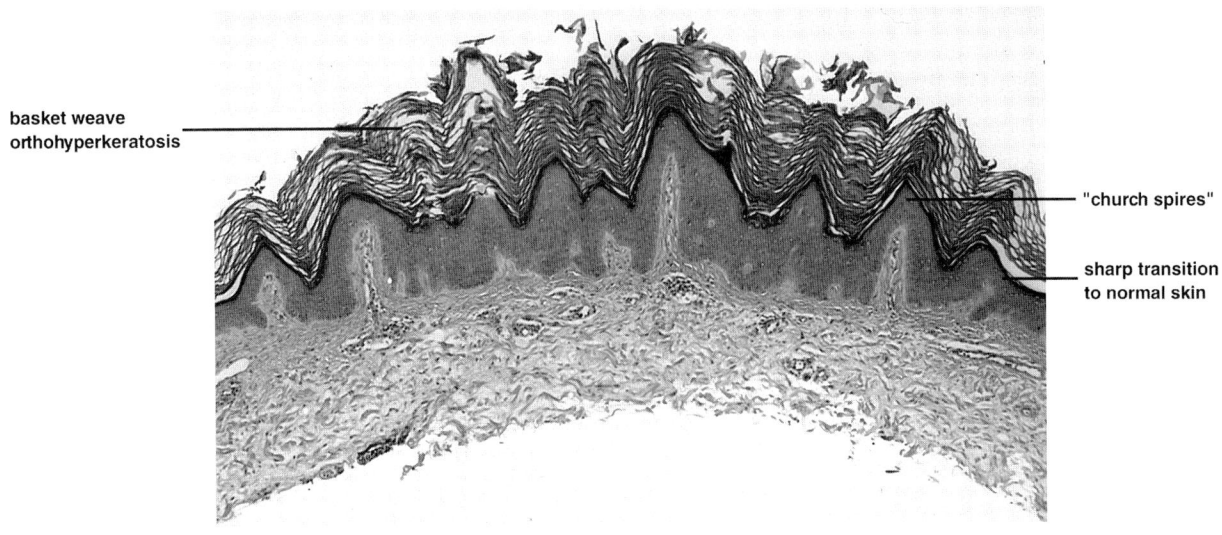

Figure 15-15. Acrokeratosis verruciformis. This is the prototype of church spire-like papillomatosis in a small lesion.

The epidermis is either normal or reveals light-induced changes. In the dermis is marked solar elastosis and often calcification.[110]

3. *Focal acral hyperkeratosis*: this disorder is clinically identical to acrokeratoelastoidosis and may also be autosomal dominantly inherited or occur sporadically.[111]

Sections show focal orthohyperkeratosis often with some epidermal atrophy, in a clavus or corn pattern. No elastic fiber changes are present.

4. *Hyperkeratosis lenticularis perstans* (Flegel's disease): numerous compact tiny scaly papules are concentrated over the dorsal feet and ankles, but may occur elsewhere.[112]

Histologic diagnosis is usually possible by recognition of a circumscribed focus with vertically arranged layers comprised by (1) compact hyperkeratosis, (2) epidermal atrophy, and (3) lichenoid infiltrate.

ACKNOWLEDGMENT

Professor H. Traupe, M.D., Münster, Germany, generously allowed me to review his extensive collection of skin biopsy specimens from patients with various ichthyoses, and patiently answered many questions.

REFERENCES

1. Smack DP, Korge BP, James WD: Keratin and keratinization. J Am Acad Dermatol 30:85, 1994
2. Williams ML, Elias PM: From basket weave to barrier: unifying concepts for the pathogenesis of the diseases of cornification. Arch Dermatol 129:626, 1993
3. Traupe H: The Ichthyoses. Springer-Verlag, Berlin, 1989
4. Novice FM, Collison DW, Burgdorf WHC, Esterly NB: Handbook of Genetic Skin Disorders. WB Saunders, Philadelphia, 1994
5. Williams ML, Elias PM: Genetically transmitted, generalized disorders of cornification. The ichthyoses. Dermatol Clin 5:155, 1987
6. Frost P, Van Scott EJ: Ichthyosiform dermatoses. Arch Dermatol 94:113, 1966
7. Mevorah B, Krayenbuhl A, Bovey EH, van Melle GD: Autosomal dominant ichthyosis and X-linked ichthyosis: comparison of their clinical and histological phenotypes. Acta Derm Venereol 71:431, 1991
8. Anton-Lamprecht I: Electron microscopy in the early diagnosis of genetic disorders of the skin. Dermatologica 157:65, 1978
9. Holbrook KA, Smith LT, Elias S: Prenatal diagnosis of genetic skin disease using fetal skin biopsies. Arch Dermatol 129:1437, 1993
10. Ackerman AB: Histopathologic concept of epidermolytic hyperkeratosis. Arch Dermatol 102:253, 1970
11. Anton-Lamprecht I, Curth HO, Schnyder UW: Zur Ultrastruktur hereditärer Verhornungsstörungen. II. Ichthyosis hystrix Typ Curth-Macklin. Arch Dermatol Forsch 246:77, 1973
12. Traupe H, Kolde G, Hamm H, Happle R: Ichthyosis bullosa of Siemens: a unique type of epidermolytic hyperkeratosis. J Am Acad Dermatol 14:1000, 1986
13. Mills CM, Marks R: Acral epidermolytic hyperkeratosis. Br J Dermatol 128:342, 1993
14. Sahn EE, Weimer CE Jr, Garen PD: Annular epidermolytic ichthyosis: a unique phenotype. J Am Acad Dermatol 27:348, 1992

15. Hirone T, Fukushiro R: Disseminated epidermolytic acanthoma. Acta Derm Venereol 53:393, 1973
16. Ackerman AB, Reed RJ: Epidermolytic variant of solar keratosis. Arch Dermatol 107:104, 1973
17. Feinstein A, Ackerman AB, Ziprkowski L: Histology of autosomal dominant ichthyosis vulgaris and X-linked ichthyosis. Arch Dermatol 101:524, 1970
18. Anton-Lamprecht I, Hofbauer U: Ultrastructural distinction of autosomal dominant ichthyosis vulgaris and X-linked recessive ichthyosis. Hum Genet 15:261, 1972
19. Fartasch M, Haneke E, Anton-Lamprecht I: Ultrastructural study of the occurrence of autosomal dominant ichthyosis vulgaris in atopic eczema. Arch Dermatol Res 279:270, 1987
20. Anton-Lamprecht I, Kahlke W: Zur Ultrastruktur hereditärer Verhornungsstörungen. V. Ichthyosis beim Refsum-Syndrom (Heredopathia atactica polyneuritiformis). Arch Dermatol Forsch 250:185, 1974
21. Price VH, Odom RB, Ward WH, Jones FT: Trichothiodystrophy: sulfur-deficient brittle hair as a marker for a neuroectodermal symptom complex. Arch Dermatol 116:1375, 1980
22. Kolde G, Happle R: Histologic and ultrastructural features of the ichthyotic skin in X-linked dominant chondrodysplasia punctata. Acta Derm Venereol 64:389, 1984
23. Williams ML, Elias PM: Heterogeneity in autosomal recessive ichthyosis: clinical and biochemical differentiation of lamellar ichthyosis and nonbullous congenital ichthyosiform erythroderma. Arch Dermatol 121:477, 1985
24. Niemi K-M, Kanerva L, Kuokkanen K, Ignatius J: Clinical, light and electron microscopic features of recessive congenital ichthyosis type 1. Br J Dermatol 130:626, 1994
25. Arnold ML, Anton-Lamprecht I, Melz-Rothfuss B, Hartschuh W: Ichthyosis congenita type III: clinical and ultrastructural characteristics and distinction within the heterogeneous ichthyosis congenita group. Arch Dermatol Res 280:268, 1988
26. Kolde G, Happle R, Traupe H: Autosomal-dominant lamellar ichthyosis: ultrastructural characteristics of a new type of congenital ichthyosis. Arch Dermatol Res 278:1, 1985
27. Roberts LJ: Long-term survival of a harlequin fetus. J Am Acad Dermatol 21:335, 1989
28. Fleck RM, Barnadas MD, Schulz WW et al: Harlequin ichthyosis: an ultrastructural study. J Am Acad Dermatol 21:999, 1989
29. Eng AM, Leischner RP, Hill D: Harlequin fetus. J Cutan Pathol 6:519, 1979
30. Williams ML, Koch TK, O'Donnell JJ et al: Ichthyosis and neutral lipid storage disease. Am J Med Genet 20:711, 1985
31. Langer K, Konrad K, Wolff K: Keratitis, ichthyosis and deafness (KID) syndrome: report of three cases and review of the literature. Br J Dermatol 122:689, 1990
32. Silverman AK, Ellis CN, Beals TF, Woo TY: Continual skin peeling syndrome: an electron-microscopic study. Arch Dermatol 122:71, 1986
33. Hofer PA, Jagell S: Sjögren-Larsson syndrome: a dermato-histopathological study. J Cutan Pathol 9:360, 1982
34. Levisohn D, Dintiman B, Rizzo WB: Sjögren-Larsson syndrome: case reports. Pediatr Dermatol 8:217, 1991
35. Gewirtzman GB, Winkler NW, Dobson RL: Erythrokeratodermia variabilis: a family study. Arch Dermatol 114:259, 1978
36. Mevorah B, Frenk E, Brooke EM: Ichthyosis linearis circumflexa comel: a clinicostatistical approach to its relationship with Netherton's syndrome. Dermatologica 149:201, 1974
37. Krafchik B: Netherton syndrome. Pediatr Dermatol 9:157, 1992
38. Levy SB, Goldsmith LA: The peeling skin syndrome. J Am Acad Dermatol 7:606, 1982
39. Burge SM, Wilkinson JD: Darier-White disease: a review of the clinical features in 163 patients. J Am Acad Dermatol 27:40, 1992
40. Munro CS: The phenotype of Darier's disease: penetrance and expressivity in adults and children. Br J Dermatol 127:126, 1992
41. Peck GL, Kraemer KH, Wetzel B et al: Cornifying Darier disease—a unique variant. Arch Dermatol 112:495, 1976
42. Sato A, Anton-Lamprecht I, Schnyder VW: Ultrastructure of dyskeratosis in Morbus Darier. J Cutan Pathol 4:173, 1977
43. Graham JH, Helwig EB: Isolated dyskeratosis follicularis. Arch Dermatol 77:377, 1958
44. Tanaya A, Mehregan AH: Warty dyskeratoma. Dermatologica 138:155, 1969
45. Price M, Russell Jones R: Familial dyskeratotic comedones. Clin Exp Dermatol 10:147, 1985
46. Grover RW, Rosenbaum R: The association of transient acantholytic dermatosis with other skin diseases. J Am Acad Dermatol 11:253, 1984
47. Chalet M, Grover R, Ackerman AB: Transient acantholytic dermatosis. Arch Dermatol 113:431, 1977
48. Ackerman AB: Focal acantholytic dyskeratosis. Arch Dermatol 106:702, 1972
49. Brownstein MH: Acantholytic acanthoma. J Am Acad Dermatol 19:783, 1988
50. Coppola G, Muscardin LM, Piazza P: Papular acantholytic dyskeratosis. Am J Dermatopathol 8:364, 1986
51. Itin PH: Classification of autosomal dominant palmoplantar keratoderma: past-present-future. Dermatology 185:163, 1992
52. Lucker GP, van de Kerkhof PC, Steijlen PM: The hereditary palmoplantar keratoses: an updated review and classification. Br J Dermatol 131:1, 1994
53. Stevens HP, Kelsell DP, Bryant SP et al: Linkage of an American pedigree with palmoplantar keratoderma and malignancy (palmoplantar ectodermal dysplasia type III) to 17q24: literature survey and proposed updated classification of the keratodermas. Arch Dermatol 132:640, 1996
54. Küster W, Zehender D, Mensing H et al: Keratosis palmoplantaris diffusa Vörner: klinische, formalgenetische und molekularbiologische Untersuchungen bei 22 Familien. Hautarzt 47:705, 1995
55. Rustad OJ, Vance JC: Punctate keratoses of the palms and soles and keratotic pits of the palmar creases. J Am Acad Dermatol 22:468, 1990
56. Feinstein A, Friedman J, Schewach-Millet M: Pachyonychia congenita. J Am Acad Dermatol 19:705, 1988

57. Su WP, Chun SI, Hammond DE, Gordon H: Pachyonychia congenita: a clinical study of 12 cases and review of the literature. Pediatr Dermatol 7:33, 1990

58. Tidman MJ, Wells RS, MacDonald DM: Pachyonychia congenita with cutaneous amyloidosis and hyperpigmentation—a distinct variant. J Am Acad Dermatol 16:935, 1987

59. Drachtman RA, Alter BP: Dyskeratosis congenita: clinical and genetic heterogeneity. Report of a new case and review of the literature. Am J Pediatr Hematol Oncol 14:297, 1992

60. Ogden GR, Connor E, Chisholm DM: Dyskeratosis congenita: report of a case and review of the literature. Oral Surg Oral Med Oral Pathol 65:586, 1988

61. Ling NS, Fenske NA, Julius RL et al: Dyskeratosis congenita in a girl simulating chronic graft-vs-host disease. Arch Dermatol 121:1424, 1985

62. Freire-Maia N, Pinheiro M: Ectodermal Dysplasias: a Clinical and Genetic Study. Alan R. Liss, New York, 1984

63. Gilgenkrantz S, Blanchet-Bardon C, Nazzaro V et al: Hypohidrotic ectodermal dysplasia: clinical study of a family of 30 over three generations. Hum Genet 81:120, 1989

64. Upshaw BY, Montgomery H: Hereditary anhidrotic ectodermal dysplasia. Arch Dermatol Syphiligr 60:1170, 1949

65. Lambert WC, Bilinski DL: Diagnostic pitfalls in anhidrotic ectodermal dysplasia: indications for palmar skin biopsy. Cutis 31:182, 1983

66. Happle R: What is a nevus? A proposed definition of a common medical term. Dermatology 191:1, 1995

67. Happle R: Mosaicism in human skin: understanding the patterns and mechanisms. Arch Dermatol 129:1460, 1993

68. Nazzaro V, Ermacora E, Santucci B et al: Epidermolytic hyperkeratosis: generalized form in children from parents with systematized linear form. Br J Dermatol 122:417, 1990

69. Paller AS, Snyder AJ, Chan YM et al: Genetic and clinical mosaicism in a type of epidermal nevus. N Engl J Med 331:1408, 1994

70. Solomon LM, Esterly NB: Epidermal and other congenital organoid nevi. Curr Prob Pediatr 6:2, 1976

71. Rogers M: Epidermal nevi and the epidermal nevus syndrome: a review of 233 cases. Pediatr Dermatol 9:342, 1992

72. Wilson Jones E, Heyl T: Naevus sebaceus. Br J Dermatol 82:99, 1970

73. Leppard B, Marks R: Comedone naevus: a report of nine cases. Trans St. Johns Hosp Dermatol Soc 59:45, 1973

74. Cestari TF, Rubim M, Valentini BC: Nevus comedonicus: case report and brief review of the literature. Pediatr Dermatol 8:300, 1991

75. Kim SC, Kang WH: Nevus comedonicus associated with epidermal nevus. J Am Acad Dermatol 21:1085, 1989

76. Altman J, Mehregan AH: Inflammatory linear verrucose epidermal nevus. Arch Dermatol 104:385, 1971

77. de Jong E, Rulo HF, van de Kerkhof PC: Inflammatory linear verrucous epidermal nevus (ILVEN) versus linear psoriasis: a clinical, histological and immunohistochemical study. Acta Derm Venereol 71:343, 1991

78. Hebert AA, Esterly NB, Holbrook KA, Hall JC: The CHILD syndrome: histologic and ultrastructural studies. Arch Dermatol 123:503, 1987

79. Happle R, Mittag H, Küster W: The CHILD nevus: a distinct skin disorder. Dermatology 191:210, 1995

80. Rogers M, McCrossin I, Commens C: Epidermal nevi and the epidermal nevus syndrome. A review of 131 cases. J Am Acad Dermatol 20:476, 1989

81. Happle R: How many epidermal nevus syndromes exist? A clinicogenetic classification. J Am Acad Dermatol 25:550, 1991

82. Su WPD: Histopathologic varieties of epidermal nevus. Am J Dermatopathol 4:161, 1982

83. Alessi E, Wong SN, Advani HH et al: Nevus sebaceus is associated with unusual neoplasms. Am J Dermatopathol 10:116, 1988

84. Mehregan AH, Pinkus H: Life history of organoid nevi. Arch Dermatol 91:574, 1965

85. Cambiaghi S, Brusasco A, Grimalt R, Caputo R: Acantholytic dyskeratotic epidermal nevus as a mosaic form of Darier's disease. J Am Acad Dermatol 32:284, 1995

86. Munro CS, Cox NH: An acantholytic dyskeratotic epidermal nevus with other features of Darier's disease on the same side of the body. Br J Dermatol 127:168, 1992

87. Rahbari H, Cordero AA, Mehregan AH: Linear porokeratosis. Arch Dermatol 109:526, 1974

88. Brownstein MH, Silverstein L, Lefing W: Lichenoid epidermal nevus: "Linear lichen planus." J Am Acad Dermatol 20:913, 1989

89. Jurecka W, Neumann RA, Knobler RM: Porokeratoses: immunohistochemical, light and electron microscopic evaluation. J Am Acad Dermatol 24:96, 1991

90. Chernosky ME, Freeman RG: Disseminated superficial actinic porokeratosis (DSAP). Arch Dermatol 96:611, 1967

91. Neumann RA, Knobler RM, Jurecka W, Gebhart W: Disseminated superficial actinic porokeratosis: experimental induction and exacerbation of skin lesions. J Am Acad Dermatol 21:1182, 1989

92. McCallister RE, Estes SA, Yarbrough CL: Porokeratosis plantaris, palmaris, et disseminata. J Am Acad Dermatol 13:598, 1985

93. Wade TR, Ackerman AB: Cornoid lamellation: a histologic reaction pattern. Am J Dermatopathol 2:5, 1980

94. Ito M, Fujiwara H, Maruyama T et al: Morphogenesis of the cornoid lamella: histochemical, immunohistochemical and ultrastructural study of porokeratosis. J Cutan Pathol 18:247, 1991

95. Shumack S, Commens C, Kossard S: Disseminated superficial actinic porokeratosis: a histological review of 61 cases with particular reference to lymphocytic inflammation. Am J Dermatopathol 13:26, 1991

96. Reed RJ, Leone P: Porokeratosis: a mutant clonal keratosis of the epidermis. Arch Dermatol 101:340, 1970

97. Gray MH, Smoller BS, McNutt NS: Carcinogenesis in porokeratosis: evidence for a role relating to chronic growth activation of keratinocytes. Am J Dermatopathol 13:438, 1991

98. Brown J, Winkelmann RK: Acanthosis nigricans: a study of 90 cases. Medicine (Baltimore) 47:33, 1968

99. Curth HO: Classification of acanthosis nigricans. Int J Dermatol 15:592, 1976

100. Schwartz RW: Acanthosis nigricans. J Am Acad Dermatol 31:1, 1994

101. Hall JM, Moreland A, Cox GJ et al: Oral acanthosis nigricans: report of a case and comparison of oral and cutaneous pathology. Am J Dermatopathol 10:68, 1988
102. Bonnekoh B, Wevers A, Spangenberger H et al: Keratin pattern of acanthosis nigricans in syndromelike association with polythelia, polycystic kidneys, and syndactyly. Arch Dermatol 129:1177, 1993
103. Ellis DL, Kafka SP, Chow JC et al: Melanoma, growth factors, acanthosis nigricans, the sign of Leser-Trelat, and multiple acrochordons. N Engl J Med 317:1582, 1987
104. Hamilton D, Tawafoghi V, Shafer GC, Hambrick GW: Confluent and reticulated papillomatosis of Gougerot and Carteaud. J Am Acad Dermatol 2:401, 1980
105. Hirokawa M, Matsumoto M, Iizuka H: Confluent and reticulated papillomatosis: a case with concurrent acanthosis nigricans associated with obesity and insulin resistance. Dermatology 188:148, 1994
106. Jimbow M, Talpash O, Jimbow K: Confluent and reticulated papillomatosis: clinical, light and electron microscopic studies. Int J Dermatol 31:480, 1992
107. Waisman M: Verruciform manifestations of keratosis follicularis. Arch Dermatol 81:1, 1960
108. Panja RK: Acrokeratosis verruciformis (Hopf): a clinical entity? Br J Dermatol 96:643, 1977
109. Highet AS, Rook A, Anderson JR: Acrokeratoelastoidosis. Br J Dermatol 106:337, 1982
110. Jordaan HF, Rossouw DJ: Digital papular calcific elastosis: a histopathological, histochemical and ultrastructural study of 20 patients. J Cutan Pathol 17:358, 1990
111. Dowd PM, Harman RRM, Black MM: Focal acral hyperkeratosis. Br J Dermatol 109:97, 1983
112. Frenk E, Tapernoux B: Hyperkeratosis lenticularis perstans (Flegel). Dermatologica 153:253, 1976

16

DERMAL MALFORMATIONS, ALTERATIONS, AND DEPOSITS

Many unrelated clinical disorders are characterized by dermal changes. They are identified by an excess or deficit of normal dermal collagen or elastic fibers, by abnormalities of these fibers, or by the replacement of the normal dermal structures by other materials such as bone, calcium, mucin, or amyloid.

Abnormalities of dermal structure may be very subtle. It is extremely helpful to have normal dermis from the same patient for comparison. One method to obtain such tissue is to perform an elliptical excision that includes both normal and abnormal skin along its long axis. The tissue is then oriented to contain both tissues in the same section. For some diseases, especially atrophoderma, the transition from normal to abnormal skin is crucial, so such a biopsy specimen is required. However, the specimen may be embedded or sectioned incorrectly, or it may be difficult to determine which region is normal. Thus, we recommend the submission of two full-thickness punch or excisional biopsy specimens, one from diseased skin and the other from contralateral normal skin.

The range of dermal abnormalities is so great that it is often difficult to determine with the light microscope whether the dermis is abnormal, much less to accurately identify the abnormality and disease. If the clinical history suggests dermal thickening or thinning and routine sections are not diagnostic, elastic fiber stains should be done. Often the changes are very subtle and difficult to appreciate. For example, both a connective tissue nevus in which collagen is increased and skin from a patient with Ehlers-Danlos syndrome in which collagen is decreased most often look normal under the microscope.

DIAGNOSTIC APPROACH TO DERMAL DISORDERS

An overall diagnostic or algorithmic approach to dermal disorders is difficult to construct. If the dermis appears qualitatively normal, one must decide whether it is thickened or thinned and how well the appendages are represented. A thickened dermis suggests

Scleroderma
Morphea
Eosinophilic fasciitis
Sclerodermoid disorders
Connective tissue nevus
Angiofibroma
Pachydermoperiostitis
Scar
Keloid

When mucin is associated with dermal thickening, scleromyxedema and scleredema should be considered, but mucin is often sparse in the latter.

A thinned dermis is seen with

Radiation dermatitis
Focal dermal hypoplasia
Aplasia cutis congenita
Ehlers-Danlos syndrome
Cutis laxa
Striae
Anetoderma
Acrodermatitis chronica atrophicans
Scar

Despite its name, atrophoderma is usually characterized by a sharp drop at the transition from normal to lesional skin without striking histologic atrophy.

Qualitative dermal abnormalities are slightly easier to approach. Collagen and elastin stain abnormally with hematoxylin and eosin (H&E) in

Pseudoxanthoma elasticum
Reactive perforating collagenosis
Solar elastosis
Elastosis perforans serpiginosa
Ochronosis (*and other exogenous deposits*)

Mucin dominates the picture in

Pretibial myxedema
Scleromyxedema
Mucocele
Myxoma
Digital mucous cyst

In addition, lupus erythematosus may show only dermal mucin, while mucin is a minor part of myxedema and scleredema.

Exogenous deposits include bone and calcified material, while cartilage may be in the wrong place or damaged. The dermis is discolored in ochronosis, hemochromatosis, and argyria, although the latter changes are very subtle. Foamy deposits suggest a xanthoma, but cutaneous xanthomas are found in normolipemic patients following trauma and in several rare disorders. Finally, amorphous dermal deposits include amyloidosis, colloid milium, gout, lipoid proteinosis, and nodular solar elastosis. These differential diagnostic suggestions should point one in the right direction, but a detailed history and special stains are often required to obtain the correct answer.

CONNECTIVE TISSUE DISORDERS

Dermal Thickening and Hypertrophy

Scleroderma and Related Conditions

Dermal sclerosis is a manifestation of many disorders. The histopathologic differences between diseases as clinically unlike as progressive systemic sclerosis (SS) and sclerodermoid porphyria cutanea tarda are minimal. Thus, the clinical history is of great importance. The following disorders have prominent dermal sclerosis and are generally indistinguishable microscopically. Their histopathologic features are discussed together at the end of the section.

Scleroderma

Scleroderma (SS) is a multisystem disorder that most often involves the skin, gastrointestinal tract, lungs, and kidneys.

Clinical Features. In the skin, typical clinical findings include cutaneous sclerosis, perioral tightening, Raynaud's phenomenon, and acral ulcerations.[1,2] Telangiectases and cutaneous calcinosis are more common in the CREST syndrome, but they also occur in SS patients. CREST is an acronym for *c*alcinosis, *R*aynaud's phenomenon, *e*sophageal disorders, *s*clerodactyly, and *t*elangiectases. Sclerosis may be a part of several connective tissue overlap syndromes, including mixed connective tissue disease.

Clinicopathologic Correlation. Nearly all patients with SS have serum antinuclear antibodies. Antibodies against Scl-70 identify diffuse disease, whereas anticentromere antibodies are most often positive in CREST syndrome.

Pathophysiology. The etiology of SS and other forms of dermal sclerosis remains unknown. Both immunologic and vascular factors appear to play a role, and mast cells and eosinophils may be important mediators. In late 1989 and early 1990, L-tryptophan ingestion was implicated as a cause of the eosinophilia-myalgia syndrome, which can include cutaneous sclerosis or eosinophilic fasciitis, as well as cutaneous mucin deposition.[3]

Morphea

Morphea is a strictly cutaneous disorder characterized by plaques of thickened skin.

Clinical Features There are several types of morphea. In the ordinary form, the patient has one or several white to tan sclerotic plaques, often with a slowly expanding violaceous border. Only rarely is there clinical overlap between morphea and SS. Variants of morphea include

1. *Linear morphea (or linear scleroderma)*: usually a single limb is involved by sclerosis that results in obvious thinning secondary to loss of fat and dermal tightening. Because a major joint is often involved by contractures, there may be significant disability.
2. *Coup de sabre*: these patients have a vertical scar on the forehead and scalp that has been likened to the slash of a saber. The major clinical disease to be differentiated is Romberg's hemifacial atrophy in which there is less dermal sclerosis and deeper involvement of fat and muscles.
3. *Disabling pansclerotic morphea*: this widespread cutaneous disease is often disabling or life-threatening because of contractures around joints or around vital structures. There are none of the systemic clinical features or serologic changes that occur in SS.
4. *Deep morphea* (morphea profunda): the sclerotic process may extend to involve not only the subcutaneous fat but also the fascia and muscles.

Pathophysiology. There have been suggestions that morphea in some cases may be caused or precipitated by *Borrelia burgdorferi*, but the association appears weak.

Clinicopathologic Correlation. About 50% of morphea patients have a positive antinuclear antibody test against a human substrate or antibodies against single-stranded DNA. It may also be appropriate to do a *Borrelia* serology.

Differential Diagnosis. One disease that is clinically and histologically confused with morphea is lichen sclerosus et atrophicus. This disorder tends to have ivory white plaques with an erythematous to violaceous border most often on the genitalia, an uncommon site for morphea. However, when lichen sclerosus et atrophicus is on the trunk, it may closely resemble morphea. Microscopically, lichen sclerosus et atrophicus has ortho-hyperkeratosis with follicular plugging, epidermal atrophy, upper dermal edema, and a lichenoid infiltrate, all of which are absent in morphea. In overlap situations, the biopsy specimen may be less helpful, for the characteristic atrophy and inflammation of lichen sclerosus et atrophicus may be missing and only dermal sclerosis is present. Lichen sclerosus et atrophicus tends to have reduced dermal elastin.[4]

Atrophoderma

Atrophoderma of Pasini and Pierini is an idiopathic sclerotic, atrophic disorder most common in young women.

Clinical Features. Atrophoderma is characterized by blue-brown plaques that are depressed below the normal skin surface and have a distinct edge. The lesions are neither indurated nor inflamed but thinned without visible epidermal atrophy. The back and lumbosacral area of young women are the most common sites.

Differential Diagnosis. Controversy exists whether atrophoderma is distinct from morphea.[5] Atrophoderma may be impossible to diagnose unless full-thickness adjacent normal skin is available for comparison. Morphea may show more inflammation.[6] Atrophoderma also refers to patulous atrophy around hair follicles, which is considered in the discussion of elastolysis.

Eosinophilic Fasciitis

Eosinophilic fasciitis (Shulman syndrome) is an idiopathic inflammation of the dermis, fat, and deep fascia whose exact relationship to SS is unclear.

Clinical Features. A typical history of a patient with eosinophilic fasciitis is overuse of a body part (e.g., painting a house) followed by painful swelling of the abused part (arm in this example). The involved skin is initially puffy and edematous rather than sclerotic.[7] Eosinophilic fasciitis is also a manifestation of the L-tryptophan eosinophilia-myalgia syndrome.

Histopathologic Features. These diverse disorders are virtually identical histologically. There is a normal epidermis that overlies a dermis that at first glance may also appear normal. However, some of the following changes are present: (1) thickening of the collagen—the individual bands of collagen are thickened, and the midpower view is relatively acellular with fewer fibroblasts (Fig. 16-1A); (2) entrapment of appendageal structure (Fig. 16-1B)—eccrine glands may seem to be higher up in the dermis than their usual location near the dermal-fat junction because of expansion of the lower dermis; (3) destruction of appendages—the most common sign is the "naked" arrector pili muscle (Fig. 16-2), either no hair follicle or a vertical scar along with the prominent smooth muscle band.

As the active border of morphea and the acute redness of eosinophilic fasciitis suggest, inflammatory changes are also present. Probably the most specific is the presence of eosinophils at the dermal-subcutaneous junction (Fig. 16-3). This change is expected in eosinophilic fasciitis and can be seen in SS but is uncommon in other forms of sclerosis. Perivascular inflammation is a common finding, but true vasculitis is rare. Typically lymphocytes admixed with plasma cells and eosinophils are found around normal to swollen vessels. The elastic fibers are usually normal.

It is important to sample the dermal-subcutaneous junction in all cases of suspected scleroderma. If eosinophilic fasciitis is a clinical concern, an even deeper incisional biopsy to include the fascia should be performed. The fascial thickening is so striking that it can be diagnosed at low power (Fig. 16-4). In addition, the infiltration of eosinophils will be even more intense. Also, even in ordinary SS eosinophils may be seen in small groups along the junction and in the fat. Panniculitis is also present in some cases of SS.

Sclerodermoid Disorders or Pseudoscleroderma

In addition to scleroderma, morphea, and all their variants, many other disorders may present with clinical or histologic features of dermal sclerosis. Included in this group are

1. Chemically induced sclerosis either from systemic sources such as L-tryptophan, Spanish toxic oil, bleomycin, or vinyl chloride or local injections such as bleomycin or pentazocine. The role of silicones as a triggering event remains unclear.
2. Pseudoscleroderma: many diseases can mimic scleroderma; some are discussed in this chapter; others are discussed elsewhere in the text. They can mimic various forms of sclerosis[8]:
   a. Edematous (scleredema, scleromyxedema, myxedema, diabetic stiff-hand syndrome)
   b. Indurative (carcinoid, phenylketonuria, porphyria cutanea tarda, chronic graft-versus-host disease, POEMS syndrome, acromegaly, pachydermoperiostitis, stasis dermatitis [lipodermatosclerosis] and many forms of panniculitis)
   c. Atrophic (acrodermatitis chronica atrophicans, lipoatrophy, lichen sclerosus et atrophicus, various premature aging syndromes, and some forms of poikiloderma)

Scleredema

Scleredema is a dermal thickening most often associated with insulin-dependent diabetes.

Clinical Features

Scleredema (scleredema of Buschke) is an uncommon disorder of unclear origin.[9] In adults, it is limited almost exclusively to patients with diabetes mellitus who develop thickened skin, most often on the back. The disease is rarely acral in contrast to SS. The old name of *scleredema adultorum* is not appropriate because the disease also affects children. In children, the disease may be postinfectious with no relationship to diabetes. Atrophy, bound-down skin, and scarring are not seen.

Histopathologic Features

The epidermis is normal, whereas the dermis is expanded to two or three times its usual thickness and may resemble SS

Figure 16-1. Morphea. **(A)** Deep punch biopsy from forearm showing marked thickening and relative acellularity of the dermis and entrapped eccrine glands. **(B)** Eccrine glands are entrapped by thick, compacted bands of collagen with few fibroblasts among them.

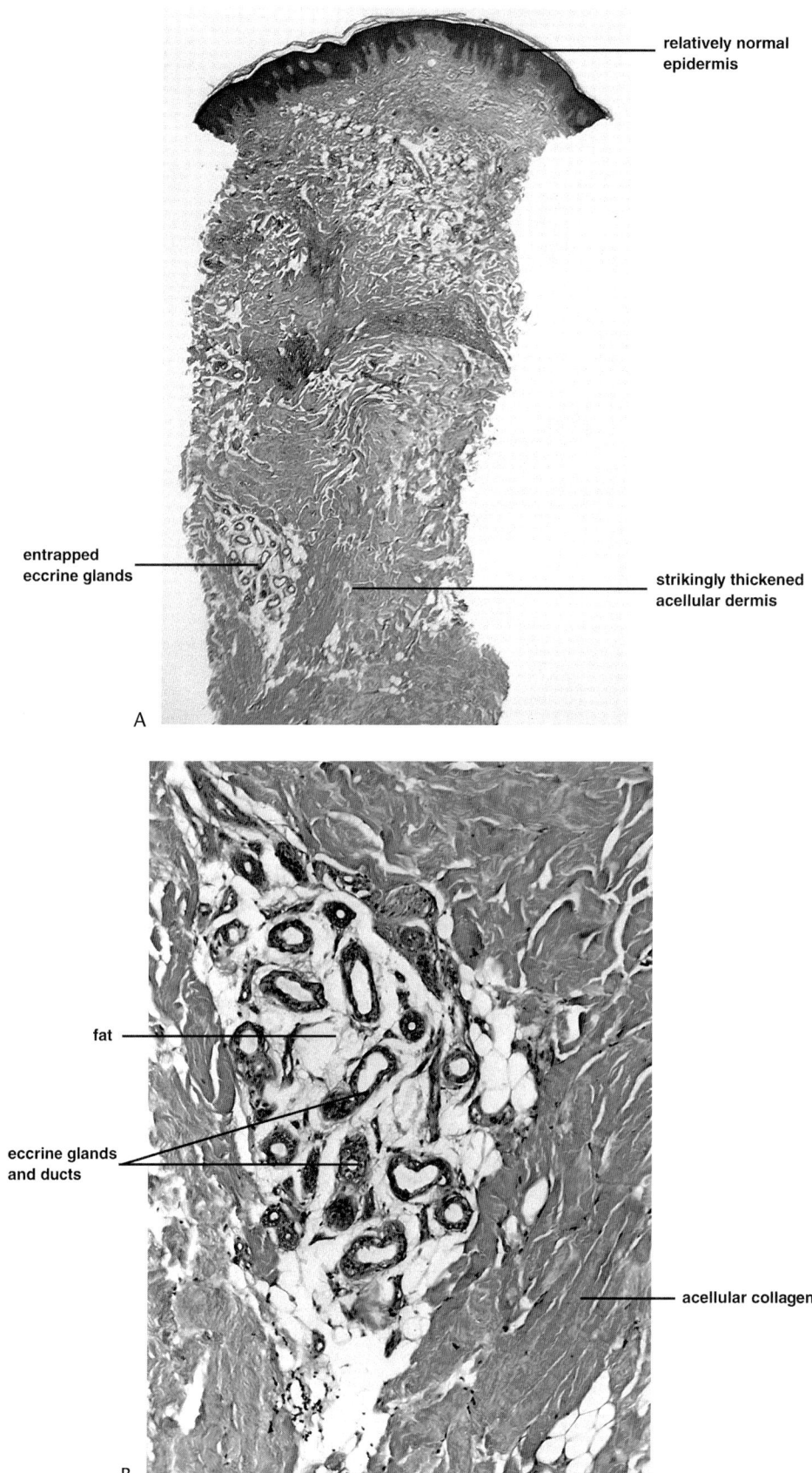

relatively normal epidermis

entrapped eccrine glands

strikingly thickened acellular dermis

A

fat

eccrine glands and ducts

acellular collagen

B

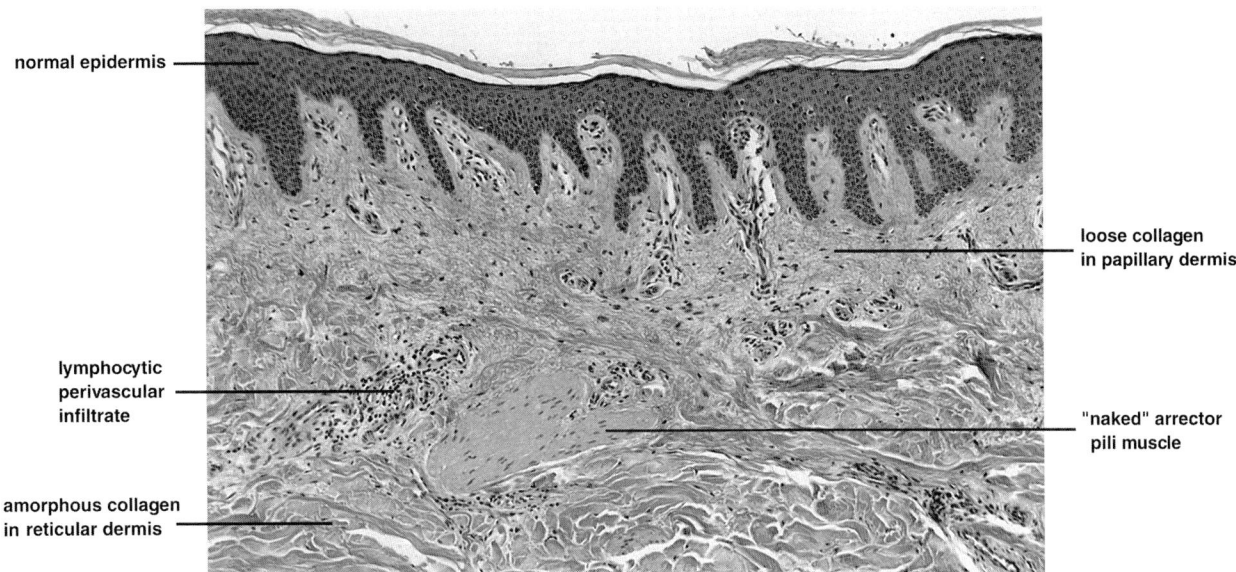

normal epidermis

loose collagen
in papillary dermis

lymphocytic
perivascular
infiltrate

"naked" arrector
pili muscle

amorphous collagen
in reticular dermis

Figure 16-2. Morphea. The epidermis is normal. There is a lymphocytic perivascular infiltrate in the superficial dermis, and an arrector pili muscle is seen without an associated follicular unit.

Figure 16-3. Morphea. There is a lobule of fat entrapped by dense collagen. In addition, numerous inflammatory cells are seen at the dermal-subcutaneous junction.

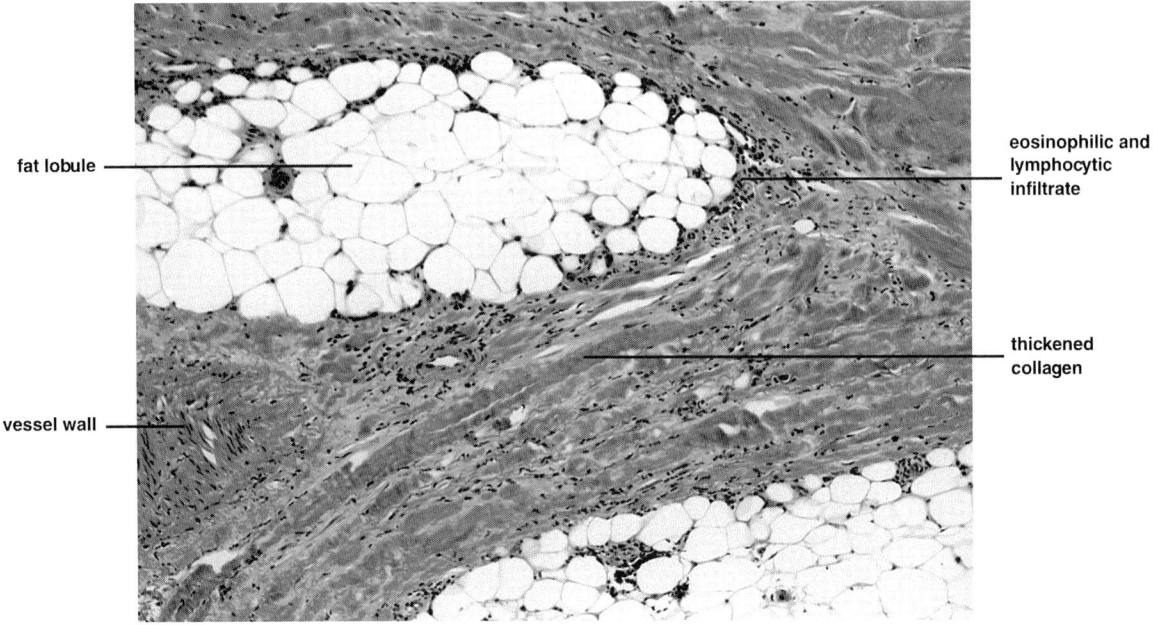

fat lobule

eosinophilic and
lymphocytic
infiltrate

thickened
collagen

vessel wall

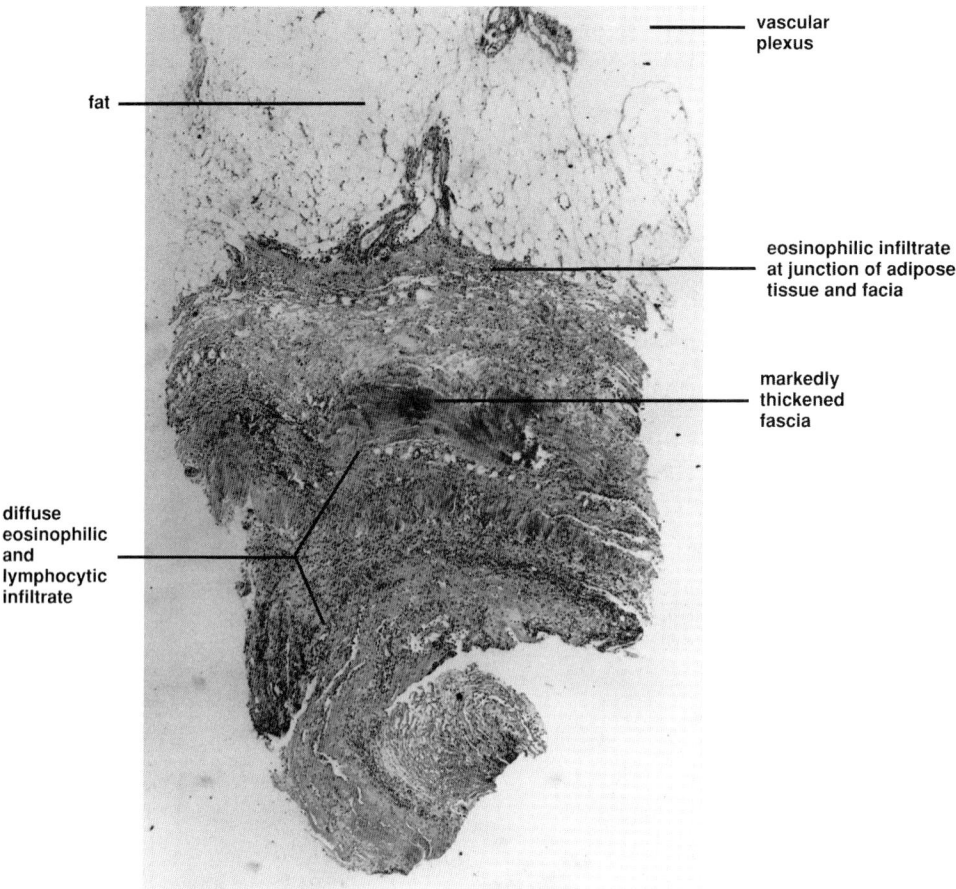

fat

vascular plexus

eosinophilic infiltrate at junction of adipose tissue and facia

markedly thickened fascia

diffuse eosinophilic and lymphocytic infiltrate

Figure 16-4. Eosinophilic fasciitis. This is the bottom of a deep biopsy that had overlying dermal sclerosis. The layer of fat is normal, but the thickened fibrous tissue at the base should be two or three cell layers thick rather than being bulky, as seen here. It is also infiltrated by inflammatory cells, including eosinophils.

on cursory examination. The collagen fibers are normal in thickness, and the appendages are not damaged (Fig. 16-5). However, a metachromatically staining amorphous substance, which is primarily hyaluronic acid, is deposited between the collagen bundles. This material stains best with toluidine blue at pH 7.0 or with colloidal iron.[10] In some cases it may be difficult to identify the mucin. In addition, mucin can also be found in scleroderma.[11] The clinical diagnosis can usually be substantiated simply by demonstrating marked dermal thickening.

Clinicopathologic Correlation

Dermal sclerosis in diabetes has been associated with abnormalities of the aldase reductase cycle, but such changes have not been demonstrated in scleredema.[12] The fibroblasts show a highly activated phenotype that persists for years.[13]

Differential Diagnosis

In contrast to SS, appendages are not damaged, although they may be displaced. Inflammation at the dermal-subcutaneous junction does not occur.

Scleromyxedema

Scleromyxedema represents the cutaneous deposition of mucin associated with a monoclonal gammopathy.

Clinical Features

Scleromyxedema begins as small lichenoid papules that coalesce to form plaques and eventuate as thickened hardened skin. The preferred name *scleromyxedema* includes both the mucin and the sclerosis.[14,15] *Lichen myxedematosus* only describes the papular stage. Patients may also have acral sclerosis and facial tightening that resembles SS.

Histopathologic Features

The dermis is replaced by an amorphous stringy mucinous material that pushes apart the collagen fibers (Fig. 16-6). The amount of mucin is highly variable. In some cases it is minimal, and in others almost no normal dermal collagen is present. There is an increased number of fibroblasts within the connective tissue matrix. Despite the lichenoid clinical appearance, inflammation at the basement membrane zone is uncommon.

Any standard mucin stain will stain the mucinous material, which is primarily hyaluronic acid. Possible stains include Hale colloidal iron, Alcian blue, and toluidine blue. When the collagen is closely examined or elastin and reticulin silver stains done, there is a relative decrease in collagen with retained or increased elastin and reticulin (or early collagen).

Differential Diagnosis

Although scleromyxedema mimics lichenoid and sclerodermoid disorders clinically, the histologic differential diagnosis involves the cutaneous mucinoses and is discussed in that section.

Pathophysiology

The gammopathy is usually an IgG λ type. The cause of the clonal proliferation and how it relates to the mucin deposition is unclear, but most evidence suggests that the immunoglobulin or another serum factor stimulates the fibroblasts to produce mucin.

Scars and Keloids

A scar is an area of damaged epidermis and dermis that has healed. A keloid is a scar that has overgrown its original boundaries.[16]

Clinical Features

Most clinicians can recognize a scar and a keloid, so biopsies are rarely done to establish these diagnoses. Occasionally the question will arise if a nodule in a treated tumor site is a recurrence or a scar. Sometimes both hypertrophic scars and keloids will be submitted after they have been treated by surgical excision, but rarely is there any clinical question. Scars may be either hypertrophic or atrophic, both clinically and histopathologically.

Histopathologic Features

The prototypic change in a scar is reorganization of the dermal collagen (Fig. 16-7A). Elastic fibers are diminished or absent. Myofibroblasts may be an important component, especially in keloids.[17] The fibers run parallel to the wound surface or line of tension. There are few if any appendages. The overlying epidermis is atrophic with a flattened pattern of papillae and rete ridges. There may be separation at the junction as well as incontinence of pigment. If the scar is recent and has been created by destructive surgery, signs of electrocautery, Monsel's solution, gelfoam, or even a foreign body response may be seen. Early scars may also contain abundant mucin.

The histologic distinction between a hypertrophic scar and a keloid is difficult. In simplest terms, a keloid should have more proliferation of collagen with more disarray. At low power, the keloid may appear as a nodule arising above the adjacent skin (Fig. 16-7B). The collagen fibers are thickened and arranged in swirls or in a haphazard fashion, not necessarily parallel to the epidermis (Fig. 16-7C). Both keloids and hypertrophic scars tend to have nodules or whorls of thickened collagen rather than an organized pattern.[18,19]

Radiation Dermatitis

Radiation dermatitis is a combination of clinical changes that occur after exposure of skin to ionizing radiation.

Figure 16-5. Scleredema. The dermis is markedly thickened. A small amount of mucin is present in the spaces between the collagen bundles. The dermal-subcutaneous junction has a normal scalloped profile.

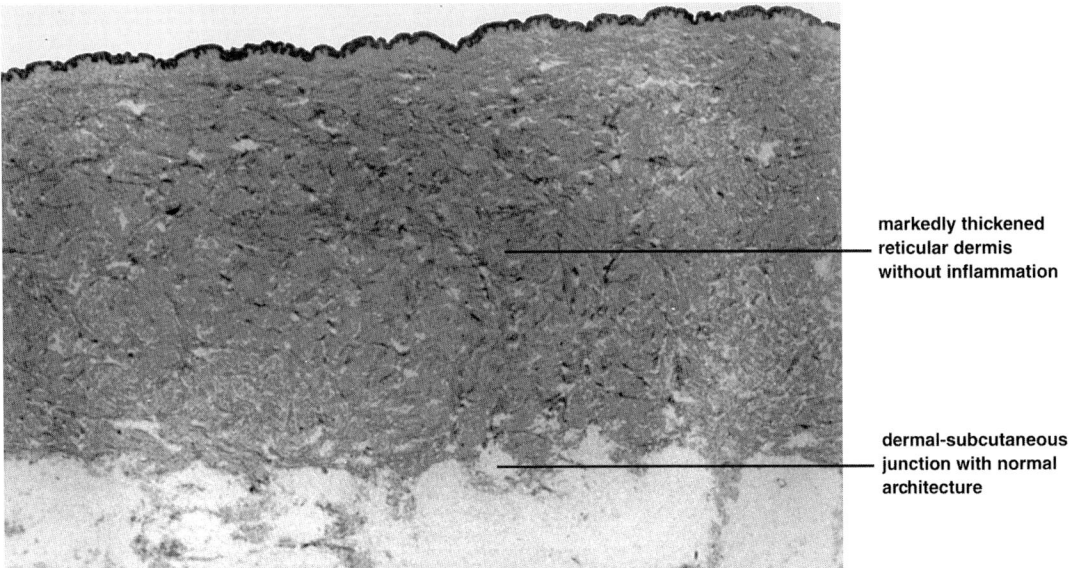

markedly thickened reticular dermis without inflammation

dermal-subcutaneous junction with normal architecture

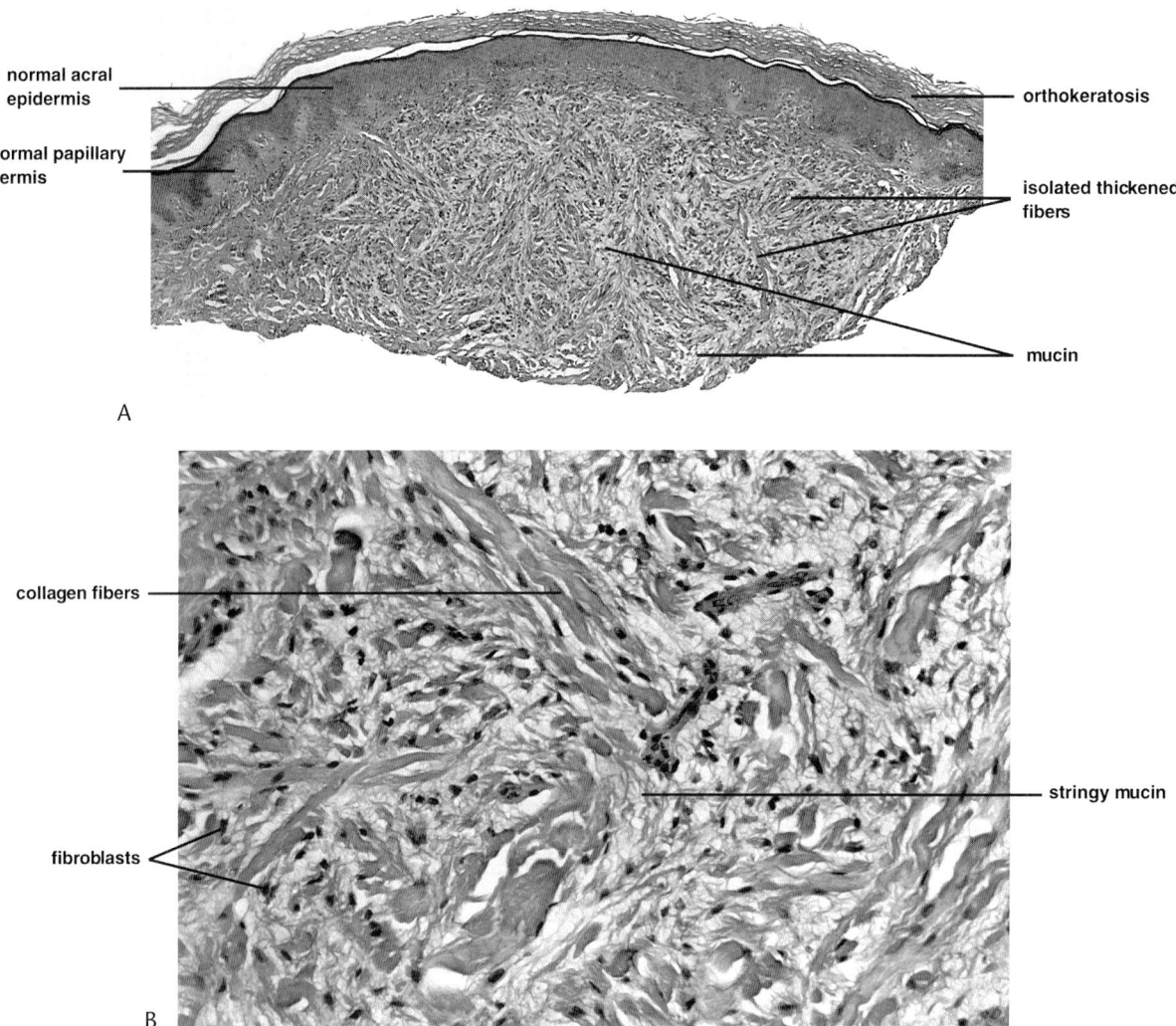

Figure 16-6. Scleromyxedema. **(A)** This is a nodule of lichen myxedematosus in a patient with a monoclonal gammopathy. The epidermis is normal for acral skin. In the dermis there are bands of collagen separated by amorphous stringy material. **(B)** A higher power view showing to better advantage the strands of collagen being pushed apart by stringy material. Note also the increased number of fibroblasts among the collagen bundles.

Clinical Features

Many changes occur after the skin has been exposed to ionizing radiation. Because of improvement in the delivery systems, cutaneous damage after deep radiation is much less common today than in the past. Similarly, treatment regimens for cutaneous tumors are now fractionated to avoid skin damage. However, even these regimens may occasionally result in skin changes. Many patients are also seen who in the past had cutaneous malignancies treated by the insertion of radium needles. This modality typically produces markedly telangiectatic scars.

Acute radiation dermatitis resembles any other erythematous eruption, except that it is confined to a radiation port. It can mimic acute graft-versus-host disease.[20] Chronic radiation damage can take several forms. Generally, it is poikilodermatous be-

cause of the combination of telangiectasia, incontinentia pigmenti, loss of appendages, and dermal sclerosis. Such skin is the likely site for the development of radiation-induced cutaneous malignancies.

Histopathologic Features

Acute radiation dermatitis is rarely biopsied. Its histologic features include spongiosis, dermal edema, and varying degrees of epidermal necrosis. The vessels may be dilated, and the deeper ones have thickened walls.

Chronic radiation dermatitis is more frequently a problem. As with scars, often the clinical question is whether a tumor has recurred. Radiation dermatitis is characterized by dilated vessels superficially and large thick-walled deep vessels with

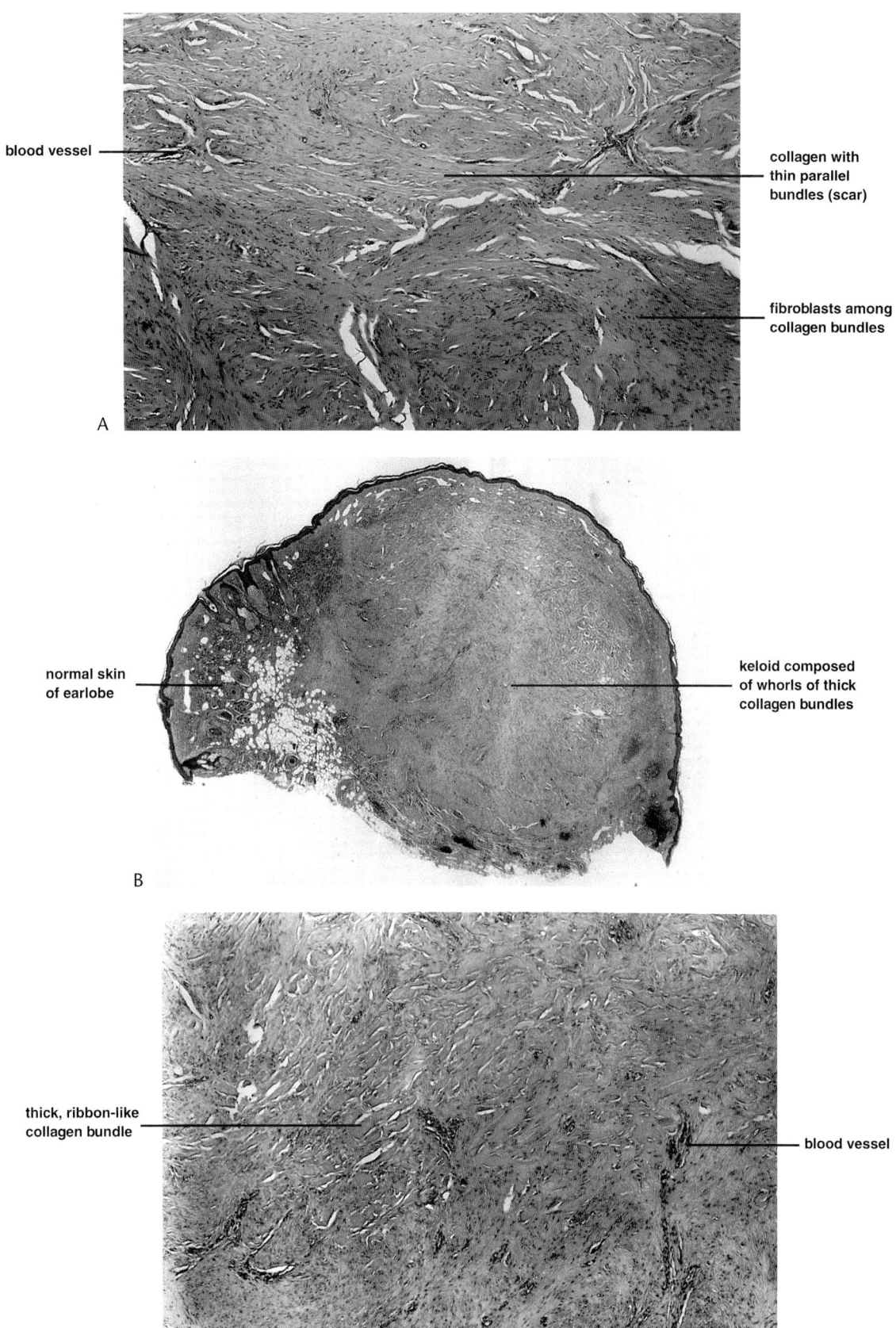

Figure 16-7. Keloid. **(A)** The fibrous tissue in the upper part of the figure is arranged in relatively parallel bands, whereas the lower half shows large thick bands of collagen arranged in more of a swirled pattern. Several of the collagen fibers are markedly thickened and homogenous. There is increased vascularity. **(B)** Earlobe keloid. There is a nodule that is demarcated from the normal skin of the earlobe. It is composed of broad, hyalinized collagen bundles that are arranged in swirls. **(C)** Earlobe keloid. Higher magnification of characteristic thick collagen bundles.

occluded lumina (Fig. 16-8). There is marked collagen proliferation often with giant bizarre fibroblasts (Fig. 16-9). Eventually there is dermal sclerosis. Incontinentia pigmenti is often present. The epithelial changes are similar to a scar with atrophy and loss of appendages. However, some degree of epidermal atypia that ranges from atrophy or benign hyperplasia to dyskeratotic changes to carcinoma in situ may be seen.[21]

Pachydermoperiostitis

Pachydermoperiostitis is a disorder characterized by thickening of the skin and bony changes.

Clinical Features

Pachydermoperiostitis (Touraine-Solente-Golé syndrome) is a rare autosomal dominant genodermatosis. Patients have thickened furrowed skin especially on the face, hands, and feet. The scalp changes are identical to cutis verticis gyrata. The digits often are clubbed, and radiographic examination shows periosteal bone formation especially of acral and long bones. Identical changes have been described in secondary or pulmonary hypertrophic osteoarthropathy associated with bronchogenic carcinoma. Patients may also have palmar-plantar hyperkeratosis, cutaneous mucin deposition and monoclonal gammopathy.[22]

Histopathologic Features

If the biopsy specimen is generous and crosses skin furrows, the answer is simplified, for the furrows can be seen. Otherwise, there is hyperplasia of both elastic fibers and collagen. One feature somewhat unique to pachydermoperiostitis is a proliferation of sebaceous or eccrine glands. Some lesions may show mucinous deposition; they are microscopically identical to scleromyxedema.[23]

Connective Tissue Nevus

Connective tissue nevus is a localized abnormality of collagen and elastin.[24]

Clinical Features

A connective tissue nevus can occur in several clinical settings. The most common is the shagreen patch of tuberous sclerosis. This bumpy pebbly patch usually on the trunk occurs in at least 25% of tuberous sclerosis patients. It often is the first sign of the disorder. Isolated connective tissue nevi also occur; solitary lesions are usually sporadic, while multiple lesions are most often familially inherited in an autosomal dominant pattern.[25] Lesions may range in size from tiny papules to large plaques or exophytic tumors.[26]

In Buschke-Ollendorff syndrome (connective tissue nevus-osteopoikilosis syndrome, dermatofibrosis lenticularis disseminata) patients have asymptomatic bony lesions seen on radio-

Figure 16-8. Chronic radiation dermatitis. The epidermis exhibits benign hyperplasia and hyperkeratosis. There are dilated vessels in the papillary dermis. The deeper dermis is sclerotic.

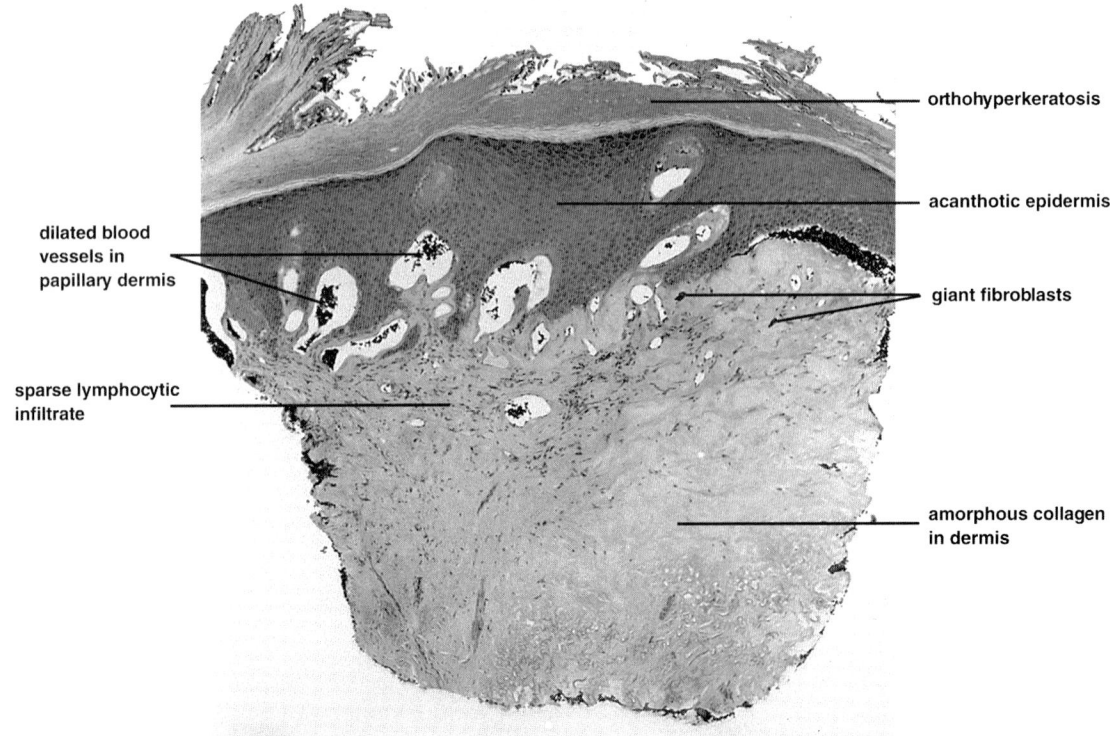

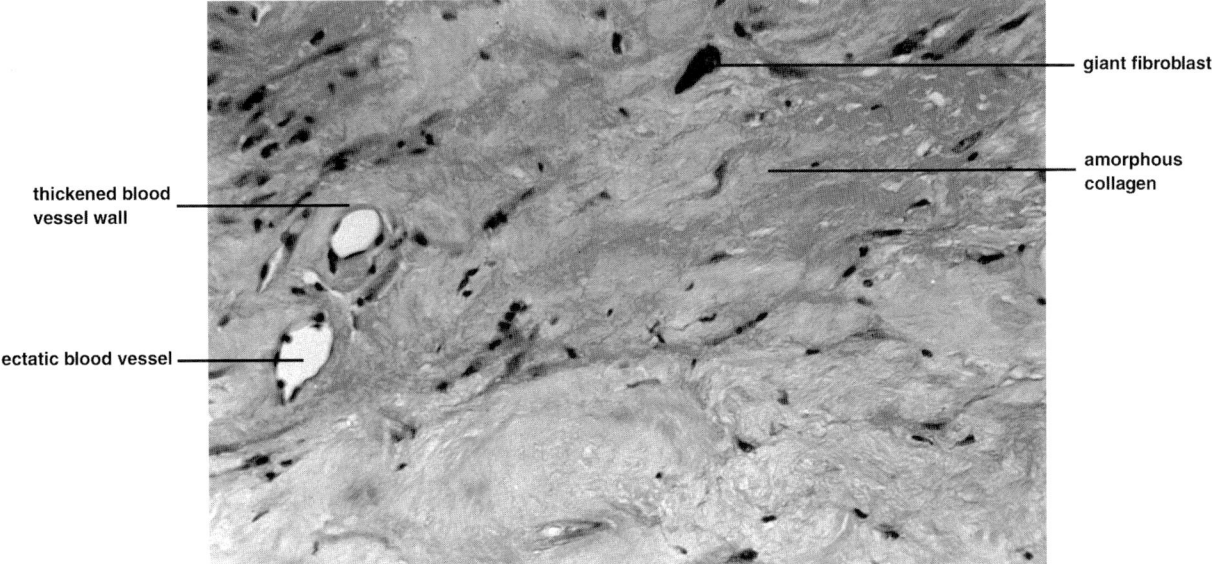

Figure 16-9. Chronic radiation dermatitis. Vessels with thickened walls are seen, as well as large atypical fibroblasts.

graphic examination as densities in acral and long bones (osteopoikilosis) along with connective tissue nevi that present as multiple papules and nodules.[27]

Histopathologic Features

Lesions have been assigned an array of names (*elastoma, collagenoma*, and *connective tissue nevus*) based on which dermal component appeared increased in the histologic study. Also, some state that as elastic fibers increase, collagen decreases and vice versa. We believe that all connective tissue nevi, no matter what their clinical background, show increases in elastic fibers or collagen, or both, and need not be further classified.

The epidermis is invariably normal, and the dermis may appear normal or somewhat sclerotic on routine light microscopy. Elastic fiber and collagen stains should be done on both the lesion and contralateral normal skin. In assessing connective tissue nevi, it is crucial to have a control specimen taken from the same patient because a diagnosis is often impossible without a normal comparison.

There may be an obvious increase in elastic fibers or collagen. When collagen fibers are present in excess, they may be identified on routine examination as coarse, thickened trabeculae (Fig. 16-10). In contrast to SS, clumps or bundles of thickened fibers are seen without destruction of appendages. A loss of collagen is singularly difficult to assess. Elastic fiber abnormalities are rarely seen with H&E stains and are best appreciated with special stains. Sometimes thickened fibers are seen. In other cases, there may be a loss of elastic fibers, especially in the papillary dermis. Elastic fibers are usually thickened and entrap collagen in the lesions of Buschke-Ollendorff syndrome.[28]

Angiofibroma

An angiofibroma is a papule characterized by both dermal fibrosis and increased number of blood vessels.

Clinical Features

Angiofibromas occur in a number of clinical settings. They may be a marker for tuberous sclerosis, in which case they are called *adenoma sebaceum*. The periungual Koenen tumor may be a very fibrous angiofibroma. Pearly penile papules, tiny papules about the corona in many normal men, are also angiofibromas. Women have similar lesions about the introitus, but they are less often biopsied. The most common solitary angiofibroma is the fibrous papule of the nose. This is a small, dome-shaped, skin-colored papule on the nose or in the nasolabial fold.

Histopathologic Features

The epidermis may be normal or slightly hyperplastic. There may be an increased number of enlarged melanocytes in the basal zone, and melanophages may be present in the stroma. In the dermis there are dilated and sometimes thick-walled vessels that may be surrounded by concentric fibrosis. There are also large stellate fibroblasts dispersed throughout the diffusely fibrotic dermis[29] (Fig. 16-11). All angiofibromas look similar histologically, and the history and site determine the diagnosis.

The origin of fibrous papule of the nose is controversial, as some have suggested that fibrous papules are involuting melanocytic nevi.[30] Histologically in most instances one sees a large angiofibroma, although occasionally scattered melanocytes are found. Almost all lesions are fibrous proliferations rich in factor XIIIa-positive dermal dendritic cells.[31]

Dermal Thinning, Atrophy, and Dystrophy

Focal Dermal Hypoplasia

Focal dermal hypoplasia (Goltz syndrome) is an X-linked dominant genodermatosis characterized by areas of dermal thinning and periorificial papules as well as ocular, skeletal, and central nervous system defects.[32]

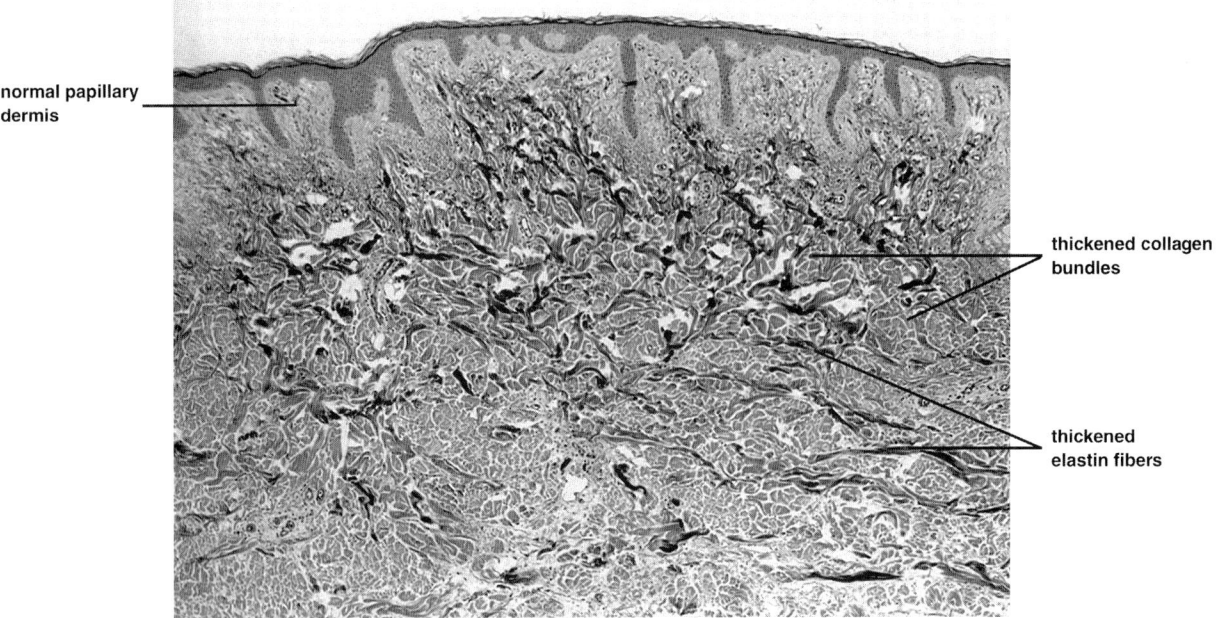

normal papillary dermis

thickened collagen bundles

thickened elastin fibers

Figure 16-10. Connective tissue nevus. The epidermis is normal. In the dermis there are thickened bundles of collagen. Some of the large dark refractile fibers stained positive for elastin.

Clinical Features

Focal dermal hypoplasia occurs primarily in females. It has linear cutaneous lesions thought to represent lyonization that also occur in incontinentia pigmenti and other X-linked dominant disorders. The lesions are erythematous and usually show atrophy and bulging of lower dermal structures and fat, which imparts a yellow hue. The papillomas are most common around the mouth and anus. They are usually mistaken for warts until the entire syndrome is identified. A valuable diagnostic aid, especially in young children, is the presence of osteopathia striata, linear streakings of the periarticular long bones on radiographic examination. Other problems include ocular, skeletal, and central nervous system abnormalities.

Figure 16-11. Fibrous papule of the nose. There are ectatic vessels and coarse collagen bundles with plump and stellate fibroblasts among them.

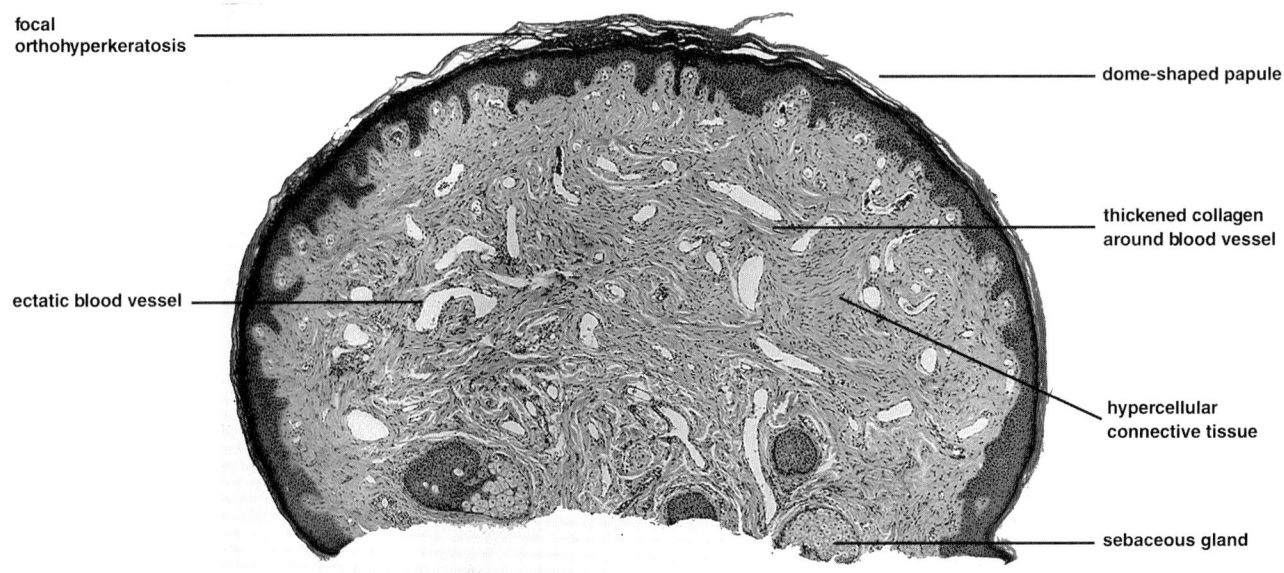

focal orthohyperkeratosis

dome-shaped papule

thickened collagen around blood vessel

ectatic blood vessel

hypercellular connective tissue

sebaceous gland

Histopathologic Features

As the name suggests, focal dermal hypoplasia is characterized by a paucity of dermis in the skin biopsy specimen (Fig. 16-12). The basic defect appears to be dermal hypoplasia with secondary herniation of fat,[33,34] although some believe that there may be active lobular expansion of fat.[35] Occasionally an initial inflammatory phase is seen.[36] In any event, a normal epidermis, a thin to absent dermis, and much fat are seen—whether a papilloma or a herniated lesion is biopsied.

Differential Diagnosis

Nevus lipomatosus of Hoffmann and Zurhelle usually occurs in young women on the trunk as multiple areas of herniated fat. Nevus lipomatosus has a lobular perivascular expansion of fat into the dermis without the profound dermal attenuation. Also, neonatal skin may show high dermal fat, as can old nevi or neurofibromas that have undergone extensive fatty degeneration.

Aplasia Cutis Congenita

Aplasia cutis congenita is a focal absence of the skin that usually occurs on a line of embryologic fusion.

Clinical Features

Aplasia cutis congenita generally occurs on the scalp. It is present at birth as an erosion, is often incorrectly blamed on forceps trauma, and heals with a scar. The disorder is subdivided based primarily on associated findings.[37]

Histologic Features

Aplasia cutis congenita is rarely diagnosed by biopsy. In the acute phase, an erosion with underlying exposed fat or fascia is seen. Rarely, heterotopic brain tissue may be found. In a healed lesion, a scar is seen, with an atrophic epidermis, thin to absent dermis, no appendages, and, if the biopsy specimen is deep enough, relatively less deep fat and muscle.

Ehlers-Danlos Syndrome

Ehlers-Danlos syndrome is a collection of at least 11 different genodermatoses that have different clinical appearances and various defects in collagen synthesis. For some variants, the exact molecular defect has been identified.

Clinical Features

The classic features of Ehlers-Danlos syndrome are loss of cutaneous elasticity, formation of abnormal scars, and hyperextensibility of joints. These changes are seen primarily in types I, II, and III. In the other forms, often fragile translucent skin with prominent vessels and frequent ecchymoses may dominate. Systemic features are dependent on the type of Ehlers-Danlos syndrome. Not all types of Ehlers-Danlos syndrome have distensible skin and hypermobile joints; some present only with severe orthopaedic or ocular abnormalities.[38]

Histopathologic Features

A biopsy is not a helpful way to diagnose or classify Ehlers-Danlos syndrome. The skin is almost always normal by routine light microscopic examination. Even special stains for collagen and elastic fiber usually have no pathognomonic features. Sometimes the skin looks "young" with immature collagen and elastin.

A group of 21 patients with at least six subtypes of Ehlers-Danlos syndrome were studied.[39] Dermal thickness in Ehlers-Danlos syndrome was similar to controls, and no consistent abnormalities of collagen or elastic fibers were found. In type I, there may be wide variation in the thickness of collagen fibrils,

Figure 16-12. Focal dermal hypoplasia. A normal epidermis is seen in immediate proximity to fat. There is nothing left of the dermis except for perhaps a series of small blood vessels just beneath the epidermis.

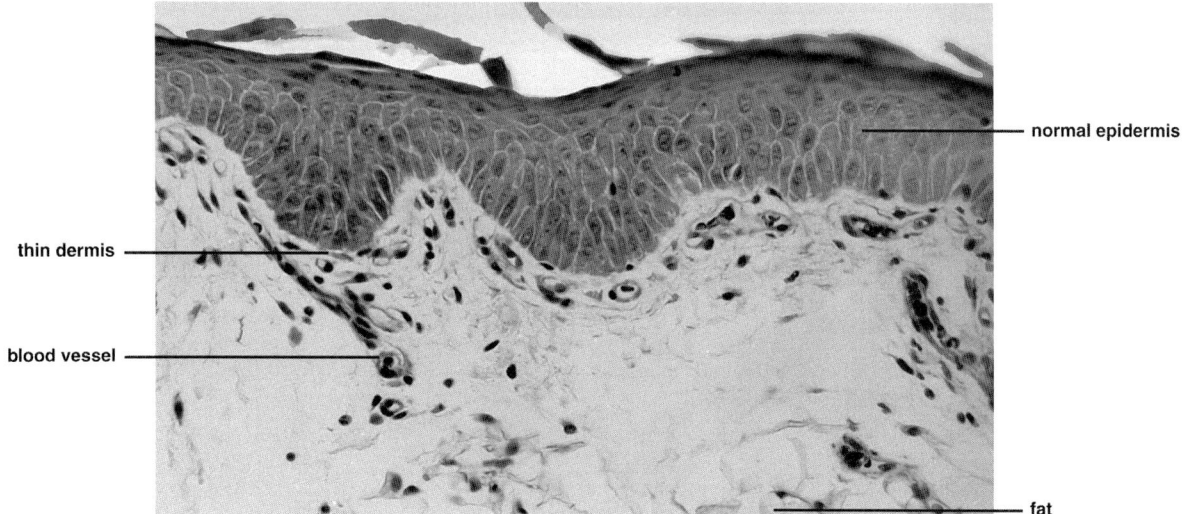

as seen with the electron microscope.[40] Type IV Ehlers-Danlos syndrome has a defect in type III collagen that results in dermal thinning and an apparent increase in elastic fibers.[41] In our experience, routine histology is not a helpful way to study Ehlers-Danlos syndrome.

Reactive Perforating Collagenosis

Reactive perforating collagenosis is an abnormality in dermal collagen metabolism manifested by transepidermal elimination of damaged collagen.

Clinical Features

In children, reactive perforating collagenosis is usually inherited, most often in an autosomal dominant fashion. A typical history is that in response to minimal trauma papules develop, most often on the arms and legs. They soon become umbilicated with a central adherent keratotic plug. In adults, the disorder is acquired and usually secondary to pruritic dermatoses.[42] Rarely a focal area of reactive perforating collagenosis develops in response to trauma; this is called *collagenoma perforans verruciforme*.[43]

Patients with chronic renal disease, especially associated with diabetes mellitus, also develop pruritic crusted papules which have been given many names. The term *perforating disorder of hemodialysis* seems most appropriate. In some instances transepidermal elimination of both collagen and elastin has been described.[44]

Histopathologic Features

There is epidermal ulceration with a thick compact crust that contains inflammatory cells, debris and degenerating collagen fibers (Fig. 16-13). In the dermis beneath the crust is an accumulation of degenerating basophilic collagen. As the lesions mature, the umbilicated plug contains serum, cell debris, and damaged collagen. Occasionally basophilic collagen fibers can be seen extending vertically from the dermis into the crust.[45]

Differential Diagnosis

There are a number of diseases in which transepidermal elimination or perforation is seen. They have little else in common and are discussed elsewhere in this text. Table 16-1 shows the classification proposed by Goette.[46]

Pseudoxanthoma Elasticum

Pseudoxanthoma elasticum is a group of genodermatoses characterized by cutaneous and systemic changes in elastic tissue.

Clinical Features

Pseudoxanthoma elasticum patients develop yellow patches or plaques in flexural areas such as the side of neck, axillae, and popliteal fossae that resemble plucked chicken skin. In the plaques, the hair follicles are prominent. Often focal firm areas of calcification develop. Epidermal ulceration with discharge of this chalky material may also occur. In most cases, the pattern of inheritance is

autosomal recessive. Systemic involvement varies with the pedigree but includes primarily vascular and retinal damage.[47]

Acquired pseudoxanthoma elasticum most often occurs on the breasts and around the umbilicus of black, obese, multiparous women. The patients have no other stigmata of pseudoxanthoma elasticum and develop their cutaneous lesions later in life. Clinically, the lesions are more papular and keratotic than the usual "chicken skin" of familial pseudoxanthoma elasticum. In addition, chronic occupational exposure to calcium salts and penicillamine therapy may produce pseudoxanthoma elasticum-like lesions.[48] Finally, similar dermal changes occur in papillary dermal elastolysis, an age-related change.[49]

Histopathologic Features

Sections show a normal epidermis that overlies a dermis in which there are bluish clumped dermal fibers, most prominent in the mid-dermis. They can be easily identified on routine H&E

Table 16-1. Classification of Perforating Disorders According to Substance Eliminated

I. Elimination of altered connective tissue
  A. Without features of necrobiotic granuloma
    1. Elastosis perforans serpiginosa
    2. Reactive perforating collagenosis
    3. Perforating folliculitis
    4. Perforating papules of diabetic dialysis patients
    5. Perforating pseudoxanthoma elasticum
    6. Chondrodermatitis nodularis chronica helicis
    7. Perforating solar elastosis
    8. Elimination of damaged collagen after intracutaneous steroid injections
    9. Perforating cutaneous amyloidosis
    10. Kyrle's disease
    11. Porokeratosis of Mibelli
  B. Necrobiotic material within palisading granulomas
    1. Perforating granuloma annulare
    2. Perforating necrobiosis lipoidica
    3. Perforating rheumatoid nodules
II. Elimination of particulate matter
  A. Perforating calcinosis cutis
  B. Perforating necrobiosis lipoidica
  C. Perforating rheumatoid nodules
III. Elimination of nonpalisading granulomas, cell aggregates, or tumors
  A. Perforating sarcoidosis
  B. Malignancies: malignant melanoma (primary or metastatic), mycosis fungoides, Woringer-Kolopp disease, Paget's disease, epidermotrophic eccrine carcinoma, and others
  C. Benign tumors: perforating ossified trichilemmal cyst, pilomatricoma, perforating verruciform angioma, and others
IV. Elimination of infectious organisms
  A. Chromomycosis
  B. North American blastomycosis
  C. Cryptococcosis
  D. Leishmaniasis
  E. Botryomycosis

(From Goette,[46] with permission.)

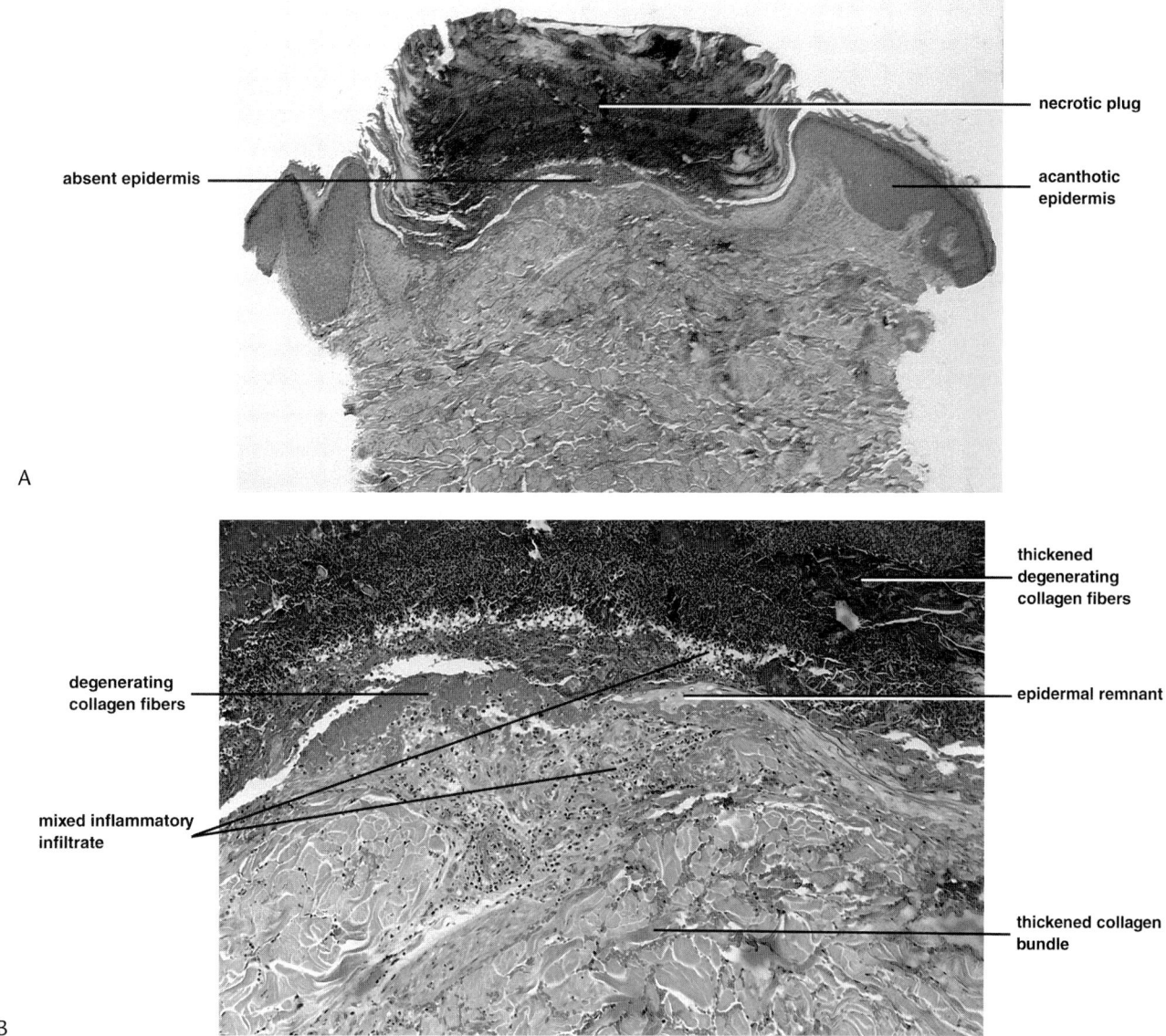

absent epidermis

necrotic plug

acanthotic epidermis

A

thickened degenerating collagen fibers

degenerating collagen fibers

epidermal remnant

mixed inflammatory infiltrate

thickened collagen bundle

B

Figure 16-13. Reactive perforating collagenosis. **(A)** Centrally there is absence of epidermis with a compact, well-circumscribed crust flanked by hyperplastic epidermis. **(B)** This is the base of the crust in the superficial dermis. Inflammatory cells, debris, and thickened collagen fibers are seen. Some degenerating collagen fibers are present within the crust.

sections, but either an elastic fiber or a calcium stain makes them more visible and confirms the diagnosis (Fig. 16-14). Electron microscopy reveals calcified pleomorphic elastic fibers, even in nonlesional skin. The collagen fibrils appear normal but are disorganized in lesional skin.[50] Occasionally the abnormal elastic fibers will be extruded through the skin. This change has been incorrectly called "elastosis perforans serpiginosa," but the latter is a different process. Perforating lesions are more common in acquired pseudoxanthoma elasticum. The elastic fibers in penicillamine-related pseudoxanthoma elasticum have a thickened bramble bush or "lumpy-bumpy" pattern.[48]

If a patient is suspected of having pseudoxanthoma elasticum, either because of systemic findings or because the patient is a member of a pedigree at risk, but does not have cutaneous lesions, a biopsy specimen of a scar is more likely to show the elastic fiber abnormalities than a specimen of normal skin.[51] Ultrastructural evaluation can allow an early or "preclinical" diagnosis.[52]

Clinicopathologic Correlation

Controversy still persists as to whether abnormal elastic fibers are calcified or whether calcium damages normal elastic fibers. The etiology of pseudoxanthoma elasticum remains unclear. Most of the known genes for elastic fiber components have been excluded through genetic linkage analysis.

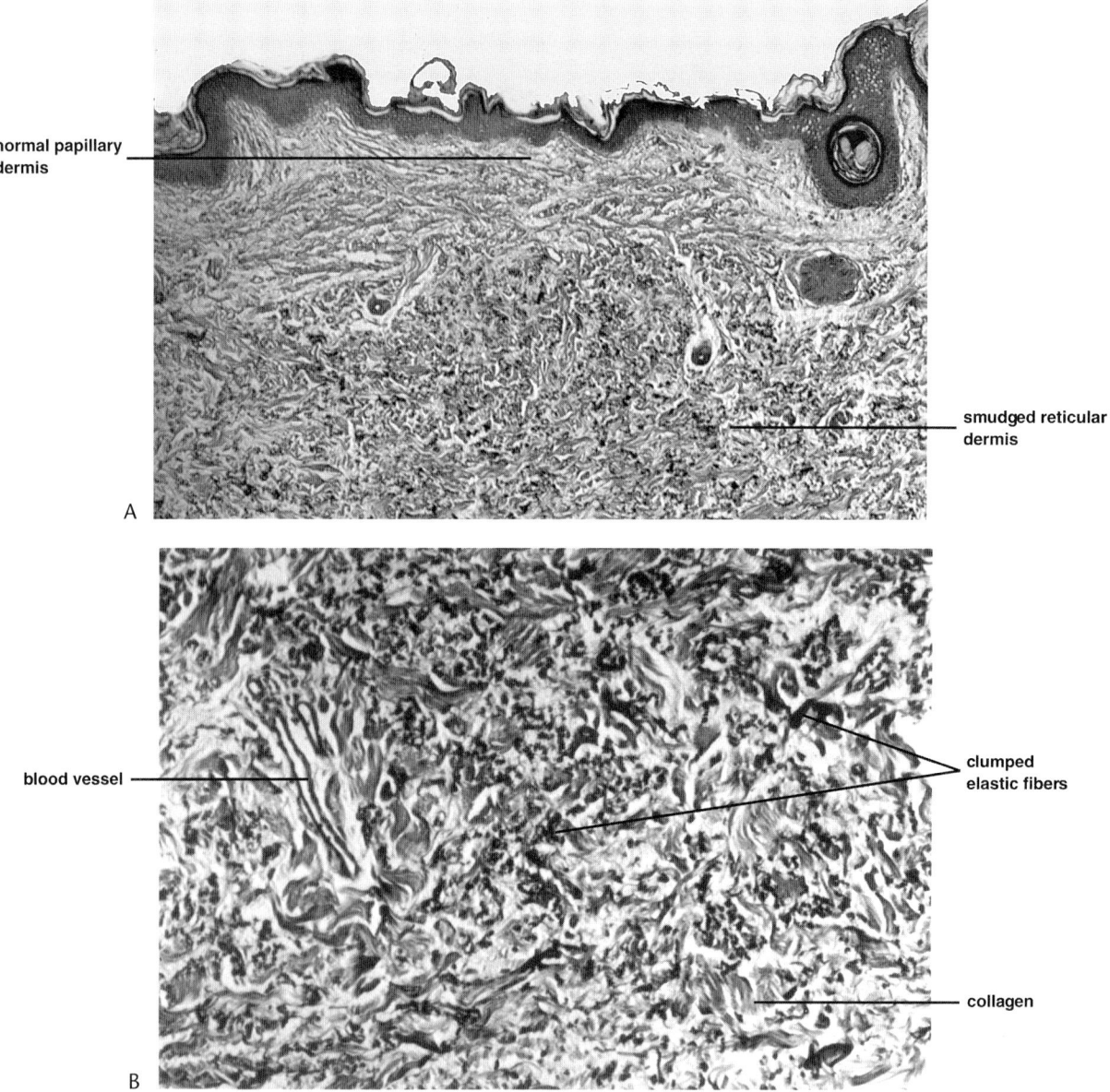

normal papillary
dermis

smudged reticular
dermis

A

blood vessel

clumped
elastic fibers

collagen

B

Figure 16-14. Pseudoxanthoma elasticum. (**A**) The epidermis is normal. In the dermis even at low power with an H&E stain the abnormal elastic fibers can be appreciated. (**B**) At higher power with an elastin stain the abnormal elastic fibers are more readily seen.

Pitfalls

Occasionally, very thin skin with prominent follicles, as in solar damage, poikiloderma, and other connective tissue disorders such as Ehlers-Danlos syndrome, may be mistaken for the chicken skin of pseudoxanthoma elasticum. However, the histology of pseudoxanthoma elasticum is usually unmistakable.

Cutis Laxa

Cutis laxa is a rare group of genodermatoses with striking abnormalities of elastic tissue.

Clinical Features

Cutis laxa patients develop marked sagging of the skin as their elastic fibers become damaged or diminished. Thus, the weight of the skin and other distending forces are not corrected by the spring back of elastic fibers. The patient develops a "basset hound" look and premature aging. The elastic fibers of internal organs such as the heart and great vessels, lungs, and joints may also be damaged.[53,54]

There are several types of cutis laxa in which different defects in the elastin gene have been identified. In addition to inherited cutis laxa, there is acquired cutis laxa,[55] in which patients develop similar clinical features after following severe inflammation, usually a drug reaction (Marshall syndrome)[56]; apparently the invading neutrophils release large amounts of elastases that damage elastic fibers.

Histopathologic Features

The routine sections in cutis laxa resemble normal skin (in contrast to pseudoxanthoma elasticum in which the elastic fiber damage can be seen with routine stains). However, elastic fiber stains reveal diminution of elastin fibers throughout the dermis as well as clumping and thickening. Eventually, most elastic fibers may be lost and leave only positive granules.[57] The inflammatory stage of acquired cutis laxa is often characterized by neutrophils and eosinophils whose products may be responsible for the elastolysis.

Anetoderma

Anetoderma, or macular atrophy, is a localized, usually acquired, defect in dermal elastic fibers.

Clinical Features

Anetoderma is characterized by the circumscribed loss of normal skin elasticity. As a result, a soft pouch is created that may extrude above the skin surface but can also be pressed below the surface. The sensation is comparable to palpating a small hernia. The trunk is the most common site. Anetoderma is usually classified as idiopathic either with or without a preceding inflammatory stage or following a well-defined inflammatory disease such as acne or varicella. However, this is an artificial distinction because both types of anetoderma have an inflammatory stage during which elastin is destroyed.[58,59] Anetoderma has been described in association with early human immunodeficiency virus infection and autoimmune abnormalities.

Histopathologic Features

Routine sections often show no abnormalities. However, with an elastic fiber stain there will be diminution or absence of fibers[60] (Fig. 16-15). In addition, early lesions often have an inflammatory lymphocytic infiltrate. The dominant cells are T-helper cells that presumably secrete lymphokines, which damage elastic fibers. Macrophages can be found that envelop fragmented elastic fibers,[61] but this is a nonspecific finding.[62]

Differential Diagnosis

Both cutis laxa and anetoderma are types of elastolysis. There are many other disorders that also have reduced or absent elastic fibers, including follicular atrophoderma and mid-dermal elastolysis. In addition, some connective tissue nevi have been described as lacking elastin (nevus anelasticus) or containing fragmented elastin (papular elastorrhexis).[63] Their relationship to elastolytic disorders remains confusing. Finally, some older patients develop fine white papules on the neck and upper trunk that histologically reveal reduced elastin, often with dystrophic fibers mimicking pseudoxanthoma elasticum.[49]

Follicular Atrophoderma

Follicular atrophoderma consists of patulous follicles, most often on the back of the hand or cheeks. In some cases, they result from elastin damage.

Clinical Features. Follicular atrophoderma may be isolated or associated with a variety of disorders, including

1. Keratosis pilaris and other disorders with plugged follicles, sometimes known as *atrophoderma vermiculatum*
2. Perifollicular scars after acne
3. Chondrodysplasia punctata, CHILD syndrome, and other X-linked dominant disorders
4. Bazex syndrome—follicular atrophoderma associated with multiple basal cell carcinomas, hypohidrosis, and hypotrichosis[64]

Histopathologic Features. In follicular atrophoderma a large dilated pore or follicle is seen. Special stains may show reduction in peripheral elastic fibers. This supports the concept of perifollicular elastolysis. Rarely scarring adjacent to the atrophic area is seen. In contrast to an acne comedo, the patulous follicle is empty and lacks inflammation.

Mid-Dermal Elastolysis

Clinical Features. Patients acquire sharply marginated finely wrinkled plaques usually on the trunk that resemble aged skin.

Histopathologic Features. Elastic fibers are normal in the papillary and deep dermis but absent in the middle regions. The changes are similar to cutis laxa. Inflammatory cells are not seen.[65]

Acrodermatitis Chronica Atrophicans

Acrodermatitis chronica atrophicans is a chronic disease, caused by *Borrelia burgdorferi* (subtype *B. afzelii*) and characterized by striking cutaneous atrophy.

Clinical Features

Acrodermatitis chronica atrophicans has long been identified in outdoor workers in central Europe. Initially patients develop a puffy erythematous periarticular eruption that often follows a tick bite. This phase may be associated with a variety of neurologic symptoms, especially a polyneuropathy (Bannwerth syndrome). If left untreated, over a period of years the involved skin becomes cigarette-paper thin so that dermal vessels and other structures can easily be seen. In addition, either in such areas or independent of them, nodules of lymphoid hyperplasia develop.[66]

Histopathologic Features

The early phase of acrodermatitis chronica atrophicans has few distinguishing features; a lymphocytic perivascular infiltrate and edema are most often seen. By contrast, later or well-developed

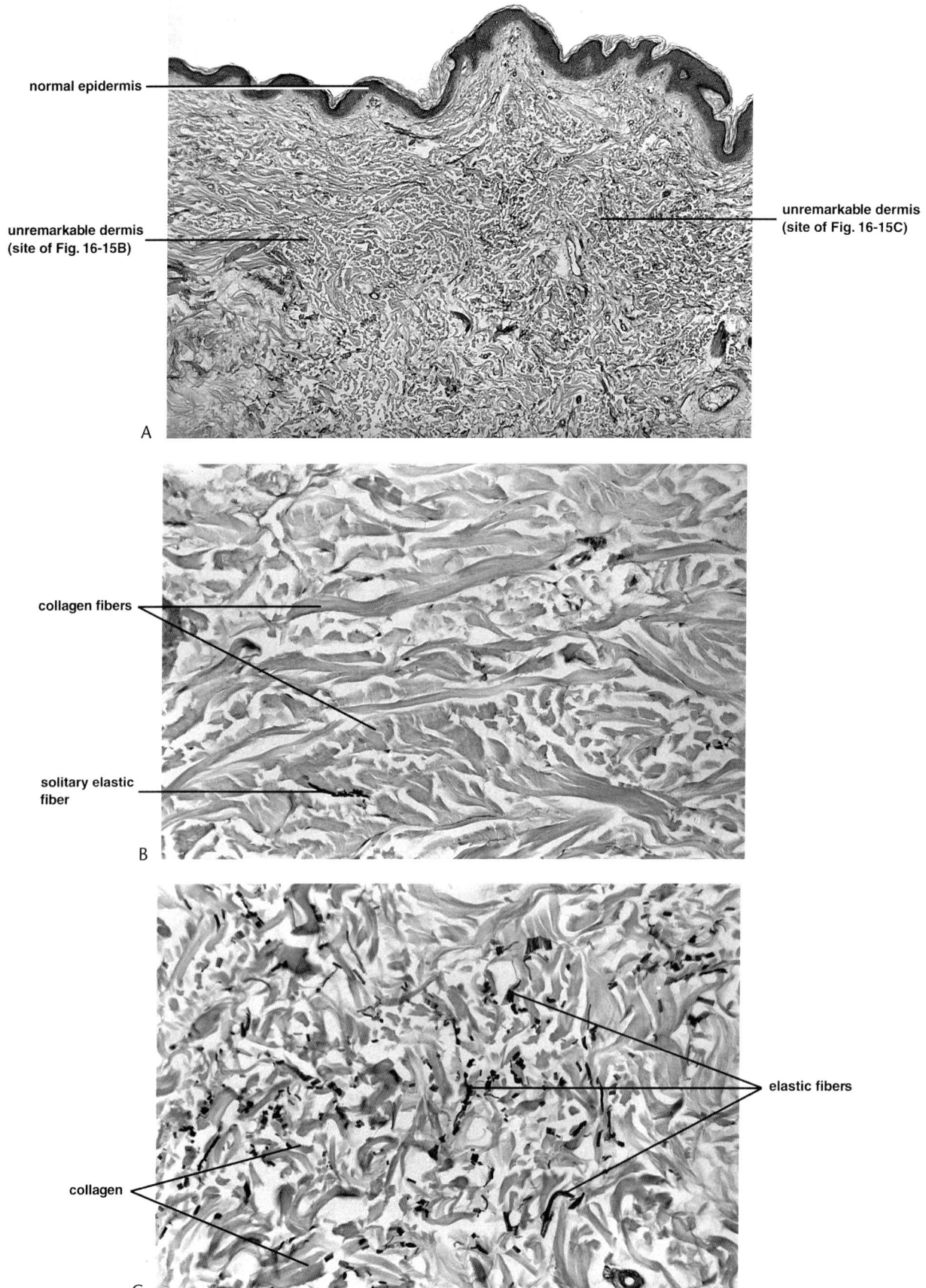

Figure 16-15. Anetoderma. (**A**) On the left, there is virtually no elastin in the otherwise normal dermis. On the right, fragments of elastin can be seen. (**B**) At higher magnification no elastic fibers can be seen. (**C**) Here elastic fibers are present. (Elastin stains.)

acrodermatitis chronica atrophicans is as distinctive histologically as it is clinically. The H&E sections show three layers: (1) an atrophic epidermis, (2) a zone of sclerotic, acellular dermis, and (3) a band-like lymphocytic infiltrate rich in plasma cells arranged around vessels and across the mid-dermis (Fig. 16-16). The dermis is also abnormal with elastic fiber staining. The papillary dermal fibers are usually normal, but beneath them there is a sclerotic and inflammatory band with markedly reduced elastic fibers, and, finally, the deeper fibers are relatively normal or even increased in number. Organisms can be found in about two-thirds of biopsy specimens most easily in infiltrated and nodular lesions.[67] Occasionally it may be difficult to separate acrodermatitis chronica atrophicans and morphea histologically.[68]

A variety of tumors may arise in acrodermatitis chronica atrophicans. Both basal cell carcinomas and squamous cell carcinomas may appear, but they do not have unique histologic features. The lymphocytic nodules must be analyzed like any other cutaneous lymphocytic infiltrate. Although most often they are reactive and benign, lymphomas have been identified in some cases. They may contain *Borrelia* organisms.

Striae

Striae are acquired dermal defects associated with both mechanical stretching and hormonal influences.

Clinical Features

Striae or stretch marks and their cause are usually identified by the patient. Occasionally, when the usual predisposing factors (pregnancy, weight gain, exogenous anabolic steroids, muscle building) are missing or the clinical location is atypical, a lesion may be biopsied.

Histopathologic Features

The best way to identify striae is to obtain a long elliptical specimen across the lesion so that normal skin is on both sides of the cutaneous defect. The central area clinically suspected of being a stretch mark will show a distortion of normal dermal architecture (Fig. 16-17). The main finding is fine straight bundles of collagen parallel to the skin surface. Elastic fibers in relatively recent striae are very fine and appear diminished.[69] They may thicken in older lesions[70,71] (Fig. 16-18). Some striae may be linear across the midback. They usually show increased elastic fibers and may represent a different process.[72]

Solar Elastosis

Solar elastosis is acquired damage to dermal collagen caused by chronic solar exposure.

Clinical Features

Solar elastosis is the most common type of dermal damage, but it is not well understood. Skin from sun-exposed areas in adults shows a variety of clinical changes. In addition to actinic keratoses, there may be speckled hyperpigmentation on the sides of the neck (poikiloderma of Civatte), tiny cysts and comedones (Favre-Racouchot, nodular elastoidosis with cysts and comedones), stellate pseudo scars, and amorphous papules and nodules (nodular elastosis and elastotic nodules of the ear), as well as many other even less common forms.[73] Although the histologic finding of solar elastosis often does not produce a specific clinical appearance, it can be expected in biopsy specimens taken from sun-exposed or sun-damaged skin.

One peculiar possible variant of solar elastosis is the papules that arise along the facing borders of the thumb and index finger. Their terminology is confusing, as they were initially called *degenerative collagenous plaques* and later *keratoelastoidosis marginalis*. Because they contain basophilic elastotic masses that are frequently calcified, the name *digital papular calcific elastosis* has also been suggested.[74] Other patients may have similar lesions with hyperplasia of elastin (acrokeratoelastoidalis) or marked hyperkeratosis and a normal dermis (focal acral hyperkeratosis).

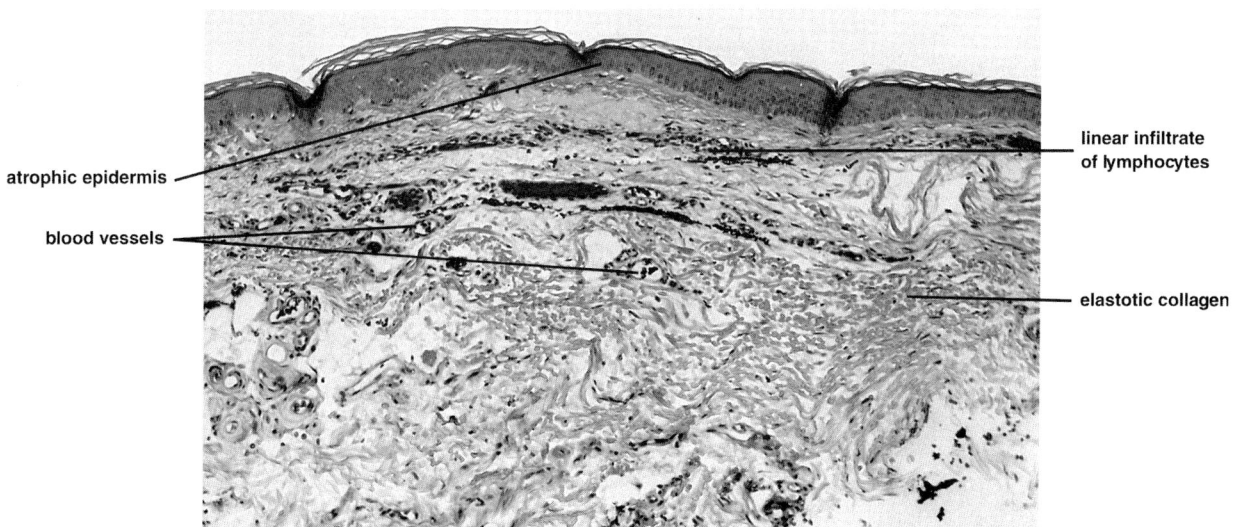

Figure 16-16. Acrodermatitis chronica atrophicans. The epidermis is atrophic. There is a small band of sclerotic dermis beneath which is a lymphocytic perivascular infiltrate and an increased number of vessels. The middle reticular dermis shows elastosis.

atrophic epidermis

blood vessels

linear infiltrate of lymphocytes

elastotic collagen

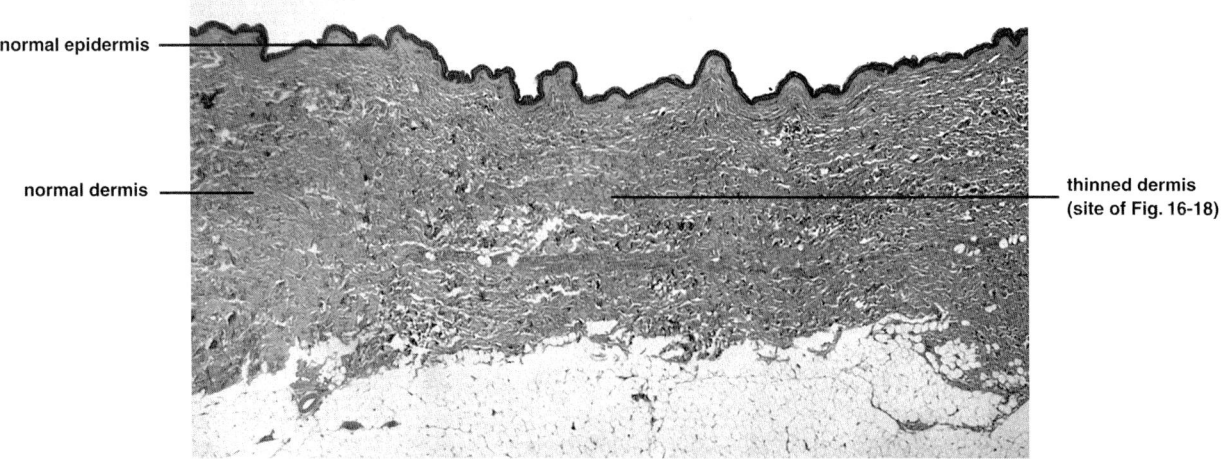

normal epidermis

normal dermis

thinned dermis
(site of Fig. 16-18)

Figure 16-17. Striae. Centrally the dermis is thinned but otherwise normal.

Histopathologic Features

In solar elastosis, the normal pink-staining dermal collagen is replaced by a blue, somewhat amorphous material, which is primarily damaged collagen, although altered elastic fibers may also be present. Peculiarly, the papillary dermis (although closer to the sun) is relatively spared, but the reticular dermis shows varying degrees of abnormally staining fibers. Most often there will be strands and clumps of blue material intermixed with residual pink-staining fibers (Fig. 16-19). In the extreme case, nodular elastosis, a large circumscribed part of the dermis stains abnormally.[75]

Clinicopathologic Correlation

The presence of solar elastosis indicates that the specimen comes from a sun-exposed area. It is usually overlooked as a tumor is searched for. Nodular solar elastosis may occasionally be clinically mistaken for a basal cell carcinoma and thus biopsied. Frequently other signs of solar damage, such as a cyst of Favre-Racouchot disease, appear in the same section.

It is puzzling that elastic fibers decrease in aged, sun-protected skin, leading to sagging and wrinkling, but increase in a dysfunctional way in sun-exposed skin. Furthermore, elastic fibers usually comprise only a small part of the dermis, so it is puzzling how they come to dominate the picture. Some have suggested that the amorphous material is collagen that has been altered to accept an elastic fiber stain while others favor overproduction of elastic fibers.[76] The issue remains unclear.

Differential Diagnosis

Solar elastosis when dispersed through bands of normal collagen can be mistaken for mucin. The elastic fiber stain will resolve the issue. Nodular solar elastosis may be confused with

Figure 16-18. Striae. The elastic fibers seem to be running parallel to the epidermal surface. (Elastin stain.)

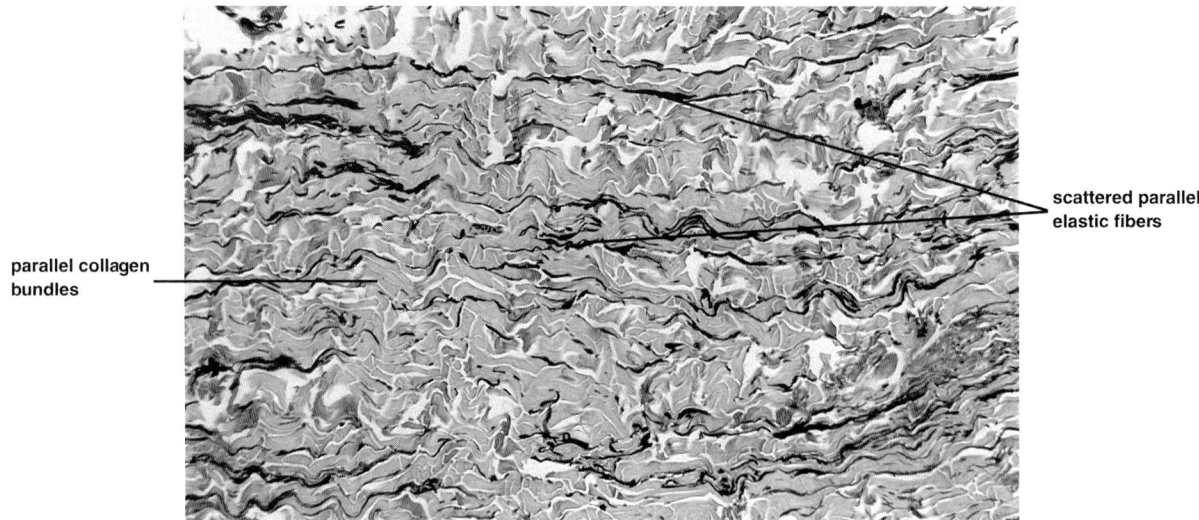

scattered parallel
elastic fibers

parallel collagen
bundles

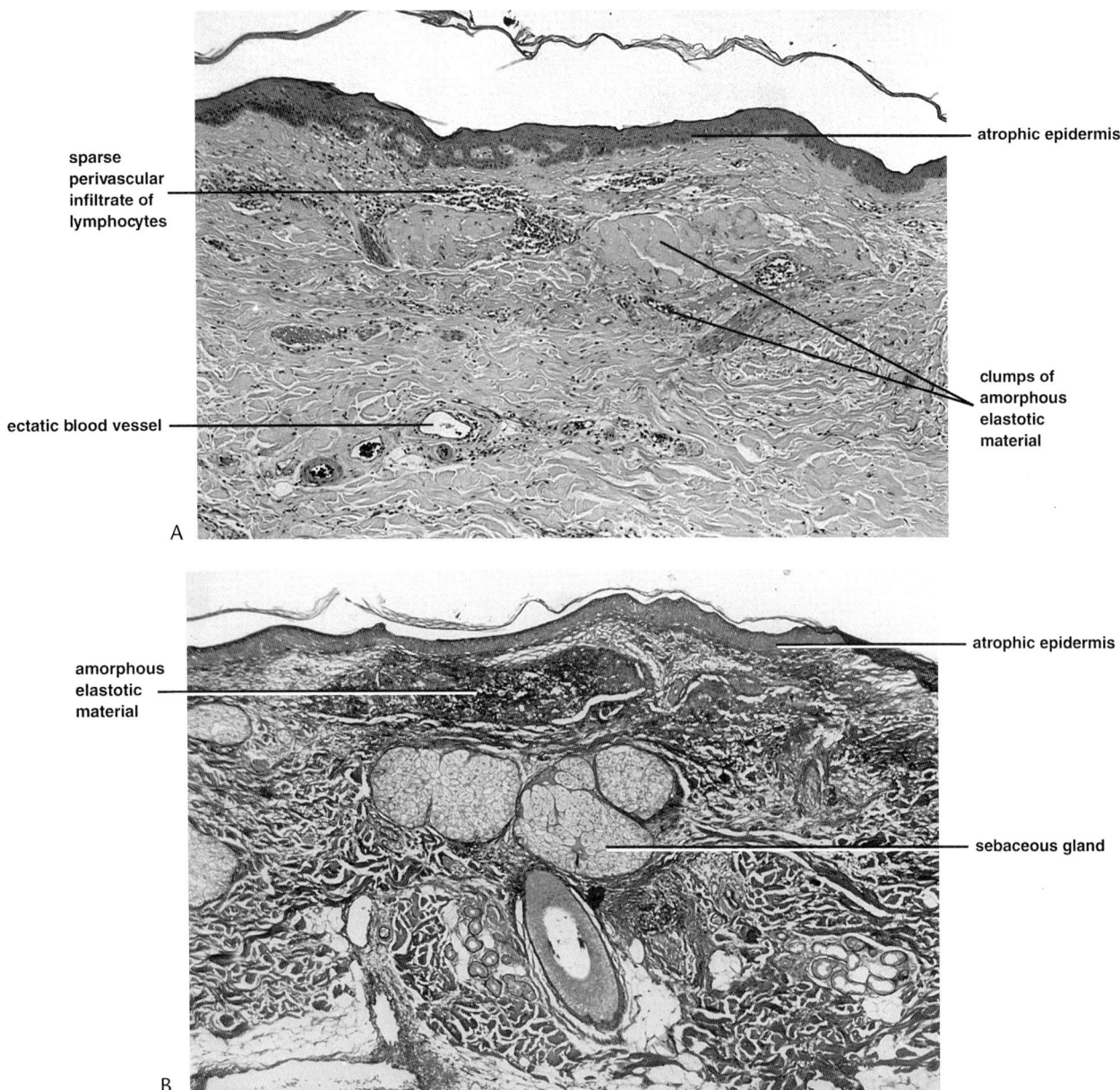

sparse
perivascular
infiltrate of
lymphocytes

atrophic epidermis

clumps of
amorphous
elastotic
material

ectatic blood vessel

A

amorphous
elastotic
material

atrophic epidermis

sebaceous gland

B

Figure 16-19. Solar elastosis. (**A**) There are two nodules of amorphous dermis seen in an otherwise unremarkable section. (**B**) This is a similar area stained with an elastin stain.

colloid milium (and in fact the two entities may be variations on the same theme). Once again, the elastic fiber stain is definitive.

Elastosis Perforans Serpiginosa

Elastosis perforans serpiginosa represents the extrusion of abnormal elastic fibers through the epidermis.

Clinical Features

Elastosis perforans serpiginosa is a clinically distinct lesion with an annular, semicircular, or serpiginous arrangement of small papules, often on the nape of the neck. It may be present in patients with Down syndrome, other connective tissue disorders (Marfan syndrome, Ehlers-Danlos syndrome, osteogenesis imperfecta, pseudoxanthoma elasticum), and in otherwise normal persons. It is also induced by the administration of penicillamine.

Histopathologic Features

The histologic picture is unique. There is a focal area of epidermal damage through which there is an extrusion of abnormally staining dermal fibers mixed with keratin and inflammatory cells (Fig. 16-20). There is often a unique snake-like channel of reactive epidermis that extends into the dermis. Special stains

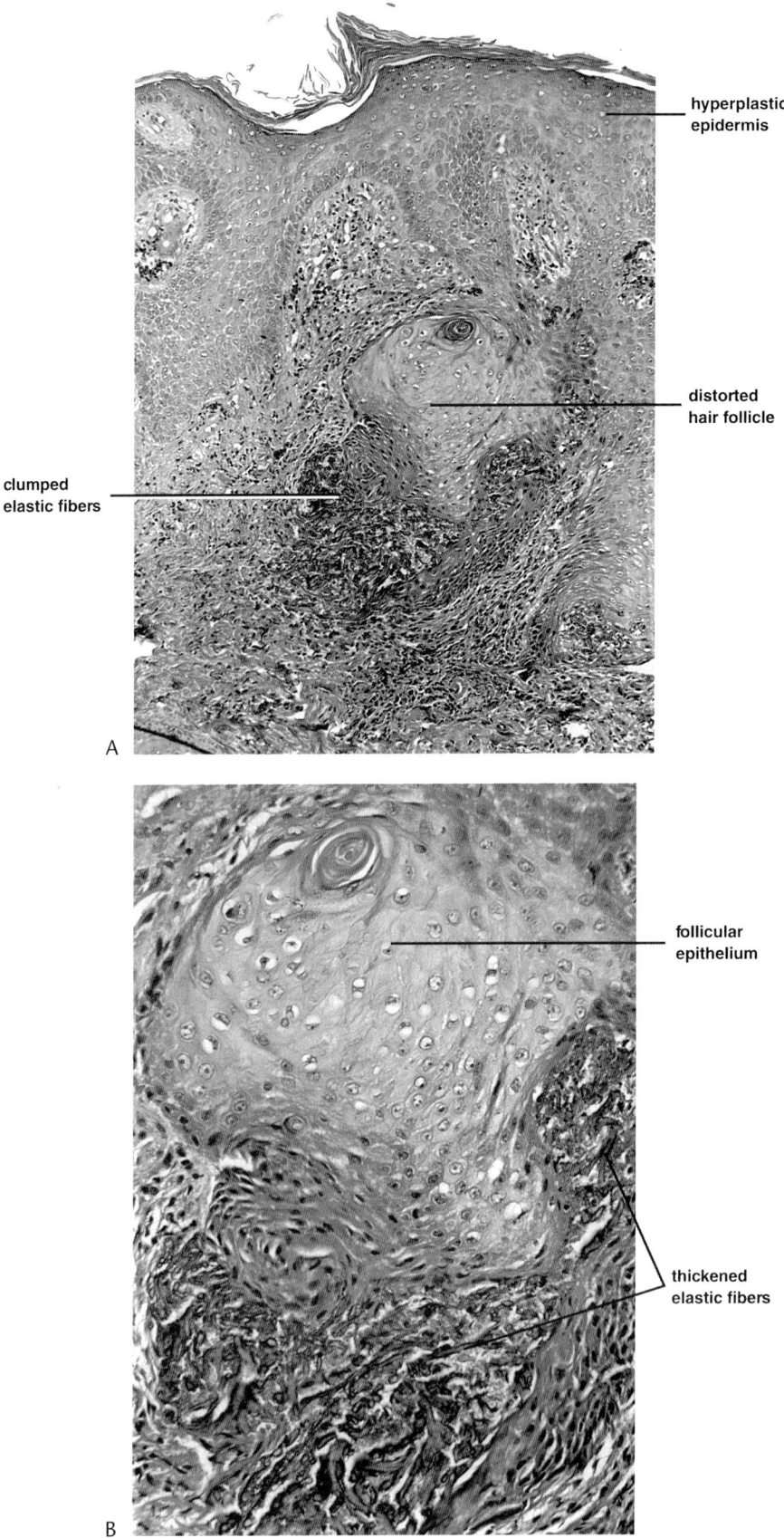

Figure 16-20. Elastosis perforans serpinosa. (**A**) An acanthotic epidermis shown with a central follicle. At the base of the follicle enlarged elastin fibers are seen. (**B**) At higher power the abnormal elastic fibers are more easily visualized.

confirm that the discharged material is elastic fibers; those at the base of the channel are more likely to be positive than those in the extruded debris.[77] This can be confirmed with electron microscopic studies. The elastic fibers in "natural" elastosis perforans serpiginosa are ultrastructurally different from those induced by penicillamine. The former are simply thickened, while the latter have lateral buds that have been compared to the twigs of a "bramble bush."[48]

EXOGENOUS DEPOSITS

In addition to the abnormalities of the normal dermal components, the skin can be altered by the dermal deposition of materials from elsewhere in the body or from exogenous sources.

Xanthomas

A xanthoma is the deposition of lipid substances in the skin or other tissues.

Clinical Features

Xanthomas are yellow papules and nodules rich in lipids. They often have an erythematous component as a result of a host inflammatory response. Although many xanthomas reflect a hyperlipidemic state, there are also normolipemic xanthomas in which either other aspects of fat metabolism are abnormal or lipids are deposited in the absence of identifiable systemic disease. The classification of xanthomas is based on their location, rapidity of onset, and clinical appearance.[78] The most common types are

1. Xanthelasma: plaques on eyelids
2. Eruptive xanthomas: tiny nodules usually on an erythematous background
3. Palmar xanthomas: papules in the palmar and plantar creases
4. Tuberous xanthomas: larger tumors, often over tendons or large joints

Although the clinical type of xanthoma may correlate with the underlying lipid abnormality to some extent, it is far simpler to obtain a blood lipid profile once a xanthoma has been identified than to attempt a subclassification based on cutaneous findings and pathology.

There are some rare disorders that are normolipemic but histologically are associated with xanthomas.[79] Included in this group are (1) xanthoma disseminatum, (2) plane xanthoma with myeloma, (3) papular xanthoma, (4) eruptive histiocytoma, and (5) progressive nodular histiocytosis. In none of these conditions are the xanthomas histologically distinct.

Histopathologic Features

Xanthomas can often be subtle. The lipids are often extracted by processing and difficult to see. In addition, only small amounts of lipids may be present. Thus, a xanthoma may fall into the differential diagnosis of an "invisible" tumor.

Xanthomas also evolve through several stages. Initially, as lipids leak from vessels and deposit in the dermis, an eruptive xanthoma may be indistinguishable from leukocytoclastic vasculitis, as the host response to lipids mounts (Fig. 16-21). Eruptive xanthoma may also contain urate-like crystals and be mistaken for early gout.[80] As more deposition occurs, lipid-laden foamy macrophages can be seen. At one end of the spectrum, a xanthoma may mimic a clear cell tumor (Fig. 16-22) and at the other end, a histiocytic lesion. Even later in the course, the foamy cells may disappear, and reactive macrophages are left that may evolve into Touton giant cells whose nuclei are arranged in a ring or wreath around a compact center with a peripheral foamy cytoplasm.

Lipid droplets can be stained with fat stains if they are preserved. Some xanthomas may also polarize; those with large amounts of cholesterol are more likely to do so, because cholesterol better resists processing. Frozen sections are ideal for visualizing xanthomas but rarely obtained.

Pitfalls

If a foamy lesion is from very thin skin or has numerous sebaceous glands or if one surface is mucosal or if striated muscle is seen, it may well represent xanthelasma.

Verruciform Xanthoma

Verruciform xanthoma is a traumatic xanthoma, usually on the oral mucosa.

Clinical Features

Verruciform xanthomas are verrucous papules that most often occur on the lips but can develop elsewhere in the oral cavity,[81,82] the genitalia, and rarely the skin.[83] The changes of verruciform xanthomas are seen in long-standing lesions of CHILD syndrome.

Histopathologic Features

Sections show a papilloma that at first glance may be mistaken for a wart. However, granular layer inclusions are absent, and the dermal papillae are filled with foamy cells (Fig. 16-23).

Amyloidosis

Amyloidosis results from the transformation of a variety of proteins into fibrillar material that is deposited in tissues.

Pathophysiology

To understand amyloid, the structure of the protein and the means of identifying it must be considered before proceeding to clinical issues. Many reviews are available.[84] Amyloid is not a single substance, but a variety of unrelated proteins with several common characteristics:

1. *Antiparallel β-sheet conformation*: this conformation of proteins is highly resistant to degradation and explains why amyloid is so persistent in tissue and not removed. The standard protein structure is an α-helix with a twisted

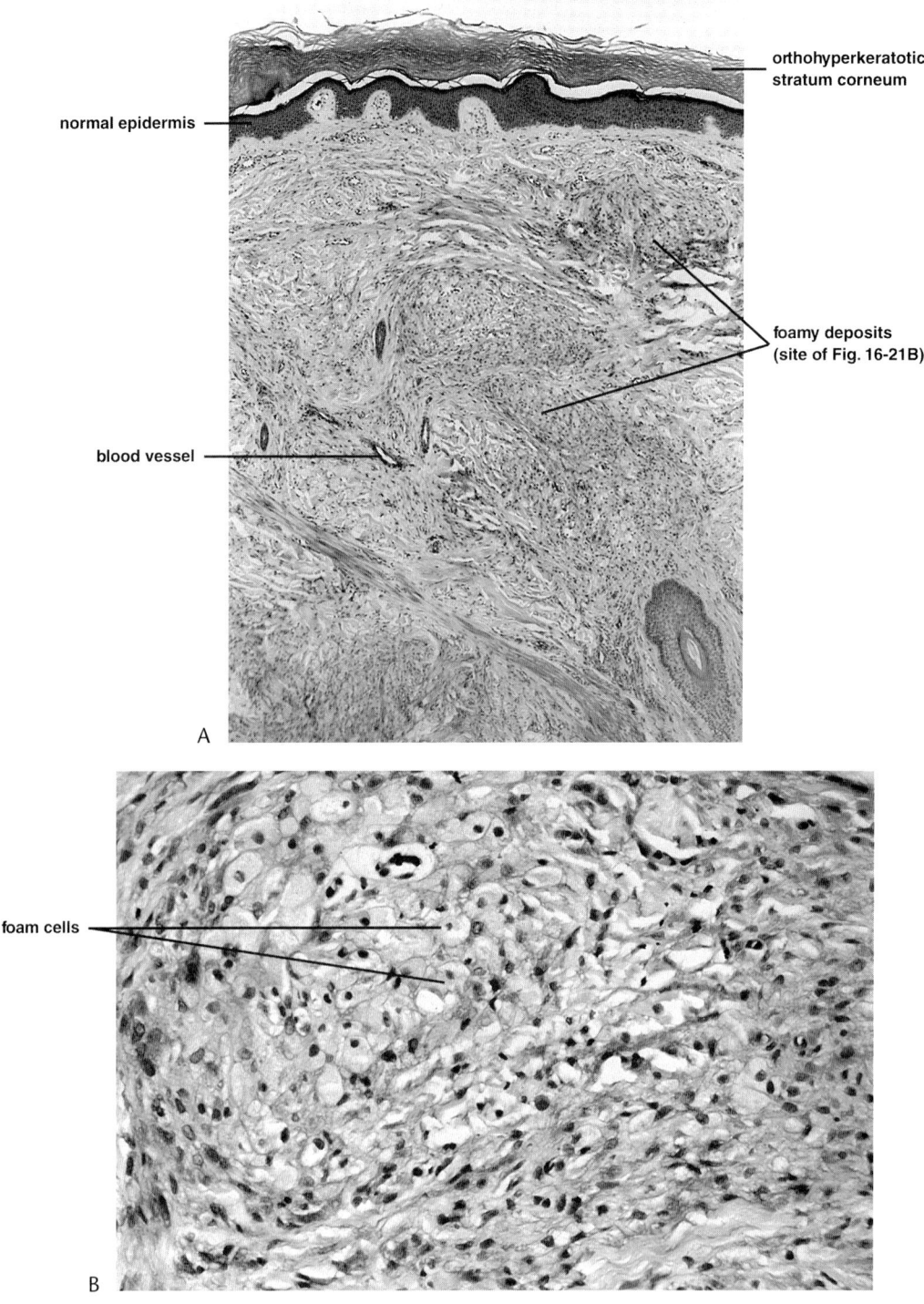

Figure 16-21.   Xanthoma. (**A**) Deposits of perivascular lipid are seen throughout the dermis. (**B**) Foam cells at higher power.

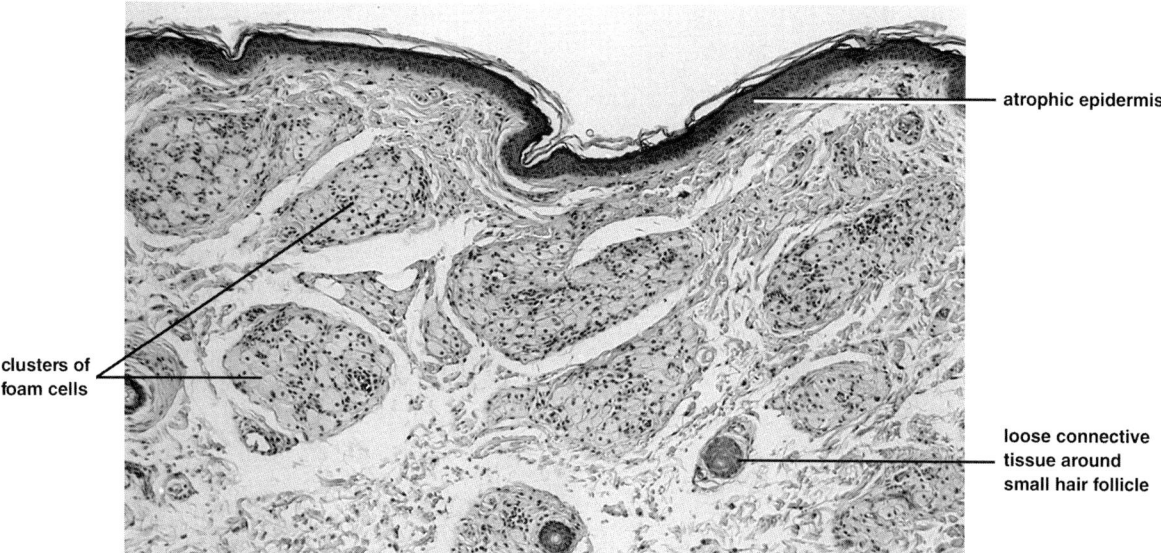

clusters of foam cells

atrophic epidermis

loose connective tissue around small hair follicle

Figure 16-22. Xanthelasma. The deposits of foamy lipids have a sharper border. The epidermis is very thin, giving a possible clue that this is from the eyelid.

Figure 16-23. Verruciform xanthoma. At midpower view one can see elongated dermal papillae, the absence of a granular layer, and increased vascularity (suggesting that this is from the oral mucosa), as well as foamy deposits in the papillae.

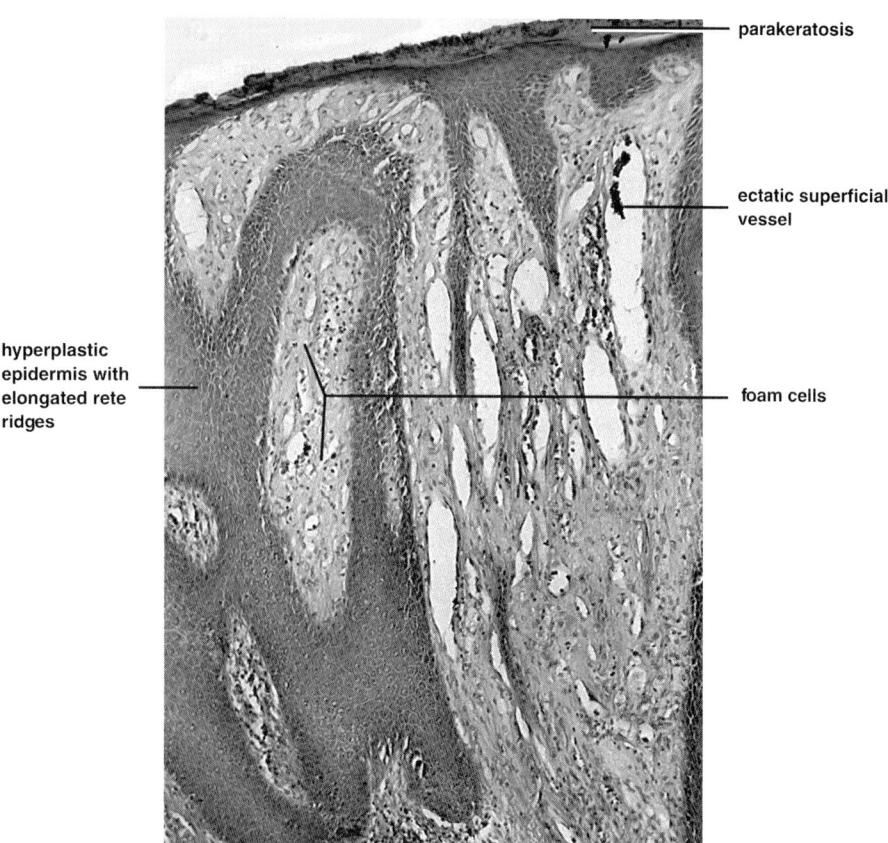

parakeratosis

ectatic superficial vessel

hyperplastic epidermis with elongated rete ridges

foam cells

Table 16-2. Staining Characteristics of Amyloid

Stain	Characteristics
H&E	Amorphous eosinophilic extracellular aggregates; clefts result from shrinkage during processing
PAS with diastase	Purple masses; probably result from presence of glycoprotein P component
Methyl violet and crystal violet	Reddish metachromasia; best used on unfixed frozen sections
Thioflavine-T	Yellowish fluorescence; sensitive, but not specific
Congo red, Sirius red (cotton dyes)	Most specific and characteristic stain for amyloid; apple-green birefringence in polarized light (dichroism); may faintly stain colloid milium, lipoid proteinosis, porphyria cutanea tarda

(From Norwood,[200] with permission.)

molecule with hydrogen bonds that stabilize a single polypeptide. In the β-sheet, adjacent polypeptides are laid down side by side with hydrogen bonds between them; depending on the direction of the adjacent polypeptides, they are called *parallel* or *antiparallel*. Other examples of antiparallel β-sheets are fibroin (silk protein), feathers, and hooves

2. *Distinct structure on electron microscopy*: amyloid fibrils are rigid nonbranching structures, 50 to 150 Å in width and 600 to 8,000 Å in length

3. *Well-defined staining characteristics* (Table 16-2)

The sources of amyloid (Table 16-3) include

1. Light chains (AL)
2. Serum amyloid A protein (SAA), an acute phase reactant and precursor of AA amyloid, the "wear and tear" amyloid, as well as the amyloid deposited in familial Mediterranean fever
3. Familial amyloid (AF) proteins, which are heterogeneous but usually prealbumin molecules
4. Amyloid of hemodialysis (AH), which primarily β2 microglobulin
5. Endocrine amyloid (AE), which results from deposition of hormonal polypeptides such as calcitonin
6. Senile amyloid (AS), which includes a variety of poorly defined proteins deposited primarily in the heart and brain
7. Cutaneous amyloid (AD), which arises from the rearrangement of tonofilaments derived from keratinocytes

In addition, most amyloids are accompanied by glycosoaminoglycans and amyloid P component derived from serum amyloid P protein, a pentraxin or doughnut-shaped pentamer closely related to C-reactive protein. Amyloid P component is normally seen in the dermis and basement membranes of cutaneous vessels and appendages but not the dermoepidermal junction. It is bound to amyloid in a calcium-dependent manner.

Clinical Features

Primary amyloidosis (immunocytic amyloidosis) represents the deposition of light chains; its most common symptoms are weight loss, weakness, and general malaise. Initial findings may include ankle edema, macroglossia, and hepatomegaly, as well as bilateral carpel tunnel syndrome.[85] Initial cutaneous findings include[86]

1. Purpura: eyelid purpura or pinch purpura is most common. Postproctoscopic palpebral purpura is fairly typical. A

Table 16-3. Types of Amyloid

Abbreviation	Type	Chemical Composition
	Systemic	
AA	Secondary (reactive, acquired)	AA (amyloid protein A) immunoglobulin light chains or fragments
AL	Primary; multiple myeloma-associated	
AF	Heredofamilial	
	Familial amyloid polyneuropathy	Prealbumins
	Hereditary cerebral angiopathy	Cystatin C
	Familial Mediterranean fever	AA (amyloid protein A)
AH	Hemodialysis associated	β2 microglobulin
	Localized	
AE	Endocrine	
	Thyroid	Precalcitonin
	Pancreas	Calcitonin gene-related protein
AS	Senile	
	Brain (Alzheimer, Down)	B protein
	Heart	Prealbumin
AD	Skin	Keratin or precursor

(From Cohen,[84] with permission.)

biopsy specimen shows deposition of amyloid in vessel walls with hemorrhage.

2. Infiltrated waxy plaques: typically seen on the eyelids, face, oral cavity, and about the anus; they reveal unmistakable diffuse sheets of amorphous material through the dermis.

3. Bullous amyloidosis: these may develop usually with separation just above papillary dermal deposits.[87]

4. Elastotic lesions: these may also develop perhaps triggered by an interaction between elastic fibers and the amyloid P component.[88]

Skin changes occur in 20% to 40% of primary amyloidosis patients. In approximately 50% of cases without cutaneous findings, a blind biopsy specimen of the rectal mucosa, gingiva, or clinically normal skin may demonstrate perivascular deposits of amyloid (Fig. 16-24). Subcutaneous fat can be aspirated and stained to search for the same changes with perhaps a higher positive yield.[89]

Reactive Amyloidosis

A variety of chronic diseases such as tuberculosis, lepromatous leprosy, rheumatoid arthritis, and many neoplasms may cause deposition of amyloid in the liver, spleen, and kidney. Cutaneous deposition is rare and cutaneous lesions even rarer. A blind biopsy as with primary amyloidosis is recommended. Familial Mediterranean fever has an erysipelas-like erythema during attacks but does not have cutaneous amyloid deposits.

Cutaneous Amyloidosis

There are three major types of cutaneous amyloidosis: macular amyloidosis, lichen amyloidosus, and nodular amyloidosis.[90,91] There are also several rare types of familial cutaneous amyloidosis; the best known is the Muckle-Wells syndrome in which

renal amyloidosis, deafness, and recurrent urticaria are inherited in an autosomal dominant fashion.

Macular Amyloidosis

Clinical Features

Macular amyloidosis is almost invariably intrascapular and characterized by intense itching and mottled hyperpigmentation,[92] suggesting an overlap with notalgia paresthetica.[93] It may occur elsewhere and rarely in association with other diseases such as pachyonychia congenita.[94] Biphasic forms have been described that show an overlap between macular amyloidosis and lichen amyloidosus.[95]

Histopathologic Features

The microscopic features of macular amyloidosis are subtle. The epidermis may be normal or thinned. There is usually some damage at the basal layer with incontinentia pigmenti. In the dermal papillae there are faint amorphous pale-staining deposits (Fig. 16-25). They are often most difficult to stain with amyloid stains. Crystal violet may be the most reliable.

Lichen Amyloidosus

Clinical Features

Lichen amyloidosus is an intensely pruritic eruption characterized by small skin-colored to violaceous papules. The most common location is on the anterior shins, but the lesions may occur anywhere. This disorder is common in some Oriental groups, especially Malaysians.[96] In some intensely itchy dermatoses such as primary biliary cirrhosis, lichen amyloidosus develops and suggests that the sequence is pruritus-epidermal cell damage-amyloid. It has also been described in multiple endocrine neoplasia type II.[97]

Figure 16-24.   Primary amyloidosis. A vessel in the fat whose wall has been infiltrated by an amorphous material that is amyloid.

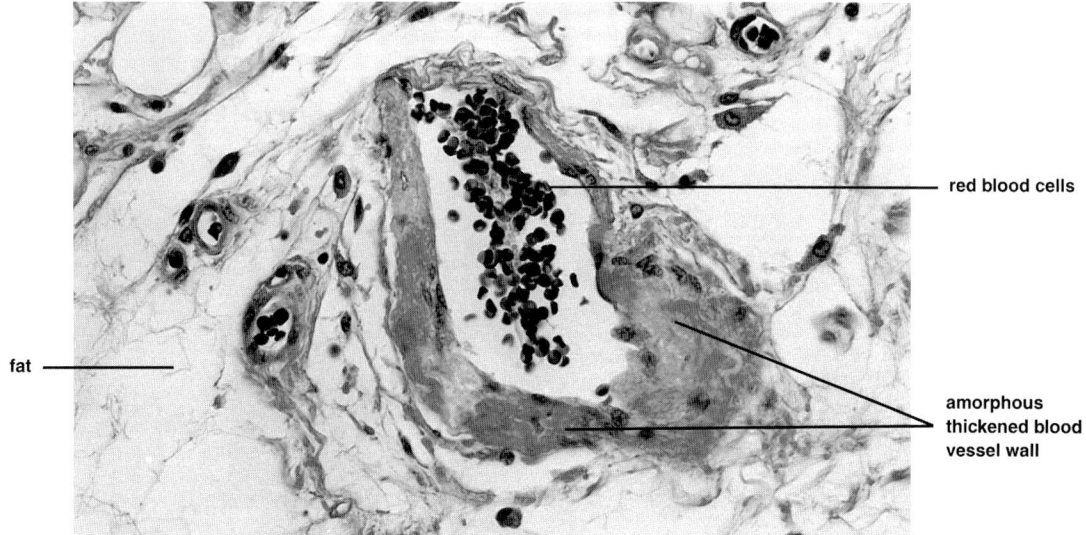

fat

red blood cells

amorphous thickened blood vessel wall

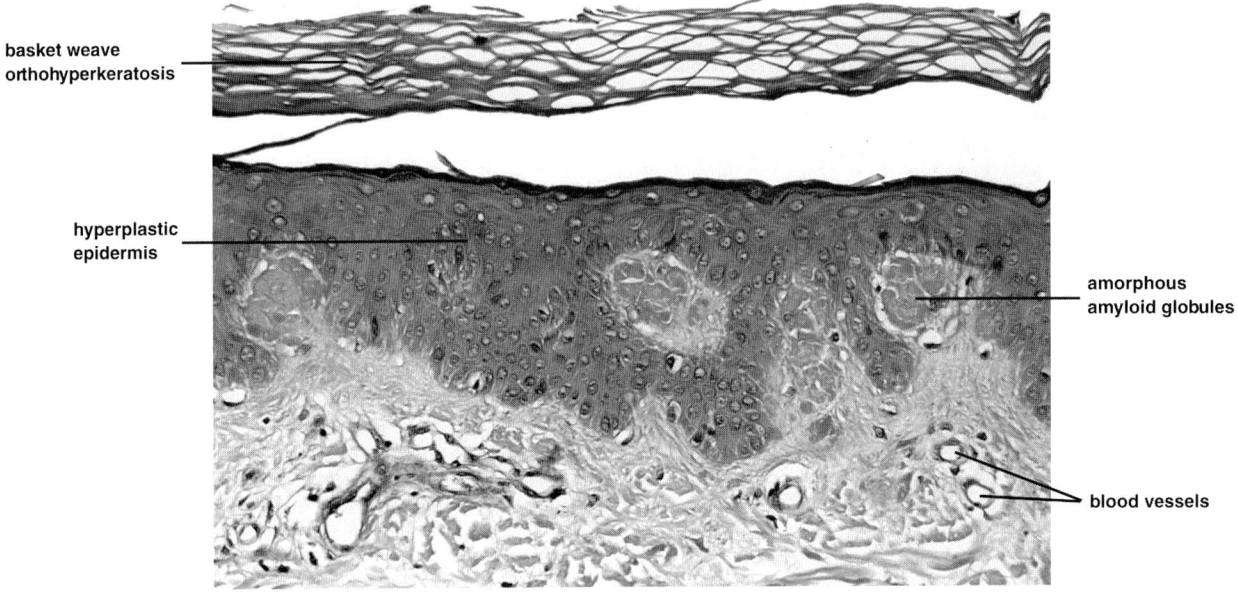

basket weave orthohyperkeratosis

hyperplastic epidermis

amorphous amyloid globules

blood vessels

Figure 16-25. Macular amyloidosis. Beneath a slightly hyperplastic epidermis there are tiny amorphous deposits in the dermal papillae.

Histopathologic Features

Sections show reactive epidermal change with orthohyperkeratosis especially in troughs between papillomatous projections of the epidermis. In the dermis, despite the clinical appearance, lichenoid inflammation is absent. Instead, there is an amorphous deposition of amyloid in the dermal papillae (Fig. 16-26). Lichen amyloidosus can be visualized as macular amyloidosis with lichen simplex chronicus superimposed.[98]

Nodular Amyloidosis

Clinical Features

Nodular amyloidosis consists of large waxy nodules in most areas of the body. They are identical to the infiltrates in primary amyloidosis and usually consist of light chains; some of these patients progress to systemic amyloidosis.

Histopathologic Features

The normal epidermis and dermis are displaced by a large amorphous nodule (Fig. 16-27). Often there are giant cells at the periphery along with plasma cells and calcification. Thus, in this type of amyloidosis, the body seems to recognize the material as foreign.[99,100] Sometimes dialysis patients develop subcutaneous nodules consisting of β-2 microglobulin.[101]

Differential Diagnosis

The differential diagnosis of a large amorphous dermal nodule includes nodular amyloidosis, colloid milium, gout, and nodular solar elastosis (Table 16-4). The light microscopic distinction is difficult. Colloid milium may display more elastic fiber damage than solar elastosis. Colloid milia may evolve into sizable lesions.

Pathophysiology

From the perspective of a dermatopathologist, amyloid can present in the skin with four patterns:

1. Vessel wall infiltration with purpura
2. Large nodules and sheets in dermis

Table 16-4. Large Amorphous Dermal Deposits

	Solar Elastosis	Giant Cells	Polarization	Calcium	Clefts	Crystals	Special Stains	Electron Microscopy
Nodular amyloidosis	−	+	−	−	−	−	Amyloid + +	Light chains
Colloid milium	+	±	−	+	+	−	Amyloid +	Damaged elastin
Gout	−	+ + +	+	+	+	+	—	—
Nodular solar elastosis	+ + +	±	−	−	+	−	Elastin + +	Damaged elastin and collagen

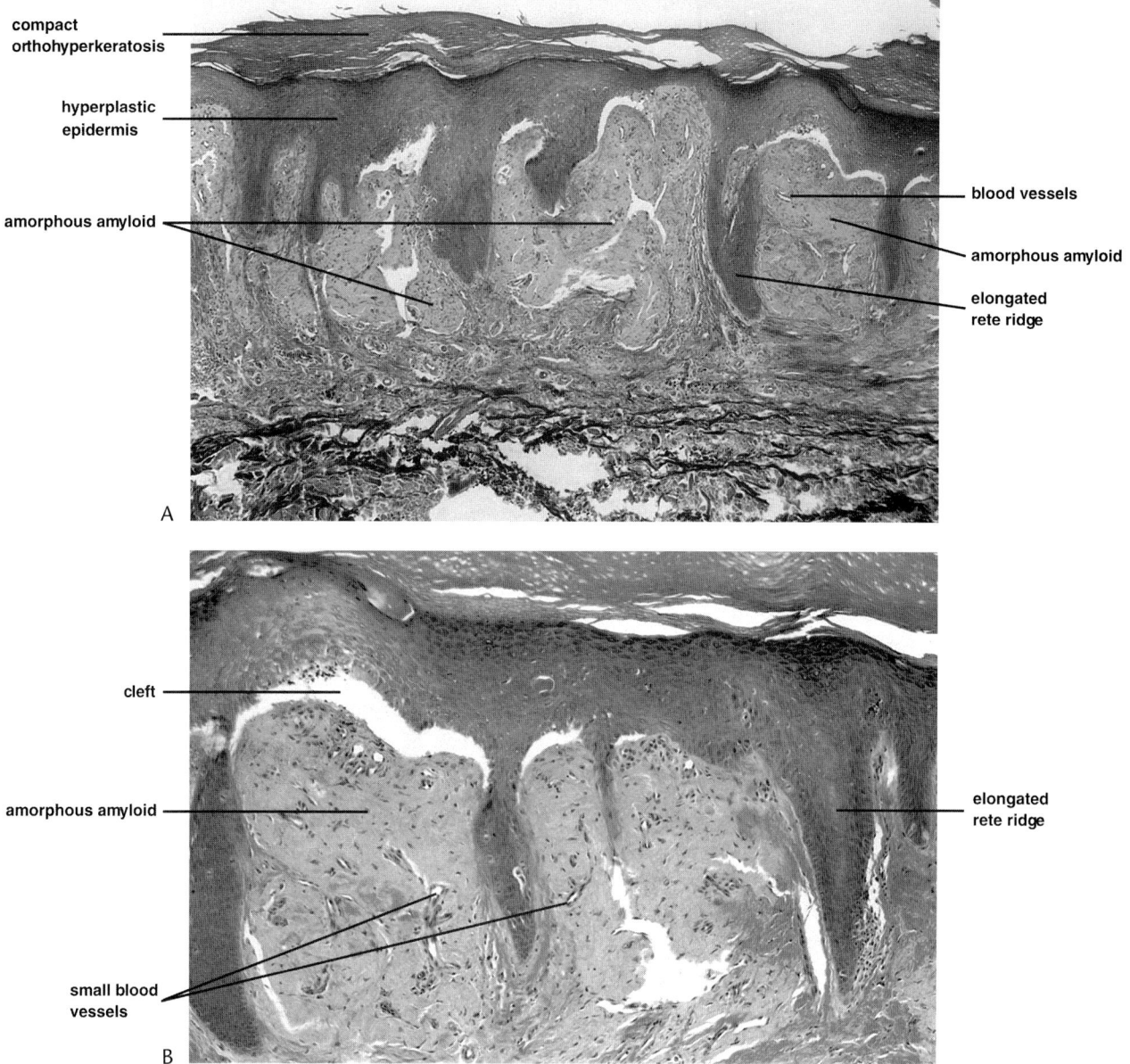

Figure 16-26. Lichen amyloidosus. **(A)** There is orthohyperkeratosis and epidermal hyperplasia. In the dermal papillae there are somewhat larger deposits of amorphous material than seen in macular amyloidosis. There is little if any infiltrate, but there is separation at the dermoepidermal junction. **(B)** At higher power squamatization of the basal layer overlying the globules of amyloid is evident. Note the stellate fibroblasts interposed among the amyloid deposits.

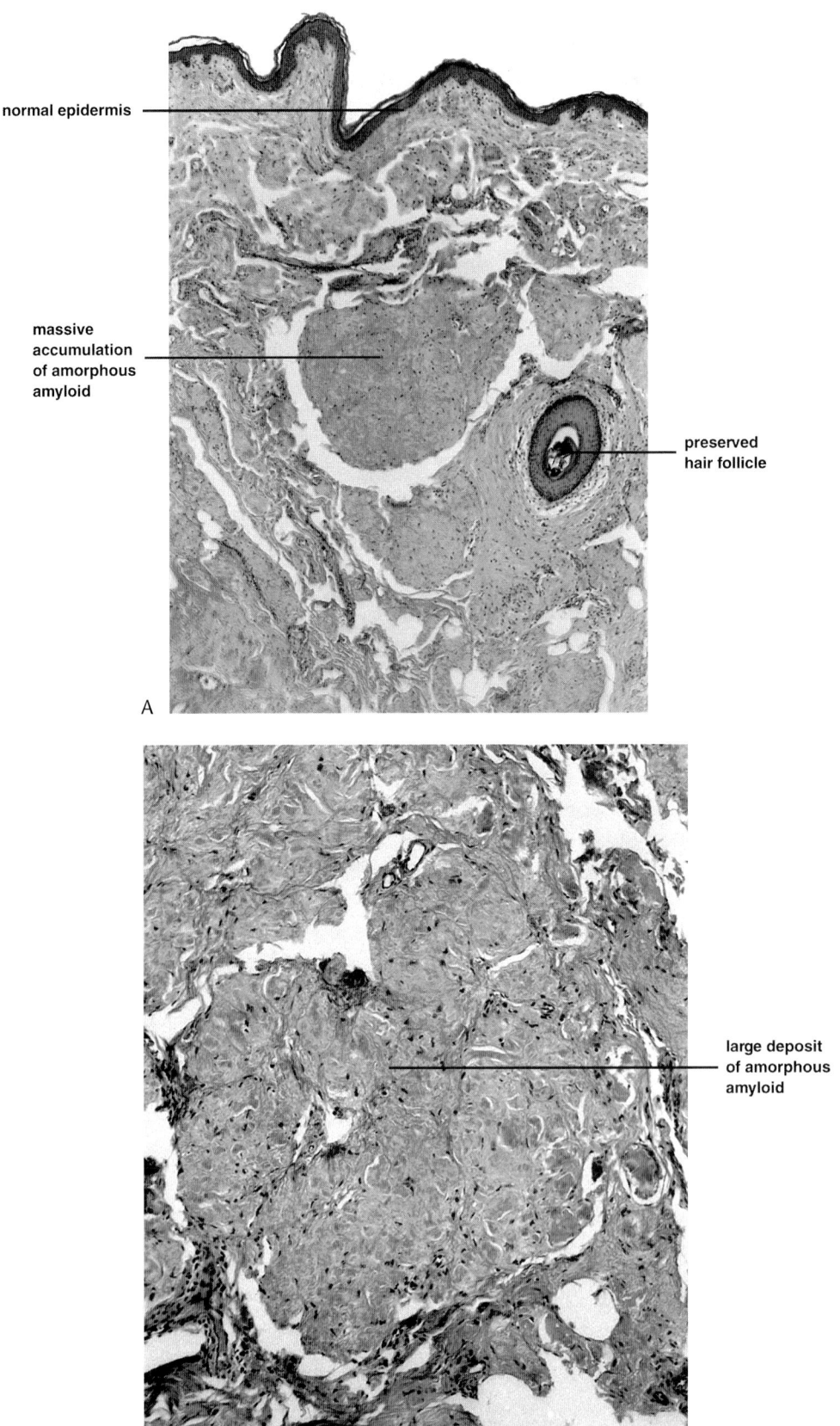

normal epidermis

massive
accumulation
of amorphous
amyloid

preserved
hair follicle

A

large deposit
of amorphous
amyloid

B

Figure 16-27. Nodular amyloidosis. (**A**) There are large bulky amorphous deposits in the dermis. The rest of this specimen is otherwise normal. There is very little foreign body reaction in this section, although occasionally that is seen in nodular amyloidosis. (**B**) The amorphous nature and great size of the deposits are evident.

3. Subtle deposition at dermoepidermal junction
4. As an innocent bystander accompanying many cutaneous tumors

In primary cutaneous amyloid, Hashimoto[102,103] has shown that the keratinocyte is the source of the amyloid and has suggested the term *K amyloid*. Damage to the epidermis from scratching, inflammation, ultraviolet light, and many other sources disrupts the normal maturation and upward migration of keratinocytes.[104] they undergo degenerative changes, and keratin drops into the dermis where it is processed by macrophages. Both histochemical and ultrastructural examinations have shown amyloid fibers in degenerating basal cells that pass into the dermis. In the process of conversion to amyloid, the α-pattern of human keratin is changed to the β-sheet. Cutaneous amyloid may be stained by monoclonal antikeratin antibodies, and in nodular amyloidosis, light chains may be identified.[100]

Amyloid deposits are frequently seen around basal cell carcinomas. Often they are readily visible; when searched for diligently, they can be found in 50% of the tumors.[105] The amyloid about basal cell carcinomas is derived from keratin. Similar deposits can be found adjacent to squamous cell carcinomas, seborrheic keratoses, and many other tumors.

Colloid Milium

Colloid milium is a waxy papule or nodule caused by an amorphous dermal deposit.

Clinical Features

Several types of colloid milium have been identified:

1. colloid milium: waxy papules in sun-damaged skin, usually on the back of the hands or the face.[106]
2. nodular or en plaque colloid degeneration: larger, fewer in number, deeper deposits

3. juvenile colloid milium: multiple papules mainly on the head and neck in children, arising before sun damage can be a factor and extremely rare.[107]

Histopathologic Features

Colloid milia have a domed surface with epidermal thinning and large amorphous dermal deposits with clefts. Solar elastosis is always present (Fig. 16-28). Nodular colloid degeneration is similar but has even larger deposits. The nature of the colloid is difficult to determine. It is most easily distinguished from amyloid based on the size of the deposits, but this does not work when contrasting nodular amyloidosis and nodular colloid degeneration. Colloid is usually negative with amyloid stains but occasionally may be weakly positive.[108] However, ultrastructural studies show an amorphous substance with fine 2-nm filaments that are the end stage of elastic degeneration.[109,110]

Juvenile colloid milium differs. While it appears identical by light microscopy and with special stains, it contains densely packed 8- to 10-nm filaments believed to represent abnormal keratin filaments from degenerating keratinocytes.[107]

Lipoid Proteinosis (Hyalinosis Cutis et Mucosae; Urbach-Wiethe Disease)

Lipoid proteinosis is a multisystem disorder characterized by the deposition of a hyaline protein in the skin, oral mucosa, and larynx. It is inherited in an autosomal recessive manner.

Clinical Features

Patients with lipoid proteinosis have beaded nodules along their eyelids as well as facial plaques. Their skin acquires a pitted or pigskin appearance. Rarely are other areas such as knees, elbows, and axillae involved. These patients also tend to be hoarse

Figure 16-28.   Colloid milium. There are amorphous deposits in the superficial dermis with numerous clefts and little inflammatory response. There is solar elastosis at the base.

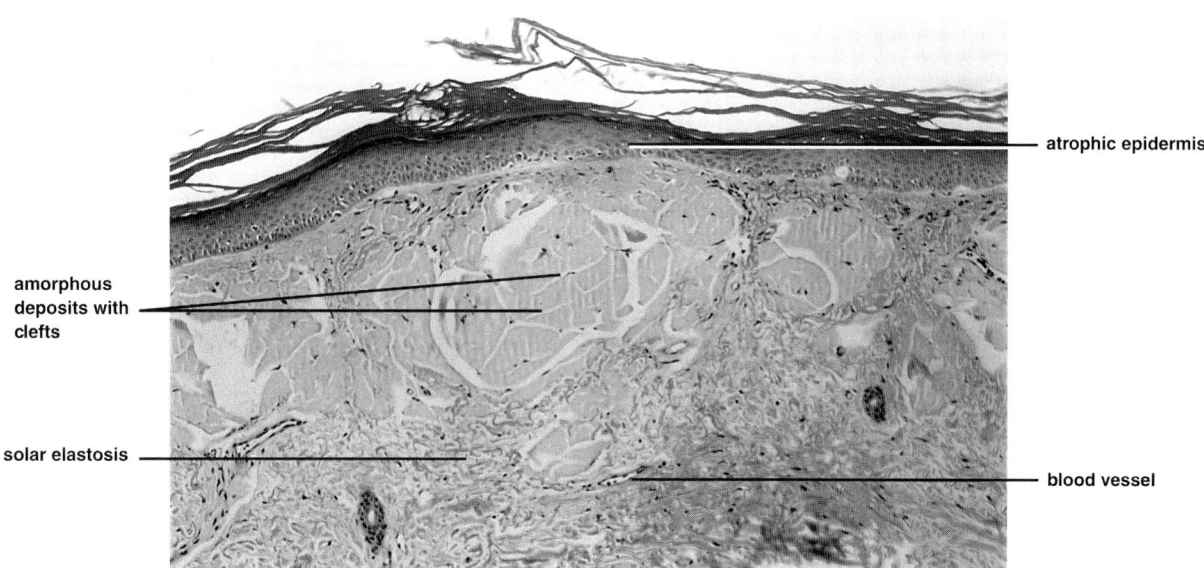

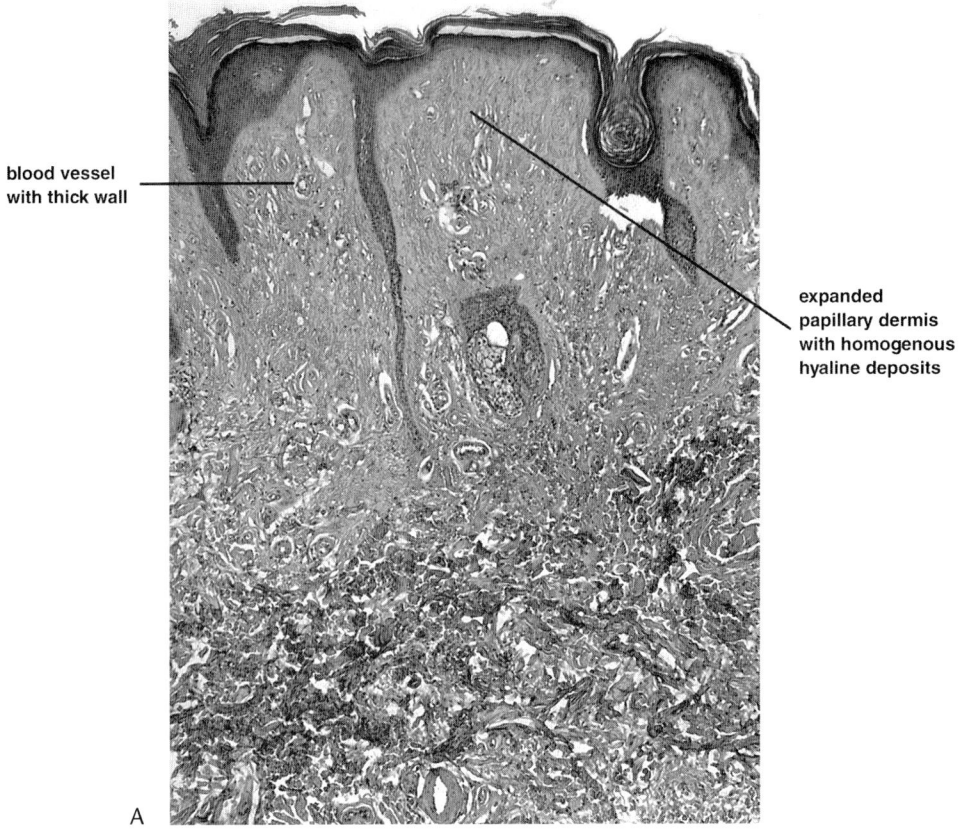

blood vessel
with thick wall

expanded
papillary dermis
with homogenous
hyaline deposits

A

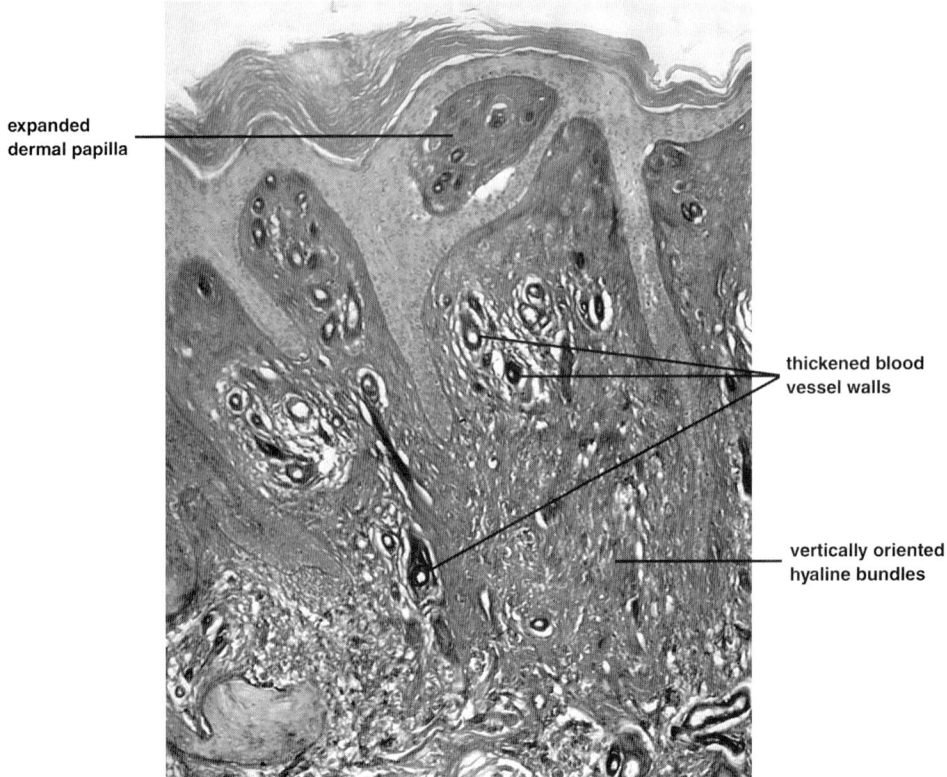

expanded
dermal papilla

thickened blood
vessel walls

vertically oriented
hyaline bundles

B

Figure 16-29. Lipoid proteinosis. (**A**) The superficial dermis is replaced by amorphous material that pushes apart the rete ridges and obliterates the collagen. (**B**) PAS shows the prominent vessels in the papillae to better advantage. (Histologic material courtesy of Gerald E. Pierard, M.D., Liege, Belgium.)

because of laryngeal nodules. Other systemic findings include diffuse infiltration of the tongue. Seizures have also been described.[111–113]

Histopathologic Features

An amorphous protein is deposited around blood vessels and as thick bundles in the dermis (Fig. 16-29). They typically are perpendicular to the skin surface. *Hyaline* means amorphous or glassy. The material is periodic acid–Schiff (PAS) positive and diastase resistant. Other stains are less conclusive. Sometimes lipid stains such as oil red O or scarlet red are positive and reveal lipid droplets throughout the hyaline material. Stains for amyloid and mucin are unpredictable and not helpful.

Ultrastructural examination reveals a complex protein produced by fibroblasts with excessive duplications of basal laminae around capillaries, appendages, nerves, and muscles. These are rich in type IV collagen. Aberrations in collagen metabolism are not the entire answer, as the deposits also contain glycoproteins.[114,115]

Differential Diagnosis

When perivascular infiltrates are seen, both porphyria (which also has duplicated basal laminae) and primary amyloidosis are suggested. The larger amorphous deposits may resemble those lesions listed in Table 16-4, but both the clinical history and the results of ultrastructural studies are different.

Gout

Gout is a systemic disturbance of uric acid metabolism.

Clinical Features

Some patients with gout have subcutaneous nodules. Gouty lesions are rarely biopsied unless the history is incomplete or inaccurate.

Histopathologic Features

Uric acid crystals are destroyed by formalin fixation, so ethanol fixation is ideal.[116] This is rarely used, so the "ghost image" of a gouty deposit is usually encountered. Nonetheless, it is quite distinct, as amorphous masses are seen with tiny clefts and shadows, surrounded usually by an intense foreign body reaction (Fig. 16-30). If alcohol fixation has been used, refractive crystals can be seen with polarization. Even formalin-fixed gout crystals polarize to a limited extent.

Differential Diagnosis

Hemodialysis patients may develop calcium oxalate crystals, which appear almost identical to gout tophi with the light microscope but can be separated by a variety of laboratory techniques.[117]

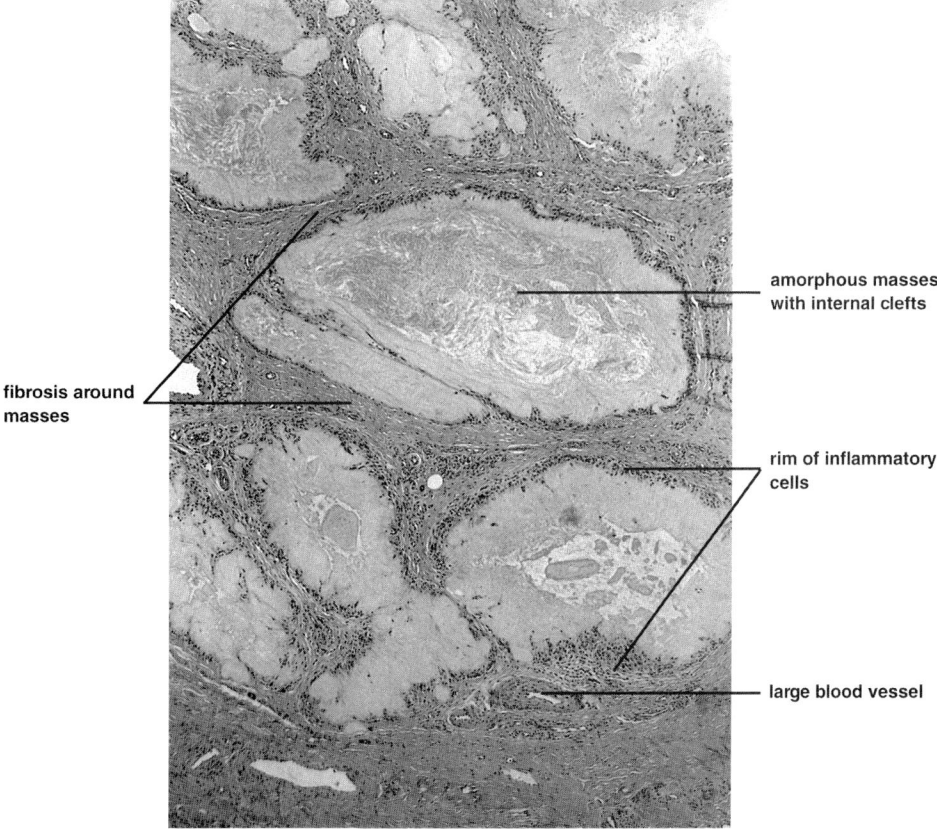

Figure 16-30. Gout. The large amorphous masses are surrounded by palisading inflammatory cell response and show the typical internal swirls and clefting.

amorphous masses with internal clefts

fibrosis around masses

rim of inflammatory cells

large blood vessel

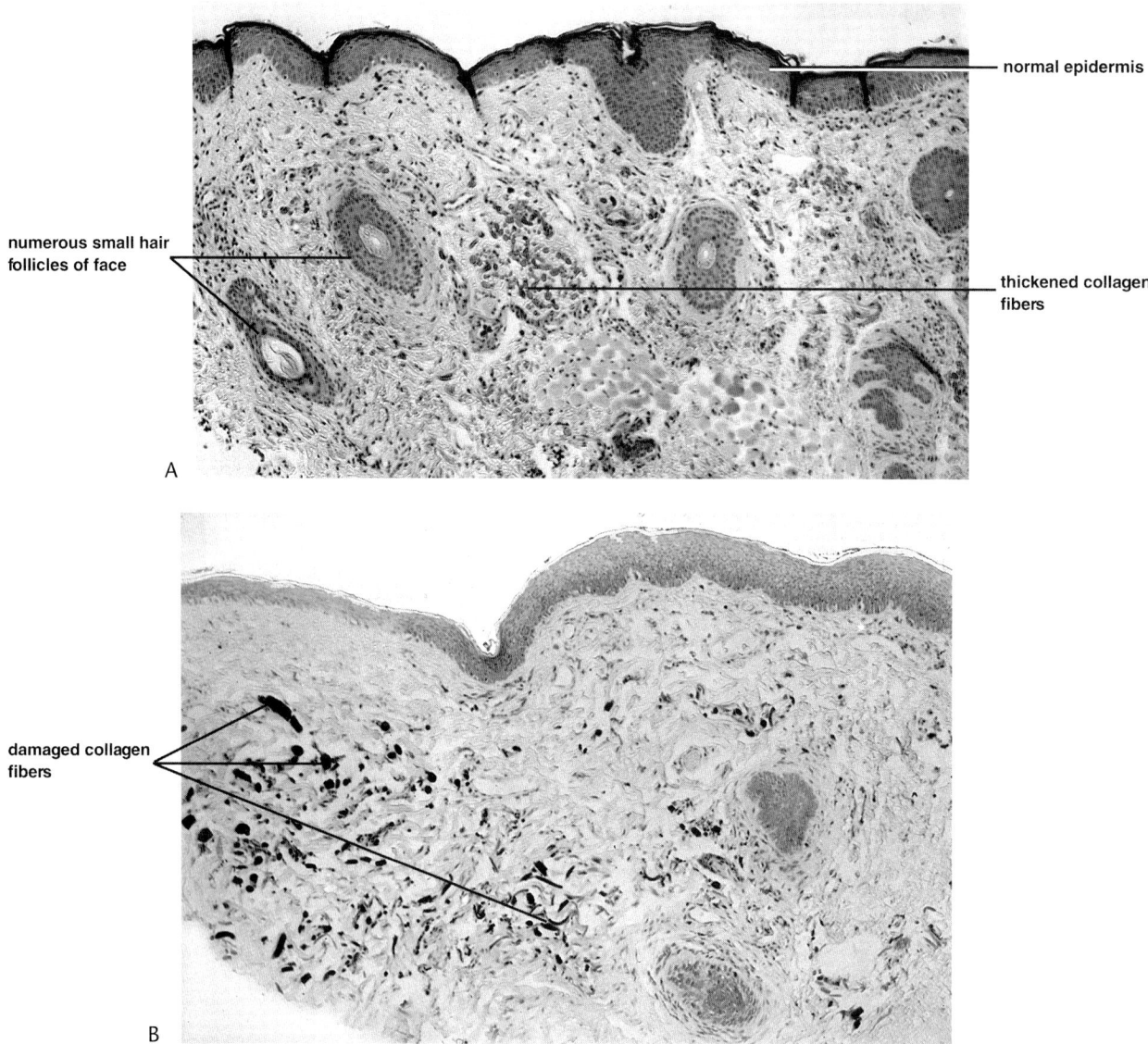

Figure 16-31. Ochronosis. (**A**) There are amorphous thickened bundles seen in the dermis. (**B**) Methylene blue stain highlights the altered collagen bundles.

Ochronosis

Ochronosis is an autosomal recessive inherited disturbance of homogentistic acid metabolism. In the skin, exogenous damage to dermal fibers may mimic the inherited disease.

Clinical Features

Endogenous ochronosis is characterized by the deposition of homogentistic acid in cartilage, ligaments, tendons, and sclerae. In the dermis and in ear cartilage, it causes a brown pigmentation. Application of topical hydroquinone produces a similar picture locally as the hydroquinone blocks homogentistic acid oxidase and the acid accumulates in the skin.[118] Caviar-like dark papules may develop, known as *ochronotic* or *pigmented colloid milium*.[119]

Histopathologic Features

The skin biopsy specimen is identical in both types. Large irregular collagen bundles are seen. With H&E staining they appear yellow-brown but are enhanced and blackened by crystal violet or methylene blue stain[120] (Fig. 16-31). The papules are filled with damaged stained collagen, which may be eliminated via follicles.[119] Ultrastructural studies show that the homogentistic acid polymerizes and accumulates in collagen as well as elastin. Rare exogenous lesions may develop a granulomatous response.[121]

Mucinoses

The terminology of the mucins is confusing and not easily clarified. We define mucin as a polysaccharide bound to varying

Table 16-5. Mucin Histochemistry

Stain	Dermal Mucins	Epithelial or Sialomucins
Alcian blue		
pH 2.5	Blue	Blue
pH 0.5	−	−
Colloidal iron	Blue	Blue
Toluidine blue	Magenta	−
Mucicarmine	Red	Red
PAS	−	Red
Hyaluronidase labile	+	−

amounts of protein that stains pale blue on ordinary H&E stains and has a vacuolated or stringy pattern.

Pathophysiology

There are many different types of mucin, characterized by the nature of the sugars and proteins, as well as the degree of sulfation and hydroxylation. The mucins are all rich in water. Routine preservation removes the water and leaves behind basophilic strands. The mucin is secreted by fibroblasts that often become stellate shaped and have been called *mucoblasts*. The main mucin in the skin is hyaluronic acid. In addition, epithelial or sialomucins can be present in oral mucous cysts and in cutaneous metastases or extensions of gastrointestinal tumors.

The major stains for cutaneous mucins used in formalin-fixed, paraffin-embedded tissue are shown in Table 16-5. The best approach to identifying mucins is to make the diagnosis on H&E-stained tissue and then confirm the diagnosis with a single special stain. Only when mucin is found within glands whose origin is unclear does histochemistry become an issue.

There are many forms of cutaneous mucinosis.[122] An initial helpful approach is to identify the pattern first:

1. Diffuse mucin: mucin scattered in an infiltrative pattern throughout the dermis
2. Localized mucin or myxoma: focal deposit of mucin in a papule or nodule.

However, these distinctions are artificial because some diffuse mucinoses (e.g., scleromyxedema) may present with papules (lichen myxedematosus). The many forms of cutaneous mucin deposition are summarized in Table 16-6.

Generalized Mucinoses

Pretibial Myxedema

Clinical Features. Thickened plaques occur in the skin of patients with hyperthyroidism, usually in association with exophthalmos and thyroid acropathy. The pretibial myxedema may persist after treatment so the patient may be euthyroid. Most patients have long-acting thyroid stimulator in their serum. The lesions are thickened, waxy plaques, often with a pale or yellow color. The anterior shin is the most common site.[123] Other patients have no sign of thyroid disease but significant stasis der-

Table 16-6. Mucin in the Skin

Primary
  Focal cutaneous mucinosis
  Myxoma
  Reticulated erythematous mucinosis (plaque-like mucinosis)
  Rare variants (many solitary case reports describe variants of focal cutaneous
    mucinosis, based on location, age, sex, or country of origin)
Secondary
  Thyroid disease
    Pretibial myxedema
    Generalized myxedema
    Focal cutaneous mucinosis
  Gammopathy
    Scleromyxedema and lichen myxedematosus
  Metabolic disorders
    Hunter's disease (light microscopy)
    Many (ultrastructural)
  Connective tissue disorders
    Lupus erythematosus
    Dermatomyositis
    Lichen sclerosus et atrophicus
  Lymphocytic infiltrates
    Jessner's disease
    Alopecia mucinosa
  Reactive processes
    Scars and keloids
    Mucinous syringometaplasia

Cysts and pseudocysts
  Mucocele
  Digital mucous cyst
  Penile mucous cyst
Dermatoses
  Degos' disease
  Scleredema
  Granuloma annulare
Tumors
  Skin
    Squamous cell carcinoma
    Basal cell carcinoma
    Neurofibroma
    Mucinous eccrine carcinoma
    Paget's disease
    Metastatic carcinoma
    Histiocytoma (some variants)
    ± Others
  Oral mucosa
    Mucoepidermoid carcinoma
    ± Others
  Soft tissue
    Intramuscular myxoma
    Lipoblastoma
    Myxoid liposarcoma
    Myxoid chondrosarcoma
    Myxoid malignant fibrous histiocytoma

matitis,[124] while ichthyosiform plaques with papillary dermal mucin have been described in euthyroid Japanese patients with Sjögren syndrome.[125]

Histopathologic Features. Large amounts of mucin replace the normal dermis (Fig. 16-32). Sometimes much of the mucin is lost in fixation, and only empty spaces are seen. At other times, mucin will be seen admixed with collagen. Usually increased numbers of small superficial vessels with thickened walls are present and indicate origin from the leg. The presence of a relatively normal papillary dermis strongly suggests association with thyroid disease, while proliferation of small vessels and mucin in the papillary dermis point toward a connection with stasis.[124]

Generalized Myxedema

Clinical Features. Patients with hypothyroidism have doughy, puffy skin. The puffiness is usually widespread, but sometimes may be confined to face.

Histopathologic Features. The dermal mucin is scant, easily overlooked, and often missed on special stains.[126]

Reticular Erythematous Mucinosis (Plaque-Like Mucinosis)

Clinical Features. The typical patient is a young to middle-aged woman with a pruritic, erythematous, telangiectatic plaque on the midchest or upper back.[127–129]

Histopathologic Features. The picture of reticular erythematous mucinosis is more complex than myxedema. In addition to the expected mucin, numerous new small vessels and a lymphocytic perivascular and periappendageal infiltrate are

seen. Vacuolar basal cell layer damage is not present (Fig. 16-33).

Differential Diagnosis. Reticular erythematous mucinosis has clinical and histologic overlaps with lupus erythematosus. The serology is more important than the histologic features. The lupus band test on direct immunofluorescent examination is negative in reticular erythematous mucinosis.

Connective Tissue Disorders

The cutaneous lesions of both lupus erythematosus and dermatomyositis may contain mucin. In lupus erythematosus it may be the presenting problem, as patients will notice nodules or plaques.

Histopathologic Features. The pattern can range from scattered mucin among dermal collagen in which case the mucin is a clue to widespread replacement of dermal collagen.[130] In some cases of lupus panniculitis, there may be deep dermal mucin with little if any overlying changes. Other signs of lupus erythematosus or dermatomyositis can usually be found elsewhere in the biopsy specimen.

Mucopolysaccharidoses

Clinical Features. Hunter syndrome patients may have pebbly plaques on their shoulders that resemble connective tissue nevi.

Histopathologic Features. These plaques may have mucin admixed with collagen.[131] Intracellular mucopolysaccharides can be identified on electron microscopic evaluation of skin

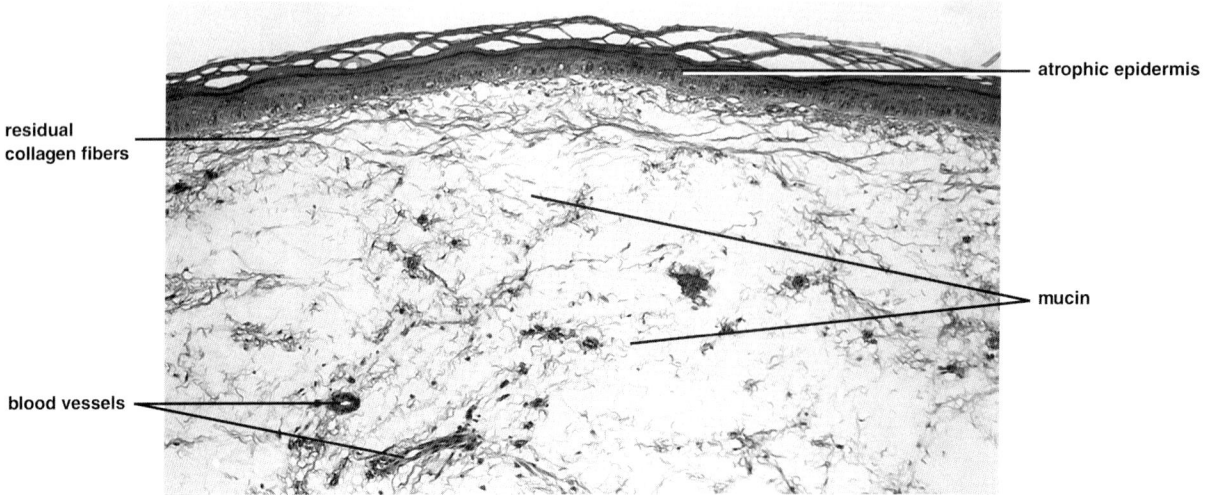

Figure 16-32. Pretibial myxedema. The dermis is almost entirely replaced by stringy mucinous material. Only a few scattered bands of collagen and vessels are seen. Large stellate fibroblasts are scattered throughout the mucinous connective tissue.

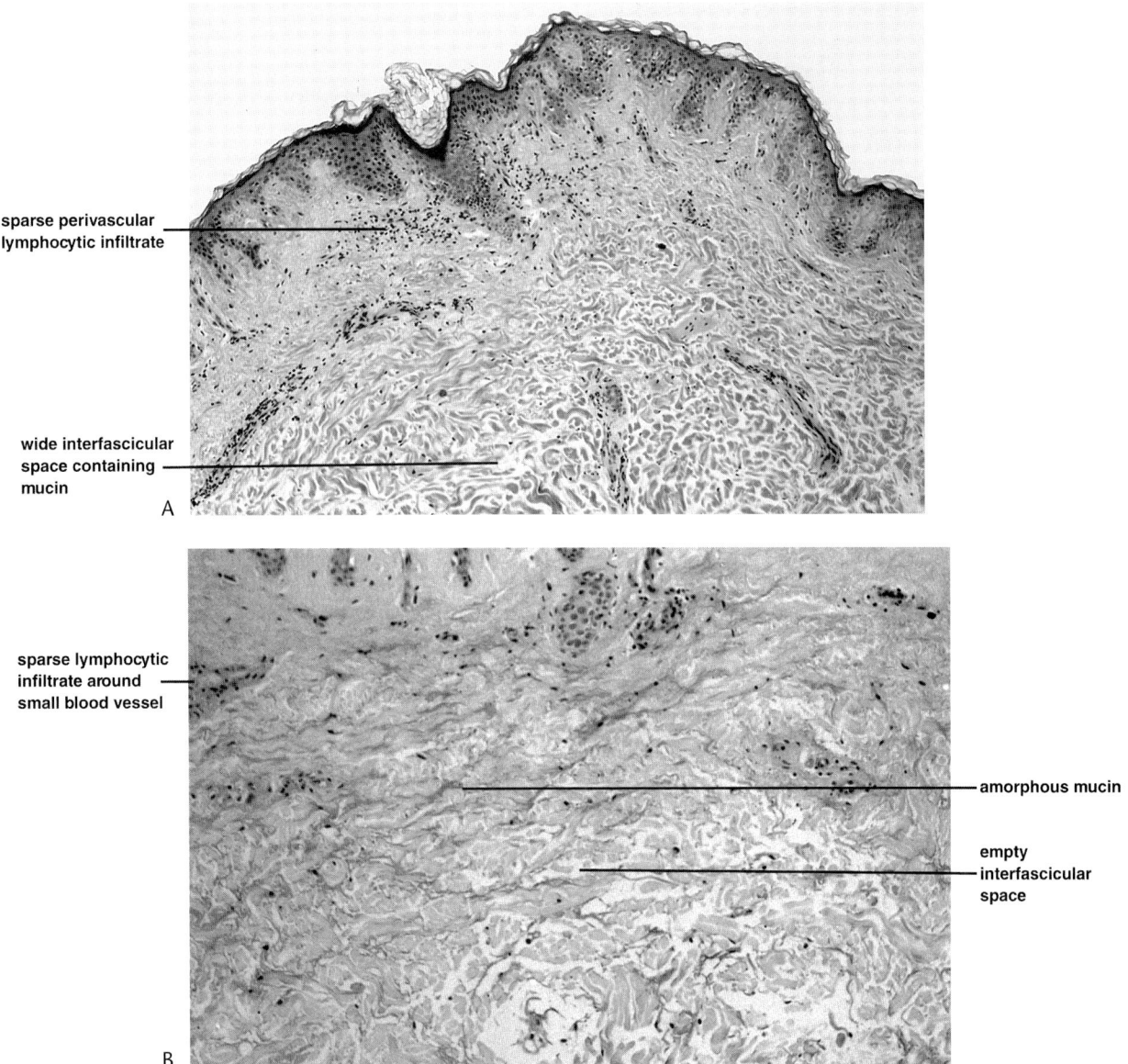

sparse perivascular
lymphocytic infiltrate

wide interfascicular
space containing
mucin

A

sparse lymphocytic
infiltrate around
small blood vessel

amorphous mucin

empty
interfascicular
space

B

Figure 16-33. Reticulated erythematous mucinosis. (**A**) At low power a relatively normal epidermis is seen. In the superficial dermis there is a lymphocytic perivascular and perifollicular infiltrate with some increase in vascularity. Strands of collagen are pushed apart, but it is difficult to see any mucin. (**B**) Colloidal iron stain reveals the amorphous mucin among the collagen bundles.

biopsy specimens in a variety of mucopolysaccharidoses and other lysozymal disorders.

Localized Mucinoses

Cutaneous Focal Mucinosis (Cutaneous Myxoma)

Clinical Features. Patients have a solitary or a few papules that are clinically nondistinct. Occasionally a gammopathy or thyroid disease may be found, but most patients are normal.[132,133]

Many unusual variants of focal mucinosis have been de-

scribed that can be identified clinically or histologically. They include

1. Myxedema of the upper lip[134]
2. Self-healing juvenile cutaneous mucinosis[135]
3. Infantile cutaneous mucinosis[136]
4. Mucinous variant of progressive nodular histiocytosis[137]
5. Acral persistent papular mucinosis[138]
6. Cutaneous emboli from an atrial myxoma, appearing as intravascular deposits that may also have extravasation of mucin into dermis with inflammation.[139]

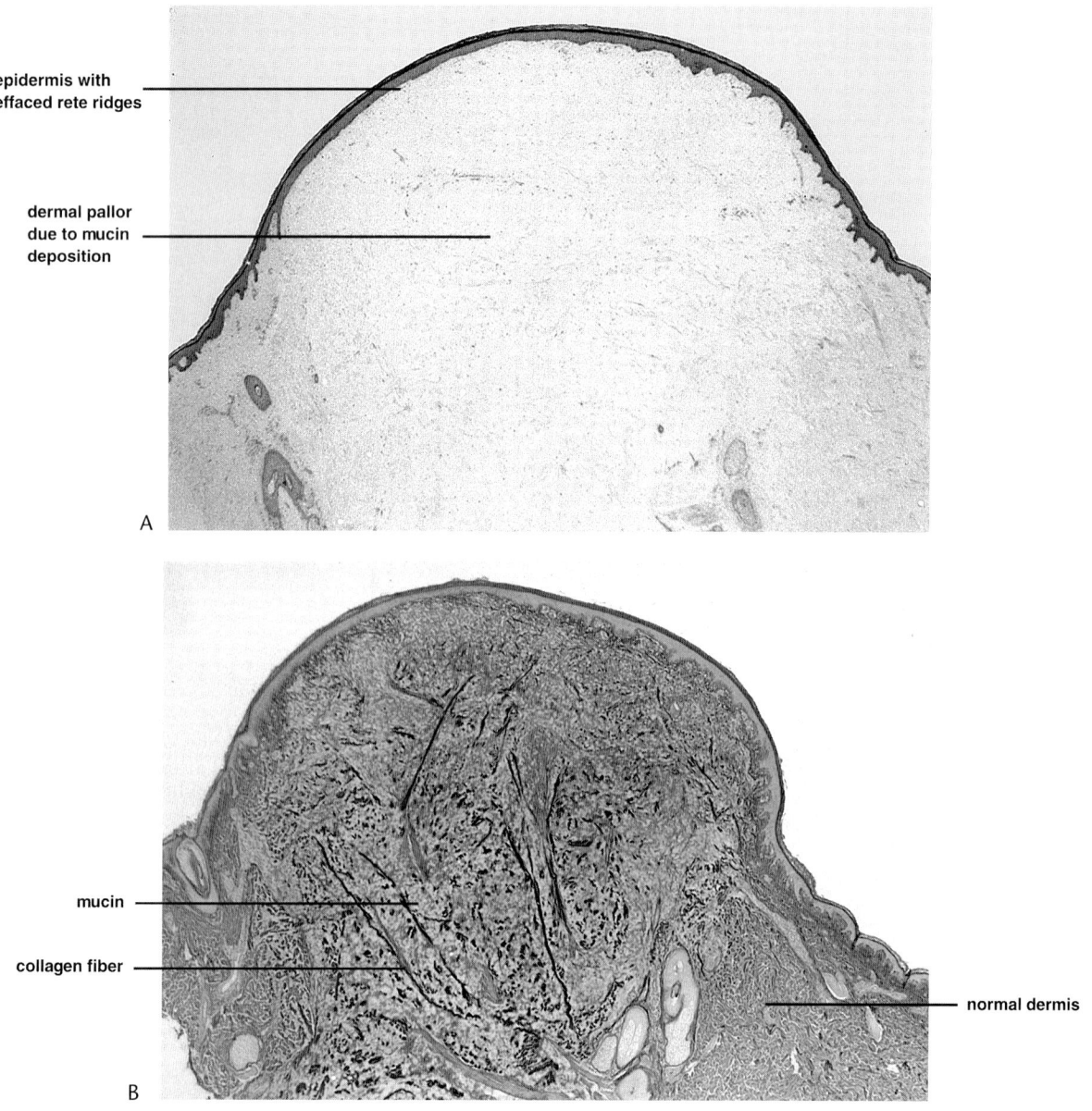

Figure 16-34. Focal cutaneous mucinosis. **(A)** There is effacement of the rete ridges of the epidermis. In the dermis there is pale amorphous material infiltrating between strands of collagen. This was a solitary papule. **(B)** Colloidal iron stain demonstrates the amorphous and stringy mucin among the collagen bundles.

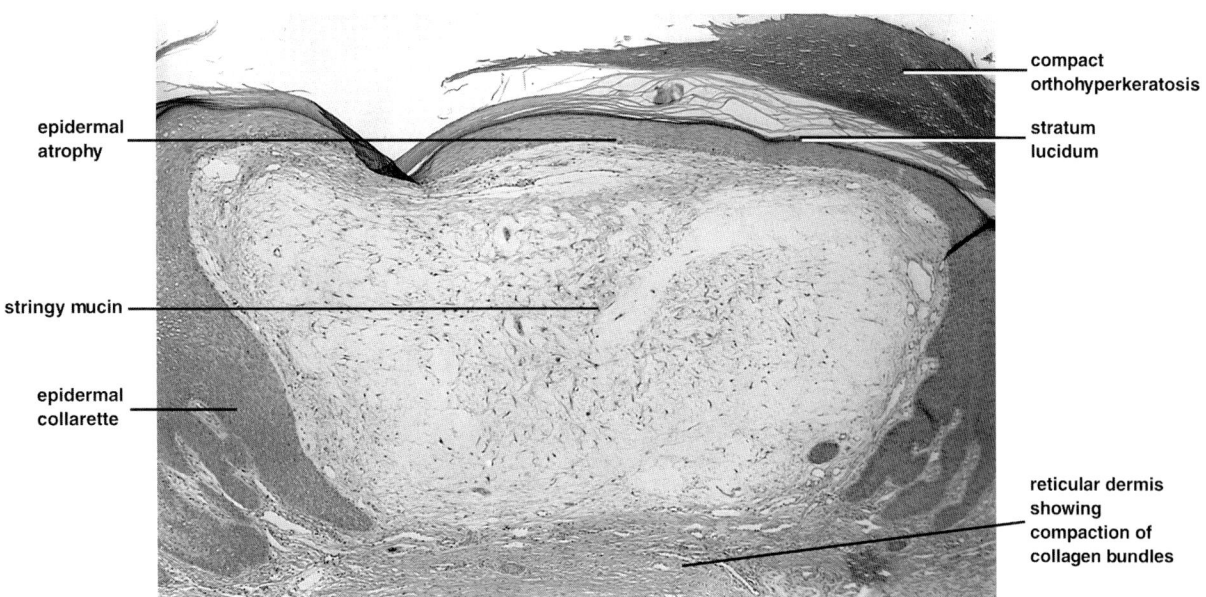

epidermal
atrophy

compact
orthohyperkeratosis

stratum
lucidum

stringy mucin

epidermal
collarette

reticular dermis
showing
compaction of
collagen bundles

Figure 16-35. Digital mucous cyst. The overlying epidermis is orthohyperkeratotic and acral. A focal expansion of mucinous material pushes apart the rete ridges. Large, plump fibroblasts are present in the mucinous matrix. There is increased vascularity. No cyst wall is present.

Histopathologic Features. There is a dome-shaped papule with the dermis infiltrated by mucin (Fig. 16-34). Sometimes there is mucin high in the dermis in the pattern of pretibial myxedema; in other cases the mucin is dispersed among collagen. No host response is seen. The low power view of a solitary lesion is most helpful.[140]

Digital Mucous Cyst

Clinical Features. A soft papule is seen on the digit usually adjacent to the nail fold. Mucin exudes from the cyst as thick clear jelly when an incision is made.

Histopathologic Features. Large amounts of mucin are found in a focal area of the dermis. Usually a good clue is the overlying acral skin with a stratum lucidum. A cyst wall is not present; sometimes a foreign body granuloma reaction develops at the periphery of the mucin[141] (Fig. 16-35).

Clinicopathologic Correlation. Controversy remains over whether digital mucous cysts are connected to the synovium. Although scientifically the issue is clouded, practically it does not matter in diagnosis or management.

Mucocele

Mucocele or mucous extravasation phenomenon is a pseudocyst created by the leakage of mucus from a damaged minor salivary gland duct.

Clinical Features. The most common location for a mucocele is the lower lip, but the lesion may arise anywhere in the oral cavity where minor salivary glands and trauma co-exist. The lesions are painless smooth bumps that are most common in children and young adults. Rarely a sialolith may obstruct a salivary duct and produce a true mucous retention cyst behind the plug as the duct is expanded.

Histopathologic Features. A lake of mucin spills into the lamina propria. There is no cyst wall but instead a granulomatous response. Minor salivary glands or ducts may be found in the biopsy specimen[142] (Fig. 16-36). In superficial variants, mucin is found just below the epithelium.[143] In a mucous retention cyst, the mucin is with the duct.

Hemochromatosis

Hemochromatosis or iron storage disease is characterized by the deposition of large amounts of iron in many organs.

Clinical Features

Primary hemochromatosis is an autosomal recessive disorder characterized by increased intestinal absorption of iron. Heterozygotes rarely have clinical problems, although they may have increased liver iron stores. Secondary hemochromatosis occurs in a variety of anemias. The classic clinical features of bronze diabetes include diabetes, liver disease, and heart failure as well as cutaneous hyperpigmentation. The skin is brown or slate-gray, with the color changes more pronounced in sun-exposed areas.[144]

Histopathologic Features

Despite the deposition of iron, the increased pigment is caused by melanin. The melanin is localized primarily in the basal layer. Any iron stain, such as Perls' stain, will show the iron as blue-staining granules, especially around sweat glands.[145] In an interesting experiment of nature, patients with hemochromatosis and vitiligo were studied.[146] Their

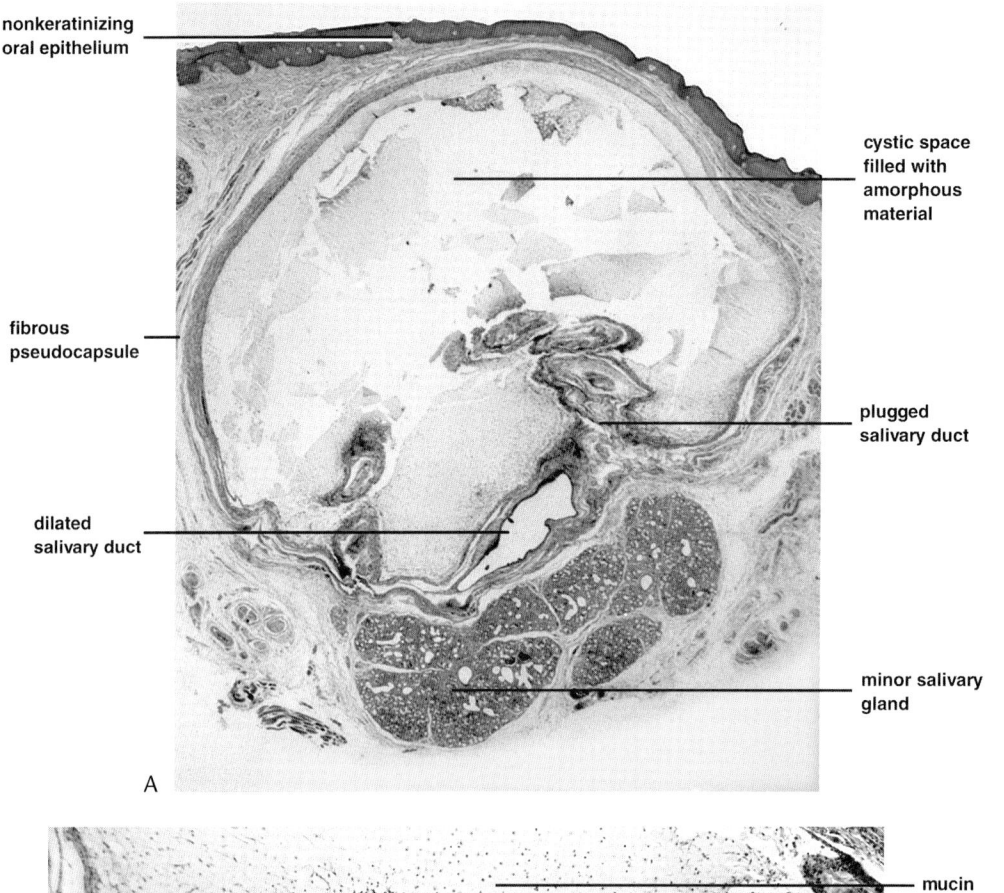

nonkeratinizing
oral epithelium

cystic space
filled with
amorphous
material

fibrous
pseudocapsule

plugged
salivary duct

dilated
salivary duct

minor salivary
gland

A

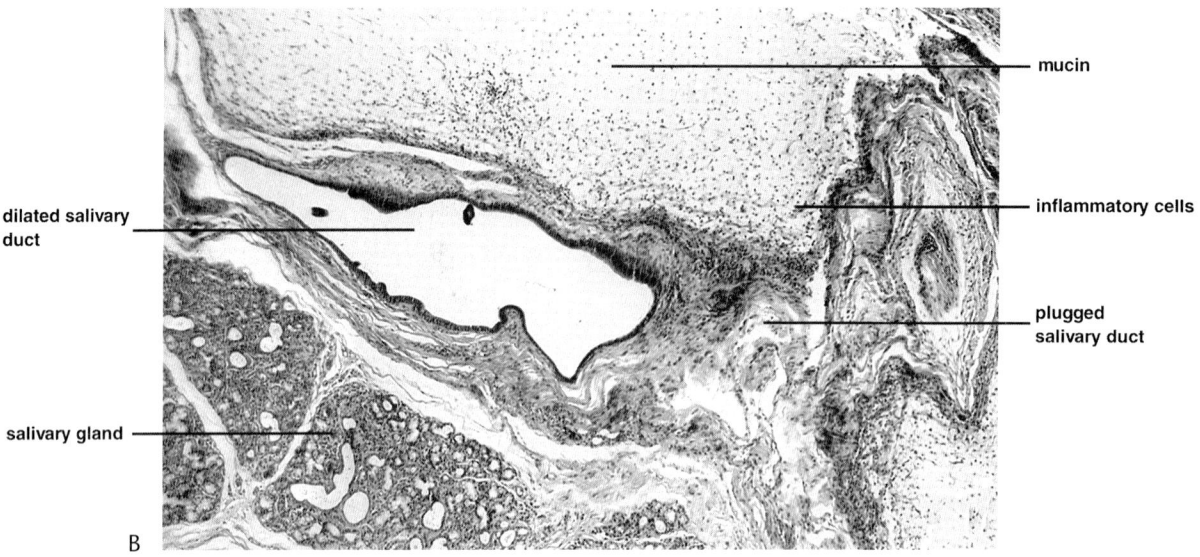

mucin

dilated salivary
duct

inflammatory cells

plugged
salivary duct

salivary gland

B

Figure 16-36. Mucocele. (**A**) There is overlying mucosa rather than epidermis. The cyst is in close proximity to a minor salivary gland, and the dilated duct leading to it is easily seen. (**B**) At higher power, the lack of a cyst wall, the presence of salivary glands, and the duct leading into the extravasated mucin are seen to better advantage.

clinically white patches were rich in iron but lacked melanin. Epidermoid cysts in hemochromatosis patients are often dark.[147]

Argyria and Other Metals

Argyria is the deposition of silver salts in the skin.

Clinical Features

Argyria is caused by prolonged systemic or topical exposure to silver salts. When silver is ingested, the entire skin may develop a blue-gray tint.[148] After topical use, the changes may be either circumscribed or, rarely, widespread. Sun-exposed skin tends to be darker.

Histopathologic Features

Skin in patients with argyria appears generally normal. The only abnormal feature is the presence of numerous tiny granules in the basement membrane zone around sweat ducts (Fig. 16-37). They are also scattered throughout the dermis. The silver granules have an affinity for elastic fibers. The granules are better seen when a dark-field examination is done; they also polarize and are easily seen with ultrastructural study.[149]

Differential Diagnosis

Other metals may be deposited in the skin, including gold and mercury:

Gold: after the use of gold salts, patients may acquire a blue-gray hyperpigmentation similar to argyria. The gold salts are larger and usually found in macrophages.

Mercury: application of topical mercury salts can cause reticulate hyperpigmentation, especially on the face. Irregular large black granules are found throughout the dermis.

The mystery in hemochromatosis, argyria, and most other metallic depositions is how the metal and its salts interact with the melanin system and sunlight to produce hyperpigmentation. No convincing explanations are available.

CALCIUM, BONE, AND CARTILAGE

Calcium

Cutaneous calcium deposition may be suspected either because a patient has a systemic disease in which calcium metabolism is abnormal, or because of the presence in the skin of chalky white to yellow particles or chunks. *Calcinosis cutis* is a nonspecific term and will be taken as a synonym for *cutaneous calcification*.[150,151] The following types of calcification are seen:

1. Metastatic calcification: deposition of calcium occurs secondary to high serum levels of calcium or phosphate ions
2. Dystrophic calcification: deposition occurs in the presence of normal calcium levels but onto damaged cutaneous components, such as in connective tissue disorders, after trauma, or in cutaneous neoplasms
3. Idiopathic calcification: serum calcium and phosphate levels are normal, and no abnormal nidus for calcification is identified

Histologic Features

Calcium is readily identified by its blue color on routine H&E stains. Most often the pattern is amorphous, although sometimes calcium outlines other structures such as vessels, glands,

Figure 16-37. Argyria. Thousands of tiny granules of silver are seen in the basement membranes around the sweat glands.

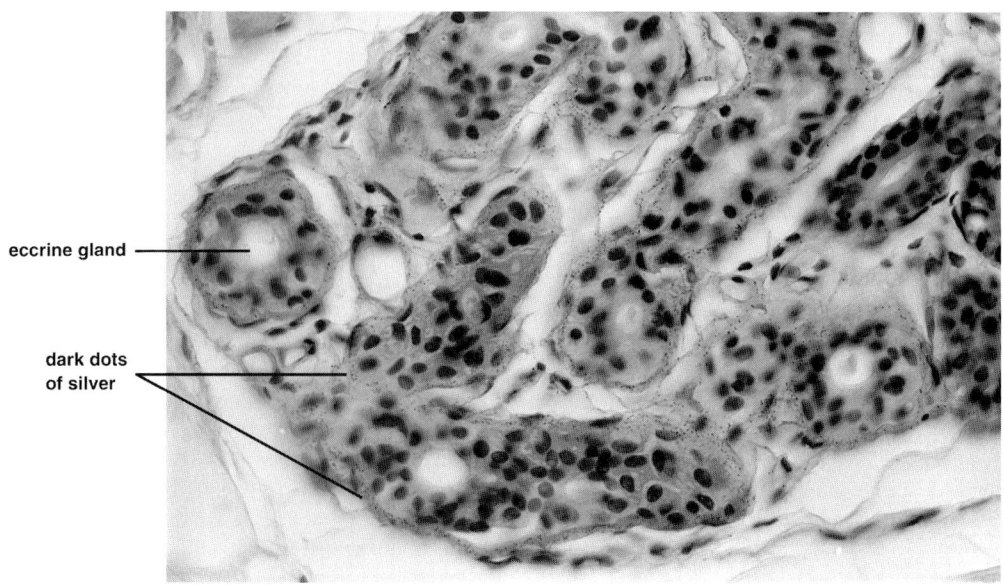

eccrine gland

dark dots of silver

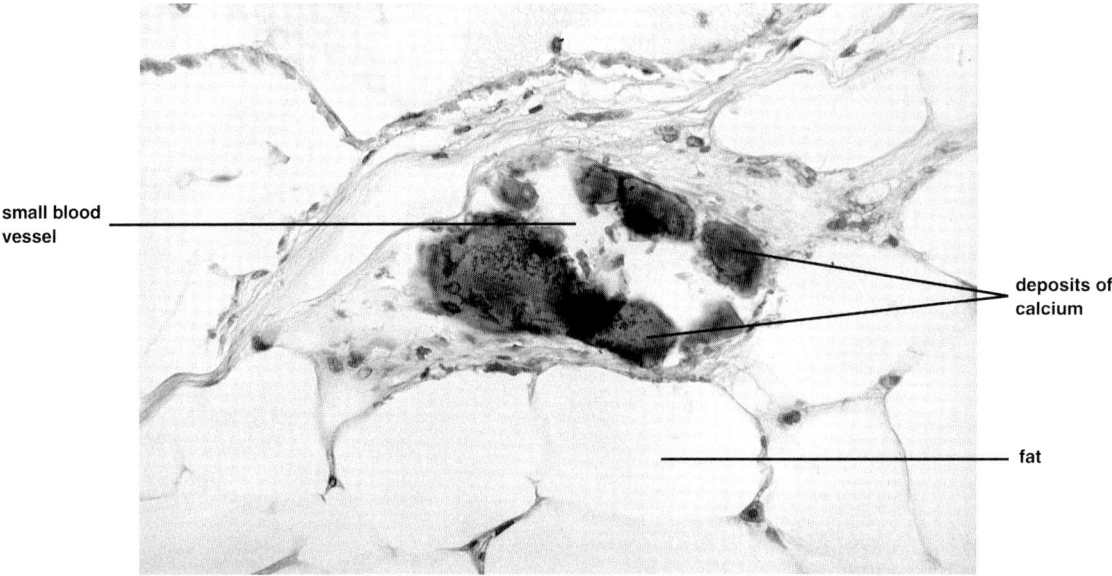

small blood vessel

deposits of calcium

fat

Figure 16-38. Metastatic calcification. Calcium is seen in the small blood vessels in a patient with chronic renal disease. The patient developed cutaneous necrosis.

or muscles. Thus, the individual histologic pictures of various forms of cutaneous calcification are discussed only when they have unique features. Calcium's presence can be confirmed with several stains. The traditional von Kossa stain is actually a silver reduction stain that identifies anionic salts such as phosphate and carbonate salts. Because almost all such material is bound to calcium, the von Kossa stain is an indirect but specific calcium stain. A true calcium stain is the dye lake reaction with alizarin red S, which, at pH 4.2, complexes only with calcium.[152]

Metastatic Calcification

Metastatic calcification is a relatively unimportant cause of cutaneous calcification. Cutaneous changes are extremely uncommon in primary hyperparathyroidism, secondary hyperparathyroidism, sarcoidosis, and Paget's disease of bone. Even when soft tissue calcification is identified, cutaneous calcification is not usually seen. However, on occasion, the skin will have nodules or plaques of calcium deposition. Metastatic calcification can be a rare cause of cutaneous necrosis because the vessel walls are the most common site of mineral deposition (Fig. 16-38). This rare event occurs most often in patients with renal failure and secondary hyperparathyroidism.[153,154] The term *calciphylaxis*, suggested by Hans Selye in a totally different context, is often applied to this dramatic deposition of calcium.

Dystrophic Calcification

The four main forms of dermal damage that serve as a nidus for dystrophic calcification are trauma, degenerative disorders, connective tissue diseases, and neoplasms. When the calcification is not too extensive, the "cause" can usually be identified in the section. In other situations, only widespread dermal calcinosis may be seen. The history and other diagnostic tools must be used to identify the underlying disorder.

Trauma

Many types of minor trauma can produce cutaneous calcification. If the trauma is coupled with topical application or systemic administration of calcium, Selye's concept of calciphylaxis is more closely reproduced, in which trauma is coupled with hypercalcific states. Causes include heel sticks (Fig. 16-39), electroencephalography and fetal monitor trauma, cold damage (especially neonatal fat necrosis), intramuscular and intravascular injections, and occupational exposure to calcium salts.

Degenerative Disorders

Two diseases, discussed elsewhere in this section, often calcify. Calcification of elastic fibers is the hallmark of pseudoxanthoma elasticum, while calcified nodules are seen after trauma in some forms of Ehlers-Danlos disease.

Connective Tissue Disorders

Calcification can occur in dermatomyositis, SS, and lupus erythematosus but in varying degrees and in different clinical settings. In dermatomyositis, cutaneous and soft tissue calcification is common, often massive, and occurs about the proximal limb muscles. It is frequently disabling.[155] In SS, the calcification is usually acral, associated with Raynaud's phenomenon, and troublesome but not serious. If the CREST syndrome and SS are considered as separate disorders, calcification occurs

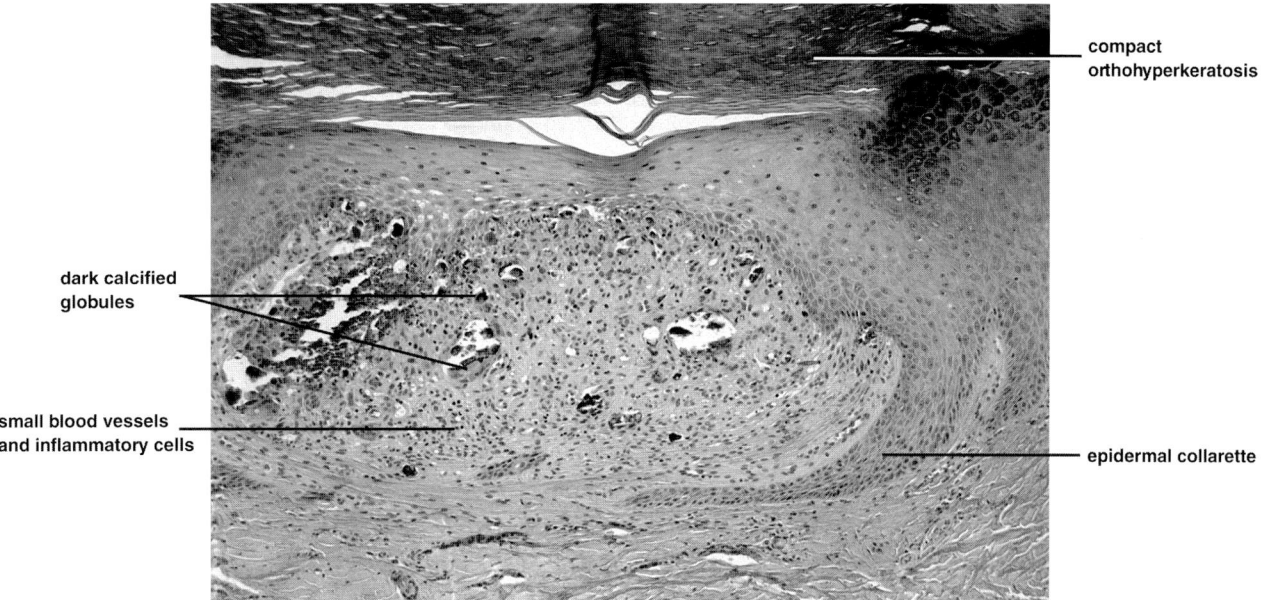

compact
orthohyperkeratosis

dark calcified
globules

small blood vessels
and inflammatory cells

epidermal collarette

Figure 16-39. Dystrophic calcification. The skin is acral because of the thick stratum corneum. There is collarette formation of the epidermis surrounding the calcium deposits in the upper dermis. In a circumscribed area of the superficial dermis there are many small calcified areas. This was heel stick calcification in a neonate.

only in the CREST group and not in SS or morphea.[156] Calcification in lupus erythematosus is rare.[157]

Tumors

Not surprisingly, the most common skin tumor is the one that calcifies the most. Basal cell carcinomas frequently contain calcium and also may contain bone. Pilomatricomas almost always calcify; in one series, calcium was seen in 80% of cases, pilar cysts calcify in about 25% of cases, while calcium is rare (less than 1%) in epidermoid cysts. Epidermoid cysts in Gardner syndrome may have pilomatricomal areas and calcify somewhat more frequently. Almost any skin tumor can calcify.

Idiopathic Calcification

The most dramatic form of idiopathic calcification is tumoral calcinosis.[158] These patients have massive subcutaneous deposits of calcium. The calcified tumoral masses may be reached through the skin and thus identified in a skin biopsy specimen, but tumoral calcinosis is otherwise not a cutaneous disorder. Several localized forms of idiopathic calcification are less dramatic but of more practical importance to the dermatologist.

Idiopathic Scrotal Calcification

Clinical Features. Patients have one to many firm white nodules in their scrotal or, rarely, penile skin.

Histopathologic Features. Amorphous masses of calcium are found in the dermis usually without any evidence of a precursor lesion.[159] However, in many cases, the calcified masses

are round, suggesting that a cyst might have been present, and occasionally a calcifying cyst can be identified.[160]

Subepidermal Calcified Nodule

Clinical Features. Single or multiple small nodules occur most often on the face. They may be congenital or acquired.

Histopathologic Features. The dermis is replaced by calcium, often in the shape of small balls or nests[161–163] (Fig. 16-40). Sweat glands, sebaceous glands, hair follicles, and nevus cells may serve as the nidus for calcification. When the eccrine sweat gland (in which calcium salts may be concentrated) calcifies, a miliaria-like disease can occur.[164]

Differential Diagnosis and Pitfalls

When the dermatopathologist sees cutaneous calcification, the following approach is suggested:

1. A history should be obtained of
   A. Abnormalities of calcium or phosphate metabolism
   B. Trauma or precursor disease
2. A precursor structure that has calcified should be sought
3. Adjacent skin should be examined for signs of any of the precursor lesions to dystrophic calcification
4. Dermal and subcutaneous vessels should be examined
5. If all of the above are negative, either subepidermal calcified nodule or scrotal calcinosis is diagnosed, based on location

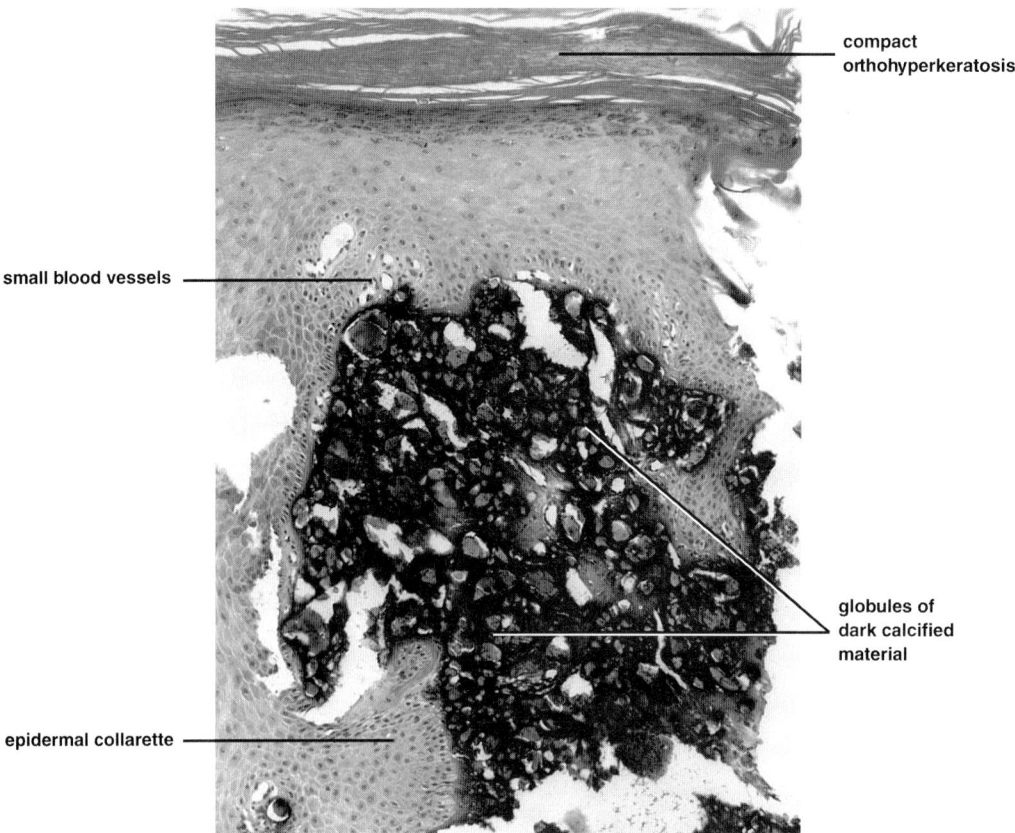

compact
orthohyperkeratosis

small blood vessels

globules of
dark calcified
material

epidermal collarette

Figure 16-40. Idiopathic calcification. There are numerous tiny globular structures lying in the dermis of acral skin. This was a subepidermal calcified nodule whose etiology remains unclear.

Bone

Cutaneous bone formation is a complicated process that requires precursor matrix (osteoid or osteoid-like substance or cartilage) and appropriate amounts of calcium and phosphate salts. Thus, any condition that predisposes to cutaneous calcification may also lead to cutaneous bone formation. Strictly speaking, osteogenesis is the formation of bone, while ossification refers to the conversion of nonosseous tissues such as skin into bone. Cutaneous ossification can be subdivided as shown in Table 16-7. For a pathologist, the question is, is just a piece of bone present in the skin, or are there other clues suggesting precursor or associated conditions?[165–168]

Histopathologic Features

Bone has few if any distinctive features in the skin. All structures present in normal bone can be seen, including haversian canals, osteoblasts, and osteoclasts. The presence of a foreign body response is variable. Frequently the bone arises in close approximation to fat (Fig. 16-41).

Primary Osteoma Cutis

Primary osteoma cutis implies cutaneous bone formation without an underlying nidus, although there is frequently a predisposing disorder. The most common is Albright syndrome (pseudohypoparathyroidism).[169,170] The osteomas are simply dermal and subcutaneous pieces of otherwise normal bone. When an associated underlying disease is absent, one is truly dealing with a primary osteoma.[171] A unique variant is the plate-like cutaneous osteoma in which bone develops in sheets or plates at the dermal-subcutaneous junction[172]; when this is more extensive, it is known as *progressive osseous heteroplasia*.[173]

Probably the most common so-called primary osteoma is the subungual osteoma. It usually presents as a friable nodule adjacent to or eroding the nail usually of the great toe. Radiographic examination usually reveals a connection to the underlying bone, so the lesion is really an exostosis and not an osteoma.[174,175]

Secondary Osteoma Cutis

With secondary osteoma cutis, all bone looks similar in the skin and is always abnormal. If it is found, associated or predisposing causes should be sought. The three major categories are tumors, trauma, and inflammation.

Table 16-7. Cutaneous Ossification

I. Primary cutaneous ossification without demonstrable cutaneous pathology
  A. Albright's hereditary osteodystrophy (pseudohypoparathyroidism and pseudopseudohypoparathyroidism)
  B. Osteoma cutis
    1. Idiopathic
    2. Plate-like
    3. Subungual exostosis
II. Secondary or metaplastic cutaneous ossification
  A. Secondary to cutaneous tumors
    1. Pilomatricoma
    2. Basal cell carcinoma
    3. Appendageal tumors
    4. Chondroid syringoma
    5. Melanocytic proliferations
    6. Fibrohistiocytic proliferations
  B. Secondary to trauma
    1. Scar
    2. Multiple postacne facial osteomas
    3. Chronic venous stasis
  C. Secondary to inflammatory conditions
    1. Myositis ossificans
    2. All forms of cutaneous calcification
  D. Secondary to noncutaneous malignant tumors
  E. Secondary to cartilaginous tumors

Tumors

Tumors are the most common cause of cutaneous bone formation. Pilomatricomas, especially in persons more than 40 years of age, are likely to calcify and then ossify. Ossification may be so complete that a pre-existing pilomatricoma may be difficult to identify.[176] Mixed tumors of skin, which almost always have some areas of chondroid matrix, are also likely to ossify.[177] Basal cell carcinomas and other appendageal tumors also may rarely contain bone. Ossification of melanocytic nevi is puzzling. The phenomenon seems to occur almost exclusively on the face (the nevus of Nanta)[178] (Fig. 16-42). Over 95% are located on the face.[179] Both dermatofibromas and their oral cousin, peripheral ossifying fibroma, may also contain bone.

Noncutaneous tumors rarely cause cutaneous bone deposits. It is rare for osteosarcomas or other malignant bone tumors to metastasize to the skin.[180] Occasionally cutaneous metastases from other sites may induce bone formation.[181] Malignant degeneration has been identified in heterotopic bone in dermatomyositis.[182] The rare cutaneous chondroma may occasionally ossify.

Trauma

Vertical scars near the xiphoid and pubis most often ossify.[183] Multiple facial osteomas may follow acne[184]; sometimes no antecedent acne is described, and then the preferred designation is *miliary primary osteomas*.[185] Chronic venous stasis with phleboliths and extravascular calcification may also ossify.[186]

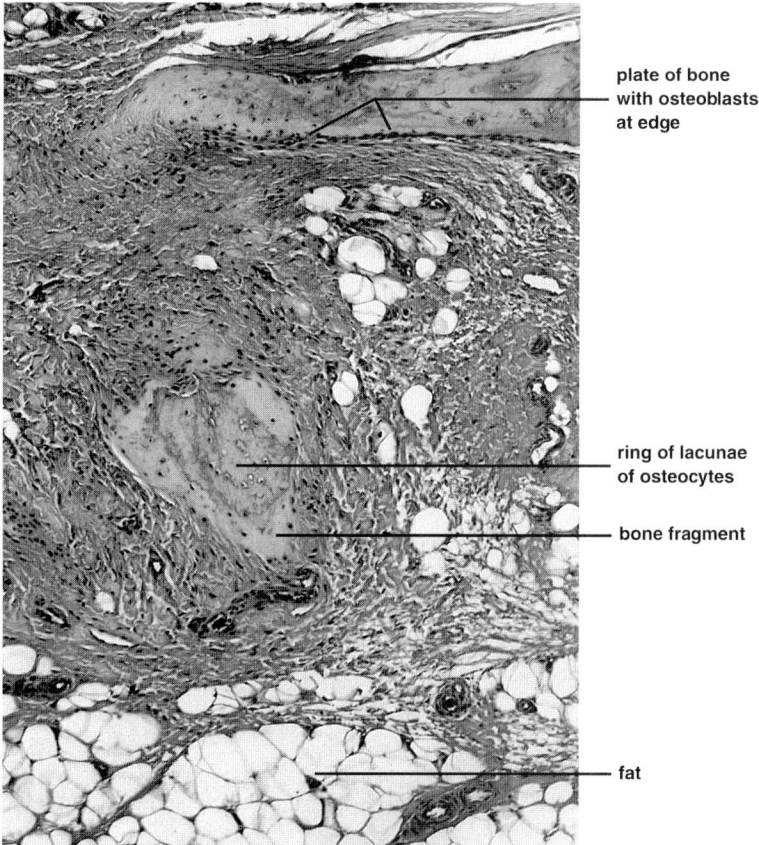

plate of bone with osteoblasts at edge

ring of lacunae of osteocytes

bone fragment

fat

Figure 16-41. Primary osteoma cutis. Two fragments of bone are seen. They are developing in close proximity to fat. Haversian canals can be seen with osteocytes in lacunae and occasional osteoclasts. The superficial piece is developing parallel to the surface of the skin, as has been seen in plaque-like cutaneous osteoma.

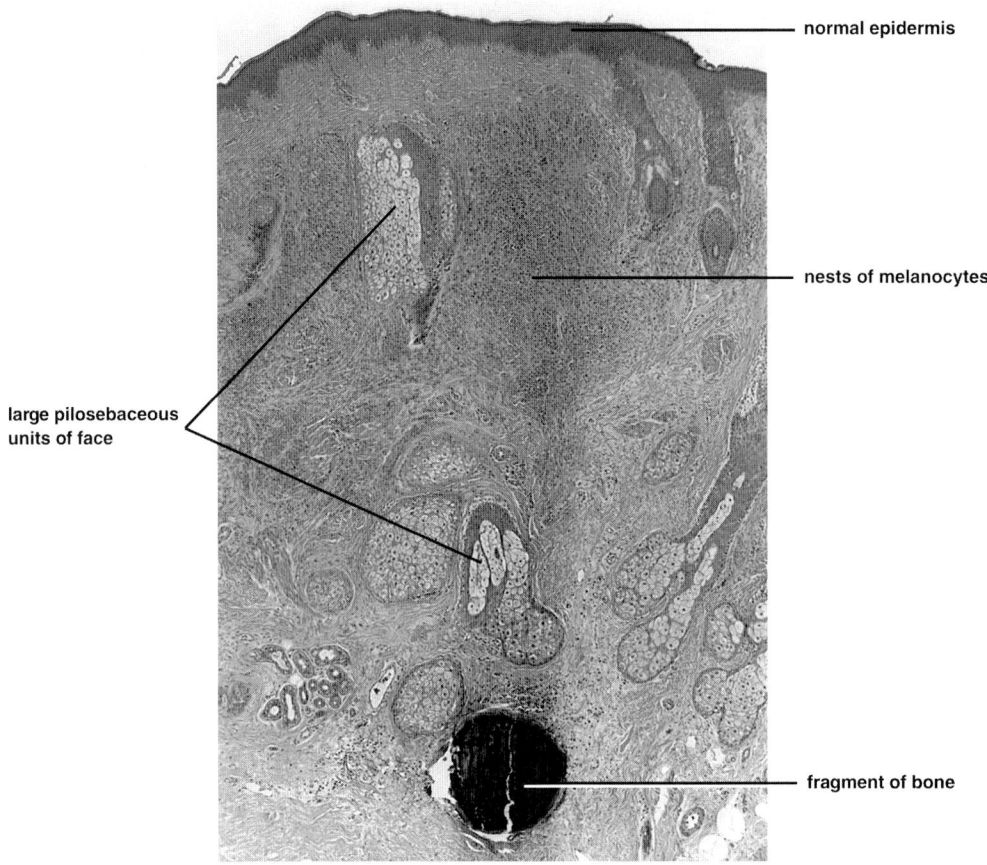

normal epidermis

nests of melanocytes

large pilosebaceous units of face

fragment of bone

Figure 16-42. Nevus of Nanta. This is a deep facial lesion as seen by the large thick sebaceous glands. The nevus cells are intradermal and banal. There is a calcified nodule of bone at the base.

Figure 16-43. Accessory tragus. There are numerous hairs in this transverse section of skin. The cartilage is in the center, while the prominent fibrous septae of the subcutaneous fat is easily appreciated.

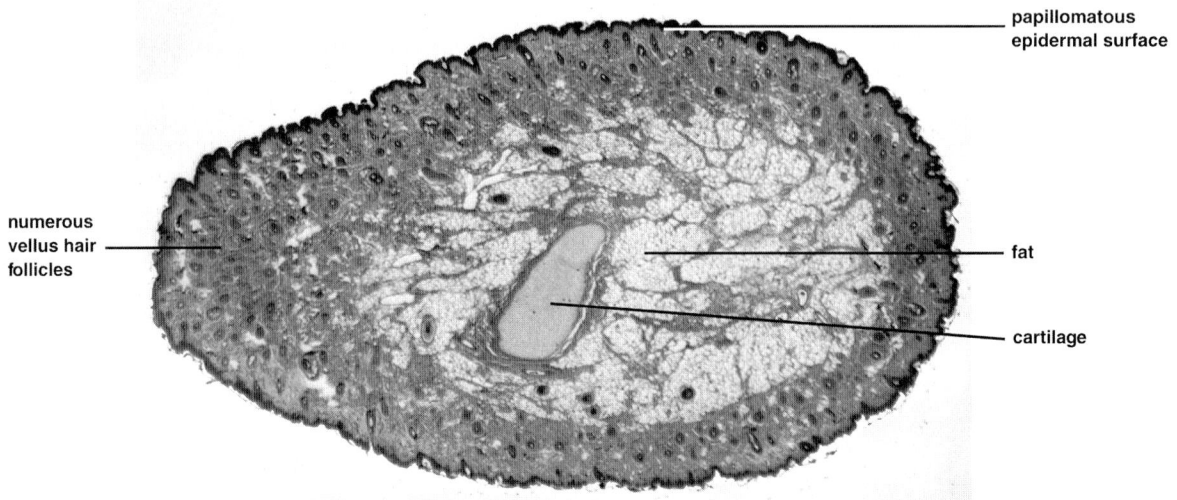

papillomatous epidermal surface

numerous vellus hair follicles

fat

cartilage

Cartilage

Cartilage in the skin is much rarer than calcium or bone. However, there are a number of anatomic situations in which cartilage is close to the skin surface, especially in the ear, so dermatopathologists may deal with diseases of cartilage.

Accessory Tragus

Accessory tragus is an embryonic abnormality formed of auricular cartilage and skin.

Clinical Features

An accessory tragus is usually just anterior to the normal tragus. It is a small skin-colored papule that is usually present at birth.

Histopathologic Features

A small piece of normal cartilage is seen in the middle of a papule or nodule. The overlying skin is usually rich in vellus hairs and sebaceous glands but has no other abnormalities. The fibrous connective tissue framework of the subcutaneous fat is prominent[187] (Fig. 16-43).

Chondrodermatitis Nodularis Helicis

Chondrodermatitis nodularis helicis is an acquired painful condition of the helix.

Clinical Features

Chondrodermatitis nodularis helicis usually presents as a small papule or nodule on the apex of the helix. The right ear is involved more often than the left. Typical lesions are crusted and tender, especially when trying to sleep on the involved side (sleeper's nodules). Clinically, a basal cell carcinoma and elastotic nodule of the ear may come into question.

Histopathologic Features

Chondrodermatitis nodularis helicis has a zonal arrangement. Most superficially, there is reactive epidermal hyperplasia that surrounds a dell filled with parakeratotic debris. Beneath this indentation is degenerated dermis, then granulation tissue, and finally cartilage (Fig. 16-44). The dermis usually shows solar elastosis, but collagen degeneration has also been identified. The cartilage is usually not inflamed, but may be damaged. The superficial changes are sufficient for the diagnosis; cartilage need not be present (Fig. 16-45). A follicular origin for chondrodermatitis nodularis helicis has been proposed, but remains controversial.[188] We believe chondrodermatitis nodularis helicis is a pressure-related perforating dermatosis independent of follicle changes.[189]

Relapsing Polychondritis

Relapsing polychondritis is an idiopathic multisystem disease with inflammation of cartilage.

Figure 16-44. Chondrodermatitis nodularis helicis. At low power one can see a superficial dell with cartilage extending very close to the surface. The cartilage beneath the ulcerated epidermis shows loss of chondrocytes and degenerative changes.

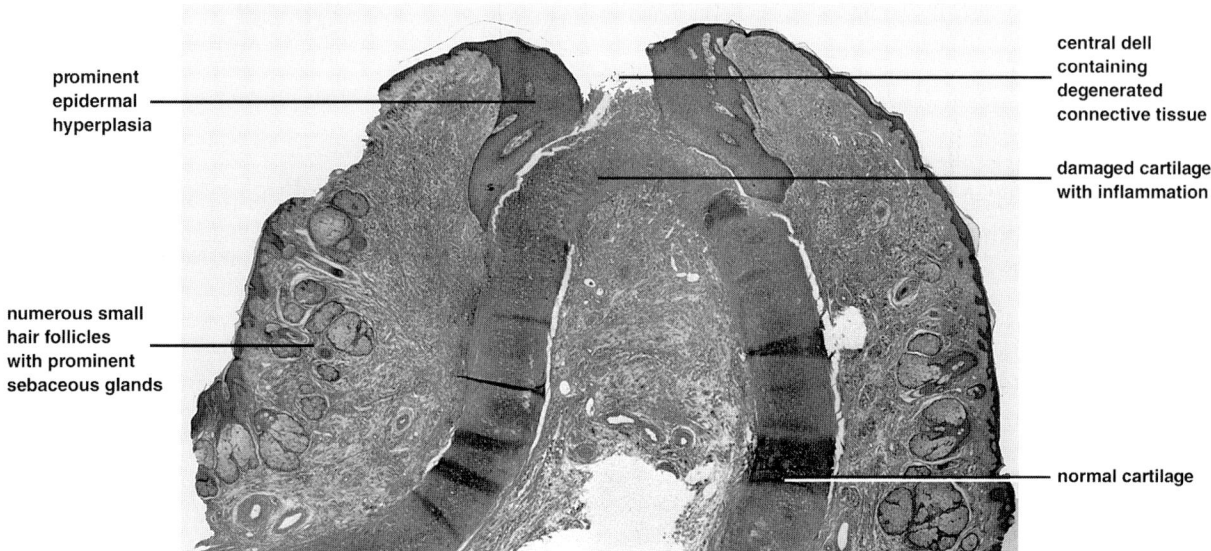

prominent epidermal hyperplasia

numerous small hair follicles with prominent sebaceous glands

central dell containing degenerated connective tissue

damaged cartilage with inflammation

normal cartilage

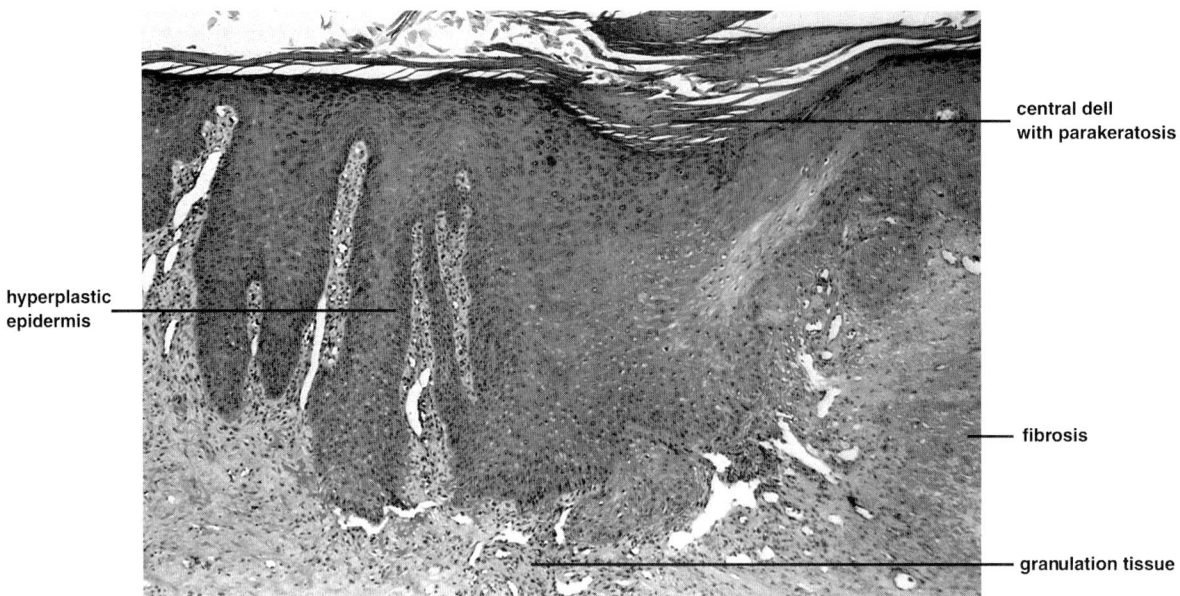

central dell with parakeratosis

hyperplastic epidermis

fibrosis

granulation tissue

Figure 16-45. Chondrodermatitis helicis nodularis. The superficial dell can be seen with parakeratotic scale and debris. The epidermis is hyperplastic without atypia. There is granulation tissue beneath the altered epidermis. There is fibrosis peripheral to the granulation tissue.

Clinical Features

Patients with relapsing polychondritis may have arthritis, ocular inflammation, and inflammation of the nasal or auricular cartilage. More than 50% of patients present with a red swollen ear or painful nose. Other organ involvement may include the larynx, internal ear, and heart. Additional cutaneous lesions include aphthous ulcers, vasculitis, urticaria, and erythema nodosum.[190]

Histopathologic Features

The skin of the red ear is usually normal or shows only edema and perivascular inflammation. The cartilage must be sampled by deep wedge biopsy, which reveals a dense neutrophilic infiltrate and degenerative changes with loss of staining[191] (Fig. 16-46). Occasionally vasculitis may be found in the adjacent dermis. Antibodies to type II collagen may be found by immunofluorescent examination.[192]

Differential Diagnosis

Occasionally cutaneous vasculitis may present with red ears, as may cold injuries. Thus, if just vasculitis and no cartilage damage is seen, relapsing polychondritis cannot be diagnosed.

Auricular Pseudocyst

Auricular pseudocyst is a post-traumatic intracartilaginous swelling of the auricle.

Clinical Features

Auricular pseudocyst is perhaps best known as the cauliflower ear of a pugilist. When the auricle is traumatized, it can acutely form a cystic mass. After multiple traumatic events, calcification or reactive hyperplasia (or both) may occur.

Histopathologic Features

When an acute lesion is biopsied, there is drainage of an oily degenerated material from a pseudocyst. As the lesion matures there may be replacement of the cartilage by fibrous tissue with focal calcification and degeneration.[193,194]

Differential Diagnosis

A perichondrial hematoma or seroma is above the cartilage rather than within it.

Chondroma

Chondroma is a tumor composed of cartilage.

Clinical Features

Cutaneous chondromas are extremely rare. Soft tissue chondromas are somewhat more common and are usually acral nodules.

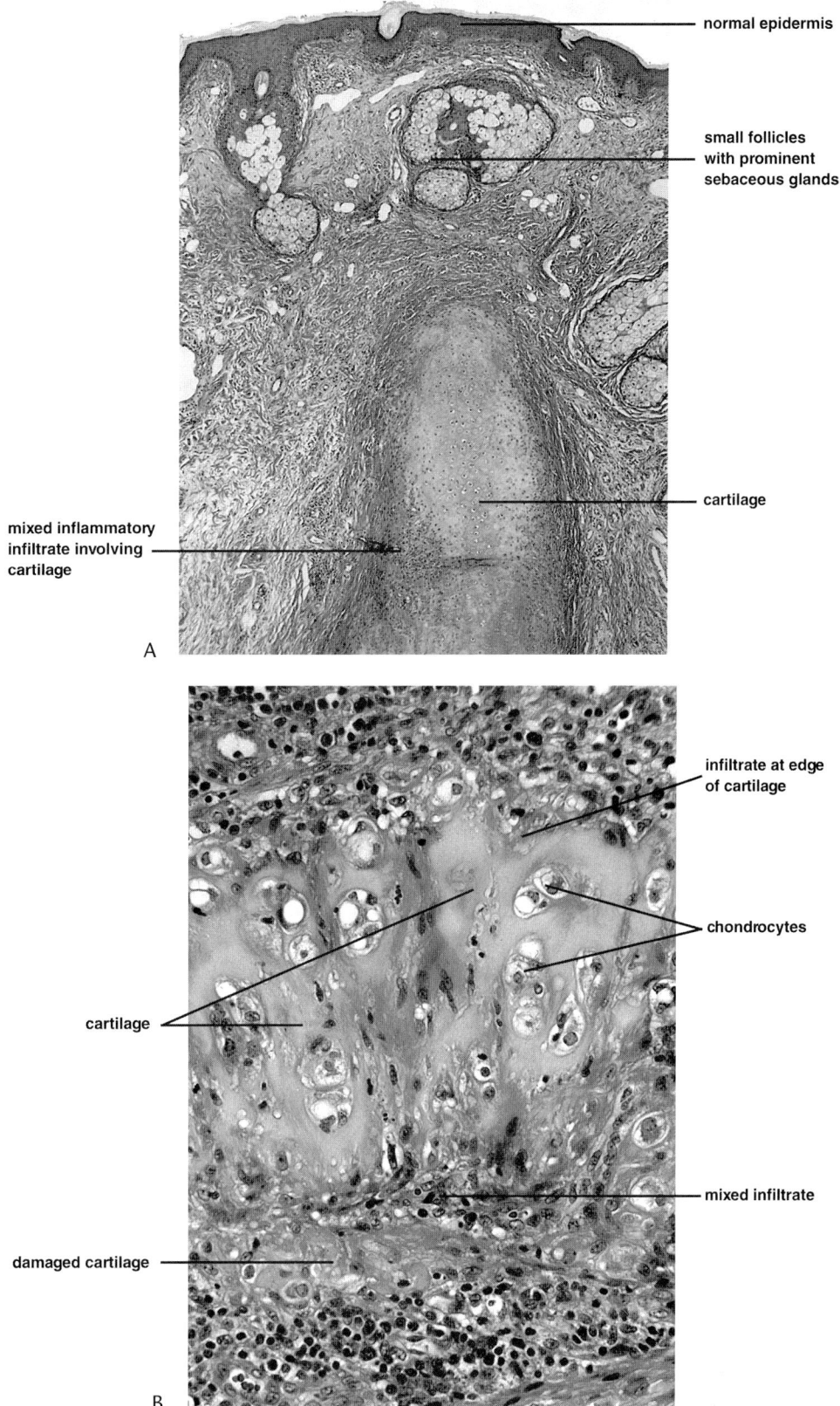

Figure 16-46. Relapsing polychondritis. (**A**) The epidermis is normal. In the dermis there is edema and a prominent blood vessel but without true vasculitis. There is an inflammatory infiltrate about the cartilage. (**B**) The cartilage is amorphous and is surrounded by a mixed infiltrate of inflammatory cells. In relapsing polychondritis inflammatory cells must be seen in the cartilage, whereas this is not a feature of chondrodermatitis helicis nodularis.

Histopathologic Features

Some chondromas simply look like a normal piece of cartilage in the wrong place. Others may be calcified, have a fibrous capsule, or show nuclear atypia. Despite this, metastases are not known to occur.[195–198]

Differential Diagnosis

The most common disorder to be mislabeled as cutaneous chondroma is the cartilaginous part of a subungual exostosis. Rarely a chondrosarcoma may metastasize to the skin.[199]

REFERENCES

1. Krieg T, Meurer M: Systemic scleroderma. Clinical and pathophysiologic aspects. J Am Acad Dermatol 18:457, 1988
2. Perez MI, Kohn SR: Systemic sclerosis. J Am Acad Dermatol 28:525, 1993
3. Silver RM, Heyes MP, Maize JC et al: Scleroderma, fasciitis and eosinophilia associated with the ingestion of tryptophan. N Engl J Med 322:874, 1990
4. Rahbari H: Histochemical differentiation of localized morphea-scleroderma and lichen sclerosus et atrophicus. J Cutan Pathol 16:342, 1989
5. Kencka D, Blaszczyk M, Jablonska S: Atrophoderma Pasini-Pierini is a primary atrophic abortive morphea. Dermatology 190:203, 1995
6. Büchner SA, Rufli T: Atrophoderma of Pasini and Pierini. Clinical and histopathological findings and antibodies to *Borrelia burgdorferi* in thirty-four patients. J Am Acad Dermatol 30:441, 1994
7. Barnes L, Rodnan GP, Medsger TA, Short D: Eosinophilic fasciitis. A pathologic study of twenty cases. Am J Pathol 96:493, 1979
8. Young EM Jr, Barr RJ: Sclerosing dermatoses. J Cutan Pathol 12:426, 1985
9. Venencie PY, Powell FC, Su WP, Perry HO: Scleredema: a review of thirty-three cases. J Am Acad Dermatol 11:128, 1984
10. Cole HG, Winkelmann RK: Acid mucopolysaccharide staining in scleredema. J Cutan Pathol 17:211, 1990
11. Rongioletti F, Gambini C, Micalizzi C et al: Mucin deposits in morphea and systemic scleroderma. Dermatology 189:157, 1994
12. Kapoor A, Sibbitt WL Jr: Contractures in diabetes mellitus: the syndrome of limited joint mobility. Semin Arthritis Rheumatism 18:168, 1989
13. Varga J, Gotta S, Li L et al: Scleredema adultorum: case report and demonstration of abnormal expression of extracellular matrix genes in skin fibroblasts in vivo and in vitro. Br J Dermatol 132:992, 1995
14. Gabriel SE, Perry HO, Oleson GB, Bowles CA: Scleromyxedema: a scleroderma-like disorder with systemic manifestations. Medicine 67:58, 1988
15. Dinneen AM, Dicken CH: Scleromyxedema. J Am Acad Dermatol 33:37, 1995
16. Murray JC, Pollack SV, Pinnel SR: Keloids: a review. J Am Acad Dermatol 4:461, 1981
17. James WD, Besanceney CD, Odom RB: The ultrastructure of a keloid. J Am Acad Dermatol 3:50, 1980
18. Knapp TR, Daniels JR, Kaplan EN: Pathological scar formation. Am J Pathol 86:47, 1977
19. Muir IFK: On the nature of keloids and hypertrophic scars. Br J Plast Surg 43:61, 1990
20. LeBoit PE: Subacute radiation dermatitis: a histologic im-
itator of acute cutaneous graft-versus-host disease. J Am Acad Dermatol 20:236, 1989
21. Hood IC, Young JEM: Late sequelae of superficial irradiation. Head Neck Surg 7:65, 1984
22. Hambrick GW, Carter DM: Pachydermoperiostosis. Arch Dermatol 94:594, 1966
23. Lindmaier A, Raff M, Seidl G, Jurecka W: Pachydermoperiostose. Hautarzt 40:752, 1989
24. Uitto J, Santa Cruz DJ, Eisen AZ: Connective tissue nevi of the skin. J Am Acad Dermatol 3:441, 1980
25. Uitto J, Santa Cruz DJ, Eisen AZ: Familial cutaneous collagenoma: genetic studies on a family. Br J Dermatol 101:185, 1979
26. Fork HE, Sanchez RL, Wagner RF Jr, Raimer SS: A new type of connective tissue nevus: isolated exophytic elastoma. J Cutan Pathol 18:457, 1991
27. Verbov J, Graham R: Buschke-Ollendorff syndrome—disseminated dermatofibrosis with osteopoikilosis. Clin Exp Dermatol 11:17, 1986
28. Cole GW, Barr RJ: An elastic tissue defect in dermatofibrosis lenticularis disseminata. Arch Dermatol 118:44, 1982
29. Bhawan J, Edelstein L: Angiofibromas in tuberous sclerosis: a light and electron microscopic study. J Cutan Pathol 4:300, 1977
30. Meigel WN, Ackerman AB: Fibrous papule of face. Am J Dermatopathol 1:329, 1979
31. Cerio R, Rao BK, Spaull J, Wilson-Jones E: An immunohistochemical study of fibrous papule of the nose: 25 cases. J Cutan Pathol 16:194, 1989
32. Goltz RW, Henderson RR, Hitch JM et al: Focal dermal hypoplasia syndrome. Arch Dermatol 101:1, 1970
33. Ishii N, Baba N, Kanaizuka I et al: Histopathological study of focal dermal hypoplasia (Goltz syndrome). Clin Exp Dermatol 17:24, 1992
34. Büchner SA, Itin P: Focal dermal hypoplasia in a male patient. Report of a case and histologic and immunohistochemical studies. Arch Dermatol 128:1078, 1992
35. Howell JB, Freeman RG: Cutaneous defects of focal dermal hypoplasia: an ectomesodermal dysplasia syndrome. J Cutan Pathol 16:237, 1989
36. Mann M, Weintraub R, Hashimoto K: Focal dermal hypoplasia with an initial inflammatory phase. Pediatr Dermatol 7:278, 1990
37. Frieden IJ: Aplasia cutis congenita: a clinical review and proposal for classification. J Am Acad Dermatol 14:646, 1986
38. Steinmann B, Royce PM, Superti-Furga A: The Ehlers-Danlos syndrome. p. 351. In Royce PM, Steinman B (eds): Connective Tissue and Its Heritable Disorders. Wiley-Liss, New York, 1993
39. Sulica VI, Cooper PH, Pope FM et al: Cutaneous histo-

logic features in Ehlers-Danlos syndrome. Arch Dermatol 115:40, 1979

40. Pope FM, Nicholls AC, Narcisi P et al: Type III collagen mutations in Ehlers-Danlos syndrome type IV and other related disorders. Clin Exp Dermatol 13:285, 1988

41. Vogel A, Holbrook KA, Steinmann B, et al: Abnormal collagen fibril structure in the gravis form (type I) of the Ehlers-Danlos syndrome. Lab Invest 40:201, 1979

42. Faver IR, Daoud MS, Su WP: Acquired reactive perforating collagenosis. Report of six cases and review of the literature. J Am Acad Dermatol 30:575, 1994

43. Woringer F, Laugier P: Collagenoma perforans verruciforme. Dermatol Wochenschr 147:64, 1963

44. Rapini RP, Herbert AA, Drucker CR: Acquired perforating dermatosis. Evidence for combined transepidermal elimination of both collagen and elastic fibers. Arch Dermatol 125:1074, 1989.

45. Mehregan AH, Schwartz OD, Livingood CS: Reactive perforating collagenosis. Arch Dermatol 96:277, 1967

46. Goette DK: Transepithelial elimination disorders. J Assoc Military Derm 11:28, 1985

47. Neldner KH: Pseudoxanthoma elasticum. Clin Dermatol 6:1, 1988

48. Bolognia JL, Braverman I: Pseudoxanthoma elasticum-like skin changes induced by penicillamine. Dermatology 184:12, 1992

49. Rongioletti F, Rebora A: Fibroelastolytic patterns of intrinsic skin aging: pseudoxanthoma elasticum-like papillary dermal elastolysis and white fibrous papulosis of the neck. Dermatology 191:19, 1995

50. Lebwohl M, Schwartz E, Lemlich G et al: Abnormalities of connective tissue components in lesional and non-lesional tissue of patients with pseudoxanthoma elasticum. Arch Dermatol Res 285:121, 1993

51. Lebwohl M, Phelps RG, Yannuzzi L et al: Diagnosis of pseudoxanthoma elasticum by scar biopsy in patients without characteristic skin lesions. N Engl J Med 317:347, 1987

52. Hausser I, Anton-Lamprecht I: Early preclinical diagnosis of dominant pseudoxanthoma elasticum by specific ultrastructural changes of dermal elastic and collagen tissue in a family at risk. Hum Genet 87:693, 1991

53. Goltz RW, Hult AM, Goldfarb M et al: Cutis laxa. Arch Dermatol 92:373, 1965

54. Thomas WO, Moses MH, Craver RD et al: Congenital cutis laxa: a case report and review of loose skin syndromes. Ann Surg 30:252, 1993

55. Koch SE, Williams ML: Acquired cutis laxa: case report and review of disorders of elastolysis. Pediatr Dermatol 2:282, 1985

56. Lewis PG, Hood AF, Barnett NK, Holbrook KA: Postinflammatory elastolysis and cutis laxa. A case report. J Am Acad Dermatol 22:40, 1990

57. Mehregan AH, Lee SC, Nabai H: Cutis laxa (generalized elastolysis). J Cutan Pathol 5:116, 1978

58. Venencie PY, Winkelmann RK, Moore BA: Anetoderma: clinical findings, associations and long-term follow-up evaluations. Arch Dermatol 120:1032, 1984

59. Karrer S, Szeimies R-M, Stolz W, Landthaler M: Primary anetoderma in children: report of two cases and literature review. Pediatr Dermatol 13:382, 1996

60. Venencie PY, Winkelmann RK: Histopathologic findings in anetoderma. Arch Dermatol 120:1040, 1984

61. Zaki I, Scerri L, Nelson H: Primary anetoderma: phagocytosis of elastic fibers by macrophages. Clin Exp Dermatol 19:388, 1994

62. Barnhill RL, Goldenhersh MA: Elastophagocytosis: a non-specific reaction pattern associated with inflammatory processes in sun-protected skin. J Cutan Pathol 16:199, 1989

63. Sears JK, Stone MS, Argenyi Z: Papular elastorrhexis: a variant of connective tissue nevus. Case reports and review of the literature. J Am Acad Dermatol 19:409, 1988

64. Goeteyn M, Geerts ML, Kint A, DeWeert J: The Basex-Dupre-Christol syndrome Arch Dermatol 130:337, 1994

65. Kim JM, Su WP: Mid dermal elastolysis with wrinkling. Report of two cases and review of the literature. J Am Acad Dermatol 26:169, 1992

66. Åsbrink E, Brehmer-Andersson E, Hovmark A: Acrodermatitis chronica atrophicans—a spirochetosis. Clinical and histopathological picture based on 32 patients; course and relationship to erythema chronicum migrans Afzelius. Am J Dermatopathol 8:209, 1986

67. deKoning J, Tazelaar DJ, Hoogkamp-Korstanje JA, Elema JD: Acrodermatitis chronica atrophicans: a light and electron microscopic study. J Cutan Pathol 22:23, 1995

68. Aberer E, Klade H, Hobisch G: A clinical, histological and immunohistochemical comparison of acrodermatitis chronica atrophicans. Am J Dermatopathol 13:334, 1991

69. Sheu HM, Yu HS, Chang CH: Mast cell degranulation and elastolysis in the early stage of striae distensae. J Cutan Pathol 18:410, 1991

70. Zheng P, Lavker RM, Kligman AM: Anatomy of striae. Br J Dermatol 112:185,1985

71. Suji T, Sawabe M: Elastic fibers in striae distensae. J Cutan Pathol 15:215, 1988

72. Burket JM, Zelickson AS, Padilla RS: Linear focal elastosis (elastotic striae). J Am Acad Dermatol 20:633, 1989

73. Calderone DC, Fenske NA: The clinical spectrum of actinic elastosis. J Am Acad Dermatol 32:1016, 1995

74. Jordaan HF, Rossouw DJ: Digital papular calcific elastosis: a histopathological, histochemical and ultrastructural study of 20 patients. J Cutan Pathol 17:358, 1990

75. Matsuta M, Izaki S, Ide C et al: Light and electron microscopic immunohistochemistry of solar elastosis. J Dermatol 14:364, 1987

76. Uitto J, Fazio MJ, Olsen DR: Molecular mechanisms of cutaneous aging. Age-associated connective tissue alterations in the dermis. J Am Acad Dermatol 21:614, 1989

77. Mehregan AH: Elastosis perforans serpiginosa. A review of the literature and report of 11 cases. Arch Dermatol 97:381, 1968

78. Cruz PD, East C, Bergstresser PR: Dermal, subcutaneous, and tendon xanthomas: diagnostic markers for specific lipoprotein disorders. J Am Acad Dermatol 19:95, 1988

79. Burgdorf WHC, Kusch SL, Nix TE Jr, Pitha J: Progressive nodular histiocytoma. Arch Dermatol 117:644, 1981

80. Walsh NM, Murray S, D'Intino Y: Eruptive xanthomas with urate-like crystals. J Cutan Pathol 21:350, 1994

81. Buchner A, Hansen LS, Merrill PW: Verruciform xanthoma of the oral mucosa. Arch Dermatol 117:563, 1981

82. Mostafa KA, Takata T, Ogawa I et al: Verruciform xanthoma of the oral mucosa: a clinicopathological study with immunohistochemical findings relating to pathogenesis. Virchows Arch A Pathol Anat 423:243, 1993

83. Smith KJ, Skelton HG, Angritt P: Changes of verruciform xanthoma in an HIV–1+ patient with diffuse psoriasiform skin disease. Am J Dermatopathol 17:185, 1995

84. Cohen AS: Amyloidosis. pp. 1427–1448. In McCarty DJ (ed): Arthritis and Allied Conditions. 12th Ed. Lea & Febiger, Philadelphia, 1993

85. Gertz MA, Kyle RA: Primary systemic amyloidosis—a diagnostic primer. Mayo Clin Proc 64:1505, 1989

86. Brownstein MH, Helwig ED: The cutaneous amyloidoses. II. Systemic forms. Arch Dermatol 102:20, 1970

87. Robert C, Aractingi S, Prost C et al: Bullous amyloidosis. Report of 3 cases and review of the literature. Medicine (Baltimore) 72:38, 1993

88. Sepp N, Pichler E, Breathnach SM et al: Amyloid elastosis: analysis of the role of the amyloid P component. J Am Acad Dermatol 22:27, 1990

89. Libbey CA, Skinner M, Cohen AS: Use of abdominal fat tissue aspirate in the diagnosis of systemic amyloidosis. Arch Intern Med 143:1549, 1983

90. Brownstein MH, Helwig EB: The cutaneous amyloidoses. I. Localized forms. Arch Dermatol 102:8, 1970

91. Wong CK, Breathnach SM (eds): Cutaneous amyloidoses. Clin Dermatol 8:1, 1990

92. Brownstein MH, Hashimoto K: Macular amyloidosis. Arch Dermatol 106:50, 1972

93. Goulden V, Highet AS, Shamy HK: Notalgia paresthetica—report of an association with macular amyloidosis. Clin Exp Dermatol 19:346, 1994

94. Tidman MJ, Wells RS, MacDonald DM: Pachyonychia congenita with cutaneous amyloidosis and hyperpigmentation—a distinct variant. J Am Acad Dermatol 16:935, 1987

95. Brownstein MH, Hashimoto K, Greenwald G: Biphasic amyloidosis: link between macular and lichenoid forms. Br J Dermatol 88:25, 1973

96. Looi LM: Primary localized cutaneous amyloidosis in Malaysians. Austral J Dermatol 32:39, 1991

97. Gagel RF, Levy ML, Donovan DT et al: Multiple endocrine neoplasia type 2a associated with cutaneous lichen amyloidosus. Ann Intern Med 111:802, 1989

98. Jambrosic J, From L, Hanna W: Lichen amyloidosus. Am J Dermatopathol 6:151, 1984

99. Masuda C, Mohri S, Nakajima H: Histopathological and immunohistochemical study of amyloidosis cutis nodularis—comparison with systemic amyloidosis. Br J Dermatol 119:33, 1988

100. Horiguchi Y, Takahashi C, Imamura S: A case of nodular cutaneous amyloidosis. Amyloid production by infiltrating plasma cells. Am J Dermatopathol 15:59, 1993

101. Floege J, Brandis A, Nonnast-Daniel B et al: Subcutaneous amyloid tumor of beta-2 microglobulin origin in a long-term hemodialysis patient. Nephron 53:73, 1989

102. Hashimoto K, Kobayashi H: Histogenesis of amyloid in the skin. Am J Dermatopathol 2:165, 1980

103. Ito K, Hashimoto K: Antikeratin autoantibodies in the amyloid deposits of lichen amyloidosis and macular amyloidosis. Arch Dermatol Res 281:377, 1989

104. Hashimoto K: Nylon brush macular amyloidosis. Arch Dermatol 123:633, 1987

105. Satti MB, Azzopardi JG: Amyloid deposits in basal cell carcinoma of the skin. J Am Acad Dermatol 22:1082, 1990

106. Innocenzi D, Barduagni F, Cerio R, Wolter M: UV-induced colloid milium. Clin Exp Dermatol 18:347, 1993

107. Handfield-Jones SE, Atherton DJ, Black MM et al: Juvenile colloid milium: clinical, histological and ultrastructural features. J Cutan Pathol 19:434, 1992

108. Stone MS, Tschen JA: Colloid milium. Arch Dermatol 122:711, 1986

109. Hashimoto K, Black M: Colloid milium: a final degeneration product of actinic elastoid. J Cutan Pathol 12:147, 1985

110. Matsuta M, Kunimoto M, Kosegawa G: Electron microscopic study of the colloid-like substance in solar elastosis. J Dermatol 16:191, 1989

111. Pierard GE, Van Cauwenberge D, Budo J, Lapière CM: A clinicopathologic study of six cases of lipoid proteinosis. Am J Dermatopathol 10:300, 1988

112. Farolan MJ, Ronan SG, Solomon LM, Loeff DS: Lipoid proteinosis: case report. Pediatr Dermatol 9:264, 1992

113. Konstantinov K, Kabakchiev P, Karchev T et al: Lipoid proteinosis. J Am Acad Dermatol 27:293, 1992

114. Newton JA, Rasbridge S, Temple A: Lipoid proteinosis—new immunological observations. Clin Exp Dermatol 16:350, 1991

115. Muda AO, Paradisi M, Angelo C: Lipoid proteinosis: clinical, histologic and ultrastructural investigations. Cutis 56:220, 1995

116. King DF, King LA: The appropriate processing of tophi for microscopy. Am J Dermatopathol 4:239, 1982

117. Isonokami M, Nishida K, Okada N, Yoshikawa K: Cutaneous oxalate granulomas in a haemodialysed patient: report of a case with unique clinical features. Br J Dermatol 128:690, 1993

118. Phillips JI, Isaacson C, Carman H: Ochronosis in black South Africans who used skin lighteners. Am J Dermatopathol 8:14, 1986

119. Jordaan HF, Van Niekerk DJ: Transepidermal elimination in exogenous ochronosis. A report of two cases. Am J Dermatopathol 13:418, 1991

120. Tidman MJ, Horton JJ, MacDonald DM: Hydroquinone-induced ochronosis: light and electron-microscopic features. Clin Exp Dermatol 11:224, 1986

121. Jordaan HF, Mulligan RP: Actinic granuloma-like change in exogenous ochronosis: case report. J Cutan Pathol 17:236, 1990

122. Truhan AP, Roenigk HH: The cutaneous mucinoses. J Am Acad Dermatol 14:1, 1986

123. Fatourechi V, Pajouhi M, Fransway AF: Dermopathy of Graves disease (pretibial myxedema). Medicine (Baltimore) 73:1, 1994

124. Somach SC, Helm TN, Lawlor KB et al: Pretibial mucin. Histologic patterns and clinical correlation. Arch Dermatol 129:1152, 1993

125. Yamazaki S, Katayama I, Satog T et al: Acral ichthyosiform mucinosis in association with Sjögren's syndrome: a peculiar form of pretibial myxedema? J Dermatol 20:715, 1993

126. Forgie JC, Highet AS, Kelly SA: Myxoedematous infiltrate of the forehead in treated hypothyroidism. Clin Exp Dermatol 19:168, 1994

127. Perry HO, Kierland RR, Montgomery H: Plaque-like form of cutaneous mucinosis. Arch Dermatol 82:980, 1960

128. Steigleder GK, Gartmann H, Linker U: REM-syndrome: reticular erythematous mucinosis (round-cell erythematosis), a new entity? Br J Dermatol 91:191, 1974

129. Braddock SW, Davis CS, Davis RB: Reticular erythematous mucinosis and thrombocytopenic purpura: report of a case and review of the world literature, including plaque-like cutaneous mucinosis. J Am Acad Dermatol 19:859, 1988

130. Weigand DA, Burgdorf WHC, Gregg LJ: Dermal mucinosis in discoid lupus erythematosus. Arch Dermatol 117:735, 1981

131. Freeman RG: A pathological basis for the cutaneous papules of mucopolysaccharidosis II (the Hunter syndrome). J Cutan Pathol 4:318, 1977

132. Farmer ER, Hambrick GW, Shulman LE: Papular mucinosis—clinicopathologic study of four patients. Arch Dermatol 118:9, 1982

133. Wilk M, Schmoeckel C: Cutaneous focal mucinosis—a histopathological and immunohistochemical analysis of 11 cases. J Cutan Pathol 21:446, 1994

134. Nödl F, Zaun H: Euthyreote zirkumskripte symmetrische Myxodermie der Oberlippe. Hautarzt 34:27, 1983

135. Pucevich MV, Latour DL, Bale GF, King LE Jr: Self-healing juvenile cutaneous mucinosis. J Am Acad Dermatol 11:327, 1984

136. Stokes KS, Rabinowitz LG, Segura AD, Esterly NB: Cutaneous mucinosis of infancy. Pediatr Dermatol 11:246, 1994

137. Bork K, Hoede N: Hereditary progressive mucinous histiocytosis in women. Arch Dermatol 124:1225, 1988

138. Flowers SL, Cooper PH, Landes HB: Acral persistent papular mucinosis. J Am Acad Dermatol 21:293, 1989

139. Reed RJ, Utz MP, Terezakis N: Embolic and metastatic cardiac myxoma. Am J Dermatopathol 11:157, 1989

140. Johnson WC, Helwig EB: Cutaneous focal mucinosis: a clinicopathologic and histochemical study. Arch Dermatol 93:13, 1966

141. Johnson WC, Graham JH, Helwig EB: Cutaneous myxoid cyst: a clinicopathologic and histochemical study. JAMA 191:15, 1965

142. Lettanand A, Johnson WC, Graham JH: Mucous cyst (mucocele). Arch Dermatol 101:673, 1970

143. Jensen JL: Superficial mucoceles of the oral mucosa. Am J Dermatopathol 12:88, 1990

144. Dadone MM, Kushner JP, Edwards CQ et al: Hereditary hemochromatosis. Am J Clin Pathol 78:196, 1982

145. Cawley EP, Hsu YT, Wood BT et al: Hemochromatosis of the skin. Arch Dermatol 100:1, 1969

146. Perdrup A, Poulsen H: Hemochromatosis and vitiligo. Arch Dermatol 90:34, 1964

147. Leyden JL, Lockshin NA, Kriebel S: The black keratinous cyst. A sign of hemochromatosis. Arch Dermatol 106:379, 1972

148. Johansson EA, Kanerva L, Niemi KM et al: Generalized argyria. Clin Exp Dermatol 7:169, 1982

149. Hönigsmann H, Konrad K, Wolff K: Argyrose (Histologie und Ultrastruktur). Hautarzt 24:24, 1973

150. Mehregan AH: Calcinosis cutis: a review of the clinical forms and report of 75 cases. Semin Dermatol 3:53, 1984

151. Bucko AD: Cutaneous calcification. Sect. 12-2. In Demis DJ (ed): Clinical Dermatology. Lippincott-Raven, Philadelphia, 1997

152. McGee-Russell SM: Histochemical methods for calcium. J Histochem Cytochem 6:22, 1958

153. Hafner J, Keusch G, Wahl C et al: Uremic small-artery disease with medial calcification and intimal hyperplasia (so-called calciphylaxis): complication of chronic renal failure and benefit from parathyroidectomy. J Am Acad Dermatol 33:954, 1995

154. Ivker RA, Woosley J, Briggaman RA: Calciphylaxis in three patients with end-stage renal disease. Arch Dermatol 131:63, 1995

155. Muller SA, Winkelmann RK, Brunsting LA: Calcinosis in dermatomyositis. Arch Dermatol 79:699, 1959

156. Muller SA, Brunsting LA, Winkelmann RK: Calcinosis cutis: its relationship to scleroderma. Arch Dermatol 80:15, 1959

157. Quismorio FP, Dubois EL, Chandor SB: Soft tissue calcification in systemic lupus erythematosus. Arch Dermatol 111:352, 1975

158. Gal G, Metzker A, Garlick J et al: Head and neck manifestations of tumoral calcinosis. Oral Surg Oral Med Oral Pathol 74:158, 1994

159. Song DH, Lee KH, Kang WH: Idiopathic calcinosis of the scrotum: histopathologic observations of fifty-one nodules. J Am Acad Dermatol 19:1095, 1988

160. Swinehart JM, Golitz LE: Scrotal calcinosis: dystrophic calcification of epidermoid cysts. Arch Dermatol 118:985, 1982

161. Winer LH: Solitary congenital nodular calcification of the skin. Arch Dermatol 66:204, 1952

162. Shmunes E, Wood MG: Subepidermal calcified nodules. Arch Dermatol 105:593, 1972

163. Weigand DA: Subepidermal calcified nodule: report of a case with apparent hair follicle origin. J Cutan Pathol 3:109, 1976

164. Eng AM, Mandrea E: Perforating calcinosis cutis presenting as milia. J Cutan Pathol 8:247, 1981

165. Roth SI, Stowell RE, Helwig EB: Cutaneous ossification: report of 120 cases and review of the literature. Arch Pathol 76:56, 1963

166. Burgdorf W, Nasemann T: Cutaneous osteomas: a clinical and histopathologic review. Arch Dermatol Res 260:121, 1977

167. Orlow SJ, Watsky KL, Bolognia JL: Skin and bones. I. J Am Acad Dermatol 25:205, 1991

168. Orlow SJ, Watsky KL, Bolognia JL: Skin and bones. II. J Am Acad Dermatol 25:447, 1991

169. Prendiville JS, Lucky AW, Mallory SB et al: Osteoma cutis as a presenting sign of pseudohypoparathyroidism. Pediatr Dermatol 9:11, 1992

170. Trueb RM, Pannizon RG, Burg G: Cutaneous ossification in Albright's hereditary osteodystrophy. Dermatology 186:205, 1993

171. Cottoni F, Dell' Orbo C, Quacci D, Tedde G: Primary os-

teoma cutis. Clinical, morphological and ultrastructural study. Am J Dermatopathol 15:77, 1993

172. Sanmartin O, Alegre V, Martinez-Aparicio A et al: Congenital platelike osteoma cutis: case report and review of the literature. Pediatr Dermatol 10:182, 1993

173. Kaplan FS, Craver R, MacEven GD et al: Progressive osseous heteroplasia: a distinct developmental disorder of heterotopic ossification. J Bone Joint Surg (Am) 76:435, 1994

174. Landon GC, Johnson KA, Dahlin DC: Subungual exostoses. J Bone Joint Surg (Am) 61:256, 1979

175. Woo TY, Rasmussen JE: Subungual osteocartilaginous exostosis. J Dermatol Surg Oncol 11:534, 1985

176. Forbis R, Jr, Helwig EB: Pilomatrixoma (calcifying epithelioma). Arch Dermatol 83:606, 1961

177. Hirsch P, Helwig EB: Chondroid syringoma: mixed tumor of skin, salivary gland type. Arch Dermatol 84:177, 1961

178. Culver W, Burgdorf WHC: Malignant melanoma arising in a nevus of Nanta. J Cutan Pathol 20:375, 1993

179. Moulin G, Souquet D, Balme B: Naevus pigmentaires et ossifications cutanées. A propos de 125 cas d'osteonaevus. Ann Dermatol Venereol 118:199, 1991

180. Cerroni L, Soyer HP, Smolle J, Kerl H: Cutaneous metastases of a giant cell tumor of bone: case report. J Cutan Pathol 17:59, 1990

181. Bettendorf U, Remmele W, Laaff H: Bone formation by cancer metastases. Virchows Arch Klin Chir 369:359, 1976

182. Eckardt JJ, Ivins JC, Perry HO et al: Osteosarcoma arising in heterotopic ossification of dermatomyositis: case report and review of the literature. Cancer 48:1256, 1981

183. Lehrman A, Pratt JH, Parkhill EM: Heterotopic bone in laparotomy scars. Am J Surg 104:591, 1962

184. Moritz DL, Elewski B: Pigmented postacne osteoma cutis in a patient treated with minocycline: report and review of the literature. J Am Acad Dermatol 24:851, 1991

185. Boneschi V, Alessi E, Brambilla L: Multiple miliary osteomas of the face. Am J Dermatopathol 15:268, 1993

186. Lippman HI, Goldin RR: Subcutaneous ossification of the legs in chronic venous insufficiency. Radiology 74:279, 1960

187. Satoh T, Tokura Y, Katsumata M et al: Histological diagnostic criteria for accessory tragi. J Cutan Pathol 17:206, 1990

188. Hurwitz RM: Painful papule of the ear: a follicular disorder. J Dermatol Surg Oncol 13:270, 1987

189. Santa Cruz DJ: Chondrodermatitis nodularis helicis: a transepidermal perforating disorder. J Cutan Pathol 7:70, 1980

190. McAdam LP, O'Hanlan MA, Bluestone R et al: Relapsing polychondritis: prospective study of 23 patients and a review of the literature. Medicine 55:193, 1976

191. Feinerman LK, Johnson WC, Weiner J et al: Relapsing polychondritis. Dermatologica 140:369, 1970

192. Foidart JM, Abe S, Martin GR et al: Antibodies to type II collagen in relapsing polychondritis. N Engl J Med 299:1203, 1978

193. Glamb R, Kim R: Pseudocyst of the auricle. J Am Acad Dermatol 11:58, 1984

194. Grabski WJ, Salasche SJ, McCollough ML, Angeloni VL: Pseudocyst of the auricle associated with trauma. Arch Dermatol 125:528, 1989

195. Dahlin DC, Salvador AH: Cartilaginous tumors of the soft tissues of the hands and feet. Mayo Clin Proc 49:721, 1974

196. Chung EB, Enzinger FM: Chondroma of soft parts. Cancer 41:1414, 1978

197. Hsueh S, Santa Cruz DJ: Cartilaginous lesions of the skin and superficial soft tissue. J Cutan Pathol 9:405, 1982

198. Ando K, Goto Y, Hirabayashi N et al: Cutaneous cartilaginous tumor. J Dermatol Surg Oncol 21:339, 1995

199. King DT, Gurevitch AW, Hirose FM: Multiple cutaneous metastases of a scapular chondrosarcoma. Arch Dermatol 114:584, 1978

200. Norwood C: Amyloidosis. J Assoc Military Derm 11:74, 1985

17

TUMORS OF THE EPIDERMIS

SEBORRHEIC KERATOSIS

Clinical Features

Seborrheic keratosis lesions are often multiple, oval, raised, and may or may not be pigmented. Their colors are usually brown or black, and they have a classic stuck-on appearance. They generally occur after age 40 on the back, chest, head, and neck, including the scalp. Spared are the palms and soles. The total number of seborrheic keratoses increases with increasing age of the patient. The sudden eruptive appearance of hundreds of pruritic seborrheic keratoses is known as *the sign of Leser-Trelat*. This is a sign of systemic malignancy such as adenocarcinoma of lung, colon, or breast, mycoses fungoides, and so forth.[1–7] A diminutive form of seborrheic keratosis, dermatosis papulosa nigra, occurs in blacks as small soft skin tag-like lesions on the face and torso. The microscopic features are the same as those of larger seborrheic keratoses.

Histopathologic Features

Five histologic types of seborrheic keratosis are recognized: acanthotic, keratotic, adenoid, clonal, and irritated. All histologic types of seborrheic keratosis show an abrupt change when compared with adjacent epidermis. There is abrupt acanthosis, hyperkeratosis, and papillomatosis, usually with the presence of horned cysts. The overall configuration or silhouette is nodular or verrucoid and raised above the back of the adjacent epidermis. The cellular composition is medium-sized keratinocytes and basal cells along with varying degrees of pigment. Melanophages may be present below the lesion in the dermis.[8]

The most common form of seborrheic keratosis is *acanthotic* (Fig. 17-1). The lesion forms a raised papule or nodule above the epidermis. The keratinocytes form blunt interconnecting projections that contain horn pseudocysts.

The *keratotic* form of seborrheic keratosis displays less acanthosis or papillomatosis, but instead hyperkeratosis is the most prominent feature. The squamous cells continue to be medium

sized but do not form acanthotic projections. The keratin present is orthokeratin, but, if ulcerated or inflamed, parakeratin will result.

The reticulated or *adenoid seborrheic keratosis* displays thin projections of keratinocytes that project downward into the dermis. They may broaden in some areas to accommodate small horn pseudocysts. These may originate from solar lentigines (Fig. 17-2).

The nested or *clonal seborrheic keratosis* shows small islands or nests of atypical keratinocytes that are distinct from their surrounding neighbors. The cytoplasm is clear, pale, or eosinophilic compared with adjacent tumor (Fig. 17-3). These can sometimes be seen as a component of any seborrheic keratosis. Dermis below is usually moderately inflamed with mononuclear cells.

The inflamed or *irritated seborrheic keratosis* shows squamous eddies as its characteristic feature (Fig. 17-4). These present as small or large whorls of squamous cells that are present in the broad acanthotic bands. The cells within the eddies can have enlarged atypical nuclei and even show mitoses. The degree of squamous eddies and streaming of keratinocytes can be alarming, but the overall outline of the lesion is maintained as a seborrheic keratosis. Regardless of subtype, all seborrheic keratoses are cytokeratin positive.[9]

Differential Diagnosis

The main diagnostic distinction to be made is that of squamous cell carcinoma (SCC). The irritated or inflamed seborrheic keratosis can be alarming because of the atypia accompanying squamous eddies and the streaming of keratinocytes. Overall, the architecture is preserved above a line connecting the two ends of the adjacent epidermis (string sign). An inflamed seborrheic keratosis does not show the atypia, atypical mitoses, or dyskeratosis seen in SCC. Verruca vulgaris may also cause some difficulty, but verruca displays inward bending of rete toward a central point. This is not a feature found in seborrheic keratosis. Koilocytes when found are present only in verruca. Horn pseudocysts are found only in seborrheic keratosis.

439

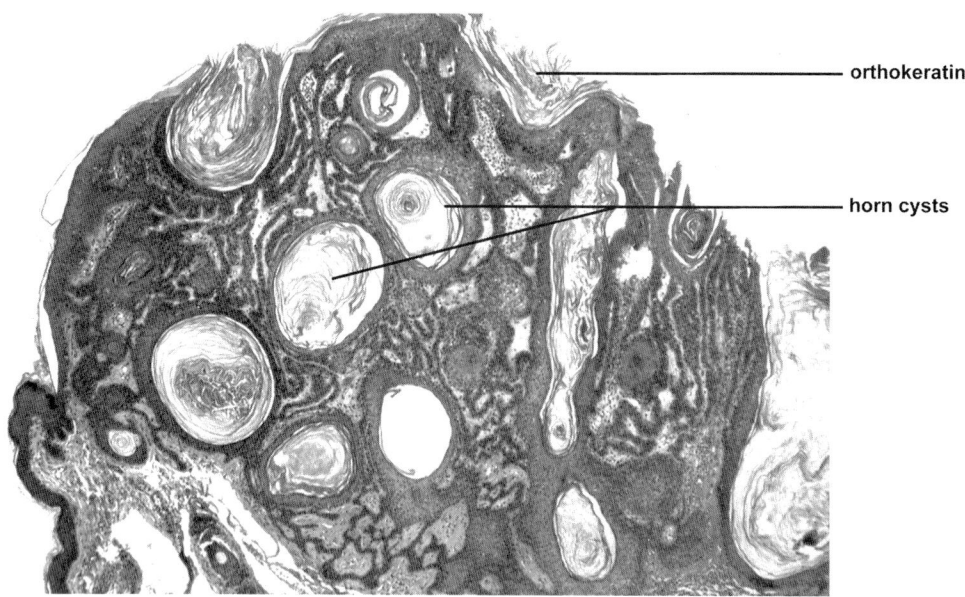

orthokeratin

horn cysts

Figure 17-1. Acanthotic seborrheic keratosis. Numerous horn pseudocysts are present. The tumor rises above the level of the adjacent epidermis, "the string sign." (H&E, × 40.)

It is important to note that basal cell carcinomas (BCCs) can occur in continuity with seborrheic keratoses. There has also been a recent report of SCCs and BCCs associated with seborrheic keratoses.[10,11] Reports such as these indicate that care should be taken in the examination of seborrheic keratoses. It has also been noted that some seborrheic keratoses occurring in anogenital regions contain DNA for human papillomavirus (HPV) and are therefore actually condyloma.[12]

EPIDERMAL NEVI

Congenital malformations of the skin are termed *epidermal nevi*. Two major subcategories exist: those that involve only the epidermis and those that involve epidermis as well as adnexae (the nevus sebaceus). In the study of Soloman et al,[13] 78% of patients with epidermal nevi had one other abnormality: skeletal system, 67%; central nervous system 48%. In another study, one-third of the patients with epidermal nevi had abnormalities in other systems: nervous system, 15%, skeletal system, 15%. The larger epidermal nevi are the ones that are more often associated with abnormalities in other organs and are on the same body side as the epidermal nevi.

Clinical Features

Epidermal nevi are pigmented, roughened areas of warty skin arranged in a linear or zosteriform pattern. They involve the distribution of Blaschko's lines. They are usually present at birth, infancy, or childhood. The lesions are congenital, but not clearly hereditary. There is neither a gender nor an ethnic predilection.[14–17]

Other cutaneous findings associated with epidermal nevi include reports of bathing trunk nevi, blue nevi, aplasia cutis, café-au-lait spots, hypopigmentation, and hypertrichosis. Neu-

rologic manifestations have included seizures, mental retardation, and developmental delay. Electroencephalograms in such patients have been abnormal. Other neurologic abnormalities include macrocephaly, hydrocephaly, focal cortical atrophy, hemiparesis, cortical blindness, and visual field defects. Skeletal abnormalities associated with epidermal nevi include hemihypertrophy, incomplete development of the talus, clubfoot, brachydactyly, and syndactyly. Miscellaneous associations include ocular abnormalities and oral abnormalities, specifically odontodysplasia.

Histopathologic Features

The nevus sebaceus shows epidermal irregularities and corrugation, which develops progressively with age. There is superficial location and duplication of sebaceous glands, hair follicles, and apocrine glands (Fig. 17-5). The nevus sebaceus is the only one of the epidermal nevi that is associated with the late development of tumors, BCC, and syringocystoadenoma papilliferum.[18]

The other epidermal nevi can be divided into several histologic types depending on their predominant appearance. Forms have been described as seborrheic keratosis-like, psoriasiform (inflammatory linear epidermal nevus [ILVEN]), verrucoid (wart-like), porokeratosis-like, acantholytic dyskeratosis-like, epidermolytic hyperkeratosis-like, and acrokeratosis verruciformis-like (Fig. 17-6). Some would include the nevus comedonicus.[19–22] All show extensive hyperkeratosis, and some form of epidermal corrugation. The various individual names describe specific shapes within the epidermis or other changes within the epidermis. Thus, the names indicate similarities with seborrheic keratosis, psoriasis, porokeratosis, verruca, and so forth. Follicular units are usually rudimentary in the malformation.

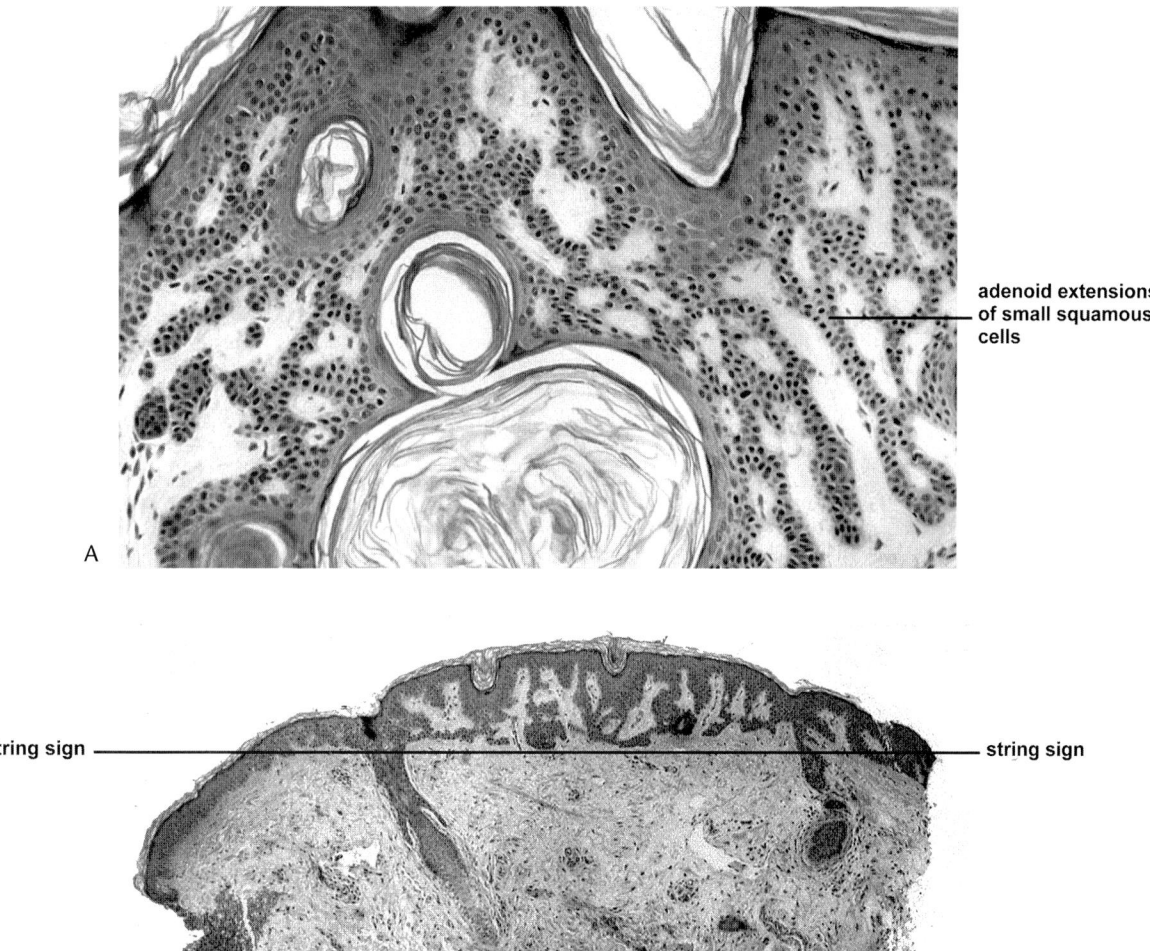

adenoid extensions
of small squamous
cells

A

string sign ———————————————————————— string sign

B

Figure 17-2. (**A & B**) Adenoid seborrheic keratosis. This lesion is characterized by elongate extensions of small cells in a reticulated or adenoid pattern extending from the surface. Occasionally they expand to accommodate horn pseudocysts. (H&E, × 100.) A very small developing adenoid seborrheic keratosis is present (Fig. A). These arise through enlargement of some lentigines. (H&E, × 40.)

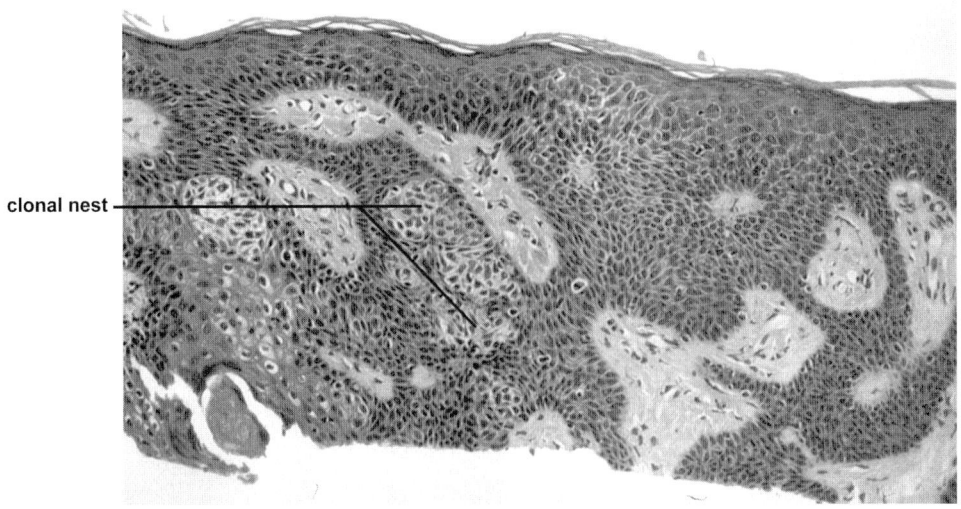

clonal nest

Figure 17-3. Flat, partially clonal seborrheic keratosis. The small, pale-staining islands within the broad intersecting rete are the clonal areas. All seborrheic keratoses are benign lesions.

Differential Diagnosis

The clinical history and appearance are extremely important in making the diagnosis of the epidermal nevi. When only a biopsy is taken it is extremely easy to make a misdiagnosis of psoriasis, seborrheic keratosis, or other in the absence of clinical history. In fact, we have recently had the experience of making the diagnosis of multiple fibroepithelial polyps from the currettings of an epidermal nevus when no clinical history was given. By contrast, a nevus sebaceus can be easily diagnosed because of the multiple abnormal and superficially placed sebaceous glands, which are present in intimate association with the corrugated epidermis. Rarely have malignancies developed in epidermal nevi, making their examination necessary.[23–26]

TUMOR OF THE FOLLICULAR INFUNDIBULUM

The tumor of the follicular infundibulum (TFI) was first described by Mehregan and Butler in 1961. It is a rare but benign adnexal tumor that is usually solitary, but there is also an eruptive variant in which there are many lesions.

Clinical Features

The TFI is usually described as a yellow or darker pigmented tumor of the face or scalp. Clinical diagnoses are often that of seborrheic keratosis or basal cell carcinoma. When multiple, the lesions appear as hypopigmented macules. While the scalp and face are the most common sites, the lesions are also found in a mantle distribution as well as other body sites. Patients are in their 40s to 60s. TFI has been associated with Cowden's disease and nevus sebaceus.[27–31]

Histopathologic Features

The only difference between solitary and eruptive TFIs is in clinical presentation. The histopathologic features are the same.[32] The characteristic histologic features consist of a plate-like or shelf-like horizontal proliferation of glycogen-containing keratinocytes parallel to, but below, the epidermis. This shelf-like configuration is connected to the overlying epidermis by thin strands and columns of similar cells (Fig. 17-7). The lesion interrupts elastic fibers, and there is a prominence of elastic fibers that surround the tumor. The tumor also interrupts follicular units in the area. TFI was found negative for reactivity to HPV.[33]

Differential Diagnosis

The TFI presents a distinctive silhouette in histologic pattern. The chief entity in the differential diagnosis is the fibroepithelioma of Pinkus. The surrounding meshwork of dense elastic fibers is distinctive to the TFI and is not seen in the fibroepithelioma of Pinkus. TFI is a benign lesion that possesses only cosmetic annoyance.

BOWENOID PAPULOSIS

Clinical Features

Bowenoid papulosis lesions are characterized by multiple pink papules in the anogenital region. They are small, usually 1 cm or less. They are found in young patients and may spontaneously regress. Clinically the lesions can resemble seborrheic keratoses, condyloma, or nevi. It has been well-established that they are associated with HPV types 16 and 18.[34–37]

Histopathologic Features

The histologic features of bowenoid papulosis, Bowen's disease, and squamous carcinoma in situ are very similar. Bowenoid papulosis displays full-thickness loss of maturation. The nuclei are crowded and irregular without normal arrangement. Hyperchromatism and mild pleomorphism are noted.

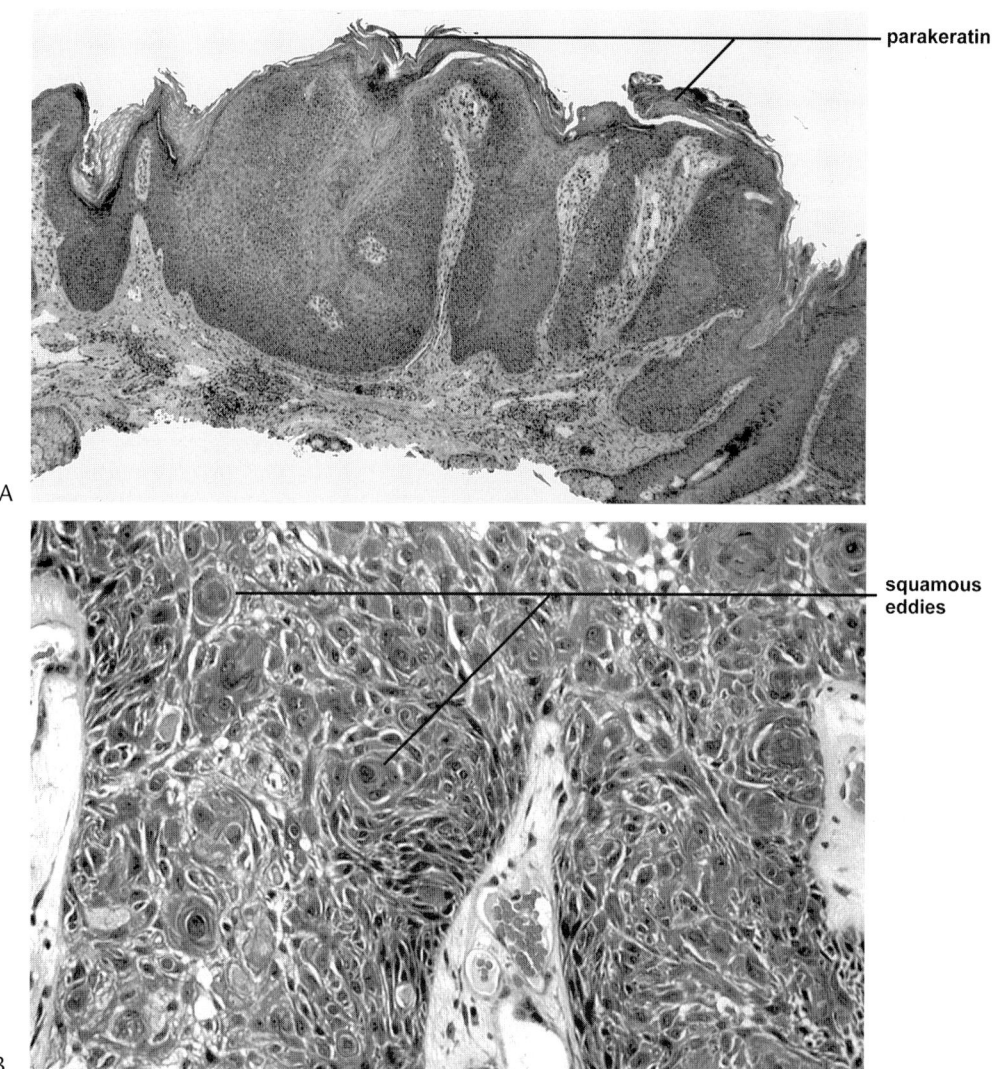

parakeratin

squamous
eddies

Figure 17-4. Inflamed or irritated seborrheic keratosis. (**A**) These lesions are often more keratotic than usual. They also display irregularly shaped acanthotic extensions of keratinocytes in the dermis. An underlying inflammatory infiltrate is noted. (**B**) Numerous squamous eddies with keratinization are identified. Nuclear atypia and mitoses may be present. Nonetheless, the overall silhouette is that of a seborrheic keratosis with a string sign.

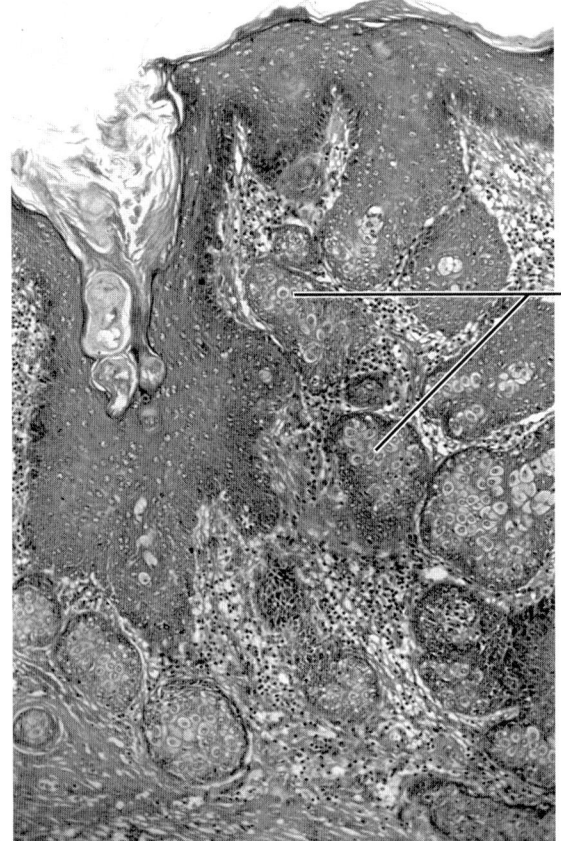

abnormal superficial
sebaceous units

A

clefts of
syringocyst-
adenoma
papilliforum

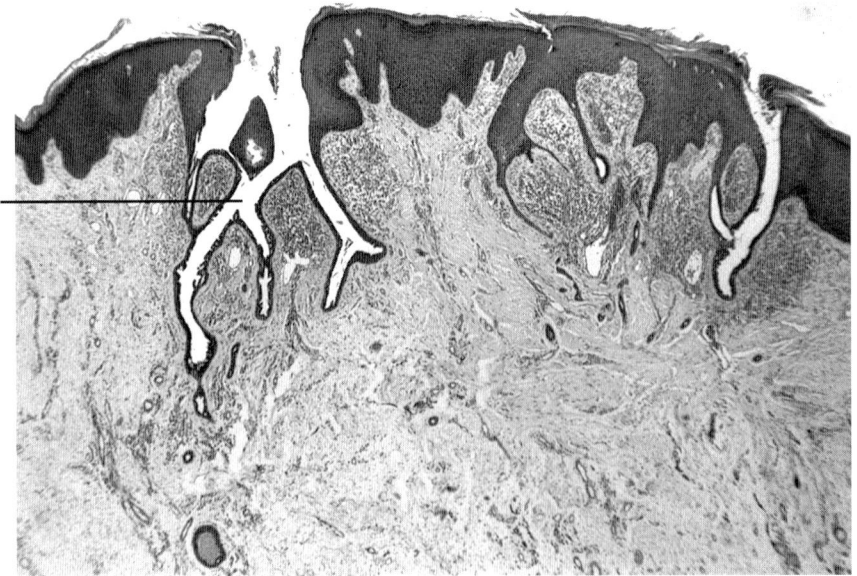

B

Figure 17-5. (**A**) Young nevus sebaceus. The epidermis is corrugated, and there are numerous abnormally formed and superficially placed sebaceous lobules. (H&E, × 40). (**B**) Nevus sebaceus showing the cleft-like extension into the dermis of an associated syringocystadenoma papilliforum.

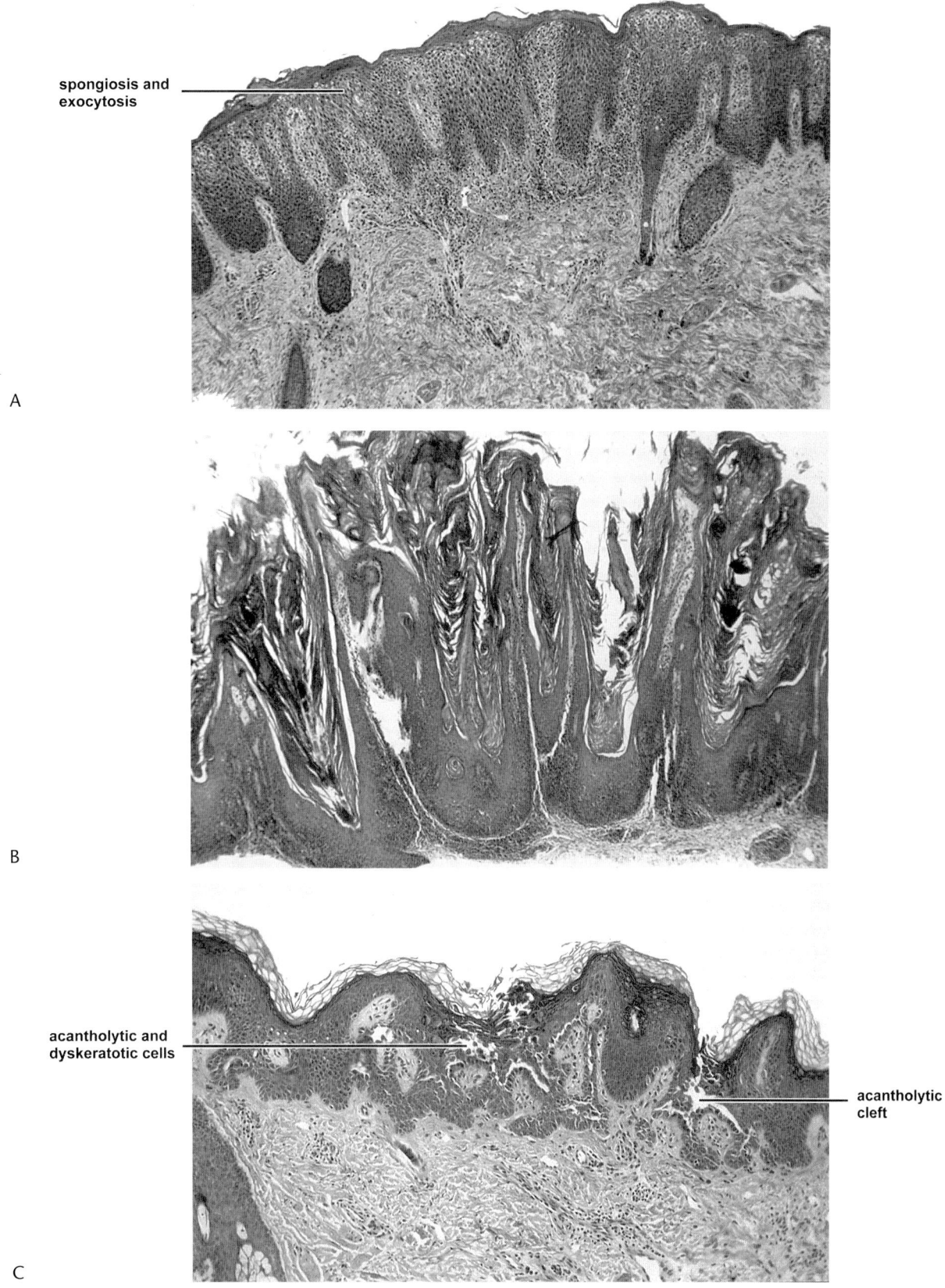

spongiosis and
exocytosis

acantholytic and
dyskeratotic cells

acantholytic
cleft

A

B

C

Figure 17-6. Three forms of epidermal nevus. (**A**) Inflammatory linear epidermal nevus. There is acanthosis with exocytosis and extensive spongiosis. (**B**) Wart-like or seborrheic keratosis-like epidermal nevus. (**C**) Corrugated epidermis with extensive acantholytic dyskeratosis. This form of epidermal nevus is less common than the others. (H&E, × 100.)

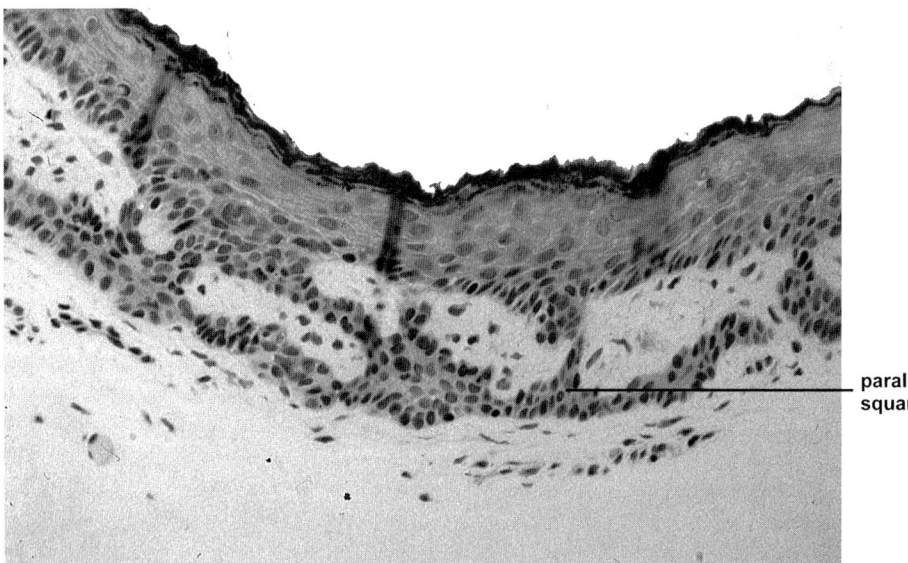

parallel plates of
squamous cells

Figure 17-7. The tumor of follicular infundibulum is characterized by parallel plate-like extensions of epidermis into the dermis. This is an easily overlooked and often unrecognized tumor. (H&E, × 100.)

Atypical mitoses and dyskeratotic cells are present near the surface of the epidermis (Fig. 17-8).

Differential Diagnosis and Clinicopathologic Correlation

The distinction of bowenoid papulosis from Bowen's disease and squamous carcinoma in situ is best made on clinicopathologic grounds. The age of the patient and body site of occurrence must be included. In a study comparing the two lesions, it was noted that the age of onset of Bowen's disease is on average 55.6 years, while that of bowenoid papulosis is 33.2 years.[38] Bowenoid papulosis is clinically related to condyloma acuminatum. It is also important to note that invasive carcinoma arising from Bowen's disease may occur in up to 28% of cases, while with bowenoid papulosis it only occurs 2.6% of the time.[38] In another study involving morphometry and DNA analysis, it was noted that aneuploidy was present in both diseases but that the degree of aneuploidy was higher in Bowen's disease than in bowenoid papulosis. On the basis of morphometry it was found that the morphologic grade of bowenoid papulosis was lower than that for Bowen's disease. Thus, the size of the cells in bowenoid papulosis is usually smaller than that in Bowen's disease or squamous carcinoma in situ. It is believed that bowenoid papulosis is a low-grade carcinoma in situ, lower grade than that of Bowen's disease.[39,40]

VERRUCA/CONDYLOMA

Warts are caused by HPV and occur on skin and mucous membranes. At least four morphologic types of warts have been established: the common wart (verruca vulgaris), the plantar wart (verruca plantaris), the flat wart (verruca plana), and the genital wart (condyloma acuminata).[41] The association of HPV with warts has been well established using molecular techniques.

Specific types predominate in specific body sites. It is well established that types 16, 18, and 33 are associated with the development of squamous carcinoma of the anogenital region.[42,43]

Histopathologic Features

Verruca vulgaris has an endophytic/exophytic shape. The base of the lesion is crescent shaped with curved broad rete extending into the dermis. The peripheral rete show a curvature toward the central portion of the lesion. The epidermal surface of the lesion shows numerous pointed parakeratotic spires that contain hemorrhage (Fig. 17-9). Koilocytic change of keratinocytes is often present in the upper half of the epidermis along with prominent hypergranulosis. Viral inclusion bodies or prominent nucleoli may also be seen. A perivascular mononuclear infiltrate is frequently present below the lesion. A lichenoid infiltrate may be seen in those lesions undergoing involution. This takes the form of a lichen planus-like keratosis.

The verruca plana is neither endophytic nor exophytic. It displays mild koilocytosis in an epidermis that is slightly thicker than adjacent uninvolved epidermis. The verruca plantaris displays changes expected because of its location. Greatly thickened stratum corneum is composed of both ortho- and parakeratin. There may be slight extension of the lesion above the surface of the adjacent epidermis, and there is deep extension of the inward bending wart rete into the dermis. Secondary features are the same as those in verruca vulgaris.

The condyloma acuminata has a more rounded shape than the jagged parakeratotic spires of the verruca vulgaris (Fig. 17-10). The stratum corneum is generally orthokeratin, but where it abuts viable epidermis there are usually enlarged parakeratotic nuclei that sometimes have koilocytic features. The shape of the lesion is asymmetric and lacks inward bending of the rete seen in verruca vulgaris. The lesions seen on the uterine cervix

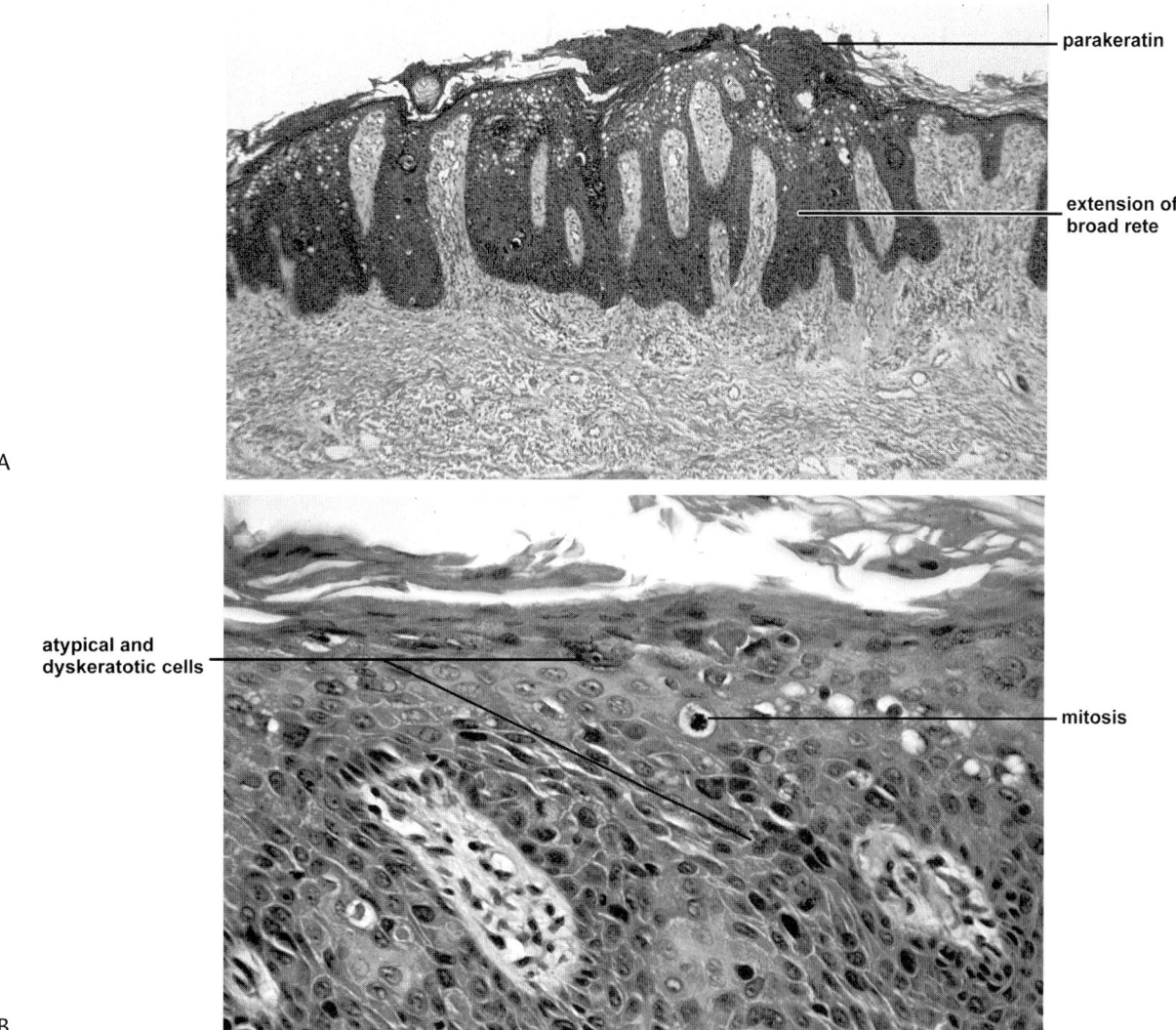

parakeratin

extension of
broad rete

atypical and
dyskeratotic cells

mitosis

Figure 17-8. (**A**) Small lesion of bowenoid papulosis. There is broadening and extension of the epidermal rete into the dermis. There is a surrounding inflammatory infiltrate. The overlying stratum corneum is parakeratin. (H&E, × 40.) (**B**) Full-thickness loss of maturation of keratinocytes. Mitoses and dyskeratotic cells are present near the surface of the epidermis. The cells involved are slightly smaller than those in Fig. 17-25. (H&E, × 150.)

Figure 17-9. (**A**) The usual fili-form wart has an endophytic/exo-phytic component. Abundant parakeratin is present at the sur-face, often in individual spires. Hemorrhage is present in the parakeratin. An equally character-istic finding is that of inward bending of the rete toward a cen-tral point near the middle of the lesion. (H&E, × 40.) (**B**) High power view of a single spire of parakeratin containing hemor-rhage. This is a very characteristic feature of a wart. (H&E, × 100.)

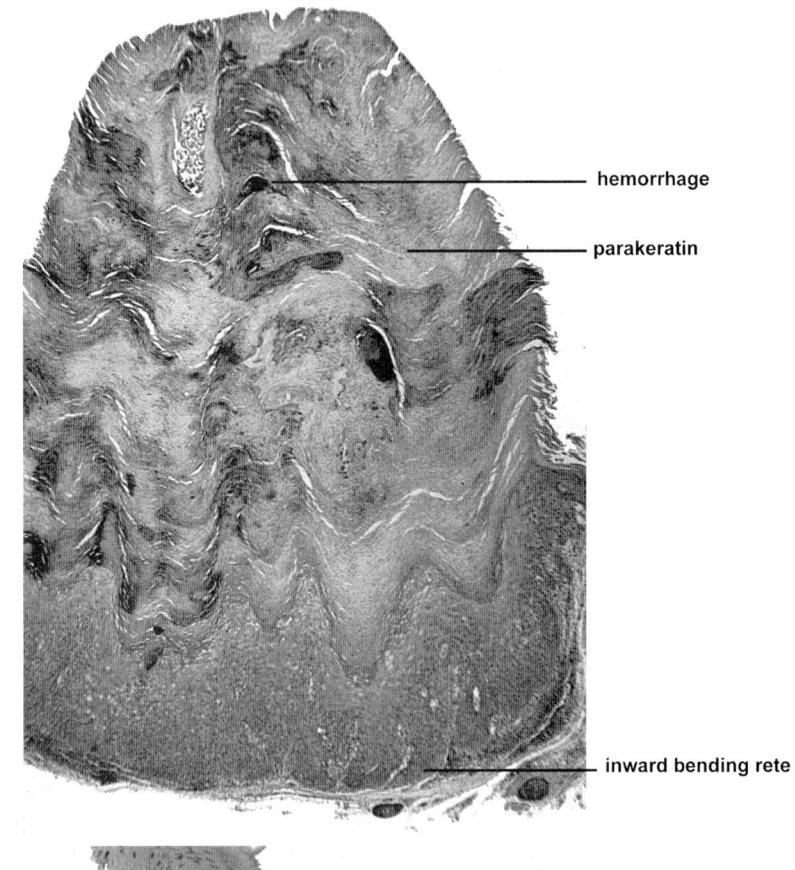

hemorrhage

parakeratin

inward bending rete

A

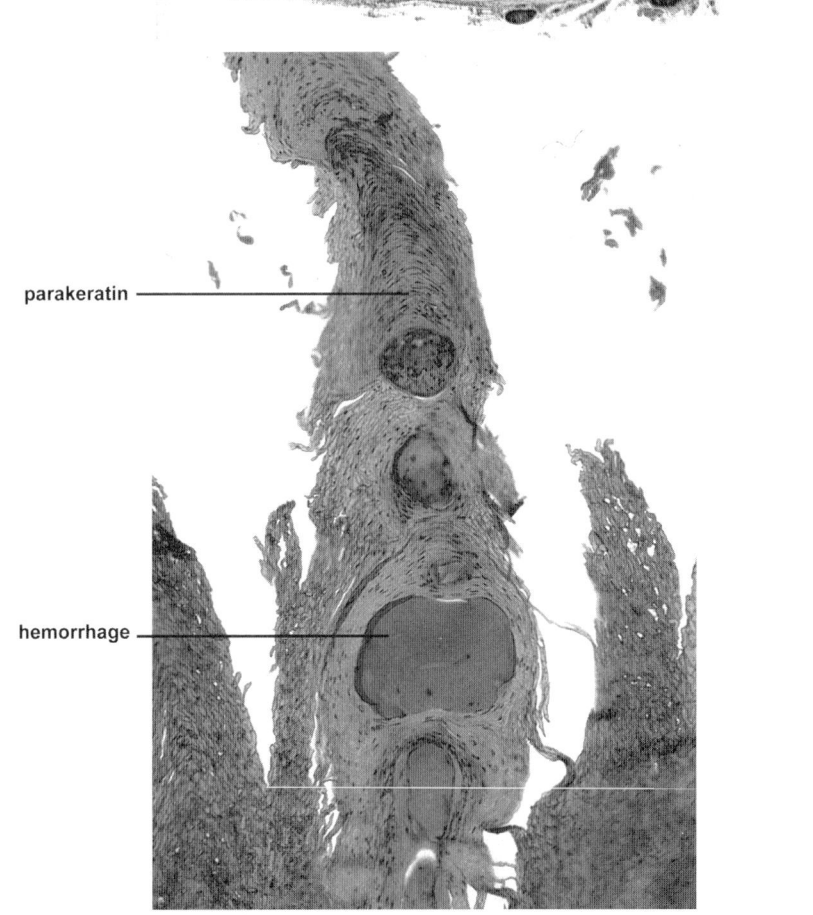

parakeratin

hemorrhage

B

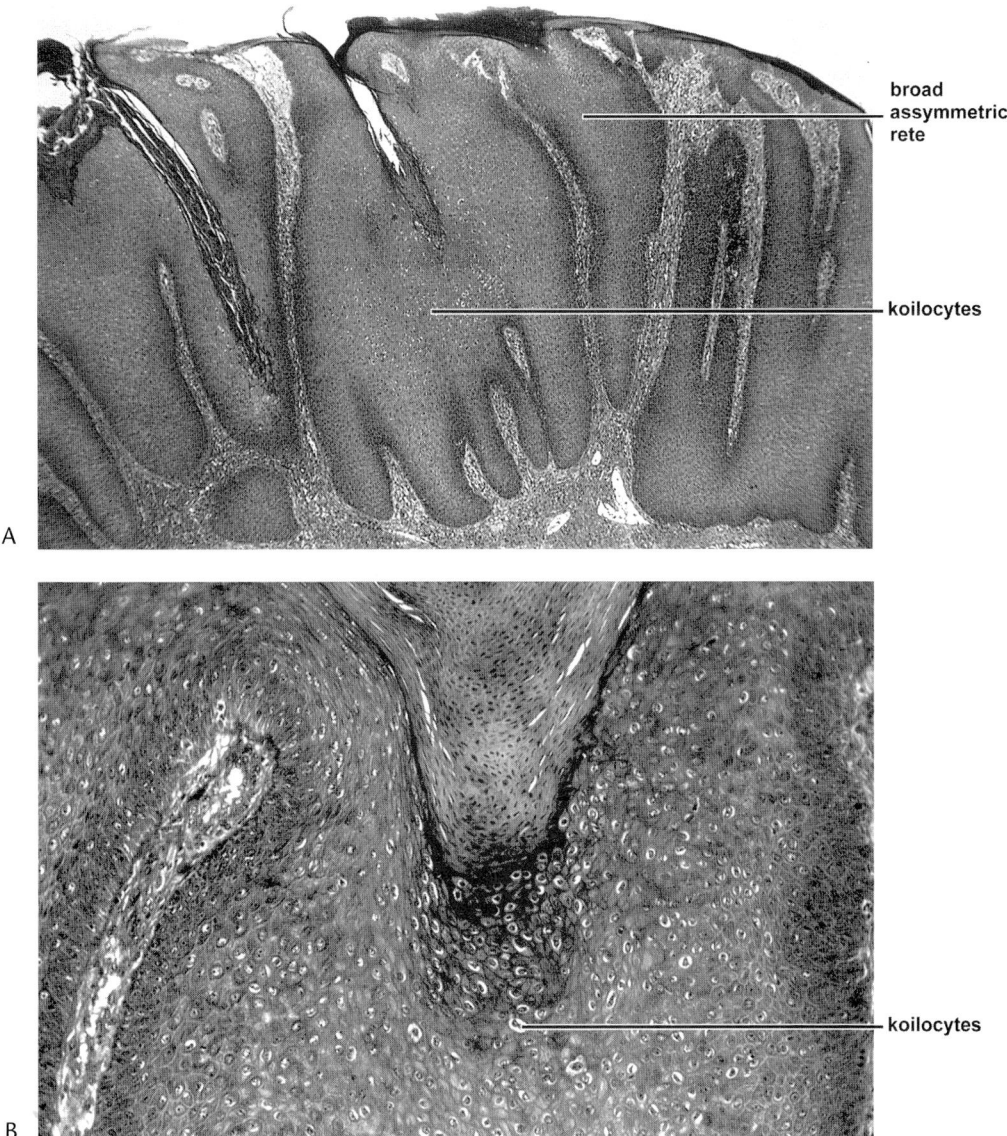

Figure 17-10.   The condyloma acuminatum is not as graceful or symmetric as a verruca. (**A**) Asymmetric acanthosis. (**B**) Koilocytic change in the keratinocytes can be identified. Koilocytic change is never as prominent in the skin as it can be in the uterine cervix. (H&E, × 150.)

and vagina show more prominent koilocytosis than on epidermis.

Clinicopathologic Correlation

Verruca vulgaris presents no problem other than cosmetic. Condyloma acuminata produced by HPV types 16,18,31, and 33 have a significant association with the development of invasive squamous carcinoma. The association with uterine cervical carcinoma has been well established.[44,45] Spontaneous regression in all forms of common warts has been reported, including those of condyloma.[46] Epidermoid carcinoma can develop in the site of nongenital warts, particularly in patients with epidermodysplasia verruciformis or in renal transplant patients. In patients with epidermodysplasia verruciformis, cancer may develop as early as age 13 years. Their flat warts are associated with HPV types 3 and 10.[47,48]

CLEAR CELL ACANTHOMA

Clear cell acanthoma, also known as Degos' acanthoma, is rare. Clinically it presents as a 1 cm red crusted nodule with peripheral scale. The lesion usually occurs on the lower extremities but has been reported anywhere. It is asymptomatic, occurs in either gender, and is slow growing. Whereas the usual lesion is single, unusual multiple eruptive forms, sometimes associated with ichthyosis or varicose veins, are very rare.[49–53]

Histopathologic Features

The lesion is an area of thickened epidermis composed of pale, edematous (clear) keratinocytes. It is clearly demarcated from adjacent epidermis. The basal area is unremarkable. There is a sprinkling of neutrophils throughout the thickened epidermis of clear cells (Fig. 17-11). There is scant overlying stratum

Figure 17-11. (**A**) The clear cell acanthoma is characterized by spongiotic, clear keratinocytes that form a distinct papule in the epidermis. There is also a characteristic sprinkling of neutrophils, which can vary in number. (**B**) The neutrophils are noted both in the epidermis and in the papillary dermis.

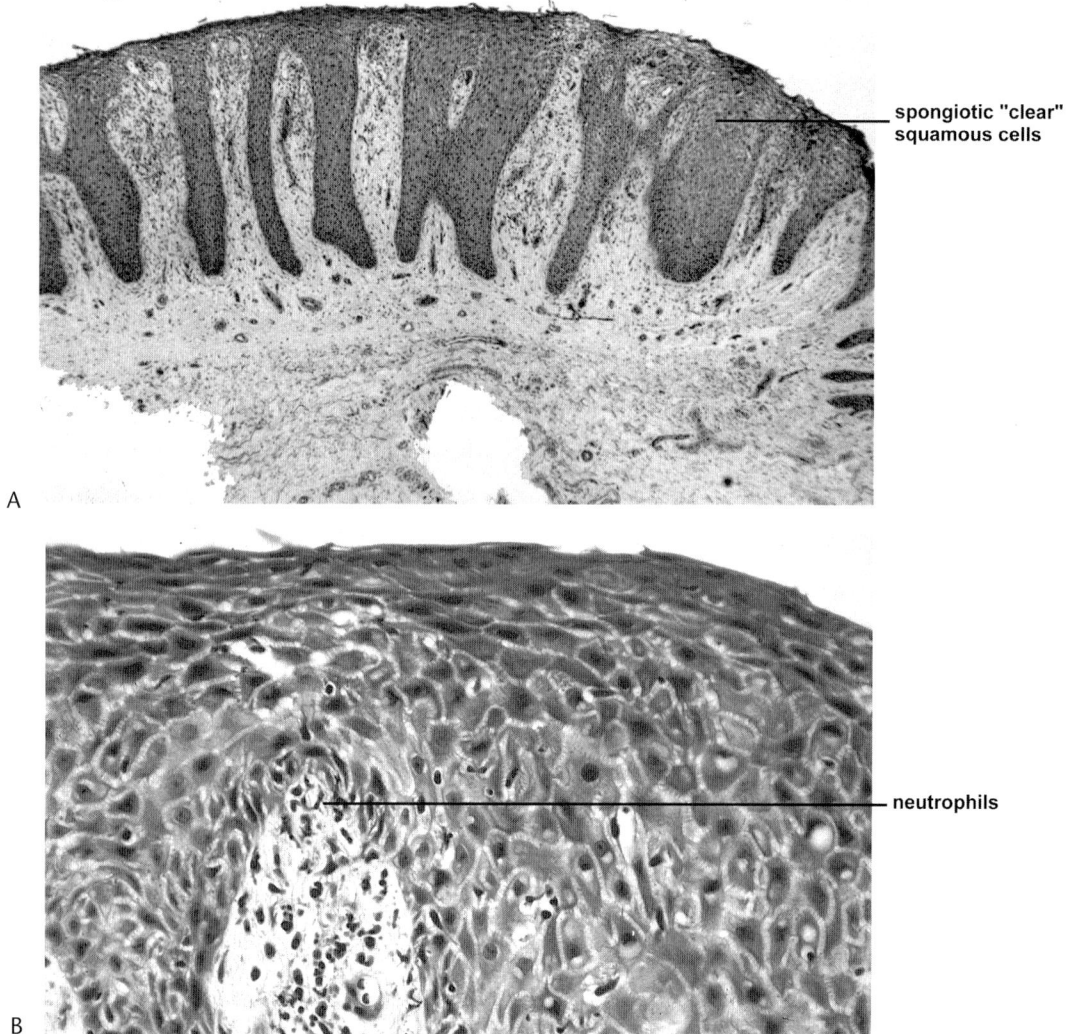

spongiotic "clear" squamous cells

neutrophils

corneum. Periodic acid–Schiff (PAS) stain will show that the clear keratinocytes contain abundant glycogen. There is increased vascularity in the underlying dermis.

The clear cell acanthoma shows positive staining for involucrin and keratin, while it is negative for carcinoembryonic antigen. These markers indicate that it is most likely of epidermal origin (keratinocytes) and not of sweat duct origin, as once believed. Similar conclusions have been drawn from lectin binding.[54] Some lesions contain S-100 positive dendritic melanocytes and are also clinically pigmented.[55]

Differential Diagnosis

This lesion should be differentiated from eccrine poroma and from clear cell hidradenoma (eccrine acrospiroma). While clear cell acanthoma and eccrine poroma both occur on the lower extremities, they generally have different silhouettes. The clear cell acanthoma appears as a thickened area of epidermis, whereas the eccrine poroma more often is a significant tumor mass that extends into the dermis. The clear cell acanthoma is negative for carcinoembryonic antigen, whereas eccrine poroma is positive. On a hematoxylin and eosin (H&E) basis, the clear cell acanthoma displays clear or pale cells while the eccrine poroma possesses basophilic cytoplasm, and eccrine ducts can be found within the masses of small cuboidal cells.

Similarly, the nodular hidradenoma forms a mass of variable kinds of epithelium that extends into the dermis and may or may not be connected with the epidermis. While both can possess clear or pale cells, only the clear cell acanthoma shows a simple thickening of the epidermis with a sprinkling of neutrophils.

Actinic keratosis may also be included in the differential diagnosis but seldom possesses the pale clear cells and the neutrophils.

WARTY DYSKERATOMA

The warty dyskeratoma presents as a red-brown papule with a yellow central keratotic plug. It is most frequently found as a lesion of the head and neck and upper torso (scalp, neck, face), but nearly all body sites have been reported.[56–59] The lesions are nearly always single, but one case report of multiple lesions exists.[60] Interestingly, reports of occurrence on the oral mucosa have all been on the left side. In the oral cavity the lesion occurs in sites of friction and trauma.[61,62]

Histopathologic Features

The lesion is distinctively flask shaped. The epidermal invagination extends into the dermis and sometimes deeper with a surrounding rim of fibrosis. There is a characteristic suprabasilar clefting with acanthotic keratinocytes forming grains and corps ronds. The complex extensions of adjacent keratinocytes into the connective tissue and their transection by the microtome blade produces villi (Fig. 17-12).

Differential Diagnosis

The atypical and acanthotic squamous cells in the warty dyskeratoma must be carefully distinguished from SCC. A cursory examination of the lesion resembles the pattern of infiltrating squamous carcinoma into a desmoplastic stroma; however, the overall silhouette of the warty dyskeratoma is characteristically flask shaped (either Erlenmeyer or Florence). The early lesion may be impossible to distinguish from the individual lesions of Darier's disease. Both types of lesions arise from the warty dyskeratoma and are centered on hair follicles, but the warty dyskeratoma is much larger. Both are likely genetically predetermined and are found in patients with similar dermatoglyphic patterns.[63] Similar ultrastructural findings are noted in warty dyskeratoma and in the individual lesions of Darier's disease.[64]

CARCINOMAS OF THE SKIN

Carcinomas of the skin are the most frequently seen malignancies in clinical medicine. Indeed, regardless of their realm of specialty practice, most physicians regularly encounter patients with such lesions.

This chapter presents an outline of the pathologic features of three common skin cancers, namely, basal cell carcinoma (BCC), squamous cell carcinoma (SCC) and keratoacanthoma (KA). In addition, a relative "newcomer" to dermatopathology—primary neuroendocrine carcinoma of the skin (PNCS)—is discussed.

Histogenesis is a nebulous term, since it is virtually impossible to determine the cellular derivation of any neoplasm in vivo. Hence, we shall not expend much effort on a consideration of this topic. Rather, the lines of differentiation toward target cell types in BCC, SCC, and PNCS are elucidated in the following discussion.

The three specified neoplasms occur in a spectrum of clinical settings, and the latter are briefly enumerated as well. Finally, histopathologic differential diagnoses are considered, with commentaries on the use of specialized techniques in difficult cases.

Basal Cell Carcinoma

Historical Perspective

Krompecher[65] is generally accorded recognition for having given certain cutaneous carcinomas ("epitheliomas") the designation of *basal cell*, with the implication that their constituent cells resembled the basal cells of the epidermis. In Hyde and Montgomery's[66] text on diseases of the skin, published in 1897, one may recognize BCC easily, as described under the title of "superficial epithelioma" and "rodent ulcer" (clinical) or "tubular epithelioma" (histopathologic). It is also notable that the behavior and treatment of BCC were accurately understood at that time. In the intervening 90 years, a great deal of literature has accrued on the origin and growth of this tumor, as well as its variant microscopic patterns. Accordingly, it is now generally accepted that *basal cell carcinoma* exhibits a spectrum of biologic behavior[67,68] and that the latter can be related to histopathologic features.

Histopathologic Features

As is true of many carcinomas, BCC displays a considerable diversity of appearances under the microscope. These may be divided into *nodulocystic*, *superficial*, *adenoid*, *morpheaform*, *infiltrative*, *keratotic*, and *pigmented* forms, as well as rarer variants.[69,70]

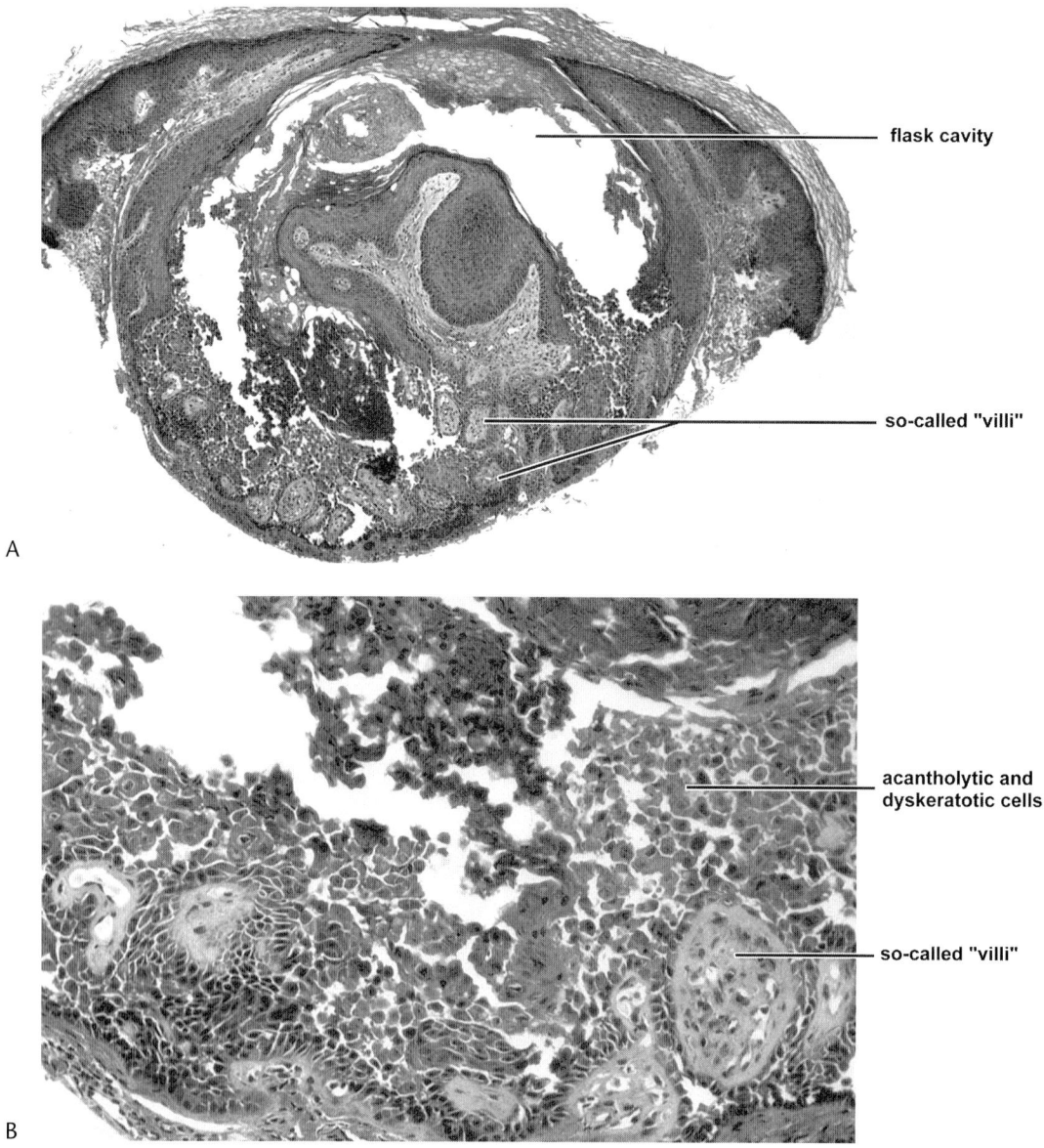

Figure 17-12. (**A**) Flask shape of the warty dyskeratoma. It extends into the dermis and has a distinct rounded silhouette. (H&E, × 40.) (**B**) Base of the lesion with the "villi." There are numerous acantholytic and dyskeratotic cells present within the flask-shaped space of the lesion.

Nodulocystic BCC

The nodulocystic form of BCC is the most frequent (approximately 70% of cases) and is composed of rounded or bluntly branched lobules of small hyperchromatic cells, which are connected to the overlying epidermis by narrow cords or broad trabeculae (Fig. 17-13). These cellular clusters vary slightly to moderately in size and shape; however, they are typified by the roughly parallel alignment of peripheral nuclei at right angles to those in the center of the nodules, peripheral palisading. The tumor cells themselves are uniform in size and polygonal in shape, with generally oval nuclei and inconspicuous nucleoli. Exceptionally, spindled or "giant" dysplastic nuclear forms may be ob-

served; these appear to have no prognostic significance.[71] Cytoplasm is scanty and amphophilic, and mitotic activity is variable. From zero to two division figures are typically seen per high power (× 400) field, but up to 10 may be observed in selected neoplasms. The stroma adjacent to this form of BCC characteristically exhibits a retraction from tumor cell nodules, and basophilic material is present in the clefts. Peritumoral actinic elastosis is invariably seen in the surrounding dermis. Not uncommonly, centrilobular necrosis in nodular BCCs accounts for their "cystic" quality, clinically and microscopically. Necrotic areas in adjacent cellular lobules may become confluent, yielding broad areas of anucleate debris. Calcifications may be present in the necrotic areas. The overlying epidermis may or may not be ulcerated.

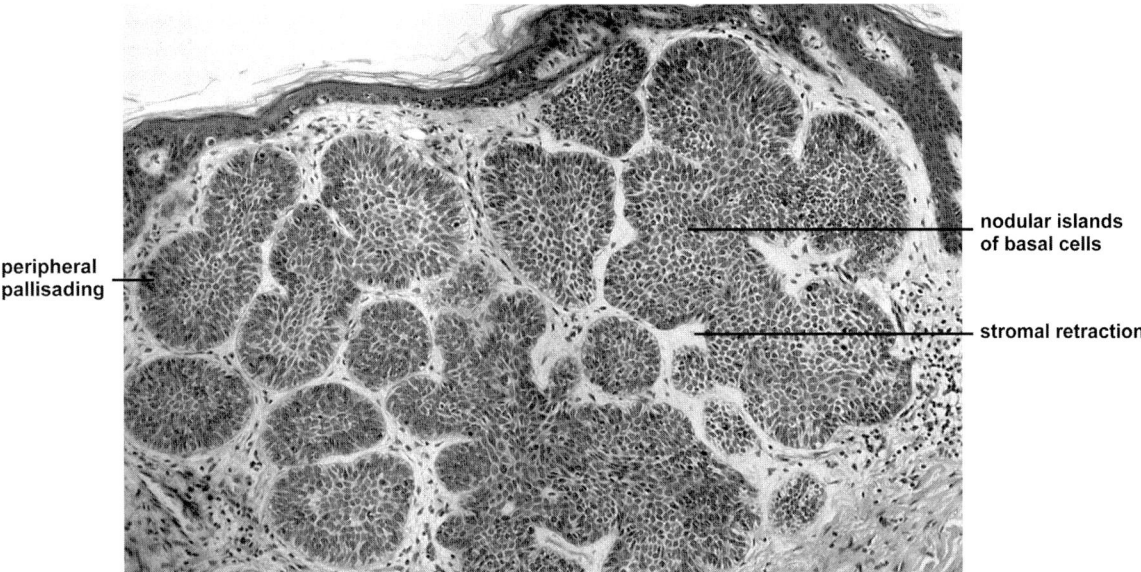

Figure 17-13. Nodular basal cell carcinoma. The numerous nests are characterized by peripheral palisading of the small basophilic cells forming the nests. The cells on the interior of the nests are the same size but display increased intercellular space.

Superficial BCC

Superficial BCC differs from the foregoing description in being multifocal in a high percentage of cases and in showing a small bud-like growth of tumor lobules from the basal epidermis (Fig. 17-14). These seldom extend more deeply than the papillary dermis, but have the same cellular composition as that of nodulocystic lesions. The surrounding stroma is less likely to manifest fibromyxoid change in superficial-multifocal BCC, but dermal elastosis is again common. Small retraction clefts may be present. Overlying ulceration is infrequently observed, but epidermal atrophy is often seen. Although acantholysis is generally uncommon in BCC, Mehregan[72] has suggested that the superficial subtype is most likely to demonstrate this finding.

Adenoid BCC

Roughly 20% of BCCs display a reticulated cribriform and gland-like growth pattern within tumor cell clusters (Fig. 17-15). Not all cellular lobules show such changes, but a pseudoglandular appearance should be readily apparent on low power microscopy to classify a BCC as "adenoid." The spaces formed

Figure 17-14. Superficial, multicentric-type basal cell carcinoma. The lesion manifests as a small bud of basaloid cells that extends slightly into the papillary dermis. There is often little inflammatory or stromal reaction to their presence.

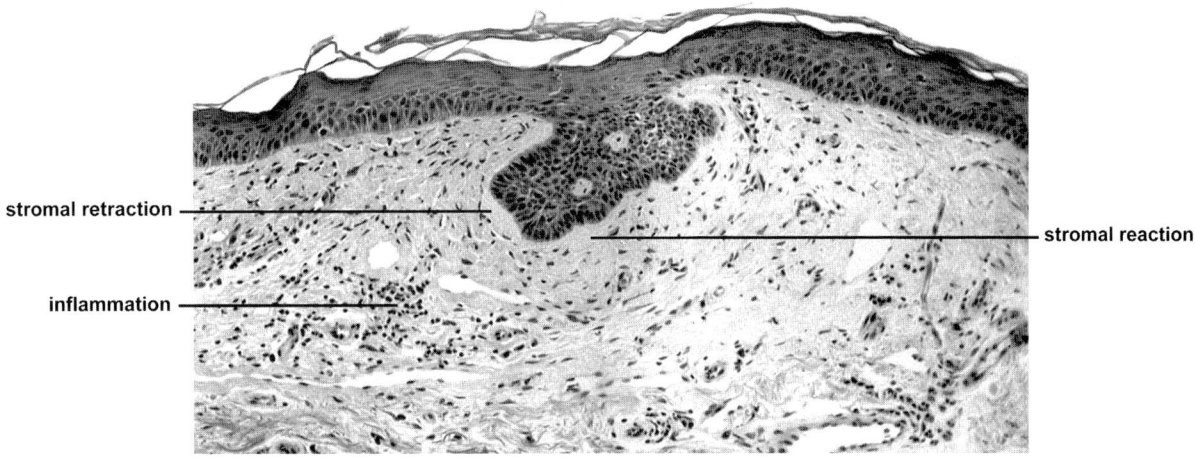

Figure 17-15. The adenoid basal cell carcinoma is characterized by multiple gland-like formations. Like other forms of basal cell carcinoma it usually has an attachment to the epidermis. The glands and spaces display basophilic stromal mucin as well as retraction. (H&E, × 100.)

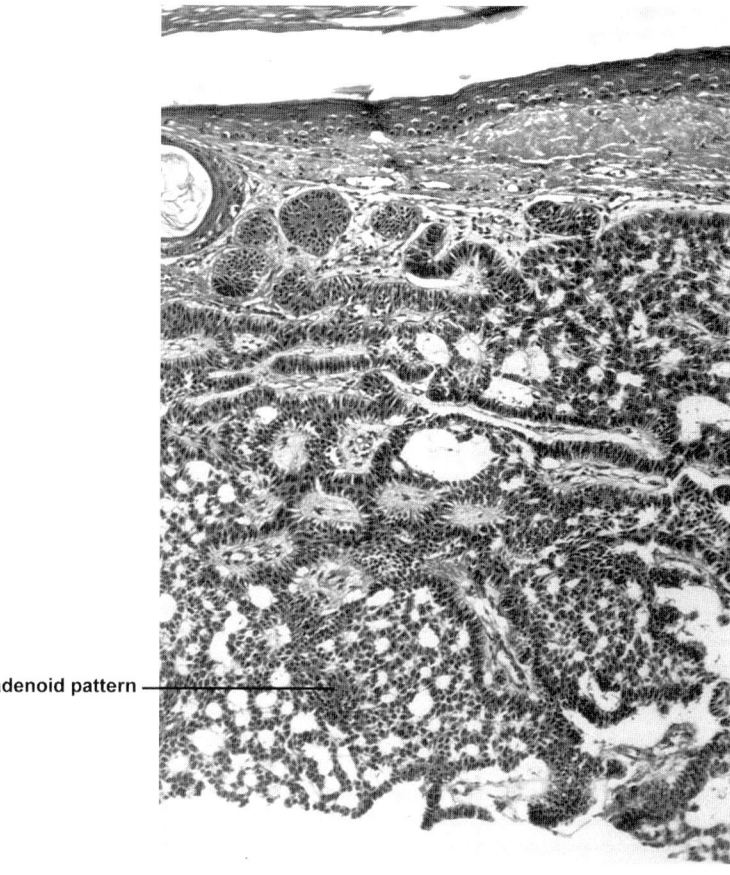

adenoid pattern ———

in these lesions contain an amorphous, granular, or colloid-like basophilic material. Connections between the dermal tumor mass and the overlying epidermis are invariably present in adenoid BCC, but they are more focal than in other variants; step sections may be required through the paraffin-embedded specimen to document their locations. The most helpful features in distinguishing this form of BCC from true glandular tumors of the skin are its retention of peripheral nuclear palisading and stromal retraction containing basophilic myxoid material.

Morpheaform BCC

Morpheaform BCC accounts for approximately 15% of all BCCs. This variant is so named because of the intense stromal fibrous proliferation (morphea-like) that is an integral part of its growth. Tumor cells are found in narrow linear cords, which are commonly branched (Fig. 17-16). Peripheral nuclear palisading is not readily apparent, and stromal retraction is likewise inconspicuous. Step sections may be required to demonstrate a connection between the tumor and the epidermis, since they are usually focal. Morpheaform BCC is characterized by its deep invasion of the dermis or the subcutis. The overlying skin surface may be ulcerated or relatively normal in appearance.

Infiltrative BCC

Infiltrative BCCs are "hybrids" of the nodulocystic and morpheaform varieties in that they show a combination of expansile solidly cellular, branched, sharply angulated, and linear cell groupings.[73] The irregular and acutely tapered profiles of tumor islands in this lesion have been described as "spiky" by Jacobs et al.[74] Deep dermal invasion is typical, and epidermal ulceration is not infrequent (Fig. 17-17).

The stroma is more fibrous than that of nodulocystic BCC, but less than in morphea-like tumors. The stroma is more cellular and fibroblast-rich than that seen in other variants, and it is more intimately attached to basaloid cell clusters. As a result, artifactual stromal retraction is not particularly notable in such lesions, and palisading of cells around the islands may not be well developed.

Keratotic BCC

Some BCCs that are otherwise identical to the nodulocystic variety contain keratinaceous ("horn") cysts and clusters of parakeratotic cells, which are interspersed throughout these tumors. The parakeratotic element possesses more abundant and eosinophilic cytoplasm than that of the basaloid tumor cells and often surrounds the accumulations of anucleate keratin, which may become densely calcified. There are no granular keratinocytes between the horn cysts and parakeratotic cells in this form of BCC. The contents of the cysts often assume a concentrically lamellated, whorled appearance and are commonly apparent on low-power examination. In light of these features, keratotic BCC is also known as *pilar* BCC because of a similarity between the complexes just mentioned and developing hair follicles. This contention is also supported by the presence of citrulline in keratotic BCC.[75]

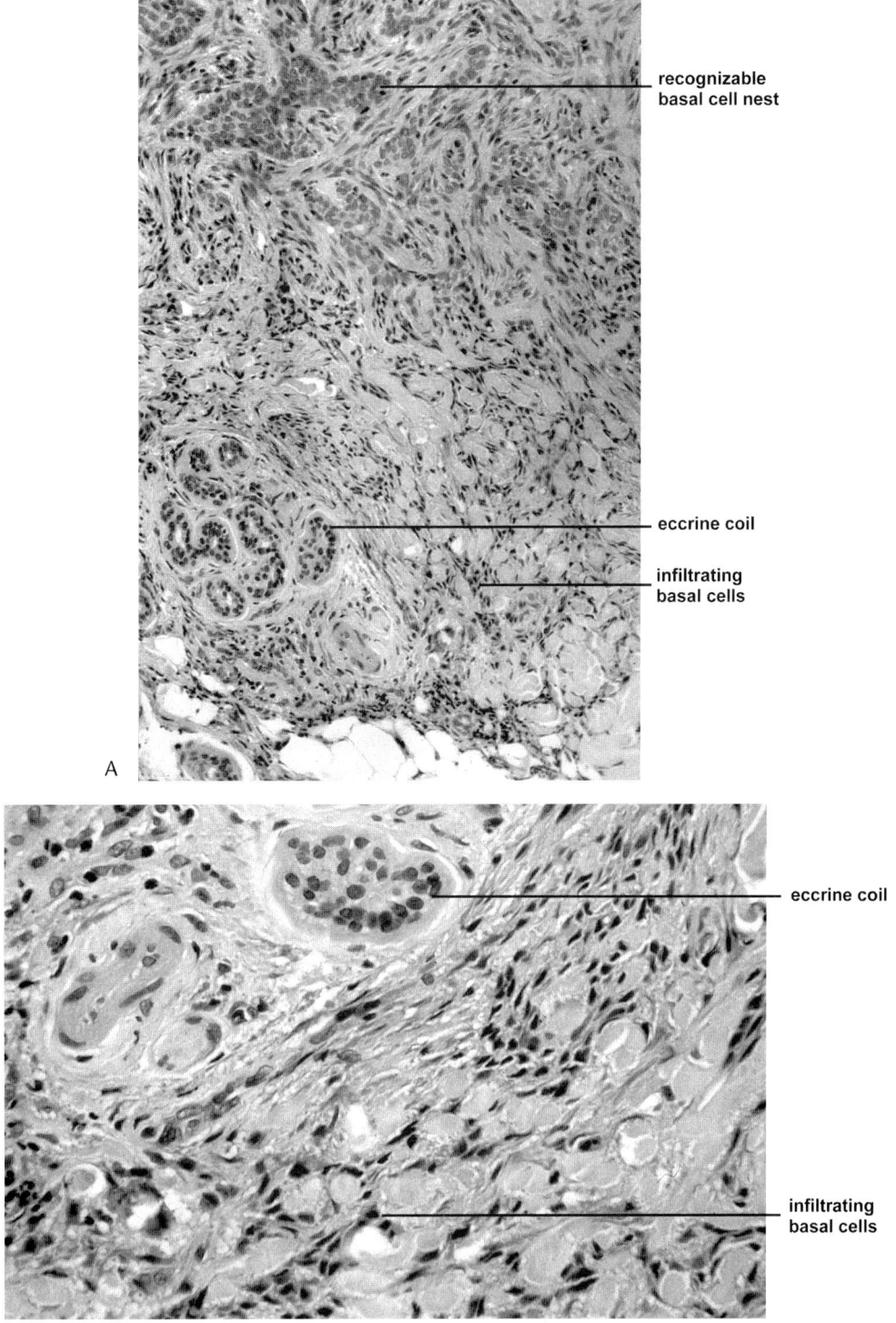

recognizable
basal cell nest

eccrine coil

infiltrating
basal cells

A

eccrine coil

infiltrating
basal cells

B

Figure 17-16. Morphea basal cell carcinoma. (**A**) Low power view showing well-formed recognizable nests of basal cell carcinoma near the surface. In the deeper portion of the lesion, near the subcutis, there are smaller single cell strands or Indian filing of basal cells. These can be difficult to recognize histologically and difficult to treat. (**B**) Higher power view showing the small dark nuclei extending between collagen bundles that represent the infiltrating tumor.

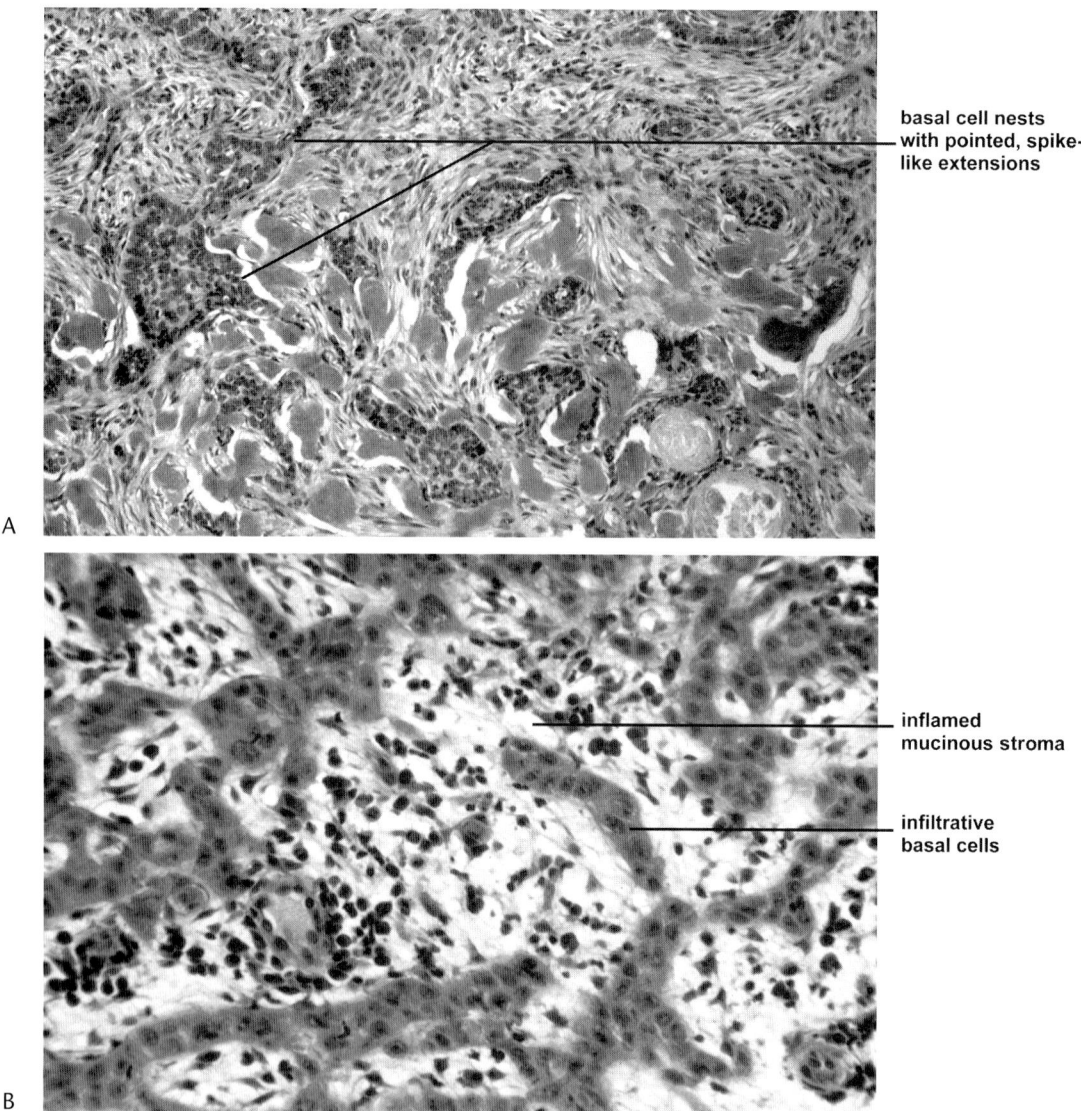

basal cell nests with pointed, spike-like extensions

inflamed mucinous stroma

infiltrative basal cells

Figure 17-17. The infiltrative basal cell carcinoma. **(A)** Pointed or spike-like extensions of small basal cells extending through dermal collagen. (H&E, × 100.) **(B)** Elongate extension of the infiltrative basal cell carcinoma in a mucinous, inflamed dermis. This category is often diagnosed simply as basal cell carcinoma, aggressive growth pattern.

Pigmented BCC

An additional special feature of some BCCs with a nodulocystic growth pattern is the presence of abundant intratumoral melanocytes[76,77] (Fig. 17-7).

These are apparently an integral part of such neoplasms. The melanocytic elements are usually evenly admixed with nonpigmented tumor cells, but have more dendritic profiles. In addition, pigment-containing melanophages are numerous in the stroma, accounting for most of the gross coloration.[78]

"Basosebaceous" BCC

Rare examples of BCC express another line of ectodermal differentiation, namely, the presence of mature sebaceous cells. These are abruptly interposed among otherwise-typical basaloid

cell nests, without transitional forms. Neoplasms displaying this morphologic pattern are otherwise most like nodulocystic BCCs.[79]

Basosebaceous BCC should not be confused diagnostically with true sebaceous carcinoma, which characteristically displays global nuclear atypia in its sebaceous elements and has a more aggressive biologic potential.[79]

"Fibroepitheliomatous" BCC

A peculiar cutaneous tumor manifests the combined features of intracanalicular fibroadenoma of the breast, seborrheic keratosis of the skin, and superficial BCC and has been named *fibroepithelioma*. It is now generally accepted that lesions having such attributes are variants of BCC.[69] They are characterized by elongated, branched, and trabecular strands of basaloid cells, with connections to the epidermis, which may contain "horn cysts" (Fig. 17-18). Fibromyxoid matrix is enclosed by these cellular arrays in a geographic pattern, yielding a reticulated appearance. Nuclear palisading is not a conspicuous finding in fibroepitheliomatous BCC, nor is stromal retraction prominent. Profiles of tumor cells in this variant seldom extend past the midreticular dermis.

"Adamantinoid" BCC

Lerchin and Rahbari[76] have documented several examples of a BCC subtype with a resemblance to adamantinoma of long bones or ameloblastoma of the jaws. This variant is characterized by solid nodular masses of basaloid cells in the corium, with epidermal attachments and peripheral palisading, like banal BCC. However, the proliferating cells are stellate rather than polygonal and are attached to one another by thin connecting bridges, enclosing an amorphous, amphophilic, intercellular material. The remainder of the stroma is fibromyxoid and shows retraction from the epithelial cell clusters. Histologic aspects of this form of BCC do not appear to represent merely a degenerative change, since Alcian blue, PAS, and aldehyde fuchsin stains are reactive with the intercellular matrix.[76]

"Basosquamous" BCC

There is some controversy in the literature on BCC as to which tumors of this type should be classified as "basosquamous." Some authors include cases that show a gradual transition between basaloid elements and cell nests with more abundant eosinophilic cytoplasm, larger nuclei, and a concentric arrangement ("pearls"), whereas others restrict the term to lesions with distinct but admixed components of BCC and overt squamous carcinoma.[80–84] The squamous carcinomatous element of basosquamous carcinoma should demonstrate nuclear anaplasia, dyskeratosis, nucleolar prominence, and mitotic activity to avoid confusion with areas of simple squamous metaplasia in BCC (Fig. 17-19). The basocellular component of such neoplasms may exhibit nodulocystic, adenoid, superficial, or infiltrative growth patterns. This variant of BCC is quite rare (less than 0.5% of all cases), if the foregoing criteria are observed.

"Metatypical" BCC

Similarly, "metatypical" BCC has been defined in various fashions by several authors.[69,80,81,85] This term is intended to describe variants of basal cell carcinoma that lack peripheral palisading within cellular lobules, have larger nuclei and more abundant eosinophilic cytoplasm, and display a bluntly spindle cell growth pattern with focally prominent intercellular bridges. Cell nests are more elongated than those in nodulocystic BCC, and the stroma is variably fibroblastic. Hence, metatypical BCC integrates certain of the features of the infiltrative and adamantinoid subtypes; in addition, De Faria[81] has suggested that metatypical BCC is cytologically intermediate to nodulocystic BCC and squamous carcinoma. Perineural and lymphatic permeation is seen more commonly in cases of metatypical BCC, relative to other variants.

"Dedifferentiated" (Carcinosarcomatous) BCC

Quay et al[86] and Dawson[87] have reported two cases of basal cell carcinoma that were intimately associated with malignant mesenchymal tissues within the same tumor masses. Each example exhibited the presence of fibrosarcoma and osteosarcoma in addition to nodulocystic BCC, and one case manifested chondrosarcomatous and synoviosarcomatous growth as well.[86] In analogy to dedifferentiation of chondrosarcoma, squamous carcinoma, and other tumors, repeated recurrence appears to be an etiologic factor in the clonal divergence of some BCCs (Fig. 17-20).

BCC Arising in Association with Other Lesions

BCC has been reported to arise in transition from, or in contiguity with, several other cutaneous lesions. These include nevus sebaceous of Jadassohn, dermatofibroma, congenital nevus, linear epidermal nevus, onchocercoma, and seborrheic keratosis.[77,88–92] These concurrences are rare (with the possible exception of nevus sebaceous) and may represent the simple coincidence of a relatively common neoplasm (BCC) with other cellular proliferations of the skin. With respect to dermatofibroma, Goette and Helwig[77] have indicated that many overlying BCC-like lesions actually represent basaloid forms of pseudoepitheliomatous hyperplasia. Nonetheless, they also reported several indisputable examples of true BCC in this context.

Specialized Pathologic Features

Because of the prevalence of BCC and its corresponding familiarity to most pathologists and dermatologists, specialized pathologic studies are not usually necessary for diagnosis. Nevertheless, occasional cases of BCC may simulate adnexal carcinomas of the skin, such as adenoid cystic carcinoma of eccrine glands[93] and basaloid sebaceous carcinoma.[94] In such circumstances, conventional special stains, electron microscopy, immunohistochemistry, or step sections can be employed to resolve interpretative difficulties.

Conventional Special Stains

BCC contains a negligible amount of glycogen, as demonstrated by relative nonreactivity with a PAS stain. The mucicarmine reaction is seen focally in examples of "apocrine" BCC, as well as in tumors containing "signet ring" cells; the same neoplasms display diastase-resistant PAS positivity. Similarly, the colloidal iron technique can be used to label the epithelium-related mucosubstance in adenoid BCC and will also stain the stroma of most BCCs faintly.

Hyaluronidase digestion will abolish the latter but not the former of these reactivities. The Movat stain also labels the contents of pseudoglandular profiles in adenoid neoplasms, but they are PAS negative. This constellation of results differs from that of true glandular tumors of the skin. Lipid stains (oil red O and Sudan IV) are nonreactive with conventional BCC, but amyloid can be detected by the Congo red, Lieb, or thioflavine-T techniques in up to 70% of such neoplasms.[95–97] The latter finding appears to be independent of histologic subtype and may be related to a relatively high degree of tumor cell apoptosis.

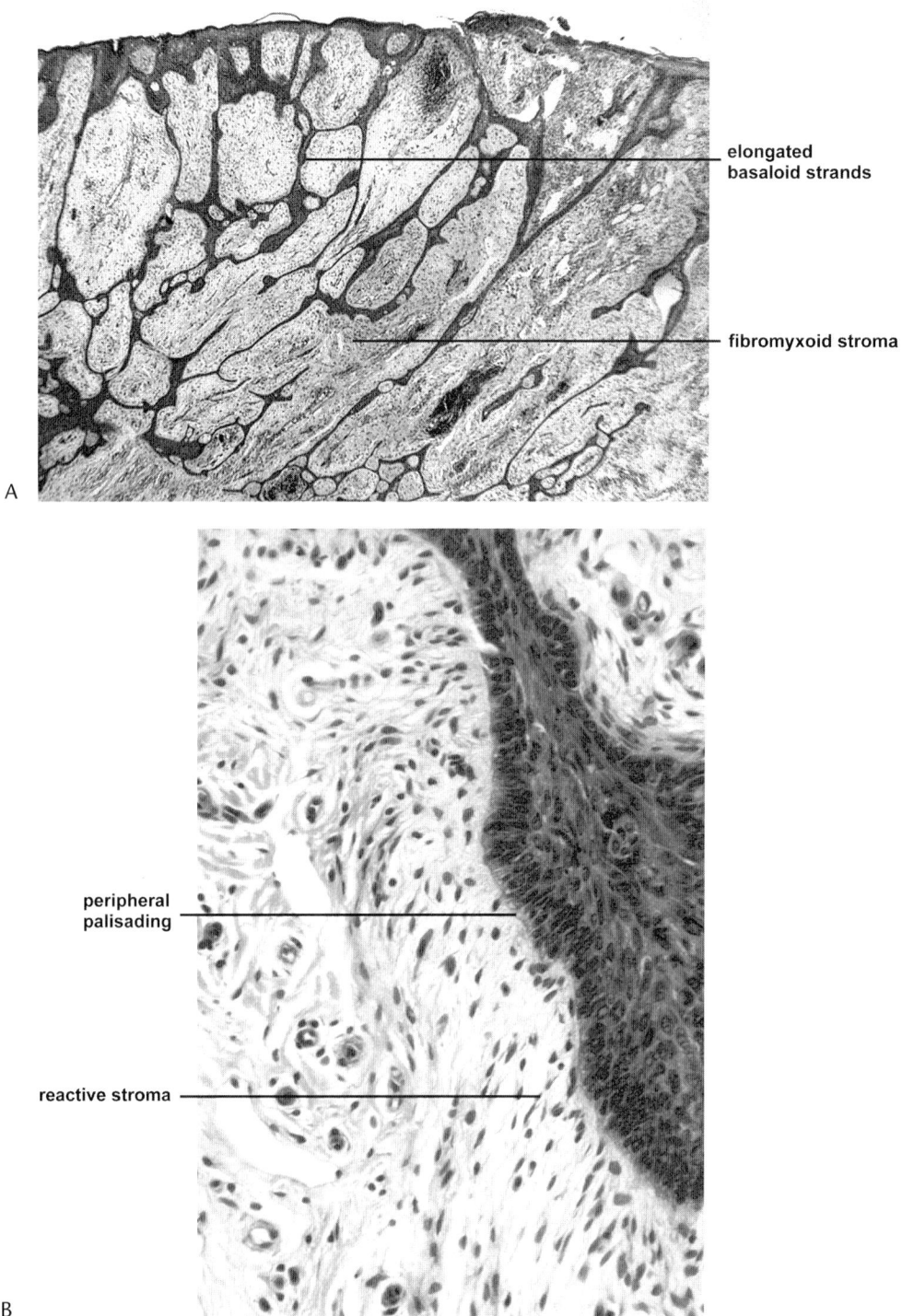

elongated
basaloid strands

fibromyxoid stroma

peripheral
palisading

reactive stroma

Figure 17-18. (**A**) The fibroepitheliomatous form of basal cell carcinoma. The elongated trabecular strands have connections to the epidermis and enclose a fibromyxoid matrix. (**B**) The edge of one of the strands with faint peripheral nuclear palisading. Note the fibromyxoid matrix. (H&E, × 250.)

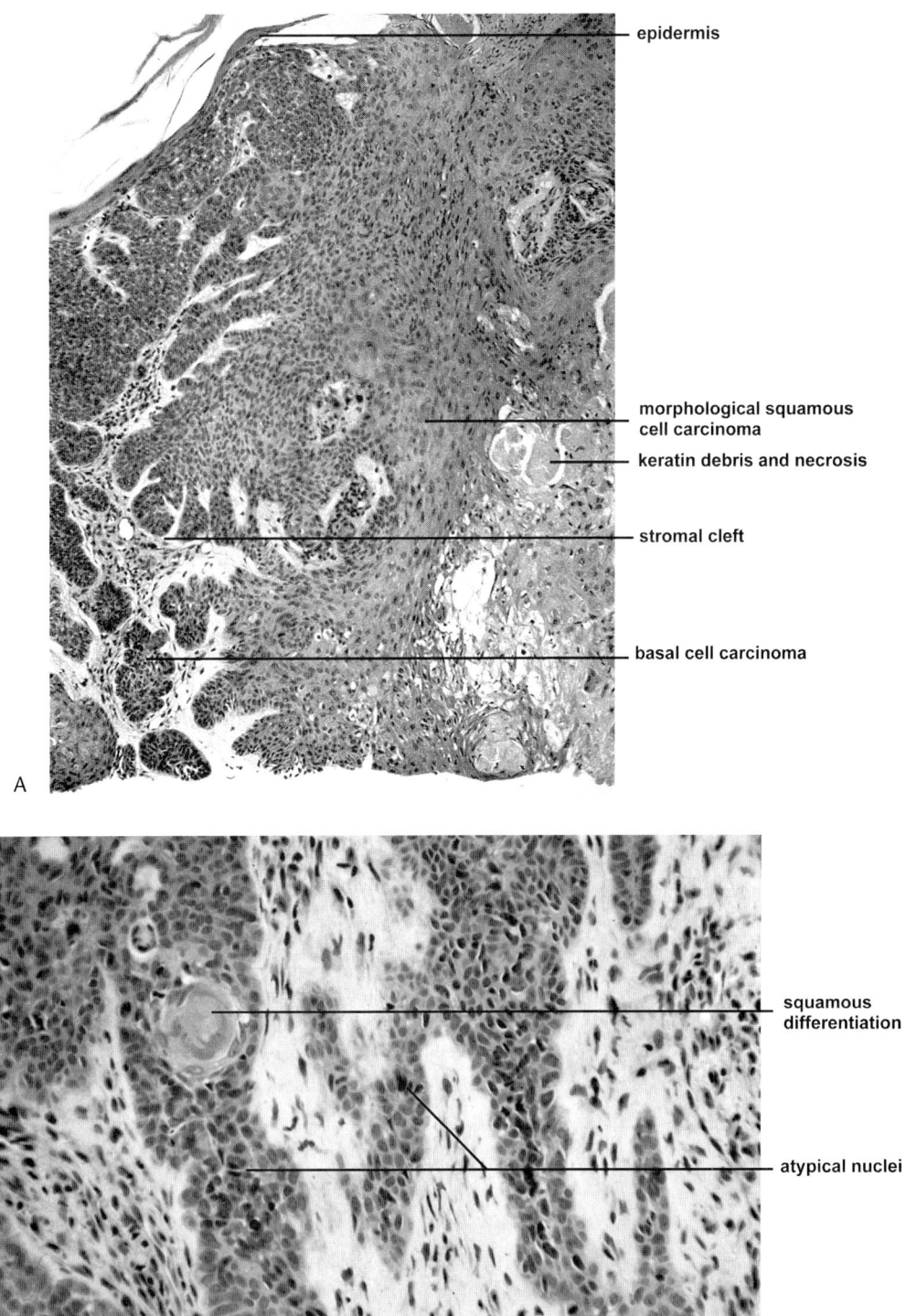

epidermis

morphological squamous cell carcinoma

keratin debris and necrosis

stromal cleft

basal cell carcinoma

A

squamous differentiation

atypical nuclei

B

Figure 17-19. (**A**) Basosquamous form of basal cell carcinoma. The definition of this lesion is not accepted by all and is poorly characterized in the literature. Continuity between two areas typical of basal cell carcinoma, and squamous cell carcinoma is shown. (H&E, × 50.) (**B**) Metatypical form of basal cell carcinoma with slightly enlarged nuclei containing nucleoli. The nests of basal cells lack peripheral palisading, and there are central foci of squamous differentiation. Some would contend that both basosquamous and metatypical basal cell carcinoma are simply forms of basal cell carcinoma showing squamous differentiation. (H&E, × 100.)

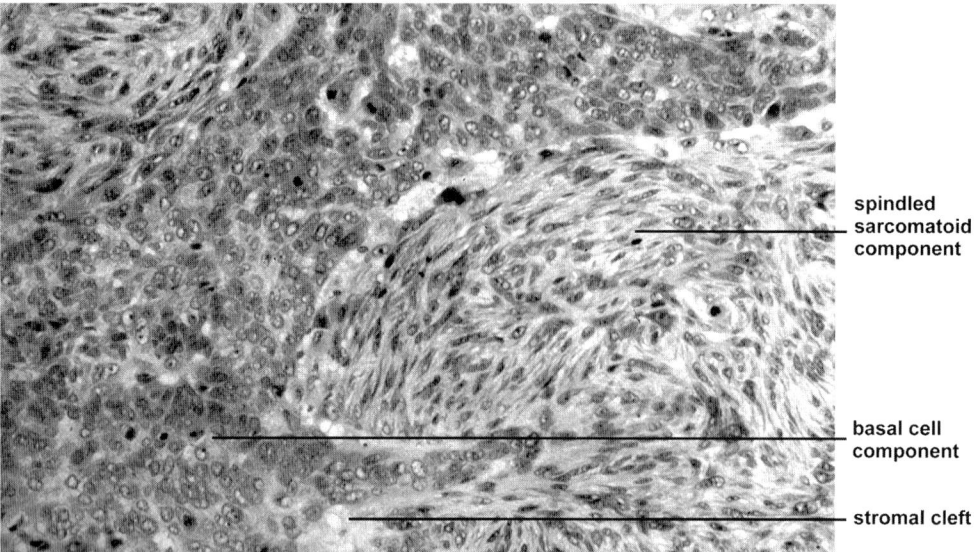

spindled
sarcomatoid
component

basal cell
component

stromal cleft

Figure 17-20. Sarcomatoid basal cell carcinoma. There is an area characteristic of basal cell carcinoma that blends imperceptibly into a spindled sarcoma-like lesion. The spindle cell component maintained immunophenotypic markers of basal cell carcinoma. (H&E, × 50.)

Electron Microscopy

BCC tumor cells have been divided into three types by some authors, based on their ultrastructural features—so-called light, intermediate, and dark.[98] One can indeed discern a heterogeneous population of cells in such tumors by electron microscopy. These form a continuum, ranging from elements with a paucity of intracytoplasmic organelles (rough endoplasmic reticulum, Golgi bodies, lysosomes, mitochondria, broad keratin filaments ["tonofibrils"], keratohyaline granules, and sphaerida-like nuclear inclusions) to other cells with an abundance of cellular contents.[99–103] Likewise, the density of pericellular basal lamina and desmosomal attachments between tumor cells varies greatly within the same lesion.[104] Cytoplasmic lipid and true microvillous modifications of plasmalemmae are not evident in BCC lacking apoecrine or sebaceous differentiation.

Immunohistochemistry

Among all malignant neoplasms of the skin, those showing cellular differentiation toward keratinocytes (BCC and squamous carcinoma) are immunohistochemical "have nots." They lack most specialized determinants other than cytokeratin polypeptides[105] and a restricted group of cell membrane-related cell products. Specifically, epithelial membrane antigen, other human milk fat globule proteins, Leu M1, salivary-type amylase, S-100 protein, and carcinoembryonic antigen are not observed in BCCs.[78,106] Thomas and colleagues[107] have demonstrated that normal epidermal basal cells and BCCs display selective immunoreactivity for low molecular weight (40 to 46 kilodalton [kd]) keratin proteins.[107] By contrast, other keratinocytes, pilar tumors, and squamous carcinomas exhibit staining for a broad spectrum of cytokeratins (45 to 65 kd). These observations may

be useful in separating trichoepithelioma or small cell squamous carcinoma (see below) from BCC. However, they do not allow for a similar distinction between BCCs and sudoriferous or sebaceous tumors, since these adnexal lesions also have a typically restricted (low molecular weight) keratin profile.[94,105,108] Immunostains for the other cell products listed in the previous paragraph may attain value in the differential diagnosis. Additional cell membrane determinants that have been detected in BCC are of little diagnostic use.[78,106,108–110]

As a final note on this topic, it is of interest that many BCCs incite an inflammatory response in the surrounding dermis. Reactive hematopoietic cells consist primarily of lymphocytes, which have been shown to manifest a predominance of T-cell immunophenotypes.[111] More specific subclassification of these elements (as suppressor or helper cells) has not yet been accomplished.

Clinical Spectrum: Correlations Between Histology and Biology

Several clinical subtypes of BCC are well known to dermatologists, including papulonodular, pigmented, morphea-like, fibroepitheliomatous, and superficial forms.[68,112,113]

Although BCC is overwhelmingly seen in sun-exposed skin, numerous reports have documented its occurrence in protected cutaneous sites in some patients.[114–116] Some, but not all, of these individuals had had prior radiotherapy to the tumor site for unrelated conditions. Other rare clinical presentations include the bilateral symmetric growth of multiple BCCs and associations with hidradenitis suppurative, stasis dermatitis, smallpox vaccinations, amputation stumps, lupus vulgaris, cutaneous gummata, and onchocerciasis.[69,88,117,118]

Some publications have attempted to identify histologic features that can be correlated with frequent recurrence and tenacious growth of BCC so that appropriately extirpative surgery can be undertaken from the outset.[67,74,119,120] Lang and Maize[119] and Jacobs et al[74] showed that tumors with an infiltrative or micronodular pattern at first excision often pursued an aggressive clinical course. In addition, BCCs in which peripheral nuclear palisading was irregular or absent manifested a tendency to recur in several series.[67,119,120] The same propensity has been associated with basosquamous carcinomas; moreover, these tumors appear to metastasize more frequently than other subtypes of BCC.[80,81]

Metastases are rare. Approximately 0.1% of all BCCs lacking squamous differentiation exhibit distant spread beyond the skin.[121] Regional lymph nodes, lungs, and bones are most frequently involved in such cases, less than 200 of which may be found in the literature.[85,115,121–123] Numerous studies have correlated clinical or histologic features of conventional BCC with risk of metastasis. It would appear that large, neglected lesions are most likely to display metastatic behavior, especially in immunocompromised or malnourished patients.[121] Lymphatic, hematogenous, and interstitial ("in transit") routes for distant spread have been proposed, all of which probably pertain to selected cases. BCC also is included among cutaneous neoplasms with a potential for perineural invasion, which may result in neuropathies.[124] By contrast, approximately 5% of BCCs demonstrate spontaneous regression, as reported by Curson and Weedon.[125] This is rarely if ever complete and is associated with heavy peritumoral lymphocytic infiltration and abundant apoptosis, microscopically.

BCC is an essential diagnostic element of the autosomal dominant basal cell nevus syndrome (BCNS).[126–128] This complex features multiple cutaneous basal cell lesions, multifocal keratocysts of the jawbones, bifid ribs, neurologic abnormalities (including neoplasms of the central nervous system), cutaneous epidermoid inclusion cysts, palmar and plantar "pits," and characteristic facies.[128] Although BCC rarely occurs in children and adolescents,[129] many cases of this neoplasm in pre-adult patients are attributable to the BCNS; hence, BCC in a pediatric-age individual should prompt a thorough examination of the familial pedigree. Histologic examination of a single BCC in patients with this constellation will show no microscopic features unique to the BCNS.[127]

The Bazex, linear unilateral basal cell nevus, and xeroderma pigmentosum syndromes are also associated with BCC.[69,130,131]

Differential Diagnosis

Several other primary cutaneous neoplasms enter into differential diagnosis with BCC variants. These include conventional trichoepithelioma (which resembles keratotic BCC), desmoplastic trichoepithelioma [DTE] with similarities to morpheaform BCC),[132] small cell squamous carcinoma,[133] basaloid sebaceous carcinoma[94] (which mimic nodulocystic BCC), and adenoid cystic eccrine carcinoma (simulating adenoid or "eccrine" BCC).[93]

In general, trichoepitheliomas exhibit a much more organoid growth pattern than BCC, with more equally sized cellular lobules. Also broad connections to the epidermis are rare in dermal hair sheath tumors (except via pilosebaceous units), whereas they are regularly observed in cases of BCC. Finally, the fibro-

myxoid stroma of BCC is not recapitulated by the fibrous matrix of trichoepithelioma, nor is stromal retraction a feature of the latter tumor. In difficult cases, immunohistochemical determinations of cytokeratin profiles may be employed diagnostically to separate these lesions, as described above.[107]

DTE can be distinguished from morphea-like BCC by the uniform observation of horn cysts in the former, along with an absence of expansile cell nests and the nearly universal presence of epidermal hyperplasia. Also, DTE occurs in a younger patient population than typical cases of morpheaform BCC.[132]

Small cell squamous carcinoma lacks nuclear palisading, as well as the fibromyxoid stroma of BCC. Moreover, tumor cell nuclei in small cell squamous carcinoma are vesicular with prominent nucleoli, as opposed to the generally compact, anucleolated forms seen in BCCs.[133]

Basaloid sebaceous carcinoma must be distinguished from "basosebaceous" BCC. This separation is particularly difficult, since the distribution of obvious areas of sebaceous differentiation may be similar in both lesions, and each has the capacity for nuclear palisading.[94] Pagetoid involvement of the epidermis favors an interpretation of sebaceous carcinoma, but is not invariably present. Sebaceous carcinomas display diffuse positivity for epithelial membrane antigen and fat stains,[79,108] whereas basosebaceous BCC is reactive only in areas of obvious sebaceous differentiation. Ultrastructural studies will reveal the widespread presence of intracytoplasmic lipid droplets only in sebaceous carcinoma.[94]

Adenoid cystic sweat gland carcinoma lacks the epidermal connections of adenoid or "eccrine" BCC. Immunostains for carcinoembryonic and epithelial membrane antigens are extremely helpful, since they are consistently positive in adenoid cystic carcinoma and negative in BCC.[93,108] In addition, electron microscopy demonstrates true glandular (microvillous) differentiation in adenoid cystic eccrine tumors, which is not apparent in BCC.

Actinic Keratosis

Clinical Features

Actinic keratoses are found on exposed skin, commonly on the face, neck, backs of hands, and forearms. They may occur in any area that is chronically sun exposed. Differing appearances are possible. They may be either flat or raised, multiple or single, pigmented or pale. Hypertrophic keratotic types with cutaneous horns are most common on the forearms and hands. The lesions are usually less than 1 cm in diameter. Actinic keratoses have also been called *senile keratoses* or *solar keratoses*. While they are nearly always due to chronic sun exposure, they may also be found in young individuals who are exposed to large quantities of solar radiation.[134–136]

Histopathologic Features

The definition of actinic keratosis could be as simple as cutaneous squamous cell atypia that is less than full-thickness change. Full-thickness change by definition should be carcinoma in situ, Bowen's disease. The stratum corneum overlying the area of keratinocyte atypia displays parakeratosis, often compounded with scale-crust. The epidermis is formed

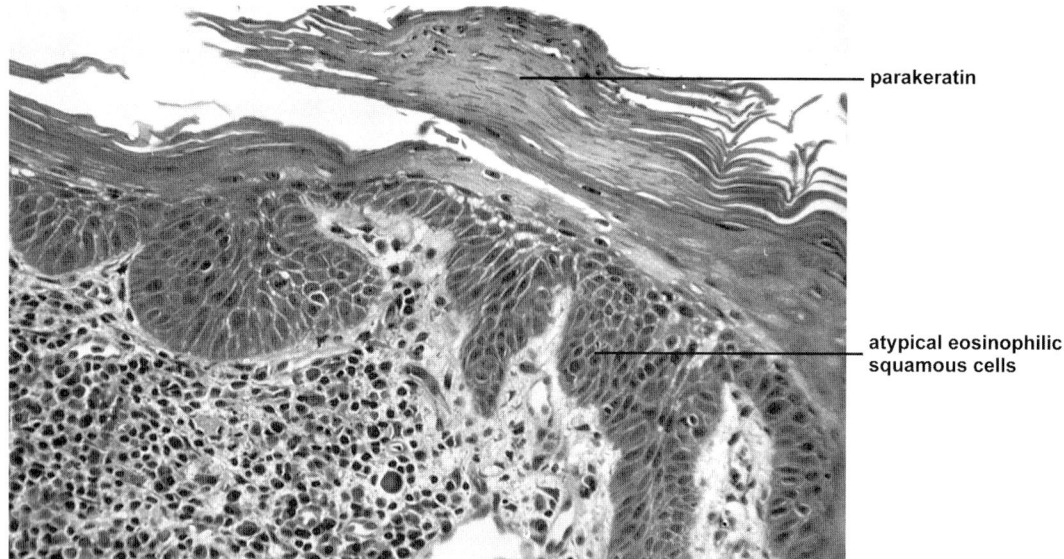

Figure 17-21. The actinic keratosis is characterized by atypia in keratinocytes. In this example, parakeratosis overlies an epidermal lesion characterized by partial loss of maturation (less than full thickness) as well as basilar budding of eosinophilic atypical ker-

by keratinocytes that possess nuclei that are larger than usual and possess clumped chromatin and often display atypical mitoses. Quite often, budding at the inferior portion of the epidermis is present. The buds of an actinic keratosis are composed of relatively large eosinophilic cells and never have an adjacent dermal cleft or dermal mucin (Fig. 17-21). There is usually an underlying inflammatory infiltrate composed of lymphocytes. Histologically, actinic keratoses can be characterized as hypertrophic, atrophic, acantholytic, and pigmented lesions.

The hypertrophic actinic keratosis displays prominent hyperkeratosis with parakeratosis. The epidermis is hyperplastic with irregular downward extension of broad rete. The basement membrane is intact. Despite the thickness of the epidermis, the disordered maturation and atypia of keratinocytes only involve a fraction of the epidermal thickness. Maturation is present in the superficial portions. Individual keratinocytes display enlarged, atypical, and lobate nuclei often with nucleoli. Atypical mitoses can be identified within the epidermis. These changes involve the interfollicular epidermis and spare the follicles. Buds of atypical eosinophilic cells extend from the base of the epidermis into the dermis. These maintain a rounded pushing configuration.

In atrophic actinic keratosis, not only is the epidermis thin, but the rete pattern is attenuated. The atypia is most distinct in the cells of the lower half of the epidermis. Those cells display nuclear pleomorphism, enlargement, and chromatin clumping (Fig. 17-22).

The acantholytic actinic keratosis has similarities to the hypertrophic type but also shows suprabasilar clefting and acantholysis of keratinocytes. Atypical cells similar to those elsewhere within the lesion may be found within the acantholytic cleft (Fig. 17-23). Again, eosinophilic buds of atypical cells

may extend from the lower part of the epidermis into the dermis, but they maintain a rounded silhouette.

The pigmented actinic keratosis has prominent melanin in the basal layer. Numerous melanophages are present in the underlying elastotic dermis.

Significant elastosis of the dermis is present below all forms of actinic keratosis. There is also a variable lymphoplasmacytic infiltrate that is variably periadnexal, perivascular, and interstitial. Because actinic keratoses, SCCs, and BCCs arise in the same sun-exposed skin, and, because their clinical appearances can be similar, multiple step sections may be needed to exclude the possibility of a lesion more significant than actinic keratosis. The distinction between actinic keratosis and invasive SCC is a fine line, namely, the basement membrane (Fig. 17-24). If the basement membrane is violated, then the lesion has shown its biologic potential to invade. Such invasion can be morphologically identified by a ragged or irregular border where it enters the dermis usually accompanied by intense mononuclear inflammation. The buds of noninvasive actinic keratosis, however, maintain a rounded smooth silhouette. Once a lesion has invaded the dermis, it often shows slightly different characteristics, namely, paradoxical keratinization and increased cytoplasmic eosinophilia. It should be remembered that some squamous carcinomas, particularly of the leg, show very little atypia and yet can be invasive.

Another important variant of actinic keratosis is the lichen planus-like keratosis. This lesion is an actinic keratosis, a seborrheic keratosis, or some other keratinocytic lesion in combination with an underlying intense lichenoid infiltrate. There are numerous dead keratinocytes or Civatte bodies at the base. Irregular parakeratosis can be present, thus excluding the diagnosis of lichen planus. These lesions are often removed because of clinical similarity to BCC.[137]

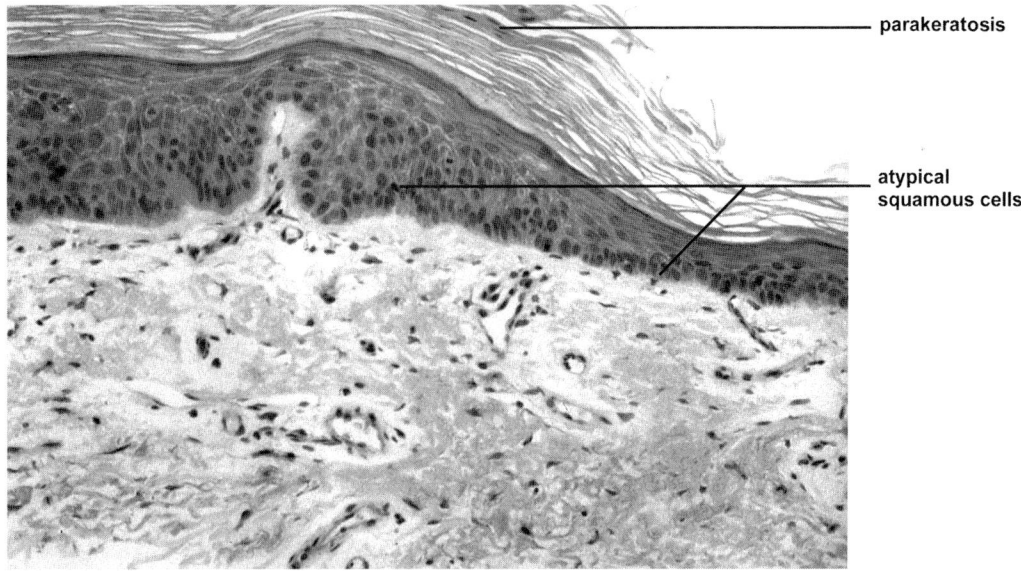

parakeratosis

atypical
squamous cells

Figure 17-22. The atrophic form of actinic keratosis displays a thinned epidermis with loss of proper maturation. Only the lower portion of the epidermis displays the keratinocytes with enlarged nuclei. The keratinocytic atypia is much less than the back-to-back atypical cells found in squamous carcinoma in situ. (H&E, × 80.)

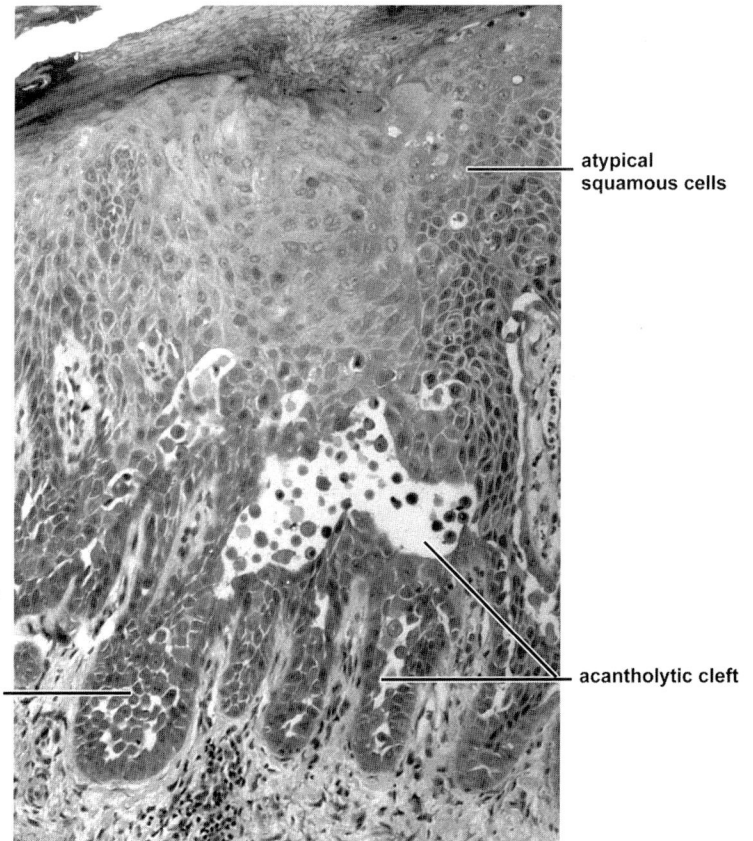

atypical
squamous cells

acantholytic cells

acantholytic cleft

Figure 17-23. Acantholytic actinic keratosis is characterized by spaces within the elongate atypical rete. Within the spaces there are sloughed, acantholytic keratinocytes. Atypia within the keratinocytes is evident. (H&E, × 100.)

Figure 17-24. Rarely, invasive squamous carcinoma can be noted arising from an actinic keratosis that is much less than an in situ lesion. In this example, there are infiltrating atypical squamous cells extending into the epidermis below an actinic keratosis. This example illustrates the importance of the biopsy in evaluating an actinic keratosis. (H&E, × 150.)

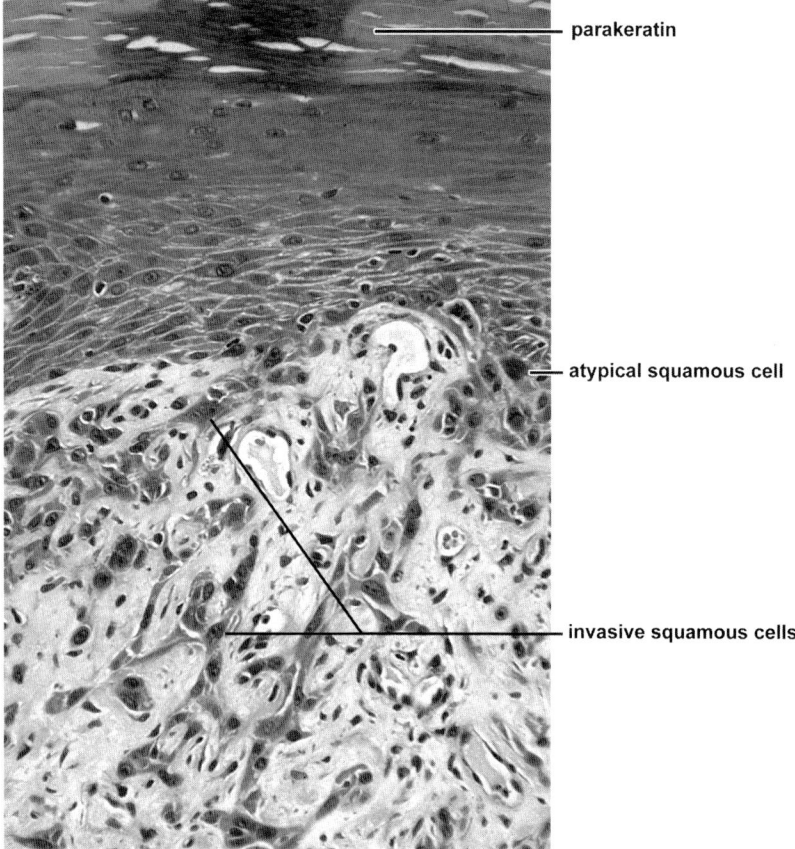

parakeratin

atypical squamous cell

invasive squamous cells

Differential Diagnosis

The main differential diagnosis for actinic keratosis is that of superficial BCC. Sometimes, with pale stains a superficial BCC can mimic the eosinophilic bud of an actinic keratosis. It is necessary to be aware of this situation and to obtain appropriate step sections and different staining. The superficial BCC will somewhere display a cleft and the underlying mucin or fibromyxoid stroma. These features are not seen in actinic keratosis. The atrophic form of actinic keratosis can resemble lupus erythematosus but lacks the concomitant features such as follicular plugging and extension of the inflammatory infiltrate to involve the deep plexus. Also, a colloidal iron stain should be positive in the deep dermis in lupus erythematosus, but not in actinic keratosis.

Clinicopathologic Correlation

Actinic keratosis serves as a clinical marker for the risk of squamous carcinoma. Conversion of these lesions to squamous carcinoma in an individual lesion is uncommon and was estimated at 1 per 1,000 per year.[134] Marks et al[138,139] suggested that the yearly incidence of squamous carcinoma occurring in individuals with actinic keratoses was 0.24%. In 1991, Dodson et al[140] made some important extrapolations. They estimated the average patient possessed 7.7 actinic keratoses. They noted that the probability of actinic keratoses converting to squamous carcinoma in 1 year was

0.0014. Conversely, the probability that an average actinic keratosis would not transform in 1 year was 0.9986. Furthermore, they noted that the probability that at least one of the 7.7 lesions would transform in 10 years was 0.1020, or 10.2%. In that mathematical model is the justification for treatment of individual actinic keratoses. The relationship between epidemiology of this lesion and solar radiation is well established.[138–141]

Squamous Cell Carcinoma

Historical Aspects

Like BCC, SCC has been recognized as a distinctive entity for several decades. Early publications on this neoplasm gave it the clinical designation of *deep*, *papillary*, or *tubercular* epithelioma; pathologically, it was known as *lobular* epithelioma.[66] The ability of SCC to metastasize to lymph nodes has been well known for many years, as well as its tendency to invade deeply into fascia, muscle, and other structures underlying the skin.

Histopathologic Features

SCC of the skin is capable of assuming a diversity of histologic growth patterns, again like BCC. These include conventional, adenoid, spindled pleomorphic, small cell, clear cell, and verrucous variants.[69,133,142–151] Also, this neoplasm can be graded according to its level of nucleocytoplasmic differentiation and

observed in a minority of cases; most manifest surface ulceration.

Spindle cell and pleomorphic SCC characteristically occur in sun-damaged skin. In common with other poorly differentiated cutaneous squamous neoplasms, deep infiltration of the dermis, subcutis, and underlying fascia is frequently observed.[153] They maintain keratin positivity whereas other spindle cell lesions such as melanoma and atypical fibroxanthoma lack keratin positivity.

Small Cell SCC

Rare cases of poorly differentiated cutaneous squamous carcinoma manifest a purely small cell appearance, superficially resembling one of the variants of Merkel cell carcinoma (see below).[133] This likeness is heightened in that both neoplasms may contain foci of keratinization and may be associated with overlying Bowen's disease.[161,162] However, the cells of small cell SCC typically contain more abundant cytoplasm and have nuclei with prominent nucleoli. Regional necrosis and abundant mitotic activity may be present in either small cell SCC or Merkel cell carcinoma. Involvement of the epidermis by the small cell proliferation favors a diagnosis of SCC, since this feature is seen in less than 10% of Merkel cell carcinomas.[133]

Clear Cell (Hydropic) SCC

Kuo[148] was the first to call attention to a variant of SCC composed of clear, nonvacuolated cells. At first glance, this neoplasm may be confused with clear cell eccrine carcinoma or sebaceous carcinoma. Any of these three lesions may contain foci of keratinization. Nevertheless, invasive clear cell SCC usually has broad connections to the epidermis in contrast to eccrine or sebaceous carcinomas. Because it appears that the cytoplasmic clarity in the first of these tumors is due to the degenerative ac-

cumulation of intracellular fluid, clear cell squamous carcinoma is also known as *hydropic* SCC.

Verrucous SCC

Squamous carcinomas that grossly simulate giant condylomata or verrucae have been diversely described as "giant condyloma of Buschke and Loewenstein,"[163] "carcinoma cuniculatum,"[147] or "verrucous carcinoma"[143,164] based on their anatomic locations. Basically, all of these lesions are nearly identical and can be considered as a group.

Verrucous SCC (VSCC) displays marked papillomatosis and acanthosis, often with "church-spiring" of the neoplastic epidermis. As a rule, cytologic atypia is only slight in this neoplasm, mitotic activity is scant, and dyskeratosis is less marked than in other forms of SCC.[147] Infiltration of the dermis occurs in broad, blunt cellular tongues rather than the jagged profiles seen in conventional squamous carcinoma. Reactive fibrosis and inflammation are minimal. Vascular and perineural invasion are seen only rarely (Fig. 17-31).

The criteria just given should be rigorously met before labeling a squamous carcinoma as verrucous. This is so because other forms (such as conventional SCC) may occasionally demonstrate verrucoid growth, but do not behave as indolently as true verrucous carcinoma. In particular, tumors displaying marked cellular atypia and abnormal mitotic figures should not be classified as VSCC. Differentiation from pseudoepitheliomatous hyperplasia may be impossible unless a long strip biopsy is obtained, which should show deep extension of blunt rete below the level of adjacent normal epidermis in VSCC.

Cutaneous Lesions Associated with SCC

Squamous carcinoma may arise in association with several other cutaneous disorders. These include linear epidermal nevus, nevus sebaceous of Jadassohn, epidermodysplasia

Figure 17-30. Spindled or sarcomatoid squamous cell carcinoma can barely be recognized as squamous in origin. Such lesions have a connection with the epidermis, or multiple step sections will show characteristic squamous features. This particular example maintained keratin immunophenotyping.

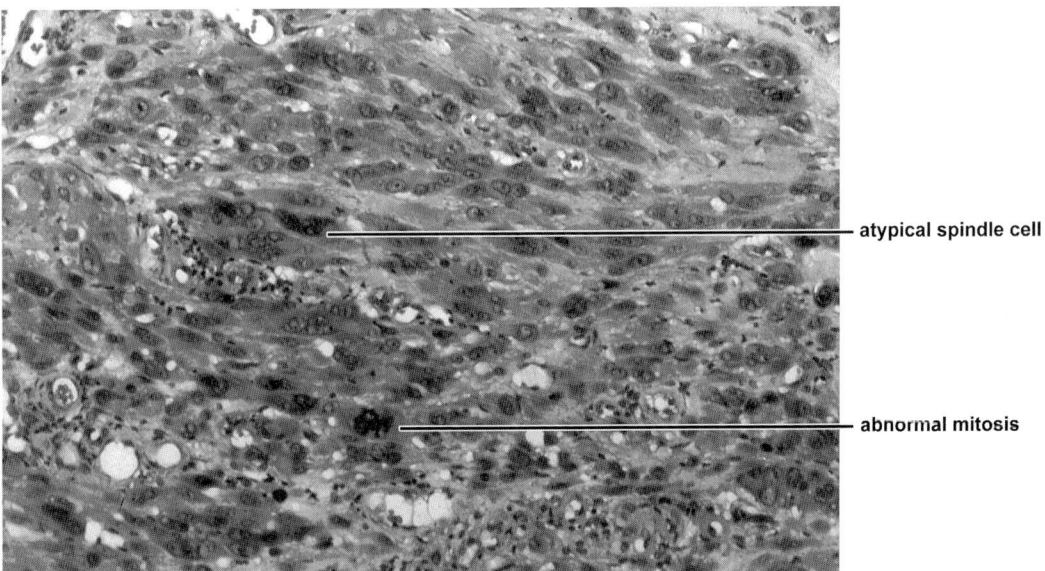

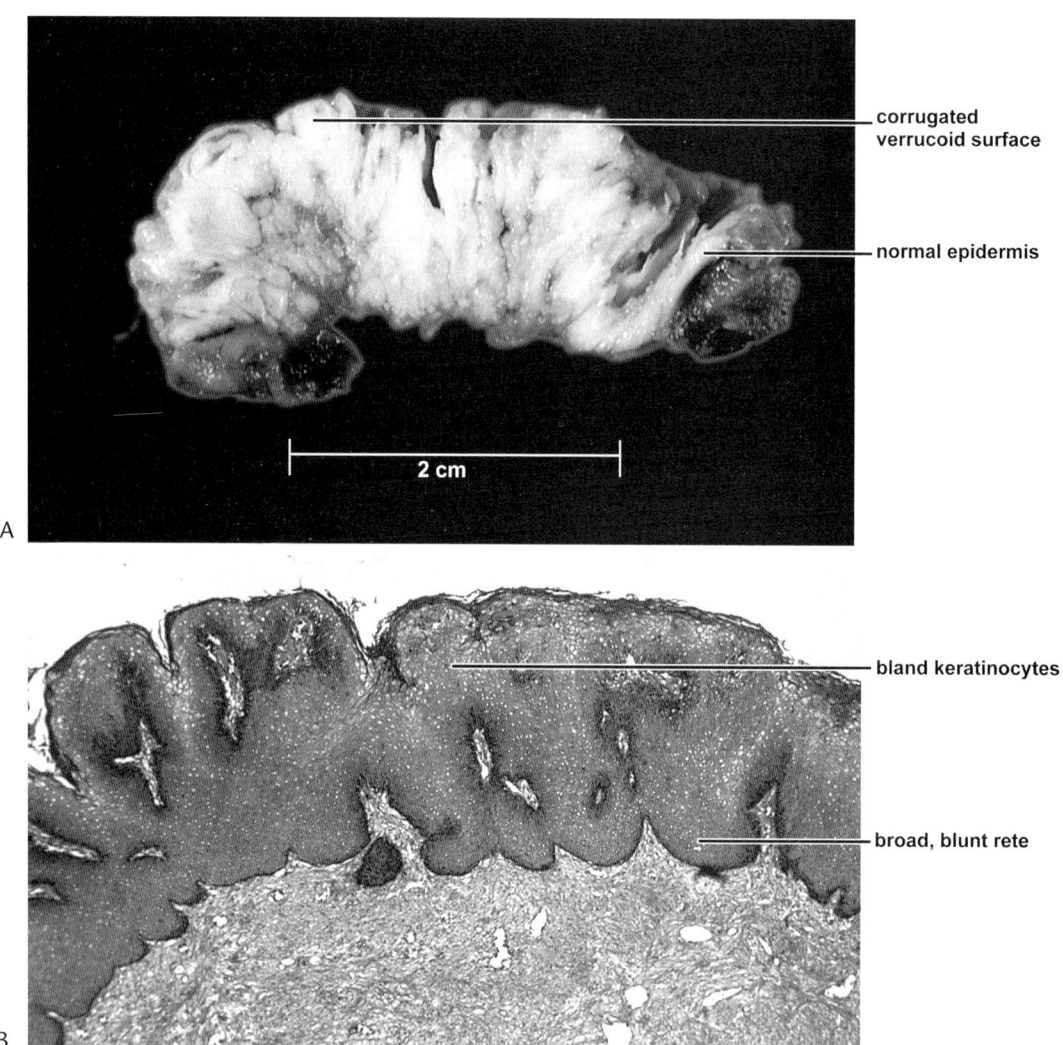

Figure 17-31. Verrucous carcinoma. (**A**), Gross specimen (slice) from a very large lesion. The cut section shows the rough, verrucoid character. The lesions are most common in the oral cavity and genital region. (**B**) Microscopic view. There are broad, blunt rete of very bland keratinocytes that extend into the dermis. Close inspection fails to reveal a well-formed basement membrane. Accurate diagnosis depends on having a specimen that includes adjacent normal epidermis. Broad, pushing rete.

verruciformis, epidermolysis bullosa, xeroderma pigmentosum, seborrheic keratosis, verruca vulgaris, hidradenitis suppurative, condyloma accuminatum, lichen planus, discoid lupus erythematosus, actinic porokeratosis, extramammary Paget's disease, epidermoid cysts, and lupus vulgaris.[69,89, 165–170] Moreover, it is now generally accepted that sites of chronic epithelial regeneration due to recalcitrant infections, radiodermatitis, or burn scars carry a definite risk of malignant transformation to SCC.[69] With respect to sinuses draining underlying foci of osteomyelitis, the name of "Marjolin's ulcers" has been appended to carcinomas originating in this context. Although they are well differentiated histologically, these tumors may pursue an aggressive clinical course.

Special Pathologic Studies

Conventional Special Stains

Conventional histochemical staining methods are of limited use in the diagnostic definition of SCC. The PAS method yields variable reactivity with this neoplasm; however, if a clear cell cutaneous tumor fails to contain glycogen, metastatic renal cell carcinoma and eccrine carcinoma may be excluded from consideration and hydropic SCC assumes greater importance in the differential diagnosis.[148] Mucin stains are nonreactive with SCC, as are the Alcian blue and colloidal iron techniques. These findings may be of some assistance in discriminating between adenoid squamous carcinoma and sweat gland tumors.

Electron Microscopy

Ultrastructural studies of SCC have shown that this tumor possesses the features of keratinocytes,[142,145,147,148,150,171] including prominent desmosomal intercellular attachments, tonofibrils, keratohyaline granules, and rough endoplasmic reticulum. Cytoplasmic lipid droplets, glycogen pools, neurosecretory granules, and glandular differentiation are uniformly lacking. It is true that the density of intracellular organelles decreases with increasing tumor grade, but careful analysis of electron microscopic specimens invariably demonstrates the presence of diagnostic features of SCC even in poorly differentiated lesions.

Immunohistochemistry

As noted earlier in the discussion of BCC, SCC of the skin demonstrates reactivity for medium- and high-molecular-weight cytokeratins.[107] Poorly differentiated tumors typically express low-molecular-weight keratin as well.[108] Spindle cell and pleomorphic squamous carcinomas manifest the facultative ability to re-express vimentin, the intermediate filament seen in virtually all embryonic cells and in mature mesenchymal tissues. Thus, reliance on vimentin immunostains alone is not a valid means of separating spindle cell carcinomas from true sarcomas. Similarly, α_1-antichymotrypsin, which has been touted as a marker for "fibrohistiocytic" neoplasms, is also present in pleomorphic SCC and should not be used exclusively in diagnosis in the absence of intermediate filament stains.[108]

An interesting trend in immunoreactivity may be seen with antibodies to epithelial membrane antigen in the analysis of SCC of varying grades. Well-differentiated cutaneous tumors lack epithelial membrane antigen, moderately differentiated SCC expresses it patchily, and high-grade neoplasms are diffusely positive for this determinant.[108,149] Other antigens of interest in dermatopathology, such as S-100 protein, carcinoembryonic antigen, neuron-specific enolase, and salivary-type amylase are uniformly absent.

Clinicopathologic Correlation

The likelihood that squamous carcinoma of the skin will recur locally or metastasize is directly related to its anatomic location, association with other cutaneous disorders, histologic grade, depth of invasion, and the immunocompetence of the host.[69,152,153] Bowen's disease without an infiltrative component never metastasizes, but may recur if inadequately excised. As an aside, it should be noted that considerable attention has been given to the premise that Bowen's disease may be a cutaneous marker for internal malignancy.[159] However, recent publications have concluded that this relationship is not statistically significant.[158]

Squamous carcinomas arising from solar keratoses metastasize only rarely (0.5%),[171] whereas histologically identical tumors associated with burn scars, draining sinuses, and radiodermatitis show distant spread in 20% to 30% of cases.[172] In like manner, those located at the vermilion border of the lower lip and other "modified" skin sites (e.g., vulva, glans penis) demonstrate more aggressive behavior than that of actinic SCC. Squamous carcinomas in immunosuppressed patients exhibit inexorable growth and metastasis in many cases, despite a low-grade appearance.

Evans and Smith[153] showed that the clinical courses of spindle cell and pleomorphic forms of SCC are intimately related to depth of invasion. Those lesions involving the deep dermis and subcutis metastasized much more frequently than others with superficial invasion of the corium. This trend is generally true of all cutaneous squamous carcinomas with Broders' grades higher than 2.

VSCC rarely metastasizes, although this possibility is not unknown.[151] Rather, VSCC is typified by repeated recurrence and locally destructive growth. A report by Perez-Mesa et al[164] documented the dedifferentiation of verrucous carcinoma following radiotherapy. The latter modality of treatment has been proscribed ever since, but the actual incidence of such transformations is unknown.

Differential Diagnosis

Due to its potential variability of appearance, SCC of the skin may be confused microscopically with several other cutaneous neoplasms and pseudoneoplastic proliferations, including extramammary Paget's disease, pseudoepitheliomatous hyperplasia, keratoacanthoma, sweat gland carcinoma, epithelioid angiosarcoma, atypical fibroxanthoma, spindle cell amelanotic melanoma, Merkel cell carcinoma, BCC, basaloid sebaceous carcinoma, and small cell eccrine carcinoma. The distinguishing points between these differential diagnostic considerations and SCC variants are outlined in Tables 17-1 to 17-4.

Keratoacanthoma

Keratoacanthoma (KA) is a common dermatologic tumor and the nemesis of pathologists. It was first described by Jonathan Hutchinson[173] in 1889. KA is usually an exophytic, nodular, or wart-like lesion found on sun-exposed skin. The hand and arm are common sites in men while the lower leg is a common site in women; however, virtually all body sites have been af-

Table 17-1. Differential Diagnosis of Well-Differentiated Squamous Cell Carcinoma

Histologic Feature	WDSCC	PEH	KA
Horn-filled central crater	0	0	+
Intraepithelial abscesses	0	0	+
Cytoplasmic lucency	0	0	+
Mitotic activity	V	0	V
Cellular atypia	V	0	V
Apoptosis and dyskeratosis	+	0	V
Sharply angulated cell profiles at lesional base	+	V	0
Dermal fibrosis and chronic inflammation	V	V	Va
Perineural invasion in dermis	V	0	Va

Abbreviations: WDSCC, well-differentiated squamous cell carcinoma; PEH, pseudoepitheliomatous hyperplasia; KA, keratoacanthoma; +, consistently present; 0, consistently absent; V, variably present; a, regressing KAs may demonstrate perilesional fibrosis (rare examples are neuroinvasive).

Table 17-2. Differential Diagnosis of Cutaneous Bowen's Disease

Histologic Feature	Pagetoid BD	EPD
Acantholysis involving atypical intraepidermal cells	0	+
Cytoplasmic lucency	V	+
Dyskeratosis and apoptosis	+	0
Global atypia of keratinocytes	+	0
Immunoreactivity for carcinoembryonic antigen and/or gross cystic disease fluid protein-15	0	+

Abbreviations: BD, Bowen's disease; EPD, extramammary Paget's disease; 0, consistently absent; +, consistently present; V, variably present.

Table 17-4. Differential Diagnosis of Spindle Cell and Pleomorphic Squamous Cell Carcinoma

Histologic Feature	SC-PSCC	MM	AFX
Continuity of tumor cells with epidermis	V	V	0
Junctional melanocytic atypia	0	+	0
Immunoreactivity for keratin	+	0	0
Immunoreactivity for vimentin	V	+	+
Immunoreactivity for S-100 protein	0	+	0
Immunoreactivity for α_1-antichymotrypsin	V	V	+

Abbreviations: SC-PSCC, spindle cell and pleomorphic squamous cell carcinoma; MM, malignant melanoma; AFX, atypical fibroxanthoma; 0, consistently absent; +, consistently present; V, variably present.

fected.[174–176] The exact incidence is unknown, but in a study from Kauai, Hawaii, the rate was 104 per 100,000 residents. The average age in that group was 63.5 years. It is generally accepted that the tumor increases in incidence with increasing age.[177]

Clinical Features

The clinical features can be divided into three stages. In the proliferative stage a rapidly growing papule or nodule develops that can reach a size of 2 cm or more. The border is erythematous. The mature form is volcano shaped with a central keratinous core. The involutional form appears after several months and leaves a depressed hypopigmented scar.

There are also many different clinical presentations of KA. KA is usually solitary, and other solitary forms have been reported as KA centrifugum marginatum, giant KA, subungual

Table 17-3. Differential Diagnosis of Cutaneous Tumors Containing Glandular or Pseudoglandular Spaces

Histologic Feature	ASCC	EAS	SGC
Continuity of cells in gland-like spaces with epidermis	+	0	V (rare +)
Erythrocytes in gland-like spaces	0	+	0
Mucin/PAS positivity	0	0	+
Keratin immunoreactivity	+	0	+
Binding of *Ulex europaeus* I lectin	V	+	V
Immunoreactivity for carcinoembryonic antigen, S-100 protein, amylase, or Leu M1	0	0	+

Abbreviations: ASCC, adenoid squamous cell carcinoma; EAS, epithelioid angiosarcoma; SGC, sweat gland carcinoma; 0, consistently absent; +, consistently present; V, variably present.

KA, and oral/mucous membrane KA. Multiple forms include the multiple KAs of Ferguson-Smith and the generalized eruptive keratoacanthomas of Grzybowski.[174] KAs have been associated with demure Muir-Torre syndrome, xeroderma pigmentosum, and nevus sebaceus of Jadassohn. KAs may occur following radiation as well as benign inflammatory conditions such as herpes zoster, lichen planus, discoid lupus erythematosus, psoriasis, pemphigus, and epidermolysis bullosa. Similarly, KAs may occur following trauma and contact with coal tar or pitch. Multiple KAs may also occur at various body sites in immunosuppressed patients.

Histopathologic Features

KA is thought to arise from hair follicles. Thus, the glassy character of the keratin in the volcano-shaped lesion is reminiscent of follicular keratin maturation. In the early stage of a KA, there is a keratin-filled invagination of the epidermis (Fig. 17-32). The overall silhouette of the lesion is nodular, circumscribed, and has distinct borders. There is hyperkeratosis, acanthosis, and sudden or premature keratinization. Around the periphery of the lesion there are irregularly shaped strands of atypical squamous cells that are definitely carcinoma-like. The atypical squamous cells form small groups and nodules as well as individual cell infiltration patterns. Mitoses are present, but atypical mitoses are generally not found. There is a mixed inflammatory infiltrate that is peripheral to the atypical squamous cells. Eosinophils and neutrophils are present in the mixed infiltrate as well as in small microabscesses that are associated with the keratin as well as small nodules of atypical squamous cells. Collagen and elastin fibers are noted within the tumor tentacles.[178] Perineural invasion and intravascular spread may also be seen, but does not portend a poor prognosis.[174,179] The lesion does not extend below the level of the eccrine sweat coils (Fig. 17-33). The fully developed KA is volcano shaped and has peripheral buttresses or lips along the perimeter. Within those buttresses of near-normal epidermis there is abundant hyalin keratin, which overlies the atypical squamous cell proliferation. In the regressed stage foreign

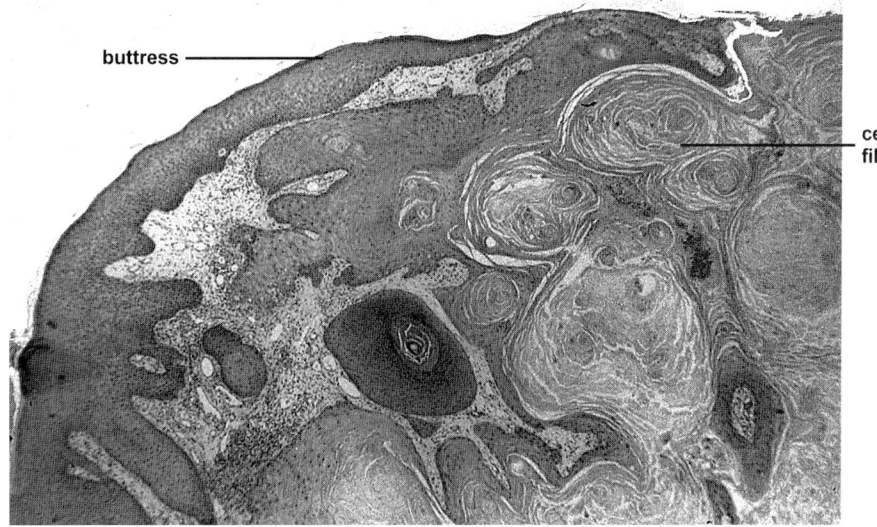

Figure 17-32. Half of a keratoacanthoma displaying the buttress and the keratin-filled crater. The glassy keratin and the buttress can be used to identify this lesion. (H&E, × 40.)

body granulomata, multinucleated histiocytes, and a lichenoid inflammation can be seen in the dermis. If there is any remnant of KA there is granulation and fibrosis (scar) beneath it (Fig. 17-34). The remnant KA may consist of nothing more than hyperkeratotic irregularly shaped epidermis.

Differential Diagnosis

The diagnosis of KA is made chiefly on the presence of the proper shape and silhouette of the lesion. The lesion should be crater or volcano shaped and possess lateral buttresses or lips. The atypical squamous cell proliferation at the base should not extend below the eccrine coils. There is an underlying mixed inflammatory infiltrate as well as small neutrophilic microabscesses within the keratin and within some of the atypical squamous cell nodules. The chief distracting diagnosis is SCC. SCCs arise usually in sun-damaged skin in association with actinic keratoses. They lack the characteristic silhouette and shape. They usually lack the hyalin keratin in the central crater of the lesion. SCCs may have extreme atypia and atypical mitoses, which are seldom found in KAs. Overall, SCCs arise in an irregular shape over a broad area. The most important feature in the diagnosis of KA is the volcano shape with lateral buttresses. It is written that actinically damaged elastic fibers are increased within the epithelial cells of KA.[178] A homogeneous staining pattern for transforming growth factor-α also favors KAs.[180] Also, squamous carcinoma shows a diffuse staining pattern for proliferating cell nuclear antigen while KA stains only on the periphery.[181]

It is sometimes necessary because of the lack of a full-thickness biopsy to make the diagnosis "probable KA, SCC cannot be excluded." A well-known dermatopathologist often makes the diagnosis of KA extending to the base of the biopsy. Another designation that has been used is "SCC of the KA type." In summary, we believe that KA is a keratinocidic neoplasm with borderline, albeit very low, malignant potential.

Primary Neuroendocrine Carcinoma of the Skin ("Merkel Cell" Carcinoma)

Since its relatively recent recognition, primary neuroendocrine carcinoma of the skin has been the subject of intensive clinicopathologic study. Because this neoplasm demonstrates neuroepithelial differentiation like that of normal Merkel cells of the skin ("Tastzellen"), the alternative term *Merkel cell carcinoma* is also widely used in reference to it.

Historical Aspects and Nomenclature

In 1972, Toker[182] described a small cell cutaneous neoplasm that tended to occur in elderly patients in sun-exposed skin areas. It resembled malignant lymphoma or metastatic oat cell carcinoma microscopically. Local recurrence, regional lymph node metastasis, and a lengthy survival in some cases made it evident that the lesion was primary in the skin. Because he observed a ribboning growth pattern in some instances, Toker designated this neoplasm as *trabecular carcinoma*. In the interim, various other diagnostic labels were applied to it, such as those mentioned above as well as *small cell carcinoma of the skin*,[183] *endocrine carcinoma of the skin*,[162] and *undifferentiated carcinoma of the skin*.[184]

The premise that such lesions exhibit Merkel cell differentiation is based on indirect morphologic and immunohistochemical data. Warner et al[185] have outlined the ultrastructural similarities between PNCS and normal Merkel cells. The

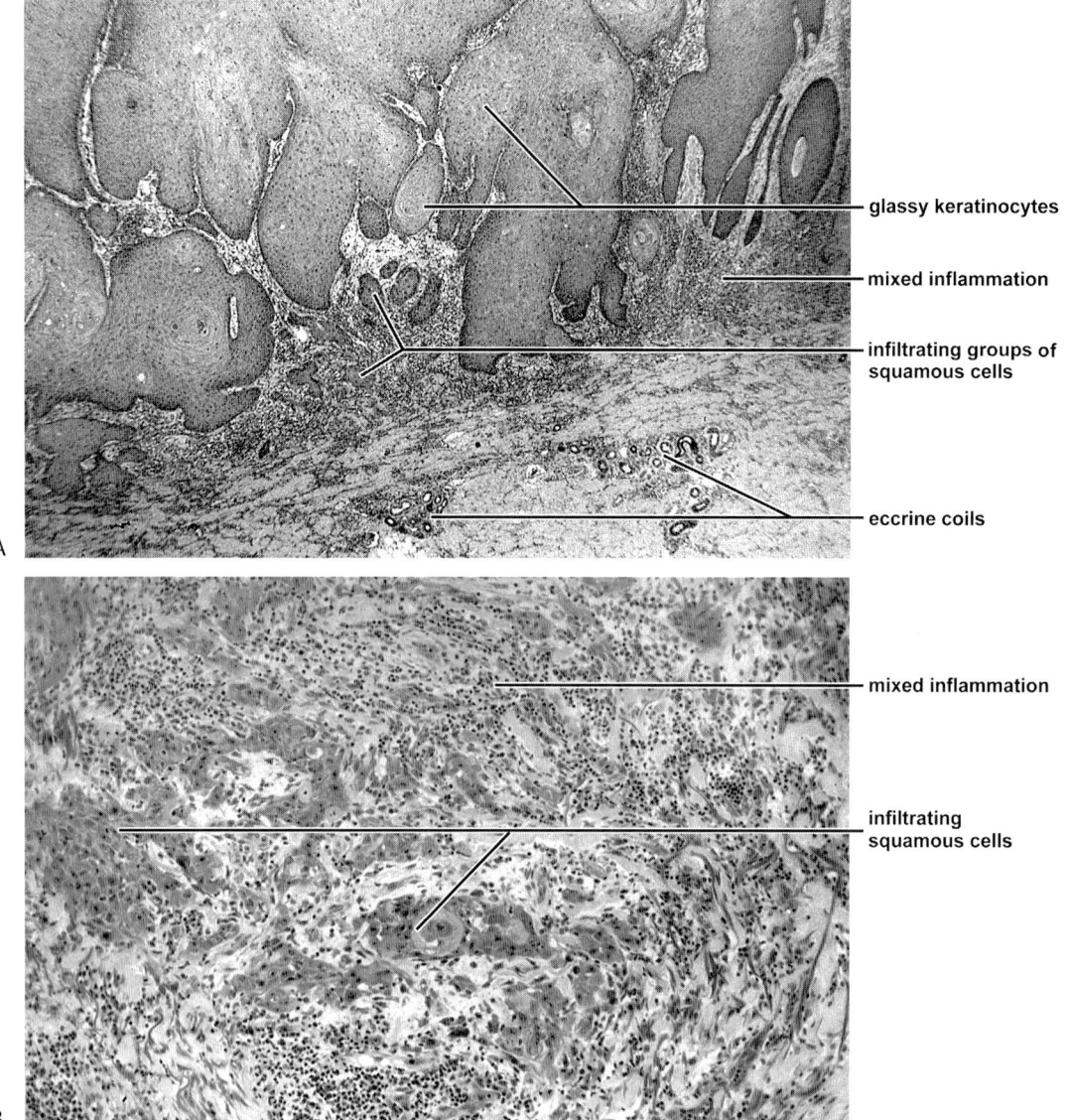

glassy keratinocytes

mixed inflammation

infiltrating groups of
squamous cells

eccrine coils

A

mixed inflammation

infiltrating
squamous cells

B

Figure 17-33. (A) Extension of the broad bands and small infiltrating groups of glassy keratinocytes into the dermis below a keratoacanthoma. The lesion never extends below the level of the eccrine coils. There is an underlying mixed inflammatory infiltrate which includes eosinophils. (B) Higher power view of the edge of a keratoacanthoma. There is a remarkable similarity to squamous cell carcinoma. The diagnosis must be made on low power silhouette of a volcano-shaped lesion with buttresses and a fairly distinct deep border. (H&E, × 250.)

work of Hartschuh and colleagues[186] and Sibley and Dahl[187] demonstrates that certain secretory cell products are common to both.

Nevertheless, the normal anatomic distribution of Merkel cells (epidermal) predominantly in the digits[185,188] is not recapitulated by the topography of PNCS.[133] Moreover, one of the intermediate filament polypeptides, neurofilament protein, is often present in PNCS[187,189] but not in normal merkelocytes.[190] Therefore, the nomenclature attending this neoplasm is arbitrary.

Histopathologic Features

Typical PNCS is characterized by the medullary, organoid, or trabecular growth of small oval cells in the dermis, with various degrees of intercellular cohesion (Fig. 17-35). A grenz zone is usually present, but the epidermis may be involved focally in approximately 10% of cases. Dermal appendages are usually spared, but permeative growth into the subcutis is often apparent. Adipocytes may be entrapped by tumor cells, yielding an appearance simulating that of lymphoma cutis. Regional coag-

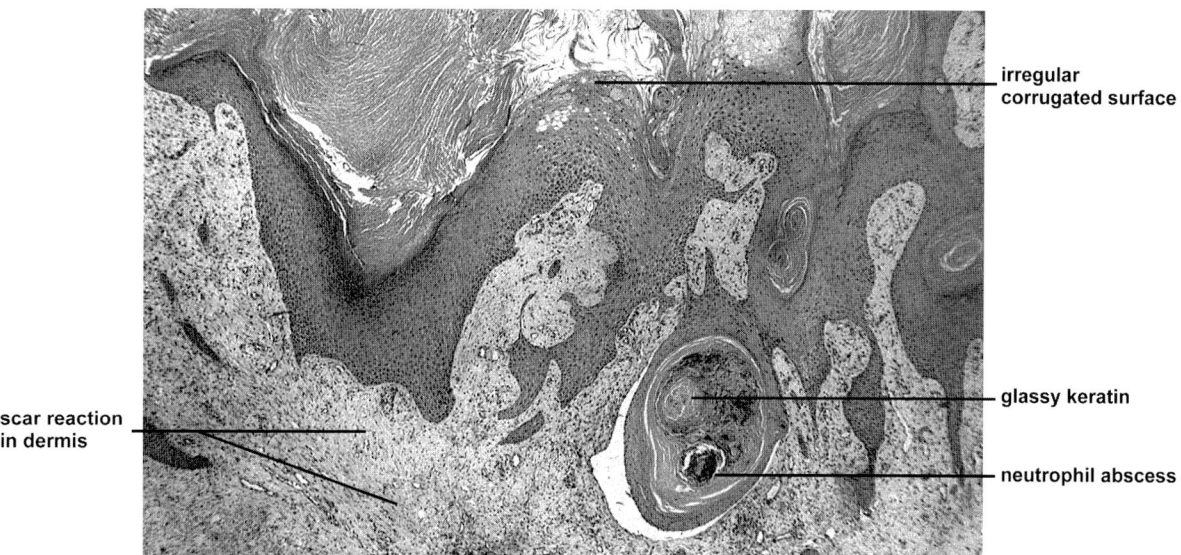

Figure 17-34. An almost entirely resolved keratoacanthoma. There is irregular epidermis, still with glassy keratin. The jagged remnants of atypical keratinocytes extend into a scarred, fibrotic dermis. Foreign body giant cells, often containing keratin remnants, are present in the dermis. (H&E, × 40.)

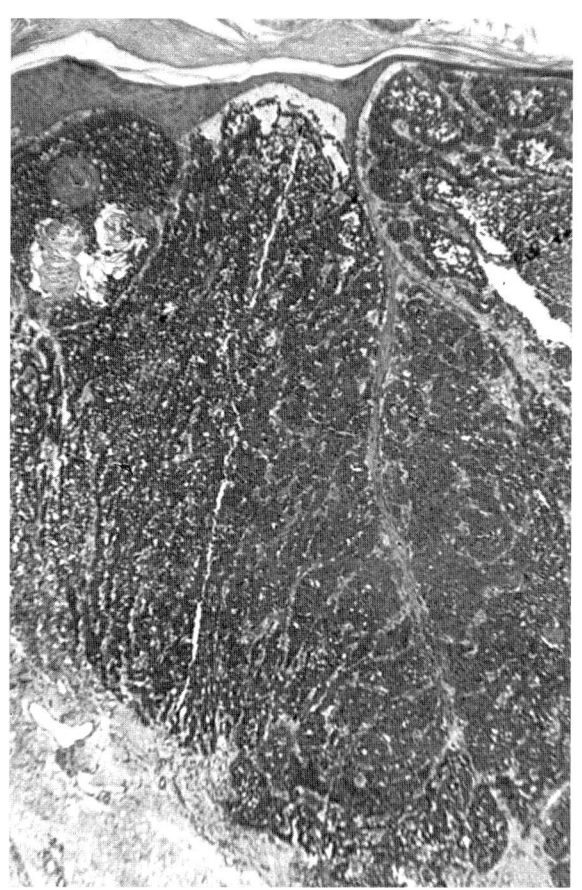

Figure 17-35. Merkel cell carcinoma of the skin is characterized by a sometimes ulcerated broad mass of small basaloid cells. The basaloid cells can be present in sheets or trabeculae. (H&E, × 50.)

ulative necrosis and apoptosis are common within PNCS.[133,162,191] Nuclei are round to oval, with evenly dispersed chromatin, inconspicuous nucleoli, and abundant mitoses (up to 12 per high power field) (Fig. 17-36). Cytoplasm is scanty and amphophilic, and cellular borders are indistinct. The stroma of PNCS may be focally sclerotic and is richly endowed with capillary- or venule-sized vessels, which may be dilated. Lymphatic invasion is apparent in 20% of cases, and variably intense stromal lymphoplasmacytic inflammation is evident in most examples.[162]

Variations on the histopathologic description just given include lesions showing scattered uninucleated tumor "giant" cells, formation of Homer-Wright rosettes, myxoid stroma, spindle cell growth, and foci of squamous or glandular differentiation.[133,162] Another subtype of PNCS is the "oat cell" variant, displaying nests of small, hyperchromatic, partially crushed tumor cells with prominent nuclear molding. The microscopic similarities between the latter and metastatic pulmonary small cell neuroendocrine carcinoma are obvious[189,192]; however, the "Azzopardi" phenomenon common in metastatic oat cell carcinoma of the lung (DNA encrustation of intratumoral blood vessels) is not observed in PNCS.

A spectrum of differentiation in PNCS, including "intermediate" and "large-cell" subtypes have been documented.[193] It is probable that cases of "primary cutaneous carcinoid" are actually PNCS.[194,195]

PNCS Associated with Other Skin Lesions

The association between PNCS and squamous carcinoma is now well recognized.[161] Roughly 25% of patients with neuroendocrine skin cancer have had squamous carcinoma in the same cutaneous region, or have it metachronously. Both invasive

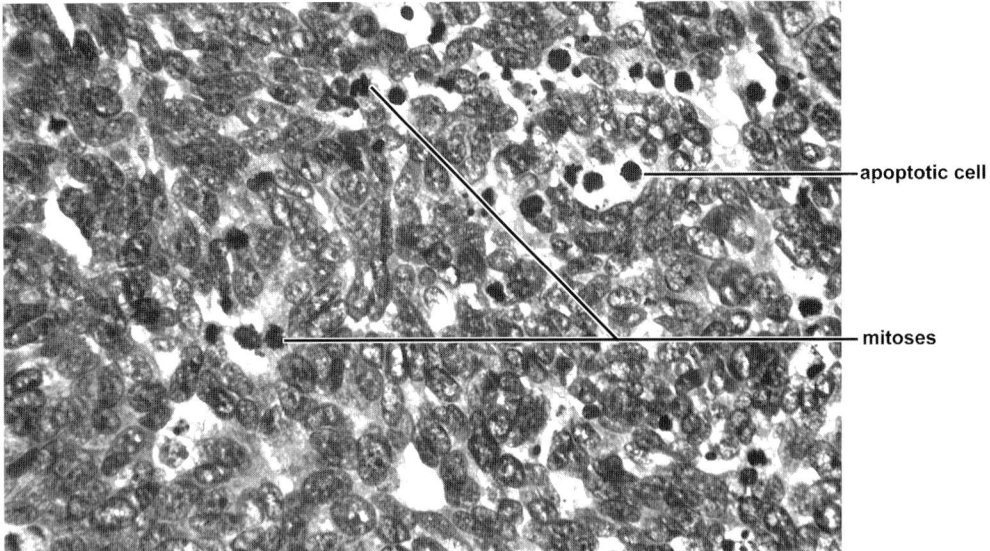

Figure 17-36. Individual cells of a Merkel cell carcinoma have a high nuclear/cytoplasmic ratio and display many mitoses and frequent apoptosis. They are characteristically neuron-specific enolase positive. Although not illustrated here, small foci of squamous differentiation may be scattered within the tumor. (H&E, × 300.)

SCC and Bowen's disease have been documented in this context. Silva et al[162] described a case in which overt sweat gland carcinoma and PNCS were admixed. We have observed one example of cutaneous neuroendocrine carcinoma arising in a background of hypohidrotic ectodermal dysplasia; the patient also had multifocal BCCs and trichoepitheliomas in the same skin field.[196] In the M.D. Anderson Hospital experience with this neoplasm, 9 of 67 cases showed the concurrence of PNCS and adjacent BCC.[162]

Special Pathologic Studies

Conventional Special Stains

The PAS method may demonstrate scanty glycogen in less than 15% of cases. The mucicarmine stain is consistently negative, but Alcian blue and colloidal iron techniques sometimes result in labeling of the tumoral stroma. Argyrophil stains (e.g., Grimelius, Churukian-Schenk) are positive in less than 10% of cutaneous neuroendocrine carcinomas that have been formalin fixed, but preservation in Bouin's solution yields silver reactivity in most cases.[188] Argentaffin and amyloid stains are uniformly negative.

Electron Microscopy

Ultrastructurally, tumor cells in PNCS are invested focally by basal lamina and bound to one another by maculae adherens-type junctions. Nuclear chromatin is evenly distributed, with small chromocenters. Cytoplasmic contents include scanty glycogen, small numbers of mitochondria, free ribosomes, focally prominent Golgi bodies, occasional lysosomes, and short profiles of rough endoplasmic reticulum.[162]

The diagnostic electron microscopic elements in this neoplasm are twofold. First, dense-core neurosecretory granules measuring 80 to 120 nm in diameter are evident in the cytoplasm, within both cell bodies and blunt cellular extensions. Second, paranuclear whorls and skeins of intermediate filaments are consistently detectable, in which neurosecretory granules are embedded.[133,183] Rare intracellular microlumina have been described in PNCS by Silva et al.[162] Premelanosomes are always absent.

Immunohistochemistry

PNCS is typified by consistent reactivity for cytokeratin in diffuse or globular/paranuclear patterns.[183,189,197] The second of these is diagnostic of neuroendocrine differentiation in a cutaneous small cell tumor, but is seen in only 40% to 50% of cases.[197] Concomitant positivity for neurofilament protein can be detected in 33% with a similar cytoplasmic distribution. Epithelial membrane antigen is positive in 75% of cases.[198]

The most sensitive "endocrine" marker for PNCS is neuron-specific enolase (NSE).[108,133,197] Although NSE is seen in all tumors of this type, it is not specific for PNCS. Rare BCCs and sweat gland carcinoma express this protein as well. The latter finding is not unexpected, since Haimoto et al[199] have demonstrated NSE in normal eccrine glands. Chromogranin, a very specific indicator of neuroendocrine differentiation, is seen in 33% of PCNS cases.[189] In addition, 5% to 30% exhibit focal reactivity for vasoactive intestinal polypeptide, calcitonin, pancreatic polypeptide, adrenocorticotropic hormone, gastrin, insulin, or somatostatin.[187,198,200] S-100 protein, carcinoembryonic antigen, and salivary-type amylase are consistently lacking in PNCS.[108,187,200]

Clinicopathologic Correlation

PNCS is an aggressive neoplasm, with a cumulative mortality rate of up to 50% in some series.[162,191] Several pathologic features have been identified that putatively predict those lesions at risk for pursuing an aggressive clinical course. These include a gross size of greater than 2 cm, more than 10 mitoses per high power field, lymphatic invasion, and the presence of the "oat cell" PNCS growth pattern. It has been recommended that such cases be subjected to prophylactic regional lymphadenectomy, subsequent to primary tumor removal. If the resected lymph nodes contain tumor, adjuvant radiotherapy to the tumor bed and remaining local lymphoid tissue would appear to be indicated.

Multifocality has been documented at initial diagnosis in 12 patients with PNCS.[162,196,201] Because such a clinical presentation is much more suggestive of metastasis to the skin of a visceral carcinoma, a great deal of caution should be exercised before accepting a diagnosis of PNCS in cases with more than one lesion. The spontaneous regression of cutaneous neuroendocrine carcinoma has been described by O'Rourke and Bell.[202] In light of the large number of recognized cases of PNCS, this phenomenon must be extremely rare; moreover, the biologic mechanisms underlying it are unknown.

Differential Diagnosis

The differential diagnosis of small cell neoplasms of the skin is extensive. Small cell SCC, eccrine carcinoma, and malignant melanoma must be included in this group, as well as malignant lymphoma, metastatic neuroendocrine carcinoma from visceral sites, peripheral neuroepithelioma, and Ewing's sarcoma. Ultrastructural and immunohistochemical studies are extremely useful in this context.

REFERENCES

1. Chiba T, Shitomi I, Nakano O et al: The sign of Leser-Trelat associated with esophageal carcinoma. Am J Gastroenterol 91:802, 1996
2. Cohen JH, Lessin SR, Vowels BR et al: The sign of Leser-Trelat in association with Sezary syndrome: simultaneous disappearance of seborrheic keratoses and malignant T-cell clone during combined therapy with photopheresis and interferon alpha. Arch Dermatol 129:1213, 1993
3. Jones-Caballero M, Penas PF, Buezo GF et al: Malignant melanoma appearing in a seborrheic keratosis. Br J Dermatol 133:1016, 1995
4. Cohn MS, Classen RF: The sign of Leser-Trelat associated with adenocarcinoma of the rectum. Cutis 51:255, 1993
5. Vignale R, Espasandin J, Deneo H et al: Halo keratosis associated with colon carcinoma. Int J Dermatol 32:846, 1993
6. Ikari Y, Ohkura M, Morita M et al: Leser-Trelat sign associated with Sézary syndrome. J Dermatol 22:62, 1995
7. Schwartz RA: Sign of Leser-Trelat. J Am Acad Dermatol 35:88, 1996
8. Maize JC, Snider RL: Nonmelanoma skin cancers in association with seborrheic keratoses. Clinicopathologic correlations. Dermatol Surg 21:960, 1995
9. Nindle M, Nakagawa H, Furue M et al: Simple epithelial cytokeratin-expression in seborrheic keratosis. J Cutan Pathol 19:415, 1992
10. Rao BK, Freeman RG, Poulos EG et al: The relationship between basal cell epithelioma and seborrheic keratosis. A study of 60 cases. J Dermatol Surg Oncol 20:761, 1994
11. Helm TN, Helm F, Marsico R et al: Seborrheic keratoses with occult underlying basal cell carcinoma. J Am Acad Dermatol 29:791, 1993
12. Li J, Ackerman AB: "Seborrheic keratoses" that contain human papillomavirus are condylomata acuminata. Am J Dermatopathol 16:398, 1994
13. Solomon LM, Fretzin DF, Dewald RL: The epidermal nevus syndrome. Arch Dermatol 97:273, 1968
14. Eichler C, Flowers FP, Ross J: Epidermal nevus syndrome: case report and review of clinical manifestations. Pediatr Dermatol 6:316, 1989
15. Happle R: How many epidermal nevus syndromes exist? J Am Acad Dermatol 25:550, 1991
16. Rogers M: Epidermal nevi and the epidermal nevus syndromes: a review of 233 cases. Pediatr Dermatol 9:342, 1992
17. Hodge JA, Ray MC, Flynn KJ: The epidermal nevus syndrome. Int J Dermatol 30:91, 1991
18. Mehregan AH, Pinkus H: Life history of organoid nevi. Arch Dermatol 91:574, 1965
19. Su WPD: Histopathologic varieties of epidermal nevus. Am J Dermatol 4:161, 1982
20. Dupré A, Christol B: Inflammatory linear verrucose epidermal nevus. Arch Dermatol 113:767, 1977
21. Hodge SJ, Barr JM, Owen LG: Inflammatory linear verrucose epidermal nevus. Arch Dermatol 114:436, 1978
22. Kim SC, Kang WH: Nevus comedicus associated with epidermal nevus. J Am Acad Dermatol 21:1085, 1989
23. Taki T, Izawa Y, Usuda T, Kozuka S et al: Basal cell epithelioma occurring in an epidermal nevus. Acta Pathol Jpn 34:859, 1984
24. Levin A, Amazon K, Rywlin AM: A squamous cell carcinoma that developed in an epidermal nevus. Report of a case and a review of the literature. Am J Dermatopathol 6:51, 1984
25. Cramer SF, Mandel MA, Hauler R et al: Squamous cell carcinoma arising in a linear epidermal nevus. Arch Dermatol 117:222, 1981
26. Horn MS, Sausker WF, Pierson DL: Basal cell epithelioma arising in a linear epidermal nevus. Arch Dermatol 117:247, 1981
27. Mehregan AH: Tumor of follicular infundibulum. Dermatologica 142:177, 1971
28. Horn TD, Vennos EM, Bernstein BD et al: Multiple tumors of follicular infundibulum with sweat duct differentiation. J Cutan Pathol 22:281, 1995
29. Trunnell TN, Waisman M: Tumor of the follicular infundibulum. Cutis 24:317, 1979
30. Koch B, Rufli T: Tumor of follicular infundibulum. Dermatologica 183:68, 1991
31. Alessi E, Wong SN, Advani HH et al: Nevus sebaceous is associated with unusual neoplasms. Am J Dermatopathol 10:116, 1988

32. Kossard S, Finley AG, Poyzer K et al: Eruptive infundibulomas: A distinctive presentation of the tumor of follicular infundibulum. J Am Acad Dermatol 21:361, 1989

33. Starink TM, Hausman R: The cutaneous pathology of facial lesions in Cowden's disease. J Cutan Pathol 11:331, 1984

34. Stafford EM, Greenberg H, Miles PA: Cervical intraepithelial neoplasia III in an adolescent with bowenoid papulosis. J Adolesc Health Care 11:523, 1990

35. Rogozinski TT, Janniger CK: Bowenoid papulosis. Am Fam Phys 38:161, 1988

36. Wade TR, Kopf AW, Ackerman AB: Bowenoid papulosis of the penis. Cancer 42:1890, 1978

37. Schwartz RA, Janniger CK: Bowenoid papulosis. J Am Acad Dermatol 24:261, 1991

38. de Belilovsky C, Lessana-Leibowitch M: Bowen's disease and bowenoid papulosis: comparative clinical, viral, and disease progression aspects. Contracep Fertil Sexual 21:231, 1993

39. Olemans C, Pierard-Franchimont C, Delvenne P et al: Comparative karyometry in Bowen's disease and bowenoid papulosis. Derivation of a nuclear atypia index. Anal Quant Cytol Histol 16:284, 1994

40. Bocking A, Chatelain R, Salterberg A et al: Bowenoid papulosis. Classification as a low-grade in a situ carcinoma of the epidermis on the basis of histomorphologic and DNA ploidy studies. Anal Quant Cytol Histol 11:419, 1989

41. Bolton RA: Nongenital warts: classification and treatment options. Am Fam Phys 43:2049, 1991

42. Laimins LA: The biology of human papillomaviruses: from warts to cancer. Infect Agents Dis 2:74, 1993

43. Downey GO, Okagaki T, Ostrow RS et al: Condylomatous carcinoma of the vulva with special reference to human papillomavirus DNA. Obstet Gynecol 72:68, 1988

44. Nyeem R, Wilkinson EJ, Grover LJ: Condylomata acuminata of the cervix: histopathology and association with cervical neoplasia. Int J Gynecol Pathol 1:246, 1982

45. Fu YS, Huang I, Beaudenon S et al: Correlative study of human papillomavirus DNA, histopathology and morphometry in cervical condyloma and intraepithelial neoplasia. Int J Gynecol Pathol 7:297, 1988

46. Kossard S, Xenias SJ, Palestine RF et al: Inflammatory changes in verruca vulgaris. J Cutan Pathol 7:217, 1980

47. Euvrard S, Chardonnet Y, Hermier C et al: Warts and epidermoid carcinoma after renal transplantation. Ann Dermatol Venereol 116:201, 1989

48. Lutzner MA: Epidermodysplasia verruciformis: an autosomal recessive disease characterized by viral warts and skin cancer. A model for viral oncogenesis. Bull Cancer 65:169, 1978

49. Innocenzi D, Barduagni F, Cerio R, Wolter M: Disseminated eruptive clear cell acanthoma—a case report with review of the literature. Clin Exp Dermatol 19:249, 1994

50. Burg G, Wursch T, Fah J et al: Eruptive hamartomatous clear-cell acanthomas. Dermatology 189:437, 1994

51. Grunwald MH, Rothem A, Halevy S: Atypical clear cell acanthoma. Int J Dermatol 30:848, 1991

52. Desmons F, Breuillard F, Thomas P et al: Multiple clear-cell acanthoma: histochemical and ultrastructural study of two cases. Int J Dermatol 16:203, 1977

53. Hashimoto T, Inamoto N, Nakamura K: Two cases of clear cell acanthoma: an immunohistochemical study. J Cutan Pathol 15:27, 1988

54. Akiyama M, Hayakawa K, Watanabe Y et al: Lectin-binding sites in clear cell acanthoma. J Cutan Pathol 17:197, 1990

55. Langer K, Wuketich S, Konrad K: Pigmented clear cell acanthoma. Am J Dermatopathol 16:134, 1994

56. Anneroth A, Isacsson G: Warty dyskeratoma. Acta Dermato-Venereol 55:227, 1975

57. Niren NM, Waldman GD, Barsky S: Warty dyskeratoma. Cutis 29:79, 1982

58. Duray PH, Merino MJ, Axiotis C: Warty dyskeratoma of the vulva. Int J Gynecol Pathol 2:286, 1983

59. Kambic V, Gale N, Radsel Z: Warty dyskeratoma of the vocal cord: First reported case. Arch Otolaryngol 108:385, 1982

60. Azuma Y, Matsukawa A: Warty dyskeratoma with multiple lesions. J Dermatol 20:374, 1993

61. Laskaris G, Sklavounou A: Warty dyskeratoma of the oral mucosa. Br J Oral Maxillofac Surg 23:371, 1985

62. Kaugars GE, Lieb RJ, Abbey LM: Focal oral warty dyskeratoma. Int J Dermatol 23:123, 1984

63. Raff M, Szilvassy J: Specific dermatoglyphic patterns: a characteristic manifestation of acantholytic dyskeratotic dermatoses. J Am Acad Dermatol 21:958, 1989

64. Newland JR, Leventon GS: Warty dyskeratoma of the oral mucosa. Correlated light and electron microscopic study. Oral Surg Oral Med Oral Pathol 58:176, 1984

65. Krompecher E: Der Basalzellenkrebs. Jena, Fischer, 1903

66. Hyde JN, Montgomery FH: Diseases of the Skin. p. 669. 4th Ed. Lea Brothers, Philadelphia, 1897

67. Dellon AL: Host-tumor relationships in basal cell and squamous cell cancer of the skin. Plast Reconstr Surg 62:37, 1978

68. Hauben DJ, Zirkin H, Mahler D, Sacks M: The biologic behavior of basal cell carcinoma: part I. Plast Reconstr Surg 69:103, 1982

69. McGibbon DH: Malignant epidermal tumors. J Cutan Pathol 12:224, 1985

70. Wade TR, Ackerman AB: The many faces of basal cell carcinoma. J Dermatol Surg Oncol 4:23, 1978

71. Okun MR, Blumenthal G: Basal cell epithelioma with giant cells and nuclear atypicality. Arch Dermatol 89:598, 1964

72. Mehregan AH: Acantholysis in basal cell epithelioma. J Cutan Pathol 6:280, 1979

73. Siegle RJ, MacMillan J, Pollack SV: Infiltrative basal cell carcinoma: a nonsclerosing subtype. J Dermatol Surg Oncol 12:830, 1986

74. Jacobs GH, Rippey JJ, Altini M: Prediction of aggressive behavior in basal cell carcinoma. Cancer 49:533, 1982

75. Holmes EJ, Bennington JL, Haber SL: Citrulline-containing basal cell carcinomas. Cancer 22:663, 1968

76. Lerchin E, Rahbari H: Adamantinoid basal cell epithelioma: a histological variant. Arch Dermatol 111:586, 1975

77. Goette DK, Helwig EB: Basal cell carcinomas and basal cell carcinoma-like changes overlying dermatofibromas. Arch Dermatol 111:589, 1975

78. Ono T, Fallas VH, Higo J: Basal cell epithelioma with dermal melanocytes. J Dermatol 13:63, 1986

79. Rulon DB, Helwig EB: Cutaneous sebaceous neoplasms. Cancer 33:82, 1974

80. Borel DM: Cutaneous basosquamous carcinoma: review of the literature and report of 35 cases. Arch Pathol 95:293, 1973

81. DeFaria JL: Basal cell carcinoma of the skin with areas of squamous cell carcinoma: a basosquamous cell carcinoma? J Clin Pathol 38:1273, 1985

82. Gertler W: Zur Epithelverbundenheit der Basaliome. Dermatol Wochenschr 151:673, 1965

83. Montgomery H: Basal squamous cell epithelioma. Arch Dermatol Syphilol 18:50, 1928

84. Silverberg JW, Sherman G, Krause CJ: Cutaneous basosquamous carcinoma of the head and neck: a comparative analysis. Otolaryngol Head Neck Surg 87:420, 1979

85. Farmer ER, Helwig EB: Metastatic basal cell carcinoma: a clinicopathologic study of seventeen cases. Cancer 46:748, 1980

86. Quay SC, Harrist TJ, Mihm MC Jr: Carcinosarcoma of the skin: case report and review. J Cutan Pathol 8:241, 1981

87. Dawson EK: Carcinosarcoma of the skin. JR Coll Surg (Edinb) 17:242, 1972

88. Abram H, Barsky S: Pigmented basal cell epithelioma arising in the scar of an onchocerciasis nodule. Int J Dermatol 23:658, 1984

89. Domingo J, Helwig EB: Malignant neoplasms associated with nevus sebaceous of Jadassohn. J Am Acad Dermatol 1:545, 1979

90. Goldberg HS: Basal cell epitheliomas developing in a localized linear epidermal nevus. Cutis 25:295, 1980

91. Mikhail GR, Mehregan AH: Basal cell carcinoma in seborrheic keratosis. J Am Acad Dermatol 6:500, 1982

92. Rosenblum GA: Large basal cell carcinoma in a congenital nevus. J Dermatol Surg Oncol 12:166, 1986

93. Wick MR, Swanson PE: Primary adenoid cystic carcinoma of the skin. Am J Dermatopathol 8:2, 1986

94. Wolfe JT III, Wick MR, Campbell RJ: Sebaceous carcinomas of the oculocutaneous adnexa and extraocular skin. p. 77. In Wick MR (ed): Pathology of Unusual Malignant Cutaneous Tumors. Marcel Dekker, New York, 1985

95. Hashimoto K, Browenstein MH: Localized amyloidosis in basal cell epitheliomas. Acta Dermatol (Stockh) 53:331, 1973

96. Looi LM: Localized amyloidosis in basal cell carcinomas: a pathologic study. Cancer 52:1833, 1983

97. Masu S, Hosokawa M, Seiji M: Amyloid in localized cutaneous amyloidosis: immunofluorescence studies with anti-keratin antiserum, especially concerning the difference between systemic and localized cutaneous amyloidosis. Acta Dermatol (Stockh) 61:381, 1981

98. Brody I: Contributions to the histogenesis of basal cell carcinoma. J Ultrastruct Res 33:60, 1970

99. Dardi LE, Memoli VA, Gould VE: Neuroendocrine differentiation in basal cell carcinomas. J Cutan Pathol 8:335, 1981

100. Eusebi V, Mambelli V, Tison V et al: Endocrine differentiation in basal cell carcinoma. Tumori 65:191, 1979

101. Ishibashi A, Kasuga T, Tsuchiya E: Electron microscopic study of basal cell carcinoma. J Invest Dermatol 56:298, 1971

102. Kumakiri M, Hashimoto K: Ultrastructural resemblance of basal cell epithelioma to primary epithelial germ. J Cutan Pathol 5:53, 1978

103. Rupec M, Kint A, Himmelmann GW: On the occurrence of sphaeridia in basalioma cells and the basal cells of the overlying epidermis. Arch Dermatol Res 256:33, 1976

104. Kobayasi T: Dermo-epidermal junction in basal cell carcinoma. Acta Dermatol (Stockh) 50:401, 1970

105. Miettinen M, Lehto VP, Virtanen I: Antibodies to intermediate filament proteins: the differential diagnosis of cutaneous tumors. Arch Dermatol 121:736, 1985

106. Gatter KC, Pulford KAF, Van Stapel MJ et al: An immunohistological study of benign and malignant skin tumours: epithelial aspects. Histopathology 8:209, 1984

107. Thomas P, Said JW, Nash G, Banks-Schlegel S: Profiles of keratin proteins in basal and squamous cell carcinomas of the skin: an immunohistochemical study. Lab Invest 50:36, 1984

108. Wick MR, Kaye VN: The role of diagnostic immunohistochemistry in dermatology. Semin Dermatol 5:136, 1987

109. Dahl M: Beta-2-microglobulin in skin cancer. J Am Acad Dermatol 5:698, 1981

110. Jiminez FJ, Burchette JL Jr, Grichnik JM, Hitchcock MG: Ber-EP4 immunoreactivity in normal skin and cutaneous neoplasms. Mod Pathol 8:854–858, 1995

111. Claudy AL, Viac J, Schmitt D et al: Identification of mononuclear cells infiltrating basal cell carcinomas. Acta Dermatol (Stockh) 56:361, 1976

112. Kuflik EG: Basal cell carcinoma: an unusual clinical and histologic variant. J Dermatol Surg Oncol 6:730, 1980

113. Kuflik EG: Clinical variants of basal cell carcinoma. Cutis 28:403–408, 1981

114. Mehregan AH: Aggressive basal cell epithelioma on sunlight-protected skin: report of eight cases, one with pulmonary and bone metastases. Am J Dermatopathol 5:221, 1983

115. Perrone T, Twiggs LB, Adcock LL, Dehner LP: Vulvar basal cell carcinoma: an infrequently metastasizing neoplasm. Int J Gynecol Pathol (in press)

116. Robins P, Rabinovitz HS, Rigel D: Basal cell carcinomas on covered or unusual sites of the body. J Dermatol Surg Oncol 7:803, 1981

117. Black MM, Walkden VM: Basal cell carcinomatous changes on the lower leg: a possible association with chronic venous stasis. Histopathology 7:219, 1983

118. Peled IJ, Wexler MR: Symmetric basal cell carcinoma of the auricles. J Dermatol Surg Oncol 11:164, 1985

119. Lang PG Jr, Maize JC: Histologic evolution of recurrent basal cell carcinoma and treatment implications. J Am Acad Dermatol 14:186, 1986

120. Sloane JP: The value of typing basal cell carcinoma in predicting recurrence after surgical excision. Br J Dermatol 96:127, 1977

121. Dormarus HV, Stevens PJ: Metastatic basal cell carcinoma: report of five cases and review of 170 cases in the literature. J Am Acad Dermatol 10:1043, 1984

122. Menz J, Sterrett G, Wall L: Metastatic basal cell carcinoma associated with a small primary tumor. Aust J Dermatol 26:121, 1985

123. Scanlon EF, Volkmer DD, Oviedo MA et al: Metastatic basal cell carcinoma. J Surg Oncol 15:171, 1980

124. Morris JGL, Joffe R: Perineural spread of cutaneous basal and squamous cell carcinomas: The clinical appearance of spread into the trigeminal and facial nerves. Arch Neurol 40:424, 1983

125. Curson C, Weedon D: Spontaneous regression in basal cell carcinomas. J Cutan Pathol 6:432, 1979

126. Donatsky O, Hjorting-Hansen E, Philipsen HP, Fejerskov O: Clinical, radiologic, and histopathologic aspects of 13 cases of nevoid basal cell carcinoma syndrome. Int J Oral Surg 5:19, 1976

127. Lindeberg H, Jepsen FL: The nevoid basal cell carcinoma syndrome: histopathology of the basal cell tumors. J Cutan Pathol 10:68, 1983

128. Southwick GJ, Schwartz RA: The basal cell nevus syndrome. Cancer 44:2294, 1979
129. Rahbari H, Mehregan AH: Basal cell epithelioma (carcinoma) in children and adolescents. Cancer 49:350, 1982
130. Bleiberg J, Brodkin RH: Linear unilateral basal cell nevus with comedones. Arch Dermatol 100:187, 1969
131. Plosila M, Kiistala R, Niemi KM: The Bazex syndrome: follicular atrophoderma with multiple basal cell carcinomas, hypotrichosis, and hypohidrosis. Clin Exp Dermatol 6:31, 1981
132. Brownstein MH, Shapiro L: Desmoplastic trichoepithelioma. Cancer 40:2979, 1977
133. Wick MR, Scheithauer BW: Primary neuroendocrine carcinoma of the skin. p. 107. In Wick MR (ed): Pathology of Unusual Malignant Cutaneous Tumors. Marcel Dekker, New York, 1985
134. Sober AJ, Burstein JM: Precursors to skin cancer. Cancer 72:645, 1995
135. Beacham BE: Solar-induced epidermal tumors in the elderly. Am Fam Phys 42:153, 1990
136. Picascia DD, Robinson JK: Actinic cheilitis: a review of the etiology, differential diagnosis, and treatment. J Am Acad Dermatol 17:255, 1987
137. Priesto VG, Casal M, McNutt NS: Lichen planus-like keratosis. A clinical and histological reexamination. Am J Surg Pathol 17:259, 1993
138. Marks R, Rennie G, Selwood TS: Malignant transformation of solar keratoses to squamous cell carcinoma. Lancet 1:795, 1988
139. Marks R, Rennie G, Selwood T: The relationship of basal cell carcinomas and squamous cell carcinomas to solar keratoses. Arch Dermatol 124:1039, 1988
140. Dodson JM, DeSpain J, Hewett JE et al: Malignant potential of actinic keratoses and the controversy over treatment. A patient-oriented perspective. Arch Dermatol 127:1029, 1991
141. Marks R: The role of treatment of actinic keratoses in the prevention of morbidity and mortality due to squamous cell carcinoma. Arch Dermatol 127:1031, 1991
142. Battifora H: Spindle-cell carcinoma: ultrastructural evidence of squamous origin and collagen production by the tumor cells. Cancer 37:2275, 1976
143. Brownstein MH, Shapiro L: Verrucous carcinoma of skin: epithelioma cuniculatum plantare. Cancer 38:1710, 1976
144. Eusebi V, Ceccarelli C, Piscioli F et al: Spindle-cell tumours of the skin of debatable origin: an immunocytochemical study. J Pathol 144:189, 1984
145. Feldman PS, Barr RJ: Ultrastructure of spindle-cell squamous carcinoma. J Cutan Pathol 3:17, 1976
146. Johnson WC, Helwig EB: Adenoid squamous cell carcinoma. Cancer 19:1639, 1966
147. Kao GF, Graham JH, Helwig EB: Carcinoma cuniculatum (verrucous carcinoma of the skin): a clinicopathologic study of 46 cases with ultrastructural observations. Cancer 49:2395, 1982
148. Kuo TT: Clear-cell carcinoma of the skin: a variant of the squamous cell carcinoma that simulates sebaceous carcinoma. Am J Surg Pathol 4:573, 1980
149. Kuwano H, Hashimoto H, Enjoji M: Atypical fibroxanthoma distinguishable from spindle-cell carcinoma in sarcoma-like skin lesions. Cancer 55:172, 1985
150. Lichtiger B, Mackay B, Tessmer CF: Spindle-cell variant of squamous cell carcinoma: a light and electron microscopic study of 13 cases. Cancer 26:1311, 1970
151. McKee PH, Wilkinson JD, Corbett MF et al: Carcinoma cuniculatum: a case metastasizing to skin and lymph nodes. Clin Exp Dermatol 6:613, 1981
152. Broders AC: Squamous cell epithelioma of the skin. Ann Surg 73:141, 1921
153. Evans HL, Smith JL: Spindle-cell squamous carcinomas and sarcoma-like tumors of the skin: a comparative study of 38 cases. Cancer 45:2687, 1980
154. Strayer DS, Santa Cruz DJ: Carcinoma in situ of the skin: a review of histopathology. J Cutan Pathol 7:244, 1980
155. Jones RE Jr, Austin C, Ackerman AB: Extramammary Paget's disease: a critical reexamination. Am J Dermatopathol 1:101, 1979
156. Steffen C, Ackerman AB: Intraepidermal epithelioma of Borst-Jadassohn. Am J Dermatopathol 7:5, 1985
157. Fulling KH, Strayer DS, Santa Cruz DJ: Adnexal metaplasia in carcinoma in situ of the skin. J Cutan Pathol 8:79, 1981
158. Callen JP, Headington JT: Bowen's disease and non-Bowen's squamous intraepidermal neoplasia of the skin. Arch Dermatol 116:422, 1980
159. Graham JH, Helwig EB: Bowen's disease and its relationship to systemic cancer. Arch Dermatol 80:133, 1959
160. Lever WF: Adenoacanthoma of sweat glands. Arch Dermatol Syphilol 56:157, 1947
161. Gomez LG, DiMaio S, Silva EG, Mackay B: Association between neuroendocrine (Merkel cell) carcinoma and squamous carcinoma of the skin. Am J Surg Pathol 7:171, 1983
162. Silva EG, Mackay B, Goepfert H, et al: Endocrine carcinoma of the skin (Merkel cell carcinoma). Pathol Annu 19:1, 1984
163. Balazs M: Buschke-Lowenstein tumour: a histologic and ultrastructural study of six cases. Virchows Arch Pathol Anat 410:83, 1986
164. Perez-Mesa CA, Kraus FT, Evans JC, Powers WE: Anaplastic transformation in verrucous carcinoma of the oral cavity after radiation therapy. Radiology 86:108, 1966
165. Chernosky ME, Rapini RP: Squamous cell carcinoma in lesions of disseminated superficial actinic porokeratosis: a report of two cases. Arch Dermatol 122:853, 1986
166. Davidson TM, Bone RC, Kiessling PJ: Epidermoid carcinoma arising from within an epidermoid inclusion cyst. Ann Otol Rhinol Laryngol 85:417, 1976
167. Garret AB: Multiple squamous cell carcinomas in lesions of discoid lupus erythematosus. Cutis 36:313, 1985
168. Grussendorf EI, Gahlen W: Metaplasia of a verruca vulgaris into spinocellular carcinoma. Dermatologica 150:295, 1975
169. Levin A, Amazon K, Rywlin AM: A squamous cell carcinoma that developed in an epidermal nevus: report of a case and review of the literature. Am J Dermatopathol 6:51, 1984
170. Peralta OC, Barr RJ, Romansky SG: Mixed carcinoma in situ: an immunohistochemical study. J Cutan Pathol 10:350, 1983
171. Fukamizu H, Inoue K, Matsumoto K et al: Metastatic squamous cell carcinomas derived from solar keratoses. J Dermatol Surg Oncol 11:518, 1985
172. Moller R, Reymann F, Hou-Jensen K: Metastases in dermatological patients with squamous cell carcinoma. Arch Dermatol 115:703, 1979
173. Hutchinson J: Morbid growth and tumors. 1. The "crateriform ulcer of the face" a form of acute epithelial cancer. Trans Pathol Soc Lond 40:275, 1889

174. Schwartz RA: Keratoacanthoma. J Am Acad Dermatol 30:1, 1994

175. Habel G, O'Regan B, Eissing A et al: Intra-oral keratoacanthoma: an eruptive variant and review of the literature. Br Dent J 170:336, 1991

176. Lovett JE, Haines TA, Bentz ML et al: Subungual keratoacanthoma masquerading as a chronic paronychia. Ann Plast Surg 34:84, 1995

177. Chuang TY, Reizner GT, Elpern DJ et al: Keratoacanthoma in Kauai, Hawaii. The first documented incidence in a defined population. Arch Dermatol 129:317, 1993

178. Jordan RC, Kahn HJ, From L et al: Immunohistochemical demonstration of actinically damaged elastic fibers in keratoacanthomas: an aid in diagnosis. J Cutan Pathol 18:81, 1991

179. Calonje E, Jones EW: Intravascular spread of keratoacanthoma. An alarming but benign phenomenon. Am J Dermatopathol 14:414, 1992

180. Ho T, Horn T, Finzi E: Transforming growth factor alpha expression helps to distinguish keratoacanthomas from squamous cell carcinomas. Arch Dermatol 127:1167, 1991

181. Phillips P, Helm KF: Proliferating cell nuclear antigen distribution in keratoacanthoma and squamous cell carcinoma. J Cutan Pathol 20:424, 1993

182. Toker C: Trabecular carcinoma of the skin. Arch Pathol 105:107, 1972

183. Kuhajda FP, Olson JL, Mann RB: Merkel cell (small cell) carcinoma of the skin: immunohistochemical and ultrastructural demonstration of distinctive perinuclear cytokeratin aggregates and a possible association with B-cell neoplasms. Histochem J 18:239, 1986

184. Stern JB: "Murky cell" carcinoma (formerly trabecular carcinoma). Am J Dermatopathol 4:517, 1982

185. Warner TFCS, Uno H, Hafez R et al: Merkel cells and Merkel cell tumors. Ultrastructure, immunocytochemistry, and review of the literature. Cancer 52:238, 1983

186. Hartschuh W, Weihe E, Yanihara N, Reinecke M: Immunohistochemical localization of vasoactive intestinal polypeptide (VIP) in Merkel cells of various animals: evidence for a neuromodulator function of the Merkel cell. J Invest Dermatol 81:361, 1983

187. Sibley RK, Dahl D: Neuroendocrine (Merkel cell?) carcinoma of the skin. II. An immunohistochemical study of 21 cases. Am J Surg Pathol 9:109, 1985

188. Frigerio B, Capella C, Eusebi V et al: Merkel cell carcinoma of the skin: the structure and function of normal Merkel cells. Histopathology 7:229, 1983

189. Battifora H, Silva EG: The use of antikeratin antibodies in the immunohistochemical distinction between neuroendocrine (Merkel cell) carcinoma of the skin, lymphoma, and oat-cell carcinoma. Cancer 58:1040, 1986

190. Saurat JH, Didierjean L, Skalli O et al: The intermediate filament proteins of rabbit normal epidermal Merkel cells are cytokeratins. J Invest Dermatol 83:431, 1984

191. Sibley RK, Dehner LP, Rosai J: Neuroendocrine (Merkel cell?) carcinoma of the skin. I. Clinicopathologic and ultrastructural study of 43 cases. Am J Surg Pathol 9:95, 1985

192. Wick MR, Millns JL, Sibley RK et al: Secondary neuroendocrine carcinomas of the skin: an immunohistochemical comparison with primary neuroendocrine carcinomas of the skin ("Merkel cell carcinomas"). J Am Acad Dermatol 13:134, 1985

193. Gould VE, Moll R, Moll I et al: Neuroendocrine (Merkel) cells of the skin: hyperplasias, dysplasias, and neoplasms. Lab Invest 52:334, 1985

194. Van Dijk C, Ten Seldam REJ: A possible primary cutaneous carcinoid. Cancer 36:1016, 1975

195. Smith PA, Chappell RH: Another possible primary carcinoid tumor of skin? Virchows Arch Pathol Anat 408:99, 1985

196. Wick MR, Thomas JR III, Scheithauer BW, Jackson I: Multifocal Merkel's cell tumors associated with a cutaneous dysplasia syndrome. Arch Dermatol 119:409, 1983

197. Hoefler H, Kerl H, Rauch HJ, Denk H: New immunocytochemical observations with diagnostic significance in cutaneous neuroendocrine carcinoma. Am J Dermatopathol 6:525, 1984

198. Drijkoningen M, DeWolf-Peeters C, Van Limberger E, Desmet V: Merkel cell tumor of the skin: an immunohistochemical study. Hum Pathol 17:301, 1986

199. Haimoto H, Takahashi Y, Koshikawa T et al: Immunohistochemical localization of gamma-enolase in normal human tissues other than nervous and neuroendocrine tissues. Lab Invest 52:257, 1985

200. Layfield L, Ulich T, Liao S et al: Neuroendocrine carcinoma of the skin: an immunohistochemical study of tumor markers and neuroendocrine products. J Cutan Pathol 13:268, 1986

201. Katenkamp D, Watzig V: Multiple neuroendocrine carcinomas (so-called Merkel cell tumors) of the skin: report on two cases with unique clinical course. Virchows Arch Pathol Anat 404:403, 1984

202. O'Rourke MGE, Bell JR: Merkel cell tumor with spontaneous regression. J Dermatol Surg Oncol 12:994, 1986

18

ADNEXAL TUMORS

It has been argued that as most adnexal neoplasms are benign or only locally aggressive, it is not important to know classifications which may at times seem mind-boggling. However, one has only to remember the acrospiroma, calcifying epithelioma, or spiradenoma, misidentified by the uninformed as metastatic carcinoma, to appreciate the importance of being familiar with these tumors.[1]

Ronald J. Barr

An adnexal neoplasm or malformation resembles one or more types of adnexal epithelium or stroma found in fetal or normal skin. Adnexal tumors can be solitary or multiple, benign or malignant. Some can occur as part of a syndrome (Appendix 18-1).

By light microscopy, adnexal tumors can be grouped into four major categories based on their similarity to adnexal structures: hair cortex and hair follicles, sebaceous glands, apocrine glands, and eccrine glands. However, any individual lesion can contain one or more lines of differentiation. In such a case, it is commonly classified by its dominant component(s). Depending on the clinicopathologic context, statements regarding its morphologic variations may be included, as appropriate, in a pathology report.

No classification of adnexal proliferations can capture fully the rich variation of these lesions that is seen in nature, but the essence of each category can be stated, or at least *indicated,* with some clarity. In addition to the usual solid and papillary adnexal tumors, this chapter also includes a separate section on cysts, selected lesions of the nail, and a tabular summary of syndromes containing adnexal tumors (Appendix 18-1), as well as an approach to the diagnosis of some adnexal tumors (Appendix 18-2).

ADNEXAL TUMORS WITH HAIR AND/OR HAIR FOLLICLE DIFFERENTIATION

Hair and hair follicle tumors resemble one or more portions of the hair cortex/medulla, the hair follicle,[2] and the perifollicular fibrous sheath.

Benign Hair/Hair Follicle Tumors

Proliferations Differentiated Toward All Portions of The Hair/Hair Follicle

Hair Nevi

Nevus, or hamartoma, in this context, implies that hairs are present in the proper dermal location but have an abnormal number, morphology, or relation to the adjacent normal skin. Hair nevi include a wide spectrum of lesions that range from small tumor-like malformations, to large patches or plaques in which a different morphologic type of hair is present,[3,4] to a generalized abnormality. The term *nevus* is usually applied to congenital conditions, while *hamartoma* is reserved for acquired conditions. These distinctions, however, have not been followed strictly in naming the lesions; thus, some nevi and hamartomas may overlap conceptually with lesions typically designated as neoplasms. The lesions in this short list include a few that illustrate part of spectrum and is not meant to be all inclusive. In addition, some lesions could be classified under other categories in which there is histologic similarity. Excluded from this discussion is organoid (sebaceous) nevus (discussed below) because all of its adnexal and epidermal components make it a complex nevus/hamartoma deserving special attention.

Perhaps the simplest form of hair malformation is the localized and excessive production of thick, scalp-like, terminal hairs; this is termed *nevus pilosus,* and it may be associated with a melanocytic nevus or a Becker's nevus, the latter of which is a macular lesion located usually on the trunk.[5] The pigmented macule of *Becker's nevus* contains long hairs in approximately half of the cases[6]; those with coarse, disorganized dermal smooth muscle fascicles have sometimes been termed *smooth muscle hamartomas* (see below). Some Becker's nevi may also contain acneiform lesions.[7]

Occasionally, patches of hair may have a different color or texture than surrounding normal scalp. *Poliosis* refers to a tuft of white hair in otherwise normal-colored scalp hair. The *woolly hair nevus* is a patch of tightly curled hair in normally straight scalp hair.[8–10] The reverse situation is termed *straight hair nevus*.[11,12] The growth of tightly packed miniature hairs is termed *hair follicle nevus* or *vellus hamartoma*.[13,14]

Nevus comedonicus[15–18] is a patch or plaque, often linear, that occurs most commonly on the neck, trunk, or upper limbs of young persons. Histologically, it is composed of multiple, closely packed, widened infundibula, similar to comedones. Some individual comedones may have features similar to a dilated pore (Winer). Occasionally, nevus comedonicus may coexist with a Becker's nevus, epidermolytic hyperkeratosis, or other conditions.[19,20]

Some hamartomatous conditions are complex in nature and contain follicular hamartomas as only part of the condition; such is the case of patients with *Bazex syndrome,* who have follicular atrophoderma and hypotrichosis. Histologically, a proliferation of small buds of basaloid cells is present around follicular structures.[21–23] *Haber syndrome,* by contrast, presents as a rosacea-like dermatosis with pitted lesions and similar basaloid follicular buddings.[24,25]

Patients with a *generalized hair follicle hamartoma* (basaloid follicular hamartoma)[26–29] may also have alopecia, aminoaciduria, and myasthenia gravis. Histologically, the alopecia corresponds to multiple malformed tumors connected to or replacing individual pilar units. The lesions are pan-follicular but, in individual cases, are similar to lesions within the classic trichoepithelioma and tricholemmoma groups. Rarely, localized forms with these patterns occur.[30]

Trichofolliculoma

Trichofolliculoma is a category of tumors composed of hair follicles that contain hairs. These radiate around one or more cyst-like dilation(s) that often open to the skin surface.

Trichofolliculoma often presents as a small facial nodule, sometimes covered by normal skin. At times, it may have a small central epidermal ostium. Not uncommonly, a whisker of white hair emerges from it; less commonly, large hairs may grow from the entire surface. Trichofolliculomas may develop at any age, but are most commonly diagnosed in the second decade.[31–35] Because many of these may be nodular and without an ostium, the differential diagnosis includes a wide variety of tumors and tumor-like conditions.

Microscopically, most trichofolliculomas are composed of a centrally dilated squamous epithelial-lined cyst that is occasionally connected to the epidermis. The central cyst contains lamellar, orthokeratotic keratin, and the lining has prominent granular cell layers. Hairs may be present within the cystic lumen. Although most lesions have only one cystic cavity, some are multilocular (Fig. 18-1A). Branchings, often in the pattern of a spoke-wheel, from these cysts are many well-differentiated structures with follicular differentiation, resembling any portion of the hair follicle or the sebaceous gland. These structures range from projections of mature, follicular epithelium (Fig. 18-1B) with minimal follicular germinal elements to well-formed miniature hairs, all of which may occur within a single tumor.[36] Many of these structures have secondary buddings that contain small hair germs. Small lobules of sebaceous glands may be present in a minority of the cases. On rare occasions, the development of sebaceous lobules is prominent, resulting in a lesion

with a remarkable degree of maturity, resembling a dermoid cyst and termed *sebaceous trichofolliculoma*.[37,38] Also included within the spectrum of the sebaceous variant are lesions termed *folliculosebaceous cystic hamartoma*.[39,40] At the other end of the spectrum, few hairs may be present; instead, simple squamous strands or buds are present. It is proper, however, to include such tumors within the category of pilar sheath acanthoma[41] unless prominent sebaceous or germinal portions of the hair follicle are identified.

Trichoepithelioma

Trichoepitheliomas are a spectrum of benign follicular or corticofollicular epithelial-germ-stromal tumors containing epithelial structures that are similar to all parts of a hair follicle and may include cortex in some cases. Some variants within the group, however, are composed predominantly of a particular aspect of the follicle. The spectrum consists of four principal subgroups, designated as classic, trichoblastic or germinal, tricho "adenoma" (mostly infundibular), and desmoplastic (sclerotic).

Classic Trichoepithelioma. The classic trichoepithelioma[42–44] can occur as a familial multiple form (epithelioma adenoides cysticum) or as a solitary lesion. The multiple form develops during adolescence or adulthood and usually has a central facial distribution; the gene for it maps to chromosome 9p21.[45] Solitary tumors occur anywhere on hairy skin, but the head and neck are the most common sites. Rarely, trichoepitheliomas are associated with other tumors and syndromes.[46–57]

Histologically, classic trichoepithelioma is a symmetric lesion (Fig. 18-2A) that contains a mixture of epithelial elements ranging from hair germs,[58] to small horn cysts, to lace-like reticular basaloid structures (Fig. 18-2B), and, rarely, to mature hairs. A key feature is that all portions of the follicle coexist within the lesion.

The stroma containing these structures is typically fibrotic, architecturally uniform from area to area, and directly contacts the tumor, in contrast with the retraction artifact of basal cell carcinoma. In some lesions, reactions such as keratin granulomas can occur secondary to rupture of horn cysts. Rarely, trichoepitheliomas are associated with basal cell carcinoma.

Trichoblastic Trichoepithelioma. In trichoblastic or germinal follicular tumors[59–61] the epithelial elements are predominately hair germs (trichoblasts) associated with a prominent stromal component usually. The nomenclature of the variations within this group depends on the amount of stroma, the number of hair germs, and any other epithelial elements that are present within an individual lesion.

Clinically, the lesions are solitary and frequently are located in the deep dermis or subcutis, usually on the extremities, trunk, or in the pelvic region,[62] but some involve the head and neck.[63] Most are less than 1 cm in greatest dimension, but a few are up to several centimeters in diameter.[64–66] Most are papules or dome-shaped tumors, but rarely are plaques.[63] They typically "shell out" easily and are cured by local excision. The clinical differential diagnosis is usually nonspecific.

Histologically, the lesions are almost always well circumscribed. Few tumors contain horn cysts, unlike the classic trichoepithelioma. The most primitive lesion, the *trichoblas-*

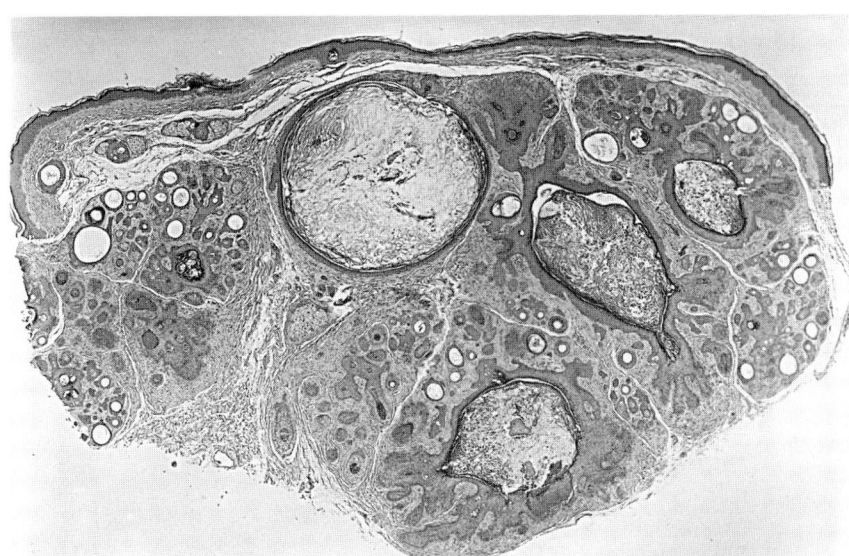

A

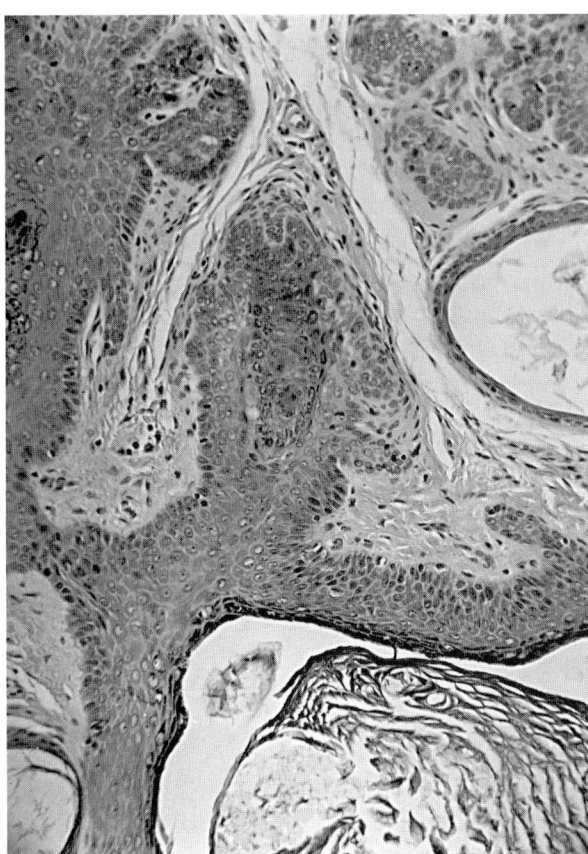

B

Figure 18-1. Trichofolliculoma. (**A**) This lesion contains several small cysts lined by infundibular epithelium and surrounded by several small vellus hair follicles. (× 36.) (**B**) Note at higher power that some of the small follicles display inner and outer sheath, while others are mostly basaloid and incompletely developed. (× 250.)

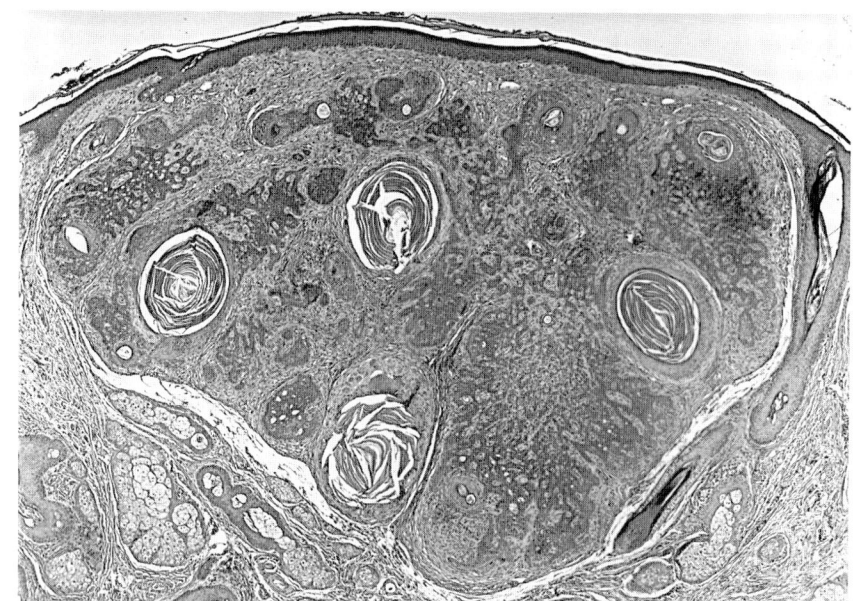

A

Figure 18-2. Trichoepithelioma, classic type. (**A**) Scanning magnification reveals a symmetric lesion of reticular, lace-like basaloid lobules as well as numerous cysts, all within a fibrous stroma demarcated from the surrounding dermis. (× 42.) (**B**) Higher power reveals the prominent lace-like pattern of the basaloid cells. Note the expanded follicular papilla. (× 300.)

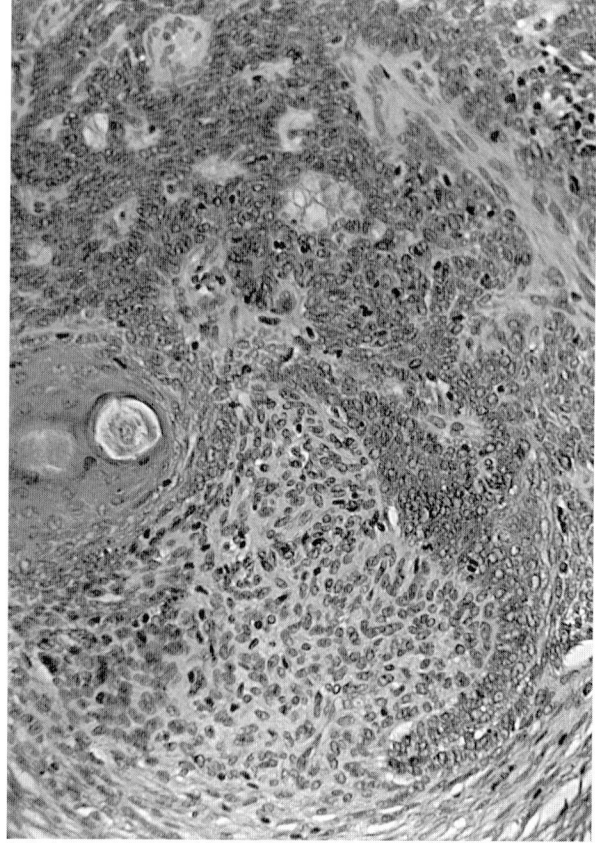

B

toma,[59] consists predominantly of basaloid hair germ-like epithelium (Fig. 18-3A). The follicular papillae are not uniformly distributed in relation to the basaloid cells (Fig. 18-3B) and can sometimes be mistaken for unusual basal cell carcinomas.[67] The *trichogerminoma*[68] is a circumscribed tumor composed of basaloid "cell balls" that are similar to follicular bulbs. They may contain foci of trichohyalin, clear cell change, and small micro-

keratocysts. *Trichoblastic fibromas*[63,69–71] are lesions with some degree of maturity (i.e., they exhibit stromal differentiation and hair germs with follicular papillae [Fig. 18-4A] so that they overlap conceptually with trichogerminoma). Trichoblastic fibromas range from those with only hair germs and stroma[72] (Fig. 18-4B) to those with stroma, hair germs, basaloid strands, and lace-like, epithelial components[73] (Fig. 18-4C). The most

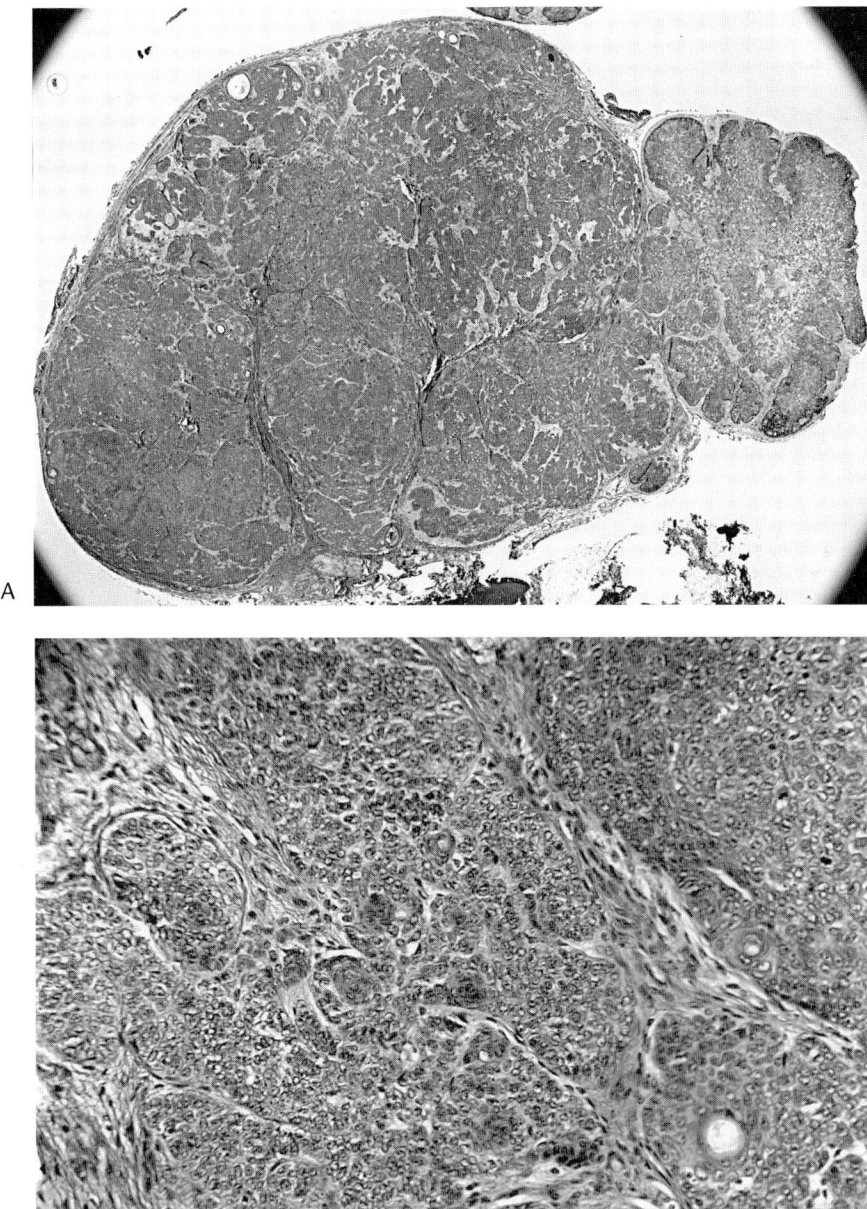

Figure 18-3. Trichoblastoma. (**A**) The scanning power of this lesion reveals a sharply circumscribed tumor composed of basaloid cells and minimal stroma. (× 12.) (**B**) At higher power, there are no clearly formed trichoblasts, but the cells have the pattern of the germ and the stroma is minimal but is similar to the perifollicular stroma. A few whirls of epithelial cells are also present. (× 250.)

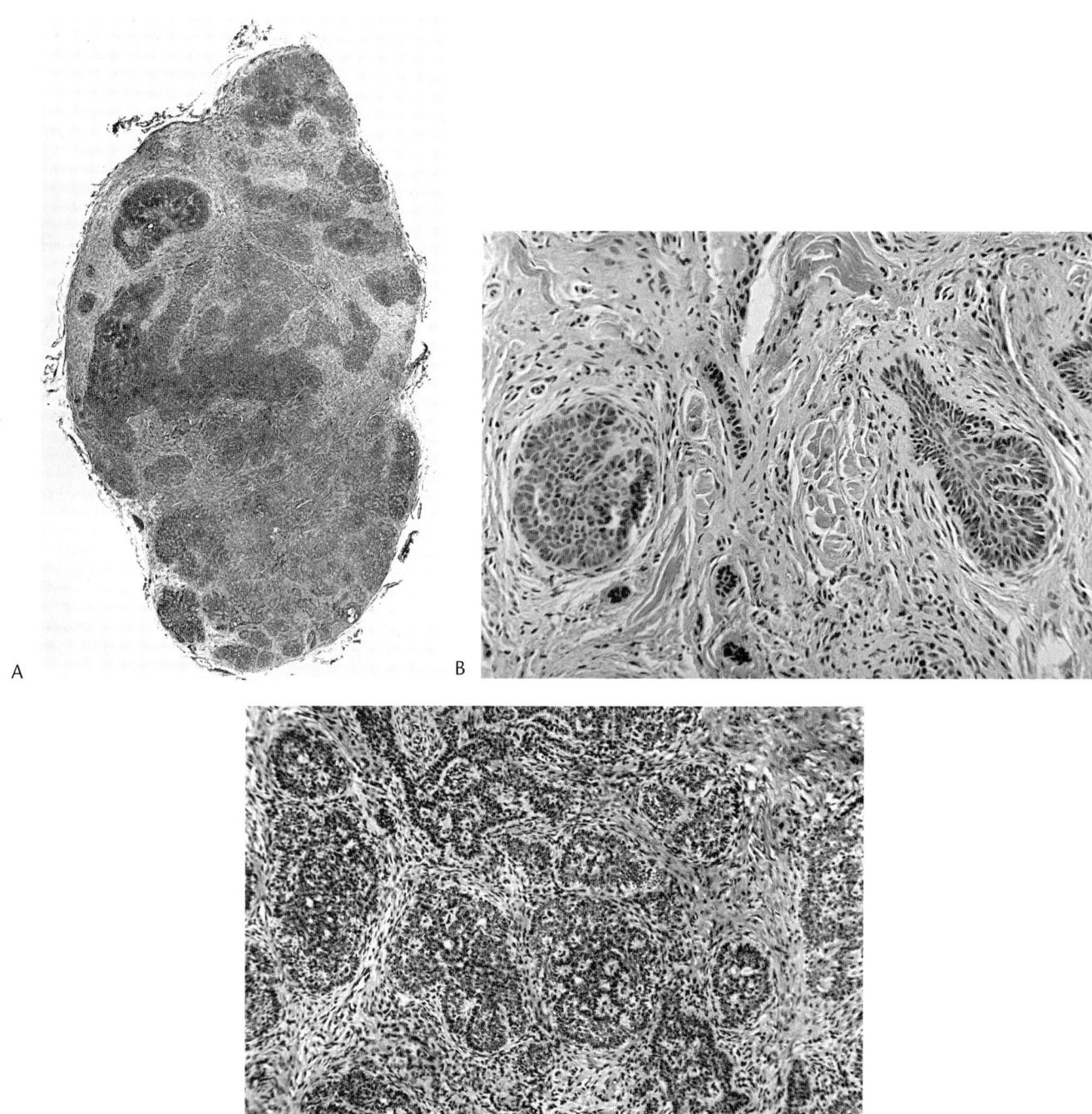

Figure 18-4. Trichoblastic fibroma. (**A**) Scanning magnification reveals a discrete nodule of fibrosis and basaloid cells, some of which have lace-like patterns. Not only are these lesions commonly located in the superficial subcutis, but they also may be found in the dermis where they often "scoop out." (× 20.) (**B**) Some trichoblastic fibromas contain mostly trichoblasts and dense stroma, such as in this example, which occurred entirely in the dermis. (× 275.) (**C**) At high power, there is often wide variation, but the lace-like epithelial zones are common and are often surrounded by layers of concentric mesenchyme similar to the follicular papilla. (× 150.)

mature tumor in the trichoblastic group is the *trichogenic trichoblastoma*,[74] which is similar to the trichoblastoma, but, in addition, contains complete hair follicles and occasionally hair cortex.[59,75] *Cutaneous lymphadenoma*[76–84] has been proposed as an unusual adamantinoid type of trichoblastoma[83,84] (Fig. 18-5), but this classification may be premature. Unusual mucinous trichoblastic lesions of the skin that also contain hair germs are termed *trichogenic myxomas* (superficial angiomyxoma)[85] (Fig. 18-6). The principal differential diagnoses for any of these lesions rest between classic trichoepithelioma and basal cell carcinomas.

Trichoadenoma (Nikolowski)[86–88] is not an adenoma, but a spectrum of follicular proliferations with prominent cystic spaces confined to a fibrotic stroma. These lesions are similar to the infundibular portion of the hair follicle, rather than the germinal portion, although germs may be present in some cases. Clinically, trichoadenomas are usually nodular or verrucous.

Histologically, trichoadenoma is a symmetric lesion with a mixture of circular horn cysts that may or may not be connected by strands of basaloid cells (Fig. 18-7). Occasionally, keratin granulomas are present if the horn cysts rupture. Sometimes the lesions are surfaced by verrucous hyperplasia.

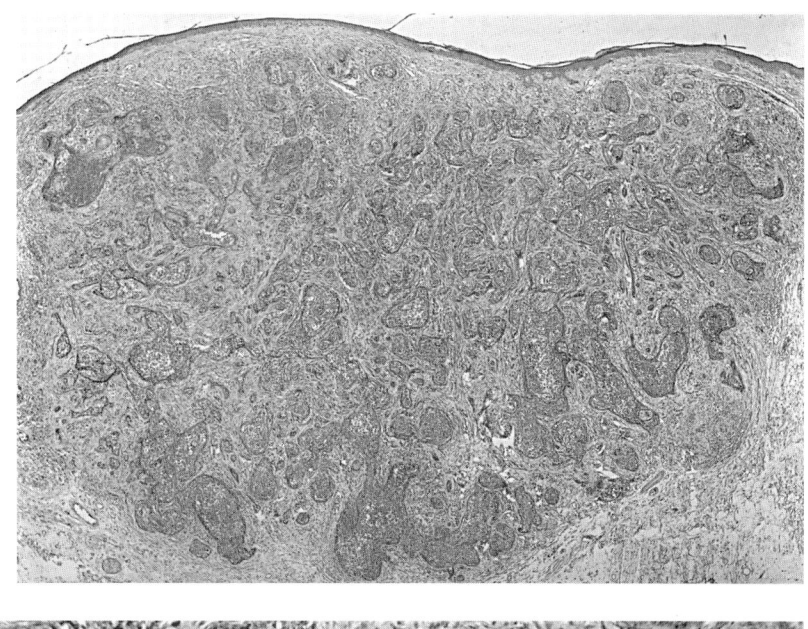

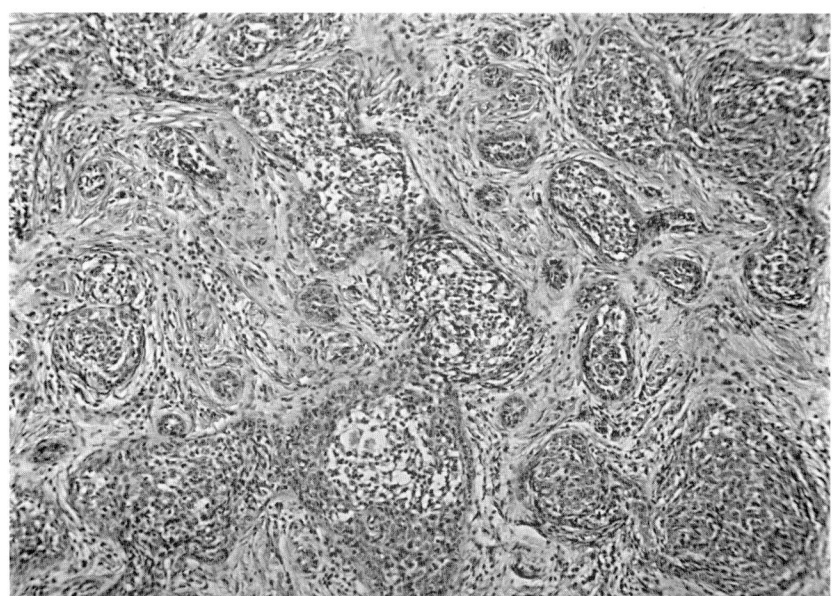

Figure 18-5. Cutaneous lymphadenoma. (**A**) On scanning magnification, the lesion is symmetric and composed of small insula of epithelial cells containing numerous lymphoid cells. (× 32.) (**B**) At high power, a thin layer of epithelial cells can be seen at the periphery of each insular nest. The desmoplastic stroma that surrounds the epithelial islands is similar to that of a trichoblastic tumor. (× 150.) (Courtesy of Evaristo Sánchez Yus, M.D., Madrid, Spain.)

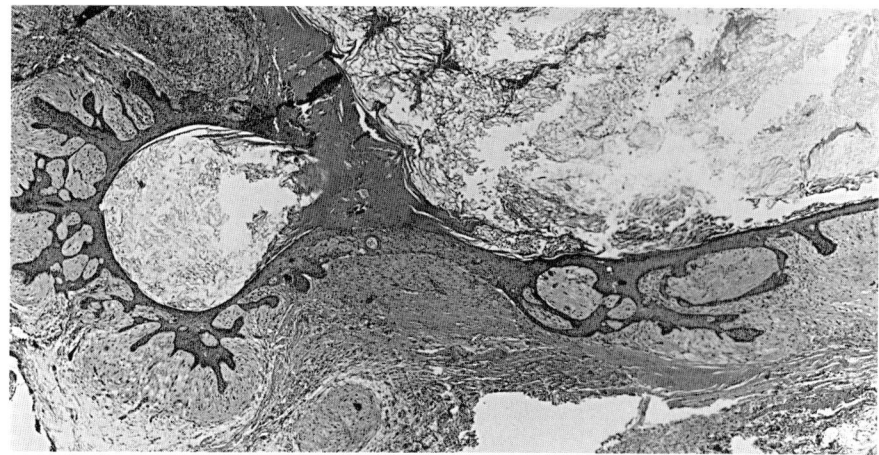

Figure 18-6. Trichogenic myxoma. This myxomatous lesion occurred in conjunction with a follicular cyst. Note the trichofolliculoma-like buddings into the mucin pools from the small cyst. (× 38.)

Desmoplastic trichoepithelioma (sclerotic epithelial hamartoma)[89,90] is a spectrum of symmetric, well-demarcated tumors composed of compressed follicular epithelium within a desmoplastic dermis. The subcutis is usually not involved.

The lesions are usually solitary, but rarely can be multiple. Familial cases of both types have been reported.[91,92] They usually occur on the cheeks of women in the third decade. Most are less than 1 cm in diameter and have a central depression or dell.[93] Local excision is curative. The principal clinical differ-

ential diagnoses include morpheic basal cell carcinoma and microcystic adnexal carcinoma.

Histologically, they are symmetric with a well-demarcated, fibrotic zone that separates the tumor from the normal skin (Fig. 18-8A). Superficially, in addition to the compressed epithelial strands, there can be small horn cysts and keratin granulomas if the cysts are ruptured. Small hair germs can be identified occasionally (Fig. 18-8B & C). Although eccrine glands can be present within the tumor, these are involved only secondarily. Im-

Figure 18-7. Tricho "adenoma." Scanning magnification reveals a tumor of infundibular and isthmic follicular epithelium with numerous, variably sized horn cysts, some of which mature through a granular zone and some of which do not. There may be occasional hair germs in such tumors, but they are not as numerous as the trichoblastic end of the trichoepithelioma spectrum. Note also that the stroma is intimately related to the epithelial structures. (× 90.)

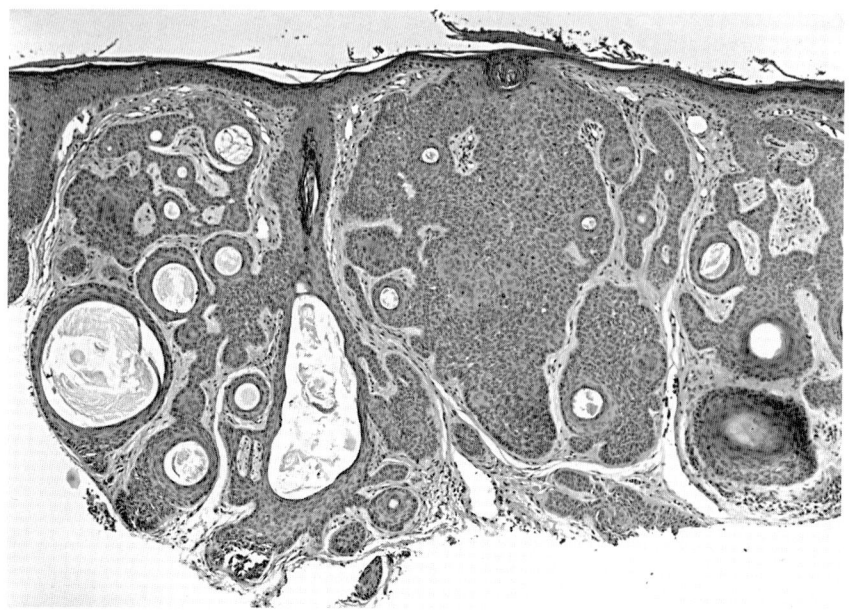

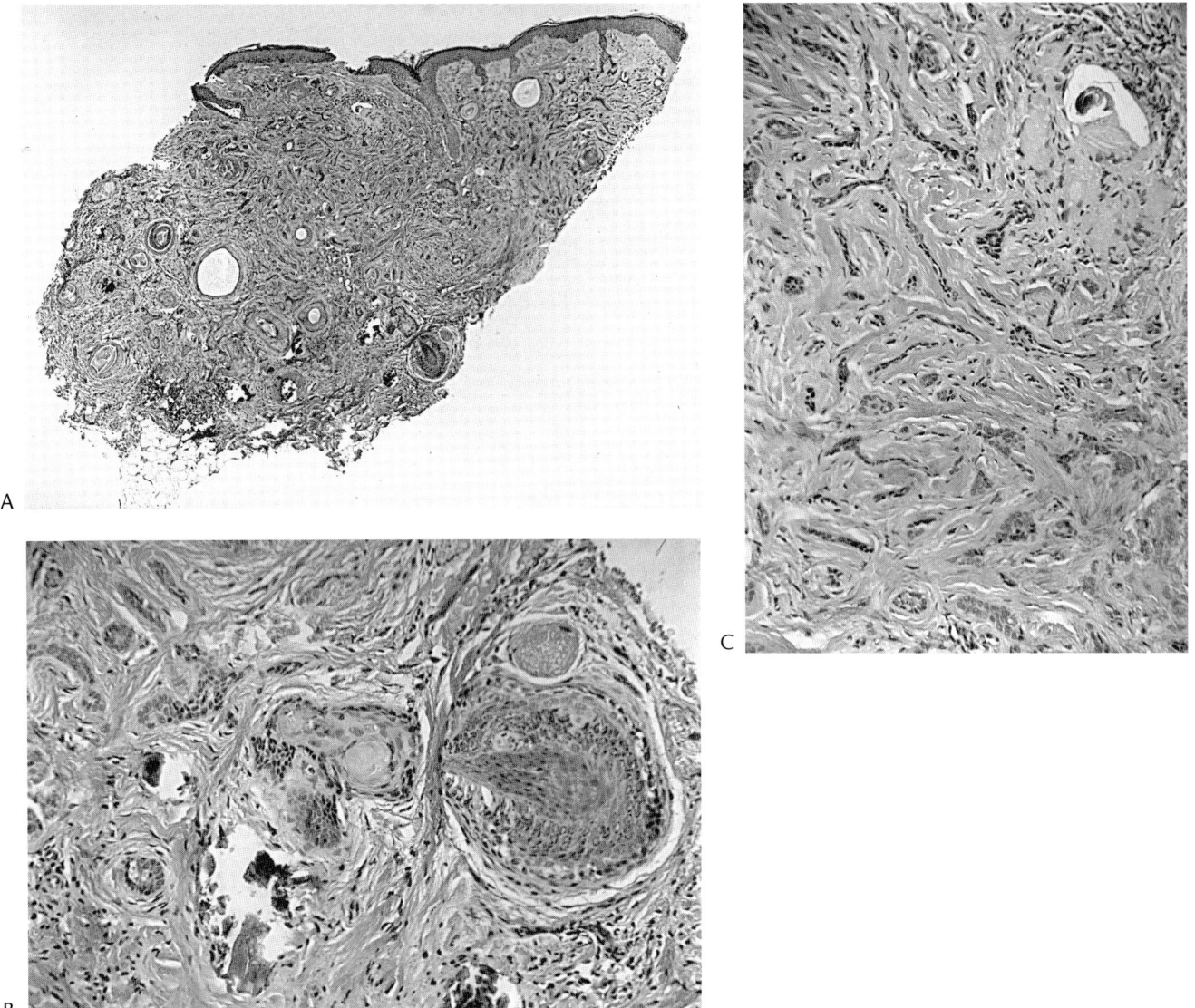

Figure 18-8. Desmoplastic trichoepithelioma. (**A**) This lesion contains uniformly compressed basaloid epithelial cords within a dense stroma. Note that there are a few horn cysts as well as focal calcification. ($\times$ 45.) (**B**) Higher power reveals a hair germ with inner and outer sheath adjacent to a focus of calcification. ($\times$ 250.) (**C**) Many of the epithelial structures are compressed, but are similar to portions of the isthmus. One small focus in this field simulates a germ. ($\times$ 250.)

munohistochemically, cytokeratins are positive in these lesions. In addition, CD34 is positive in the stroma of most desmoplastic trichoepitheliomas, an important contrast with lesions of microcystic adnexal carcinoma and morpheic basal cell carcinoma.[94] However, it should not be used as the sole criterion for diagnosis,[95] and a negative CD34 does not exclude desmoplastic trichoepithelioma.

The differential diagnosis includes morpheic basal cell carcinoma, microcystic adnexal carcinoma, and metastatic carcinoma (particularly of the breast), each of which can have asymmetry, heterogeneous patterns of dermal sclerosis, and subcutaneous involvement. The assessment of a superficial shave biopsy specimen, therefore, should be evaluated with caution because such specimens can contain areas within which benign and malignant tumors cannot be distinguished sufficiently.

Proliferations Differentiated Toward Specific Portions of The Hair/Hair Follicle

Permanent Follicular Sheath

Infundibular and isthmic tumors include a variety of lesions composed of epithelium similar to the infundibular and isthmic portions of the hair follicle. They range from widened infundibular ostia lacking pronounced epithelial proliferation (dilated pore), to vertically oriented, patulous pores combined with lobules of solid to cystic infundibular and isthmic epithelium (pilar sheath acanthoma), to cysts (seborrheic keratosis-like cyst). While these groups are often separated in the literature, the feature of infundibular and/or isthmic follicular epithelium is fundamental to them all and serves to unite them conceptually.

Tumor of The Follicular Infundibulum. Tumor of the follicular infundibulum (parallel plate-like isthmicoma)[96–103] is a plate-like proliferation of monomorphous, isthmic cells that parallels the skin surface and connects with it at intervals. Because of the isthmic differentiation pattern of these lesions, they should probably be renamed accordingly.

Clinically, the tumors are small papules or plaques that can be single or multiple,[103–110] and the latter can be associated rarely with basal cell carcinoma or Cowden's syndrome.[103,111] They are commonly located on the head and neck of elderly persons, but can also occur on the trunk. The differential diagnosis includes basal cell carcinoma, tinea versicolor, and disseminated superficial actinic porokeratosis.

Histologically, the tumors are symmetric, with a plate-like growth, and are composed of isthmic cells with a uniform nucleus and amphophilic cytoplasm (Fig. 18-9). A thick periodic acid-Schiff (PAS)-positive basement membrane typically invests the lesion. Small orthokeratotic microcavities can be present within the hyperplastic epithelium. No maturation through a granular zone is present. In reconstructions of multiple levels through these lesions, numerous perforating connections to the epidermis are observed. Ductal elements have been described in a few cases.[112] A rich elastic stroma is present just below the epithelial component. The differential diagnosis includes plaque-like seborrheic keratosis, solar keratosis, and superficial basal cell carcinoma.

Dilated Pore (Winer). Dilated pore (Winer)[113,114] refers to a sac-like lesion that is usually solitary and connects to the epidermis by a small to large, dilated follicular ostium. It usually occurs on the upper lip of adults but can be found at other sites. Rarely, it exists as a nevoid growth.[18] The clinical differential diagnosis includes a comedone and basal cell carcinoma.

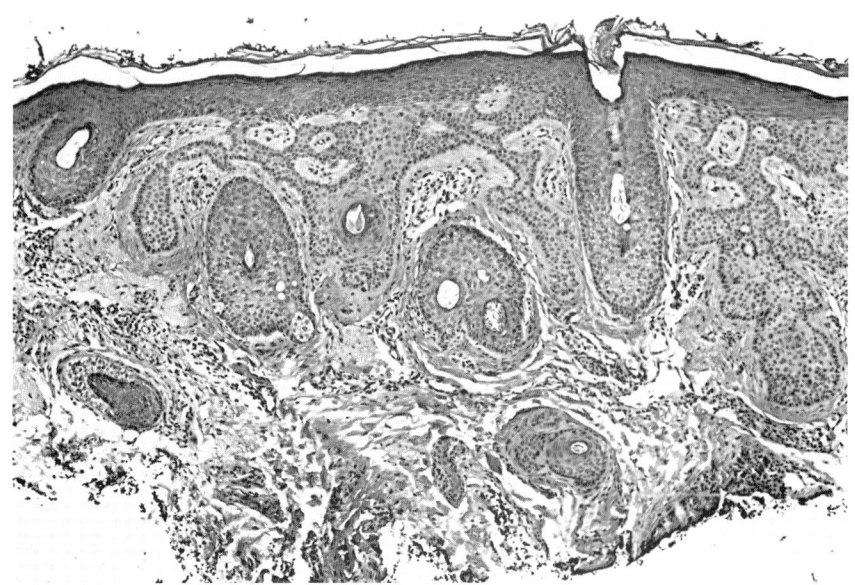

Figure 18-9. Tumor of follicular infundibulum (isthmicoma). This tumor is a hamartomatous proliferation of epithelial cells similar in quality to the isthmic portion of the hair follicle. Note the periodic connections to the surface epithelium. Three-dimensional constructions prove that such tumors have a plate-like pattern parallel to the surface epithelium. (× 90.)

Histologically, it is a simple funnel-shaped structure that is deep within the dermis, but open to the surface (Fig. 18-10). It is lined by infundibular epithelium and filled with dense, lamellar, orthokeratotic keratin. There is a range of acanthosis of the lining epithelium, but it is not pronounced in most cases.

The dilated pore should be distinguished from a comedo and unusual cases of pilar sheath acanthoma. Some tangentially sectioned cases can appear cystic and are similar to so-called seborrheic keratosis-like cysts.

Pilar Sheath Acanthoma. Pilar sheath acanthoma (lobular infundibuloisthmicoma)[41,115–122] refers to a class of lobular lesions with differentiation toward the isthmus and infundibulum. They are usually located on the face, often the lips, of adults. They must be differentiated clinically from comedo, dilated pore, and infundibular cyst.

Histologically, they are patulous follicles connected to the surface and have sheets of isthmic and infundibular epithelium radiating from a central pore (Fig. 18-11A). Some contain small orthokeratotic microcavities, but others are solid and contain small ducts similar to sebaceous ducts (Fig. 18-11B). Depending on the plane of section, the lesion can be perceived as a

Figure 18-10. Dilated pore (Winer). This dilated pore has a narrow ostium, but often the opening is as wide as the entire pore. Note the infundibular pattern of keratinization as well as the slight proliferative epithelial pattern of the deep lining similar to that of a seborrheic keratosis. When pores such as this are cut at angles, the appearance is that of a cyst. (× 32.)

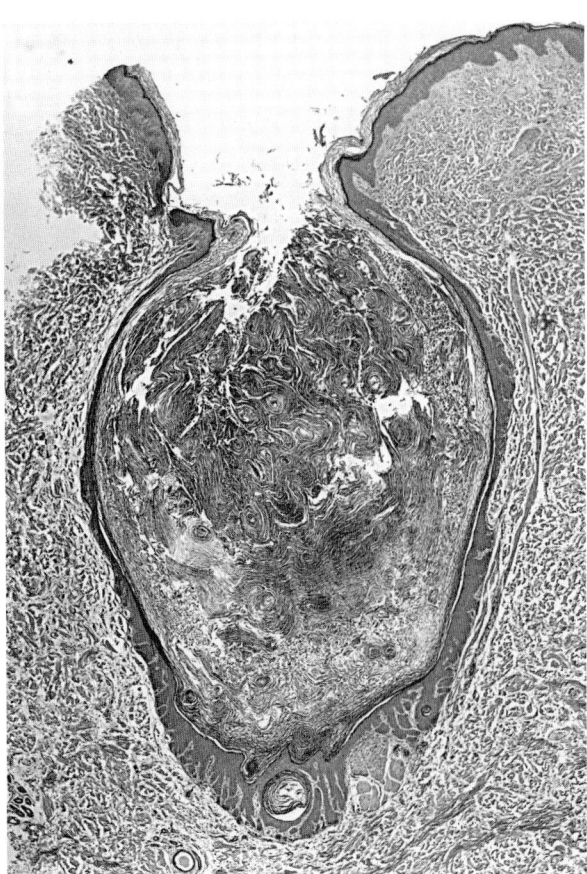

small cyst (Fig. 18-11C). The differential diagnosis includes dilated pore, trichofolliculoma, and acrospiroma.

Tricholemmal Keratosis. Tricholemmal keratosis (horn)[67, 123,124] is a proliferation of acanthotic epithelium with isthmic differentiation that often presents as a cutaneous horn and often is similar to an actinic keratosis, especially those of the extremities.

Clinically, most are solitary, slowly growing cutaneous horns that occur usually on the upper portions of the body, particularly the limbs. Some lesions may be present for many years prior to diagnosis. Persons of any age can be affected (median age, 50 years).

Histologically, there is an exophytic epithelial lesion with isthmic keratinization that may contain small cysts filled with keratin similar to isthmus-catagen (tricholemmal) cysts. The lesions may extend across a broad front as contiguous epithelial lobules that extend into the papillary dermis. The deeper portion typically has multiple cysts similar to those of a proliferative tricholemmal cyst. Immunohistochemically, the lesions are focally positive for AE1/3 and for CD34 (QBEND/10), suggesting focal differentiation toward the transient outer follicular sheath[125] in addition to the isthmic differentiation of the hematoxylin and eosin (H&E) stains.

The differential diagnosis consists of pilar sheath acanthoma (lobular infundibuloisthmicoma), isthmus-catagen (tricholemmal) cyst, proliferative tricholemmal cyst, and tricholemmal horn.

Proliferative Tricholemmal Cyst. Proliferative tricholemmal cyst (pilar tumor)[126–145] refers to a group of benign but locally destructive multilocular cystic epithelial lesions differentiated toward the isthmus or the transient outer follicular sheath of the anagen hair follicle. They are similar superficially to isthmus-catagen cysts (tricholemmal cysts), but are included in this section because their morphology and biology are often those of a solid tumor or solid and cystic tumor rather than a simple cyst.

Clinically, the lesions can occur in any sex and race, but most have been reported in older women; many have been present from months to years before diagnosis. The lesions are usually single, but sometimes are multiple,[146] and approximately 90% arise as a skin-covered or ulcerated nodule in the scalp; however, other sites may be affected.[126,133,139,141,147–155] They are characteristically well circumscribed, sharply demarcated, and lobulated. Most are a few centimeters in greatest dimension. Exceptional cases may exceed 25 cm in diameter.[133,156,157] The differential diagnosis includes isthmus-catagen (tricholemmal cyst), tricholemmal carcinoma, squamous carcinoma,[127] and rare familial[158] or hamartomatous conditions such as organoid nevi.[153]

The treatment for proliferative tricholemmal cysts is simple excision; however, a certain percentage will recur, and an even smaller percentage is capable of metastasis. It may be difficult to separate such tumors from the common benign ones based on morphologic features alone.

Pathologically, the gross lesions are lobulated and sharply circumscribed, regardless of size.[133] The overlying skin, unless ulcerated, is stretched and bosselated by bulbous projections of the underlying tumor. Usually one or more dilated, keratin-filled ostia open to the surface and communicate with cystic ar-

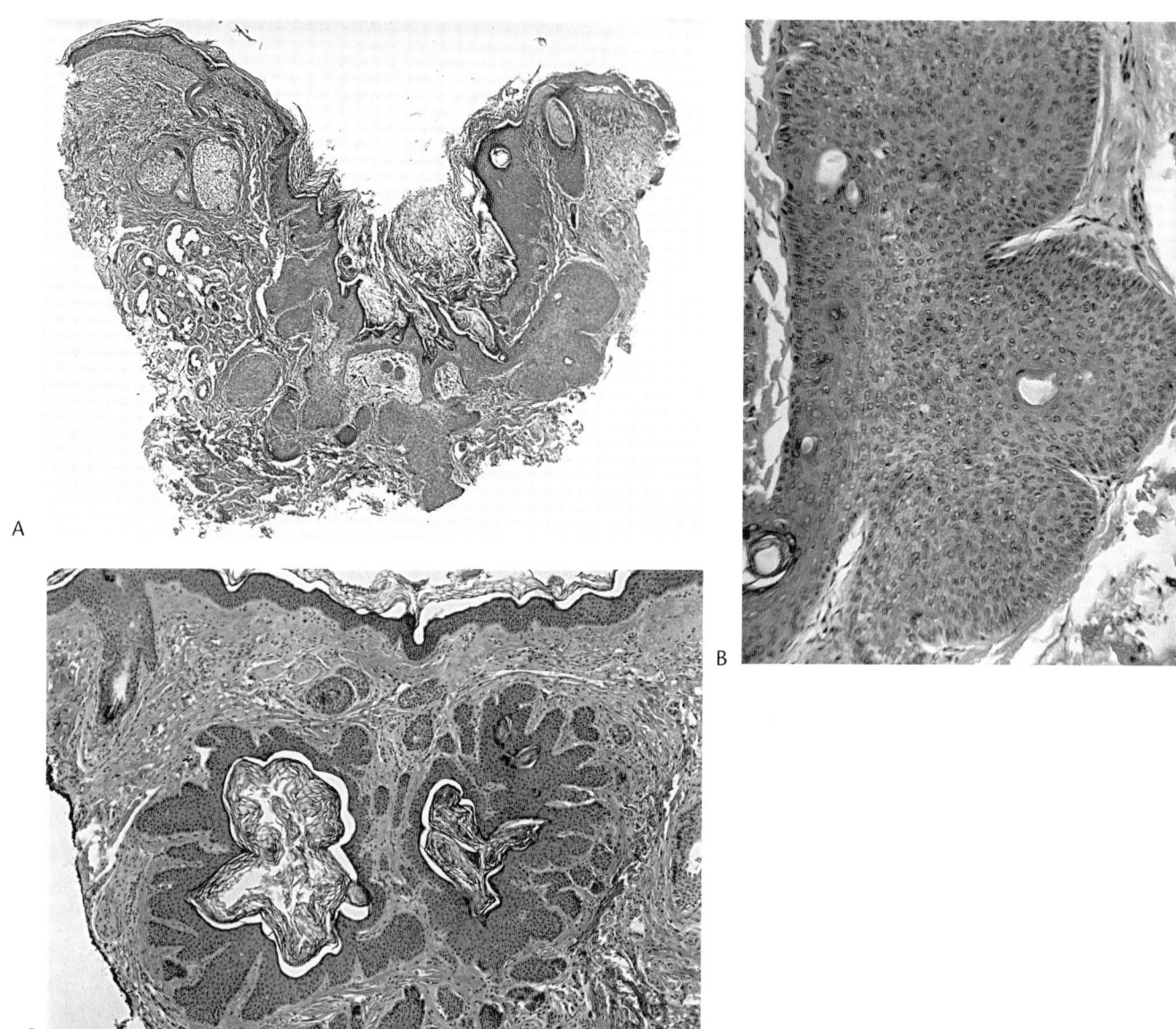

Figure 18-11. Pilar sheath acanthoma (lobular infundibuloisthmicoma). **(A)** Scanning magnification reveals a patulous follicle containing a multilobular lesion with infundibular and isthmic differentiation. (× 45.) **(B)** Higher power reveals definite isthmic differentiation with small ducts, similar to the sebaceous duct openings. (× 250.) **(C)** Slightly unusual example in that there are two small cysts filled with keratin because the lesion has been sectioned away from the ostium. Note the thickened, stellate edges of mostly isthmic epithelium that radiate from the cysts. Also note that no germinal epithelium or mesenchyme is present. (× 90.)

eas in the tumor. The cut surface is gray-white, sharply circumscribed, and lobulated, with convoluted margins extending into the subcutaneous tissue. Empty and keratin-filled spaces lined by epithelium are irregularly distributed throughout.[127]

Microscopically, the tumor usually connects with the surface epidermis through one or more dilated openings.[127] The openings are separated by septa comprised of fibrous tissue and edematous granulation tissue. The adjacent epidermis is acanthotic, often with hyperpigmented rete ridges. The lobules, which correspond to the gross cysts, are composed of irregular cysts (Fig. 18-12A) and keratin-filled follicles surrounded by hyperplastic, well-differentiated, but often anisocytotic squamous cells. Keratinized cores within epithelial evaginations are often oriented parallel to the long axis of the follicles, and keratinization usually proceeds without the formation of an intermediate granular layer (Fig. 18-12B), although one is occasionally seen focally.[149] Parakeratotic cells may be prominent in some cysts. Others may contain a granular, hyalinized material with scattered, keratinized epithelial cells. Vacuolization of keratinocytes is seen commonly. Dyskeratotic cells with pleomorphic, hyperchromatic nuclei are also

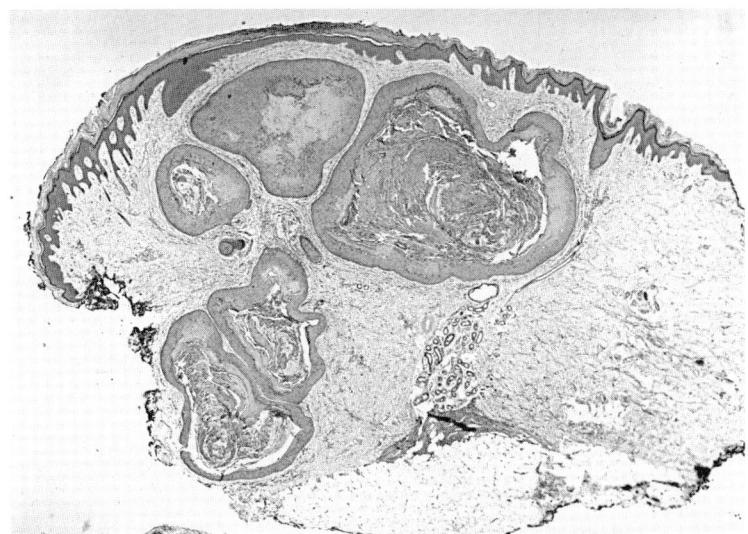

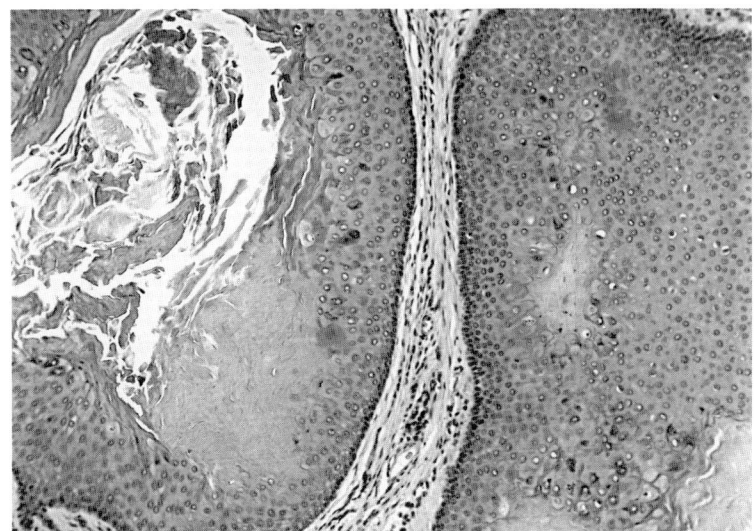

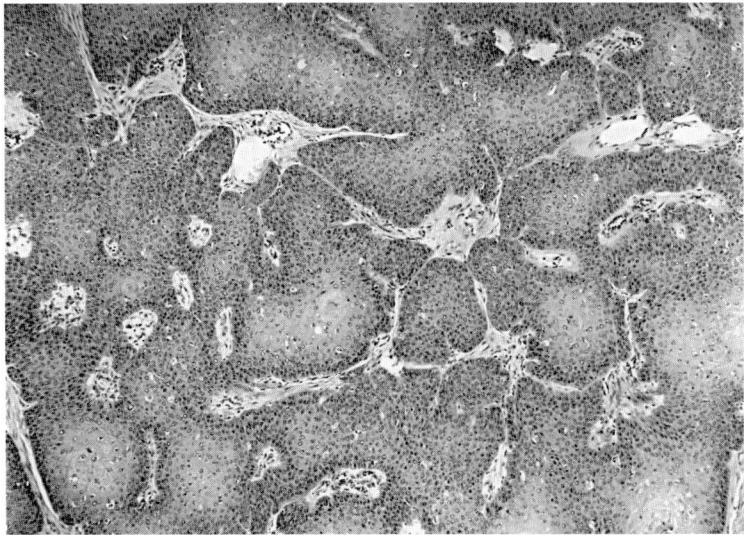

Figure 18-12. Proliferative tricholemmal cyst. (**A**) Scanning magnification reveals a multicystic lesion within the dermis. Very dense keratin fills the cysts. (× 22.) (**B**) Two adjacent cysts are present. One clearly has isthmus-catagen differentiation, lacking a granular layer. The other is a mostly solid focus of well-differentiated isthmic cells. (× 150.) (**C**) Some lesions contain solid, well-differentiated lobules of isthmic cells connected focally. This lesion contained classic cysts elsewhere. (× 90.)

common. Clear cells filled with PAS-positive, diastase labile material resembling the transient outer sheath of anagen hair follicles can be seen.[129] In some areas, the squamous cells may exhibit whorled architectural patterns simulating irritated seborrheic keratoses or inverted keratoses, but the fully developed "squamous eddies" of those lesions are not demonstrable in proliferative tricholemmal cysts.[126] Some lesions contain solid, connected, lobular patterns (Fig. 18-12C). A thick, hyalinized membrane similar to the glassy membrane of the transient outer sheath of the anagen hair follicle is present at the advancing margins of most tumors.[127] Necrosis may be focal or extensive.[126] Peripherally, small epithelial extensions of basaloid cells may protrude from the tumor, sometimes accompanied by a loose stroma, forming a hair induction pattern often seen in trichogenesis. These areas may simulate tumor invasion if any viable squamous epithelium is entrapped. Occasionally, a few sebocytes are present[141]; rarely, ducts may be present focally.[159]

Cytologically, cellular atypia of the squamous cells may vary greatly between tumors and within an individual tumor. At the advancing margins, the cells often contain scant cytoplasm and a hyperchromatic nucleus with prominent nucleoli. Mitotic figures are variable in number.

Edema and vascularized connective tissue with a mononuclear and foreign body giant cell infiltrate with occasional cholesterol clefts may surround the keratinous debris. Occasionally, neutrophilic, plasmacytic, and/or eosinophilic infiltrates, sometimes with germinal centers, may be seen[141]; this is commonly associated with areas of calcification and, rarely, ossification.[141] The multinucleated giant cells may be associated with bone resorption.[160] Rarely, shadow cells reminiscent of pilomatricoma exist within the lesion.[126] Hemosiderin-laden macrophages may also be present peripherally, presumably secondary to tumoral trauma.

Ultrastructurally, the bulk of the tumor is composed of squamous cells with numerous tonofilaments and intercellular desmosomes that may be differentiated toward sebaceous gland cells or ductal cells.[148,161] The former are characterized by numerous, closely packed cytoplasmic lipid droplets, indenting an eccentric nucleus. The latter consists of desmosomal attachments to the prickle cells; in addition, they contain many blunt, short microvilli. They also contain many cytoplasmic tonofilaments, scattered glycogen, and variable cytoplasmic lipid. The tumor stroma consists of ground substance, fusiform cells, mast cells, and condensations of collagen bundles.

Biochemical experiments have shown that extracts of keratins exhibit variation in molecular weights in proliferative tricholemmal cysts (57, 51, and 43kd) compared with keratins from plantar stratum corneum (64, 53, and 43kd). The significance of this finding is not completely clear.[162] The lack of immunostaining of the outer root sheath with anti-64kd keratin[163] as well as the application of CD34 (QBEND/10)[125] suggests that cells of the transient outer follicular sheath and the cells of proliferative tricholemmal cyst are similar, at least focally.

Preliminary studies with flow cytometry[164] and DNA image analysis[165] have shown diploid and aneuploid patterns in histologically classic cases of proliferative tricholemmal cysts.

The histologic differential diagnosis includes squamous cell carcinoma, pilomatricoma, solid or clear cell poroma (acrospiroma, hidradenoma), proliferative epidermoid (infundibular) lesions,[166] and tricholemmal cysts.

Since the initial reports of proliferative tricholemmal cysts, rare cases with metastasis have been reported.[129,145,151,167–170] In these lesions, the helpful clinicopathologic features indicating a potentially aggressive course include atypical location in one case (inguinal region),[151] numerous squamous pearls, excessive numbers of cells in mitosis (up to 35/10 high-power fields [hpf], but with areas as low as 1/10 in portions resembling the typical proliferative tricholemmal cyst),[168] multinucleated tumor giant cells, numerous apoptotic cells, and bizarre and typical mitoses. Unfortunately, overall size, focal cellular atypia, focal necrosis, and local aggressiveness do not appear to be helpful predictors of potential metastasis in most cases. Thus, rare lesions, commonly placed in this group as proliferative tricholemmal cysts, must be regarded as potentially capable of metastasis.

Fibrofolliculoma. Fibrofolliculoma is a class of follicular proliferations composed of thin strands of infundibular, isthmic, and, sometimes, sebaceous epithelium surrounded by concentric follicular stroma. They often radiate from the infundibular portion of the hair follicle. In some cases, they may be associated with small cysts. This lesion has also been regarded by some as a mantleoma[171] and related to the sebaceous glands.

Fibrofolliculomas usually occur on the head and neck of adults and may be associated with trichodiscomas and acrochordons, the Birt-Hogg-Dubé syndrome.[172] In a few cases, visceral tumors have been found in these patients.[173–175] It is not known if such an association is significant. The differential diagnosis includes fibrous papule, neurofibroma, melanocytic nevus, and tricholemmoma.

Histologically, fibrofolliculomas are similar to the infundibular and isthmic portions of the follicles. Thin strands of follicular epithelium emerge from the follicle and are associated with a prominent stromal component that forms a tight sheath around the strand (Fig. 18-13). The strands often interconnect, forming a reticulated pattern. In some cases, small milium-sized cysts are associated. In other cases, these may open to the surface like a comedo. The differential diagnosis includes mantleoma and trichofolliculoma. The former contains foci of sebaceous glands and may just be a variation of this lesion, while the latter contains fully formed hair follicles.

Transient Follicular Sheath: Tricholemmoma

Tricholemmoma is the prototype of adnexal tumors with histologic similarity to the outer follicular sheath at the level of the stem and bulb.

Tricholemmoma[176] is a category of tumors characterized by papules composed histologically of glycogen-containing clear epithelial cells and delimited by a prominent vitreous layer similar to the one observed external to the outer follicular sheath of the transient portion of the anagen hair follicle.

Clinically, tricholemmoma is solitary or multiple. It usually affects older adults, but the range varies from the second to the ninth decades. Individual lesions are usually dome-shaped, skin-colored papules less than 5 mm in diameter. Tricholemmomas are usually located on the face, particularly the nose, but the eyelids, lips, and oral cavity can also be affected.[177–179] The clinical differential diagnosis of tricholemmoma includes verruca, inverted (follicular) keratosis, and basal cell carcinoma. Treatment is by simple excision or local destruction.

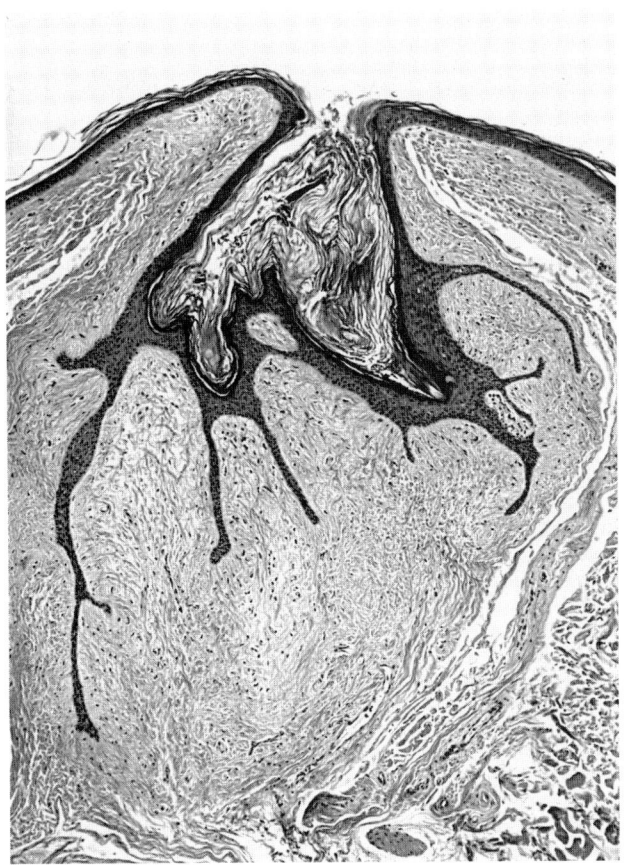

Figure 18-13. Fibrofolliculoma. This lesion was biopsied from a patient with the Birt-Hogg-Dubé syndrome. The lesion is similar to a trichofolliculoma in that it contains a cyst with radiating epithelial strands. It differs from trichofolliculoma in that it lacks all aspects of the follicle and it contains abundant stroma. (× 90.)

Multiple tricholemmomas are characteristically associated with Cowden syndrome (multiple hamartoma syndrome), defined as a spectrum of multiple cutaneous hamartomas[180–185] (tricholemmomas, verrucous keratinocytic lesions, and fibromas), visceral hamartomas,[186] and/or visceral carcinomas (particularly breast carcinoma).[187] It is an inherited, autosomal dominant disorder with high penetrance.[188] The clinical differential diagnosis for the facial lesions of Cowden syndrome includes viral warts, Darier's disease, tuberous sclerosis, trichoepitheliomas, neurofibromatosis, nevoid basal cell carcinoma syndrome, syringomas, and cylindromas.[181] The acral lesions also can resemble epidermodysplasia verruciformis, flat warts, acrokeratosis verruciformis, stucco keratoses, and punctate keratoderma.[181] Treatment must be individualized,[189] as the large number of lesions may preclude their excision or destruction.

Histologically, tricholemmoma is symmetric and typically has a bulbous, circumscribed border that is demarcated by a prominent PAS-positive vitreous membrane (Fig. 18-14). There are architectural variations ranging from follicle-like, vertically oriented lesions, to lobular, bulbous, poroma (acrospiroma)-like lesions that are devoid of eccrine or apocrine ducts, to verrucous lesions. In many cases, there is a broad connection with the sur-

face epithelium. The cells tend to form a peripheral palisaded pattern usually in the deeper portions. Less commonly, squamous eddies or orthokeratotic microcavities, similar to those of inverted keratosis, can be found. *Desmoplastic tricholemmomas*[190] have extensive stroma peripherally rimmed with epithelium and frequently located in the midst of the tumor nodule (Fig. 18-15). This variant has a spindle cell component in which the tumor cells merge with the stroma and mimic invasion. Ample areas of eosinophilic, amorphous, Alcian blue and PAS-positive, diastase-resistant material is also found; this probably represents basement membrane material. Involucrin has been identified in some lesions.[191] QBEND/10 (anti-CD34 antibody) has also been identified in tricholemmomas and compared with similar findings in controls of the outer (transient) follicular sheath of an anagen hair follicle.

In some tricholemmomas, a connection with individual hair follicles can be observed; these can be prominent clear cell epithelial proliferations in the midfollicular area. There is a variable, fibrous stroma similar to the perifollicular fibrous sheath; a mononuclear inflammatory can be present in some cases.

Although some tumors are largely subepidermal, others are verrucous.[192,193] It has been proposed that tricholemmomas, especially the ones with verrucous architecture, are aged warts.[194,195] This position has been both supported and denied.[196–199] Attempts to identify viral particles or antigens in tricholemmomas with rare exception have failed.[181,200,201,201A]

Cytologically, the epithelial cells have abundant clear cytoplasm that contains glycogen, demonstrated by the use of PAS with diastase.[176] Some lesions contain eosinophilic "intermediate" cells that lack the clear cell pattern of classic lesions and are similar to the cells of the isthmus. Some refer to these as *acrotrichomas*[202] or *follicular poromas.*[203]

The most difficult differentiation is from clear cell poroma (hidradenoma, acrospiroma), which contains duct lumens but lacks the peripheral palisading and the vitreous basement membrane of tricholemmoma. In tumors with a predominance of intermediate cells, differentiation from basal cell carcinoma or inverted (follicular) keratosis can be difficult. The desmoplastic tricholemmomas pose the additional danger of being confused with malignant neoplasms, namely, spindle cell squamous cell carcinoma and/or desmoplastic basal cell carcinoma. Large tumors composed of clear cells, often described as tricholemmomas, are probably best classified as proliferative tricholemmal cysts.[204,205]

Matrix

Pilomatricoma. Pilomatricoma (calcifying epithelioma; trichomatricoma)[206–211] is a benign dermal and subcutaneous tumor that is histologically similar to the matrical portion of the hair follicle.

Clinically, most are solitary nodules located on the head, neck, and upper limbs. They can be rubbery and pliable or hard and faceted; they usually measure 5 mm to 2 cm in diameter. Rarely, they can be multiple,[212,213] perforated,[214] or rapidly progressive. They usually occur in the first two decades of life, but can occur at any age. The differential diagnosis is usually broad unless the lesion is faceted. Rare cases are associated with myotonic dystrophy[215–217] and the Rubinstein-Taybi syndrome.[218] Simple excision is curative.

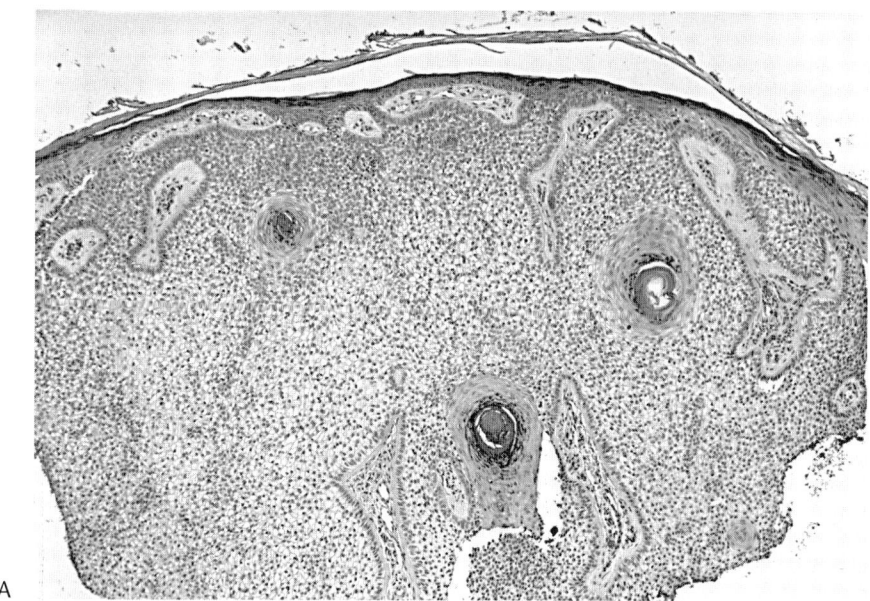

A

Figure 18-14. Tricholemmoma. (**A**) Scanning magnification reveals the classic pattern. There is a homogeneous sheet of clear cells bounded by a thickened vitreous membrane that can be appreciated fully only at higher power. (× 90.) (**B**) High-power view emphasizes the relationship of the vitreous membrane to the stroma and the tumor epithelium. (× 340.)

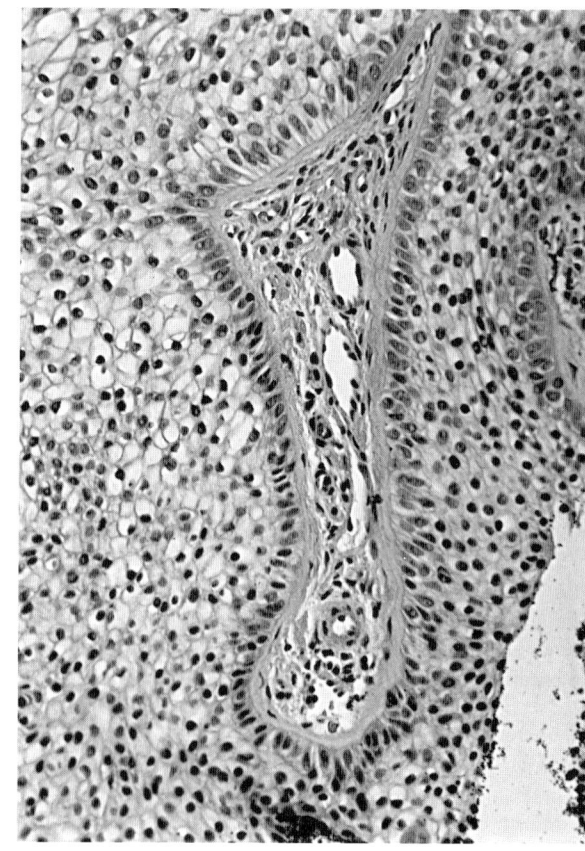

B

Histologically, the hallmark is that of lobules of basaloid cells that are contiguous, merging gradually with eosinophilic keratinous effete cells[219,220]; the latter are termed *shadow* cells (Fig. 18-16). The basaloid cells are typically homogeneous and monomorphous, similar in size to the basaloid cells of basal cell carcinoma. Many of these cells can be in mitosis in any given histologic field. The shadow cells are keratinized but retain the microscopic structure of the basaloid cells, presumably because of premature keratinization compared with normal hairs (Fig. 18-17). As a secondary finding, a giant cell infiltrate and dystrophic calcification are also usually present, presumably as a host response to the shadow cells. Lesions that contain a significant number of basaloid cells can be cystic; lesions that are devoid of basaloid cells are typically solid tumors of shadow cells, calcification, and giant cell reaction, the so-called burned-out lesions. A small number of cases contain zones of extramedullary hematopoiesis.[221–223] Pilomatricoma-like changes have been observed in cysts of Gardner syndrome[224–226] and, rarely, in organoid (sebaceous) nevi.[227] Histochemically[228] and ultrastructurally,[229] pilomatricoma is similar to the hair matrix. The histologic differential diagnosis includes basal cell carcinoma, neuroendocrine carcinoma, and proliferative tricholemmal cyst. The diagnosis is typically straightforward unless the entire lesion is composed of basaloid cells.[230]

Matricoma. The term *matricoma* has been used to describe a class of tumors with differentiation toward the matrical, supramatrical, infundibular sheath and the inner follicular sheath portions of a hair follicle. The tumors grow in multinodular aggregates that often are large clinically[231] (Fig. 18-18).

Cortex: Hair Cortex Comedo

The hair cortex comedo is a recently described lesion that consists of a simple invagination of infundibular-type epithelium containing a plug of dense, highly laminated keratin similar to a hair cortex.[232]

The two cases described occurred as single, black, well-circumscribed papules on the face and back, respectively, in two Japanese patients, both in their second decade.

Both lesions were characterized by a V-shaped invagination of infundibular epithelium that contained a dense plug of keratin that was similar to the hair cortex. Toward the surface, it developed flake-like keratin. At the base of the plug were basophilic cells, similar to matrical cells, mixed with dendrocytic melanocytes.

The differential diagnosis consists of dilated pore, pilar sheath acanthoma, and nevus comedonicus.

Tumors of Follicle-Associated Mesenchyme

Uncommonly, proliferations occur that are similar to the purported hair follicle disc, perifollicular fibrous sheath, and hair follicle-associated smooth muscle. Trichodiscoma, perifollicular fibroma, and piloleiomyoma are described in this section. Fibrofolliculoma and trichogenic myxoma are described above.

Trichodiscoma. Trichodiscomas[233] are small papules of myxoid connective tissue and Alcian blue-positive mucin

Figure 18-15. Desmoplastic tricholemmoma. This tumor contains tricholemmoma of the transitional cell type in the right half; note the thickened basement membrane. The right half gradually merges with a trabecular pattern of epithelial cells enmeshed in hyalinized stroma. This pattern can be difficult to differentiate from some squamous cell carcinomas without a proper sample of the lesion. (× 90.)

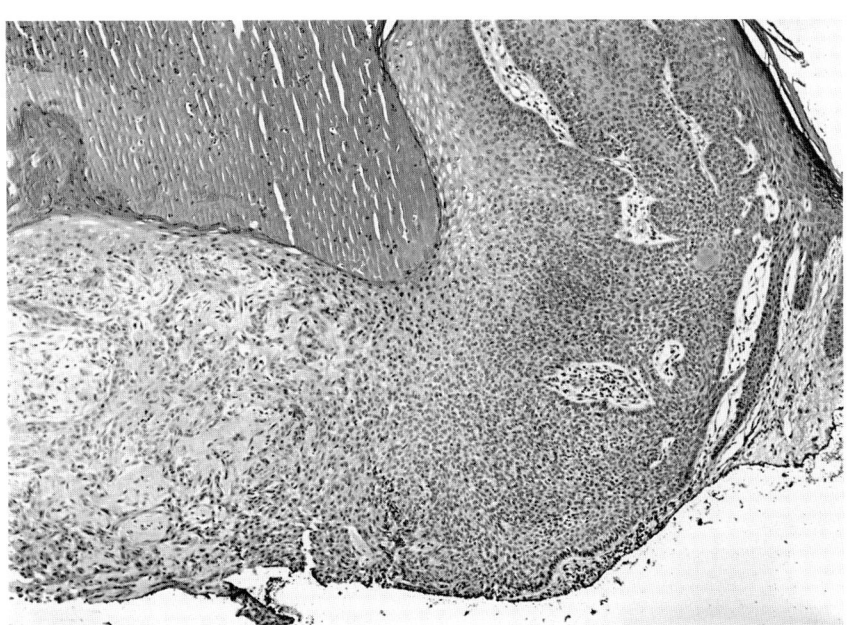

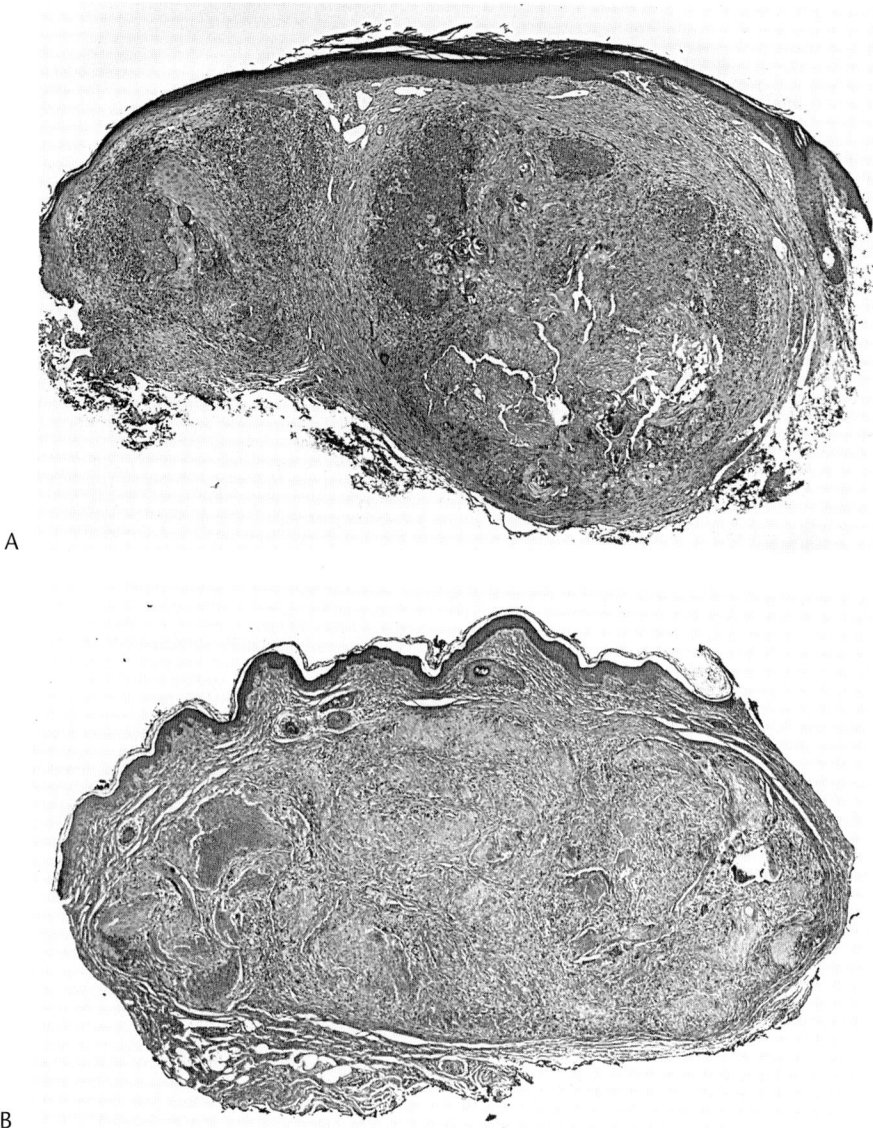

A

B

Figure 18-16. Pilomatricoma. (**A**) In this case, there are a few basaloid cell zones; much of the tumor consists of "shadow" cells. (× 39.) (**B**) This lesion contains effete matrix in the form of "shadow" cells and abundant foreign body reaction. This is a classic "burned out" pilomatricoma. (× 39.)

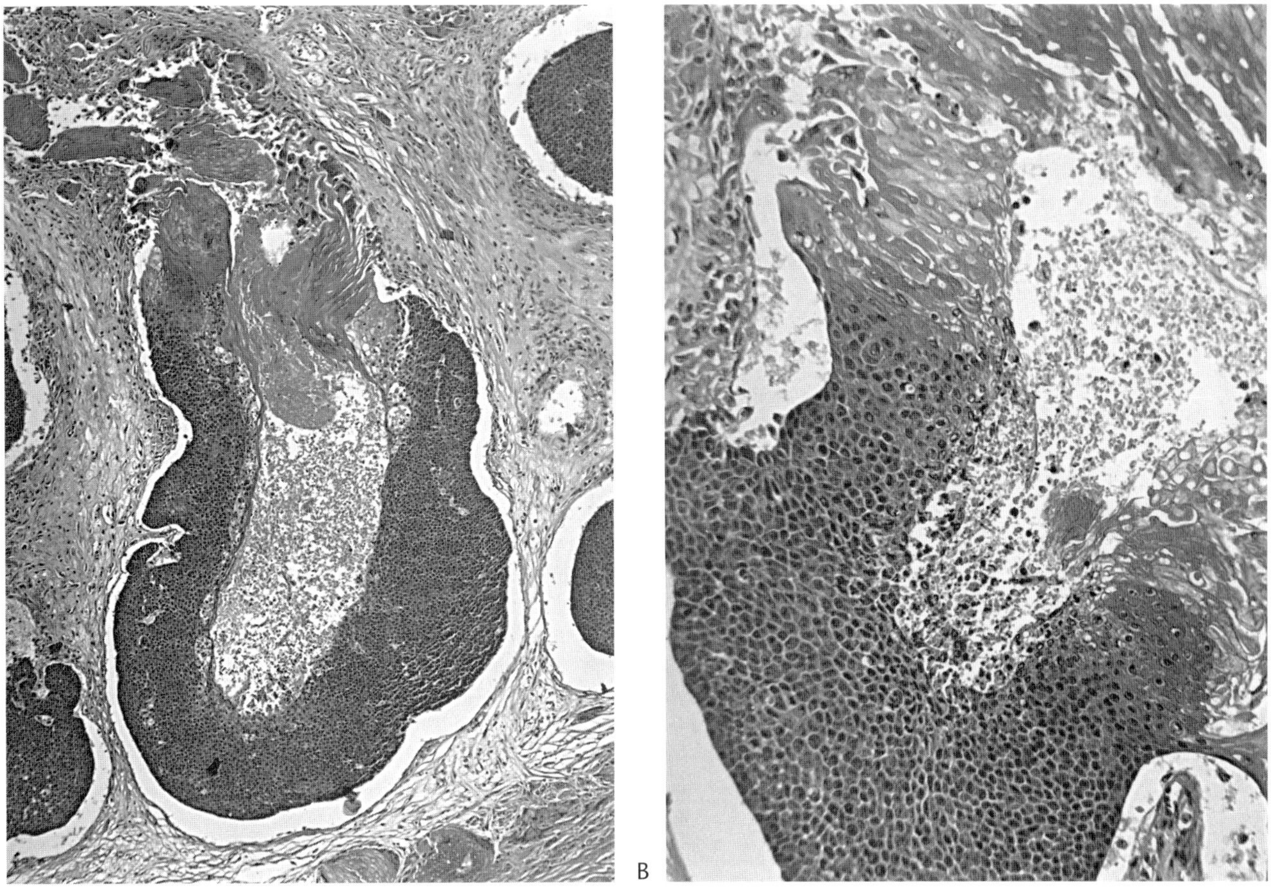

A

B

Figure 18-17. Pilomatricoma. (**A**) Medium magnification reveals a "shadow" cell keratogenous zone that is diagnostic of pilomatricoma. (× 90.) (**B**) High magnification reveals the uniformity of the matrical cells as they merge with "shadow" cells at the keratogenous zone. (× 300.)

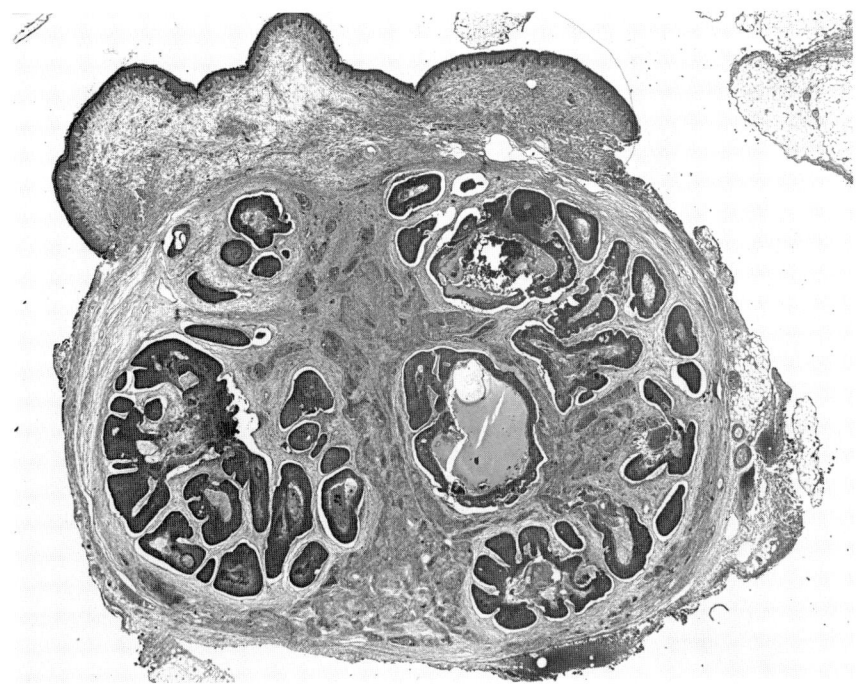

Figure 18-18. Matricoma (pilomatricoma). At scanning magnification, this is a tumor composed of basaloid cells arranged in islands and lobules. Note the prominent circumscription. There are only a few zones that contain shadow cells in this particular case. (× 12.)

Figure 18-19. Trichodiscoma. This lesion was one of several found in a patient with the Birt-Hogg-Dubé syndrome. The lesion is papular and contains a loose stroma. (× 90.)

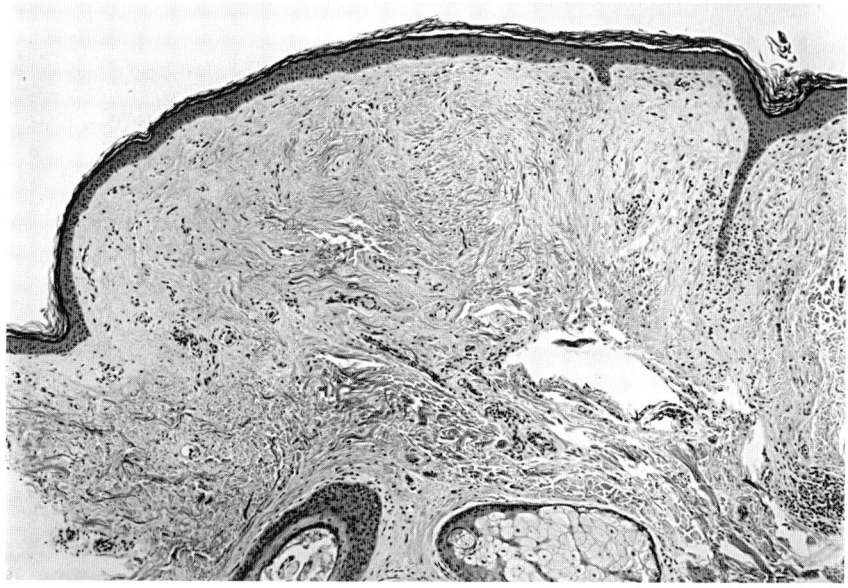

thought to be associated with hair follicles (Fig. 18-19). The occurrence of trichodiscomas with fibrofolliculomas is seen in the Birt-Hogg-Dubé syndrome.[172,173] Trichodiscomas may be nothing more than fibrofolliculomas with excessive stroma.[234]

Perifollicular Fibroma. Perifollicular fibromas are papulonodular lesions that consist histologically of hyperplasia of the mesenchymal portion of the follicular sheath. Similar changes may be seen in hair follicle nevi and fibrofolliculomas; however, the follicular epithelium in the later conditions is more prominent.[235] Some consider perifollicular fibromas to be fibrous papules.[236] A possible association of perifollicular fibromas and colon polyps has been described.[237]

Trichogenic Myxoma. Trichogenic myxoma is described above.

Follicular Myomas. *Smooth Muscle Hamartoma.* Smooth muscle hamartomas[3,238–240] are congenital and resemble Becker's nevi clinically.[241] They usually present as congenital patches or slightly indurated plaques with prominent overlying hair or rarely as patches with perifollicular papules without prominent hair. Most cases are somewhat hyperpigmented, but many are skin colored.[242] Histologically, bundles of smooth muscle are present in the dermal collagen as distinctly isolated bundles similar to the follicular muscles.[243]

Follicular Myoma. Follicular myomas (piloleiomyomas) are clinical papules that can be solitary or multiple; sometimes they can be painful. Histologically, they are similar to the arrector muscles or directly contiguous with the follicular smooth muscle[244] (Fig. 18-20). They typically blend into the background

Figure 18-20. Follicular myoma (piloleiomyoma). The leiomyoma fills the papillary dermis and extends vertically in the central portion, similar to native follicular muscle. (× 40.)

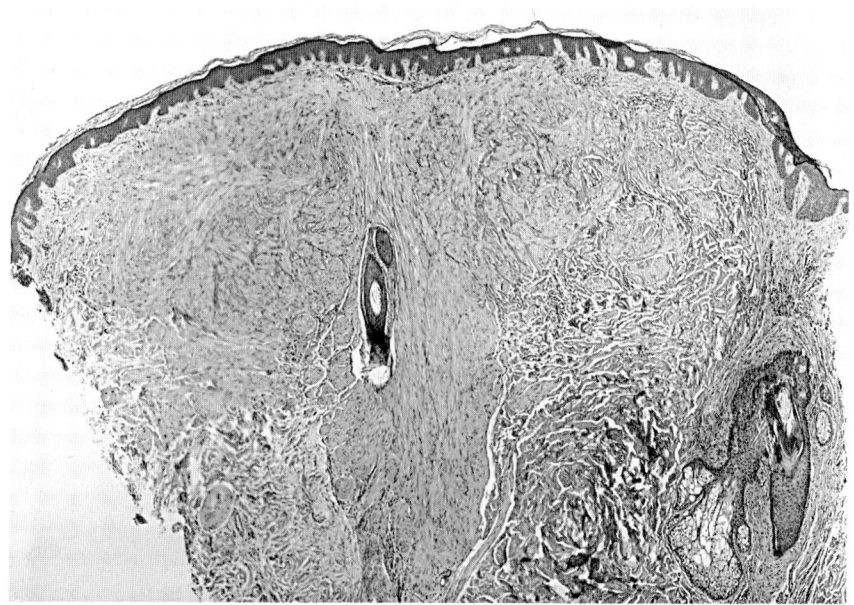

and are separate and distinct, in contrast with the hamartomas. The immunostains are typically positive with smooth muscle actin and desmin, but negative for S–100 and CD34.

Malignant Hair/Hair Follicle/Follicle Mesenchyme Tumors

Carcinomas that are similar to portions of the hair follicle are rare, and most have been reported as single cases. These have been classified broadly into carcinomas that are similar to one or more portions of the follicular sheath (tricholemmal carcinomas) or matrix (matrical carcinomas) and those with mixed mature elements associated with a malignant component.[245,246] Some of the latter cases could be considered trichoepithelial carcinomas. Although it is widely recognized that microcystic adnexal carcinomas may contain follicular differentiation,[247,248] this class of lesions is discussed in greater depth in the section on carcinomas of apocrine or eccrine glands. Follicle-related leiomyosarcomas, albeit very rare, also deserve brief mention.

Tricholemmal Carcinoma

Tricholemmal carcinoma[249–252] is a group of biologically low-grade, malignant, clear cell tumors that look similar to the outer sheath of the transient portion of the hair follicle.

Most tricholemmal carcinomas occur in sun-exposed areas of older adults. They are often exophytic papules or nodules that may be ulcerated. Rare cases have been associated with burn scars.[253] The differential diagnosis includes squamous or basal cell carcinoma. Excision is usually curative.

Histologically, the tumors are often circumscribed, although some are infiltrative. They are composed of islands and trabeculae of clear cells that connect to the epidermis superficially (Fig. 18-21). They may have areas of centrilobular necrosis, necrosis en masse, or abrupt keratinization, similar to isthmus-catagen (tricholemmal cysts) or proliferative tricholemmal cysts, and the periphery of the lobule is surrounded by a thick PAS-positive, diastase-resistant basement membrane. Cytologically, the cells are pleomorphic, often exhibiting frequent or abnormal mitoses. Occasional areas of epidermis may exhibit a pagetoid pattern of the clear cells.

The cytoplasm of the tumor cells is rich in glycogen, as evidenced by a PAS-positive, diastase-sensitive pattern. Cytokeratin antibodies have marked some tumors.[254] Mucin, epithelial membrane antigen (EMA), carcinoembryonic antigen (CEA), S-100, and HMB-45 are consistently negative.

The histologic differential diagnosis includes clear cell tu-

Figure 18-21. Tricholemmal carcinoma. **(A)** This tumor is large and circumscribed, but with an infiltrative advancing edge. It is composed of small insular epithelial structures with trabecular connections. Lucent areas in some of them correspond to zones of clear cell change, some with centrilobular necrosis or necrosis en masse. (× 9.) **(B)** Medium power reveals that there is prominent clear cell change in some of the islands. Note that there are several small infiltrative epithelial cords adjacent to the larger epithelial islands. (× 90.)

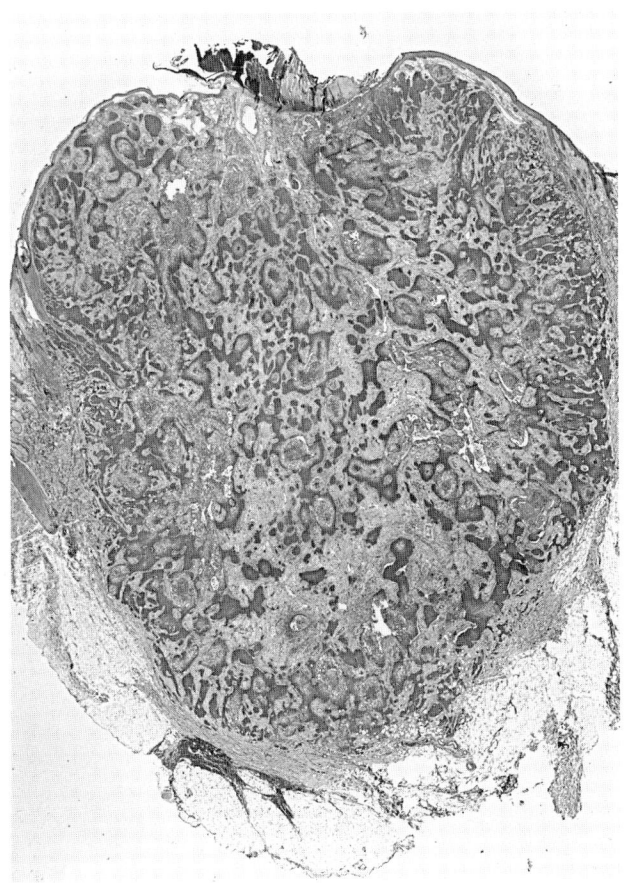

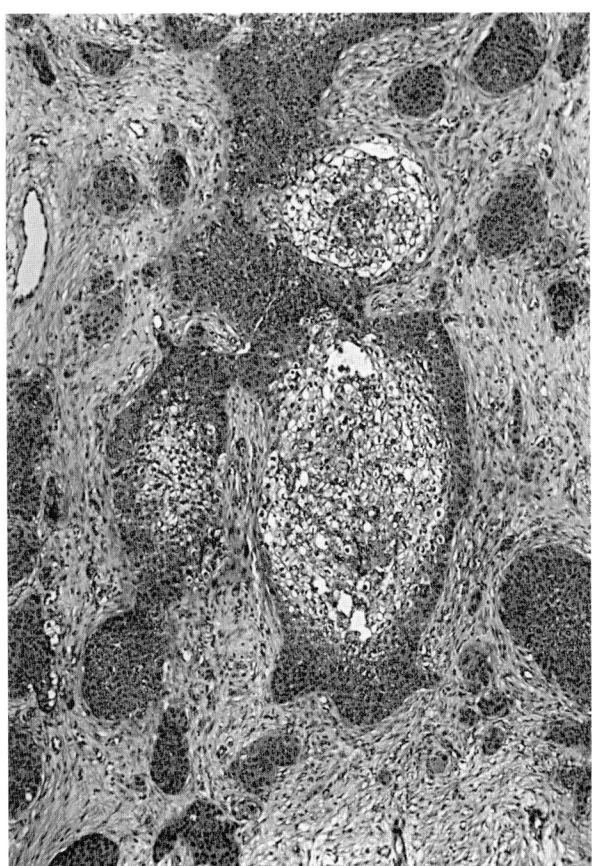

A

B

mors of the skin,[255] such as clear cell variants of squamous or basal cell carcinoma. In addition, tricholemmoma of the common or desmoplastic types, clear (pale) cell acanthoma, clear cell syringoma, porocarcinoma (acrospirocarcinoma), sebaceous carcinoma, some proliferative tricholemmal cysts, and balloon cell melanocytic nevus or melanoma should be considered. Most lesions, however, are not easily confused with tricholemmal carcinoma.

Matrical Carcinoma

Matrical carcinoma[256–260] is a family of rare malignant tumors that are similar histologically to pilomatricomas. In addition, these contain significant zones of matrical cells that exhibit infiltrative patterns of growth and biologic virulence.

The lesions occur usually on the head or neck of adults. When removed, they may extend into the subcutis, fascia, or muscle. Rarely, the lesions may metastasize, but most remain localized; about half recur after excision.

Histologically, the tumors are composed of nests and trabeculae of basaloid cells that overlap each other as observed in H&E-stained sections. They often have a growth pattern in which the cells are oriented in the same direction, similar to the hair matrix. The cells are similar to conventional pilomatricomas with the ex-

ception that the carcinomas are considerably more pleomorphic cytologically. Some clear cell foci with tricholemmal keratinization and shadow cells are usually seen, but these are less common than in conventional pilomatricomas. The stroma ranges from fibroblastic to fibrotic even when the lesions extend into the subcutis. Occasionally, neural or vascular invasion (or both) is present. The differential diagnosis includes basal cell carcinoma, tricholemmal carcinoma, and proliferative tricholemmal cyst.

Follicular Leiomyosarcoma

Cutaneous leiomyosarcomas can occur at any age and in either sex, but they are more common in middle to older age and are found usually on the extremities, particularly the lower limb. They develop usually as small (1 cm) solitary painful or tender dermal nodules. These may recur after excision, but they do not usually metastasize despite a high mitotic frequency and marked cytologic atypia[261] provided they are, in fact, cutaneous.[262] The prognosis is worse for large (over 5 cm), subcutaneous, and high-grade leiomyosarcomas.

Microscopically, they consist of poorly delineated proliferations of spindle-shaped, often pleomorphic or frankly bizarre myomatous cells arranged in interlacing fascicles that merge into collagenous stroma (Fig. 18-22). Some of these contain

Figure 18-22. Follicular leiomyosarcoma. (**A**) This lesion is highly cellular and contains areas that blend with the follicular muscle. (× 36.) (**B**) At high power, the lesion clearly merges with the follicular muscle and is much more cellular than the follicular myomas. This lesion contained an occasional mitotic figure. (× 275.)

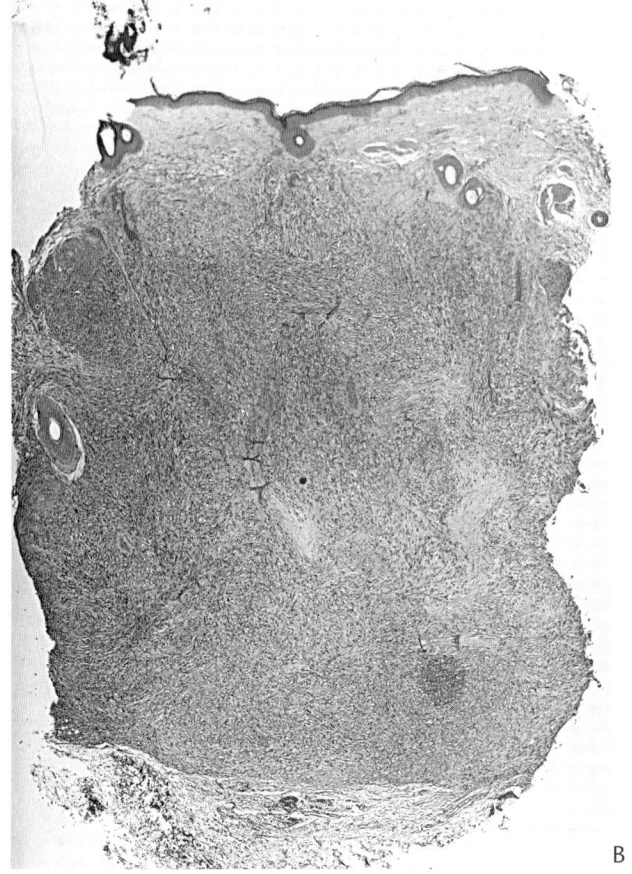

A

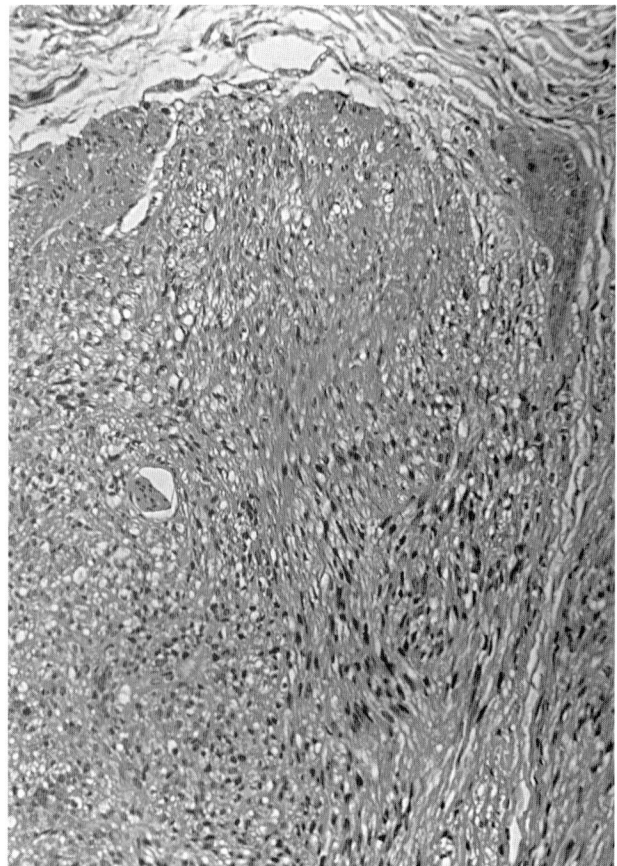

B

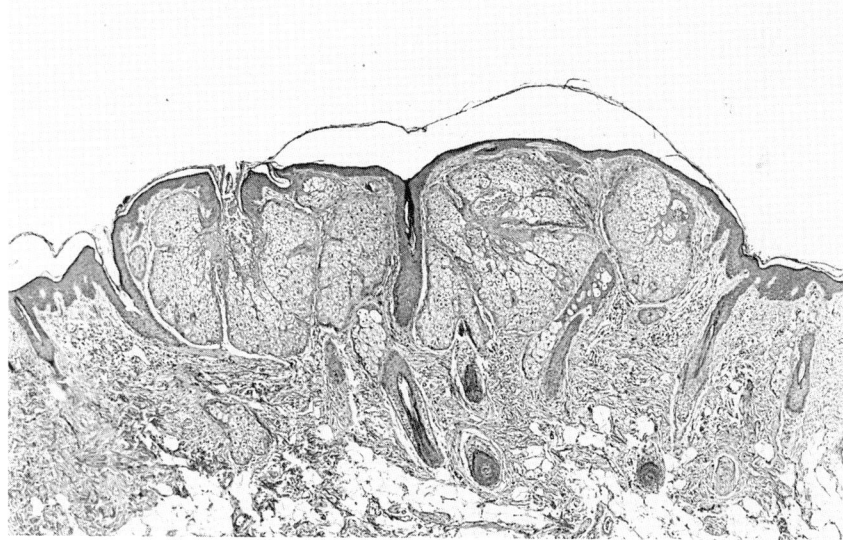

Figure 18-23. Sebaceous hyperplasia. At scanning magnification, the sebaceous lobules stand out from the background like a tumor in the superficial dermis. Note also that the epidermis protrudes above the line of adjacent epidermis. In one of the hyperplastic lobules on the left, the lobule opens almost directly to the surface. In some cases, *Demodex folliculorum* mites are present in the follicular canal. (× 45.)

myxoid areas, but necrosis is rare in the purely dermal lesions. The number of mitotic figures is variable and does not correlate well with prognosis[261]; usually there are no more than 5 mitoses/10 hpf in the most pleomorphic dermal lesions, in contrast to the subcutaneous lesions, which often have higher grades. Unusual histologic variations include those with granular cells[263] and epithelioid cells.[264] Rarely, they may be sclerotic.[265]

Immunohistochemically they are usually positive for smooth muscle actin and vimentin. About two-thirds are positive for desmin. They are negative for S-100, HMB-45, CD34, and cytokeratin. They are ultrastructurally similar to leiomyosarcomas from any site.

The differential diagnosis consists mainly of spindle cell melanoma, atypical fibroxanthoma, and selected neural lesions.

TUMORS OF GLANDS

Adnexal Tumors with Sebaceous Differentiation

Other than sebaceous hyperplasia, which is common (Fig. 18-23), the sebaceous gland tumors are relatively rare. Historically, the spectrum has been presented under a variety of terms, including *sebaceous adenoma, sebaceoma,*[266] *sebaceous epithelioma,* and *sebaceous carcinoma.* Recently described lesions, such as sebocrine adenoma,[267,268] sebaceous epithelioma with sweat gland differentiation,[268] cutaneous lymphadenoma,[77] and superficial epithelioma with sebaceous differentiation[269] may have zones containing sebaceous cells and could be included in this family. Furthermore, foci of sebaceous cells can be observed in a variety of basaloid tumors and hamartomas, most notably mantleoma, which is a basaloid proliferation containing occasional sebocytes and probably is a tumor-like cycling phase

of a sebaceous gland or a hamartoma.[171] The term *sebomatricoma*[270,271] has been proposed recently to stand for the entire spectrum of benign sebaceous neoplasms. However, the use of such a term for all lesions in the benign sebaceous tumor group is somewhat confusing because the term targets specifically the germinal layers of the sebaceous lobule and is too specific for the general class. The classic term *sebaceous adenoma* serves better for the general group designation and is truer to the general definition of an adenoma. Thus, in the classification scheme set forth here, benign sebaceous neoplasms are classified broadly as *sebaceous adenoma,* while the malignant forms are termed *sebaceous carcinoma.* The histologic dividing line between these classes is not clear in every case.

Sebaceous Adenoma

Sebaceous adenomas[266,272] are a spectrum of lobular tumors containing sebaceous cells and a germinal layer that may be prominent. These lesions are usually discrete, circumscribed, and biologically self-limited. Patients with these tumors can have associated visceral malignancies, principally of the colon, a syndrome designated the *Muir-Torre syndrome.*[273,274]

Clinically, most sebaceous adenomas are yellow, solitary tumors on the face of an adult. Most are less than 1 cm in diameter. Multiple sebaceous adenomas are common in the Muir-Torre syndrome, but the sensitivity and specificity of sebaceous adenomas for the syndrome remain unclear. There is some evidence that the presence of multiple sebaceous adenomas may have greater predictive value for the presence of visceral carcinomas than solitary sebaceous adenomas.

Histologically, the spectrum varies from small tumors with mostly mature sebaceous cells and few layers of germinal epithelium (conventional type) (Fig. 18-24) to tumors with mostly

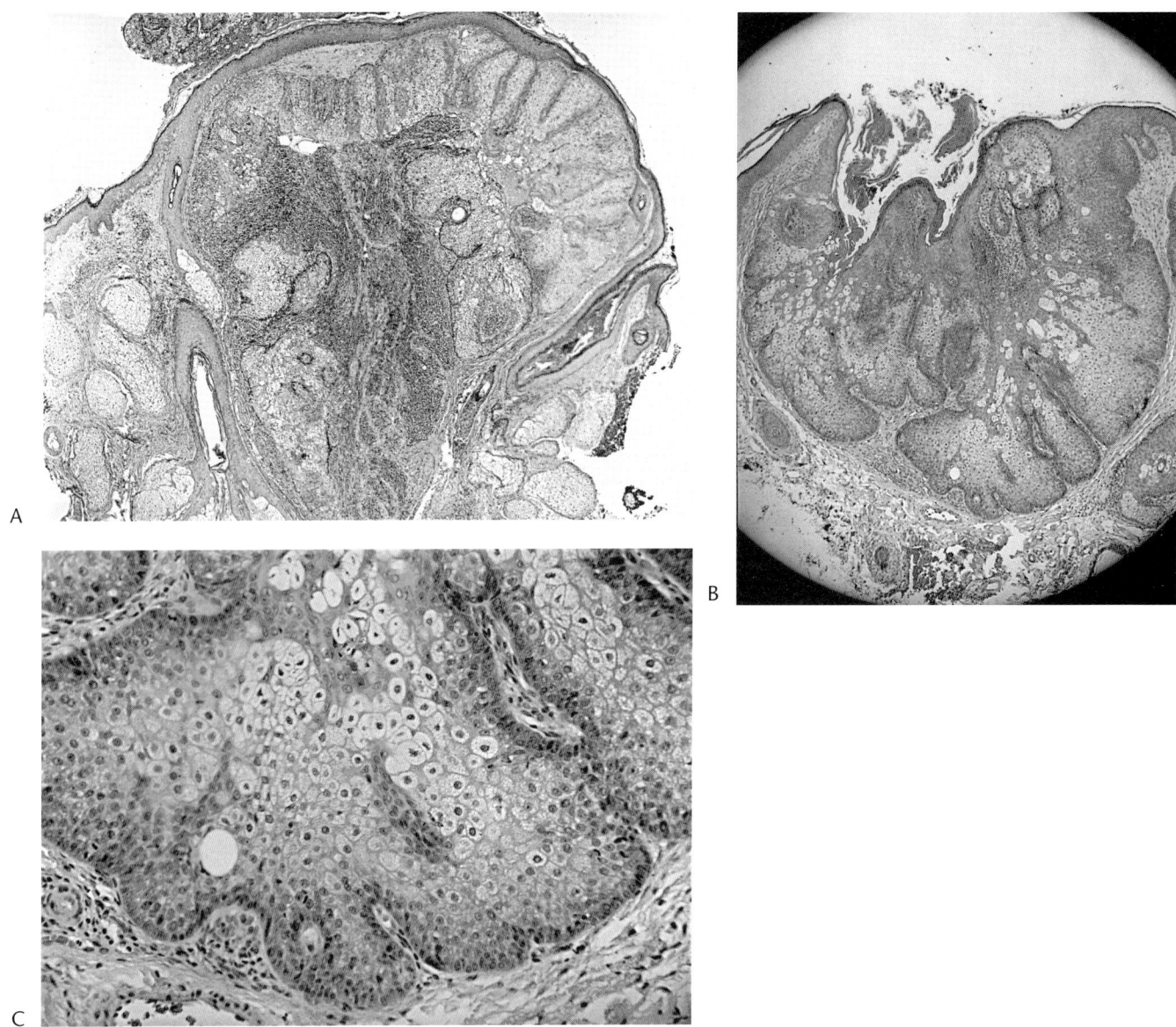

Figure 18-24. Sebaceous adenoma, classic type. (**A**) This lesion contains a tumor of sebocytes with prominent differentiation in the pyriform lobules that connect and have a vertical orientation. (× 40.) (**B**) This lesion connects to the surface by a patulous opening, but the sebaceous lobules contain increased numbers of germinal cells and have a pyriform architecture. (× 70.) (**C**) The high power of one of the lobules reveals its pyriform architecture and the increased numbers of germinal cells. (× 250.)

basaloid germinal epithelium and few mature sebaceous cells (sebomatricoma; sebaceoma) (Fig. 18-25). In the latter type, sebaceous ducts and small cysts can be present. All tumors in this class lack stromal infiltration, in contrast to the characteristics of most carcinomas. The differential diagnosis includes basal cell carcinoma and sebaceous carcinoma.

Sebaceous Carcinoma

Sebaceous carcinomas[275] are a spectrum of rare cutaneous tumors similar to sebaceous adenomas but with stromal infiltration, often pleomorphic sebocytes, and a biologically progressive course.

Historically, these tumors have been separated into ocular[276,277] and extraocular[278] types, the former of which are more common and may be confused with a chalazion. The lesions have the potential for recurrence and metastasis, but the data are insufficient to draw definitive conclusions. Elderly women are affected most commonly, although the tumors may develop at any age. These lesions may occur in patients with Muir-Torre syndrome.[273]

Histologically, the lesions are similar to benign sebaceous tumors except that they have infiltrative zones and often harbor pleomorphic cell populations of clear and/or basaloid cells

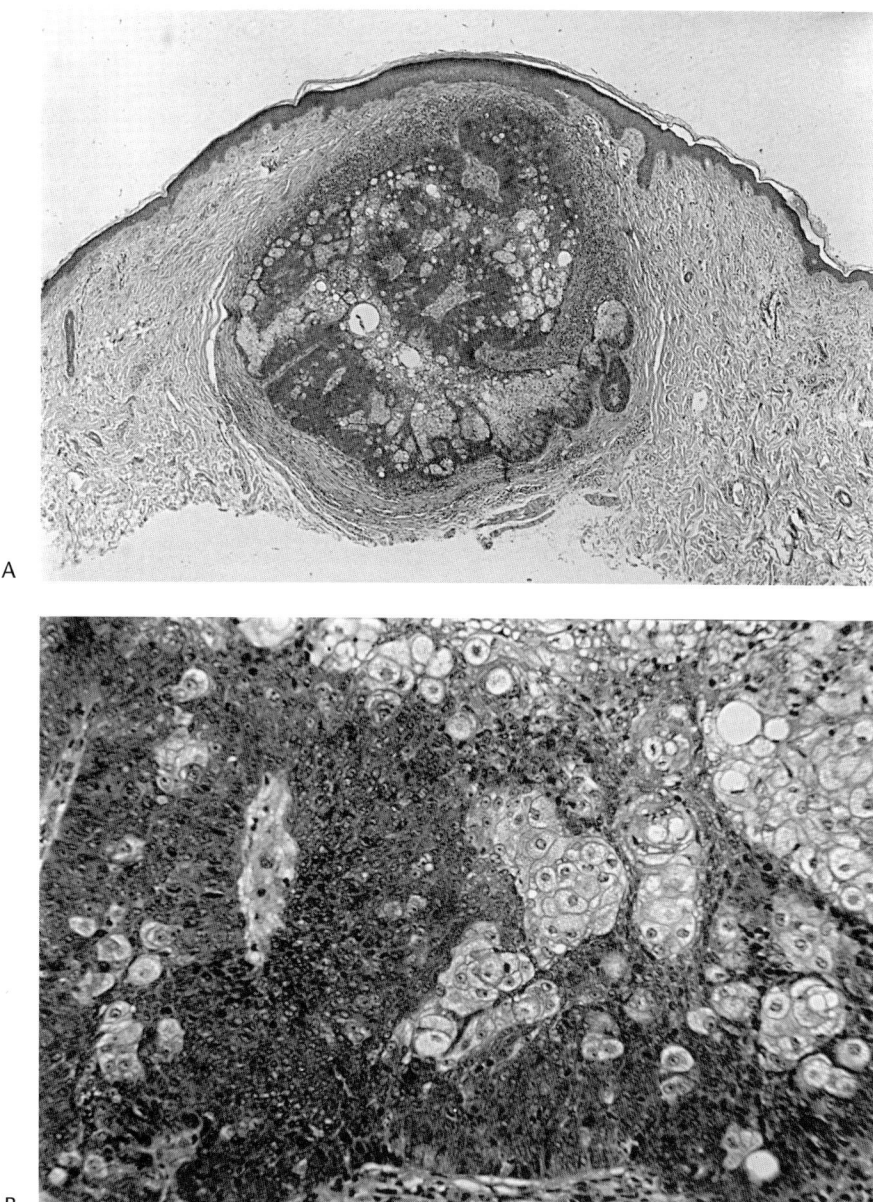

Figure 18-25. Sebaceous adenoma, cellular or germinal type (sebaceoma; sebomatricoma). **(A)** Scanning magnification reveals a circumscribed dermal lesion containing many basaloid sebocytes. The clearer zones consist of terminal sebocyte differentiation. (× 45.) **(B)** At high power, the germinal cells are much more prominent than in classic sebaceous adenomas. Small clusters of well-differentiated sebocytes are present adjacent to the basaloid cells with similarity to the matrical follicular cells. (× 250.)

(Fig. 18-26). Histologically, the growth patterns include lobular, comedo carcinoma-like, papillary, and mixed. Cytologically, if sebocytes are identified easily within such a tumor, the diagnosis is more straightforward than for many sebaceous carcinomas in which the intracytoplasmic lipid spherules are absent by H&E stains. In the latter cases, the cytology may be squamoid, basaloid, adenoid, or fusiform, raising an entire set of differential diagnoses for each pattern. Pagetoid spread in the epidermis is a feature observed occasionally in periocular

tumors (Fig. 18-27) and should not be mistaken for ductal carcinomas of apocrine or eccrine glands, malignant melanoma, or epidermotropic neuroendocrine carcinoma.[279] Special studies for intracytoplasmic lipid, such as oil red O and Sudan IV (which require fresh tissue), may be useful in aiding the diagnosis. They are especially helpful in tumors with pagetoid patterns that mimic ductal (eccrine?) or apocrine carcinomas, which typically produce intracytoplasmic mucin, in contrast with sebaceous carcinomas. Immunostains such as epithelial

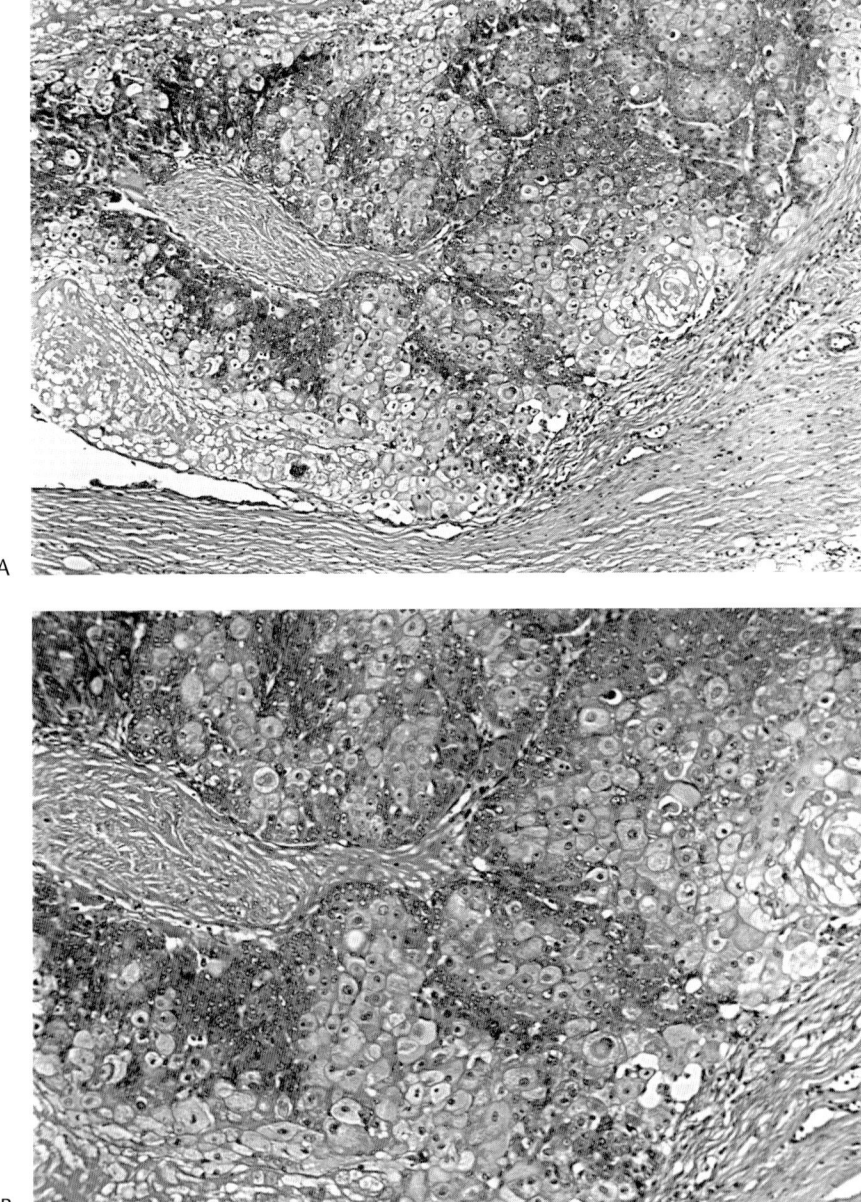

Figure 18-26.   Sebaceous carcinoma. **(A)** These tumors have a wide variety of patterns. This one has lost some of the lobular architecture of a sebaceous lobule and contains an accentuated zone of basaloid cells. Even in the better differentiated sebaceous cells, the nuclei are slightly enlarged compared with normal controls. Other areas in this tumor were more basaloid and infiltrative, similar to a general carcinoma pattern. (× 90.) **(B)** At this power, there is slight variation in the sebocyte nuclei, which is very uncommon in sebaceous adenomas. (× 150.)

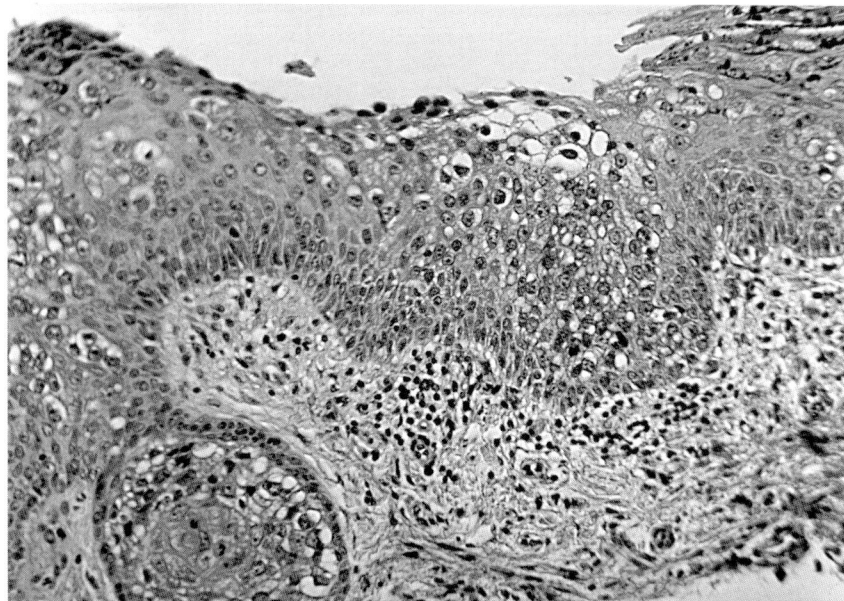

Figure 18-27. Sebaceous carcinoma, epidermotropic. This eyelid sebaceous carcinoma fills the epidermis and extends from a follicle. Note the vesicular cytoplasm within the tumor cells. (× 275.)

membrane antigen, human milk fat globulin,[280] and S-100 protein may be helpful in differentiating these lesions from porocarcinoma (acrospirocarcinoma), extramammary Paget's disease, tricholemmal carcinoma, clear cell squamous carcinoma, malignant melanoma, and basal cell carcinoma. Electron microscopy may be helpful to identify intracytoplasmic lipid in difficult cases.

Tumors of Apocrine or Eccrine Glands

Nevi and Adenomas

Historically, the ductal tumors have been divided into apocrine and eccrine. This distinction is not always straightforward as the ducts of each gland type are similar and focal apical "decapitation" can be observed in a variety of traditional "eccrine" tumors, such as those in the poroma (acrospiroma) group. As a practical matter, these should be divided into apocrine or eccrine based on their dominant features in H&E-stained sections. As a point of controversy, most lesions traditionally classified as "eccrine" do not have clearly demonstrable zones similar to the eccrine secretory coil. Therefore, this classification, with rare exception, is separated into apocrine and ductal lesions, realizing that many of the ductal adenomas probably originated in eccrine ducts.

Two types of ductal lesions, *squamous and mucinous syringometaplasia,* are not discussed in detail in this chapter. Both probably are reactive rather than neoplastic in nature. This is certainly true for squamous syringometaplasia[281–292] in which a variety of traumatic and chemical agents have been implicated in its cause. The epidemiology of mucinous syringometaplasia is not as clear for a reactive cause, as most of these lesions are solitary, often verrucous, and often associated with a clinical differential diagnosis of a tumor. The typical histologic findings of focal bland mucinous goblet cells in the distal ducts or acrosyringia suggest a localized metaplastic process.[281,293–302]

Proliferations with Ductal and Apocrine Differentiation

Tumors with distinct apocrine features comprise a narrow category of lesions. Included are those tumors that contain apocrine epithelium as a major or conspicuous component.

Apocrine Nevus. Apocrine nevus[303–306] is a spectrum of rare hamartomas that contain lobules of mature apocrine glands in a tumor-like pattern of growth. These usually occur in adults, and most affect the axilla, chest, or scalp.

Tubular Apocrine Adenoma. Tubular apocrine adenoma[307–310] includes a range of small nodular tumors composed of tubules with apocrine features. The lesions affect adults, and some can occur in association with organoid nevus (nevus sebaceus).

Histologically, the lesions are circumscribed and composed of dilated tubules usually lined by one or more layers of cells; the apical cells have apocrine features. The tubules are typically separated by a fibrous stroma (Fig. 18-28). Some have designated these lesions as *tubulopapillary hidradenomas* or *papillary tubular adenomas*[311,312] when they are composed solely of ductal epithelium[312,313] and no apocrine epithelium is present. Others have suggested that it be placed in a spectrum including papillary syringadenoma and papillary (eccrine) adenoma.[314]

Papillary Syringadenoma. Papillary syringadenomas (syringocystadenoma papilliferum)[315,316] are a spectrum of benign papillary tumors usually located on the scalp of adults and have a granular surface from which weeps serosanguinous fluid. Most are less than 2 cm in diameter. Some are associated with a nevus sebaceus.

Histologically, the lesions are usually marsupialized, although some can be cystic. As a rule, the marsupium or cyst, respectively, contains numerous rounded papillary dermal cores surrounded by a two-cell epithelial layer that may or may not

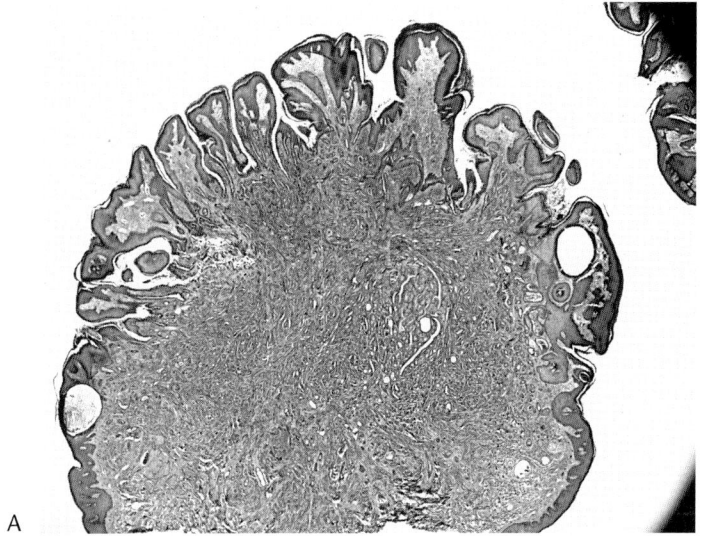

A

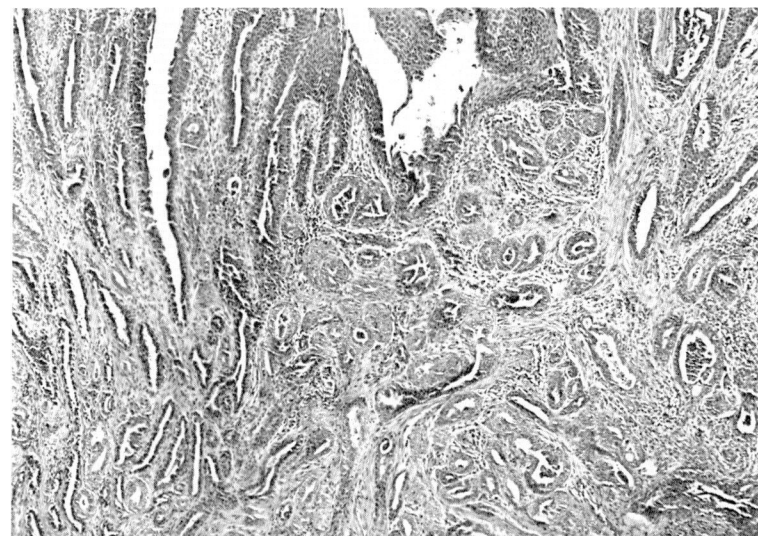

B

Figure 18-28. Tubular apocrine adenoma. (**A**) Scanning magnification from a scrotal lesion reveals a papillary surface with a complex dermal tubular pattern that slowly attenuates in the deep aspects. (× 12.) (**B**) Medium power reveals a two-cell layer tubular pattern throughout. In a few areas there was a minor degree of luminal secretion similar to apocrine glands. Most of this lesion, however, was ductal. (× 90.) (**C**) In some areas, small luminal papillations were present similar to those seen in cases of papillary (eccrine?) adenoma. It is not surprising that many have linked tubular apocrine adenoma and papillary (eccrine?) adenoma under the designation of *tubulopapillary hidradenoma* or *papillary tubular hidradenoma*. (× 90.)

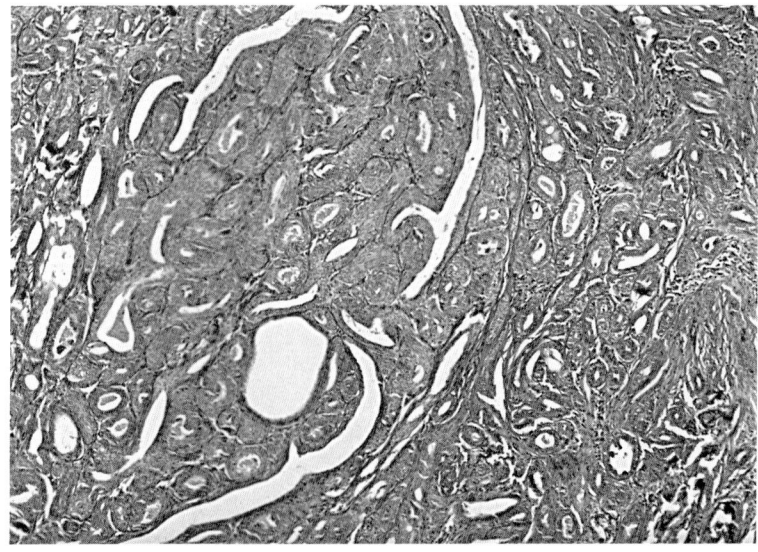

C

exhibit apocrine secretion (Fig. 18-29A). The papillary cores can contain numerous plasma cells (Fig. 18-29B), especially in marsupialized cases.

Papillary Hidradenoma. Papillary hidradenomas (hidradenoma papilliferum)[317–319] are a range of benign vulvar or perianal tumors that are usually nodular and covered by skin; however,

they are marsupialized occasionally. Occurrence in other anatomic sites is extremely rare.[320] Most lesions are 1 cm or smaller.

Histologically, most tumors are circumscribed and solid (Fig. 18-30A), but some are cystic. The growth pattern consists of a mixture of tubules and papillary tufts lined by a two-cell layer: an apical cuboidal cell and a deep myoepithelial cell (Fig. 18-30B). Distinct apocrine changes are usually observed in por-

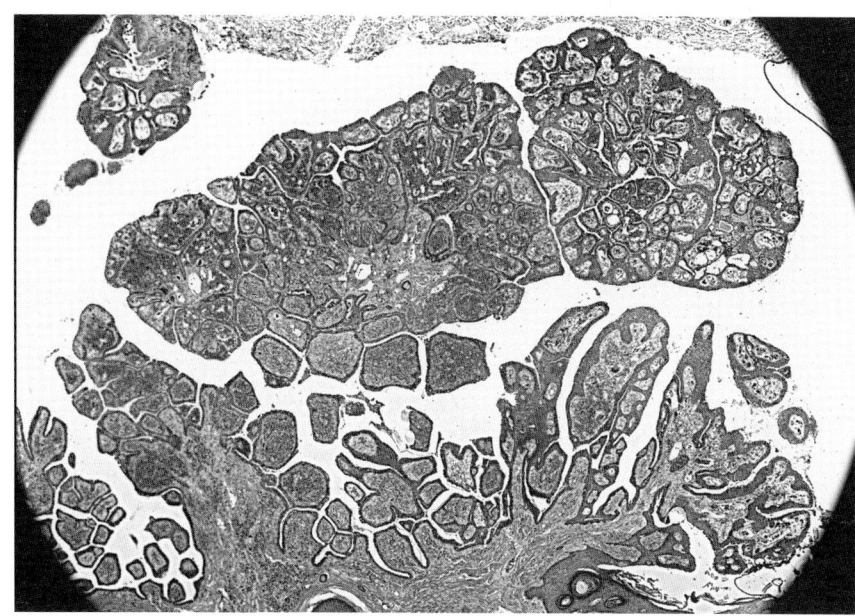

A

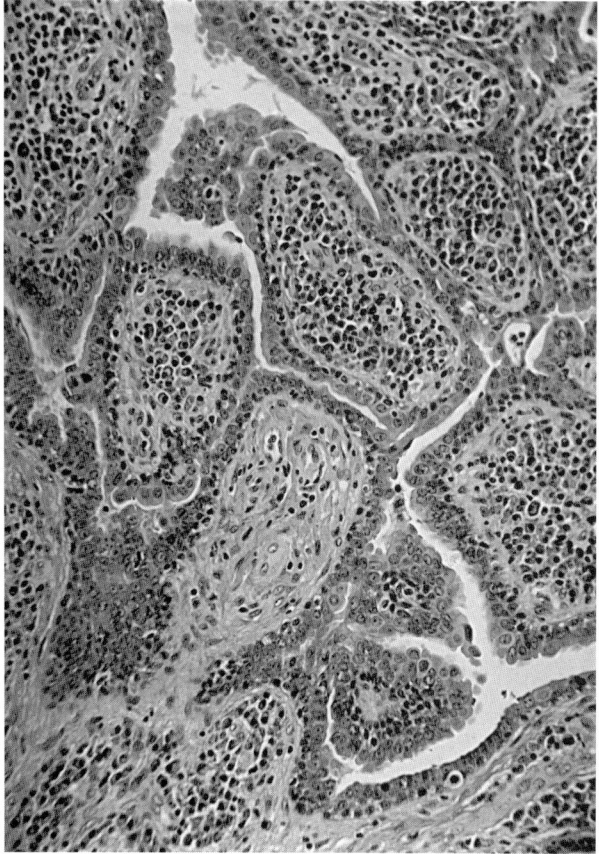

B

Figure 18-29. Papillary syringadenoma (syringocystadenoma papilliferum). (**A**) The lesion contains a papillary surface characterized by cores of fibrous tissue lined by a two-cell layer. (× 26.) (**B**) At higher power, the papillary cores are filled with mononuclear cells, principally plasma cells. There is pink apical cytoplasm in the epithelial lining cells, suggestive of apocrine differentiation. (× 250.)

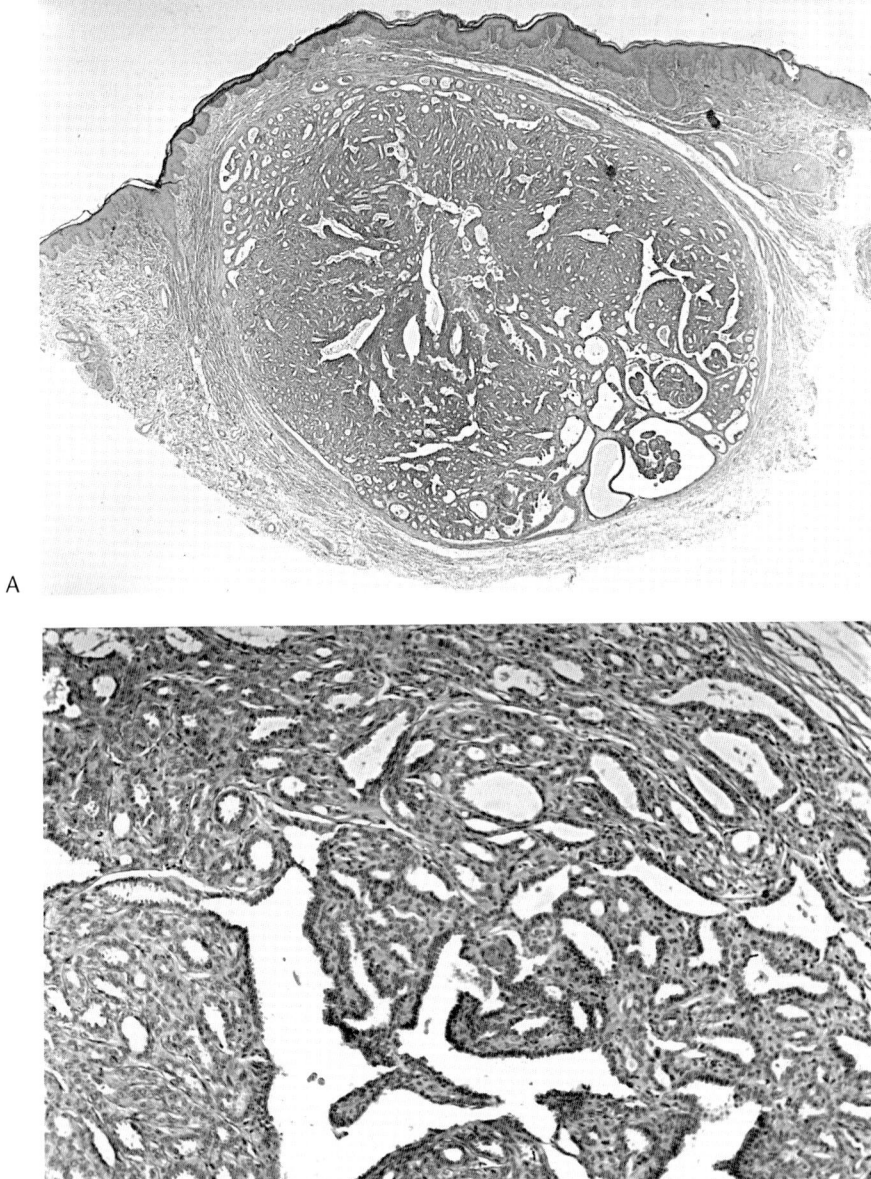

A

B

Figure 18-30. Papillary hidradenoma (hidradenoma papilliferum). (**A**) Scanning magnification reveals the spectrum within a single tumor. In much of the lesion, it exists as small tubules. In one small focus in the right lower portion, there is a papillary tuft. Some of these tumors may vary from nearly all tubular to nearly all papillary. Apocrine differentiation is seen commonly. (× 22.) (**B**) At medium power, note that most of this lesion consists of tubules. A few papillary tufts are noted. In a few areas, some of the linings contain zones of apocrine secretion. Some cases can be papillary as a predominant feature. (× 150.)

tions of the tumors, although there is considerable variation. An important differential consideration is adenocarcinoma, which can be excluded with confidence in most cases.

(Papillary) Oncocytoma.   Oncocytomas[321–323] are rare adenomas that are located usually in the eyelid and are thought to be related to Moll's (apocrine) glands. Of the few cases that

have been reported, all have occurred in older men. Excision appears to be curative.

The lesions are either cystic, papillary-cystic, or solid. The cystic or papillary portion is covered by a double layer of eosinophilic cells with granular cytoplasm. The cytoplasm is mildly PAS positive, diastase resistant. The nuclei are small and uniform. Ultrastructurally, the cytoplasm is filled with mitochondria. The differential diagnosis includes oncocytic nodular hidradenoma and granular cell tumor.[324]

Nipple Adenoma.   Nipple adenoma (florid papillomatosis of the nipple ducts)[325–329] is a spectrum of uncommon benign lesions that occur almost exclusively in women. The lesions are usually less than 1 cm in diameter; most are crusted or have a serous or serosanguinous surface, which must be differentiated from Paget's disease of the nipple.

Histologically, most nipple adenomas are circumscribed nodules composed of numerous duct-like structures lined by an inner breast-duct epithelium and an outer myoepithelial layer (Fig. 18-31A). Ductal, adenosis, or tubular patterns can be seen with or without epithelial hyperplasia (Fig. 18-31B). Variable amounts of sclerosis, apocrine secretion, or squamous metaplasia can be observed. Some occur with an associated intraductal papilloma. These lesions can rarely be associated with carcinoma.[327] Syringomatous patterns can be observed in some lesions[330,331]; these are similar to microcystic adnexal carcinomas (syringomatous carcinomas) histologically.

Fibroadenoma.   Fibroadenomas similar to those seen in the breast have been described rarely in extramammary sites.[332–338]

Most of these have occurred in the vulvar or perianal region except for one case on the arm.[339] The lesions present clinically as lumps or swellings in the affected site. Multiple lesions have been reported in one patient.[334]

Histologically, the lesions are circumscribed and contain branching glands usually lined by a two-cell layer that exhibits apocrine secretion (Fig. 18-32). The stroma is generally loose and myxoid, but can be fibrotic in some cases. The differential diagnosis may include papillary hidradenoma in some cases.

It has been postulated that these lesions arise in mammary-like glands of the vulva or perianal region.[340] An expanded list of related disorders, including lactating adenoma of the vulva, is discussed elsewhere.[340,341]

Mixed Tumor.   Benign mixed tumor (chondroid syringoma)[342–346] is a spectrum of benign ductal neoplasms, often with apocrine differentiation, and with a complex canalicular epithelial component including a myxoid and/or chondroid stroma. These tumors are histologically analogous to similar tumors in the salivary gland, but the cutaneous lesions seldom recur after excision.

Mixed tumors are solitary nodules that usually occur on the head and neck of adults. Most are small, approximately 1 to 3 cm in diameter. Rarely, giant lesions occur.[347] They have no specific clinical features.

Histologically, they are well circumscribed, located in the dermis or subcutaneous tissue, and are devoid usually of epidermal connections (Fig. 18-33). They contain mixtures of epithelial and myoepithelial patterns in a microtubular or tubular branching pattern (Fig. 18-34). The epithelium can be apocrine, but ductal-only differentiation may be identified in a significant percentage of the tumors. Some of these lesions exhibit clear cell change, linking a small population to the somewhat historic concept of clear cell myoepithelioma or its successor, the poroma (hidradenoma).[255] Rarely, shadow cells can be observed in some tumors, thus linking a minor population of these lesions to follicular differentiation. Immunostains, such as Cam

5.2 and carcinoembryonic antigen, highlight the epithelial and ductal components of these lesions. Gross cystic disease fluid protein-15 (GCDFP-15) highlights some lesions, especially those with apocrine differentiation. S-100 protein is positive for the myoepithelial components.

The stroma is fibroblastic, mucoid, myxoid, chondroid, adipose (Fig. 18-35), and, rarely, osteoid. Stromal mixtures are common in these lesions.

Because of the wide spectrum of epithelial and stromal variations in these lesions, the term *mixed tumor* is appropriate. The differential diagnosis ranges from poroma for the mostly solid tumors to myxoma for the lesions with abundant myxoid stroma. Those lesions that contain numerous small, uniform tubules can be confused with syringoma.

Poroma (Acrospiroma, Hidradenoma).   Poromas can have definite foci of apocrine differentiation (Fig. 18-36). In fact, one group of authors contends that most hidradenomas have foci of apocrine differentiation and should be classified in the apocrine group.[348] This class of lesions is discussed further below.

Proliferations with Ductal (Eccrine?) Differentiation

The benign ductal tumors can be regarded as a large class of lesions, the poroma (acrospiroma) group, and several smaller classes in which lesions are similar to specific portions of the normal eccrine apparatus.

Nevi.   Ductal (eccrine?) nevi are rare, benign lesions that are analogous to hair nevi. They consist of eccrine ductal or acinar structures located within the dermis that exist in excess number or have an abnormal relation to each other or to other skin structures. There are three main categories: eccrine angiomatous hamartoma, porokeratotic eccrine ostial and dermal duct nevus, and syringofibroadenoma.

Eccrine Angiomatous Hamartomas.   Eccrine angiomatous hamartomas[349–355] are discrete, solitary or multiple, often painful and hyperhidrotic[356] lesions that occur on the hands, feet, or trunk of young persons.

Histologically, there are increased numbers of eccrine secretory lobules around and within which are increased numbers of capillary-sized vessels, some of which can be ectatic. Local excision, including amputation of digit,[357] may be required for relief of pain in some cases.

Porokeratotic Eccrine Ostial and Dermal Duct Nevus.   Porokeratotic eccrine ostial and dermal duct nevi;[358–364] are localized to linear, pinpoint, keratotic papules that are, with rare exception,[365] congenital. They typically occur on the palms, soles, fingers, or toes, but other sites can be involved.[366,367]

Histologically, the papules correspond to cornoid lamellae that are located in numerous, adjacent, hyperplastic eccrine ductal ostia that contain foci of carcinoembryonic antigen-positive dermal ducts joining the eccrine lobule to the depths of the ostia[368]; rarely follicular ostia can also be involved.[369] The eccrine coils are spared.

Syringofibroadenoma.   Syringofibroadenoma (acrosyringeal nevus)[370–373] is clinically characterized by solitary or multiple papules, plaques, or tumors that can be linear or agminated.

Text continued on p. 518

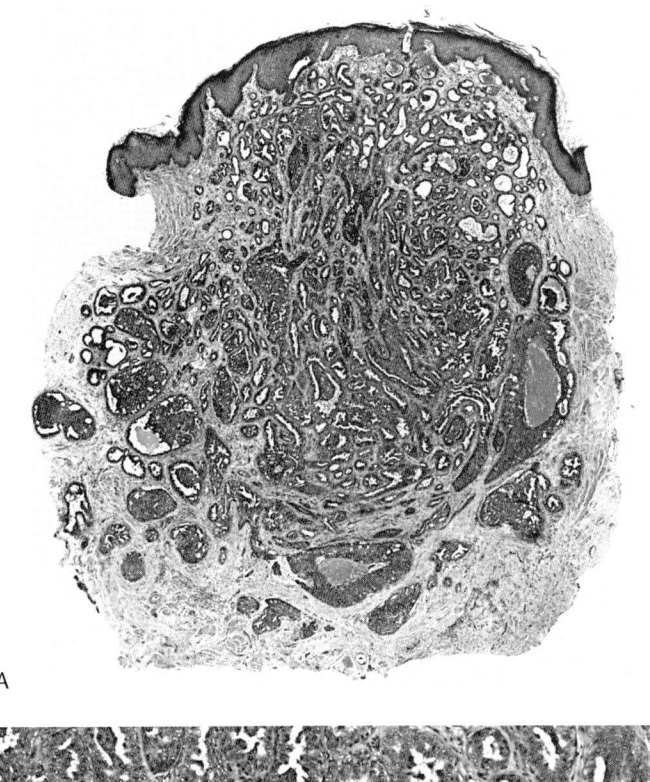

A

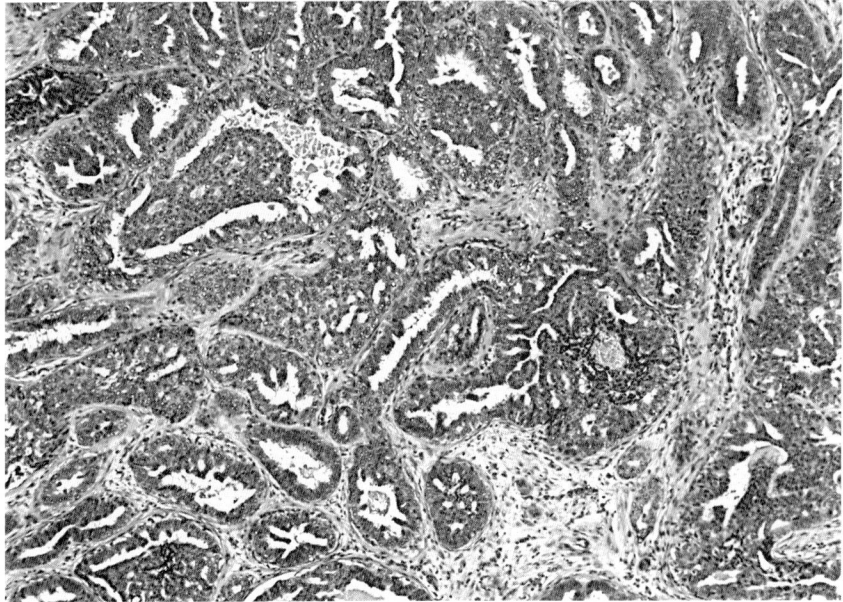

B

Figure 18-31. Nipple adenoma (florid papillomatosis of the nipple ducts). (**A**) The scanning magnification of the lesion reveals that it is just subjacent to the nipple. Some of the ducts connect to the epidermis. The ducts in the dermis have a heterogeneous pattern. Some clearly contain intraductal epithelial hyperplasia. Others are small, tubular, and relatively empty. This tumor must be differentiated from ductal carcinoma of the breast. (× 20.) (**B**) This medium-power perspective reveals the heterogeneity of the ducts within the tumor. Some are simple tubes, while others contain small tufts of ductal epithelium that extend into the lumens, while still others are virtually filled with epithelial cells. Focal apocrine secretion is present. This pattern is similar to ductal epithelial hyperplasia in the breast proper and must be differentiated from ductal carcinoma. (× 90.) (Courtesy of Charles S. Stevens, M.D., San Antonio, TX.)

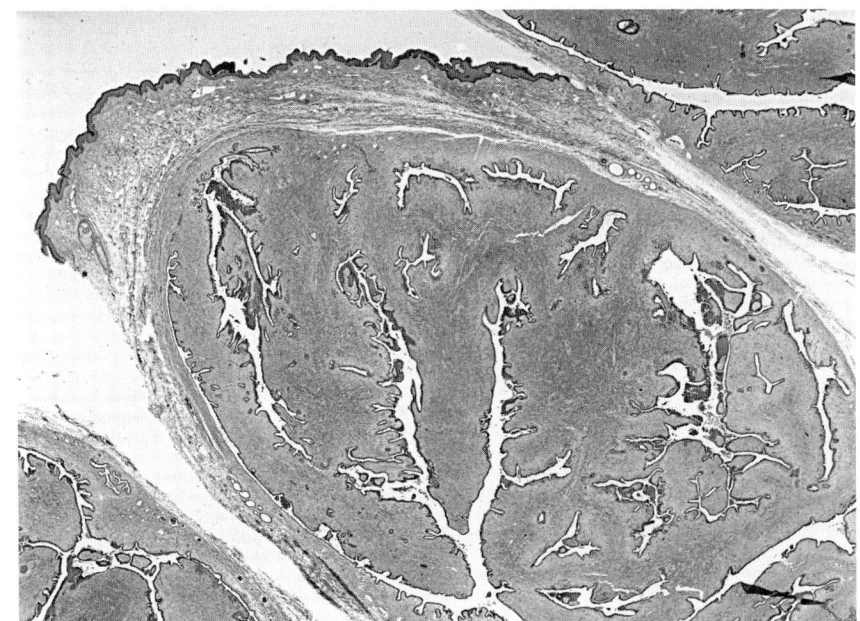

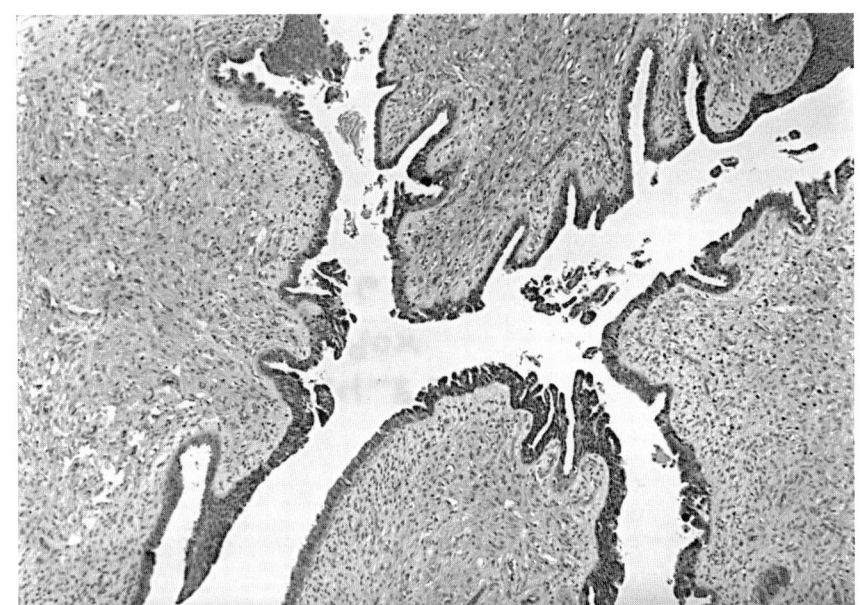

Figure 18-32. Fibroadenoma. (**A**) This lesion occurred in the vulva. Note the similarity to fibroadenomas of the breast with its abundant stroma and staghorn ducts. (× 10.) (**B**) The ducts contain papillations as well as focal apocrine differentiation. (× 90.)

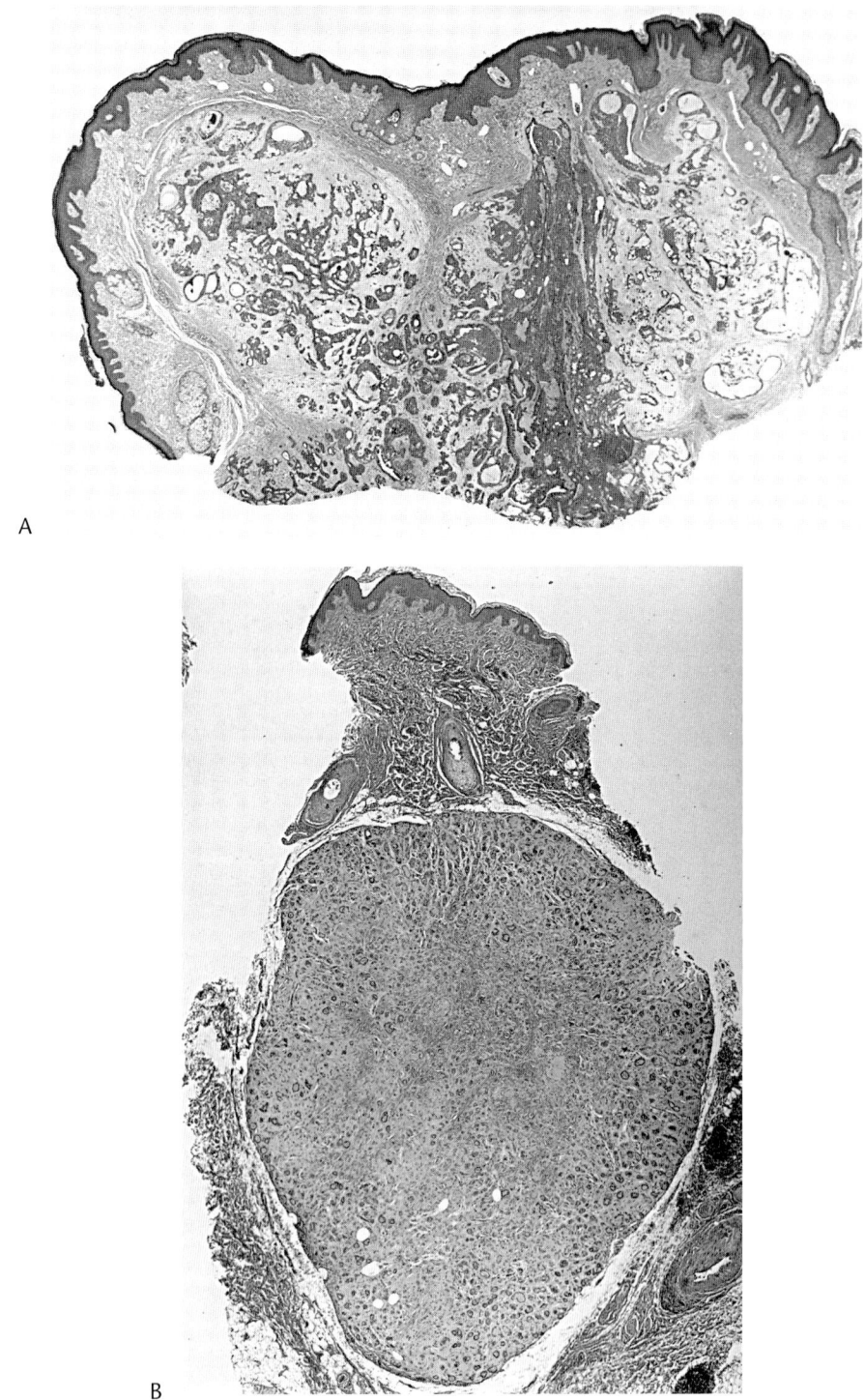

A

B

Figure 18-33. Mixed tumor. (**A**) Scanning magnification of this tumor highlights its peripheral circumscription and illustrates one end of the spectrum. The epithelial portion is somewhat heterogeneous. The branching tubular epithelial portions are enmeshed within a myxoid stroma. In some lesions, chondroid material is noted. (× 22.) (**B**) Mixed tumor, chondroid syringoma pattern. This scanning perspective reveals the opposite end of the spectrum with a sharply circumscribed dermal tumor containing small tubules of similar size that are distributed evenly throughout the tumor. (× 32.)

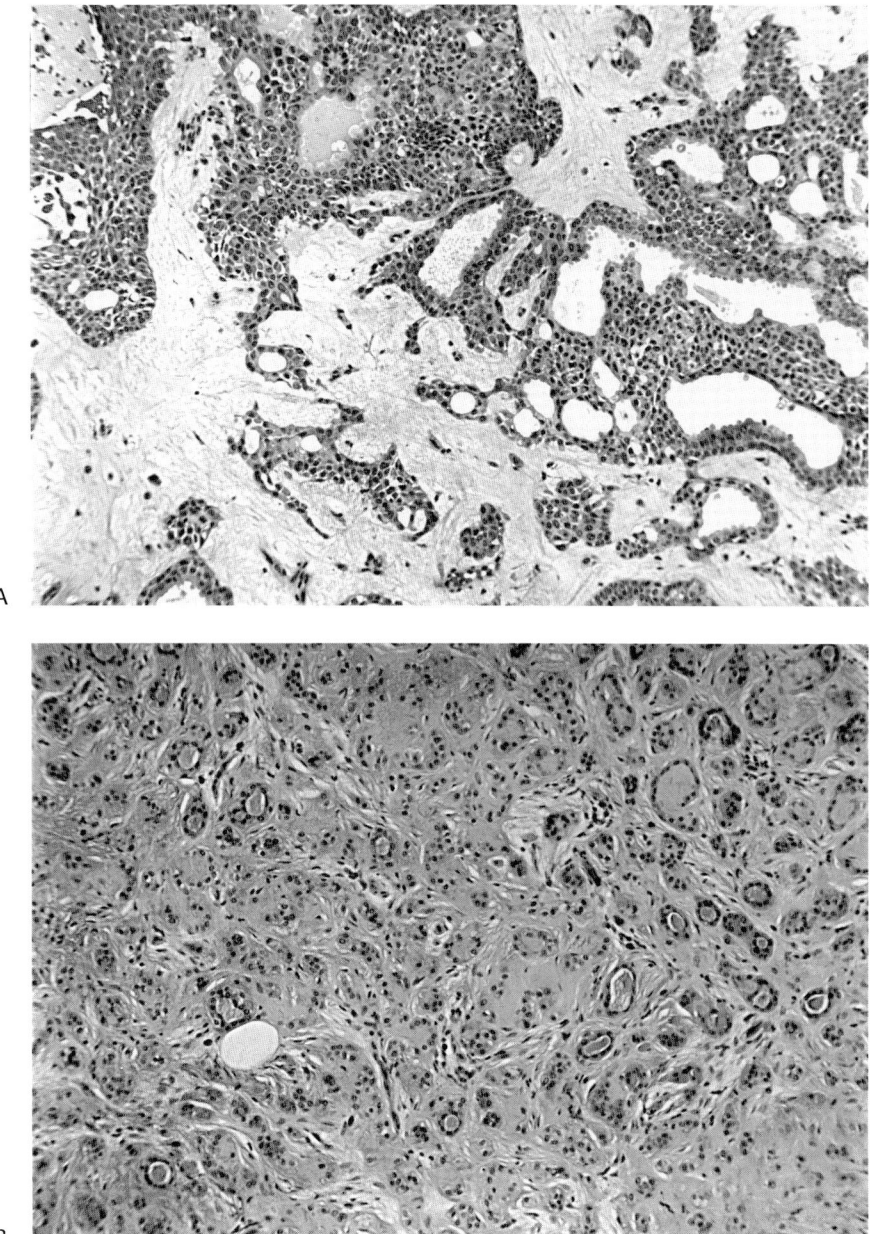

Figure 18-34. Mixed tumor. (**A**) This is a higher power perspective of the tumor shown in Fig. 18-33A. Note the branching pattern and the numerous tubules. Some are lined by apocrine epithelium in this case. The stroma is loose and myxoid. (× 150.) (**B**) Mixed tumor, chondroid syringoma pattern. This is a higher power perspective of the tumor shown in Fig. 18-33B. Note the uniformity of the tubules in the stroma. No apocrine differentiation is seen in this lesion. (× 150.)

Figure 18-35. Mixed tumor with abundant adipose stroma. Note that this lesion has quite a different pattern than the ones with a myxoid or chondroid background. However, the epithelial elements in this tumor are similar to the usual type of mixed tumor. (× 38.)

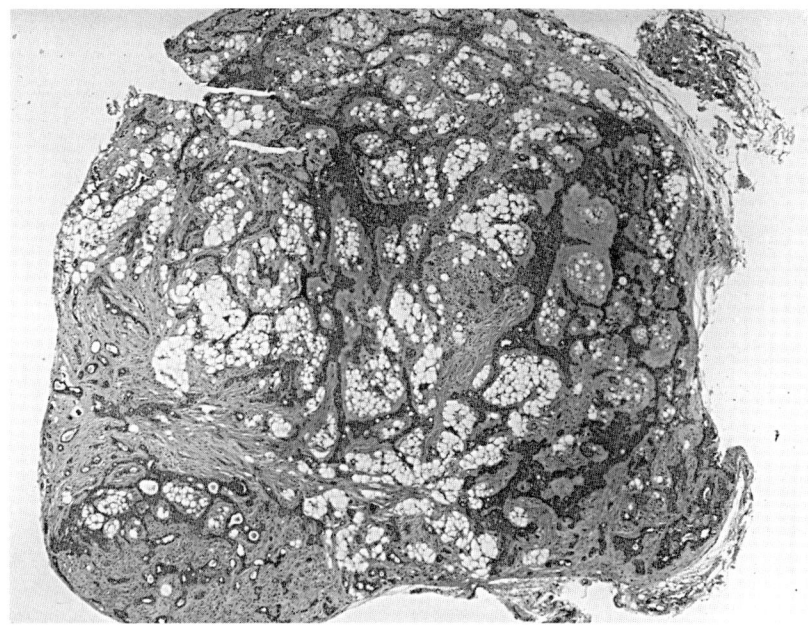

Some are moist and spongy to palpation. Most occur in older adults; some can be associated with hidrotic ectodermal dysplasia.[374]

Histologically, there are thin anastomotic epithelial strands with ductal differentiation extending from the epidermis. The myxoid stroma can be prominent in some lesions. Solitary lesions can be excised. The differential diagnosis includes reactive phenomena such as ductal proliferations around scars and keratoacanthomas.[375]

Poroma (Acrospiroma). Poromas (acrospiromas)[376,377] are a spectrum of benign, relatively monomorphous epithelial ductal tumors, some of which have focal zones of clear cell change and apocrine differentiation.[378] Historically, they were termed *poroma* because of their similarity to the cells of the intraepidermal eccrine duct.[379] However, lesions within the group are also similar to cells of the dermal duct and the coiled duct. Thus, it is reasonable to use the term *poroma* as a global designation for all architectural patterns within this class and subdivide them as described below.

Clinically, lesions in the poroma group range from a solitary plaque to exophytic papules to dermal nodules. The tumors usually occur in adults. They often occur on the sole and ooze or bleed, but they can occur at any site and are usually skin covered.

Histologically, the spectrum is separated by the location of the tumor in relation to the epidermis and by the growth pattern and cytologic pattern. Those with tumor confined principally within nests in the epidermis are termed *epidermal poroma* (acrospiroma) or *hidroacanthoma*[380,381] (Fig. 18-37). Those that involve both epidermis and dermis are termed *juxtaepidermal poroma* (acrospiroma) or just *(eccrine) poroma*[379,382] (Fig. 18-38). Those that are confined exclusively to the dermis are termed *dermal poromas* (acrospiromas), but historically have been referred to as *hidradenoma* (Fig. 18-39); those poromas (acrospiromas) with conspicuous ducts are termed *dermal duct tumors*[383] (Fig. 18-40).

Poromas are characterized by a pronounced variation in pattern and cell type. More than one type is often present in a single tumor.[384] Variable amounts of macroscopic or microscopic cysts and lumens can be observed within a given tumor. Most of these cavities are lined by cuboidal or cylindrical epithelium that, at times, has variable degrees of mucinous (goblet cell) differentiation. Focal areas of squamous metaplasia can be present. These spaces have an amorphous, proteinaceous, eosinophilic content. Tumors with epidermal contact often have solid sheets of small cuboidal cells with a uniform nucleus and scant basophilic cytoplasm. These tumors occasionally have moderate to heavy melanin pigmentation.[385,386] Similar cell types predominate in the mostly solid tumors.

Poromas commonly contain uniform polygonal cells with ample eosinophilic cytoplasm and squamoid features.[348,387] This growth pattern tends to have a concentric organization of cell aggregates. Often, the aggregates form a central lumen with cuticular differentiation. Alternatively, several centrally located cells can display cytoplasmic vacuolization, representing intracytoplasmic lumen formation that recapitulates the embryogenesis of the ducts. Rare tumors may contain oncocytes.[324] Not uncommonly lesions with such varied patterns may have foci of apocrine differentiation.[387]

Some tumors have sheets of polygonal cells with ample clear cytoplasm, a centrally located nucleus, and distinct cell membranes. This cell type can comprise part of a tumor or be responsible for most of its mass.

Occasionally, some tumors display a pattern of small, thin cords and nests. Others have rounded nests of small, regular basaloid cells, with a poroma-like intraepidermal component. Many of the tumor lobules have a central cystic, lumen-like cavity filled with eosinophilic, granular material.

Immunomarkers for carcinoembryonic antigen and a variety of cytokeratins are found commonly in poromas[388,389] and are similar to patterns found in the duct. Estrogen and progesterone receptors are generally negative.[390]

The stroma may be composed of delicate collagen fibers or, more characteristically, eosinophilic hyalinized collagen. Infrequently, an inflammatory infiltrate accompanies the peripheral

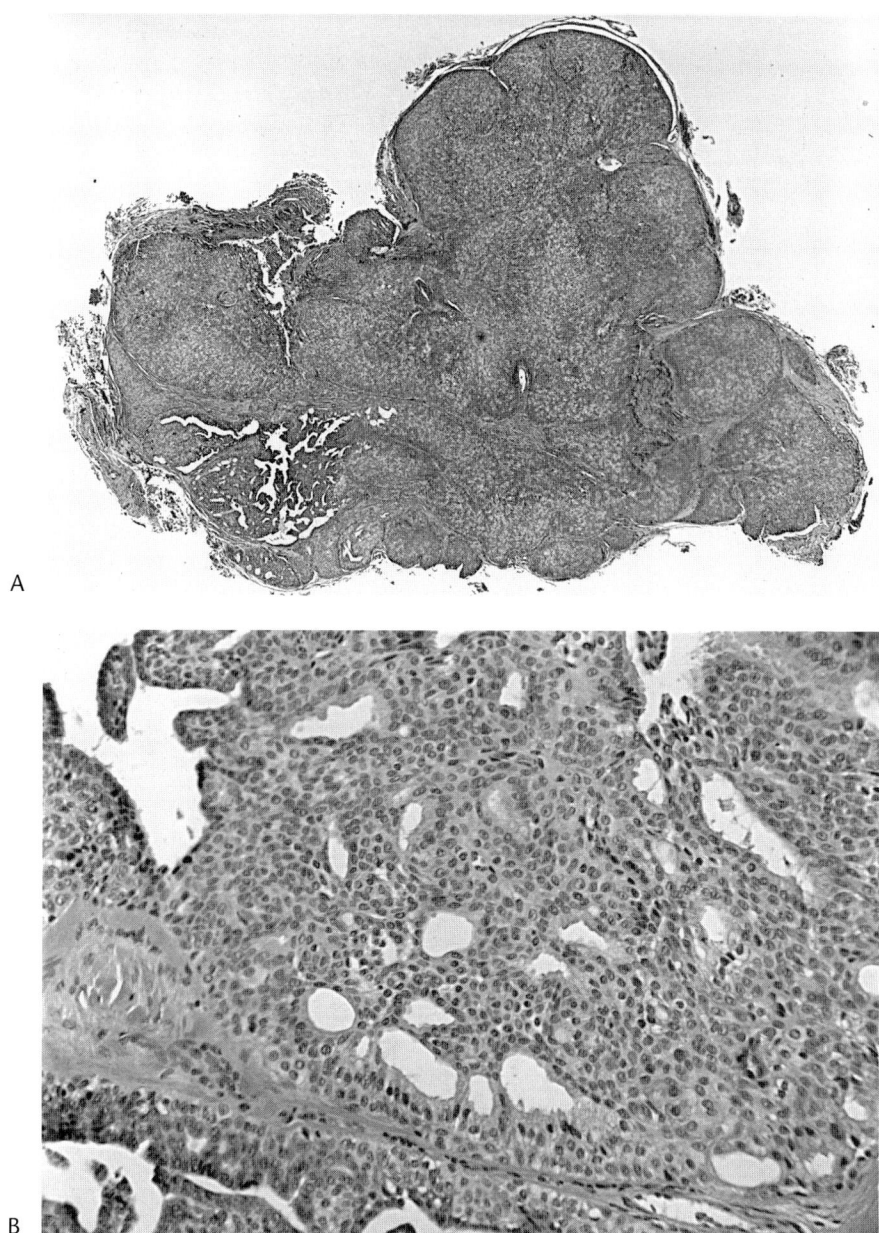

A

B

Figure 18-36. Poroma (acrospiroma, hidradenoma). (**A**) This lesion contains prominent clear cells with uniform, separate nuclei that do not overlap. Focal apocrine changes are present in this lesion. (× 21.) (**B**) Apocrine differentiation is noted in a focus from this lesion. (× 250.)

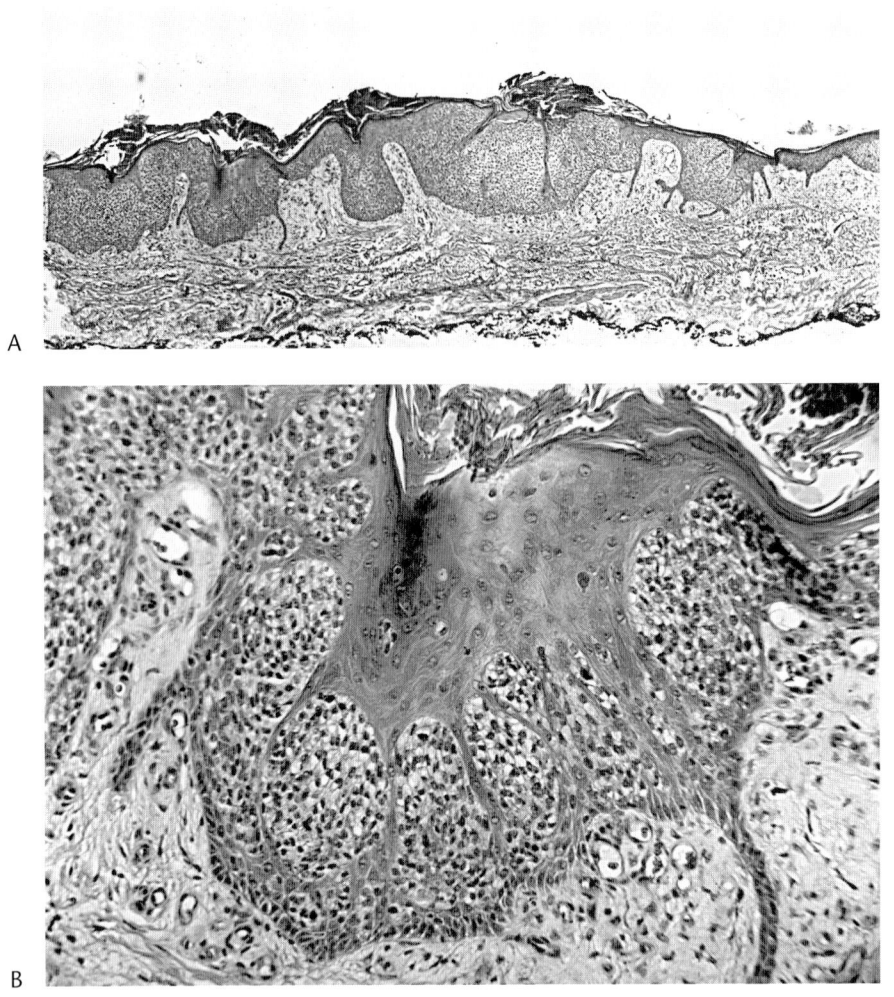

A

B

Figure 18-38. Poroma (juxtaepidermal acrospiroma, hidradenoma). Although there is focal connection to the epidermis, most of the lesion is dermal. In this case, numerous large cystic spaces are present within the tumor lobules. Note the cholesterol clefts in the lower right, signifying a reparative reaction around the tumor. (×17.)

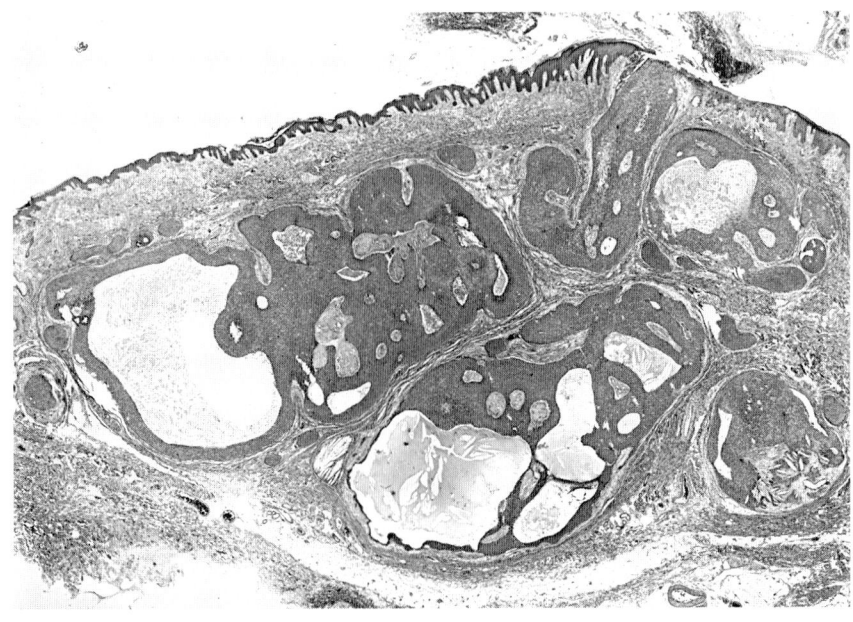

Figure 18-37. Intraepidermal poroma (hidroacanthoma simplex). (**A**) This lesion contains prominent clones of clear cells with features similar to clear cell poromas (hidradenomas), but confined to the epidermis. Occasionally, ducts are found in these lesions. (× 33.) (**B**) At higher power, the clone of clear cells is sharply demarcated from the keratinocytes. (× 250.)

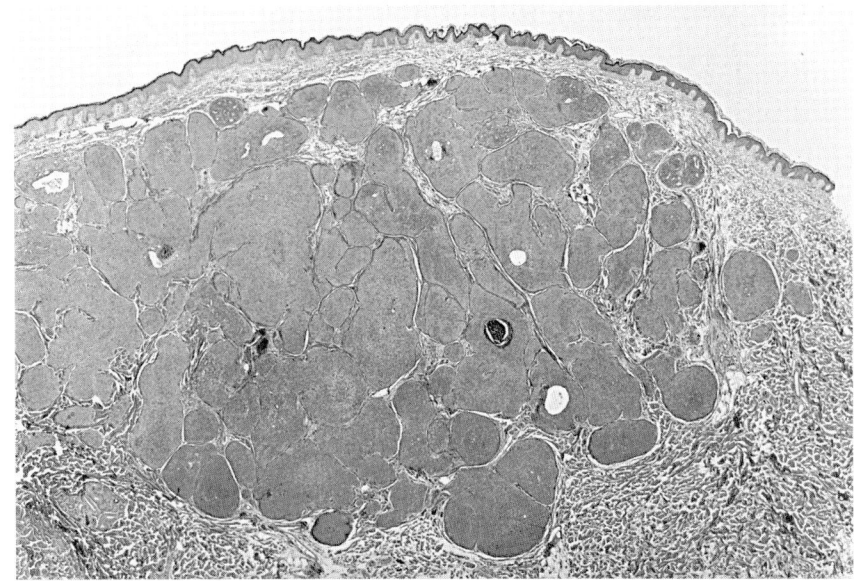

A

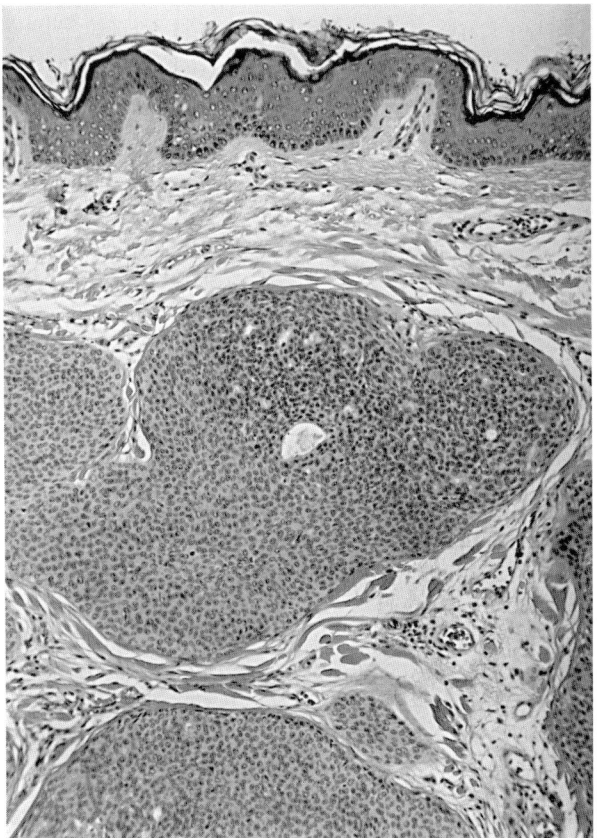

B

Figure 18-39. Poroma, dermal type (dermal acrospiroma; hidradenoma). (**A**) Scanning perspective reveals a dermal tumor containing closely apposed, discrete lobules. A few clear openings are noted in some of the lobules, but most are solid. Minimal dermal reaction is noted around the tumor. (× 20.) (**B**) Within the tumor lobule, small ducts are present. In some dermal poromas, these may be difficult to find. (× 150.)

Figure 18-40. Poroma, dermal duct type (dermal duct tumor). Scanning magnification reveals lobules of dermal poroma with prominent intraepithelial openings as well as small ducts. (× 45.)

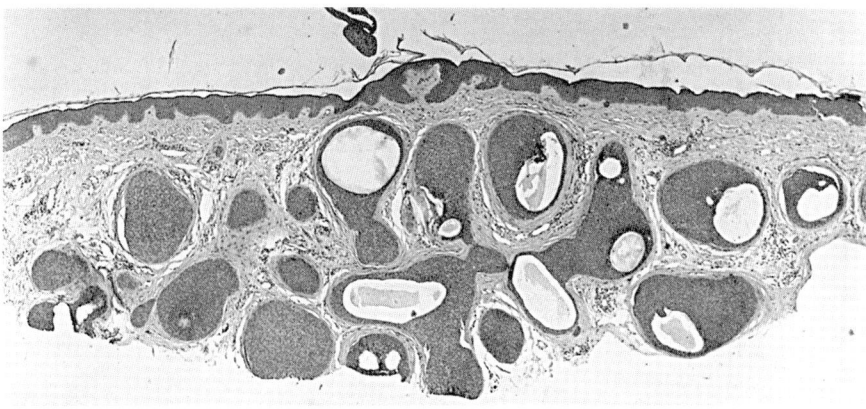

tumor lobules. Some tumors contain small, centrally located areas of necrosis en masse, especially those with monomorphous small cells.

Mitotic figures are usually sparse and may be abundant in some tumors, but these morphologic findings or their presumed immunologic correlates, such as the presence of proliferating cell nuclear antigen or p53 antigen,[391] do not necessarily confer a poor prognosis. Although the nuclei are usually regular and vesicular with finely granular chromatin, some tumors contain a few cells with a large, variably sized nucleus. This can raise a concern about the possibility of an aggressive course. However, these findings are almost always limited to only a few cells and do not appear to confer an adverse prognosis.[392]

Syringoma. Syringoma includes a spectrum of benign tumors characterized by complex, tortuous ducts. The tumors are typically skin colored. They usually occur on the head and neck of adults; they are usually multiple, but may be solitary.[393] Rarely, they are unilateral and plaque-like.[394,395] They have a predilection for the eyelids, but any site can be affected. A distinctly different pattern is that of disseminated syringomas, which may include a variety of presentations, such as eruptive[396] lichen planus-like,[397] urticaria pigmentosa-like,[398] and milia-like.[396] Some cases are familial,[399] and there is an association of syringomas in some patients with trisomy 21.[400,401]

Histologically, syringomas are interweaving nests, cords, and small cysts in the upper half of the dermis (Fig. 18-41). They seldom have epidermal contact and are enmeshed in a dense collagenous stroma. When they do join the epidermis, the lumens usually connect with small keratinizing cystic structures. The ducts of syringoma are composed of one or two layers of cuboidal cells, rarely with clear cell differentiation.[402–406] Some tumors have only a few epithelial structures, while others have hyperplastic cystic structures with luminal lamellar keratinization. Rupture of the cysts with subsequent foreign body reaction to keratin frequently occurs.

The solitary form of syringoma must be differentiated from microcystic adnexal carcinoma.[393] As a rule, syringomas do not infiltrate deeper than the mid-dermis, and they lack perineural or perivascular infiltration. In addition, syringomas are usually wider than they are deep, in contrast to microcystic carcinomas.

Papillary (Eccrine) Adenoma. Papillary (eccrine) adenoma[407–410] includes a range of benign ductal tumors composed of tubular ducts lined by a papillary cuboidal two-cell layer and separated by a fibrous stroma.

The lesions are small nodules or papules usually on the upper limbs. There are no specific clinical findings.

Histologically, the lesions are well-circumscribed, unencapsulated, dermal masses immediately subjacent to the epidermis (Fig. 18-42A). They are composed of dilated tortuous ducts of variable caliber (Fig. 18-42B). The ducts have prominent papillae, and the cells lining the ductal lumens are arranged in a double layer of uniform, cuboidal cells (Fig. 18-42C). Most ductal cell nuclei are regular, oval or round, with small nucleoli. Mitoses are rare or absent, except for rare focal changes. Focal areas of ductal cells may have apocrine patterns of secretion. The ductal lumens occasionally contain granular or amorphous eosinophilic material. Fibro-collagenous stroma surrounds the ducts.

The main differential diagnosis is tubular apocrine adenoma, which in some cases is similar to the papillary adenomas, thus accounting for the recent generic designation of *tubulopapillary hidradenoma* or *papillary tubular adenoma*.[311–313] It has also been suggested that it be placed in a spectrum including papillary syringadenoma and tubular apocrine adenoma.[314]

Adenomas with Predominantly Basaloid Epithelial Cells

Cylindroma. Cylindroma[411–413] is a spectrum of benign basaloid tumors that have a mosaic architecture and a biologically benign, but sometimes disfiguring natural history. Although their histogenesis is controversial, ductal differentiation is present in most. Apocrine differentiation is present in some. In addition, the occurrence of these tumors in the scalp suggests a conceptual link to folliculosebaceous structures.

Clinically, cylindromas can be solitary or multiple and usually occur in adults. The solitary form is the most common; it is an erythematous or skin-colored lesion on the scalp, head and neck, or trunk. It can have overlying telangiectases, but otherwise is fleshy. Some are painful. The multiple form is often referred to as the *turban tumor,* as it can cover the entire scalp. It can, on rare occasion, be associated with trichoepithelioma[49] and spiradenoma.[414] If familial, it is inherited as an autosomal dominant trait.[415]

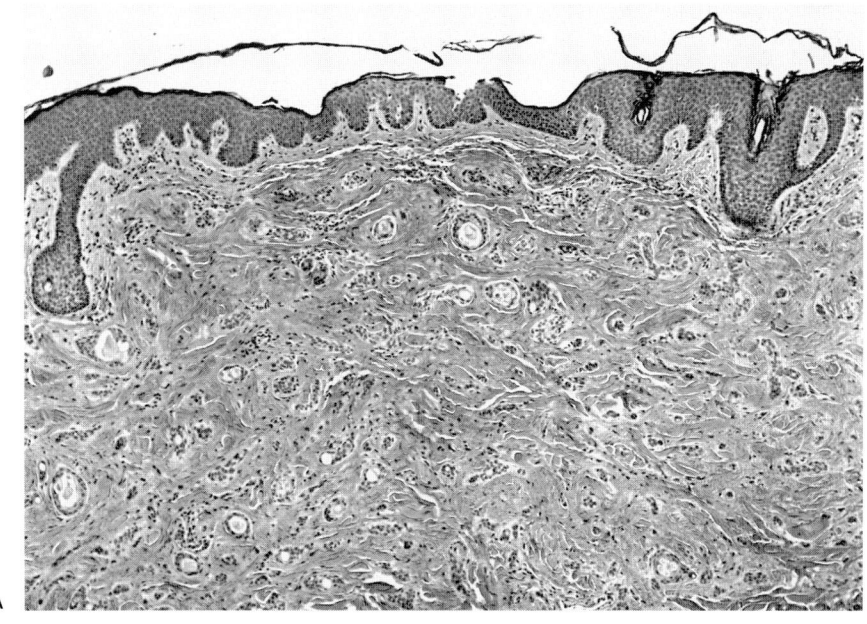

A

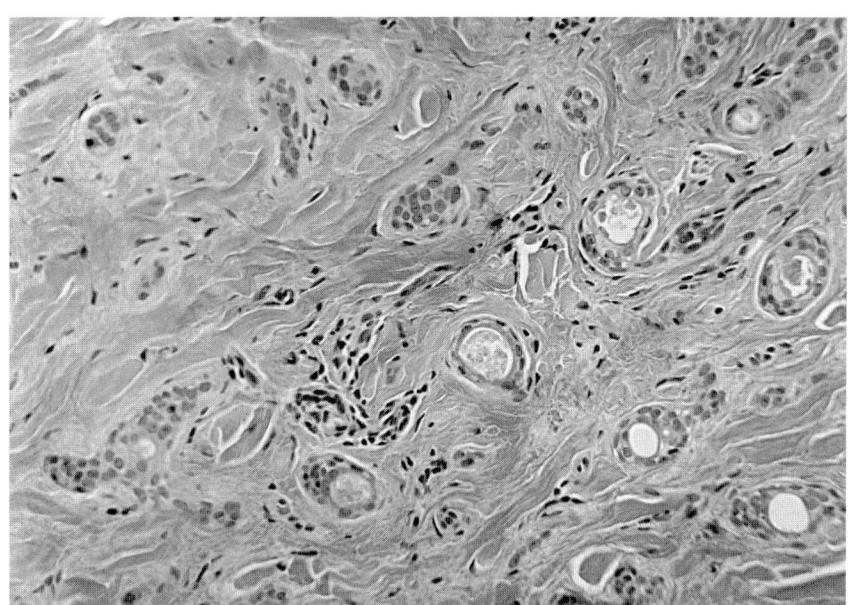

B

Figure 18-41. Syringoma. (**A**) This tumor consists of small ducts distributed within a fibrous stroma. Because there are many ducts, all coursing at different angles in the skin, any section will contain a mixture of findings, including tubules, cords, and tubules with attached cords (so-called "comma tails"). (× 90.) (**B**) Higher power clearly shows the teardrop-shaped ducts. (× 290).

Figure 18-42. Papillary (eccrine) adenoma. (**A**) Scanning magnification shows that the tumor is circumscribed and contains numerous tubules separated by stroma. (× 32.) (**B**) Medium power reveals rounded and angular tubules, some of which contain luminal projections. (× 90.) (**C**) High power reveals that the tubules have two-cell layers with intraluminal papillae. (× 250.)

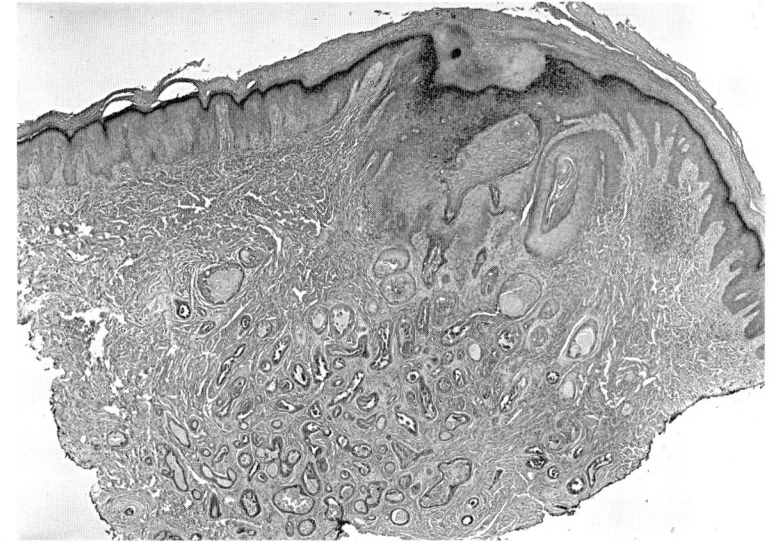

A

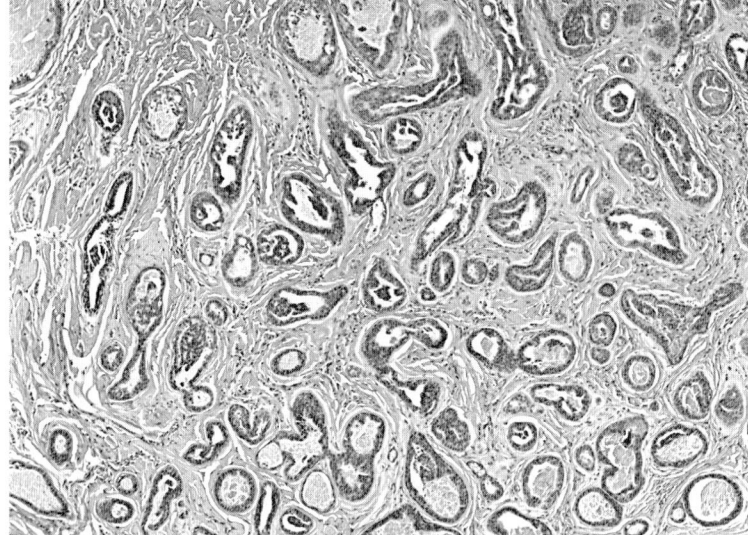

B

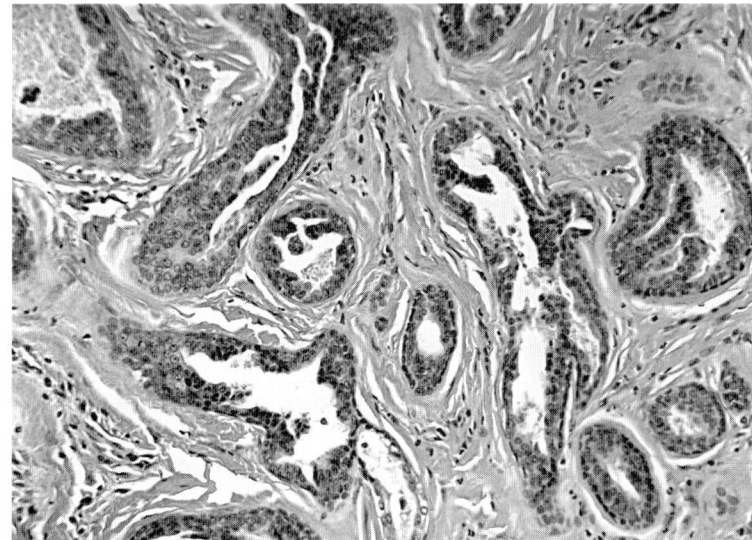

C

Histologically, the cylindroma consists of circumscribed, non-encapsulated dermal nodules composed of islands and cords of basaloid tumor cells surrounded by thick, hyalinized, PAS-positive basement membrane material. The cells are arranged in an interlocking jigsaw puzzle-like architecture (Fig. 18-43). Islands can have lumens or pseudolumens. Two cell types are characteristically present. The first is a small, dark cell, often located in the periphery of the tumor nodule; the second is a larger, lighter cell comprising the central portions of the cords. The tubules of cylindroma are often lined by an eosinophilic cuticle, although some apocrine-type secretion can be seen in some of the lumens. Some cylindromas coexist with spiradenoma and rarely with trichoepithelioma, suggesting a histogenetic link.

Spiradenoma. Spiradenomas[416–418] are a range of benign dermal tumors composed of anastomotic basaloid cells containing two distinct populations of cells. Many contain ductal elements. Some can coexist with cylindromas, and others are associated with follicular tumors.[419] Historically, spiradenomas have been classified as eccrine, but this classification appears to be too narrow. Rather than arbitrarily placing this lesion in the eccrine category, it is included in a broader category for this discussion.

The tumors are usually solitary, affect adults, and occur on the trunk, but rarely they can be congenital[420] and can occur in a variety of sites. Some lesions are painful.

Histologically, spiradenoma consists of one or more, often oval to spherical, distinct lobules located within the deep dermis

Figure 18-43. Cylindroma. (**A**) Medium power perspective reveals nests of basaloid cells with a "jigsaw puzzle" pattern. ($\times$ 30.) (**B**) Many cylindromas have only solid basaloid patterns, while others contain ducts. Basement membrane surrounds each of the tumor islands. ($\times$ 90.) (**C**) Often, cylindromas contain hyalin droplets of basement membrane material. Note the ducts in this lesion. ($\times$ 340.)

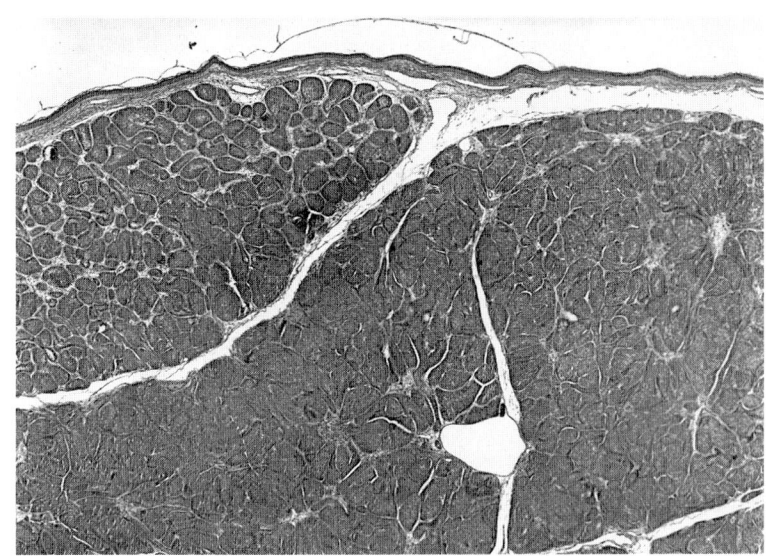

A

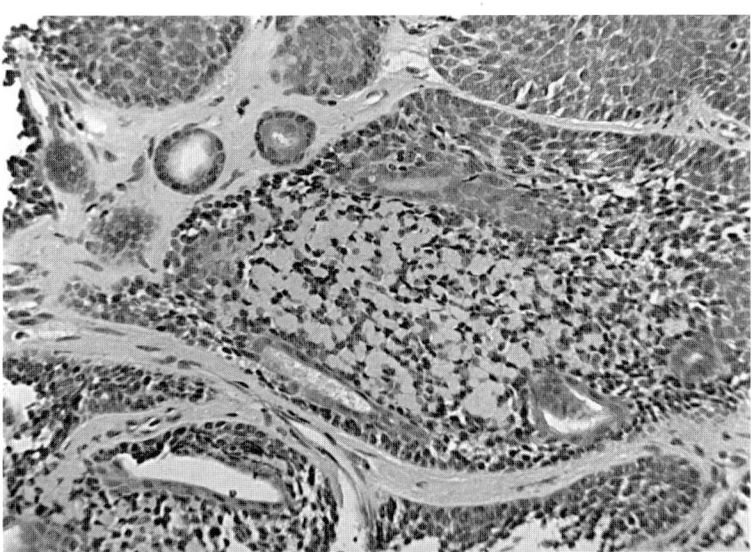

C

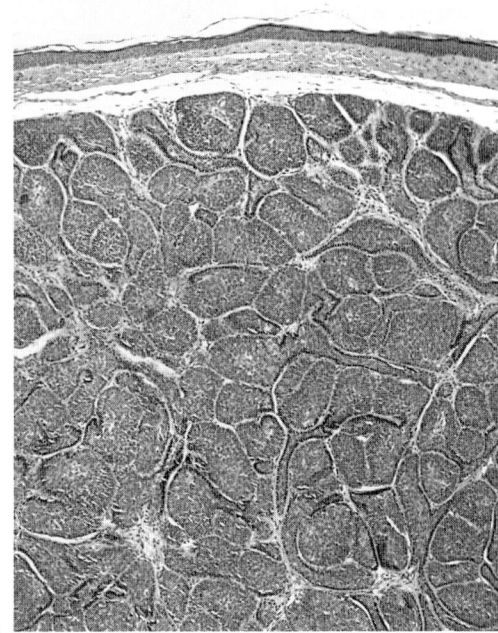

B

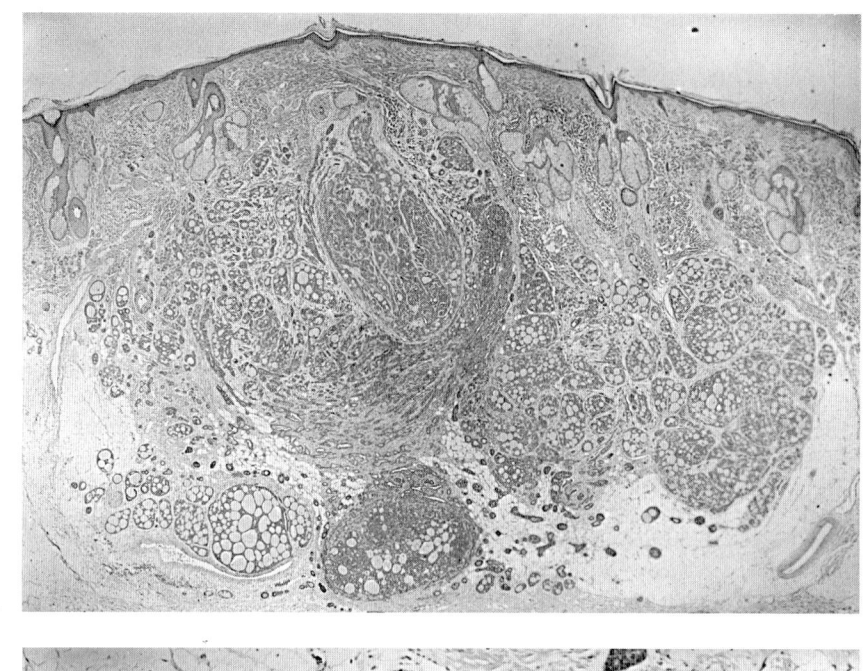

A

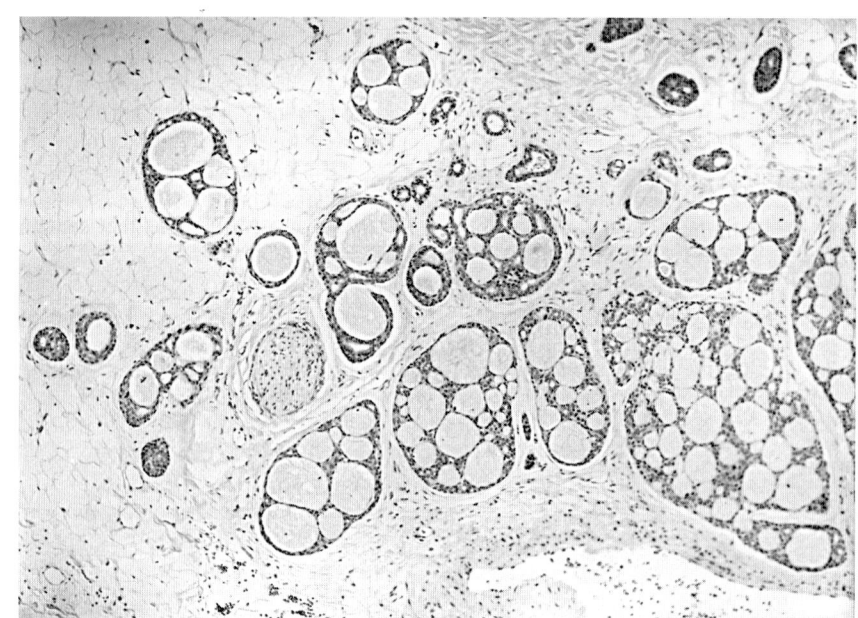

B

Figure 18-45. Adenoid cystic carcinoma. (**A**) Scanning magnification reveals large and small insula of basaloid cells containing round fenestrations. Observe how the lesion extends into the adipose tissue. (× 17.) (**B**) In a high-power perspective, note the stereotyped pattern of the fenestrated basaloid islands. Additionally, a nerve is involved by the tumor, a characteristic occurrence in such lesions. (× 90.)

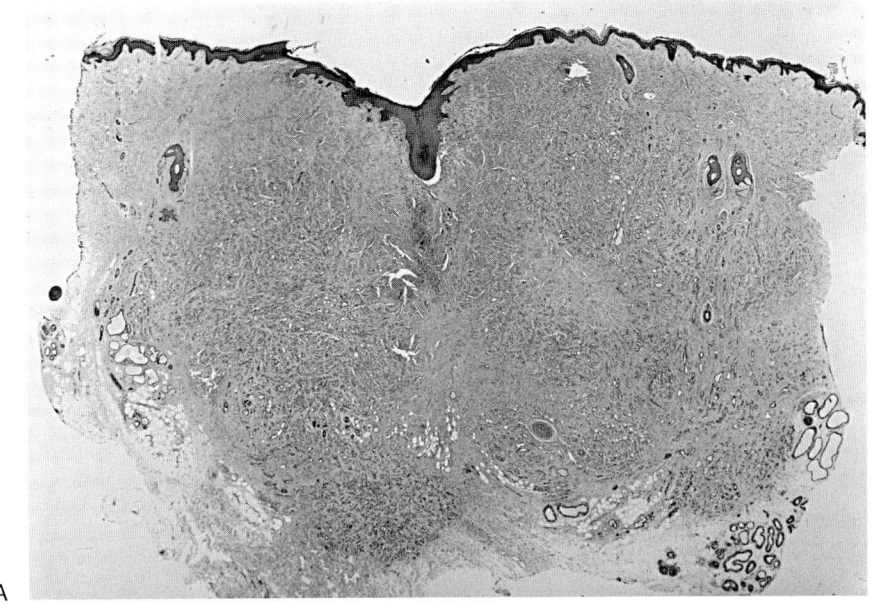

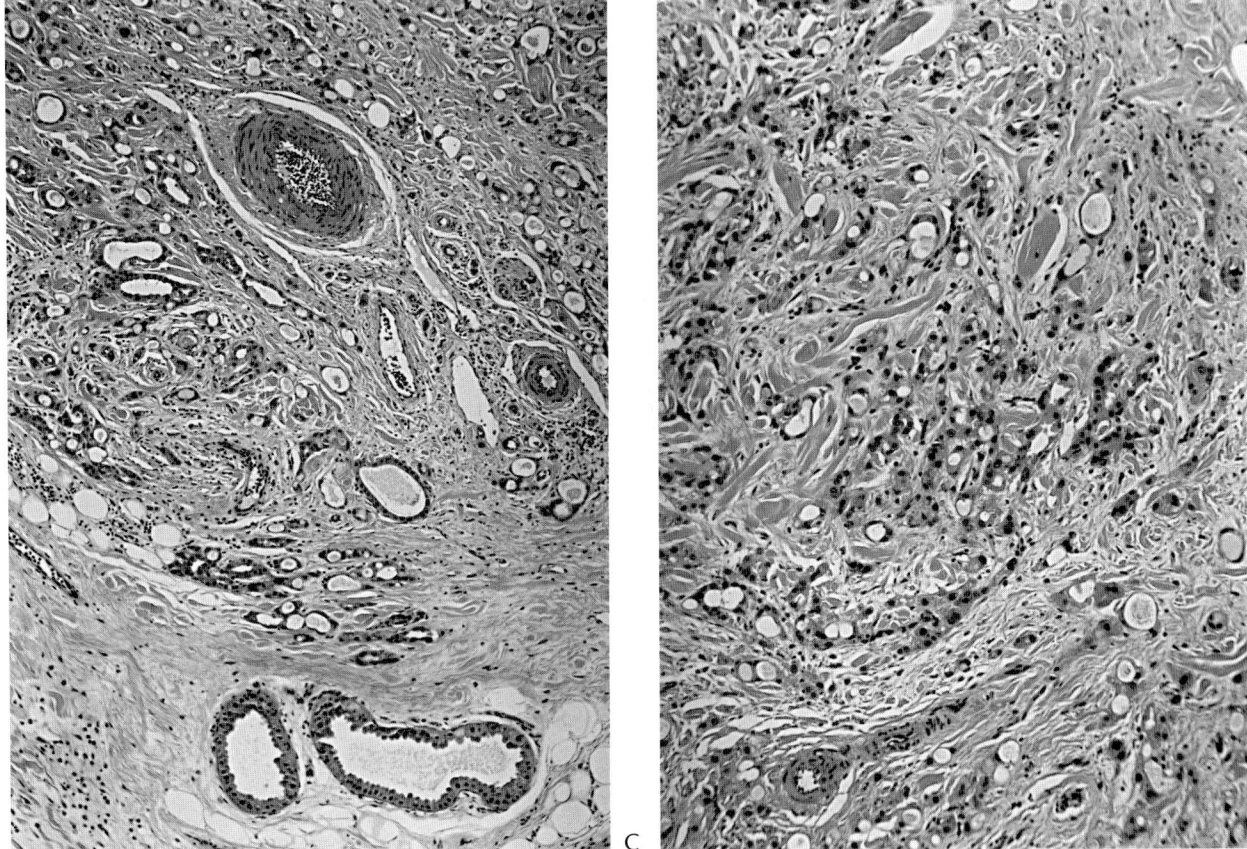

Figure 18-46. Apocrine adenocarcinoma. (**A**) Scanning magnification perspective reveals a circumscribed lesion with an infiltrative margin. It encroaches upon several large tubular apocrine glands in the periphery. This was an axillary lesion without a known breast primary. (× 12.) (**B**) In the deep portion of the tumor, one can contrast the irregular, infiltrative, tubules with the native apocrine glands. (× 90.) (**C**) High-power perspective illustrating large and small tubules, some with intracytoplasmic lumina. A small number of the tubules contain the characteristic "decapitation secretion" effect that is useful in the identification of apocrine differentiation. (× 150.)

Figure 18-47. Cylindrocarcinoma (carcinoma ex cylindroma). Medium-power perspective depicting the transition zone between the cylindromatous zones and the carcinomatous zones. Note the small cell "jigsaw puzzle" pattern adjacent to the larger cells. Obvious carcinoma was identified elsewhere in the lesion. (× 90.)

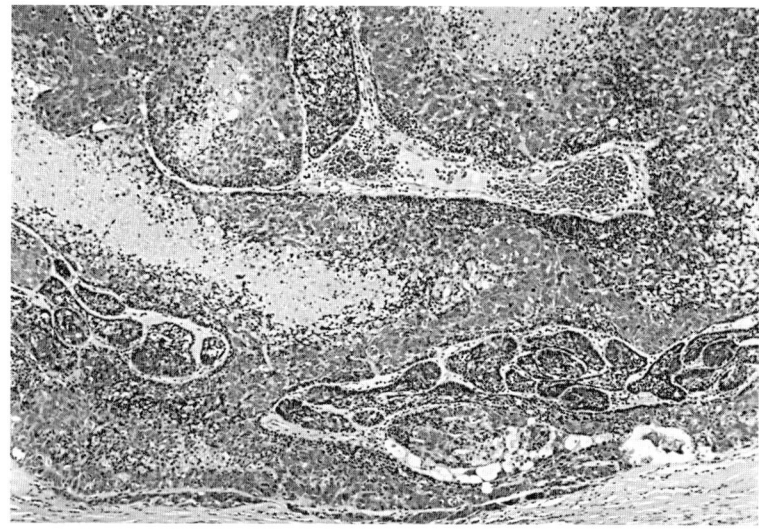

Spiradenocarcinoma

Spiradenocarcinoma[442–445] is a group of rare malignancies that resemble their benign counterparts, some of which clearly are associated with spiradenoma.

The tumors occur in adults of either sex; the anatomic location is variable. They can be associated with a solitary or multiple forms of spiradenoma. There is considerable risk for localized or metastatic disease.

Histologically, the malignant elements are similar to spiradenoma except that there is a loss of the two-cell population, architectural heterogeneity, and cytologic pleomorphism, often with tumor necrosis. Unusual cases may contain sarcomatoid features.[444] The presence of a spiradenoma aids in establishing a diagnosis. The differential diagnosis includes cylindromatous carcinoma.

Extramammary Paget's Disease

Extramammary Paget's disease[446,447] is a spectrum of malignant lesions similar histologically to mammary Paget's disease. It refers to a type of malignant tumor composed of randomly distributed individual cells, cell nests, small acini, or all of these patterns, existing within the epidermis (Fig. 18-48). These cells exhibit phenotypic attributes of adenocarcinoma. When this pattern occurs in association with a cutaneous gland (ductal) carcinoma or visceral carcinoma, commonly those originating in the urinary bladder and gastrointestinal tracts, the finding is termed the *Paget phenomenon,* and this should not be referred to as *extramammary Paget's disease.* Rather, it should be considered as pagetoid spread from a visceral carcinoma or a primary cutaneous adenocarcinoma.

Extramammary Paget's disease usually occurs in the anogenital region, axilla, or on the eyelid of adults and ranges from an erythematous patch, to a weeping, crusted plaque, to a tumor. It may be skin colored and hyper- or hypopig-

mented.[448] Women are usually affected more often than men (3:1). It is often multifocal and is unresponsive to conventional treatments for inflammatory dermatoses. While it is usually a slowly evolving process, rare cases can have a virulent course.[449] Because of the risk of a visceral tumor associated with the Paget phenomenon, it may be advisable to search for visceral tumors in selected patients. Treatment consists usually of surgical excision, but varied chemotherapeutic or radiotherapeutic treatments have been employed with limited success.

In addition to the essential histological features, Paget cells may be observed in adnexal epitheliums. Tumor gland acini may be seen as units within the surface or adnexal epithelium. A panel of special stains, including Hale's colloidal iron, carcinoembryonic antigen, Cam 5.2, and gross-cystic disease fluid protein-15 may be useful in difficult cases.[450–452] Cross-control stains to exclude other conditions in the differential diagnosis may be useful. The differential diagnosis includes malignant melanoma, pagetoid squamous carcinoma in situ (Bowen's disease), and (less likely) the epidermal phase of neuroendocrine carcinoma.

Microcystic Adnexal Carcinoma

Microcystic adnexal carcinoma[247,248,390,453–467] is a spectrum of infiltrative epithelial tumors composed of small cysts, ducts, focal follicular differentiation, and strands of basaloid cells within a fibrotic stroma. The spectrum ranges from those tumors that are mostly ductal (syringomatous carcinoma) to those that have clearly defined ductal and follicular differentiation.

Most lesions occur on the face, particularly the skin of the lips, of adults. They are usually skin-colored, indurated plaques, but can be tumorous. The lesions are locally aggressive, but complete excision may be curative. The lesions are not known to metastasize.

Histologically, there is general progression from superficial microcysts or plump morules of ductal cells to deep compressed tubules and strands (Fig. 18-49A). Microkeratocysts are usually observed in the superficial dermis (Fig. 18-49B). Solid strands of basaloid cells alternate with the cysts; some of these can harbor ducts and zones of microcalcification, although some lesions can have ductal lumens, solid cords, clear cell changes, and arborizing tubules. Combined follicular and ductal differentiation[247,248,455,456,468] is characterized by ducts as well as superficial microcysts, shadow cells, and rare sebaceous[465] and trichohyalin foci.[248] In some cases shadow cells have been described within the cysts.[248] One group of authors suggests that the keratocysts are merely the acrosyringeal portions of ducts and are not follicular.[469] In the mid-dermis, the basaloid strands

and ducts are usually dominant, while the microkeratocysts are diminished. In the deeper portions, the stroma is typically more desmoplastic, and the epithelial elements can diminish to small clusters of two to three cells. Often nerves and skeletal muscle are invaded, as many of these lesions occur on the cutaneous lip (Fig. 18-50). In most lesions few cells, if any, are in mitosis. Lesions with prominent glandular components are also seen and have been termed *sclerosing sweat duct carcinoma* or *malignant syringoma*. For practical purposes, many of the lesions described as "eccrine epithelioma" should also be considered a variation of microcystic carcinoma.[469,470]

Immunohistochemistry reveals that microcystic adnexal carcinomas have evidence of differentiation toward ducts (with

Figure 18-48. Extramammary Paget's disease. **(A)** Scanning magnification shows the confluent adenocarcinoma cells and slightly verrucous architectural pattern in this lesion. Note that the pagetoid cells are confined to the epidermis only, and most are in the lower portion of the epidermis. (× 45.) **(B)** The occasional pagetoid cell is separate from the confluence of most of the adenocarcinoma cells. No intraepidermal acini were found in this lesion, but such acini can be seen commonly. (× 250.) **(C)** In this case, the epidermis is thinner, and the pagetoid cells have a classic pagetoid or "buckshot" pattern. (× 150.)

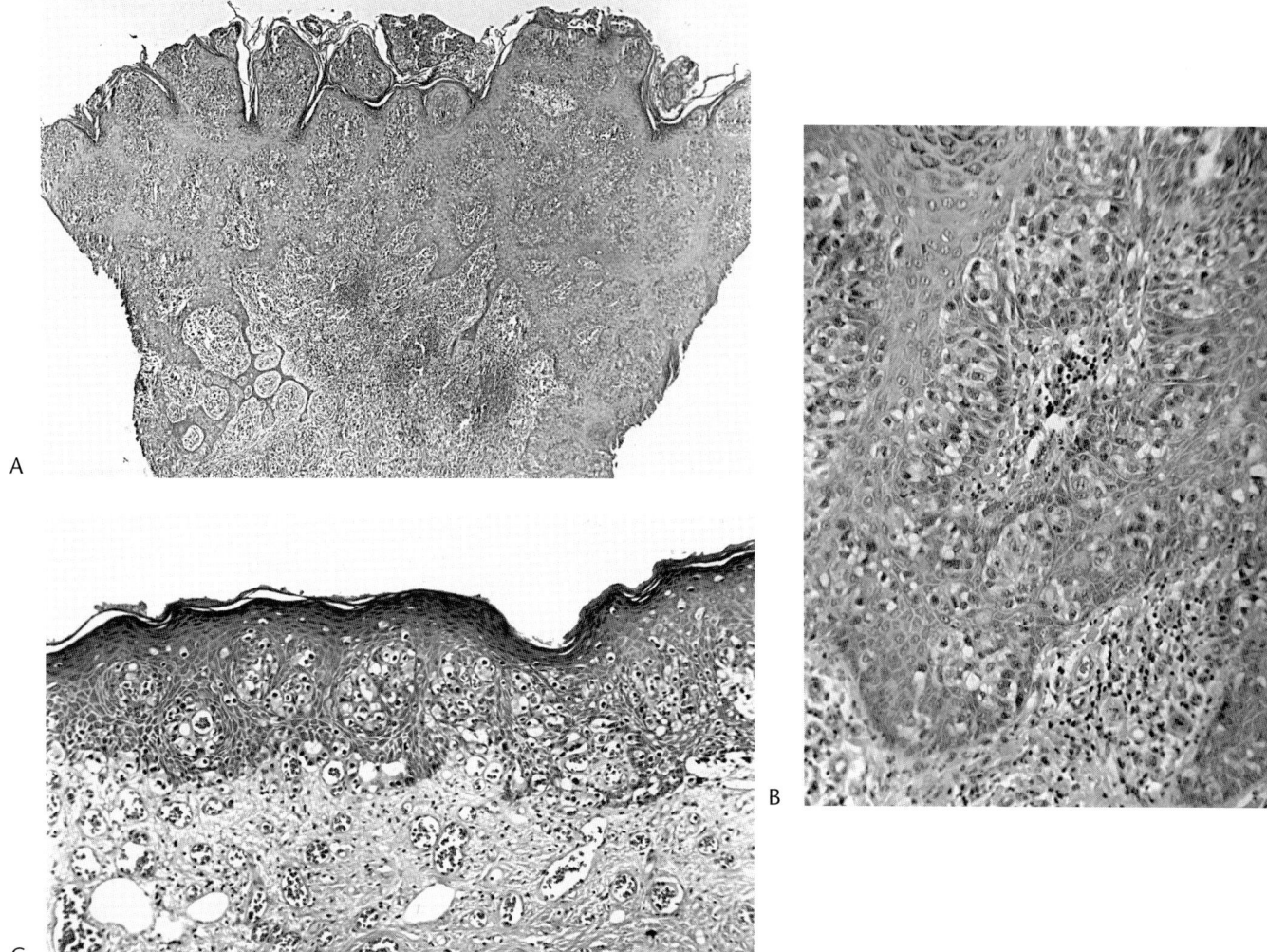

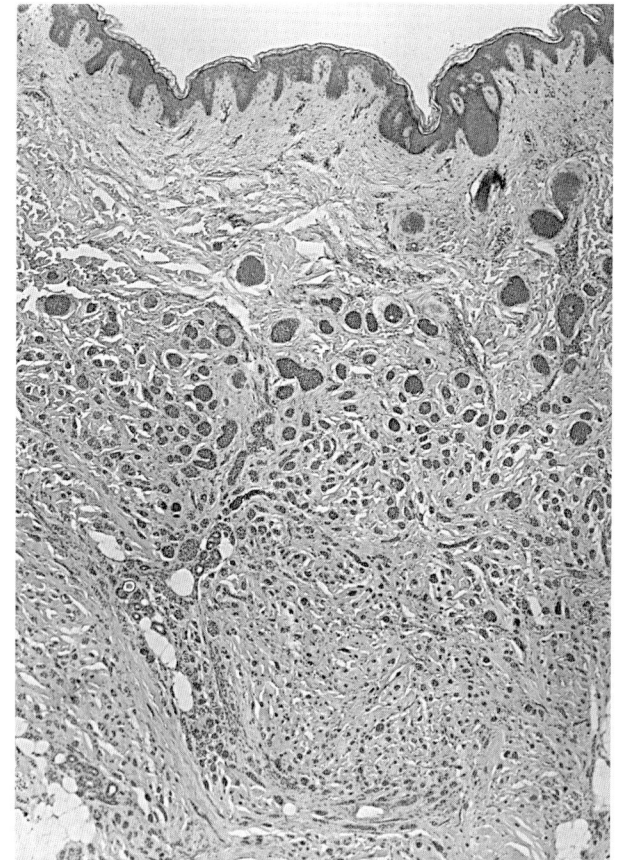

A

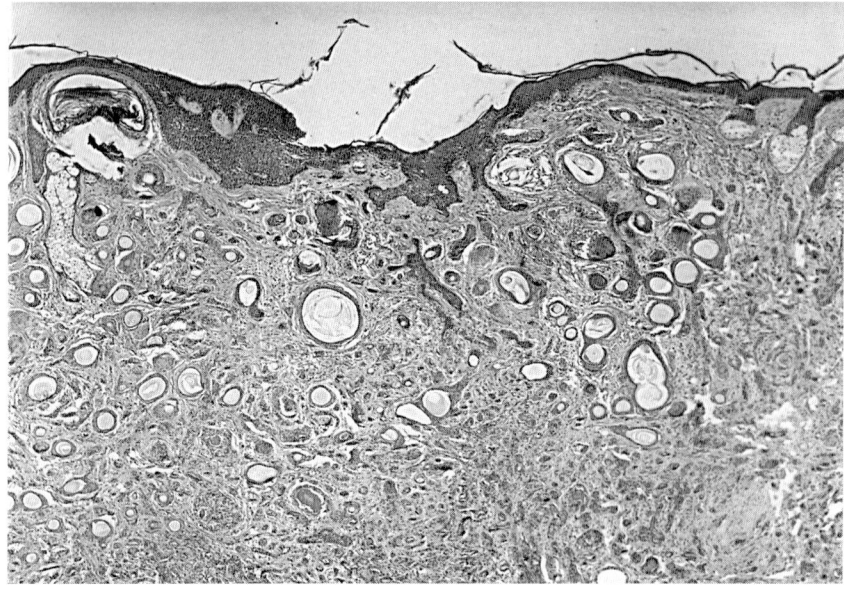

B

Figure 18-49.   Microcystic adnexal carcinoma. (**A**) Scanning magnification reveals rounded morula-like nests of tumor superficially with compressed strands and ducts deep. (× 50.) (**B**) Superficially, small cysts are seen commonly, while in the deeper portions, thin cords of infiltrative cells are present. (× 45.)

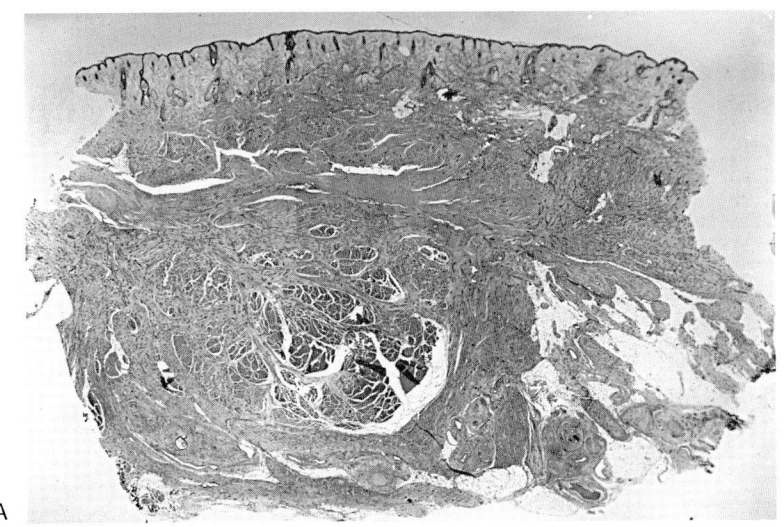

A

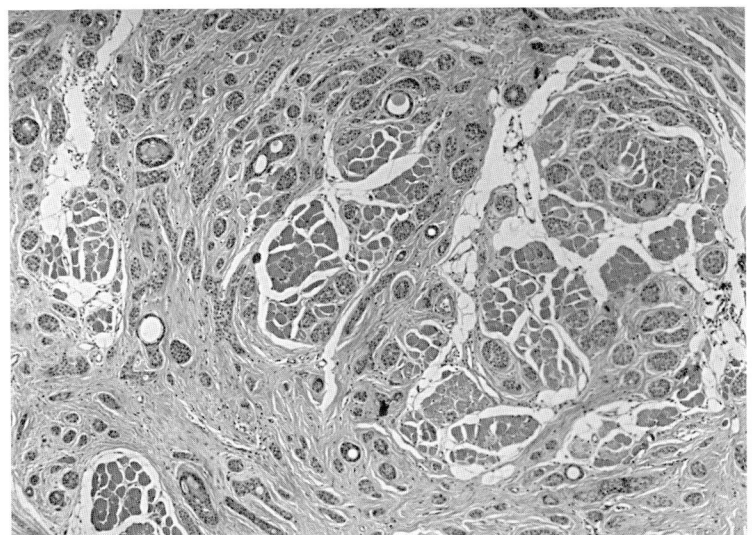

B

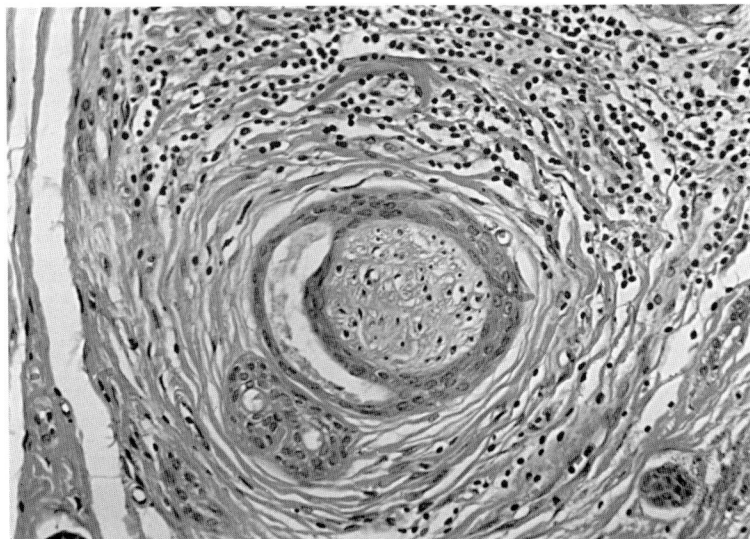

C

Figure 18-50. Microcystic adnexal carcinoma. (**A**) Scanning magnification reveals the markedly infiltrative nature of this carcinoma into skeletal muscle of the lip. (× 13.) (**B**) Medium power shows the prominent skeletal muscle invasion by small ducts and solid cords. (× 90.) (**C**) High power reveals prominent perineural invasion by the tumor. (× 350.)

carcinoembryonic antigen) as well as follicular keratin (AE1/3).[248,456] Rarely, gross cystic disease fluid protein-15, estrogen receptor, and progesterone receptor are found.[390] Immunostains for CD34 are negative in the stroma of microcystic adnexal carcinoma (as well as morpheic basal cell carcinoma), in contrast to CD34-positive stroma in 80% of desmoplastic trichoepitheliomas.[94]

The differential diagnosis includes desmoplastic trichoepithelioma, morpheic basal cell carcinoma, metastatic breast carcinoma, syringoma, and papillary eccrine adenoma.

Mucinous Adenocarcinoma

Mucinous adenocarcinoma[471,472] is a group of low-grade carcinomas characterized by large mucin pools containing aggregates of tumor cells.

The lesions are usually 3 cm or smaller, fleshy, gray, or blue. Most occur on the head, particularly around the eyelids. The male/female ratio is 2:1. Older adults are typically affected (median age, 63 years); black persons appear to have a predilection to develop these lesions (67% white, 32% black, and 4% Asian).[473] Approximately one-third of the lesions recur, but metastatic progression is rare, usually less than 4%.[473]

Histologically, most tumors are often lobular and have expansile growth with abundant pools of mucin containing small clusters or individual tumor cells (Fig. 18-51A). Virtually no stromal reaction is present. Rare cases can have solid areas[474] or infiltrative areas in addition to the characteristic mucin lakes. The cells in these tumors are cytologically homogeneous, uniform, and contain few, if any, mitotic figures (Fig. 18-51B). Mucin histochemistry substantiates sialomucin formation.[475] Immunohistochemically, carcinoembryonic antigen, S-100 protein, gross cystic disease fluid protein-15, α-lactalbumin, estrogen receptor, and progesterone receptor have been identified in the tumor cells.[476,477] Diploid DNA has been identified in one case.[478] Ultrastructurally, there is a highly differentiated pattern with mucin secretion similar to that observed in the dark (mucinous) cell of the eccrine coil.[475]

The differential diagnosis includes metastatic mucinous carcinoma and some (rare) mucinous basal cell carcinomas, which are negative for PAS. Immunohistochemistry may help differentiate primary from secondary mucinous carcinomas, except for cases of primary mucinous carcinomas of the breast metastatic to other sites.[477]

Aggressive Digital Papillary (Adenoma?) and Adenocarcinoma

Aggressive digital papillary adenoma and adenocarcinoma[479,480] is a spectrum of rare basaloid adnexal tumors with tubular and papillary patterns that occur on the digits.

Clinically, the neoplasms occur as a solitary, painless mass, almost exclusively on the fingers, toes, and adjacent skin of the palms and soles. Persons of any age can be affected, but most are middle-aged adults, and most occur in men. The lesions range from approximately 0.5 to 4.5 cm in diameter. The carcinomas have a high potential for metastasis involving the lung especially. Surgical excision is advised for these tumors, especially if they are found to erode bone or soft tissue.

Histologically, the tumors are usually dermal and subcutaneous. The characteristic features include tubuloalveolar and ductal structures with areas of papillary projections protruding

into cystic lumina. Sometimes large cystic areas are present (Fig. 18-52A). The stroma varies from thin, fibrous sepia to areas of dense, hyalinized collagen. While both lesions contain tubular and papillary areas (Fig. 18-52B), aggressive digital papillary adenocarcinoma is distinguished from aggressive digital papillary adenoma in that the former exhibits poor glandular differentiation with cribriform (Fig. 18-52C) and solid/insular (Fig. 18-52D) areas, by the presence of necrosis and necrosis en masse (Fig. 18-52E), increased cytologic pleomorphism, invasion of soft tissue and bone, and invasion of blood vessels. Mitotic figures are found easily. Immunohistochemically, S-100 protein is often positive in the epithelial cells around the nuclei and in the cytoplasm. Carcinoembryonic antigen is positive predominantly along luminal borders and sometimes around the nuclei and in the cytoplasm of the epithelial cells. Cytokeratins in the epithelial cells are usually found in a diffuse and intense pattern, especially in zones of squamous metaplasia. Ultrastructural features include light, dark, and myoepithelial cells. The former contain microvillar projections and desmosomes. The differential diagnosis includes metastatic carcinoma, such as breast carcinoma.

Porocarcinoma

Porocarcinoma (acrospirocarcinoma; clear cell hidradenocarcinoma)[423] is a broad spectrum of epidermal, juxtaepidermal, and dermal malignant ductal tumors that are characterized by nests and islands of nonkeratinized but cytologically pleomorphic cells. Foci of clear cells and distinct ductal elements can be observed.

Clinically, the poroma-like lesions occur as small, indurated, or verrucous plaques. The acrospiromas can appear as polyps, plaques, or nodules. Rarely they may be linear.[481] The lesions occur often on the lower limbs, but may involve the head and neck and upper limbs. However, any site may be affected. Most lesions occur in older adults.

Histologically, the lesions range from intraepidermal nests of pleomorphic solid or clear cells with lumens[482–488] that may involve the dermis with areas of apoptosis, necrosis en masse, and perineural and lymphatic invasion (Fig. 18-53). They can also occur as dermal tumors[389,489–499] and can have insular, sclerotic, and comedocarcinoma-type histologies. Immunomarkers such as cytokeratins, epithelial membrane antigen, and carcinoembryonic antigen are usually positive. Proliferation markers, such as proliferating cell nuclear antigen, confirm that the porocarcinomas have a higher index than the poromas (acrospiromas).[391]

Rare Adenocarcinomas

Rare adenocarcinomas include a spectrum of exceptionally rare cutaneous malignancies, including signet ring carcinoma,[500,501] malignant mixed tumor,[502,503] papillary syringadenocarcinoma,[504,505] mucoepidermoid carcinoma,[506] adenosquamous carcinoma,[507] adenocarcinoma of mammary-like glands of the valve,[508] and polymorphous sweat gland carcinoma.[509]

PAN-DIFFERENTIATION: TUMORS THAT CONTAIN ALL LINES OF DIFFERENTIATION

Some adnexal tumors contain all types of adnexal differentiation. The most notable is the organoid nevus.

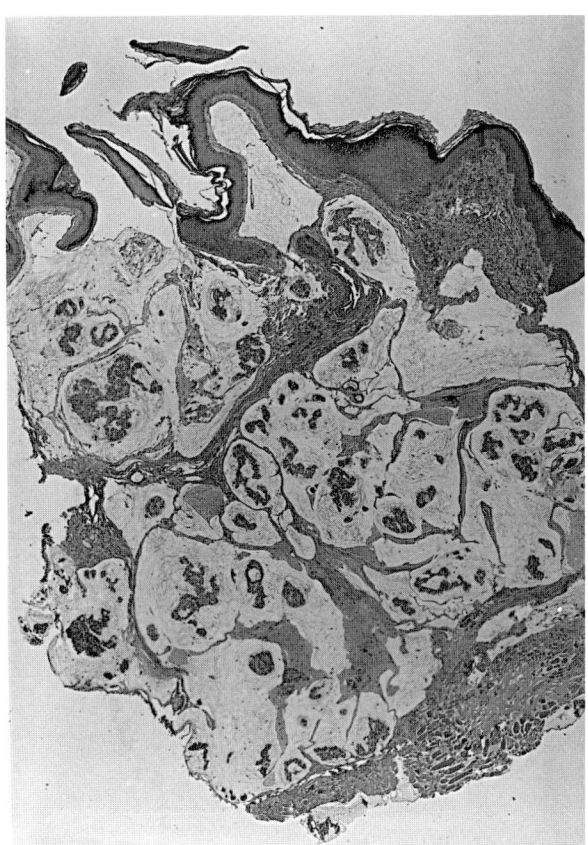

A

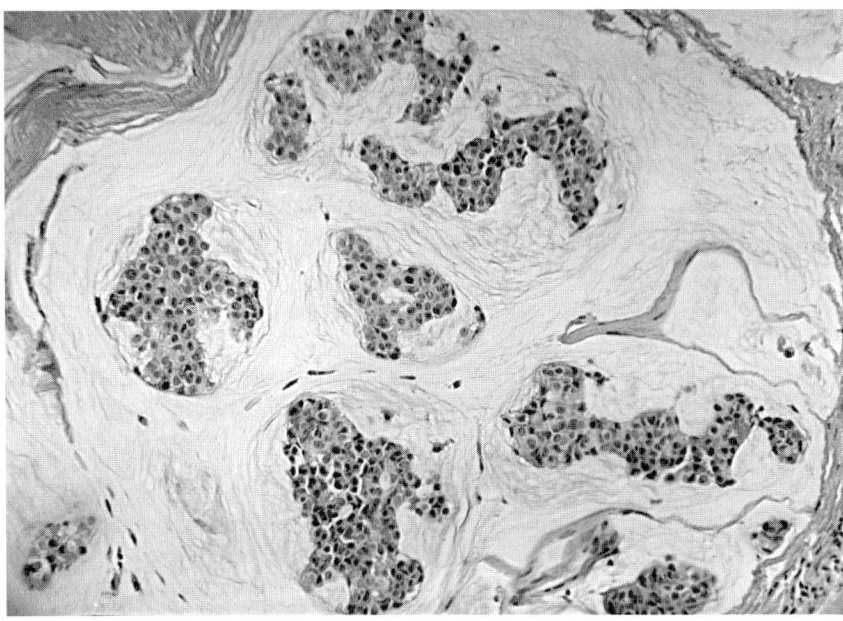

B

Figure 18-51. Mucinous adenocarcinoma. (**A**) Scanning magnification is classic for the tumor, with large mucin pools containing clusters of tumor cells. (× 38.) (**B**) High-power detail of the tumor cells within the mucin. Note the uniformity of the cells. (× 250.)

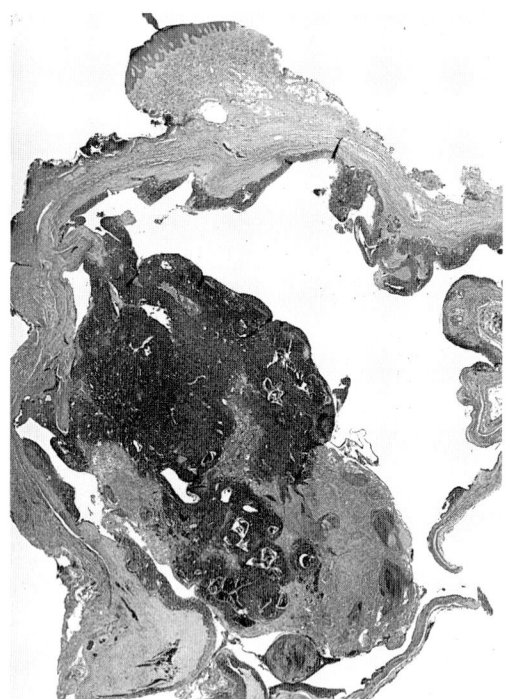

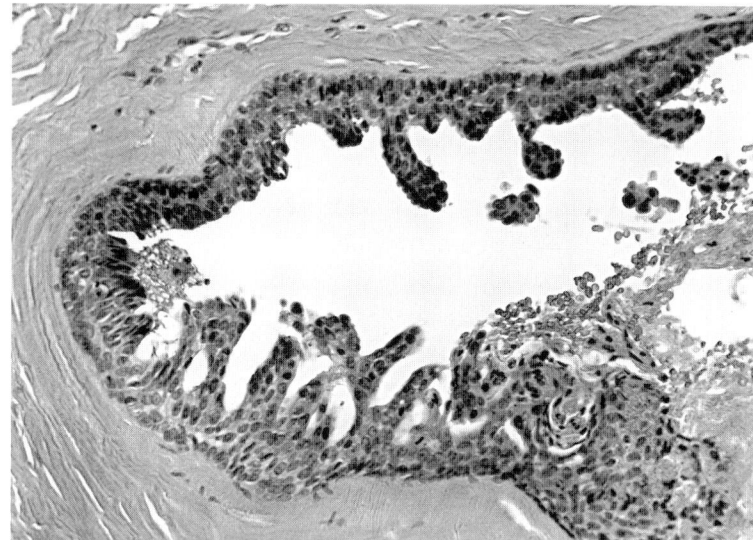

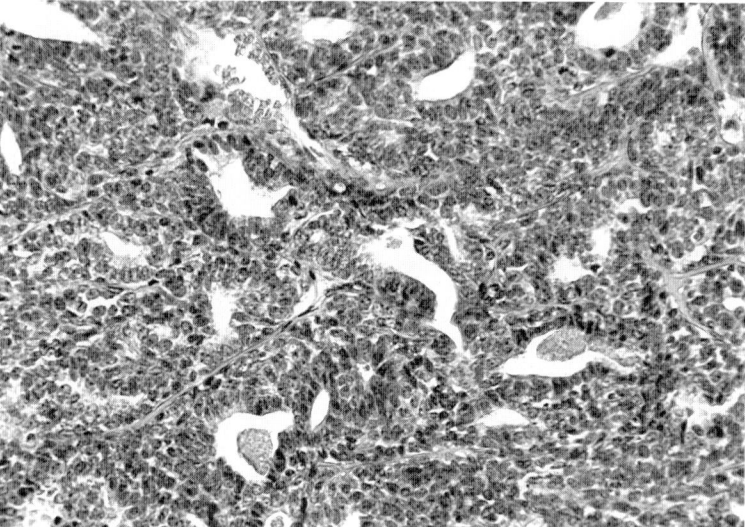

Figure 18-52. Aggressive digital papillary adenocarcinoma. (**A**) Scanning magnification reveals a largely cystic lesion with focal solid areas. The tumor is dermal. Small papillary projections are present in the deep part of the lesion. (× 9.) (**B**) The papillary areas are seen often in this lesion. Note that some of the papillae have apical cytoplasm similar to apocrine differentiation. (× 300.) (**C**) The tubular zones have a gland-in-gland arrangement. Several mitotic tumor cells are present in this field. (× 350.) (Continued)

Organoid Nevus (Nevus Sebaceus of Jadassohn)

Organoid nevus (nevus sebaceus of Jadassohn)[510–515] includes a wide spectrum of hamartomas with mostly mature elements of all lines of adnexal differentiation. Basaloid proliferations are relatively common, but malignant foci can develop uncommonly.

Organoid nevi usually occur on the head and neck, particularly the scalp, and most are yellow to skin-colored to brown, hairless, congenital linear, flat, or verrucous plaques. There are usually three phases of growth: early (childhood), middle (puberty), and late (postpuberty). Treatment is excision except in important cosmetic locations.

Histologically, the early-phase tumors consist of zones of epidermal hyperplasia with small foci of sebaceous glands, miniature hairs, and eccrine glands (Fig. 18-54). The middle-phase tumors retain the epidermal hyperplasia; in addition, basaloid proliferations are more commonly observed as well as the ap-

pearance of apocrine lobules. In the late phase, other tumors can be associated with an organoid nevus. Probably the most common observation is that of basaloid hamartomas that are often confused with basal cell carcinomas. A useful, albeit nondiagnostic, clue is the observation of "holes" within sebaceous gland lobules.[511] Additionally, almost every other type of adnexal tumor has been described within the context of nevus sebaceus. Some of the more common include tricholemmoma, papillary syringadenoma, trichoepithelioma, and hidrocystoma. Conceivably, any type of adnexal tumor combination could be observed.

CARCINOMAS PROBABLY RELATED TO ADNEXA

Basal Cell Carcinoma

Although basal cell carcinoma is not discussed in detail in this chapter, one may argue that it has a histosimilarity not only to the basal cells of the epidermis, but also to the basaloid regions of the hair follicle, particularly the follicular germ and perifollicular

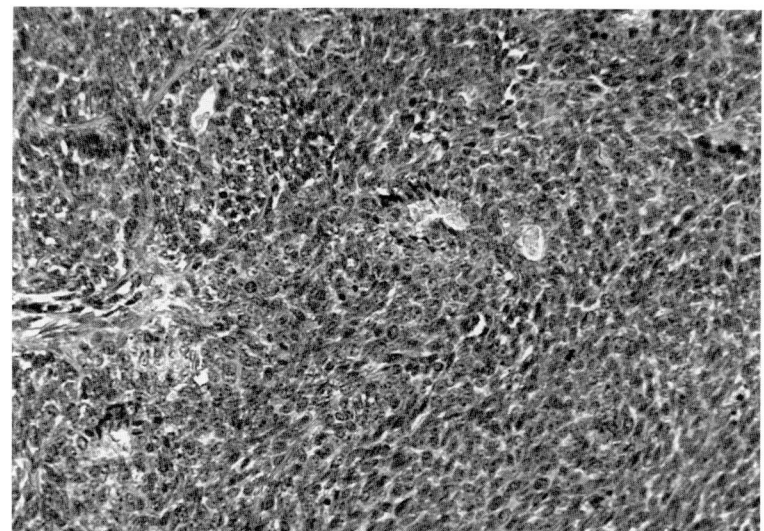

D

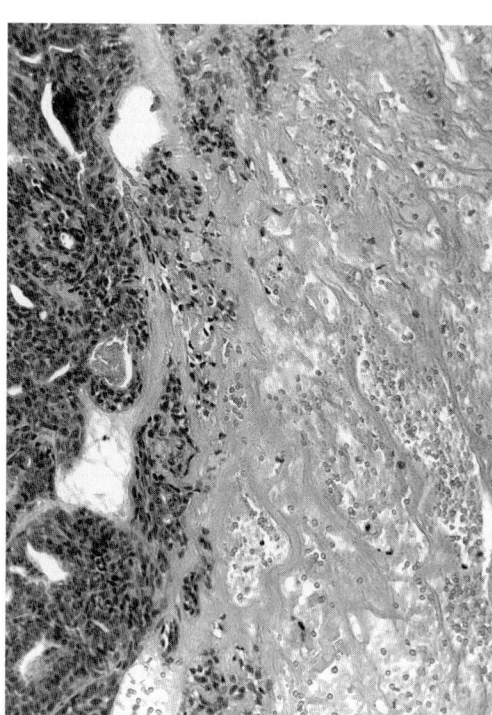

E

Figure 18-52. *(Continued)* **(D)** The solid areas have some insula. Mitotic figures are found easily in this area. (× 350.) **(E)** Several large areas of necrosis en masse are present in this lesion. (× 275.)

mesenchyme.[516] Moreover, unequivocal follicular differentiation is present in some basal cell carcinomas.[517–524] Variations of basal cell carcinoma, such as the fibroepithelioma of Pinkus,[525] suggest strongly a link between the follicular germ tumors and basal cell carcinoma (Fig. 18-55). In addition, some contain foci of matrical differentiation,[526] ductal differentiation,[527] sebaceous differentiation,[272] and neuroendocrine differentiation.[528]

Neuroendocrine Carcinoma

Cutaneous neuroendocrine carcinoma (Merkel cell carcinoma; trabecular carcinoma)[529–536] is a group of small blue cell tumors that usually occur within the dermis. The tumors have histologic features of epithelial cells and neuroendocrine cells. Some have

epidermal connections, and others have ductal and/or follicular components, but most lack these features.

Neuroendocrine carcinomas arise most commonly in older adults. There is a predilection for the upper body. The clinical differential diagnosis includes a variety of lesions, but especially basal cell carcinoma. The prognosis is variable; empirically, the larger tumors seem to recur and metastasize. In patients with visceral involvement, the outcome is uniformly fatal.

Histologically, the growth patterns range from trabecular to insular to diffuse to desmoplastic,[537] any or all of which may coexist within a particular tumor. The lesion can often fill the entire dermis, usually with sparing of the epidermis by a thin grenz zone. Uncommonly, there is epidermotropism,[538–540] Bowen's disease-like changes,[541] and ductal or follicular components.

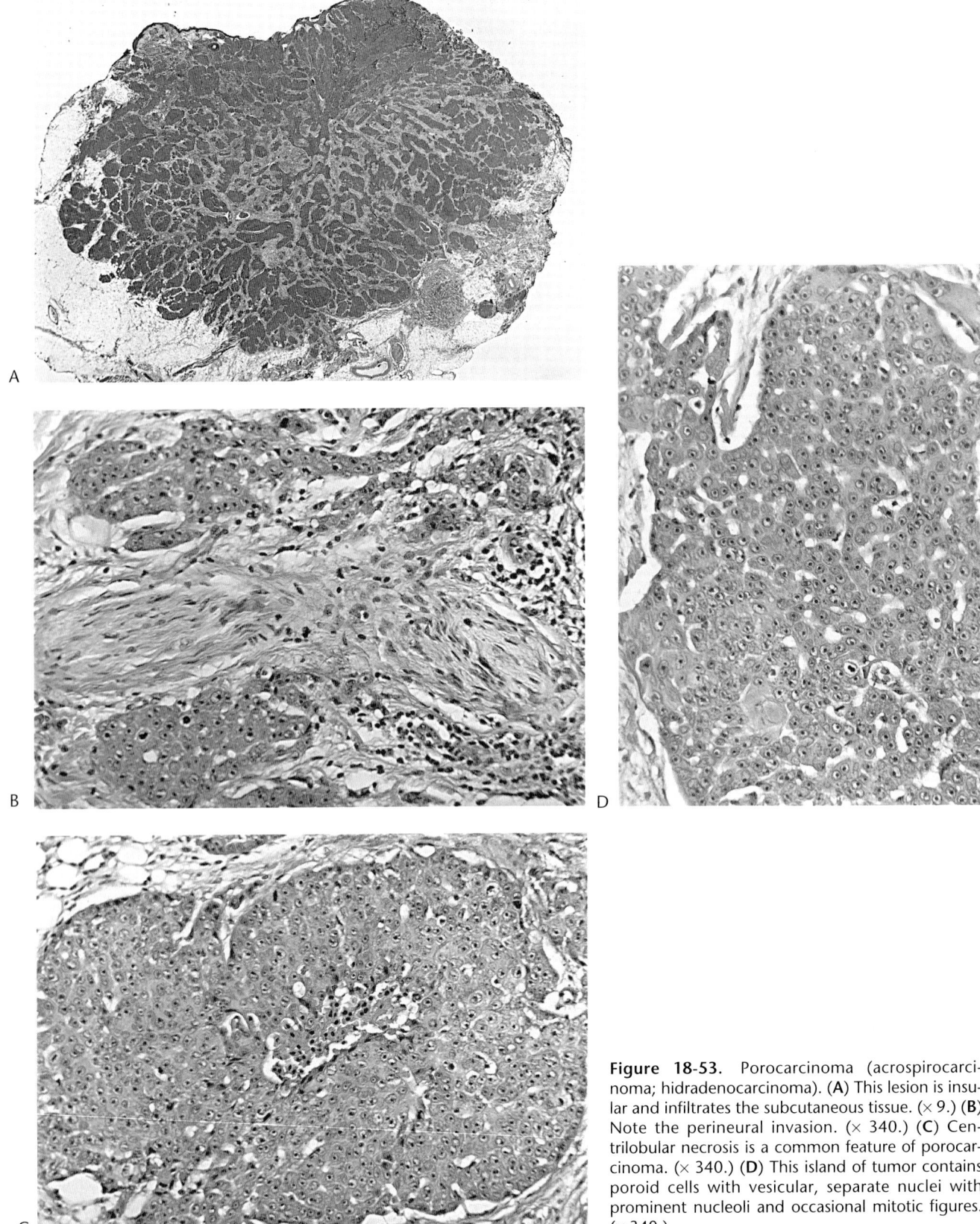

Figure 18-53. Porocarcinoma (acrospirocarcinoma; hidradenocarcinoma). (**A**) This lesion is insular and infiltrates the subcutaneous tissue. (× 9.) (**B**) Note the perineural invasion. (× 340.) (**C**) Centrilobular necrosis is a common feature of porocarcinoma. (× 340.) (**D**) This island of tumor contains poroid cells with vesicular, separate nuclei with prominent nucleoli and occasional mitotic figures. (× 340.)

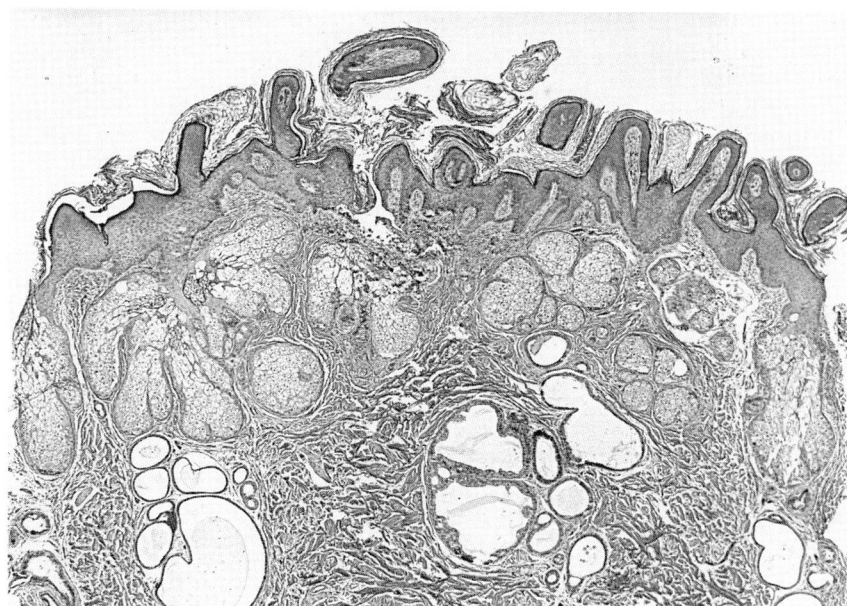

Figure 18-54. Organoid nevus (nevus sebaceus of Jadassohn). This scanning magnification reveals the characteristic epidermal hyperplasia, prominent sebaceous lobules (one containing a lobular hole), and prominent ectatic sweat glands with focal apocrine areas. Miniature hair germs are seen commonly in such lesions. Some lesions may contain secondary adnexal tumors. (× 39.)

The tumor cells are usually homogeneous. The cytoplasm is typically scant and is amphophilic to eosinophilic. The nuclei are usually homogeneous, molded, and similar to visceral small cell carcinomas, but are often preserved better than the visceral lesions. Small nucleoli are observed in most cells.

Histochemically, silver stains are usually negative, corresponding to the small numbers of neurosecretory granules in the tumor cell cytoplasm.

Immunohistochemically,[542–544] the cells contain paranuclear dot-like aggregates of filaments that are positive for low-molecular-weight keratins such as AE1 or Cam 5.2. Endothelial membrane antigen and neuron-specific enolase are positive within the cytoplasm in most tumors. S-100 protein, carcinoembryonic antigen, and lymphocyte markers are consistently negative.

Ultrastructurally, the tumor cells are joined to each other by macula adherens-type junctions. Paranuclear filaments[545–549] arranged in circular aggregates are seen; 80 to 120 nm neurosecretory granules are also observed in properly fixed specimens.

The histologic differential diagnosis includes small cell malignant melanoma, cutaneous lymphoma,[544] neuroendocrine basal cell carcinoma (rarely),[528] metastatic small cell carcinoma, and Ewing's sarcoma.

Lymphoepithelioma-Like Carcinoma

Lymphoepithelioma-like carcinoma[550–555] is a spectrum of basaloid epithelial malignancies containing abundant lymphoid stroma, similar to lesions described at visceral sites, principally the nasopharynx.

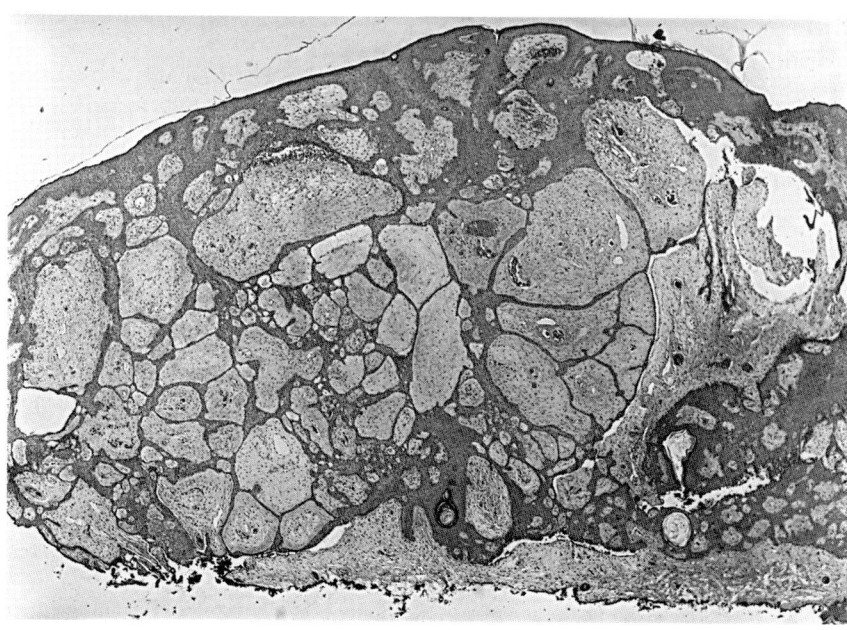

Figure 18-55. Fibroepithelioma of Pinkus. This lesion has a characteristic reticular pattern with abundant stroma and small basaloid buds that extend from the epithelial strands, suggesting differentiation toward the hair germ/follicle. (× 23.)

The tumors present in adults occur most commonly on the scalp or face and are present usually for a short time before diagnosis. Most are papules or nodules. The clinical differential diagnosis is nonspecific. Local recurrence with regional and distant metastasis has been observed rarely in these lesions.[550]

Histologically, the tumors are well circumscribed and consist of lobules of nests, trabeculae, or cords of basaloid cells surrounded and infiltrated by lymphoid cells and plasma cells. In many cases, sparse numbers of neutrophils and eosinophils are present. The tumor stroma is usually sclerotic. In some cases, structures similar to hair follicles or ducts are present,[551] but many cases lack these features. Immunohistochemistry is invariably positive for T and B lymphocytes in the lesions. In addition, cytokeratin and epithelial membrane antigen mark the tumor cells. S-100 protein highlights dendritic Langerhans cells within the tumor and stroma. The differential diagnosis includes neuroendocrine (Merkel cell) carcinoma, malignant lymphoma, poorly differentiated squamous carcinoma, and metastatic carcinoma.

CYSTS

A cutaneous cyst is defined as a saccular structure that occurs within the dermis or, uncommonly, the subcutis. It may or may not be connected to the surface or to another adnexal structure. It may have one or more types of lining epithelium, contain one or more types of adnexal structures, occur either singly or be multiple, or be associated with a clinical syndrome.

Cysts greater than 2 mm in diameter can be distinguished from milia,[556] the microcavities (less than 1 mm in diameter) of seborrheic keratoses, and the squamous "pearls" of squamous carcinoma, which are all smaller than 2 mm. With the exception of traumatic implantation cysts, which are secondary cysts whose linings almost always resemble the epidermis,[557] cysts of the skin should be regarded as idiopathic cystic malformations that should be named based on the predominant type of epithelium present in the cyst wall, although other elements can also be present in an individual case.

As a rule, the cutaneous adnexal cysts can be classified broadly as follicular, sebaceous duct (steatocystoma), apocrine, ductal (eccrine?), or mixed, depending on the similarity of any particular cyst's epithelial lining to the characteristics of normal adnexal epithelium. In addition to these, some lesions, such as the dilated pore (Winer), trichofolliculoma, fibrofolliculoma, pilomatricoma, and some poromas (acrospiromas) can be predominately cystic.

Differentiation that Includes All Adnexal Elements: Dermoid Cyst

Dermoid cysts are uncommon congenital cysts that are histologically similar to epidermis and usually located in the subcutis of the head and neck, along an embryonic closure line.[558] Histologically, the cysts contain a lining, typically infundibular, and one or more types of adnexal structures (Fig. 18-56). However, any particular cyst can contain all types (i.e., ductal [eccrine?], apocrine, follicular, and sebaceous). Smooth muscle elements can be present. Dermoid cysts are to be differentiated from teratomas that contain tissues derived from all three germ layers.

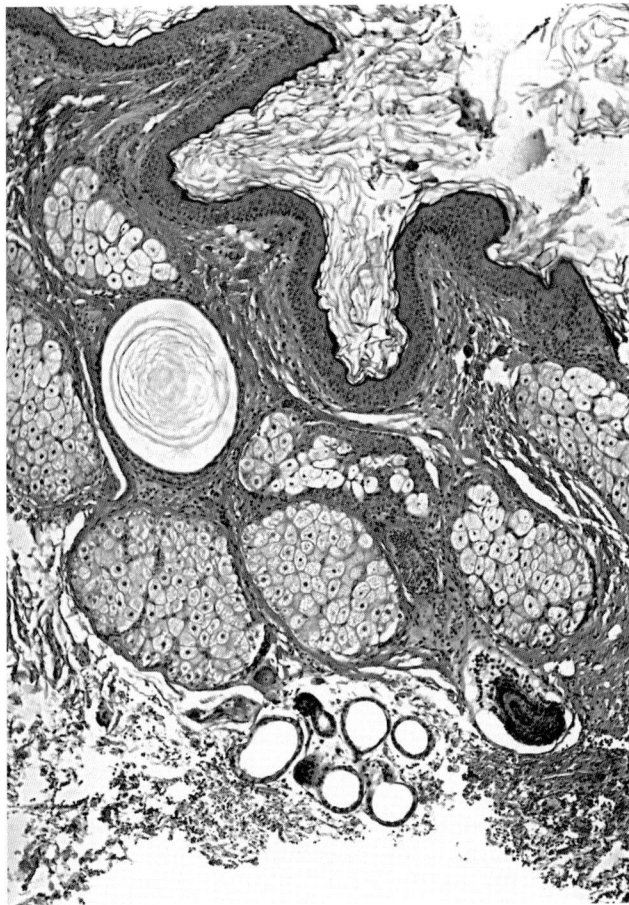

Figure 18-56. Dermoid cyst. The cyst is lined by orthokeratotic, basket-weave keratin and contains all adnexal elements (i.e., folliculosebaceous structures and sweat glands). (× 90.)

Differentiation that is Predominantly Specific

Follicular Cysts

A follicular cyst is defined as a saccular structure whose lining is similar to one or more portions of a hair follicle and is often filled with keratin.

Infundibular Cysts

Infundibular cyst (so-called epidermoid cyst) is the most common type of follicular cyst (approximately 80%). It can be located on any area of hairy skin, but usually occurs on the head, neck, or trunk.[559] Occasionally, such cysts occur in glabrous areas and are historically related to trauma. These are termed *implantation cysts* (Fig. 18-57) and can be considered true epidermal cysts rather than follicular cysts.

The infundibular cyst generally ranges in size from 2 mm to 5 cm and can be treated by simple excision. The differential diagnosis is with numerous dermal tumors. The concomitant occurrence of multiple infundibular cysts and colon polyps, desmoid tumors, and osteomas is known as Gardner syndrome.[560]

Histologically, it is usually not connected to the surface, but occasionally a small connection is present. If sectioned sequentially, it will connect to the surface in most cases. It is lined by stratified squamous epithelium that matures through a granular layer and produces basket-weave and laminated flakes of orthokeratin similar to that of the epidermis (Fig. 18-58). Occasional cysts are hyperpigmented, usually in persons with dark skin. In rare instances changes such as carcinoma in situ, molluscum contagiosum, koilocytosis from a human papillomavirus effect,[561] or acantholytic dyskeratosis is present (Fig. 18-59). If there is rupture of the cyst wall, a granulomatous reaction results.

Pigmented Follicular Cyst

Pigmented follicular cyst[562–565] is a rare, stratified squamous-lined cyst that contains laminated keratin and numerous hair shafts. It occurs on the head, neck, trunk, and, rarely, the limbs. It is usually less than 2 cm in diameter and typically has a dark hue. The clinical differential diagnosis includes blue nevus, hidrocystoma, and cystic basal cell carcinoma.

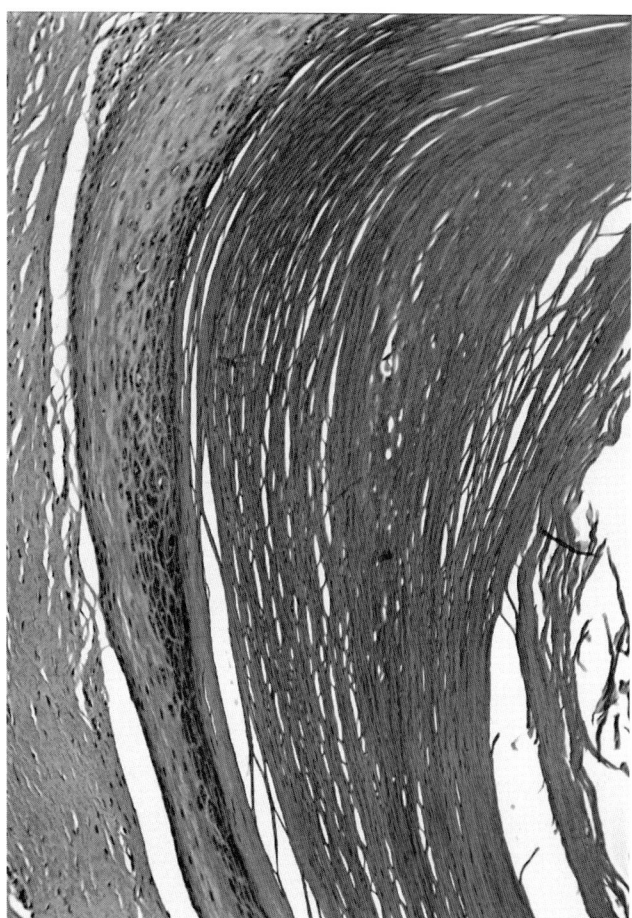

Figure 18-57. Implantation cyst. This cyst arose in a digit subsequent to trauma. These cysts contain epidermoid maturation of their linings as well as orthokeratotic keratin within the cyst. The cystic keratin is often more compact than conventional idiopathic infundibular cysts, but there is a wide variation within the histologic spectrum. (× 150.)

Histologically, it has a narrow opening to the surface. It is lined by stratified squamous epithelium that matures through a granular zone and contains laminated keratin and numerous hairs within the cyst cavity (Fig. 18-60). It is typically not associated with other appendages. Histologically, the differential diagnosis is infundibular cyst and eruptive vellus hair cyst.

Isthmus-Catagen Cyst (Tricholemmal Cyst)

Isthmus-catagen cyst (tricholemmal cyst; pilar cyst) is the second most common type of follicular cyst (approximately 10% to 15%) and historically was called *sebaceous cyst*. Clinically, an isthmus-catagen cyst almost always occurs on the scalp, but the trunk or extremities can be affected.[559] Women are more commonly affected than men. Simple excision is curative. The differential diagnosis includes a variety of dermal tumors.

Histologically, the epithelial lining exhibits a diminished or absent granular layer. The lining cells are large and contain abundant cytoplasm toward the apical portions, similar to the keratinization of the isthmic portion of the catagen hair follicle. Keratinization is abrupt and dense in contrast to the laminated keratin of the infundibular cyst (Fig. 18-61). In some, there is hyperplasia of the lining similar to proliferative tricholemmal cyst (pilar tumor), which is the primary differential diagnosis.

Matrical Cysts

Pilomatricomas, in the early phase of development,[219,220] are often cystic (Fig. 18-62). These are discussed further in the section on pilomatricoma above.

Hybrid Cysts

Hybrid (mixed) follicular cyst is a cyst with two or more types of lining epithelium, such as infundibular and isthmus-catagen,[566] but a virtually endless spectrum could be conceptualized and is being documented.[567–571] Such changes can be helpful to identify syndromes, such as Gardner syndrome, in which multiple cysts, some of which have a lining similar to epidermoid and matrical epithelium,[225] are a feature. If all cysts are examined closely, subtle mixed changes can often be identified, but it is uncommon to see distinctly different types of epithelium within a particular cyst.

Sebaceous Duct Region Cysts

Steatocystoma

Steatocystoma (sebaceous duct cyst)[572–579] is a small cyst whose lining is similar to the corrugated cuticle of the sebaceous duct. Sebaceous glands are usually associated with these cysts.

The cysts usually arise in the second through the fourth decades, most commonly at or around puberty. They are usually skin-colored to blue to black papules or nodules that range from a few millimeters to several centimeters in size. If they are incised, a white or yellow fluid often exudes. The cysts are usually multiple (steatocystoma multiplex), but can be solitary (steatocystoma simplex). They are usually located on the chest, but they can also occur on the face, back, limbs, and, rarely, other locations. There is often an autosomal dominant pattern if

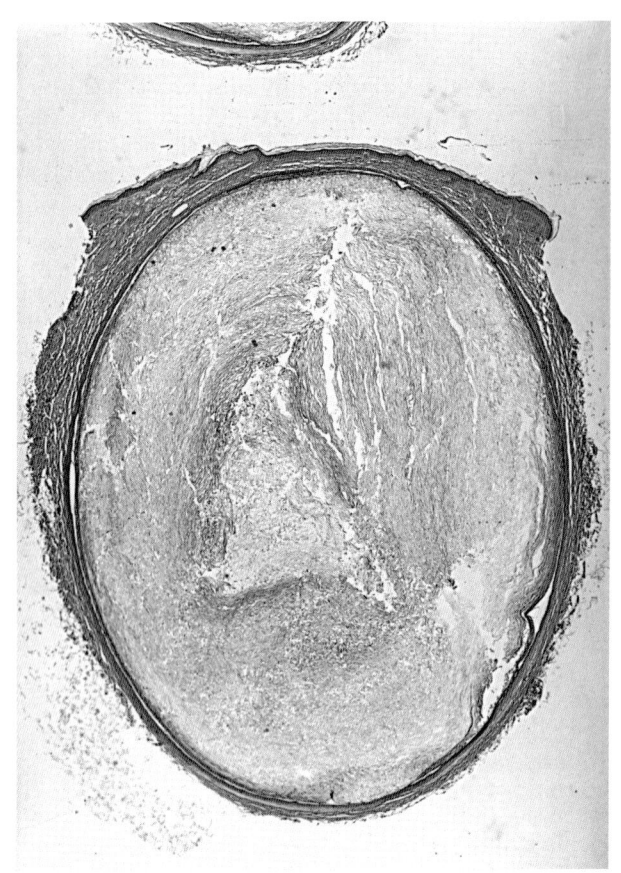

A

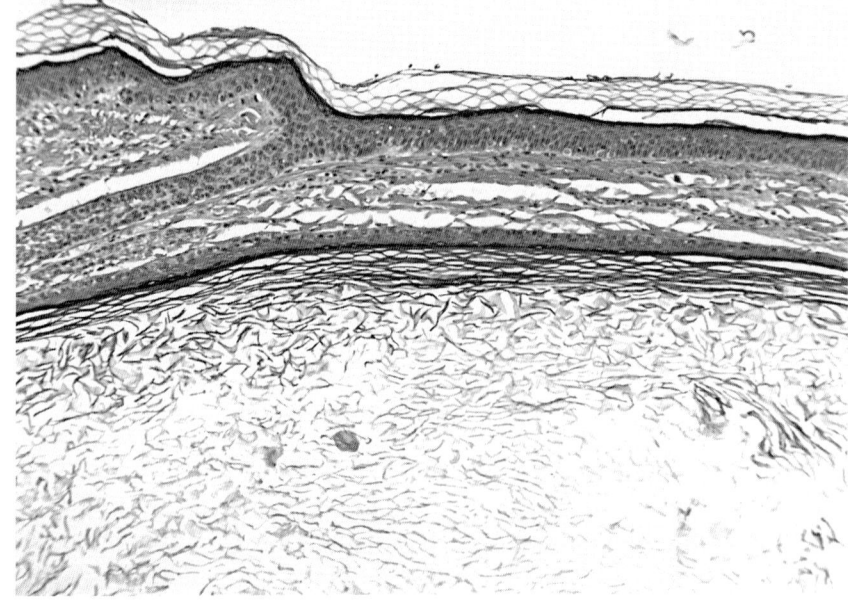

B

Figure 18-58. Follicular cyst, infundibular type. (**A**) Scanning magnification of an intact cyst reveals a thin lining and abundant keratin within. The keratin is similar to the surface keratin. This is the most common type of cyst observed in practice. (× 22.) (**B**) At high power, note that the cyst keratin (within the concavity) and the surface keratin (on the convexity) are highly similar; there is a loose, flaky pattern. Many such cases have cyst walls that contain a prominent granular layer, simulating surface maturation. (× 150.)

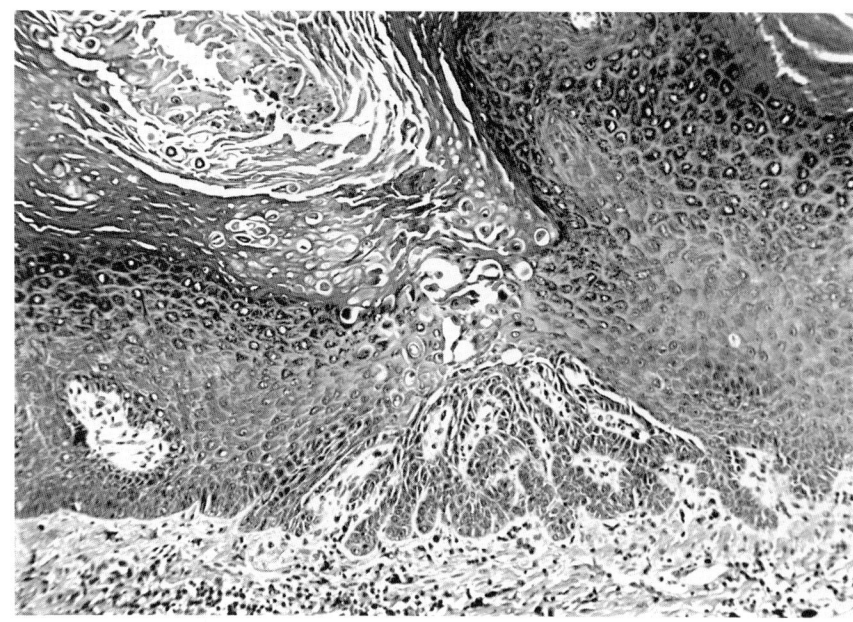

Figure 18-59. Follicular cyst, infundibular type, with focal acantholytic dyskeratosis. This cystic lesion has features similar to the pattern seen in Darier's disease. Such changes may be focal and are of no clinical significance. (× 150.)

the cysts are multiple. Sometimes steatocystoma is associated with an ectodermal dysplasia. For multiple lesions, the differential diagnosis includes eruptive vellus hair cysts, and raises the question of a number of syndromes (Appendix 18–1). For the solitary lesion, the differential diagnosis includes a wide variety of cysts and tumors. Therapy is usually unsuccessful, but oral isotretinoin[580] and cryosurgery[581] have been used with limited success.

Histologically, there is an empty cyst with a serpiginous wall lined by thin squamous epithelium and surfaced by a corrugated cuticle (Fig. 18-63). There is little to no granular layer.[576,577] There can be an abortive epithelial track extending from the cyst to the epidermal surface. Sebaceous glands are commonly adjacent to or directly contiguous with the cyst wall.[578] Occasional

vellus hairs are found within such cysts[582]; rarely a vellus hair germ is seen within the cyst wall.[577] Smooth muscle may be found subjacent to the cyst wall.[583] The differential diagnosis includes eruptive vellus hair cysts, dermoid cysts, cystic sebaceous hyperplasia, and pigmented follicular cyst.

Eruptive Vellus Hair Cyst

Eruptive vellus hair cyst[584–587] is a rare phenomenon of rapidly appearing small cysts with epidermoid maturation and numerous vellus hairs. In rare cases there may be an association with steatocystomas and conditions such as pachyonychia congenital.[588] One author considers these a variation of steatocystoma.[589]

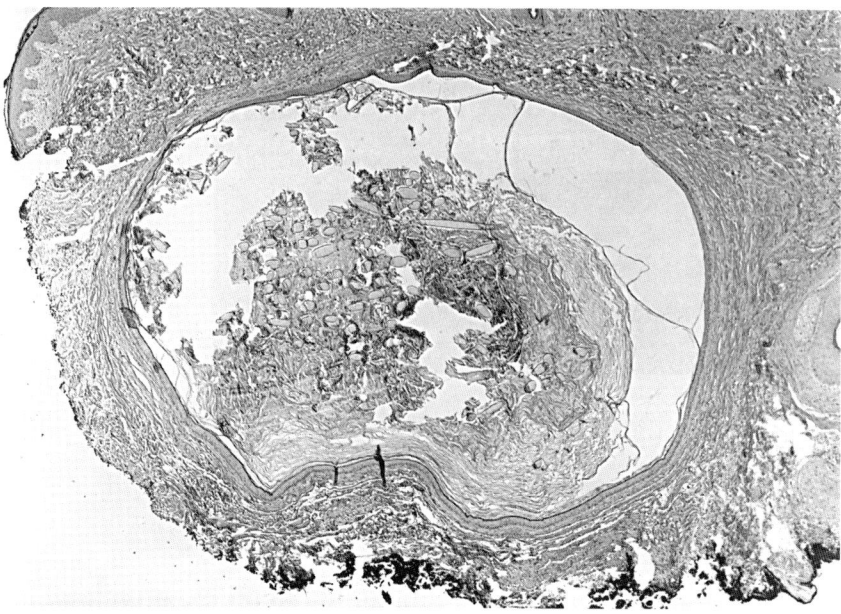

Figure 18-60. Pigmented follicular cyst. This rare cyst has infundibular maturation of the lining and contains numerous large hair shafts. (× 50.)

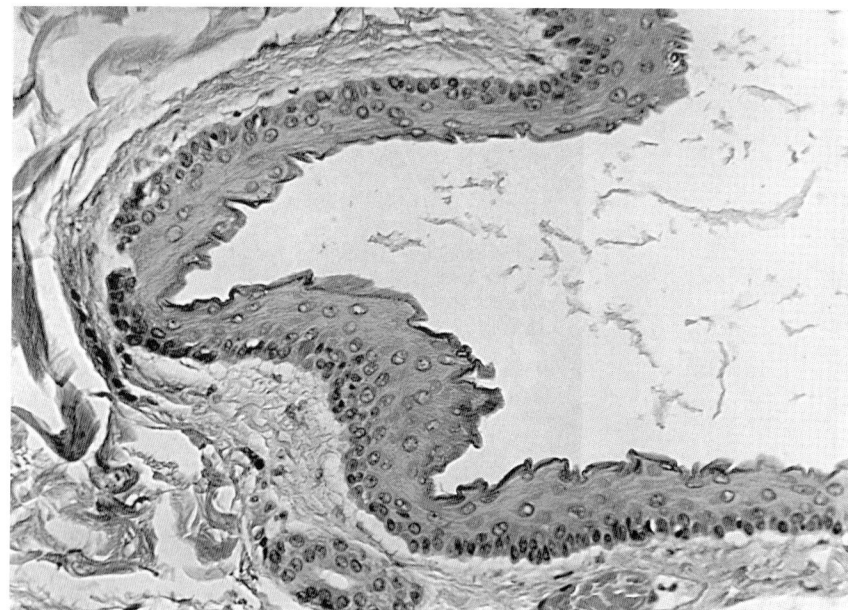

Figure 18-63. Steatocystoma. This cyst has a corrugated cuticle and is empty. Often, sebaceous glands join the cyst. (× 340.)

The cysts usually become evident within the first three decades of life. They affect white persons predominantly in the first two decades and Oriental persons in the second and third decades. Some kindreds have been affected, which suggests a genetic association in some cases.[590–592] The lesions are papules of varying color, measuring 1 to 4 mm in diameter, some of which have central umbilication. There is no sex predilection. The lesions appear, in decreasing order, on the chest, arms, face,[593] and legs. Half the patients with chest involvement have no involvement elsewhere. The clinical differential diagnosis includes acne, steatocystoma multiplex, folliculitis, keratosis pilaris, trichostasis spinulosa, perforating disorders, and milia. Most lesions are recalcitrant to therapy, but limited success has been achieved with the CO_2 laser[594] and topical retinoic acid.[595]

Histologically, there is epidermoid maturation through a granular layer. Numerous small hair shafts are seen within the cyst (Fig. 18-64). Occasionally, there are telogen follicles and, rarely, sebaceous glands or smooth muscle or both. The histologic differential diagnosis includes steatocystoma,[596,597] infundibular cyst, and pigmented follicular cyst.

Cysts of Apocrine or Eccrine Glands and Ducts

Apocrine Hidrocystoma/Cystadenoma

Apocrine hidrocystoma/cystadenoma[598,599] is a spectrum of lesions ranging from fluid-filled cysts with simple apocrine linings to cysts that contain apocrine-lined papillary structures.

Figure 18-64. Eruptive vellus hair cyst. In this cyst, one may observe a thin, stratified keratocyst containing numerous small hairs. Some of these cysts are similar to cysts of steatocystoma. (× 150.)

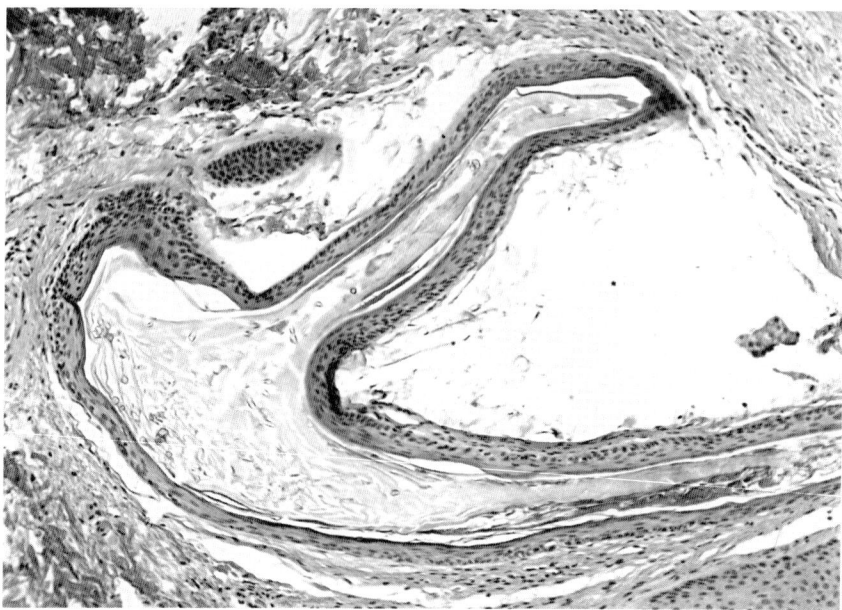

The lesions usually occur on the face, particularly the eyelid (Moll's gland cyst)[600] and head of older adults of either sex. Other sites, such as the trunk and genital region, can be affected. They are usually solitary, skin colored, or blue-black[601] and typically measure less than 2 cm in diameter. Sometimes, multiple lesions occur. The differential diagnosis includes basal cell carcinoma and certain melanocytic lesions such as blue nevi. Surgical treatment is curative.

Grossly, the lesions are uni- or multilocular cystic structures that contain a clear or brown fluid. Histologically, the cyst lining consists of a layer of high columnar cells with abundant eosinophilic, granular cytoplasm and a round, basally located nucleus (Fig. 18-65). Apocrine secretion is present. Papillary structures, if present, are lined by apocrine epithelium. Rarely, the lining epithelium can form a cribriform[598] or microcystic[602] pattern. If excessive, the epithelial proliferation can be similar to hidradenoma papilliferum or syringocystadenoma papilliferum.[603] In other areas, however, the lining can be simple cuboidal, similar to that of eccrine hidrocystoma. The apocrine cells often contain PAS-positive, diastase-resistant granules that are probably lipofuscin. Myoepithelial cells can be identified beneath the epithelial cells in some cases.[599] Immunohistochemically, gross cystic disease fluid protein-15 has been identified in these lesions, in contrast to the (eccrine?) hidrocystoma.[604] Ultrastructurally, the lining cells are similar to normal apocrine glands.[605] The differential diagnosis includes (eccrine?) hidrocystoma, apoeccrine gland,[606] cutaneous ciliated cyst,[607] and median raphe cyst of the penis.

(Eccrine) Hidrocystoma/Cystadenoma

(Eccrine) hidrocystoma/cystadenomas[608–610] are small, sometimes multiple (Robinson type), ductal cysts lined by simple epithelium. They often occur in the head and neck region of adults.

Clinically, white persons, typically women, are affected. The cysts are small, usually ranging from 1 to 3 mm in diameter, and are clear to blue. When multiple, they typically occur on the face; when solitary, they can also occur on the neck, chest, and trunk. If the cysts are multiple, the differential diagnosis includes miliaria crystallina, steatocystoma multiplex, and eruptive vellus hair cysts. If solitary, the differential diagnosis is apocrine cystadenoma, cystic basal cell carcinoma, and cutaneous ciliated cysts. Solitary cysts can be surgically removed. Patients with multiple cysts may require medical treatments, such as atropine or scopolamine.[611]

Histologically, the cysts are simple and lined by a single layer of cuboidal cells devoid of a myoepithelial layer[610,612] (Fig. 18-66). Eccrine lobules are often closely apposed,[610,613,614] and, occasionally, eccrine ducts enter the cysts.[608,612,615] No apocrine secretion or PAS-positive cytoplasmic granules are present,[610] as opposed to apocrine cystadenomas. S-100 protein and carcinoembryonic antigen are observed in some lesions,[616] but gross cystic disease fluid protein-15 is negative.[604] Ultrastructurally, the lining cells are similar to duct epithelium.[612,617,618] The differential diagnosis includes apocrine or apoeccrine cysts and cystadenomas.

Uncommon to Rare Cutaneous Cysts

A variety of uncommon to rare cutaneous cysts or cyst-like lesions have also been described.[619] These include branchial cleft cyst,[620] bronchogenic cyst (bronchogenic choristoma),[621] ciliated cyst,[607] cystic teratoma,[622–624] endometriosis[625] and endosalpingiosis,[626] digital mucous cyst,[627] folliculosebaceous cystic hamartoma,[39] median raphe cyst of the penis,[628,629] metaplastic synovial cyst,[630,631] mucocele,[632,633] omphalomesenteric duct cyst (umbilical polyp),[634–636] orbital respiratory cyst,[637] thymic cyst,[638] and thyroglossal duct cyst.[639]

TUMORS OF THE NAIL

The vast majority of tumors and tumor-like conditions that affect the nail are related to extrinsic conditions, such as myxoid cysts, melanomas, glomus tumors, verruca vulgares, or adnexal

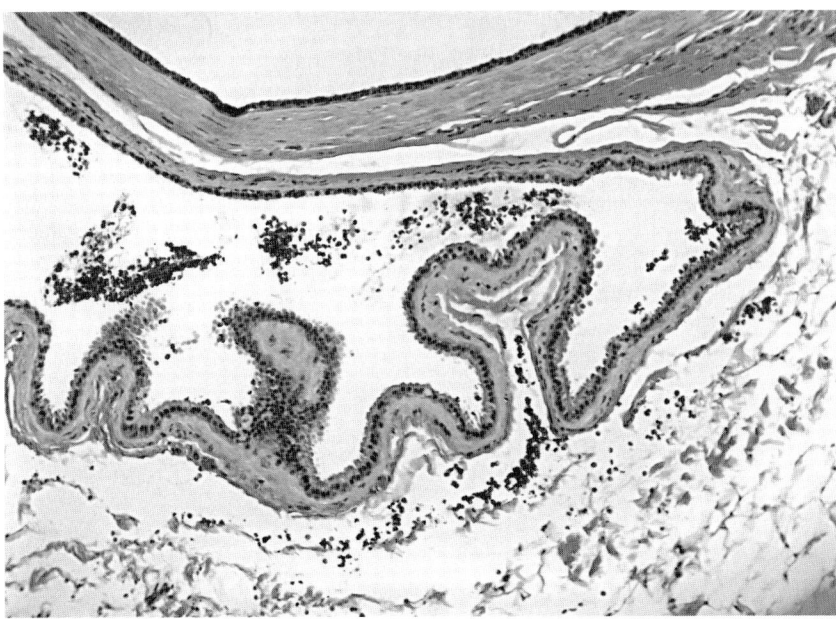

Figure 18-65. Ductal cyst, apocrine hidrocystoma/cystadenoma. This lesion is cystic, lined by a two-cell layer with prominent "decapitation" secretion. Some of these lesions contain a complex, virtually solid tumor pattern; these are often termed *cystadenomas*. (× 150.)

Figure 18-66. Ductal cyst, eccrine hidrocystoma. This is a cyst lined by a single or, rarely, a double layer of flattened cells. Note that this cyst contains inspissated material. (× 250.)

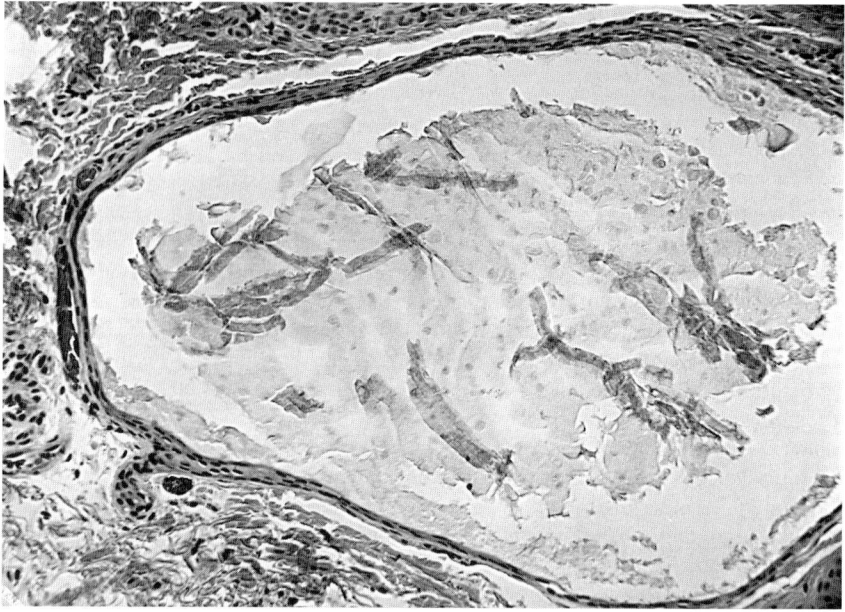

tumors that encroach on the nail from an external source. Uncommonly, epithelial lesions such as keratoacanthoma,[640] squamous carcinoma,[641] and basal cell carcinoma[642] occur in the nail bed.

Nail Matrix: Onychomatricoma

Onychomatricoma (unguioblastic fibroma) is a group of filamentous, tufted tumors differentiated toward the nail matrix.[643–645]

Clinically, onychomatricoma is characterized by a yellowish discoloration of a longitudinal segment of the nail plate with small splinter hemorrhages within the proximal portion of the nail. In addition, there is thickening with increased transverse curvature of the involved nail plate positively corresponding with the yellow discoloration. Multiple nails may be involved in a single patient. The treatment of onychomatricoma is complete excision of the tumor.

Histologically there is a papillary matrix tumor consisting of multiple fine filiform or papillary projections that extend vertically from the matrix or nail bed into the dermis (Fig. 18-67). In some areas, they may have anastomotic patterns enclosing insular zones of peritumoral stroma. The epithelial portions contain two to three layers of keratinocytes. In some areas, there are small spherical collections of parakeratotic keratinocytes. Cytologically, the matrical components are uniform and cytologi-

cally bland. The stroma is cellular with a collagenous matrix. The differential diagnosis consists of fibrokeratoma and onycholemmal horn.

Nail Bed: Cystic Onycholemmal Carcinoma

Cystic onycholemmal carcinoma[646] is a lesion analogous to cystic proliferative tricholemmal carcinomas. Because of the recent introduction of this concept, more observations will be necessary to expand the diagnostic spectrum.

ADNEXAL TUMORS AND ASSOCIATED SYNDROMES

Adnexal tumors are associated with many syndromes, and some syndromes may have one or more type of adnexal tumor. Rather than enumerate these in the text, Appendix 18-1 summarizes both.

DIAGNOSING ADNEXAL TUMORS

Appendix 18-2 shows a mostly morphologic approach to the diagnosis of adnexal tumors, beginning from the lowest power characteristics to the usual high-power features that are sufficient for the final diagnosis. It is not meant to be all-inclusive, but it should serve to indicate the diagnosis or differential diagnosis.

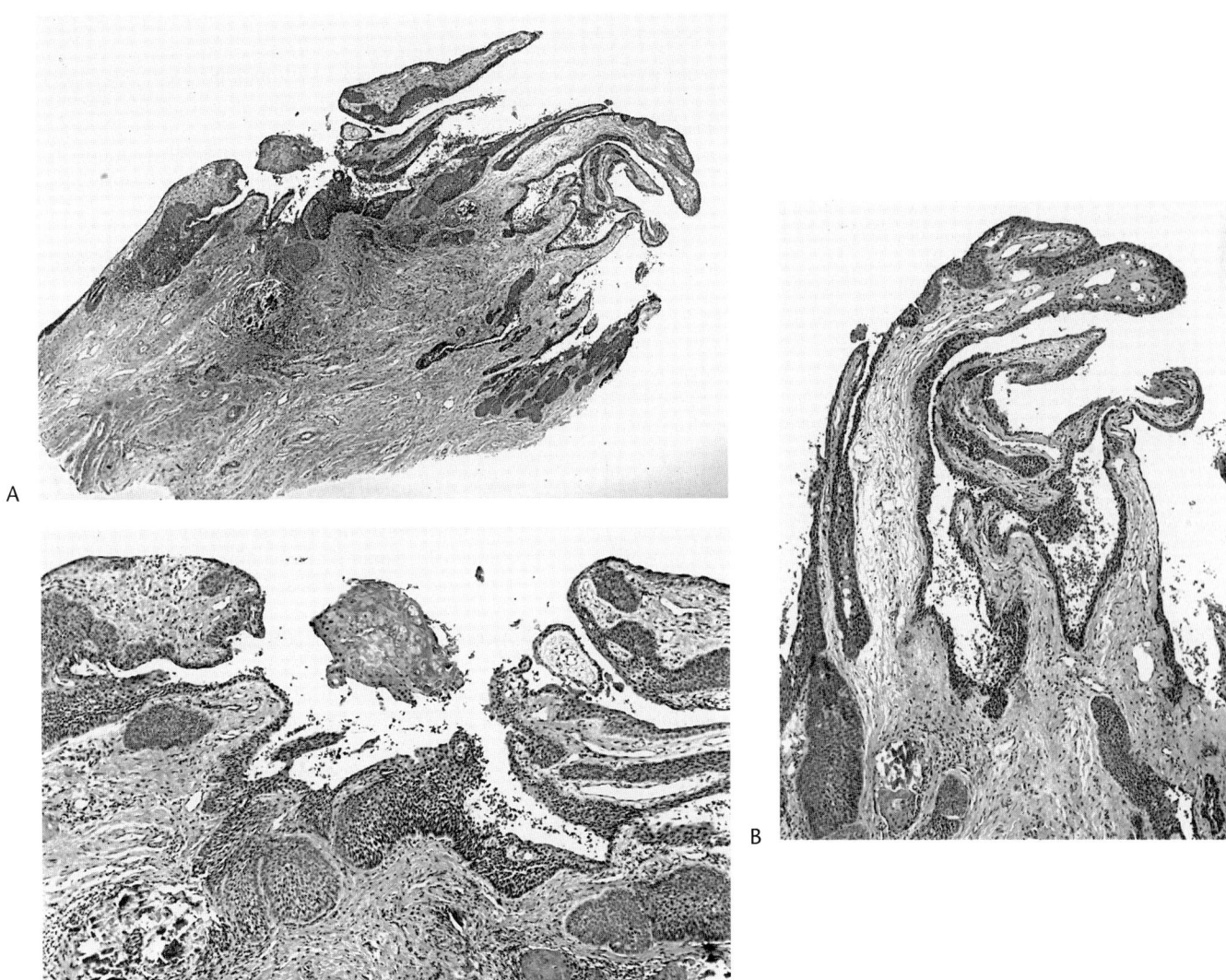

Figure 18-67. Onychomatricoma (unguioblastic fibroma). (**A**) Scanning magnification reveals a papillary tumor centrally with basaloid insular zones at each periphery. (× 38.) (**B**) The papillary zones contain filiform projections of fibrous tissue lined by two to three flattened pink cells. (× 90.) (**C**) In addition to the filiform structures, there are occasional basaloid insula within the dermis. (× 90.)

REFERENCES

1. Barr RJ: Adnexal neoplasms: introduction, comments, and controversies. J Cutan Pathol 11:347, 1984
2. Rosen LB: A review and proposed new classification of benign acquired neoplasms with hair follicle differentiation. Am J Dermatopathol 12:496, 1990
3. Haneke E: The dermal component in melanosis naeviformis Becker. J Cutan Pathol 6:53, 1979
4. Reda AM, Rogers RS III, Peters MS: Woolly hair nevus. Part 2. J Am Acad Dermatol 22:377, 1990
5. Becker SW: Concurrent melanosis and hypertrichosis in the distribution of nevus unis lateris. Arch Dermatol Syph (Chicago) 60:155, 1949
6. Tymen R, Forestier JF, Boutet B, Colomb D: Naevus tardif de Becker. A propos d'une série de 100 observations. Ann Dermatol Venereol 108:41, 1981
7. Burgreen BL, Ackerman AB: Acneform lesions in Becker's nevus. Cutis 21:617, 1978
8. Wise F: Woolly hair nevus: peculiar form of birth mark of the hair of the scalp, hitherto undescribed, with report of two cases. Med J Rec 125:545, 1927
9. Lantis SDH, Pepper MC: Woolly hair nevus. Two case reports and a discussion of unruly hair forms. Arch Dermatol 114:233, 1978
10. Amichai B, Grunwald MH, Halevy S: A child with a localized hair abnormality–woolly hair nevus (off-center fold). Arch Dermatol 132:577, 1996
11. Gibbs RC, Berger RA: The straight hair nevus. Int J Dermatol 9:47, 1970
12. Downham RF, Chapel TA, Lupulescu AP: Straight hair nevus syndrome: a case report with scanning electron microscopy findings of hair morphology. Int J Dermatol 15:438, 1976
13. Pippione M, Aloi F, Depaoli MA: Hair-follicle nevus. Am J Dermatopathol 6:245, 1984
14. Labandeira J, Peteiro C, Toribio J: Hair follicle nevus. Case report and review. Am J Dermatopathol 18:90, 1996
15. Kofman S: Ein fall von seltener localisation und verbreitung von comedonen. Arch Dermatol Syph (Berlin) 32:177, 1895
16. Selhorst SB: Naevus acneiformis unilateralis. Br J Dermatol 8:419, 1896
17. Beerman HB, Homan JB: Naevus comedonicus. Arch Klin Exp Derm 208:325, 1959
18. Resnik KS, Kantor GR, Howe NR, Ditre CM: Dilated pore nevus. A histologic variant of nevus comedonicus. Am J Dermatopathol 15:169, 1993
19. Engber PB: The nevus comedonicus syndrome: a case report with emphasis on associated internal manifestations. Int J Dermatol 17:745, 1978
20. Kim SC, Kang WH: Nevus comedonicus associated with epidermal nevus. Part 2. J Am Acad Dermatol 21:1085, 1989
21. Bazex A, Dupré A, Christol B: Atrophodermie folliculaire, proliférations basocellulaires, et hypotrichose. Ann Dermatol Syph Paris 93:241, 1966
22. Pierard J, Dohnt F, Geerts ML, Kriekemans J: Atrophodermie folliculaire, proliférations baso-cellulaires et hypotrichose. Arch Belg Dermatol Syphilol 27:55, 1971
23. Plosila M, Kiistala R, Niemi KM: The Bazex syndrome: follicular atrophoderma with multiple basal cell carcinomas, hypotrichosis and hypohidrosis. Clin Exp Dermatol 6:31, 1981
24. Sanderson KV, Wilson HTH: Haber's syndrome: familial rosacea-like eruption with intraepidermal epithelioma. Br J Dermatol 77:1, 1965
25. Seiji M, Otaki N: Haber's syndrome. Familial rosacea-like dermatosis with keratotic papules and pitted scars. Arch Dermatol 103:452, 1971
26. Brown AC, Crounse RG, Winkelmann RK: Generalized hair-follicle hamartoma. Associated with alopecia, aminoaciduria, and myasthenia gravis. Arch Dermatol 99:478, 1969
27. Mehregan AH, Hardin I: Generalized follicular hamartoma. Complicated by multiple proliferating trichilemmal cysts and palmar pits. Arch Dermatol 107:435, 1973
28. Delacrétaz J, Balsiger F: Hamartome folliculaire multiple familial. Dermatologica 159:316, 1979
29. Ridley CM, Smith N: Generalized hair follicle hamartoma associated with alopecia and myasthenia gravis: report of a second case. Clin Exp Dermatol 6:283, 1981
30. Alessi E, Azzolini A: Localized hair follicle hamartoma. J Cutan Pathol 20:364, 1993
31. Hyman AB, Clayman SJ: Hair follicle nevus. Report of a case and a review of the literature concerning this lesion and some related conditions. Arch Dermatol 75:678, 1957
32. Kligman AM, Pinkus H: The histogenesis of nevoid tumors of the skin. The folliculoma–a hair follicle tumor. Arch Dermatol 81:922, 1960
33. Gray HR, Helwig EB: Trichofolliculoma. Arch Dermatol 86:619, 1962
34. Duperrat B, Mascaro JM, Lambergeon S: Naevus annexiel en "Soie Floche": Trichofolliculome de Miescher. Bull Soc Fr Dermatol Syph 71:318, 1964
35. Ishii N, Kawaguchi H, Takahashi K, Nakajima H: A case of congenital trichofolliculoma. J Dermatol (Tokyo) 19:195, 1992
36. Kato N, Ueno H: A pedunculated follicular hamartoma: a case showing a central trichofolliculoma-like tumor with multiple trichogenic tumors. J Dermatol (Tokyo) 18:465, 1991
37. Plewig G: Sebaceous trichofolliculoma. J Cutan Pathol 7:394, 1980
38. Nomura M, Hata S: Sebaceous trichofolliculoma on scrotum and penis. Dermatologica 181:68, 1990
39. Kimura T, Miyazawa H, Aoyagi T, Ackerman AB: Folliculosebaceous cystic hamartoma. A distinctive malformation of the skin. Am J Dermatopathol 13:213, 1991
40. Yamamoto O, Suenaga Y, Bhawan J: Giant folliculosebaceous cystic hamartoma. J Cutan Pathol 21:170, 1994
41. Mehregan AH, Brownstein MH: Pilar sheath acanthoma. Arch Dermatol 114:1495, 1978
42. Brooke HG: Epithelioma adenoides cysticum. Br J Dermatol 4:269, 1892
43. Fordyce JA: Multiple benign cystic epithelioma of the skin. J Cutan Genitourin Dis 10:459, 1892
44. Gray HR, Helwig EB: Epithelioma adenoides cysticum and solitary trichoepithelioma. Arch Dermatol 87:142, 1963

45. Harada H, Hashimoto K, Ko MSH: The gene for multiple familial trichoepithelioma maps to chromosome 9p21. J Invest Dermatol 107:41, 1996
46. Ingels AE: Epithelioma adenoides cysticum with features of syringoma. Arch Dermatol Syph (Chicago) 32:75, 1935
47. Binkley GW, Johnson HH Jr: Epithelioma adenoides cysticum: basal cell nevi, agenesis of the corpus callosum and dental cysts. Arch Dermatol 63:73, 1951
48. Gross PP: Epithelioma adenoides cysticum with follicular cysts of maxilla and mandible. J Oral Surg 11:160, 1953
49. Welch JP, Wells RS, Kerr CB: Ancell-Spiegler cylindromas (turban tumors) and Brooke-Fordyce trichoepitheliomas: evidence for a single genetic entity. J Med Genet 5:29, 1968
50. Gottschalk HR, Graham JH, Aston EE IV: Dermal eccrine cylindroma, epithelioma adenoides cysticum of Brooke, and eccrine spiradenoma. Arch Dermatol 110:473, 1974
51. Rasmussen JE: A syndrome of trichoepitheliomas, milia, and cylindromas. Arch Dermatol 111:610, 1975
52. Headington JT, Batsakis JG, Beals TF et al: Membranous basal cell adenoma of parotid gland, dermal cylindromas, and trichoepitheliomas. Comparative histochemistry and ultrastructure. Cancer 39:2460, 1977
53. Cramers M: Trichoepithelioma multiplex and dystrophia unguis congenita: a new syndrome? Acta Derm Venereol (Stockh) 61:364, 1981
54. Michaëlsson G, Olsson E, Westermark P: The Rombo syndrome: a familial disorder with vermiculate atrophoderma, milia, hypotrichosis, trichoepitheliomas, basal cell carcinomas and peripheral vasodilation with cyanosis. Acta Derm Venereol (Stockh) 61:497, 1981
55. Starink TM, Lane EB, Meijer CJ: Generalized trichoepitheliomas with alopecia and myasthenia gravis: clinicopathologic and immunohistochemical study and comparison with classic and desmoplastic trichoepithelioma. Part 2. J Am Acad Dermatol 15:1104, 1986
56. Brownstein MH, Starink TM: Desmoplastic trichoepithelioma and intradermal nevus: a combined malformation. J Am Acad Dermatol 17:489, 1987
57. Lloyd KM, Lloyd JR, Fatteh S: Palmar pits and multiple trichoepitheliomas: an association. Part 1. J Am Acad Dermatol 22:1109, 1990
58. Brooke JD, Fitzpatrick JE, Golitz LE: Papillary mesenchymal bodies: a histologic finding useful in differentiating trichoepitheliomas from basal cell carcinomas. Part 1. J Am Acad Dermatol 21:523, 1989
59. Headington JT: Differentiating neoplasms of hair germ. J Clin Pathol 23:464, 1970
60. Schirren CG, Rutten A, Sander C et al: Das trichoblastom. Ein tumor mit follikulärer differenzierung. Hautarzt 46:81, 1995
61. DiLeonardo M: Trichoblastomas: small nodular vs. large nodular vs. cribriform. Dermatopathol Pract Concept 1:279, 1995
62. Tatnall FM, Wilson Jones E: Giant solitary trichoepitheliomas located in the perianal area: a report of three cases. Br J Dermatol 115:91, 1986
63. Altman DA, Mikhail GR, Johnson TM, Lowe L: Trichoblastic fibroma. A series of 10 cases with report of a new plaque variant. Arch Dermatol 131:198, 1995
64. Czernobilsky B: Giant solitary trichoepithelioma. Arch Dermatol 105:587, 1972
65. Filho GB, Toppa NH, Miranda D et al: Giant solitary trichoepithelioma. Arch Dermatol 120:797, 1984
66. Requena L, Barat A: Giant trichoblastoma on the scalp. Am J Dermatopathol 15:497, 1993
67. Headington JT: Tumors of the hair follicle. A review. Am J Pathol 85:480, 1976
68. Sau P, Lupton GP, Graham JH: Trichogerminoma. Report of 14 cases. J Cutan Pathol 19:357, 1992
69. Gilks CB, Clement PB, Wood WS: Trichoblastic fibroma. A clinicopathologic study of three cases. Am J Dermatopathol 11:397, 1989
70. Requena L, Renedo G, Sarasa J et al: Trichoblastic fibroma. J Cutan Pathol 17:381, 1990
71. Watanabe S, Torii H, Matsuyama T, Harada S: Trichoblastic fibroma. A case report and an immunohistochemical study of cytokeratin expression. Am J Dermatopathol 18:308, 1996
72. Long SA, Hurt MA, Santa Cruz DJ: Immature trichoepithelioma: report of six cases. J Cutan Pathol 15:353, 1988
73. Grouls V, Hey A: Trichoblastic fibroma (fibromatoid trichoepithelioma). Pathol Res Pract 183:462, 1988
74. Requena L, Requena I, Romero E et al: Trichogenic trichoblastoma. An unusual neoplasm of hair germ. Am J Dermatopathol 12:175, 1990
75. Imai S, Nitto H: Trichogenes trichoblastom. Hautarzt 33:609, 1982
76. Civatte J, Moulonguet-Michau I, Marinho E et al: Epitheliolymphohistiocytic tumor. Apropos of 3 cases. Ann Dermatol Venereol 117:441, 1990
77. Santa Cruz DJ, Barr RJ, Headington JT: Cutaneous lymphadenoma. Am J Surg Pathol 15:101, 1991
78. Tsang WY, Chan JKC: So-called cutaneous lymphadenoma: a lymphotropic solid syringoma? Histopathology 19:382, 1991
79. Requena L, Sánchez Yus E: Cutaneous lymphadenoma with ductal differentiation. J Cutan Pathol 19:429, 1992
80. Masouye I: Cutaneous lymphadenoma: report of 2 cases. Dermatology 185:62, 1992
81. Wechsler J, Fromont G, Andre JM, Zafrani ES: Cutaneous lymphadenoma with focal mucinosis. J Cutan Pathol 19:142, 1992
82. Botella R, Mackie RM: Cutaneous lymphadenoma: a case report and review of the literature. Br J Dermatol 128:339, 1993
83. Soyer HP, Kutzner H, Jacobson M et al: Cutaneous lymphadenoma is adamantinoid trichoblastoma. Dermatopathol Pract Concept 2:32, 1996
84. Diaz-Cascajo C, Borghi S, Rey-Lopez A, Carretero-Hernandez G: Cutaneous lymphadenoma. A peculiar variant of nodular trichoblastoma. Am J Dermatopathol 18:186, 1996
85. Allen PW, Dymock RB, MacCormac LB: Superficial angiomyxomas with and without epithelial components. Report of 30 tumors in 28 patients. Am J Surg Pathol 12:519, 1988
86. Nikolowski W: "Tricho-adenom" (organoides follikelhamartom). Arch Klin Exp Derm 207:34, 1958
87. Rahbari H, Mehregan A, Pinkus H: Trichoadenoma of Nikolowski. J Cutan Pathol 4:90, 1977
88. Jaqueti G, Requena L, Sánchez Yus E: Verrucous trichoadenoma. J Cutan Pathol 16:145, 1989

89. Brownstein MH, Shapiro L: Desmoplastic trichoepithelioma. Cancer 40:2979, 1977

90. MacDonald DM, Wilson Jones E, Marks R: Sclerosing epithelial hamartoma. Clin Exp Dermatol 2:153, 1977

91. Dervan PA, O'Hegarty M, O'Loughlin S, Corrigan T: Solitary familial desmoplastic trichoepithelioma. A study by conventional and electron microscopy. Am J Dermatopathol 7:277, 1985

92. Shapiro PE, Kopf AW: Familial multiple desmoplastic trichoepitheliomas. Arch Dermatol 127:83, 1991

93. Blanc D, Zahouani H, Rochefort A, Faivre B: Desmoplastic trichoepithelioma nosology. Reappraisal about a case developed on a varicella scar. Dermatologica 180:44, 1990

94. Kirchmann TT, Prieto VG, Smoller BR: Use of CD34 in assessing the relationship between stroma and tumor in desmoplastic keratinocytic neoplasms. J Cutan Pathol 22:422, 1995

95. Bryant D, Penneys NS: Immunostaining for CD34 to determine trichoepithelioma (correspondence). Arch Dermatol 131:616, 1995

96. Mehregan AH, Butler JD: A tumor of follicular infundibulum. Arch Dermatol 83:924, 1961

97. Mehregan AH: Tumor of follicular infundibulum. Dermatologica 142:177, 1971

98. Johnson WC, Hookerman BJ: Basal cell hamartoma with follicular differentiation. Arch Dermatol 105:105, 1972

99. Mehregan AH, Coskey RJ: Pigmented nevi of sole. A report of two cases with histologic evidence of hair follicle formation. Arch Dermatol 106:886, 1972

100. Trunnell TN, Watsman M: Tumor of the follicular infundibulum. Cutis 24:317, 1979

101. Casas JG, Palacios AM, Schroh RG, Magnin PH: Tumor del infundibulo folicular. Rev Argent Dermatol 62:223, 1981

102. Mehregan AH: Infundibular tumors of the skin. J Cutan Pathol 11:387, 1984

103. Cribier B, Grosshans E: Tumor of the follicular infundibulum: a clinicopathologic study. J Am Acad Dermatol 33:979, 1995

104. Kossard S, Kocsard E, Poyzer KG: Infundibulomatosis. Arch Dermatol 119:267, 1983

105. Mehregan AH, Baker S: Basaloid follicular hamartoma: three cases with localized and systematized unilateral lesions. J Cutan Pathol 12:55, 1985

106. Findlay GH: Multiple infundibular tumours of the head and neck. Br J Dermatol 120:633, 1989

107. Kossard S, Finley AG, Poyzer K, Kocsard E: Eruptive infundibulomas. A distinctive presentation of the tumor of follicular infundibulum. Part 2. J Am Acad Dermatol 21:361, 1989

108. Cribier B, Waskievicz W, Heid E: Infundibulomes multiples. Ann Dermatol Venereol 118:281, 1991

109. Koch B, Rufli T: Tumor of follicular infundibulum. Dermatologica 183:68, 1991

110. Kolenik III SA, Bolognia JL, Castiglione FM Jr., Longley BJ: Multiple tumors of the follicular infundibulum. Int J Dermatol 35:282, 1996

111. Schnitzler L, Civatte J, Robin F, Demay CL: Tumeurs multiples de l'infundibulum pilaire avec dégénérescence basocellulaire. A propos d'un cas. Ann Dermatol Venereol 114:551, 1987

112. Horn TD, Vennos EM, Bernstein BD, Cooper PH: Multiple tumors of follicular infundibulum with sweat duct differentiation. J Cutan Pathol 22:281, 1995

113. Winer LH: The dilated pore. A trichoepithelioma. J Invest Dermatol 23:181, 1954

114. Klovekorn G, Pinkus H, Plewig G: Dilated Pore: re-Evaluation of a Benign Tumor. American Academy of Dermatology, Chicago, December 1–6, 1979

115. Bhawan J: Pilar sheath acanthoma. A new benign follicular tumor. J Cutan Pathol 6:438, 1979

116. Smolle J, Kerl H: Pilar sheath acanthoma a benign follicular hamartoma. Dermatologica 167:335, 1983

117. Lee JY, Hirsch E: Pilar sheath acanthoma, letter. Arch Dermatol 123:569, 1987

118. Vakilzadeh F: Pilar sheath acanthoma. Hautarzt 38:40, 1987

119. Choi YS, Park SH, Bang D: Pilar sheath acanthoma–report of a case with review of the literature. Yonsei Med J 30:392, 1989

120. Ackerman AB, de Viragh PA, Chongchitnant N et al: Pilar sheath acanthoma. p. 509. In: Neoplasms with Follicular Differentiation. 1st Ed. Ackerman's Histologic Diagnosis of Neoplastic Skin Diseases: A Method by Pattern Analysis. Lea & Febiger, Philadelphia, 1993

121. DiLeonardo M: Dilated pore vs. pilar sheath acanthoma vs. trichofolliculoma. Dermatopathol Pract Concept 2:108, 1996

122. Hurt MA: Pilar sheath acanthoma (lobular infundibuloisthmicoma), abstracted. Am J Dermatopathol 18:435, 1996

123. Brownstein MH: Trichilemmal horn: cutaneous horn showing trichilemmal keratinization. Br J Dermatol 100:303, 1979

124. Poblet E, Jimenez-Reyes J, Gonzalez-Herrada C, Granados R: Trichilemmal keratosis. A clinicopathologic and immunohistochemical study of two cases. Am J Dermatopathol 18:543, 1996

125. Poblet E, Jimenez-Acosta F, Rocamora A: QBEND/10 (anti-CD34 antibody) in external root sheath cells and follicular tumors. J Cutan Pathol 21:224, 1994

126. Wilson Jones E: Proliferating epidermoid cysts. Arch Dermatol 94:11, 1966

127. Reed RJ, Lamar LM: Invasive hair matrix tumors of the scalp. Invasive pilomatrixoma. Arch Dermatol 94:310, 1966

128. Lever WF: Tumors of the epidermal appendages (Pilar tumor of the scalp). p. 561. In: Histopathology of the Skin. 4th Ed. Lippincott-Raven, Philadelphia, 1967

129. Holmes EJ: Tumors of lower hair sheath. Common histogenesis of certain so-called "sebaceous cysts," acanthomas and "sebaceous carcinomas." Cancer 21:234, 1968

130. Korting GW, Hoede N: Zum sogenannten "pilar tumor of the scalp." Arch Klin Exp Derm 234:409, 1969

131. Pinkus H, Mehregan AH: Pilar tumor. p. 446. In: A Guide to Dermatohistopathology. 1st Ed. Appleton-Century-Crofts, E. Norwalk, CT, 1969

132. Shelley WB, Beerman H: Hydatidiform keratinous cyst: clinical recognition of a benign proliferating epidermoid cyst. Br J Dermatol 83:279, 1970

133. Dabska M: Giant hair matrix tumor. Cancer 28:701, 1971

134. Christophers E, Spelberg H: Proliferierende tricholemmaleysten. Hautarzt 24:377, 1973

135. Rivera F, Matilla A, Panea P, Galera H: Quiste epidermoide

proliferante (proliferant epidermoid cyst). Morfol Norm Patol 2:311, 1978

136. Le Roux FB, Van Der Walt JJ: Proliferating tricholemmal cysts. S Afr Med J 54:833, 1978

137. Bloch PH, Müller HD: Pilartumor der kopfhaut. Hautarzt 30:84, 1979

138. Morgan RF, Dellon AL, Hoopes JE: Pilar tumors. Plast Reconstr Surg 63:520, 1979

139. Janitz J, Wiedersberg H: Trichilemmal pilar tumors. Cancer 45:1594, 1980

140. Welke S, Christophers E: Proliferierender trichilemmaltumor. Hautarzt 32:253, 1981

141. Brownstein MH, Arluk DJ: Proliferating trichilemmal cyst: a simulant of squamous cell carcinoma. Cancer 48:1207, 1981

142. Poiares Baptista A, Garcia E Silva L, Born MC: Proliferating trichilemmal cyst. J Cutan Pathol 10:178, 1983

143. Janitz J, Wiedersberg H: Proliferierende trichilemmale zysten. Eine mögliche vorstufe des pilartumors des behaarten kopfes. Pathologe 8:217, 1987

144. Bulengo-Ransby SM, Johnson C, Metcalf JS: Enlarging scalp nodule. Proliferating trichilemmal cyst (PTC). Arch Dermatol 131:721, 1995

145. Sau P, Graham JH, Helwig EB: Proliferating epithelial cysts. Clinicopathological analysis of 96 cases. J Cutan Pathol 22:394, 1995

146. Hendricks DL, Liang MD, Borochovitz D, Miller T: A case of multiple pilar tumors and pilar cysts involving the scalp and back. Plast Reconstr Surg 87:763, 1991

147. Tapernoux B, Delacrétaz J: Kyste épidermoïde papillifére. Dermatologica 143:357, 1971

148. Roberts PF, Jerrome DW: Ultrastructure of a pilar tumor. Arch Dermatol 108:399, 1973

149. Yoshikawa K, Nakanishi A: Proliferating trichilemmal cyst on the back. J Dermatol (Tokyo) 5:279, 1978

150. Buchler DA, Sun F, Chuprevich T: A pilar tumor of the vulva. Gynecol Oncol 6:479, 1978

151. Amaral ALMP, Nascimento AG, Goellner JR: Proliferating pilar (trichilemmal) cyst. Report of two cases, one with carcinomatous transformation and one with distant metastases. Arch Pathol Lab Med 108:808, 1984

152. Rubinstein N, Lijovetzky G, Knobler HY et al: Pilar tumor of the nose. Cutis 36:251, 1985

153. Rahbari H, Mehregan AH: Development of proliferating trichilemmal cyst in organoid nevus. Presentation of two cases. J Am Acad Dermatol 14:123, 1986

154. Munro JM, Hall PA, Thompson HH: Proliferating trichilemmal cyst occurring on the shin. J Cutan Pathol 13:246, 1986

155. Avinoach I, Zirkin HJ, Glazerman M: Proliferating trichilemmal tumor of the vulva. Case report and review of the literature. Int J Gynecol Pathol 8:163, 1989

156. Aliaga A, Fortea JM, Gonzalez-Fontana R et al: Kyste épidermoïde proliférant géant. Ann Dermatol Syph 102:409, 1975

157. Casas JG, Woscoff A: Giant pilar tumor of the scalp. Arch Dermatol 116:1395, 1980

158. Stranc MF, Bennett MH, Melmed EP: Pilar tumour of the scalp developing in hereditary sebaceous cysts. Br J Plast Surg 24:82, 1971

159. Sakamoto F, Ito M, Nakamura A, Sato Y: Proliferating

160. Athanasou NA, Quinn JM: Bone resorption by macrophage polykaryons of a pilar tumor of scalp. Cancer 70:469, 1992

161. Miyairi H, Takahashi S, Morohashi M: Proliferating trichilemmal cyst: an ultrastructural study. J Cutan Pathol 11:274, 1984

162. Hosokawa M, Rokugo M, Aiba S et al: Biochemical characteristics of keratins from proliferating trichilemmal cyst. Arch Dermatol Res 276:250, 1984

163. Hosokawa M, Ohkohchi K, Tagami H: Immunohistochemical staining characteristics of epidermal appendages (hair follicles and eccrine sweat glands) to anti-epidermal keratin antisera. Acta Derm Venereol (Stockh) 64:466, 1984

164. Sleater J, Beers B, Stefan M et al: Proliferating trichilemmal cyst. Report of four cases, two with nondiploid DNA content and increased proliferation index. Am J Dermatopathol 15:423, 1993

165. Chor PJ, Perkins SL, Hurt MA, Santa Cruz DJ: Malignant proliferative trichilemmal tumor: a morphologic DNA ploidy, and immunohistochemical comparison to selected trichilemmal tumors, abstracted. Mod Pathol 7:44A, 1994

166. Perwein E, Maciejewski W: Proliferating epidermoid cysts. Hautarzt 37:102, 1986

167. Saida T, Oohara K, Hori Y, Tsuchiya S: Development of a malignant proliferating trichilemmal cyst in a patient with multiple trichilemmal cysts. Dermatologica 166:203, 1983

168. Batman PA, Evans HJR: Metastasizing pilar tumour of scalp. J Clin Pathol 39:757, 1986

169. Mori O, Hachisuka H, Sasai Y: Proliferating trichilemmal cyst with spindle cell carcinoma. Am J Dermatopathol 12:479, 1990

170. Weiss J, Heine M, Grimmel M, Jung E: Malignant proliferating trichilemmal cyst. Part 2. J Am Acad Dermatol 32:870, 1995

171. Steffen C: Mantleoma. A benign neoplasm with mantle differentiation. Am J Dermatopathol 15:306, 1993

172. Birt AR, Hogg GR, Dubé WJ: Hereditary multiple fibrofolliculomas with trichodiscomas and acrochordons. Arch Dermatol 113:1674, 1977

173. Rongioletti F, Hazini R, Gianotti G, Rebora A: Fibrofolliculomas, tricodiscomas and acrochordons (Birt-Hogg-Dubé) associated with intestinal polyposis. Clin Exp Dermatol 14:72, 1989

174. Roth JS, Rabinowitz AD, Benosn M, Grossman ME: Bilateral renal cell carcinoma in the Birt-Hogg-Dubé syndrome. J Am Acad Dermatol 29:1055, 1993

175. Chung JY, Ramos-Carlo FA, Beers B et al: Multiple lipomas, angiolipomas, and parathyroid adenomas in a patient with Birt-Hogg-Dube syndrome. Int J Dermatol 35:365, 1996

176. Headington JT, French AJ: Primary neoplasms of the hair follicle. Histogenesis and classification. Arch Dermatol 86:430, 1962

177. Ingrish FM, Reed RJ: Tricholemmoma. Dermatol Int 7:182, 1968

178. Brownstein MH, Shapiro L: Trichilemmoma. Analysis of 40 new cases. Arch Dermatol 107:866, 1973

179. Möhlenbeck FW: Trichilemmoma. Eine studie von 100 fällen. Z Hautkr 49:791, 1974

180. Brownstein MH, Mehregan AH, Bikowski JB: Trichilemmomas in Cowden's disease. JAMA 238:26, 1977

181. Brownstein MH, Mehregan AH, Bikowski JB et al: The dermatopathology of Cowden's syndrome. Br J Dermatol 100:667, 1979

182. Starink TM, Hausman R: The cutaneous pathology of facial lesions in Cowden's disease. J Cutan Pathol 11:331, 1984

183. Starink TM, Hausman R: The cutaneous pathology of extrafacial lesions in Cowden's disease. J Cutan Pathol 11:338, 1984

184. Starink TM, Meijer CJ, Brownstein MH: The cutaneous pathology of Cowden's disease: new findings. J Cutan Pathol 12:83, 1985

185. Johnson BL, Kramer EM, Lavker RM: The keratotic tumors of Cowden's disease: an electronmicroscopic study. J Cutan Pathol 14:291, 1987

186. Carlson GJ, Nivatvongs S, Snover DC: Colorectal polyps in Cowden's disease (multiple hamartoma syndrome). Am J Surg Pathol 8:763, 1984

187. Lloyd KM, Dennis M: Cowden's disease: a possible new symptom complex with multiple system involvement. Ann Intern Med 58:136, 1963

188. Starink TM, van der Veen JPW, Arwert F et al: The Cowden syndrome: a clinical and genetic study in 21 patients. Clin Genet 29:222, 1986

189. Wheeland RG, McGillis ST: Cowden's disease–treatment of cutaneous lesions using carbon dioxide laser vaporization: a comparison of conventional and superpulsed techniques. J Dermatol Surg Oncol 15:1055, 1989

190. Hunt SJ, Kilzer B, Santa Cruz DJ: Desmoplastic trichilemmoma: histologic variant resembling invasive carcinoma. J Cutan Pathol 17:45, 1990

191. Hashimoto T, Inamoto N, Nakamura K, Harada R: Involucrin expression in skin appendage tumours. Br J Dermatol 117:325, 1987

192. Brownstein MH, Shapiro EE: Trichilemmomal horn: cutaneous horn overlying trichilemmoma. Clin Exp Dermatol 4:59, 1979

193. Kimura S: Trichilemmal keratosis (horn): a light and electron microscopic study. J Cutan Pathol 10:59, 1983

194. Ackerman AB: Trichilemmoma, letter. Arch Dermatol 114:286, 1977

195. Ackerman AB, Wade TR: Tricholemmoma. Am J Dermatopathol 2:207, 1980

196. Headington JT: Tricholemmoma. To be or not to be? Am J Dermatopathol 2:225, 1980

197. Reed RJ: Tricholemmoma. A cutaneous hamartoma. Am J Dermatopathol 2:227, 1980

198. Richfield DF: Tricholemmoma. True and false types. Am J Dermatopathol 2:233, 1980

199. Brownstein MH: Trichilemmoma. Benign follicular tumor or viral wart? Am J Dermatopathol 2:229, 1980

200. Penneys NS, Mogollon RJ, Nadji M, Gould E: Papillomavirus common antigens. Papillomavirus antigen in verruca, benign papillomatous lesions, trichilemmoma, and bowenoid papulosis: an immunoperoxidase study. Arch Dermatol 120:859, 1984

201. Leonardi CL, Zhu WY, Kinsey WH, Penneys NS: Trichilemmomas are not associated with human papillomavirus DNA. J Cutan Pathol 18:193, 1991

201A. Schaller J, Rohwedder A, Keminer O, Hendricks C: Detection of HPV-DNA in trichilemmomas by polymerase chain reaction (abstract). Dermatopathol Pract Concept 3(1):5, 1997

202. Duperrat B, Mascaró JM: Une tumeur bénigne developpée aux depens de l'acrotrichium du partie intraépidermique du follicule pilaire: porome folliculaire (acanthome folliculaire intraépidermique; acrotrichoma). Dermatologica 126:291, 1963

203. Oswald FH: On benign intraepidermal follicular acanthomas. Dermatologica 142:29, 1971

204. Burdick CO, Clearkin KP, Brown RK, Arakaki S: Tricholemmoma of the scalp. Arch Dermatol 95:73, 1967

205. Hanau D, Grosshans E: Trichilemmal tumor undergoing specific keratinization. "Keratinizing trichilemmoma." J Cutan Pathol 6:463, 1979

206. Ch'in K-Y: Calcified epithelioma of the skin. Am J Pathol 9:497, 1933

207. Martins AG: Tumor mumificado de Malherbe. Arq Pathol (Lisboa) 28:123, 1956

208. Forbis R Jr, Helwig EB: Pilomatrixoma (calcifying epithelioma). Arch Dermatol 83:606, 1961

209. Moehlenbeck FW: Pilomatrixoma (calcifying epithelioma). A statistical study. Arch Dermatol 108:532, 1973

210. Marrogi AJ, Wick MR, Dehner LP: Pilomatrical neoplasms in children and young adults. Am J Dermatopathol 14:87, 1992

211. Kaddu S, Soyer HP, Cerroni L et al: Clinical and histopathologic spectrum of pilomatricomas in adults. Int J Dermatol 33:705, 1994

212. Wilson Jones E, Schellander FG: Multifocal pilomatrixoma. Part of a follicular malformation. Trans St Johns Hosp Dermatol Soc 58:182, 1972

213. Aslan G, Erdogan B, Aköz T et al: Multiple occurrence of pilomatrixoma. Plast Reconstr Surg 98:510, 1996

214. Alli N, Güngör E, Artüz F: Perforating pilomatricoma. J Am Acad Dermatol 35:116, 1996

215. Chiaramonti A, Gilgor RS: Pilomatricomas associated with myotonic dystrophy. Arch Dermatol 114:1363, 1978

216. Ribera M, Calderon P, Barranco C, Ferrandiz C: Pilomatrixomas múltiples asociados a distrofia miotónica y a carcinoma medular de tiroides. Med Cutan Ibero Lat Am 17:395, 1989

217. Street ML, Rogers RS III: Multiple pilomatricomas and myotonic dystrophy. J Dermatol Surg Oncol 17:728, 1991

218. Cambiaghi S, Ermacora E, Brusasco A et al: Multiple pilomatricomas in Rubinstein-Taybi syndrome: a case report. Pediatr Dermatol 11:21, 1994

219. Schiff T, Ackerman AB: Pilomatricoma. Dermatopathol Pract Concept 1:257, 1995

220. Kaddu S, Soyer HP, Hödl S, Kerl H: Morphological stages of pilomatricoma. Am J Dermatopathol 18:333, 1996

221. Kaddu S, Beham-Schmid C, Soyer HP et al: Extramedullary hematopoiesis in pilomatricomas. Am J Dermatopathol 17:126, 1995

222. Falk S: EMH in pilomatricomas, letter. Am J Dermatopathol 18:218, 1996

223. Kaddu S, Soyer HP, Kerl H, Beham-Schmid C: EMH in pilomatricomas, reply. Am J Dermatopathol 18:219, 1996

224. Leppard BJ, Bussey HJR: Gardner's syndrome with epidermoid cysts showing features of pilomatrixomas. Clin Exp Dermatol 1:75, 1976

225. Cooper PH, Fechner RE: Pilomatricoma-like changes in the epidermal cysts of Gardner's syndrome. J Am Acad Dermatol 8:639, 1983

226. Narisawa Y, Kohda H: Cutaneous cysts of Gardner's syndrome are similar to follicular stem cells. J Cutan Pathol 22:115, 1995

227. Aloi FG, Boalino G, Pippione M: Sindrome del nevo epidermico di Solomon. Nevo verruco-sebaceo con siringocistoadenoma papillfero e pilomatricoma. Giornale Ital Dermatol Venereol 119:401, 1984

228. Hashimoto K, Nelson RG, Lever WF: Calcifying epithelioma of Malherbe. Histochemical and electron microscopic studies. J Invest Dermatol 46:391, 1966

229. McGavran MH: Ultrastructure of pilomatrixoma (calcifying epithelioma). Cancer 18:1445, 1965

230. Kaddu S, Soyer HP, Wolf IH, Kerl H: Proliferating pilomatricoma: a benign histopathologic simulator of matrical carcinoma, abstracted. J Cutan Pathol 23:53, 1996

231. Ackerman AB, de Viragh PA, Chongchitnant N et al: Pilomatricoma and matricoma. p. 477. In: Neoplasms with Follicular Differentiation. 1st Ed. Ackerman's Histologic Diagnosis of Neoplastic Skin Diseases: A Method by Pattern Analysis. Lea & Febiger, Philadelphia, 1993

232. Toshitani A, Imayama S, Urabe A et al: Hair cortex comedo. Am J Dermatopathol 18:322, 1996

233. Pinkus H, Coskey R, Burgess GH: Trichodiscoma. A benign tumor related to haarscheibe (hair disk). J Invest Dermatol 63:212, 1974

234. Ackerman AB: Trichodiscoma related to the hair disk and Merkel-cell neoplasm to Merkel cells? p. 307. In: Ackerman's Resolving Quandaries in Dermatology, Pathology, and Dermatopathology. 1st Ed. Promethean Medical Press, Philadelphia, 1995

235. Wick MR, Swanson PE, Kaye VN, Marrogi A: Hair follicle tumors. p. 113. In: Cutaneous Adnexal Tumors. A Guide to Pathologic Diagnosis. 1st Ed. ASCP Press, Chicago, 1991

236. Ackerman AB, de Viragh PA, Chongchitnant N et al: Fibrous papule. p. 207. In: Neoplasms with Follicular Differentiation. 1st Ed. Ackerman's Histologic Diagnosis of Neoplastic Skin Diseases: A Method by Pattern Analysis. Lea & Febiger, Philadelphia, 1993

237. Hornstein OP, Krickenberg M: Perifollicular fibromatosis cutis with polyps of the colon: a cutaneointestinal syndrome sui generis. Arch Dermatol Res 253:161, 1975

238. Stokes JH: Nevus pilaris with hyperplasia of nonstriated muscle. Arch Dermatol Syph (Chicago) 7:479, 1923

239. Urbanek RW, Johnson WC: Smooth muscle hamartoma association with Becker nevus. Arch Dermatol 114:104, 1978

240. Chapel TA, Tavafoghi V, Mehregan AH, Cagliardi C: Becker's melanosis: an organoid hamartoma. Cutis 27:405, 1981

241. Tsambaos D, Orfanos CE: Cutaneous smooth muscle hamartoma. J Cutan Pathol 9:33, 1982

242. Johnson MD, Jacobs AH: Congenital smooth muscle hamartoma. A report of six cases and a review of the literature. Arch Dermatol 125:820, 1989

243. Berger TG, Levin MW: Congenital smooth muscle hamartoma. Part 2. J Am Acad Dermatol 11:709, 1984

244. Fisher WC, Helwig EG: Leiomyomas of the skin. Arch Dermatol 88:510, 1963

245. Hunt SJ, Abell E: Malignant hair matrix tumor ("malignant trichoepithelioma") arising in the setting of multiple hereditary trichoepithelioma. Am J Dermatopathol 13:275, 1991

246. Rahbari H, Mehregan AH: Pilary complex carcinoma: an adnexal carcinoma of the skin with differentiation towards the components of the pilary complex. J Dermatol (Tokyo) 20:630, 1993

247. Goldstein DJ, Barr RJ, Santa Cruz DJ: Microcystic adnexal carcinoma: a distinct clinicopathologic entity. Cancer 50:566, 1982

248. LeBoit PE, Sexton M: Microcystic adnexal carcinoma of the skin. A reappraisal of the differentiation and differential diagnosis of an underrecognized neoplasm. J Am Acad Dermatol 29:609, 1993

249. Boscaino A, Terracciano LM, Donofrio V et al: Tricholemmal carcinoma: a study of seven cases. J Cutan Pathol 19:94, 1992

250. Swanson PE, Marrogi AJ, Williams DJ et al: Tricholemmal carcinoma: clinicopathologic study of 10 cases. J Cutan Pathol 19:100, 1992

251. Reis JP, Tellechea O, Cunha MF, Baptista AP: Trichilemmal carcinoma: review of 8 cases. J Cutan Pathol 20:44, 1993

252. Wong T-Y, Suster S: Tricholemmal carcinoma. A clinicopathologic study of 13 cases. Am J Dermatopathol 16:463, 1994

253. Ko T, Tada H, Hatoko M et al: Trichilemmal carcinoma developing in a burn scar: a report of two cases. J Dermatol (Tokyo) 23:463, 1996

254. Misago N, Tatsurou T, Kohda H: Trichilemmal carcinoma occurring in a lesion of solar keratosis. J Dermatol (Tokyo) 20:358, 1993

255. Suster S: Clear cell tumors of the skin. Semin Diagn Pathol 13:40, 1996

256. Green DE, Sanusi ID, Fowler MR: Pilomatrix carcinoma. J Am Acad Dermatol 17:264, 1987

257. Sau P, Lupton GP, Graham JH: Pilomatrix carcinoma. Cancer 71:2491, 1993

258. Hanly MG, Allsbrook WC, Pantazis CG et al: Pilomatrical carcinosarcoma of the cheek with subsequent pulmonary metastases. A case report. Am J Dermatopathol 16:196, 1994

259. McCulloch TA, Singh S, Cotton DWK: Pilomatrix carcinoma and multiple pilomatrixomas. Br J Dermatol 134:368, 1996

260. Prieto VG, Lugo J, McNutt NS: Intermediate- and low-molecular-weight keratin detection with the monoclonal antibody MNF116. An immunohistochemical study on 232 paraffin-embedded cutaneous lesions. J Cutan Pathol 23:234, 1996

261. Fields JP, Helwig EB: Leiomyosarcoma of the skin and subcutaneous tissue. Cancer 47:156, 1981

262. Jensen ML, Jensen OM, Michalski W et al: Intradermal and subcutaneous leiomyosarcoma: a clinicopathological and immunohistochemical study of 41 cases. J Cutan Pathol 23:458, 1996

263. Suster S, Rosen LB, Sánchez JL: Granular cell leiomyosarcoma of the skin. Am J Dermatopathol 10:234, 1988

264. Suster S: Epithelioid leiomyosarcoma of the skin and subcutaneous tissue. Clinicopathologic, immunohistochemical, and ultrastructural study of five cases. Am J Surg Pathol 18:232, 1994

265. Karroum JE, Zappi EG, Cockerell CJ: Sclerotic primary cutaneous leiomyosarcoma. Am J Dermatopathol 17:292, 1995

266. Troy JL, Ackerman AB: Sebaceoma. A distinctive benign neoplasm of adnexal epithelium differentiating toward sebaceous cells. Am J Dermatopathol 6:7, 1984

267. Zaim MT: Sebocrine adenoma. An adnexal adenoma with sebaceous and apocrine poroma-like differentiation. Am J Dermatopathol 10:311, 1988

268. Okuda C, Ito M, Fujiwara H, Takenouchi T: Sebaceous epithelioma with sweat gland differentiation. Am J Dermatopathol 17:523, 1995

269. Friedman KJ, Boudreau S, Farmer ER: Superficial epithelioma with sebaceous differentiation. J Cutan Pathol 14:193, 1987

270. Sanz Vico D, Sánchez Yus E: Adenoma sebaceo (sebomatricoma). Tres casos solitarios. Gaceta Dermatol 4:107, 1983

271. Sánchez Yus E, Requena L, Simón P, del Río E: Sebomatricoma: a unifying term that encompasses all benign neoplasms with sebaceous differentiation. Am J Dermatopathol 17:213, 1995

272. Rulon DB, Helwig EB: Cutaneous sebaceous neoplasms. Cancer 33:82, 1974

273. Cohen PR, Kohn SR, Kurzrock R: Association of sebaceous gland tumors and internal malignancy: the Muir-Torre syndrome. Am J Med 90:606, 1991

274. Schwartz RA, Torre DP: The Muir-Torre syndrome: a 25 year retrospect. J Am Acad Dermatol 33:90, 1995

275. Nelson BR, Hamlet KR, Gillard M et al: Sebaceous carcinoma. J Am Acad Dermatol 33:1, 1995

276. Doxanas MT, Green WR: Sebaceous gland carcinoma. Review of 40 cases. Arch Ophthalmol 102:245, 1984

277. Wolfe JT III, Yeatts RP, Wick MR et al: Sebaceous carcinoma of the eyelid. Errors in clinical and pathologic diagnosis. Am J Surg Pathol 8:597, 1984

278. Wick MR, Goellner JR, Wolfe JT III, Su WPD: Adnexal carcinomas of the skin. II. Extraocular sebaceous carcinomas. Cancer 56:1163, 1985

279. Russell WG, Page DL, Hough AJ, Rogers LW: Sebaceous carcinoma of meibomian gland origin. The diagnostic importance of pagetoid spread of neoplastic cells. Am J Clin Pathol 73:504, 1980

280. Ansai S, Hashimoto H, Aoki T et al: A histochemical and immunohistochemical study of extra-ocular sebaceous carcinoma. Histopathology 22:127, 1993

281. King DT, Barr RJ: Syringometaplasia: mucinous and squamous variants. J Cutan Pathol 6:284, 1979

282. Lerner TH, Barr RJ, Dolezal JF, Stagnone JJ: Syringomatous hyperplasia and eccrine squamous syringometaplasia associated with benoxaprofen therapy. Arch Dermatol 123:1202, 1987

283. Bhawan J, Petry J, Rybak ME: Histologic changes induced in skin by extravasation of doxorubicin (adriamycin). J Cutan Pathol 16:158, 1989

284. Hurt MA, Halvorson RD, Petr FC Jr et al: Eccrine squamous syringometaplasia. A cutaneous sweat gland reaction in the histologic spectrum of "chemotherapy-associated eccrine hidradenitis" and "neutrophilic eccrine hidradenitis." Arch Dermatol 126:73, 1990

285. Metcalf JS, Maize JC: Squamous syringometaplasia in lobular panniculitis and pyoderma gangrenosum. Am J Dermatopathol 12:141, 1990

286. Rongioletti F, Ballestrero A, Bogliolo F, Rebora A: Necro-

287. tizing eccrine squamous syringometaplasia presenting as acral erythema. J Cutan Pathol 18:453, 1991

287. Rongioletti F, Rebora A: Eccrine squamous syringometaplasia in chemotherapy-induced acral erythema, letter. J Am Acad Dermatol 26:284, 1992

288. Cribier B, Lipsker D, Grosshans E: Squamous syringometaplasia: an original manifestation of pathomimesis. Ann Dermatol Venereol 120:900, 1993

289. Serrano T, Saez A, Moreno A: Eccrine squamous syringometaplasia. A prospective clinicopathologic study. J Cutan Pathol 20:61, 1993

290. Wong P, Bangert JL, Levine N: A papulovesicular eruption in a man receiving chemotherapy for metastatic melanoma. Squamous syringometaplasia (squamous metaplasia) of the eccrine glands. Arch Dermatol 129:232, 1993

291. Helton JL, Metcalf JS: Squamous syringometaplasia in association with annular elastolytic granuloma. Am J Dermatopathol 17:407, 1995

292. Rios-Buceta L, Penas PF, Dauden-Tello E et al: Recall phenomenon with the unusual presence of eccrine squamous syringometaplasia. Br J Dermatol 133:630, 1995

293. Kwittken J: Muciparous epidermal tumor. Arch Dermatol 109:554, 1974

294. Mehregan AH: Mucinous syringometaplasia letter. Arch Dermatol 116:988, 1980

295. Scully K, Assaad D: Mucinous syringometaplasia. J Am Acad Dermatol 11:503, 1984

296. Walker AN, Morton BD: Acral mucinous syringometaplasia. A benign cutaneous lesion associated with verrucous hyperplasia. Arch Pathol Lab Med 110:248, 1986

297. Madison JF, Cooper PH, Burgdorf WH: Mucinous syringometaplasia with prominent epithelial hyperplasia and deep dermal involvement. J Cutan Pathol 17:220, 1990

298. Hunt SJ, Abell E: Mucinous syringometaplasia mimicked by a clear cell hidradenoma with mucinous change. J Cutan Pathol 18:339, 1991

299. Kappel TJ, Abenoza P: Mucinous syringometaplasia. A case report with review of the literature. Am J Dermatopathol 15:562, 1993

300. Trotter MJ, Stevens PJ, Smith NP: Mucinous syringometaplasia–a case report and review of the literature. Clin Exp Dermatol 20:42, 1995

301. Bergman R, David R, Friedman-Birnbaum R et al: Mucinous syringometaplasia. An immunohistochemical and ultrastructural study of a case. Am J Dermatopathol 18:521, 1996

302. Fitzgibbon JF, Googe PB: Mucinous differentiation in adnexal sweat gland tumors. J Cutan Pathol 23:259, 1996

303. Rabens SF, Naness JI, Gottlieb BF: Apocrine gland organic hamartoma (apocrine nevus). Arch Dermatol 112:520, 1976

304. Mehregan AH, Rahbari H: Benign epithelial tumors of the skin. IV: benign apocrine gland tumors. Cutis 21:53, 1978

305. Kim JH, Hur H, Lee CW, Kim YT: Apocrine nevus, letter. J Am Acad Dermatol 18:579, 1988

306. Ando K, Hashikawa Y, Nakashima M et al: Pure apocrine nevus. A study of light-microscopic and immunohistochemical features of a rare tumor. Am J Dermatopathol 13:71, 1991

307. Landry M, Winkelmann RK: An unusual tubular apocrine adenoma. Histochemical and ultrastructural study. Arch Dermatol 105:869, 1972

308. Umbert P, Winkelmann RK: Tubular apocrine adenoma. J Cutan Pathol 3:75, 1976

309. Civatte J, Belaich S, Lauret P: Adénome tubulaire apocrine (quatre cas). Ann Dermatol Venereol 106:665, 1979

310. Ansai S, Watanabe S, Aso K: A case of tubular apocrine adenoma with syringocystadenoma papilliferum. J Cutan Pathol 16:230, 1989

311. Abenoza P, Ackerman AB, Di Leonardo M: Papillary tubular adenomas. p. 353. In: Neoplasms with Eccrine Differentiation. 1st Ed. Ackerman's Histologic Diagnosis of Neoplastic Skin Diseases: A Method by Pattern Analysis. Lea & Febiger, Philadelphia, 1990

312. Tellechea O, Reis JP, Marques C, Poiares Baptista A: Tubular apocrine adenoma with eccrine and apocrine immunophenotypes or papillary tubular adenoma? Am J Dermatopathol 17:499, 1995

313. Fox SB, Cotton DWK: Tubular apocrine adenoma and papillary eccrine adenoma. Entities or unity? Am J Dermatopathol 14:149, 1992

314. Ishiko A, Shimizu H, Inamoto N, Nakmura K: Is tubular apocrine adenoma a distinct clinical entity? Am J Dermatopathol 15:482, 1993

315. Helwig EB, Hackney VC: Syringadenoma papilliferum. Arch Dermatol 71:361, 1955

316. Niizuma K: Syringocystadenoma papilliferum. Light and electron microscopic studies. Acta Derm Venereol (Stockh) 56:327, 1976

317. Anderson NP: Hidradenoma of the vulva. Arch Dermatol Syph (Chicago) 62:873, 1950

318. Meeker JH, Neubecker RD, Helwig EB: Hidradenoma papilliferum. Am J Clin Pathol 37:182, 1962

319. Woodworth H Jr, Dockerty MB, Wilson RB, Pratt JH: Papillary hidradenoma of the vulva: a clinicopathologic study of 69 cases. Am J Obstet Gynecol 110:501, 1971

320. Santa Cruz DJ, Prioleau PG, Smith ME: Hidradenoma papilliferum of the eyelid. Arch Dermatol 117:55, 1981

321. Thaller VT, Collin JRO, McCartney ACE: Oncocytoma of the eyelid: a case report. Br J Ophthalmol 71:753, 1987

322. Rodgers IR, Jakobiec FA, Krebs W et al: Papillary oncocytoma of the eyelid. A previously undescribed tumor of apocrine gland origin. Ophthalmology 95:1071, 1988

323. Fukuo Y, Hirata H, Takeda N et al: A case of oncocytoma in the eyelid. Ophthalmologica 208:54, 1994

324. Roth MJ, Stern JB, Hijazi Y et al: Oncocytic nodular hidradenoma. Am J Dermatopathol 18:314, 1996

325. Jones DB: Florid papillomatosis of the nipple ducts. Cancer 8:315, 1955

326. Brownstein MH, Phelps RG, Magnin PH: Papillary adenoma of the nipple: analysis of fifteen new cases. J Am Acad Dermatol 12:707, 1985

327. Rosen PP, Caicco JA: Florid papillomatosis of the nipple. A study of 51 patients, including nine with mammary carcinoma. Am J Surg Pathol 10:87, 1986

328. Myers JL, Mazur MT, Urist MM, Peiper SC: Florid papillomatosis of the nipple: immunohistochemical and flow cytometric analysis of two cases. Mod Pathol 3:288, 1990

329. Diaz NM, Palmer JO, Wick MR: Erosive adenomatosis of the nipple: histology, immunohistology, and differential diagnosis. Mod Pathol 5:179, 1992

330. Rosen PP: Syringomatous adenoma of the nipple. Am J Surg Pathol 7:739, 1983

331. Jones MW, Norris HJ, Snyder RC: Infiltrating syringomatous adenoma of the nipple. A clinical and pathological study of 11 cases. Am J Surg Pathol 13:197, 1989

332. Burger RA, Marcuse PM: Fibroadenoma of vulva. Am J Clin Pathol 24:965, 1954

333. Foushee JH, Pruitt AB Jr: Vulvar fibroadenoma from aberrant breast tissue. Report of 2 cases. Obstet Gynecol 29:819, 1967

334. Assor D, Davis JB: Multiple apocrine fibroadenomas of the anal skin. Am J Clin Pathol 68:397, 1977

335. Ahluwalia HS, Gopinath A, Kumaradeva S: Fibroadenoma of vulva. Med J Malaysia 32:215, 1978

336. Assor D: Multiple apocrine fibroadenomas of the anal skin, letter to the editor. Am J Clin Pathol 71:356, 1979

337. van der Putte SC: Anogential "sweat" glands. Histology and pathology of a gland that may mimic mammary glands. Am J Dermatopathol 13:557, 1991

338. Prasad KR, Kumari GS, Aruna CA et al: Fibroadenoma of ectopic breast tissue in the vulva. A case report. Acta Cytol 39:791, 1995

339. Amazon K, Glick H: Subcutaneous fibroadenoma on an arm. Am J Dermatopathol 7:127, 1985

340. van der Putte SC: Mammary-like glands of the vulva and their disorders. Int J Gynecol Pathol 13:150, 1994

341. O'Hara MF, Page DL: Adenomas of the breast and ectopic breast under lactational influences. Hum Pathol 16:707, 1985

342. Stout AP, Gorman JG: Mixed tumors of the skin of the salivary gland type. Cancer 12:537, 1959

343. Hirsch P, Helwig EB: Chondroid syringoma. Mixed tumor of the skin of salivary gland type. Arch Dermatol 84:835, 1961

344. Headington JT: Mixed tumors of the skin: eccrine and apocrine types. Arch Dermatol 84:989, 1961

345. Hassab-El-Naby HM, Tam S, White WL, Ackerman AB: Mixed tumors of the skin. A histological and immunohistochemical study published erratum appears in The American Journal of Dermatopathology 1990; 12:108. Am J Dermatopathol 11:413, 1989

346. Abenoza P, Ackerman AB, Di Leonardo M: Mixed tumors. p. 285. In: Neoplasms with Eccrine Differentiation. 1st Ed. Ackerman's Histologic Diagnosis of Neoplastic Skin Diseases: A Method by Pattern Analysis. Lea & Febiger, Philadelphia, 1990

347. Kakuta M, Tsuboi R, Yamazaki M et al: Giant mixed tumor of the face. J Dermatol (Tokyo) 23:369, 1996

348. Abenoza P, Ackerman AB, Di Leonardo M: Poromas. p. 113. In: Neoplasms with Eccrine Differentiation. 1st Ed. Ackerman's Histologic Diagnosis of Neoplastic Skin Diseases: A Method by Pattern Analysis. Lea & Febiger, Philadelphia, 1990

349. Vilanova X, Piñol Aguadé J, Castells A: Hamartome angiomateux sudoripare sécrétant. Dermatologica 127:9, 1963

350. Hyman AB, Harris H, Brownstein MH: Eccrine angiomatous hamartoma. NY State Med J 68:2803, 1968

351. Challa VR, Jona J: Eccrine angiomatous hamartoma: a rare skin lesion with diverse histological features. Dermatologica 155:206, 1977

352. Kikuchi I, Kuroki Y, Inoue S: Painful eccrine angiomatous nevus on the sole. J Dermatol (Tokyo) 9:329, 1982

353. Velasco JA, Almeida V: Eccrine-pilar angiomatous nevus. Dermatologica 177:317, 1988

354. Donati P, Amantea A, Balus L: Eccrine angiomatous hamartoma: a lipomatous variant. J Cutan Pathol 16:227, 1989

355. Wolf R, Krakowski A, Dorfman B, Baratz M: Eccrine angiomatous hamartoma. A painful step. Arch Dermatol 125:1489, 1989

356. Mayou SC, Black MM, Jones RR: Sudoriferous hamartoma. Clin Exp Dermatol 13:107, 1988

357. Gabrielsen T-Ø, Elgjo K, Sommerschild H: Eccrine angiomatous hamartoma of the finger leading to amputation. Clin Exp Dermatol 16:44, 1991

358. Marsden RA, Fleming K, Dawber RPR: Comedo naevus of the palm–a sweat duct naevus? Br J Dermatol 101:717, 1979

359. Abell E, Read SI: Porokeratotic eccrine ostial and dermal duct naevus. Br J Dermatol 103:435, 1980

360. Balato N, Cusano F, Lembo G, Ayala F: Naevus sudoral eccrine porokératosique pseudo-comédonien palmaire et plantaire. Ann Dermatol Venereol 113:921, 1986

361. Civatte J, Jeanmougin M, Denisart M et al: Naevus sudoral eccrine palmaire pseudo-comédonien. Ann Dermatol Venereol 113:923, 1986

362. Driban NE, Cavicchia JC: Porokeratotic eccrine ostial and dermal duct nevus. J Cutan Pathol 14:118, 1987

363. Moreno A, Pujol RM, Salvatella N et al: Porokeratotic eccrine ostial and dermal duct nevus. J Cutan Pathol 15:43, 1988

364. Fernández-Redondo V, Toribio J: Porokeratotic eccrine ostial and dermal duct nevus. J Cutan Pathol 15:393, 1988

365. Stoof TJ, Starink TM, Nieboer C: Porokeratotic eccrine ostial and dermal duct nevus. Report of a case of adult onset. J Am Acad Dermatol 20:924, 1989

366. Cobb MW, Vidmar DA, Dilaimy MS: Porokeratotic eccrine ostial and dermal duct nevus: a case of systematized involvement. Cutis 46:495, 1990

367. Murata Y, Nogita T, Kawashima M, Hidano A: Unilateral, systematized, porokeratotic eccrine ostial and dermal duct nevi. J Am Acad Dermatol 24:300, 1991

368. Soloeta R, Yanguas I, Lozano M et al: Immunohistochemical study of porokeratotic eccrine nevus. Int J Dermatol 35:881, 1996

369. Coskey RJ, Mehregan AH, Hashimoto K: Porokeratotic eccrine duct and hair follicle nevus. J Am Acad Dermatol 6:940, 1982

370. Mascaró J-M: Considérations sur les tumeurs fibroépithéliales: le syringofibradénome eccrine. Ann Dermatol Syph 90:143, 1963

371. Weedon D, Lewis J: Acrosyringeal nevus. J Cutan Pathol 4:166, 1977

372. Mehregan AH, Marufi M, Medenica M: Eccrine syringofibroadenoma (mascaro). Report of two cases. J Am Acad Dermatol 13:433, 1985

373. Hurt MA, Igra-Serfaty H, Stevens CS: Eccrine syringofibroadenoma (mascaró). An acrosyringeal hamartoma. Arch Dermatol 126:945, 1990

374. Nordin H, Månsson T, Svensson Å: Familial occurrence of eccrine tumours in a family with ectodermal dysplasia. Acta Derm Venereol (Stockh) 68:523, 1988

375. Requena L, Sánchez Yus E, Simón P, del Rio E: Induction of cutaneous hyperplasias by altered stroma. Am J Dermatopathol 18:248, 1996

376. Johnson BL, Helwig EB: Eccrine acrospiroma. A clinicopathologic study. Cancer 23:641, 1969

377. Hernández PE, Cestoni-Parducci R: Nodular hidradenoma and hidradenocarcinoma. A 10-year review. Part 1. J Am Acad Dermatol 12:15, 1985

378. Harvell JD, Kerschmann RL, LeBoit PE: Eccrine or apocrine poroma? Six poromas with divergent adnexal differentiation. Am J Dermatopathol 18:1, 1996

379. Pinkus H, Rogin JR, Goldman P: Eccrine poroma. Tumors exhibiting features of the epidermal sweat duct unit. Arch Dermatol 74:511, 1956

380. Smith JLS, Coburn JG: Hidroacanthoma simplex. An assessment of a selected group of intraepidermal basal cell epitheliomata and of their malignant homologues. Br J Dermatol 68:400, 1956

381. Oka K, Moroashi M, Nitto H: Hidroacanthoma simplex: an ultrastructural study and comparison with eccrine poroma. J Dermatol (Tokyo) 2:69, 1975

382. Hyman AB, Brownstein MH: Eccrine poroma. An analysis of forty-five new cases. Dermatologica 138:29, 1969

383. Winkelmann RK, McLeod WA: The dermal duct tumor. Arch Dermatol 94:50, 1966

384. Pylyser K, De Wolf-Peeters C, Marien K: The histology of eccrine poromas: a study of 14 cases. Dermatologica 167:243, 1983

385. Wilson Jones E: Pigmented nodular hidradenoma. Arch Dermatol 104:117, 1971

386. Mousawi A, Kibbi A-G: Pigmented eccrine poroma: a simulant of nodular melanoma. Int J Dermatol 34:857, 1995

387. Abenoza P, Ackerman AB, Di Leonardo M: Hidradenomas. p. 311. In: Neoplasms with Eccrine Differentiation. 1st Ed. Ackerman's Histologic Diagnosis of Neoplastic Skin Diseases: A Method by Pattern Analysis. Lea & Febiger, Philadelphia, 1990

388. Watanabe S, Mogi S, Ichikawa E et al: Immunohistochemical analysis of keratin distribution in eccrine poroma. Am J Pathol 142:231, 1993

389. Wollina U, Castelli E, Rulke D: Immunohistochemistry of eccrine poroma and porocarcinoma–more than acrosyringeal tumors? Recent Results Cancer Res 139:303, 1995

390. Wallace ML, Smoller BR: Estrogen and progesterone receptors and anti-gross cystic disease fluid protein 15 (BRST-2) fail to distinguish metastatic breast carcinoma from eccrine neoplasms. Mod Pathol 8:897, 1995

391. Tateyama H, Eimoto T, Tada T et al: p53 protein and proliferating cell nuclear antigen in eccrine poroma and porocarcinoma. An immunohistochemical study. Am J Dermatopathol 17:457, 1995

392. Cooper PH: Mitotic figures in sweat gland adenomas. J Cutan Pathol 14:10, 1987

393. Henner MS, Shapiro PE, Ritter JH et al: Solitary syringoma. Report of five cases and clinicopathologic comparison with microcystic adnexal carcinoma of the skin. Am J Dermatopathol 17:465, 1995

394. Chi H-I: A case of unusual syringoma: unilateral linear distribution and plaque formation. J Dermatol (Tokyo) 23:505, 1996

395. Rongioletti F, Semino MT, Rebora A: Unilateral multiple plaque-like syringomas. Br J Dermatol 135:623, 1996

396. Weiss E, Paez E, Greenberg AS et al: Eruptive syringomas associated with milia. Int J Dermatol 34:193, 1995

397. Zalla JA, Perry HO: An unusual case of syringoma. Arch Dermatol 103:215, 1971

398. Seifert HW: Multiple syringome mit vermehrung von mastzellen unter dem klinishen bild einer urticaria pigmentosa. Z Hautkr 56:303, 1981

399. Hashimoto K, Blum D, Fukaya T, Eto H: Familial syringoma. Case history and application of monoclonal anti-eccrine gland antibodies. Arch Dermatol 121:756, 1985

400. Butterworth T, Strean LP, Beerman H, Wood MG: Syringoma and mongolism. Arch Dermatol 90:483, 1964

401. Rhodes LE, Verbov JL: Widespread syringomata in Down's syndrome. Clin Exp Dermatol 18:333, 1993

402. Headington JT, Koski J, Murphy PJ: Clear cell glycogenosis in multiple syringomas. Description and enzyme histochemistry. Arch Dermatol 106:353, 1972

403. Yamasaki Y, Toda M, Kitamura K: Syringomas of the clear cell type–an ultrastructural observation. J Dermatol (Tokyo) 9:431, 1982

404. Furue M, Hori Y, Nakabayashi Y: Clear-cell syringoma. Association with diabetes mellitus. Am J Dermatopathol 6:131, 1984

405. Feibelman CE, Maize JC: Clear-cell syringoma. A study by conventional and electron microscopy. Am J Dermatopathol 6:139, 1984

406. Ambrojo P, Requena Caballero L, Aguilar Martínez A et al: Clear-cell syringoma. Immunohistochemistry and electron microscopy study. Dermatologica 178:164, 1989

407. Rulon DB, Helwig EB: Papillary eccrine adenoma. Arch Dermatol 113:596, 1977

408. Elpern DJ, Farmer ER: Papillary eccrine adenoma, letter. Arch Dermatol 114:1241, 1978

409. Sexton M, Maize JC: Papillary eccrine adenoma. A light microscopic and immunohistochemical study. Part 1. J Am Acad Dermatol 18:1114, 1988

410. Jerasutus S, Suvanprakorn P, Wongchinchai M: Papillary eccrine adenoma: an electron microscopic study. J Am Acad Dermatol 20:1111, 1989

411. Crain RC, Helwig EB: Dermal cylindroma (dermal eccrine cylindroma). Am J Clin Pathol 35:504, 1961

412. Munger BL, Graham JH, Helwig EB: Ultrastructure and histochemical characteristics of dermal eccrine cylindroma (turban tumor). J Invest Dermatol 39:577, 1962

413. Urbach F, Graham JH, Goldstein J, Munger BL: Dermal eccrine cylindroma. A histochemical, electron microscopic, and therapeutic (x-ray) study. Arch Dermatol 88:880, 1963

414. Goette DK, McConnell MA, Fowler VR: Cylindroma and eccrine spiradenoma coexistent in the same lesion. Arch Dermatol 118:274, 1982

415. Gerretsen AL, Beemer FA, Deenstra W et al: Familial cutaneous cylindromas: investigations in five generations of a family. Part 1. J Am Acad Dermatol 33:199, 1995

416. Kersting DW, Helwig EB: Eccrine spiradenoma. Arch Dermatol 72:199, 1956

417. Hashimoto K, Gross BG, Lever WF: Eccrine spiradenoma. Histochemical and electron microscopic studies. J Invest Dermatol 46:347, 1966

418. Mambo NC: Eccrine spiradenoma: clinical and pathologic study of 49 tumors. J Cutan Pathol 10:312, 1983

419. Weyers W, Nilles M, Eckert F, Schill W-B: Spiradenomas in Brooke-Spiegler syndrome. Am J Dermatopathol 15:156, 1993

420. Noto G, Bongiorno MR, Pravatà G, Aricò M: Multiple nevoid spiradenomas. Am J Dermatopathol 16:280, 1994

421. Cotton DW, Slater DN, Rooney N et al: Giant vascular eccrine spiradenomas: a report of two cases with histology, immunohistology and electron microscopy. Histopathology 10:1093, 1986

422. van den Oord JJ, De Wolf-Peeters C: Perivascular spaces in eccrine spiradenoma. A clue to its histological diagnosis. Am J Dermatopathol 17:266, 1995

423. Santa Cruz DJ: Sweat gland carcinomas: a comprehensive review. Semin Diagn Pathol 4:38, 1987

424. Stout AP, Cooley SGE: Carcinoma of sweat glands. Cancer 4:521, 1951

425. Miller WL: Sweat-gland carcinoma: a clinicopathologic problem. Am J Clin Pathol 47:767, 1967

426. Freeman RG, Winkelmann RK: Basal cell tumor with eccrine differentiation (eccrine epithelioma). Arch Dermatol 100:234, 1969

427. Boggio R: Adenoid cystic carcinoma of scalp, letter. Arch Dermatol 111:793, 1975

428. Headington JT, Teears R, Niederhuber JE, Slinger RP: Primary adenoid cystic carcinoma of skin. Arch Dermatol 114:421, 1978

429. Dissanayake RV, Salm R: Sweat-gland carcinomas: prognosis related to histological type. Histopathology 4:445, 1980

430. Cooper PH, Adelson GL, Holthaus WH: Primary cutaneous adenoid cystic carcinoma. Arch Dermatol 120:774, 1984

431. Wick MR, Swanson PE: Primary adenoid cystic carcinoma of the skin. A clinical, histological, and immunocytochemical comparison with adenoid cystic carcinoma of salivary glands and adenoid basal cell carcinoma. Am J Dermatopathol 8:2, 1986

432. Seab JA, Graham JH: Primary cutaneous adenoid cystic carcinoma. J Am Acad Dermatol 17:113, 1987

433. Bergman R, Lichtig C, Moscona RA, Friedman-Birnbaum R: A comparative immunohistochemical study of adenoid cystic carcinoma of the skin and salivary glands. Am J Dermatopathol 13:162, 1991

434. Eckert F, Pfau A, Landthaler M: Das adenoid-zystische schweiβdrüsenkarzinom. Eine klinisch-pathologische un immunohistochemische studie. Hautarzt 45:318, 1994

435. Chesser RS, Bertler DE, Fitzpatrick JE, Mellette JR: Primary cutaneous adenoid cystic carcinoma treated with Mohs micrographic surgery toluidine blue technique. J Dermatol Surg Oncol 18:175, 1992

436. Fukai K, Ishii M, Kobayashi H et al: Primary cutaneous adenoid cystic carcinoma: ultrastructural study and immunolocalization of types I, III, IV, V collagens and laminin. J Cutan Pathol 17:374, 1990

437. van der Kwast TH, Vuzevski VD, Ramaekers F et al: Primary cutaneous adenoid cystic carcinoma: case report, immunohistochemistry, and review of the literature. Br J Dermatol 118:567, 1988

438. Warkel RL, Helwig EB: Apocrine gland adenoma and adenocarcinoma of the axilla. Arch Dermatol 114:198, 1978

439. Paties C, Taccagni GL, Papotti M et al: Apocrine carcinoma of the skin. A clinicopathologic, immunocytochemical, and ultrastructural study. Cancer 71:375, 1993

440. Rockerbie N, Solomon AR, Woo TY et al: Malignant dermal cylindroma in a patient with multiple dermal cylindromas,

trichoepitheliomas, and bilateral dermal analogue tumors of the parotid gland. Am J Dermatopathol 11:353, 1989

441. Gerretsen AL, van der Putte SC, Deenstra W, van Vloten WA: Cutaneous cylindroma with malignant transformation. Cancer 72:1618, 1993

442. Cooper PH, Frierson HF Jr, Morrison AG: Malignant transformation of eccrine spiradenoma. Arch Dermatol 121:1445, 1985

443. Wick MR, Swanson PE, Kaye VN, Pittelkow MR: Sweat gland carcinoma *ex* eccrine spiradenoma. Am J Dermatopathol 9:90, 1987

444. McKee PH, Fletcher CDM, Stavrinos P, Pambakian H: Carcinosarcoma arising in eccrine spiradenoma. A clinicopathologic and immunohistochemical study of two cases. Am J Dermatopathol 12:335, 1990

445. Argenyi ZB, Nguyen AV, Balogh K et al: Malignant eccrine spiradenoma. A clinicopathologic study. Am J Dermatopathol 14:381, 1992

446. Helwig EB, Graham JH: Anogenital (extramammary) Paget's disease: a clinicopathologic study. Cancer 16:387, 1963

447. Jones RE Jr, Austin C, Ackerman AB: Extramammary Paget's disease: a critical reexamination. Am J Dermatopathol 1:101, 1979

448. Sawamura D, Ishikawa H, Murai T et al: Depigmented macula as an initial manifestation of extramammary Paget's disease, letter to the editor. J Dermatol (Tokyo) 23:429, 1996

449. Kato N, Matsue K, Sotodate A, Tomita Y: Extramammary Paget's disease with distant skin metastasis. J Dermatol (Tokyo) 23:408, 1996

450. Olson DJ, Fujimura M, Swanson P, Okagaki T: Immunohistochemical features of Paget's disease of the vulva with and without adenocarcinoma. Int J Gynecol Pathol 10:285, 1991

451. Helm KF, Goellner JR, Peters MS: Immunohistochemical stains in extramammary Paget's disease. Am J Dermatopathol 14:402, 1992

452. Kohler S, Smoller BR: Gross cystic disease fluid protein-15 reactivity in extramammary Paget's disease with and without associated internal malignancy. Am J Dermatopathol 18:118, 1996

453. Cooper PH, Mills SE, Leonard DD et al: Sclerosing sweat duct (syringomatous) carcinoma. Am J Surg Pathol 9:422, 1985

454. Lupton GP, McMarlin SL: Microcystic adnexal carcinoma. Report of a case with 30-year follow-up. Arch Dermatol 122:286, 1986

455. Nickoloff BJ, Fleischmann HE, Carmel J et al: Microcystic adnexal carcinoma. Immunohistologic observations suggesting dual (pilar and eccrine) differentiation. Arch Dermatol 122:290, 1986

456. Wick MR, Cooper PH, Swanson PE et al: Microcystic adnexal carcinoma. An immunohistochemical comparison with other cutaneous appendage tumors. Arch Dermatol 126:189, 1990

457. Sebastien TS, Nelson BR, Lowe L et al: Microcystic adnexal carcinoma. Part 2. J Am Acad Dermatol 29:840, 1993

458. Burns MK, Chen SP, Goldberg LH: Microcystic adnexal carcinoma: ten cases treated by Mohs' micrographic surgery. J Dermatol Surg Oncol 20:429, 1994

459. Hazen PG, Bass J: Microcystic adnexal carcinoma: success-

ful management using Mohs' micrographically controlled surgery. Int J Dermatol 33:801, 1994

460. Bier-Lansing CM, Hom DB, Gapany M et al: Microcystic adnexal carcinoma: management options based on long-term follow-up. Laryngoscope 105:1197, 1995

461. Hesse RJ, Scharfenberg JC, Ratz JL, Griener E: Eyelid microcystic adnexal carcinoma. Arch Ophthalmol 113:494, 1995

462. Hunt JT, Stack BC Jr, Futran ND et al: Pathologic quiz case 1. Microcystic adnexal carcinoma (MAC). Arch Otolaryngol Head Neck Surg 121:1430, 1995

463. Hunts JH, Patel BC, Langer PD et al: Microcystic adnexal carcinoma of the eyebrow and eyelid. Arch Ophthalmol 113:1332, 1995

464. Robinson ML, Knibbe MA, Roberson JB: Microcystic adnexal carcinoma: report of a case. J Oral Maxillofac Surg 53:846, 1995

465. Pujol RM, Su WPD: Microcystic adnexal carcinoma with extensive sebaceous differentiation, abstract ed. J Cutan Pathol 23:89, 1996

466. Billingsley EM, Fedok F, Maloney ME: Microcystic adnexal carcinoma. Case report and review of the literature. Arch Otolaryngol Head Neck Surg 122:179, 1996

467. Metze D, Grunert F, Neumaier M et al: Neoplasms with sweat gland differentiation express various glycoproteins of the carcinoembryonic antigen (CEA) family. J Cutan Pathol 23:1, 1996

468. Cooper PH: Sclerosing carcinomas of sweat ducts (microcystic adnexal carcinoma), editorial. Arch Dermatol 122:261, 1986

469. Abenoza P, Ackerman AB, Di Leonardo M: Syringomatous Carcinomas. p. 373. In: Neoplasms with Eccrine Differentiation. 1st Ed. Ackerman's Histologic Diagnosis of Neoplastic Skin Diseases: A Method by Pattern Analysis. Lea & Febiger, Philadelphia, 1990

470. McKee PH, Fletcher CD, Rasbridge SA: The enigmatic eccrine epithelioma (eccrine syringomatous carcinoma). Am J Dermatopathol 12:552, 1990

471. Mendoza S, Helwig EB: Mucinous (adenocystic) carcinoma of the skin. Arch Dermatol 103:68, 1971

472. Wright JD, Font RL: Mucinous sweat gland adenocarcinoma of eyelid. A clinicopathologic study of 21 cases with histochemical and electron microscopic observations. Cancer 44:1757, 1979

473. Snow SN, Reizner GT: Mucinous eccrine carcinoma of the eyelid. Cancer 70:2099, 1992

474. Santa Cruz DJ, Meyers JH, Gnepp DR, Perez BM: Primary mucinous carcinoma of the skin. Br J Dermatol 98:645, 1978

475. Headington JT: Primary mucinous carcinoma of skin: histochemistry and electron microscopy. Cancer 39:1055, 1977

476. Komatsu T: An immunohistochemical study of cutaneous tumors using an antibody to the breast cyst fluid protein (GCDFP-15). Nippon Hifuka Gakkai Zasshi 99:991, 1989

477. Carson HJ, Gattuso P, Raslan WF, Reddy V: Mucinous carcinoma of the eyelid. An immunohistochemical study. Am J Dermatopathol 17:494, 1995

478. Katoh N, Hirano S, Hosokawa Y et al: Mucinous carcinoma of the skin: report of a case with DNA cytofluorometric study. J Dermatol (Tokyo) 21:117, 1994

479. Kao GF, Helwig EB, Graham JH: Aggressive digital papil-

lary adenoma and adenocarcinoma. A clinicopathological study of 57 patients, with histochemical, immunopathological, and ultrastructural observations. J Cutan Pathol 14:129, 1987

480. Smith KJ, Skelton HG, Holland TT: Recent advances and controversies concerning adnexal neoplasms. Dermatol Clin 10:117, 1992

481. Hamanaka S, Otsuka F: Multiple malignant eccrine poroma and a linear epidermal nevus. J Dermatol (Tokyo) 23:469, 1996

482. Pinkus H, Mehregan AH: Epidermotropic eccrine carcinoma. A case combining features of eccrine poroma and Paget's dermatosis. Arch Dermatol 88:597, 1963

483. Akano A, Nagakawa T, Kikuchi Y: Epidermotropic eccrine carcinoma. Rynsho Hifu-Hinyokika 21:43, 1967

484. Miura Y: Epidermotropic eccrine carcinoma. Jpn J Dermatol 78:226, 1968

485. Krinitz K: Malignes intraepidermales ekkrines porom. Z Haut-Geschl Kr 47:9, 1972

486. Bardach H: Hidroacanthoma simplex with in situ porocarcinoma. A case suggesting malignant transformation. J Cutan Pathol 5:236, 1978

487. Pique E, Olivares M, Espinel ML et al: Malignant hidroacanthoma simplex. A case report and literature review. Dermatology 190:72, 1995

488. Huet P, Dandurand M, Pignodel C, Guillot B: Metastasizing eccrine porocarcinoma: report of a case and review of the literature. Part 2. J Am Acad Dermatol 35:860, 1996

489. Mohri S, Chika K, Saito I, Yagishita K: A case of porocarcinoma. J Dermatol (Tokyo) 7:431, 1980

490. Shaw M, McKee PH, Lowe D, Black MM: Malignant eccrine poroma: a study of twenty-seven cases. Br J Dermatol 107:675, 1982

491. Mehregan AH, Hashimoto K, Rahbari H: Eccrine adenocarcinoma. A clinicopathologic study of 35 cases. Arch Dermatol 119:104, 1983

492. Bottles K, Sagebiel RW, McNutt NS et al: Malignant eccrine poroma. Case report and review of the literature. Cancer 53:1579, 1984

493. Claudy AL, Garcier F, Kanitakis J: Eccrine porocarcinoma. Ultrastructural and immunological study. J Dermatol (Tokyo) 11:282, 1984

494. Abenoza P, Ackerman AB, Di Leonardo M: Porocarcinomas. p. 415. In: Neoplasms with Eccrine Differentiation. 1st Ed. Ackerman's Histologic Diagnosis of Neoplastic Skin Diseases: A Method by Pattern Analysis. Lea & Febiger, Philadelphia, 1990

495. Akiyoshi E, Nogita T, Yamaguchi R et al: Eccrine porocarcinoma. Dermatologica 182:239, 1991

496. Van Hees CLM, Van Duinen CM, Bruijin JA, Vermeer BJ: Malignant eccrine poroma in a patient with Rothmund-Thomson syndrome, correspondence. Br J Dermatol 134:813, 1996

497. Hara K, Kamiya S: Pigmented eccrine porocarcinoma: a mimic of malignant melanoma. Histopathology 27:86, 1995

498. Ujihara M, Hamanaka S, Hamanaka Y, Kamei T: A case of multiple eccrine porocarcinoma with stepping-stone distribution on the foot. J Dermatol (Tokyo) 22:450, 1995

499. Kauderer C, Clarke HD, Fatone CT: Malignant eccrine acrospiroma. A case study, letter. J Am Podiatr Med Assoc 85:116, 1995

500. Rosen Y, Kim B, Yermakov VA: Eccrine sweat gland tumor of clear cell origin involving the eyelids. Cancer 36:1034, 1975

501. Grizzard WS, Torczynski E, Edwards WC: Adenocarcinoma of the eccrine sweat glands. Arch Ophthalmol 94:2112, 1976

502. Isimura E, Iwamoto H, Kobashi Y et al: Malignant chondroid syringoma. Report of a case with widespread metastasis and review of the pertinent literature. Cancer 52:1966, 1983

503. Trown K, Heenan PJ: Malignant mixed tumor of the skin (malignant chondroid syringoma). Pathology 26:237, 1994

504. Seco Navedo MA, Fresno Forcelledo M, Orduna Domingo A et al: Syringocystadenome papillifere a evolution maligne. Presentation d'un cas. Ann Dermatol Venereol 109:685, 1982

505. Bondi R, Urso C: Syringocystadenocarcinoma papilliferum. Histopathology 28:475, 1996

506. Wenig BL, Sciubba JJ, Goodman RS et al: Primary cutaneous mucoepidermoid carcinoma of the anterior neck. Laryngoscope 93:464, 1983

507. Banks ER, Cooper PH: Adenosquamous carcinoma of the skin: a report of 10 cases. J Cutan Pathol 18:227, 1991

508. van der Putte SC, van Gorp LH: Adenocarcinoma of the mammary-like glands of the vulva: a concept unifying sweat gland carcinoma of the vulva, carcinoma of supernumerary mammary glands and extramammary Paget's disease. J Cutan Pathol 21:157, 1994

509. Suster S, Wong T-Y: Polymorphous sweat gland carcinoma. Histopathology 25:31, 1994

510. Mehregan AH, Pinkus H: Life history of organoid nevi. Arch Dermatol 91:574, 1965

511. Wilson Jones E, Heyl T: Nevus sebaceus. A report of 140 cases with special regard to the development of secondary malignant tumors. Br J Dermatol 82:99, 1970

512. Domingo J, Helwig EB: Malignant neoplasms associated with nevus sebaceus of Jadassohn. J Am Acad Dermatol 1:545, 1979

513. Morioka S: The natural history of nevus sebaceus. J Cutan Pathol 12:200, 1985

514. García Hernández MJ, Muñoz Pérez MA, Rios JJ et al: Nevus sebaceus: clinical-pathological study, abstracted. J Cutan Pathol 23:74, 1996

515. Ng WK: Nevus sebaceus with apocrine and sebaceous differentiation. Am J Dermatopathol 18:420, 1996

516. Kaserer C, Hantich B: Trichogenic tumors, letter. Arch Dermatol 131:1464, 1995

517. Tozawa T, Ackerman AB: Basal cell carcinoma with follicular differentiation. Am J Dermatopathol 9:474, 1987

518. Rosai J: Basal cell carcinoma with follicular differentiation, letter. Am J Dermatopathol 10:457, 1988

519. Ackerman AB: Basal cell carcinoma with follicular differentiation, reply. Am J Dermatopathol 10:458, 1988

520. Rosai J: Basal cell carcinoma with follicular differentiation, reply. Am J Dermatopathol 11:479, 1989

521. Ackerman AB: Basal cell carcinoma with follicular differentiation, reply. Am J Dermatopathol 11:481, 1989

522. Reed RJ: Basal cell carcinoma with follicular differentiation, letter. Am J Dermatopathol 11:497, 1989

523. Ackerman AB: Basal cell carcinoma with follicular differentiation, reply. Am J Dermatopathol 11:498, 1989

524. Sánchez Yus E, Simón P, Requena L, Ambrojo P: Basal cell carcinoma with follicular differentiation, letter. Am J Dermatopathol 11:505, 1989

525. Pinkus H: Premalignant fibroepithelial tumors of skin. AMA Arch Dermatol Syph 67:598, 1953

526. Ambrojo P, Aguilar A, Simón P et al: Basal cell carcinoma with matrical differentiation. Am J Dermatopathol 14:293, 1992

527. Nogita T, Ohta A, Hidano A et al: Basal cell carcinoma with eccrine differentiation. J Dermatol (Tokyo) 22:111, 1995

528. George E, Swanson PE, Wick MR: Neuroendocrine differentiation in basal cell carcinoma. An immunohistochemical study. Am J Dermatopathol 11:131, 1989

529. Toker C: Trabecular carcinoma of the skin. Arch Dermatol 105:107, 1972

530. Kroll MH, Toker C: Trabecular carcinoma of the skin. Further clinicopathologic and morphologic study. Arch Pathol Lab Med 106:404, 1982

531. Rosai J: On the nature and nomenclature of a primary small carcinoma of the skin exhibiting endocrine (?Merkel cell) differentiation. Am J Dermatopathol 4:501, 1982

532. Silva EG, Mackay B, Goepfert H et al: Endocrine carcinoma of the skin (Merkel cell carcinoma). Pathol Annu 19:1, 1984

533. Gould VE, Moll R, Moll I et al: Neuroendocrine (Merkel) cells of the skin: hyperplasias, dysplasias, and neoplasms. Lab Invest 52:334, 1985

534. Wick MR, Swanson PE, Kaye VN, Marrogi A: Merkel cell carcinoma. p. 169. In: Cutaneous Adnexal Tumors. A Guide to Pathologic Diagnosis. 1st Ed. ASCP Press, Chicago, 1991

535. Ratner D, Nelson BR, Brown MD, Johnson TM: Merkel cell carcinoma. Part 1. J Am Acad Dermatol 29:143, 1993

536. O'Connor WJ, Brodland DG: Merkel cell carcinoma. Dermatol Surg 22:262, 1996

537. Kossard S, Wittal R, Killingsworth M: Merkel cell carcinoma with a desmoplastic portion. Am J Dermatopathol 17:517, 1995

538. Gillham SL, Morrison RG, Hurt MA: Epidermotropic neuroendocrine carcinoma. Immunohistochemical differentiation from simulators, including malignant melanoma. J Cutan Pathol 18:120, 1991

539. LeBoit PE, Crutcher WA, Shapiro PE: Pagetoid intraepidermal spread in Merkel cell (primary neuroendocrine) carcinoma of the skin. Am J Surg Pathol 16:584, 1992

540. Smith KJ, Skelton HG III, Holland TT et al: Neuroendocrine (Merkel cell) carcinoma with an intraepidermal component. Am J Dermatopathol 15:528, 1993

541. Tang C-K, Toker C, Nedwich A, Zaman AN: Unusual cutaneous carcinoma with features of small cell (oat cell-like) and squamous cell carcinomas. A variant of malignant Merkel cell neoplasm. Am J Dermatopathol 4:537, 1982

542. Sibley RK, Dahl D: Primary neuroendocrine (Merkel cell?) carcinoma of the skin. II. An immunocytochemical study of 21 cases. Am J Surg Pathol 9:109, 1985

543. Layfield L, Ulich T, Liao S et al: Neuroendocrine carcinoma of the skin: an immunohistochemical study of tumor markers and neuroendocrine products. J Cutan Pathol 13:268, 1986

544. Wick MR, Kaye VN, Sibley RK et al: Primary neuroendocrine carcinoma and small-cell malignant lymphoma of the skin. A discriminant immunohistochemical comparison. J Cutan Pathol 13:347, 1986

545. Tang C-K, Toker C: Trabecular carcinoma of the skin. An ultrastructural study. Cancer 42:2311, 1978

546. Sidhu GS, Mullins JD, Feiner H et al: Merkel cell neoplasms. Histology, electron microscopy, biology, and histogenesis. Am J Dermatopathol 2:101, 1980

547. Wick MR, Goellner JR, Scheithauer BW et al: Primary neuroendocrine carcinomas of the skin (Merkel cell tumors). A clinical, histologic, and ultrastructural study of thirteen cases. Am J Clin Pathol 79:6, 1983

548. Sibley RK, Dehner LP, Rosai J: Primary neuroendocrine (Merkel cell?) carcinoma of the skin. I. A clinicopathologic and ultrastructural study of 43 cases. Am J Surg Pathol 9:95, 1985

549. Haneke E: Electron microscopy of Merkel cell carcinoma from formalin-fixed tissue. J Am Acad Dermatol 12:487, 1985

550. Swanson SA, Cooper PH, Mills SE, Wick MR: Lymphoepithelioma-like carcinoma of the skin. Mod Pathol 1:359, 1988

551. Wick MR, Swanson PE, LeBoit PE et al: Lymphoepithelioma-like carcinoma of the skin with adnexal differentiation. J Cutan Pathol 18:93, 1991

552. Ortiz-Frutos FJ, Zarco C, Gil R et al: Lymphoepithelioma-like carcinoma of the skin. Clin Exp Dermatol 18:83, 1993

553. Jimenez F, Clark RE, Buchanan MD, Kamino H: Lymphoepithelioma-like carcinoma of the skin treated with Mohs micrographic surgery in combination with immune staining for cytokeratins. Part 2. J Am Acad Dermatol 32:878, 1995

554. Gillum PS, Morgan MB, Naylor MF, Everett MA: Absence of Epstein-Barr virus in lymphoepitheliomalike carcinoma of the skin. Polymerase chain reaction evidence and review of five cases. Am J Dermatopathol 18:478, 1996

555. Takayasu S, Yoshiyama M, Kurata S, Terashi H: Lymphoepithelioma-like carcinoma of the skin. J Dermatol (Tokyo) 23:472, 1996

556. Epstein W, Kligman AM: The pathogenesis of milia and benign tumors of the skin. J Invest Dermatol 26:1, 1956

557. King ESJ: Post-traumatic epidermoid cysts of hands and fingers. Br J Surg 21:29, 1933

558. Brownstein MH, Helwig EB: Subcutaneous dermoid cysts. Arch Dermatol 107:237, 1973

559. McGavran MH, Binnington B: Keratinous cysts of the skin. Arch Dermatol 94:499, 1966

560. Leppard B, Bussey HJR: Epidermoid cysts, polyposis coli and Gardner's syndrome. Br J Surg 62:387, 1975

561. Soyer HP, Schadendorf D, Cerroni L, Kerl H: Verrucous cysts: histopathologic characterization and molecular detection of human papillomavirus-specific DNA. J Cutan Pathol 20:411, 1993

562. Mehregan AH, Medenica M: Pigmented follicular cysts. J Cutan Pathol 9:423, 1982

563. Pavlidakey GP, Mehregan AH, Hashimoto K: Pigmented follicular cysts. Int J Dermatol 25:174, 1986

564. Requena Caballero L, Sánchez Yus E: Pigmented follicular cyst. Part 2. J Am Acad Dermatol 21:1073, 1989

565. Sandoval R, Urbina F: Pigmented follicular cyst. Br J Dermatol 131:130, 1994

566. Brownstein MH: Hybrid cyst: a combined epidermoid and trichilemmal cyst. J Am Acad Dermatol 9:872, 1983

567. Young E, Orentreich N, Ackerman AB: The "vanilla fudge" cyst. Cutis 18:513, 1976

568. Stevens CS: Follicular cysts: how should we name them? letter. J Am Acad Dermatol 12:367, 1985

569. Satoh T, Mitoh Y, Katsumata M et al: Follicular cyst derived from hair matrix and outer root sheath. J Cutan Pathol 16:106, 1989

570. Requena L, Sánchez Yus E: Follicular hybrid cysts. An expanded spectrum. Am J Dermatopathol 13:228, 1991

571. Andersen WK, Rao BK, Bhawan J: The hybrid epidermoid and apocrine cyst. A combination of apocrine hidrocystoma and epidermal inclusion cyst. Am J Dermatopathol 18:364, 1996

572. Bosellini PL: Beitrag zur Lehre von den multipeln folliculären hautzysten. Arch Dermatol Syph (Berlin) 45:81, 1898

573. Pringle JJ: A case of peculiar multiple sebaceous cysts (steatocystoma multiplex). Br J Dermatol 11:381, 1899

574. Abdel Aziz AM, El-Khashab MM: Steatocystoma multiplex: histologic studies and histogenesis. J Egyptian Med Assoc 55:292, 1972

575. Rohde B, Jänner M, Post B, Hartmann G: Steatocystoma multiplex. Hautarzt 25:29, 1974

576. Kimura S: An ultrastructural study of steatocystoma multiplex and the normal pilosebaceous apparatus. J Dermatol (Tokyo) 8:459, 1981

577. Plewig G, Wolff HH, Braun-Falco O: Steatocystoma multiplex: anatomic reevaluation, electron microscopy, and autoradiography. Arch Dermatol Res 272:363, 1982

578. Brownstein MH: Steatocystoma simplex. A solitary steatocystoma. Arch Dermatol 118:409, 1982

579. Lee YJ, Lee SH, Ahn SK: Sebocystomatosis: a clinical variant of steatocystoma multiplex. Int J Dermatol 35:734, 1996

580. Mortiz DL, Silverman RA: Steatocystoma multiplex treated with isotretinoin: a delayed response. Cutis 42:437, 1988

581. Notowicz A: Treatment of lesions of steatocystoma multiplex and other epidermal cysts by cryosurgery. J Dermatol Surg Oncol 6:98, 1980

582. Contreras MA, Costello MJ: Steatocystoma multiplex with embryonal hair formation. Case presentation and consideration of pathogenesis. Arch Dermatol 76:720, 1957

583. Sabater-Marco V, Pérez-Ferriols A: Steatocystoma multiplex with smooth muscle. A hamartoma of the pilosebaceous apparatus. Am J Dermatopathol 18:548, 1996

584. Esterly NB, Fretzin DF, Pinkus H: Eruptive vellus hair cysts. Arch Dermatol 113:500, 1977

585. Lee S, Kim J-G: Eruptive vellus hair cyst. Arch Dermatol 115:744, 1979

586. Lee S, Kim J-G, Kang JS: Eruptive vellus hair cysts. Arch Dermatol 120:1191, 1984

587. Denoldi D, Allegra F: Congenital eruptive vellus hair cysts. Int J Dermatol 28:340, 1989

588. Moon SE, Lee YS, Youn JI: Eruptive vellus hair cyst and steatocystoma multiplex in a patient with pachyonychia congenita. Part 1. J Am Acad Dermatol 30:275, 1994

589. Ackerman AB: Eruptive vellus hair cyst? p. 111. In: Ackerman's Resolving Quandaries in Dermatology, Pathology, and Dermatopathology. 1st Ed. Promethean Medical Press, Philadelphia, 1995

590. Stiefler RE, Bergfeld WF: Eruptive vellus hair cysts—an inherited disorder. J Am Acad Dermatol 3:425, 1980

591. Piepkorn MW, Clark L, Lombardi DL: A kindred with congenital vellus hair cysts. J Am Acad Dermatol 5:661, 1981

592. Mayron R, Grimwood RE: Familial occurrence of eruptive vellus hair cysts. Pediatr Dermatol 5:94, 1988

593. Kumakiri M, Takashima I, Iju M et al: Eruptive vellus hair cysts—a facial variant. J Am Acad Dermatol 7:461, 1982

594. Huerter CJ, Wheeland RG: Multiple eruptive vellus hair cysts treated with carbon dioxide laser vaporization. J Dermatol Surg Oncol 13:260, 1987

595. Fisher DA, Bergfeld WF: Retinoic acid in the treatment of eruptive vellus hair cysts. J Am Acad Dermatol 5:221, 1981

596. Sánchez-Yus E, Aguilar-Martínez A, Cristóbal-Gil MC et al: Eruptive vellus hair cyst and steatocystoma multiplex: two related conditions? J Cutan Pathol 15:40, 1988

597. Sexton M, Murdock DK: Eruptive vellus hair cysts. A follicular cyst of the sebaceous duct (sometimes). Am J Dermatopathol 11:364, 1989

598. Mehregan AH: Apocrine cystadenoma. A clinicopathologic study with special reference to the pigmented variety. Arch Dermatol 90:274, 1964

599. Smith JD, Chernosky ME: Apocrine hidrocystoma (cystadenoma). Arch Dermatol 109:700, 1974

600. Hashimoto K, Zagula-Mally ZW, Youngberg G, Leicht S: Electron microscopic studies of Moll's gland cyst. J Cutan Pathol 14:23, 1987

601. Veraldi S, Gianotti R, Pabisch S, Gasparini G: Pigmented apocrine hidrocystoma—a report of two cases and review of the literature. Clin Exp Dermatol 16:18, 1991

602. Hunter GA, Donald GF: Apocrine cystadenoma. Aust J Dermatol 11:82, 1970

603. Schewach-Millet M, Trau H: Congenital paillated apocrine cystadenoma: a mixed form of hidrocystoma, hidradenoma papilliferum, and syringocystadenoma papilliferum. Part 2. J Am Acad Dermatol 11:374, 1984

604. Mazoujian G, Margolis R: Immunohistochemistry of gross cystic disease fluid protein (GCDFP-15) in 65 benign sweat gland tumors of the skin. Am J Dermatopathol 10:28, 1988

605. Hassan MO, Khan MA, Kruse TV: Apocrine cystadenoma. An ultrastructural study. Arch Dermatol 115:194, 1979

606. Sato K, Leidal R, Sato F: Morphology and development of an apoeccrine sweat gland in human axillae. Am J Physiol 252:R166, 1987

607. Farmer ER, Helwig EB: Cutaneous ciliated cysts. Arch Dermatol 114:70, 1978

608. Robinson AR: Hidrocystoma. J Cutan Genitourin Dis 11:293, 1893

609. Dostrovsky A, Sagher F: Experimentally induced disappearance and re-appearance of lesions of hidrocystoma. J Invest Dermatol 5:167, 1942

610. Smith JD, Chernosky ME: Hidrocystomas. Arch Dermatol 108:676, 1973

611. Clever HW, Sahl WJ: Multiple eccrine hidrocystomas: a nonsurgical treatment, letter. Arch Dermatol 127:422, 1991

612. Sperling LC, Sakas EL: Eccrine hidrocystomas. J Am Acad Dermatol 7:763, 1982

613. Wolf M, Brownstein MH: Eccrine hidrocystoma (society transactions). Arch Dermatol 108:850, 1973

614. Cordero AA, Montes LF: Eccrine hidrocystoma. J Cutan Pathol 3:292, 1976

615. Adam J: Hidrocystoma. Br J Dermatol 7:169, 1895

616. Tokura Y, Takigawa M, Inoue K et al: S-100 protein-positive cells in hidrocystomas. J Cutan Pathol 13:102, 1986

617. Ebner H, Erlach E: Ekkrine hidrozystome. Dermatol Monatsschr 161:739, 1975

618. Hassan MO, Khan MA: Ultrastructure of eccrine cystadenoma. A case report. Arch Dermatol 115:1217, 1979

619. Kurban RS, Bhawan J: Cutaneous cysts lined by nonsquamous epithelium. Am J Dermatopathol 13:509, 1991

620. Bhaskar SN, Bernier JL: Histogenesis of branchial cysts. A report of 468 cases. Am J Physiol 35:407, 1959

621. Fraga S, Helwig EB, Rosen SH: Bronchogenic cysts in the skin and subcutaneous tissue. Am J Clin Pathol 56:230, 1971

622. Camacho F: Benign cutaneous cystic teratoma. J Cutan Pathol 9:345, 1982

623. Moreno A, Muns R: A cystic teratoma in skin. Am J Dermatopathol 7:383, 1985

624. Tsai T-F, Chuan M-T, Hsiao C-H: A cystic teratoma of the skin. Histopathology 29:384, 1996

625. Tidman MJ, MacDonald DM: Cutaneous endometriosis. A histopathologic study. Part 1. J Am Acad Dermatol 18:373, 1988

626. Doré N, Landry M, Cadotte M, Schürch W: Cutaneous endosalpingiosis. Arch Dermatol 116:909, 1980

627. Johnson WC, Graham JH, Helwig EB: Cutaneous myxoid cyst. JAMA 191:15, 1965

628. Cole LA, Helwig EB: Mucoid cysts of the penile skin. J Urol 115:397, 1976

629. Asarch RG, Golitz LE, Sausker WF, Kreye GM: Median raphe cysts of the penis. Arch Dermatol 115:1084, 1979

630. Gonzalez JG, Ghiselli RW, Santa Cruz DJ: Synovial metaplasia of the skin. Am J Surg Pathol 11:343, 1987

631. Stern DR, Sexton FM: Metaplastic synovial cyst after partial excision of nevus sebaceus. Am J Dermatopathol 10:531, 1988

632. Cohen L: Mucoceles of the oral cavity. Oral Surg Oral Med Oral Pathol 19:365, 1965

633. Jensen JL: Superficial mucoceles of the oral mucosa. Am J Dermatopathol 12:88, 1990

634. Moore TC: Omphalomesenteric duct anomalies. Surg Gynecol Obstet 103:569, 1956

635. Nix TE, Young CJ: Congenital umbilical anomalies. Arch Dermatol 90:160, 1964

636. Steck WD, Helwig EB: Cutaneous remnants of the omphalomesenteric duct. Arch Dermatol 90:463, 1964

637. Eggert JE, Harris GJ, Caya JG: Respiratory epithelial cyst of the orbit. Ophthalmic Plast Reconstr Surg 4:101, 1988

638. Sanusi ID, Carrington PR, Adams DN: Cervical thymic cyst. Arch Dermatol 118:122, 1982

639. Allard RHB: The thyroglossal cyst. Head Neck Surg 5:134, 1982

640. Keeney GL, Banks PM, Linscheid RL: Subungual keratoacanthoma. Report of a case and review of the literature. Arch Dermatol 124:1074, 1988

641. Kouskoukis CE, Scher RK, Kopf AW: Squamous-cell carcinoma of the nail bed. J Dermatol Surg Oncol 8:853, 1982

642. Hoffman S: Basal cell carcinoma of the nail bed. Arch Dermatol 108:828, 1973

643. Baran R, Kint A: Onychomatrixoma. Filamentous tufted tumour in the matrix of a funnel-shaped nail: a new entity (report of three cases). Br J Dermatol 126:510, 1992

644. Haneke E, Fränken J: Onychomatricoma. Dermatol Surg 21:984, 1995

645. Barr R, Headington JT, Molne L, Ternesten-Bratel A: Unguioblastic fibroma–a histological and immunohistochemical study of a previously unrecognized neoplasm, abstracted. J Cutan Pathol 23:46, 1996

646. Alessi E, Zorzi F, Gianotti R, Parafioriti A: Malignant proliferating onycholemmal cyst. J Cutan Pathol 21:183, 1994

647. Rubin MG, Mitchell AJ: Generalized cutaneous cylindromatosis. Cutis 33:568, 1984

648. Biggs PJ, Wooster R, Ford D et al: Familial cylindromatosis (turban tumour syndrome) gene localised to chromosome 16q12–q13: evidence for its role as a tumour suppressor gene. Nat Genet 11:441, 1995

649. Berberian BJ, Sulica VI, Kao GF: Familial multiple eccrine spiradenomas with cylindromatous features associated with epithelioma adenoides cysticum of Brooke. Cutis 46:46, 1990

650. van der Putte SCJ: The pathogenesis of familial multiple cylindromas, trichoepitheliomas, milia, and spiradenomas. Am J Dermatopathol 17:271, 1995

651. Araki W, Hirose S, Mimori Y et al: Familial hypobeta-lipoproteinaemia complicated by cerebellar ataxia and steatocystoma multiplex. J Intern Med 229:197, 1991

652. Sohn D, Chin TC, Fellner MJ: Multiple keratoacanthomas associated with steatocystoma multiplex and rheumatoid arthritis. A case report. Arch Dermatol 116:913, 1980

653. Aoyagi T, Ohnishi O: Pachyonychia congenita with steatocystoma multiplex: a report of 12 cases in one family [author's transl] Nippon Hifuka Gakkai Zasshi [Jpn J Dermatol] 86:767, 1976

654. Hodes ME, Norins AL: Pachyonychia congenita and steatocystoma multiplex. Clin Genet 11:359, 1977

655. Feinstein A, Friedman J, Schewach-Millet M: Pachyonychia congenita. J Am Acad Dermatol 19:705, 1988

656. Barone JG, Brown AS, Gisser SD, Barot LR: Steatocystoma multiplex with bilateral preauricular sinuses in four generations. Ann Plast Surg 21:55, 1988

657. McDonald RM, Reed WB: Natal teeth and steatocystoma multiplex complicated by hidradenitis suppurativa. A new syndrome. Arch Dermatol 112:1132, 1976

658. King NM, Lee AM: Natal teeth and steatocystoma multiplex: a newly recognized syndrome. J Craniofac Gen Dev Biol 7:311, 1987

659. Woods KA, Larcher VF, Harper JI: Extensive naevus comedonicus in a child with Alagille syndrome. Clin Exp Dermatol 19:163, 1994

660. Schmidt KT, Ma A, Goldberg R, Medenica M: Multiple adnexal tumors and a parotid basal cell adenoma. Part 2. J Am Acad Dermatol 25:960, 1991

661. Schirren CG, Wörle B, Kind P, Plewig G: A nevoid plaque with histological changes of trichoepithelioma and cylindroma in Brooke-Spiegler syndrome. J Cutan Pathol 22:563, 1995

662. Fargnoli MC, Orlow SJ, Semel-Concepcion J, Bolognia JL: Clinicopathologic findings in the Bannayan-Riley-Ruvalcaba syndrome. Arch Dermatol 132:1214, 1996

663. Kern F, Hambrick GW Jr: Multiple trichoepithelioma and cylindroma. Birth Defects 7:332, 1971

664. Delfino M, D'Anna F, Ianniello S, Donofrio V: Multiple

hereditary trichoepithelioma and cylindroma (Brooke-Spiegler syndrome). Dermatologica 183:150, 1991

665. Burrows NP, Russell Jones R, Smith NP: The clinicopathological features of familial cylindromas and trichoepitheliomas (Brooke-Spiegler syndrome): a report of two families. Clin Exp Dermatol 17:332, 1992

666. Carney JA: Carney complex: the complex of myxomas, spotty pigmentation, endocrine overactivity, and schwannomas. Semin Dermatol 14:90, 1995

667. Yuasa T, Hanano M, Ohshima F, Tsubaki T: The association of myasthenia gravis with multiple hamartoma syndrome (Cowden disease), letter. Ann Neurol 7:591, 1980

668. Starink TM: Cowden's disease: analysis of fourteen new cases. J Am Acad Dermatol 11:1127, 1984

669. Albrecht S, Haber RM, Goodman JC, Duvic M: Cowden syndrome and Lhermitte-Duclos disease. Cancer 70:869, 1992

670. Hamby LS, Lee EY, Schwartz RW: Parathyroid adenoma and gastric carcinoma as manifestations of Cowden's disease. Surgery 118:115, 1995

671. Wilk M, Kaiser HW, Steen KH, Kreysel HW: Das sklerotische Fibrom. Hautarzt 46:413, 1995

672. Abenoza P, Ackerman AB, Di Leonardo M: Syringomas. p. 187. In: Neoplasms with Eccrine Differentiation. 1st Ed. Ackerman's Histologic Diagnosis of Neoplastic Skin Diseases: A Method by Pattern Analysis. Lea & Febiger, Philadelphia, 1990

673. Leibowitz MR, Jenkins T: A newly recognized feature of ectrodactyly, ectodermal dysplasia, clefting (EEC) syndrome: comedone naevus. Dermatologica 169:80, 1984

674. Leppard B, Thompson HR: Gardner's syndrome and steatocystoma multiplex. Two unusual genetically determined conditions occurring in same patient. J Med Genet 13:407, 1976

675. Perniciaro C: Gardner's syndrome. Dermatol Clin 13:51, 1995

676. Muir EG, Yates Bell AJ, Barlow KA: Multiple primary carcinomata of the colon, duodenum and larynx associated with keratoacanthomata of the face. Br J Surg 54:191, 1967

677. Torre D: Multiple sebaceous tumors (Society transactions). Arch Dermatol 98:549, 1968

678. Cohen PR, Kohn SR, Davis DA, Kurzrock R: Muir-Torre syndrome. Dermatol Clin 13:79, 1995

679. Cantwell AR Jr, Reed WB: Myotonia atrophica and multiple calcifying epithelioma of Malherbe. Acta Dermatovenereol (Stockh) 45:387, 1965

680. Harper PS: Calcifying epithelioma of Malherbe. Association with myotonic muscular dystrophy. Arch Dermatol 106:41, 1972

681. Graells J, Servitje O, Badell A et al: Multiple familial pilomatricomas associated with myotonic dystrophy. Int J Dermatol 35:732, 1996

682. Leppard BJ: Skin cysts in the basal cell naevus syndrome. Clin Exp Dermatol 8:603, 1983

683. Barr RJ, Headley JL, Jensen JL, Howell JB: Cutaneous keratocysts of nevoid basal cell carcinoma syndrome. J Am Acad Dermatol 14:572, 1986

684. Gorlin RJ: Nevoid basal cell carcinoma syndrome. Dermatol Clin 13:113, 1995

685. Baselga E, Dzwierzynski WW, Neuburg M et al: Cutaneous keratocyst in naevoid basal cell carcinoma syndrome. Br J Dermatol 135:810, 1996

686. Bittencourt AL, Marback R, Peralta MJ, Nascimento MC: Neuro-oculo-cutaneous syndrome with multiple sebaceous nevi. Presentation of a case [in portuguese]. Med Cutan Ibero Lat Am 11:375, 1983

687. Happle R: Epidermal nevus syndromes. Semin Dermatol 14:111, 1995

688. Dupre A, Carrere S, Bonafe JL et al: Eruptive generalized syringomas, milium and atrophoderma vermiculata. Nicolau and Balus' syndrome [author's transl] [French]. Dermatologica 162:281, 1981

689. Ashinoff R, Jacobson M, Belsito DV: Rombo syndrome: a second case report and review. J Am Acad Dermatol 28:1011, 1993

690. Schöpf E: Syndrome of cystic eyelids, palmo-plantar keratosis, hypodontia and hypotrichosis as a possible autosomal recessive trait. Birth Defects 7:219, 1971

691. Font RL, Stone MS, Schanzer MC, Lewis RA: Apocrine hidrocystomas of the lids, hypodontia, palmar-plantar hyperkeratosis, and onychodystrophy. A new variant of ectodermal dysplasia. Arch Ophthalmol 104:1811, 1986

692. Starink TM, Keijser MH: Multiple eyelid hidrocystoma, eccrine poromatosis, hypodontia, hypotrichosis syndrome ("Schöpf syndrome"). Br J Dermatol 123:543, 1990

Appendix 18–1.

ADNEXAL TUMORS AND ASSOCIATED SYNDROMES

I. Specific tumors and their associated findings or syndromes
  A. Cylindroma
     1. Brooke-Spiegler syndrome (see below)
     2. Familial cylindromatosis[647,648]
     3. Trichoepitheliomas and spiradenoma[50,419,649,650]
     4. Milia and trichoepitheliomas[51]
  B. Cysts, follicular infundibular
     1. Gardner syndrome (see below)
     2. Haber syndrome (see below)
     3. Milia with trichoepitheliomas and cylindromas[51]
     4. Milia in Nicolau Balus syndrome (see below)
     5. Nevoid basal cell carcinoma syndrome (see below)
  C. Cysts, follicular with pilomatricoma-like changes
     1. Gardner syndrome (see below)
  D. Cysts, hidrocystomas, apocrine
     1. Schöpf syndrome (see below)
  E. Cysts, steatocystoma
     1. Gardner syndrome (see below)
     2. Hyperbetalipoproteinemia and cerebellar ataxia[651]
     3. Keratoacanthomas and rheumatoid arthritis[652]
     4. Pachyonychia congenita[588,653–655]
     5. Bilateral preauricular sinuses[656]
     6. Natal or defective teeth[657,658]
  F. Fibroma, perifollicular
     1. Perifollicular fibromatosis cutis with polyps of the colon[237]
  G. Fibrofolliculomas
     1. Birt-Hogg-Dubé syndrome (see below)
  H. Follicular hamartomas, generalized
     1. Myasthenia gravis[26,29]
   I. Infundibuloma (tumor of follicular infundibulum; isthmicoma)
     1. Cowden syndrome (see below)
  J. Myxoid tumors with follicular differentiation
     1. Carney syndrome (see below)
  K. Nevus comedonicus
     1. With Alagille syndrome (see below)[659]
     2. EEC syndrome (see below)
     3. Skeletal defects, cataracts, and possible electroencephalographic abnormalities[19]
  L. Organoid nevus (nevus sebaceus)
     1. Nevus sebaceus syndrome (see below)

  M. Pilomatricoma
     1. Multiple pilomatricomas and myotonic muscular dystrophy (see below)
     2. Gardner syndrome (see below)
     3. Rubinstein-Taybi syndrome (see below)
  N. Poromatosis
     1. Hidrotic ectodermal dysplasia[374]
  O. Sebaceous adenoma
     1. Muir-Torre syndrome (see below)
  P. Sebaceous carcinoma
     1. Muir-Torre syndrome (see below)
  Q. Spiradenomas
     1. Trichoepitheliomas and cylindromas[50,419,649,650]
  R. Syringofibroadenoma
     1. Hidrotic ectodermal dysplasia[374]
  S. Syringoma
     1. Bannayan-Riley-Ruvalcaba syndrome (see below)
     2. Down syndrome (39%)[400,401]
     3. Nicolau-Balus syndrome (see below)
  T. Syringoma, clear cell type
     1. Diabetes mellitus[404]
  U. Trichodiscomas
     1. Birt-Hogg-Dubé syndrome (see below)
  V. Trichoepitheliomas
     1. Basaloid (monomorphic) adenomas of the parotid[52,660]
     2. Brooke-Fordyce disease (see below)
     3. Brooke-Spiegler syndrome (see below)
     4. Congenital nail dystrophy
     5. With dystrophia unguis congenita[53]
     6. Myasthenia gravis[55]
     7. Milia and cylindromas[51]
     8. With palmar pits (variation of nevoid basal cell carcinoma syndrome?)[57]
     9. Rombo syndrome (see below)
     10. Spiradenomas and cylindromas[50,419,649,650,661]
  W. Tricholemmoma
     1. Bannayan-Riley-Ruvalcaba syndrome (see below)
     2. Cowden syndrome (see below)
II. Specific syndromes and their associated tumors and manifestations
  A. Alagille syndrome: arteriohepatic dysplasia associated rarely with nevus comedonicus[659]

B. Bannayan-Riley-Ruvalcaba syndrome: overlap of three syndromes–Riley-Smith syndrome, Bannayan-Zonana syndrome, and Ruvalcaba-Myhre-Smith syndrome; patients may have tricholemmomas, syringomas, multiple subcutaneous lipomas, vascular malformation, penile and vulvar lentigines, verrucae, acanthosis nigricans, macrocephaly with normal ventricular size, mental retardation, central nervous system vascular malformation, intestinal polyposis, skeletal abnormalities, and thyroid tumors[662]

C. Birt-Hogg-Dubé syndrome: trichodiscomas, fibrofolliculomas, and acrochordons[172]; one family with medullary carcinoma of thyroid[172]; one patient with bilateral renal cell carcinoma[174]

D. Brooke-Fordyce disease: multiple trichoepitheliomas presenting as skin-colored papules on the face with cribriform and palisaded basaloid cells with abundant stroma[42,43]

E. Brooke-Spiegler syndrome: multiple cylindromas in combination with trichoepitheliomas[49,661,663–665]

F. Carney syndrome: myxoid follicular tumors, myxomas including atrial myxomas, spotty pigmentation, endocrine overactivity, and schwannomas[85,666]

G. Cowden syndrome (multiple hamartoma syndrome): tricholemmomas, infundibulomas (isthmicoma), acral keratoses, cutaneous fibromas (collagenomas) (76%), oral papillomas, breast carcinoma (33%), gastrointestinal polyps (60%), thyroid abnormalities (benign and malignant) (62%); possible association with Lhermitte-Duclos disease; possible association with parathyroid adenoma and gastric carcinoma; possible association with myasthenia gravis[103,180–184,187,667–671]

H. Down syndrome (trisomy 21): syringomas in 39%[400,401,672]

I. EEC syndrome: nevus comedonicus and ectrodactyly, ectodermal dysplasia, clefting[673]

J. Gardner Syndrome: follicular infundibular cysts, follicular cysts with pilomatricoma-like changes in 37%, steatocystoma, colon polyps, desmoid tumors, and osteomas[226,560,674,675]

K. Haber syndrome: familial rosacea-like dermatosis with keratotic papules, pitted scars, and infundibular cysts with basaloid proliferations[25]

L. Lhermitte-Duclos disease: peculiar proliferation of abnormal neuronal elements of the cerebellum that has features of a hamartoma and of a neoplasm. Rarely associated with Cowden syndrome[669]

M. Muir-Torre syndrome: sebaceous adenomas or carcinomas with internal malignancy, usually of the gastrointestinal tract [273,274,676–678]

N. Myasthenia gravis
  1. Follicular hamartomas, generalized[26,29]
  2. Trichoepithelioma[55]
  3. Cowden syndrome[667]

O. Myotonic muscular dystrophy: autosomal dominant myotonic phenomena with lens opacities, frontal baldness, testicular atrophy, and mild mental retardation. Rarely associated with pilomatricomas[215–217, 679–681]

P. Nevoid basal cell carcinoma syndrome: numerous basal cell carcinomas, infundibular cysts, palmar and plantar pits, keratocysts of the jaw, keratocysts of the skin (rarely), calcified dural folds, various skeletal anomalies, cleft lip and/or cleft palate, and various other neoplasms or hamartomas[682–685]

Q. Nevus comedonicus syndrome: nevus comedonicus with skeletal defects, cataracts, and possible electroencephalographic abnormalities[19]

R. Nevus sebaceus syndrome: nevus sebaceus and multiple neurologic anomalies [686,687]

S. Nicolau-Balus syndrome: eruptive syringomas of the disseminated micropapular type, milium cysts, and atrophoderma vermiculata[688]

T. Rombo syndrome: trichoepitheliomas with vermiculate atrophoderma, milia, hypotrichosis, basal cell carcinomas, and peripheral vasodilation with cyanosis[54,689]

U. Rubinstein-Taybi syndrome: peculiar facies, mental retardation, broad thumbs and first toes, rarely with multiple pilomatricomas[218]

V. Schöpf syndrome: apocrine hidrocystomas (usually eyelid) with hypodontia, palmar-plantar hyperkeratosis, and onychodystrophy[690–692]

Appendix 18–2.

DIAGNOSING ADNEXAL TUMORS*

I. Cysts
  A. Opened to surface usually and conspicuously
    1. Infundibular differentiation
      a) Single lesion usually
        (1) Dilated pore (Winer)
      b) Multiple lesions
        (1) Nevus comedonicus
    2. Containing hair cortex
      a) Hair cortex comedo
    3. Infundibular and isthmic differentiation
      a) Lobular pattern usually deep
        (1) Pilar sheath acanthoma (infundibuloisthmicoma)
  B. Unilocular
    1. Infundibular differentiation
      a) Without other adnexa
        (1) Filled with flaky keratin only
          (*a*) Lining smooth and thin
            i) Follicular infundibular cyst
          (*b*) Lining variegated or sometimes papillary
            i) Dilated pore (Winer) cut in tangential or cross section
        (2) Filled with flaky keratin and hair cortex
          (*a*) Pigmented follicular cyst
      b) With other adnexa
        (1) All types of adnexa within or around the cyst
          (*a*) Dermoid cyst
        (2) Stellate structures join the cyst at perpendicular intervals
          (*a*) Vellus hairs join the cyst
            i) Trichofolliculoma
          (*b*) Thin infundibular or isthmic epithelial structures join the cyst
            i) Fibrofolliculoma
    2. Isthmic differentiation
      a) Isthmus-catagen (tricholemmal, pilar) cyst
    3. Sebaceous duct differentiation
      a) Corrugated cuticle, cyst empty
        (1) Steatocystoma
      b) Thin, multilayered, no granular component, sometimes corrugated, containing numerous vellus hair cortices
        (1) Eruptive vellus hair cyst

    4. Simple one- or two-cell epithelial lining
      a) Without apocrine differentiation
        (1) Hidrocystoma (eccrine?)
      b) With apocrine differentiation
        (1) Apocrine hidrocystoma/cystadenoma
    5. Two to several layers of matrical lining
      a) Matrical cyst (cystic pilomatricoma)
    6. Multiple types of linings
      a) Hybrid cyst
  C. Multilocular
    1. Infundibular differentiation
      a) Joined by thin basaloid strands with occasional zones containing hair bulbs or germs
        (1) Tricho "adenoma"
      b) Stellate structures join the cyst at perpendicular intervals
        (1) Vellus hairs join the cyst
          (*a*) Trichofolliculoma
        (2) Thin infundibular or isthmic epithelial structures join the cyst
          (*a*) Fibrofolliculoma
    2. Isthmic differentiation
      a) Proliferative tricholemmal cyst
    3. Sebaceous duct differentiation (may contain sebaceous lobules in wall)
      a) Steatocystoma
II. Lesions with lobules
  A. Pink cells (isthmic)
    1. Symmetric patulous follicle with focal infundibular differentiation
      a) Pilar sheath acanthoma
  B. Pink to slate-gray cells to clear cells with ducts
    1. Epidermal only
      a) Hidroacanthoma simplex (intraepidermal poroma/acrospiroma)
    2. Epidermal and dermal
      a) Poroma (juxtaepidermal acrospiroma)
    3. Dermal
      a) Dermal poroma (acrospiroma/hidradenoma)
  C. Basaloid cells
    1. With sebocytes in lobules
      a) Sebaceous adenoma
    2. With jigsaw puzzle patterns
      a) Cylindroma
    3. With solid-cystic patterns connected by thin trabeculae
      a) Spiradenoma

---

*This outline is meant to be used as a working tool and cannot replace a good working knowledge of these lesions and the experience of having observed a great number of them.

568

III. Lesions with islands (spheres or oblong shapes)
   A. Single island
      1. Basaloid cells mostly
         a) Solid
            (1) Single-cell type, cells overlap, prominent stroma with follicular mesenchyme
               (*a*) Trichoblastoma
            (2) Small and large cells, ducts often present, sometimes large vascular spaces
               (*a*) Spiradenoma
      2. Pink or clear cells with occasional ducts
         a) Poroma (acrospiroma) group
   B. Multiple islands
      1. Basaloid cells mostly
         a) With follicular germ
            (1) Trichoblastic fibroma
         b) With numerous hyalin droplets and surrounded by thick hyalin membrane in a "jigsaw puzzle" pattern
            (1) Well differentiated
               (*a*) Cylindroma
            (2) With pleomorphic cells, necrosis, or adjacent cylindroma
               (*a*) Cylindrocarcinoma
         c) With mostly solid areas containing small and large cells with occasional ducts
            (1) Well differentiated
               (*a*) Spiradenoma
            (2) With pleomorphic cells, necrosis, or adjacent spiradenoma
               (*a*) Spiradenocarcinoma
         d) With zones of sebocyte differentiation in each island
            (1) Uniform cytology throughout
               (*a*) Sebaceous adenoma, cellular type (sebaceoma; sebomatricoma)
            (2) Pleomorphic cytology with apoptosis, necrosis, or necrosis en masse
               (*a*) Sebaceous carcinoma
         e) Matrical cells, shadow cells, and foreign body reaction
            (1) Pilomatricoma
         f) Mostly matrical cells with few shadow cells
            (1) Uniform cytology with rare shadow cells
               (*a*) Matricoma
            (2) Pleomorphic cytology with zonal or massive necrosis, destruction of adjacent structures
               (*a*) Matrical carcinoma
         g) With papillary zones, tubules, cribriform areas, and numerous mitotic figures
            (1) Papillary digital adenocarcinoma
      2. Pink or clear cells
         a) Tumor cells uniform, do not overlap, and ducts present
            (1) Uniform cytology
               (*a*) Poroma (acrospiroma)
            (2) Pleomorphic cytology with mitoses and necrosis
               (*a*) Porocarcinoma
         b) With prominent vitreous later peripherally
            (1) Uniform cytology
               (*a*) Tricholemmoma
            (2) Pleomorphic cytology with mitoses and necrosis
               (*a*) Tricholemmal carcinoma
IV. Trabecular lesions
   A. Lesions with small basaloid cells
      1. Lace-like trabeculae, occasional horn cysts, and hair germs
         a) Trichoepithelioma classic type
      2. Some trabeculae with infundibular differentiation, numerous horn cysts, few hair germs
         a) Tricho "adenoma"
      3. Perinuclear whorls and nuclei with uniform granular patterns, nuclear molding, numerous mitotic figures
         a) Neuroendocrine carcinoma (some cases)
   B. Pink cells (isthmic) with superficial parallel plate
      1. Tumor of follicular infundibulum
   C. Pink cells that form thin strands, containing ducts and acrosyringeal patterns
      1. Syringofibroadenoma
   D. Pink to slate-gray cells with ducts, cells do not overlap, with myxiod or chondroid stroma (or both)
      1. Mixed tumor
V. Lesions with tubules
   A. Small uniform tubules
      1. Stroma uniform and usually fibrous
         a) Syringoma
      2. Stroma heterogeneous myxoid or chondroid (or both) and tubules possibly associated with poroid areas
         a) Mixed tumor
   B. Occasional and somewhat inconspicuous tubules
      1. Basaloid cells
         a) "Jigsaw puzzle" patterns typically
            (1) Cylindroma
         b) Solid patterns typically
            (1) Spiradenoma
   C. Tubules change from round to cord-like from superficial to deep
      1. Prominent horn cyst-like areas superficially in many cases
         a) Microcystic adnexal carcinoma
      2. Recapitulates the apocrine lobule typically
         a) Apocrine carcinoma
      3. Sieve-like round ducts typically
         a) Adenoid cystic carcinoma
   D. Tubules big and small, some papillary structures
      1. Elongated closely arranged tubules with focal apocrine zones and focal papillary zones
         a) Papillary hidradenoma
      2. Complex pattern with epithelial hyperplasia and focal necrosis en masse in nipple
         a) Nipple adenoma
      3. Small to moderate separated tubules with apocrine change and occasional intraductal papillary tufts
         a) Tubular apocrine adenoma
      4. Small to moderate separated tubules with minimal apocrine change and prominent intraductal papillary tufts
         a) Papillary (eccrine?) adenoma

  5. Circumscribed mass similar to fibroadenoma of breast
     a) Fibroadenoma of vulva or perianal region
  E. Tubules part of a complex lesion with multiple lines of differentiation
     1. Organoid nevus (nevus sebaceus)
VI. Lesions with papillary structures
  A. Papillary surface usually
     1. Exophytic papillary structures with two-cell layer, apocrine differentiation, and plasma cells within the cores
        a) Papillary syringadenoma
     2. Exophytic and endophytic lesion with epithelial hyperplasia usually within crowded ducts in the nipple
        a) Nipple adenoma
     3. One to several pink cells with a syncytial pattern, small basaloid morules, nail location
        a) Onychomatricoma
  B. Papillary structures within the tumor usually
     1. Separate tubules containing papillary tufts, rarely apocrine differentiation
        a) Papillary (eccrine?) adenoma
     2. Internal papillary structures and some tubules with oncocytic change and apocrine differentiation, usually in eyelid
        a) Papillary oncocytoma
  C. Papillary and tubular structures common
     1. Well-formed tubules with focal papilla, often with apocrine differentiation, usually vulvar or perianal location
        a) Papillary hidradenoma
     2. Basaloid cells with sieve-like tubules, some papilla, some ducts with papillary tufts, occasional cystic spaces, mitotic figures common, necrosis en masse common, occurs on digits
        a) Papillary digital adenocarcinoma
  D. Tubulopapillary structures in a complex lesion with multiple lines of differentiation
     1. Organoid nevus (nevus sebaceus)
VII. Lesions with clear cells
  A. Lobular
     1. Prominent clear cells with thick vitreous layer surrounding the lobule
        a) Tricholemmoma
     2. Slate-gray to pink uniform cells with ducts and hyalinized stroma
        a) Poroma group lesions
     3. With clear and basaloid cells, small lipid droplets in clear cells
        a) Uniform distribution of sebocytes
           (1) Sebaceous adenoma
        b) Heterogeneous distribution of sebocytes with minor to marked degrees of pleomorphism
           (1) Sebaceous carcinoma

  B. Islands
     1. Clear cells with ducts, cells usually monotonous and separate
        a) Cytologically uniform
           (1) Poroma (acrospiroma, hidradenoma) group
        b) Cytologically pleomorphic
           (1) Porocarcinoma
     2. Clear cells surrounded by vitreous layer with cytologic pleomorphism
        a) Tricholemmal carcinoma
  C. Trabecular
     1. Clear cells with ducts, cells usually monotonous and separate, with myxoid, chondroid, or adipose stroma
        a) Mixed tumor
VIII. Lesions with pagetoid cells
  A. Large mucin-filled cells in the epidermis, in pagetoid pattern, sometimes with epidermal gland acini
     1. Extramammary Paget's disease
  B. Large intraepidermal basaloid to clear cells with small spherical cytoplasmic vacuoles
     1. Sebaceous carcinoma, particularly of the eyelid
  C. Poroid cells often in clones within the epidermis
     1. Porocarcinoma, epidermotropic
  D. Small blue cells with lentiginous or pagetoid or nested patterns in the epidermis, positive for neuroendocrine markers
     1. Neuroendocrine carcinoma, epidermotropic
  E. Zones of clear and pink cells with pagetoid pattern but not glandular (similar to pagetoid Bowen's disease)
     1. Tricholemmal carcinoma (pseudopagetoid)
IX. Desmoplastic lesions
  A. Thin strands of basaloid cells, usually extending no deeper than mid-dermis, with rare hair germs, but no ducts
     1. Desmoplastic trichoepithelioma
  B. Complex pink cells in cords and trabeculae without cytologic pleomorphism, but with focal areas suggesting peripheral bulbous tricholemmoma pattern
     1. Desmoplastic tricholemmoma
  C. Superficial cysts containing pink material, compression into tubules and cords from superficial to deep, sometimes with follicular structures, often perineural invasion
     1. Microcystic adnexal carcinoma
  D. Small single infiltrating cells within the fibrotic dermis, signet ring cytology, often on the eyelid
     1. Signet ring cell carcinoma
X. Lesions with perineural invasion commonly
  A. Microcystic adnexal carcinoma
  B. Adenoid cystic carcinoma
  C. Signet ring cell carcinoma
  D. Porocarcinoma

19

MESENCHYMAL TUMORS OF THE SKIN

With a few selected exceptions, mesenchymal neoplasms of the skin are generally uncommon. This fact, together with the wide histologic variety that such lesions may exhibit, often makes their accurate diagnosis challenging for the dermatologist and dermatopathologist alike. This chapter outlines a practical approach to the recognition and proper categorization of cutaneous benign and malignant mesenchymal neoplasms and tumorlike conditions. Inasmuch as entire textbooks have been devoted to this topic, this is not purported to provide an exhaustive, all-encompassing treatise on such lesions. Rather, those clinical and pathologic features that allow for reliable classification and management of mesenchymal proliferations are stressed.

GENERAL CLINICAL FEATURES

The clinical characteristics of cutaneous mesenchymal neoplasms are rather nondescript in most instances. Such tumors may present as plaque-like or nodular lesions that are only uncommonly ulcerated and that have generally been present for months or years. Some—such as the common dermatofibroma—are superficial, circumscribed, firm, dermal lesions that are freely mobile on palpation. More deeply seated neoplasms are fixed to underlying structures and are more ill-defined on clinical examination.

The age of the patient is important in the formulation of a tenable clinical differential diagnosis in this context. Children under the age of 1 year virtually never develop sarcomas of the skin and superficial soft tissues. Likewise, malignant tumors of this type are uncommon in other pediatric patients as well.[1] By contrast, de novo mesenchymal neoplasms in elderly individuals are biologically aggressive in a sizable proportion of cases.

The color and consistency of tumors in this category may contribute to clinical interpretation. For example, vascular neoplasms are red or violaceous, whereas others of a myofibroblastic nature commonly have a pale, white-tan, translucent appearance. Lymphangiomas and lipomas are often fluctuant, while sarcomas of various types may be "woody" on palpation. Even though the "dimple sign" (downward retraction of a lesion induced by lateral compression) is equated by many clinicians with a diagnosis of dermatofibroma, this finding is nonspecific and is observed in association with any tumor that forms a connection between the dermis and superficial subcutis. Similarly, overlying hyperpigmentation of the epidermis is seen as a reaction to many slowly growing and localized mesenchymal tumors of the corium, both benign and malignant in nature.

Multiplicity of such neoplasms offers another clue to proper diagnosis in some instances. Von Recklinghausen's disease may feature the presence of multiple cutaneous lesions, and this potential is shared by tumors with myofibroblastic, smooth muscular, and endothelial differentiation.

Pain on palpation or after minor trauma is a characteristic that is peculiar to a relatively limited set of cutaneous mesenchymal tumors. These are included among the lesions represented by the acronym *ANGEL* (*a*ngiolipoma, post-traumatic *n*euroma, *g*lomus tumor, *e*ccrine spiradenoma, and *l*eiomyoma cutis).[2]

Finally, the topographic location of such proliferations is sometimes a helpful point of differential diagnosis. Sporadic angiosarcomas and atypical fibroxanthomas are largely confined to the skin of the face and scalp in elderly patients, whereas epithelioid sarcoma and clear cell sarcoma are found almost exclusively in the extremities of young adults.

CONDITIONS THAT PREDISPOSE TO CUTANEOUS MESENCHYMAL NEOPLASIA

Several heritable conditions may predispose individuals who have them to cutaneous mesenchymal neoplasia. These include von Recklinghausen's disease (neurofibromas, vascular proliferations, neurilemmomas, and striated muscle tumors); tuberous sclerosis (angiofibromas, lipomas, connective tissue hamartomas); the Klippel-Trenaunay-Weber, "blue rubber bleb," Sturge-Weber, and Maffuci syndromes (vascular neoplasms); Gardner syndrome (fibromatoses, lipomas); Bannayan syndrome (hemangiomas and lipomas); the basal cell nevus syndrome (fetal rhabdomyomas and rhabdomyosarcomas); and familial lipomatosis. All these afflictions are autosomal dominant traits.[1]

571

Occupational conditions also can play a role in the genesis of mesenchymal tumors or tumor-like conditions. Elastofibroma dorsi is seen in those who have done heavy manual labor, whereas post-traumatic neuromas, nodular fasciitis, and palmar fibromatosis have been observed in workers handling high-vibration pneumatic devices. In addition, exposure to megavoltage irradiation—occupational or otherwise—is linked to the potential development of malignant fibrous histiocytoma, nerve sheath sarcoma, and angiosarcoma in the affected field of skin and soft tissue.[3–5]

Lastly, over the past decade the association between a particular infectious agent—the human immunodeficiency virus (HIV)—and mesenchymal neoplasia of the skin has been appreciated. The relationship between HIV infection, the resulting acquired immunodeficiency syndrome (AIDS), and the development of mucocutaneous Kaposi's sarcoma[6] is now all too familiar to physicians everywhere.

INTRODUCTION TO SPECIAL TECHNIQUES IN THE PATHOLOGIC ANALYSIS OF CUTANEOUS MESENCHYMAL TUMORS

As mentioned at several points in the ensuing discussion, mesenchymal neoplasms of the skin and other organ systems have a perplexing ability to simulate one another on conventional histologic studies. For that reason, it is not uncommon to employ specialized modalities of analysis to resolve differential diagnostic uncertainties. Those that are most often used are electron microscopy and immunohistology.

Basic Ultrastructural Features of Mesenchymal Proliferations

The electron microscope still plays a definite role in the above-cited context. It is now well recognized that well-formed intercellular junctional complexes and specialized aggregates of cytoplasmic filaments (tonofibrils) indicate the presence of epithelial differentiation at an ultrastructural level. Similarly, the presence of plasmalemmal dense plaques, bundles of thin cytoplasmic filaments and associated dense bodies, and cellular pinocytotic activity are typical of smooth muscle or myofibroblastic proliferations.[7]

Schwann cell tumors manifest long, overlapping cytoplasmic processes and pericellular basal lamina. By contrast, "fibrohistiocytic" neoplasms, which may mimic schwannian lesions on conventional microscopy, lack such characteristics and instead are composed of fibroblast-like cells with abundant rough endoplasmic reticulum, intracytoplasmic collagen fibers, and irregular plasmalemmal contours.[8] Endothelial tumors exhibit primitive intercellular junctional complexes *together* with pinocytosis and pericellular basal lamina, and a unique cytoplasmic organelle—the Weibel-Palade body—is observed in a proportion of these lesions[9,10] (Table 19-1).

Immunohistologic Studies in Mesenchymal Neoplasia

Paraffin section immunohistochemistry also represents a useful tool in the distinction between mesenchymal proliferations. The detection of keratin proteins with this technique can be equated with the presence of epithelial differentiation in like manner to the observation of cell membrane–based immunoreactivity for epithelial membrane antigen. Muscle-specific actin, desmin, and smooth muscle actin are expected in myogenous lesions. S-100 protein, the CD57 antigen, and myelin basic protein may be expressed by schwannian neoplasms, although a final interpretation of the significance of these markers is dependent on the histologic context and an *absence* of the other antigens mentioned thus far.[8] The latter caveats also apply to "endothelial" determinants, which potentially include von Willebrand factor, receptors for *Ulex europaeus* I agglutinin, and the CD31 and CD34 antigens.[11,12]

"Neuroectodermal" lineage markers are represented by neuron-specific (γ dimer) enolase, CD57, and synaptophysin, as interpreted in the context of a small round cell proliferation. Only the last of these three indicators is truly specific for neuroectodermal differentiation, but the others serve a useful screening role or contribute to ultimate diagnosis in combination with other determinants.[8]

Vimentin is ubiquitous among mesenchymal proliferations of all types, because it represents the "primordial" intermediate filament class of such lesions. Nevertheless, this marker is indeed useful as a sort of "internal control" for tissue antigenicity in general.[13] Also, if it represents the *only* determinant seen in a mesenchymal proliferation, a diagnosis of fibroblastic or "fibrohistiocytic" neoplasia is indicated.[14] With these points of submicroscopic information in mind, a directed discussion of such lesions is undertaken in the remainder of this chapter.

Biologically benign and "borderline" cutaneous mesenchymal neoplasms are sufficiently distinctive on clinicopathologic grounds that they can be considered individually as distinctive entities. However, overtly malignant tumors in this category have a propensity to demonstrate overlapping microscopic features. Therefore, they are grouped together in four generic categories: small round cell tumors, spindle cell neoplasms, epithelioid lesions, and pleomorphic tumors.

SPECIFIC CLINICOPATHOLOGIC FEATURES

Benign Neoplasms

Fibroblastic Lesions—"Fibrous Papule"/ Angiofibroma (Adenoma Sebaceum of Pringle)

Clinical Features

Fibrous papules are common lesions that occur in the midfacial skin of adults, most of whom are white. These tumors are small, firm, tan or light brown papules that are largely cosmetic nuisances.[15] These are identical tumors of tuberous sclerosis (an autosomal dominant phakomatosis characterized by cortical glial nodules, dermal connective tissue and cardiac rhabdomyomas, and subependymal giant cell hamartomas). The pearly penile papule and acquired digital fibrokeratoma are identical. Simple excision is curative.

Histopathologic Features

Whether fibrous papules are truly neoplastic is an unresolved question at present and has remained so since the original description of these lesions.[16] They are characterized by a local-

Table 19-1. Selected Electron Microscopic Features of Value in Pathologic Diagnosis of Cutaneous Neoplasms

Finding	Predominant Distribution	Diagnostic Use
Intercellular junctions	Epithelial cells; selected mesenchymal nonlymphoid tumors	Distinction between lymphoma and carcinoma
External basal lamina (pericellular)	Epithelial cells; selected mesenchymal (neural and myogenous) neoplasms	Distinction between lymphoma and carcinoma; aids recognition of some soft tissue tumors
Intra- or intercellular lumina	Glandular epithelia	Recognition of adenocarcinomas
Microvillous core rootlets	Glandular epithelia of alimentary tract	Recognition of some metastatic adenocarcinomas
Cytoplasmic tonofibrils	Squamous epithelia	Recognition of squamous cell carcinoma
Premelanosomes	Melanocytic cells	Recognition of melanomas
Neurosecretory granules	Neuroendocrine cells	Recognition of neuroendocrine carcinomas
Thick and thin filament complexes	Striated muscle cells	Recognition of rhabdomyoma and rhabdomyosarcoma
Attenuated cytoplasmic processes	Schwannian and neural cells	Recognition of peripheral nerve sheath tumors
Thin filament-dense body complexes	Smooth muscle cells	Recognition of smooth muscle tumors
Birbeck granules	Langerhans cells	Recognition of Langerhans cell proliferations
Cytoplasmic mucin	Secretory glandular epithelia	Recognition of adenocarcinomas

ized proliferation of bland fusiform fibroblasts in the reticular and papillary dermis, forming concentric densities around vessels but also hair follicles.[17] This feature accounts for one of the synonyms for fibrous papule, namely, *perifollicular fibroma*.[18] Stellate cells, which often contain melanin pigment, are also interspersed throughout these proliferations; the surrounding skin demonstrates a proliferation of telangiectatic capillaries and venules and may contain melanophages as well (Fig. 19-1). Guitart et al[19] have reported two examples in which small foci of epithelioid granular cells were apparent.

Some authors believe that a fibrous papule is merely a form of regressed intradermal nevus.[20] Based on results of immunostaining for factor XIIIa (a putative marker for "dermal dendrocytes") in fibrous papules, others have advanced the premise that they represent unique dermal mesenchymal neoplasms.[21]

Myofibroblastic Proliferations

Clinical Features

Myofibroblastic neoplasms of the skin may be solitary or multifocal and are classically placed into one of several discrete clinicopathologic categories (Table 19-1).

Infantile (congenital) myofibromatosis is a condition affecting newborn children and those under 1 year of age. They present with firm, tan-pink nodular lesions of the dermis and superficial subcutis, with no particular topographic predilection. The lesions are often multiple and may be associated with similar proliferations in the viscera and bones.[22–25] If the latter are present (disseminated myofibromatosis), the prognosis is guarded because multiorgan failure may supervene as a result of the growing tumefactions.[22] By contrast, restricted cutaneous infantile myofibromatosis is a relatively innocuous condition.

Acquired digital myofibromatosis (fibrous tumor of the digits) is observed in children, adolescents, and young adults. It affects the distal phalanges of the fingers and toes (sparing the thumbs and great toes), often has a periungual location, and is represented by solitary or multiple translucent white-pink nodules that are centered in the dermis.[26] Although such lesions may recur following conservative excision, they are entirely benign.[27,28]

Calcifying aponeurotic fibroma is another myofibroblastic proliferation that tends to localize to the distal extremities. A firm, painless, multinodular or plaque-like mass is observed in the palms or soles, most often in patients under 30 years of age. However, some cases have been observed in elderly individuals as well. Simple excision is curative.[29,30]

Hyaline fibromatosis primarily affects children, who have masses in the scalp and the mucosal surfaces. It is often observed as firm tan-pink plaques in the gingiva and may have a familial distribution.[31,32] Multifocality of the lesions is common, and therefore surgical removal may be followed by development of new masses in contiguous sites.[31]

Desmoid-type (aggressive) fibromatosis (DTF) typically involves the skin only secondarily because it is centered in the aponeuroses of deep muscle groups.[33] This lesion develops during pregnancy or the immediate postpartum period in some women, where it characteristically arises in the abdominal wall. Extra-abdominal examples of DTF can be seen in patients of all ages[34] and both sexes, with a predilection for the extremities.[33] The condition is typified by firm, ill-defined, slowly growing nodular masses that may be multifocal and slightly painful on palpation.[35] The lesion can attain a maximum size of several centimeters and has a stubborn tendency to recur after surgical removal. Rare cases are fatal because of their location in a vital

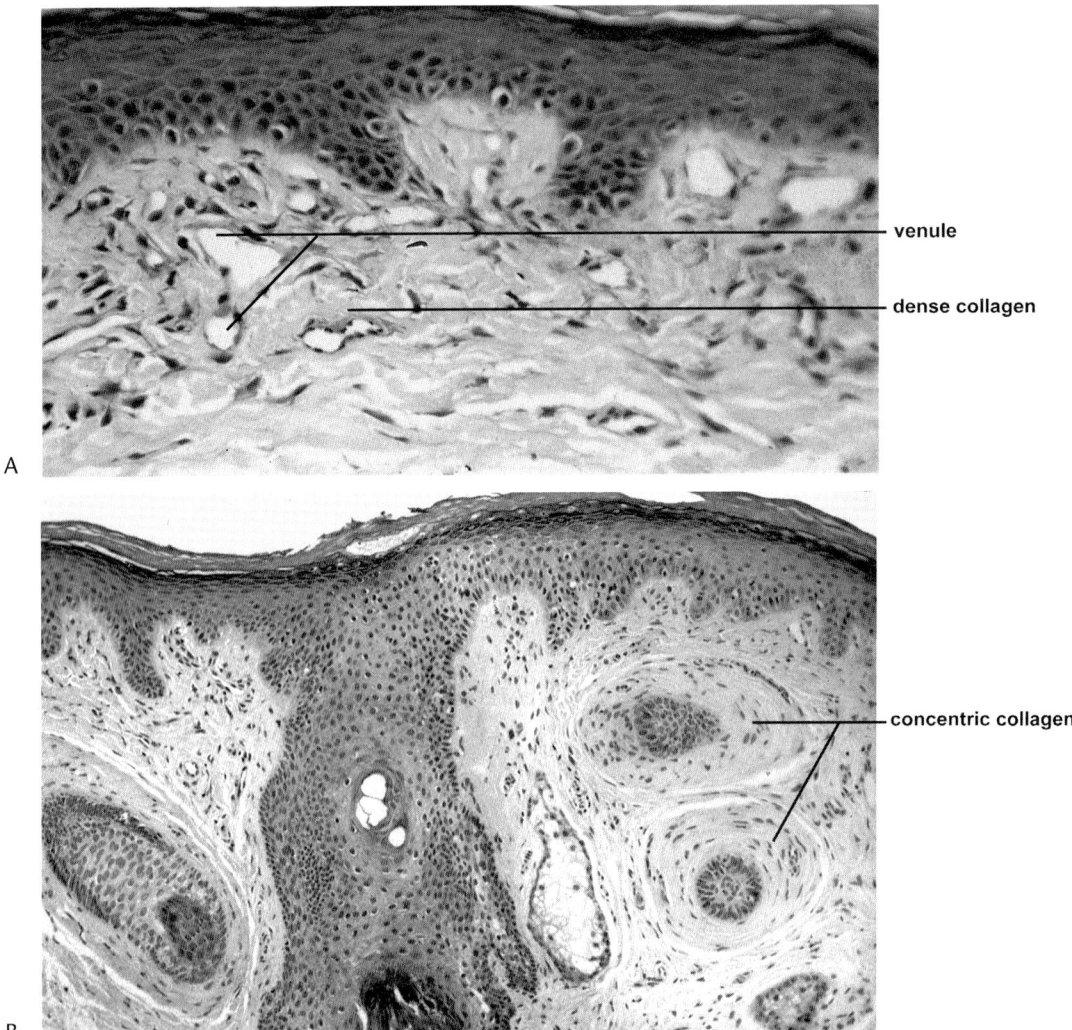

A

venule

dense collagen

B

concentric collagen

Figure 19-1. **(A)** Characteristic features of a fibrous papule. The fibrous papule displays dense dermal collagen encircling small venules of the papillary and superficial reticular dermis. Dermal dendrocytes are characteristically enlarged and reactive. **(B)** Perifollicular fibroma, another form of fibrous papule or angiofibroma. There are concentric rings of dermal collagen surrounding small pilar units.

but relatively inaccessible body site, with recalcitrant local growth.[33,36]

Solitary adult myofibromatosis is virtually identical to the infantile form of this disorder, except that it appears in postpubertal patients.[37,38] Conservative surgical removal constitutes sufficient treatment, with only rare examples of recurrence.[39] Kamino et al[40] recently reported a lesion dubbed "dermatomyofibroma," which has many clinical similarities to solitary myofibromatosis. However, it shows a striking tendency to arise only in the proximal extremities and is more plaque-like macroscopically.

Palmar-plantar fibromatosis is a common disorder that may follow trauma to the hands or feet. It takes the form of multinodular firm masses that are centered in the palmar or plantar fasciae[41,42]; patients with a long history of lesional growth may develop local contractures. Excision is curative.

Histopathologic Features

With minor alterations, the microscopic appearance of the fibromatoses is a consistent one. It features the presence of interweaving fascicles of cytologically bland spindle cells with slightly fibrillar cytoplasm set in a collagenous matrix and punctuated by a distinctive vascular network. The latter is composed of venule-sized blood vessels with thick pericytic cuffs (Fig. 19-2). Even though the stroma of the fibromatoses is often sclerotic, the lesional vascular lumina are typically open and slightly branched.[22–25,34,37–39]

The latter characteristics may lead to confusion with hemangiopericytomas (see below), particularly in infantile myofibromatosis cases.[43] Reported examples of "congenital hemangiopericytoma"[44] actually represented myofibroblastic proliferations.

Myxoid change also is frequent in the matrix around intrale-

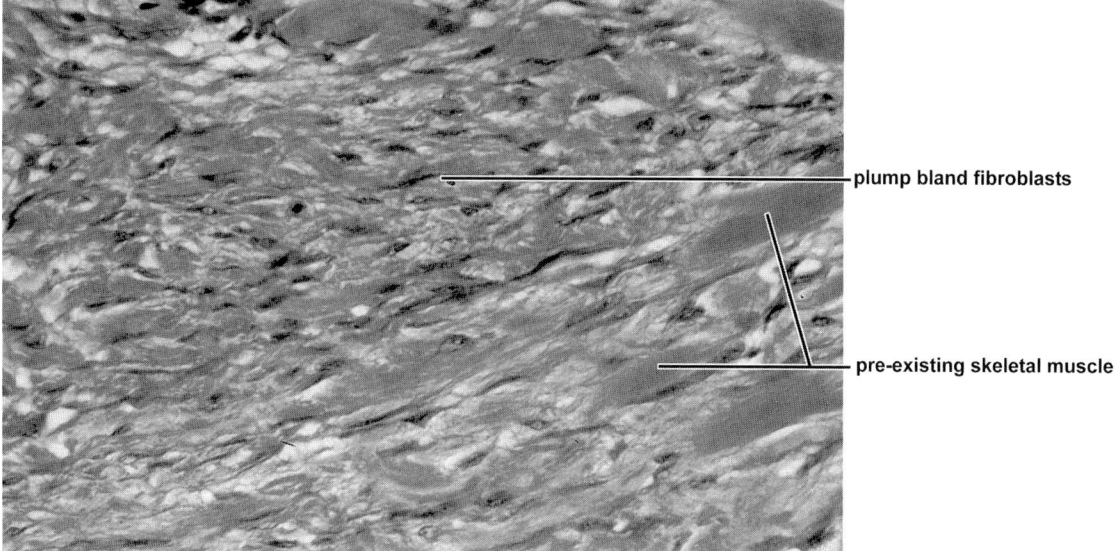

plump bland fibroblasts

pre-existing skeletal muscle

Figure 19-2. Characteristic features of an aggressive fibromatosis. Plump, small basophilic fibroblasts are seen infiltrating between skeletal muscle. Mitoses are rare. Fibromatoses enlarge and infiltrate until it seems that they reach a predetermined size or time. At that point, they mature into dense collagen. Fatalities result when they impinge on vital organs.

sional vessels, and these areas typically contain cells that are more stellate than fusiform.[45] Cellularity is variable in the myofibromatoses; hypodense zones with abundant collagenous or myxoid stroma are admixed with others that manifest closely apposed spindle cells and that may assume rounded contours.[22,37] Peripheral interfaces between these tumors and surrounding tissues are indistinct, and the lesions typically blend imperceptibly with the surrounding dermis or deeper soft tissue.[34]

Mitotic activity in the myofibromatoses is characteristically limited, and observation of more than 1 to 2 mitoses per 10 high power ($\times$ 40) microscopic fields should therefore lead one to consider an alternative diagnosis. An exception to this general rule is seen in palmar-plantar fibromatosis (Fig. 19-3), where division figures may occasionally be numerous. However, they should never assume pathologic shapes.

Specific histologic findings typify several members of this lesional category. Calcified aponeurotic fibromas are, as their name would suggest, partially calcified; the presence of focal chondroid-type matrical differentiation may be seen as well.[29,30] Hyaline fibromatosis manifests cytoplasmic lucency in proliferating myofibroblasts and zones of extreme paucicellularity, where the stroma takes on a "glassy," eosinophilic, hyaline character.[32] Acquired digital fibromatosis shows distinctive, intracytoplasmic, eosinophilic globular inclusions in the proliferating cells[26–28,46]; these have been shown to contain an actin isoform that may be unique to such lesions.[47] A peculiarity of palmar-plantar fibromatosis is its tendency toward dense cellularity in "early" lesions, together with the aforementioned capacity for brisk mitotic activity (Fig. 19-3). These findings may tempt one to make a diagnosis of sarcoma instead of fibromatosis, but this decision should be avoided at all costs if the clinical presentation is typical of the latter condition.

Fibrous Hamartoma of Infancy

Clinical Features

Fibrous hamartoma of infancy is a tan-pink, firm, nodular or plaque-like lesion that most often arises on the trunk or upper extremities in male children under 3 years of age.

Histopathologic Features

An admixture (usually triphasic) of cytologically banal fibroblastic groupings, mature lobules of adipose tissue, and zones of myxoid stroma is seen in fibrous hamartomas (Fig. 19-4). Lesional stroma may be very sclerotic, and limited mitotic activity may be observed in the constituent spindle cells.[48] The circumscription of this lesion is distinct and attests to its clinical benignity.

Leiomyomas and Angioleiomyomas

Clinical Features

Benign smooth muscle tumors of the skin may be centered in the dermis or subcutis, and they present as slowly growing and relatively nondescript tan-pink nodular lesions that may be familial in certain cases.[49–51] Some examples are painful when spontaneously traumatized or palpated, and regional multifocality is not uncommonly observed.[49,50,52] Leiomyomas of the corium are thought to be related to the arrector pili muscles ("piloleiomyomas"), whereas deeper tumors have a putative association with the muscular walls of blood vessels.[49] Special variants of leiomyomas also may be found in the mammary or genital skin, where they are presumably related to the periareolar or dartos muscles.[49]

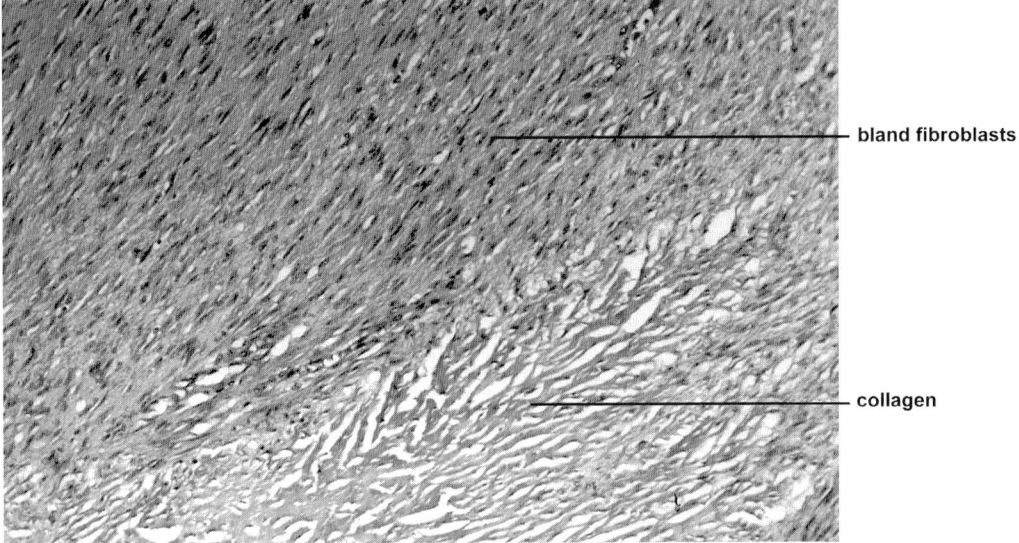

Figure 19-3. Palmar fibromatosis with basophilic proliferating fibroblasts in the upper portion of the field. The lower portion of the field shows maturation, where the process has become collagenized.

Histopathologic Features

Leiomyomas show a fascicular growth pattern, with interweaving bundles of spindle cells disposed in variable orientations to one another[53] (Fig. 19-5). When cut in cross section, many of the tumor cells demonstrate a perinuclear clear zone in the cytoplasm; this is probably an artifact of formalin fixation, but is reproducible and diagnostically helpful. Nuclei are typically described as blunt ended and "cigar shaped," with evenly dispersed chromatin and indistinct nucleoli. The cytoplasm is faintly eosinophilic and fibrillar; these attributes may be highlighted with the Masson trichrome stain, which imparts a red color to the myogenous filaments. Mitotic activity in leiomyomas should, by definition, be negligible. The observation of even a few division figures in smooth muscle tumors of the skin usually signifies a more aggressive biologic potential and equates with a diagnosis of leiomyosarcoma.[54] Leiomyomas of the skin are sharply marginated but unencapsulated; they tend to displace cutaneous adnexae rather than entrapping them.

Rare examples of cutaneous leiomyoma may be composed pre-

Figure 19-4. Fibrous hamartoma of infancy characterized by a triad mixture of myxoid tissue, adipose tissue, and intersecting trabeculae of dense fibrous tissue. All three are arranged in an organoid pattern. The entire mass forms a distinct tumor in the dermis or subcutis.

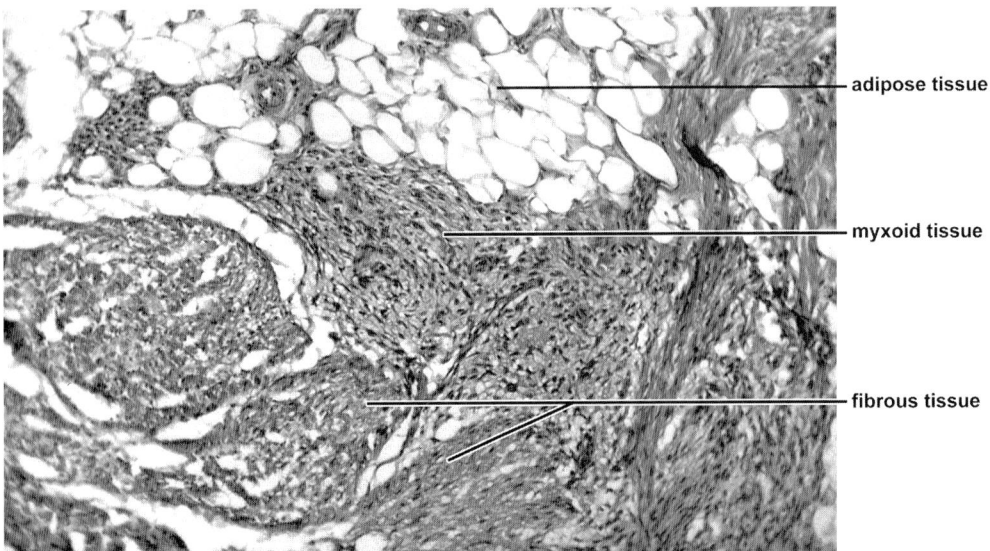

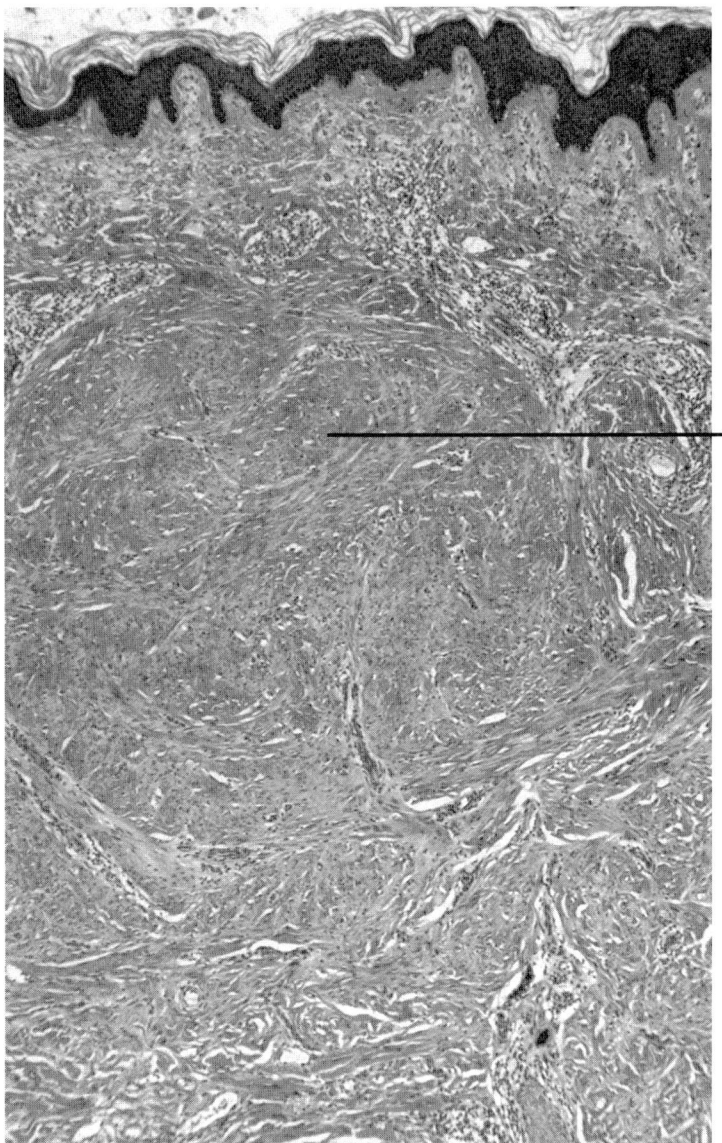
smooth muscle bundles

Figure 19-5. Leiomyoma of the skin, which often arises from arrector pili muscles. In this example, there is a distinct mass of eosinophilic smooth muscle occupying most of the reticular dermis. These lesions may be painful. In this example, there is a thin grenz zone between the tumor and the atrophic epidermis.

dominantly of epithelioid polyhedral cells rather than fusiform elements. These are potentially troublesome diagnostically unless one finds small foci of typically fascicular spindle cell growth somewhere in the mass. Serial sections may be necessary to detect such areas.

The microscopic attributes of angioleiomyomas differ from those of archetypical leiomyoma cutis, but only because the former lesions feature prominent and numerous venule-sized or capillary-like blood vessels that are admixed with the fascicular bundles of tumor cells.[55–57] Occasionally, branched vascular lumina with a "staghorn" appearance may cause one to consider a diagnosis of hemangiopericytoma.[57] Three phenomena that mimic cutaneous leiomyoma variants are Becker's nevus/ smooth muscle hamartoma and acral arteriovenous tumor

(AAVT). The first of these differential diagnostic alternatives differs from leiomyoma in that it is typically congenital and often shows overlying epidermal hyperpigmentation and dystrichosis.[58,59] AAVTs show a striking similarity to arteriovenous malformations and a passing likeness to angioleiomyomas.[60] However, AAVTs are infiltrative lesions that entrap dermal adnexal structures.[61,62] Large, distorted, interconnecting veins and arteries with thick muscular walls are observed in AAVT; nonetheless, unlike true vascular malformations, the vessels do not contain lamellae of elastic fibers.[62] Likewise, angioleiomyomas differ from AAVTs in the relative size and prominence of constituent vasculature[57]; moreover, the latter lesion does not show solid fascicular aggregates of fusiform cells.

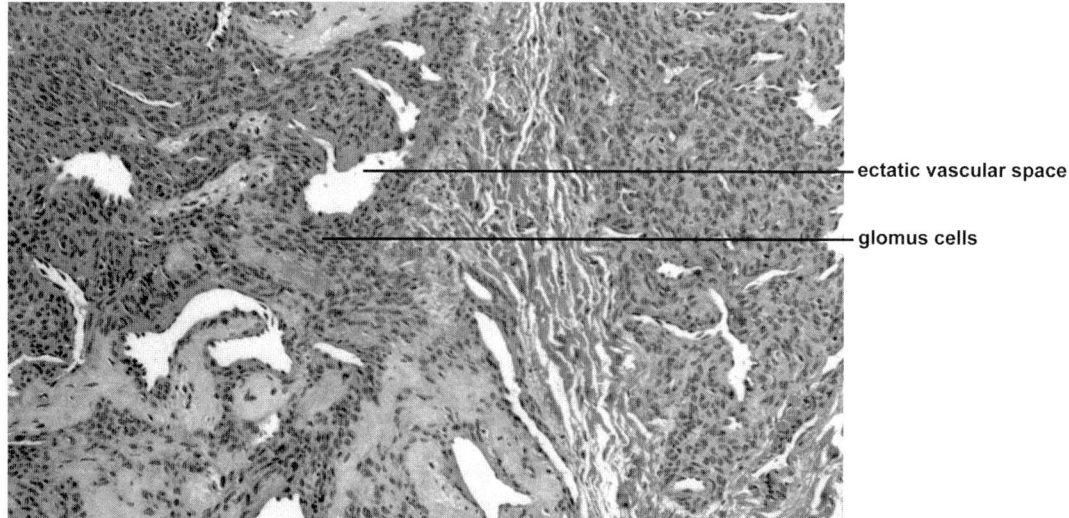

ectatic vascular space

glomus cells

Figure 19-6. Glomus tumor displaying dilated vascular spaces in association with sheets and aggregates of small, rounded cells. The cells are in intimate contact with the dilated vascular channels. Tumors with varying proportions of components are known as *glomus tumors, glomangioma,* and *glomangiomyoma.* The glomangiomyoma also includes a smooth muscle component.

Hemangiopericytoma

We do not recognize the existence of a totally benign variant of hemangiopericytoma, in the skin or elsewhere. Accordingly, this tumor type is considered elsewhere in this chapter.

Glomus Tumors

Clinical Features

Glomus tumors typically have an acral distribution, and they are papulonodular lesions that may be tan-pink, red, or blue. These neoplasms are often extremely painful with even slight compression and can occur in both children and adults.[63] They may be multifocal and inherited as an autosomal dominant condition.[64]

Histopathologic Features

Circumscribed sheets and rounded nests of small ovoid or polyhedral cells with bland oval nuclei and a moderate amount of amphophilic cytoplasm are typical of the glomus tumor. It may be located in the dermis or subcutis[63] (Fig. 19-6). The cells of glomus tumors may be arranged focally in cords or festoons, and they also may enclose vascular "lakes" of variable size.[65] When the latter formations are prominent, the term *glomangioma* is used. Mitotic activity is variable in glomus tumors, but it has little significance when present. Necrosis and nuclear pleomorphism are absent.

There is a passing similarity between glomus tumor and deep hemangiopericytoma on cytologic grounds, but the distinctively branching stromal vessels of the latter neoplasm[66] are not observed in the former lesion. Other, more pertinent differential diagnostic considerations include angiomatoid intradermal nevus and solid eccrine hidradenoma (acrospiroma) or spirade-

noma.[65] Careful attention to microscopic nuances usually allows them to be distinguished from glomus tumor or glomangioma. Interpretative difficulties may also be resolved with the use of immunostains for S-100 protein, keratin, and muscle-specific actin, only the last of which is seen in glomus tumors.[14,65]

Rhabdomyomas and Rhabdomyomatous Mesenchymal Hamartomas

Clinical Features

Rhabdomyomas are benign proliferations of striated muscle cells that may be seen in patients of all ages, although children are typically favored. Three types are recognized, known as the "adult," "fetal," and "juvenile" forms.[67–70] The first of these does not occur in the skin, but rather is confined to mucosal surfaces.[68–71] Fetal rhabdomyomas show a propensity to affect the superficial soft tissues of the proximal trunk, particularly at the base of the neck.[69] The juvenile variant has most often been observed on the extremities.[70] All of these lesions are tan-brown, firm, smooth nodules. They are cured by conservative excision.

Rhabdomyomatous mesenchymal hamartomas are polypoid lesions that appear to be confined to the facial skin of infants. Only a few examples have been reported, as pedunculated, soft, skin-colored excrescences.[72–74] As their name implies, such proliferations are thought to be malformative rather than neoplastic.

Histopathologic Features

Rhabdomyomas, in each of their variant forms, are characterized by a proliferation of large, plump, eosinophilic cells that demonstrate the cytoplasmic cross-striations typical of striated muscle. These comprise the entire neoplastic population in "adult" rhabdomyoma[67,68] (Fig. 19-7), whereas the "fetal" subtype also contains more nondescript spindle cells and compact hyperchromatic round cells in admixture.[69] Juvenile rhabdomy-

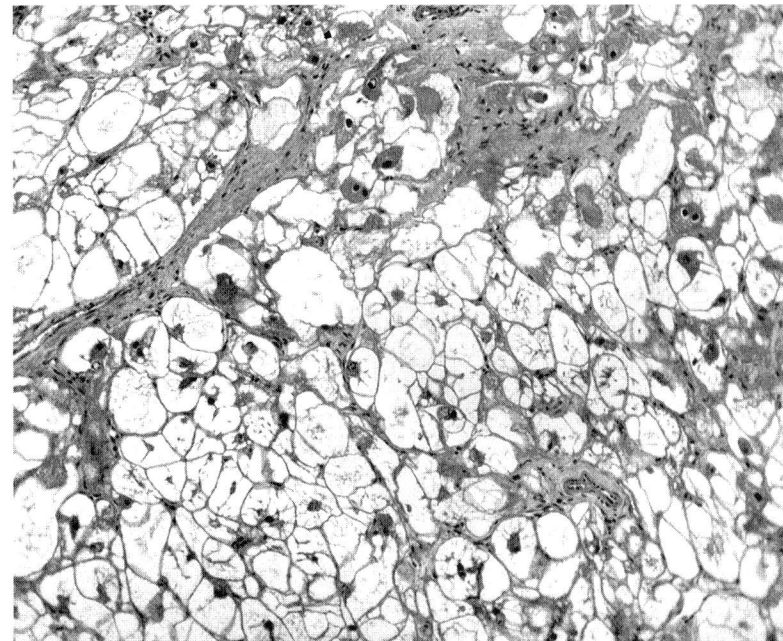

Figure 19-7. Adult form of rhabdomyoma. The tumor is characterized by polygonal cells having a pronounced vacuolated appearance, secondary to accumulation of glycogen. Characteristically, variable quantities of cytoplasm remain in the central portion of the cell. The fetal rhabdomyoma, not illustrated, has a more spindled appearance.

oma has a distinctly fascicular growth pattern and is likewise composed of overtly striated muscle cells and fusiform cells with serpiginous contours.[70] The nuclei of all cellular variants are hyperchromatic and bland, with no mitotic activity or significant pleomorphism. Unlike *malignant* striated muscle tumors, rhabdomyomas are typically well-circumscribed and may be surrounded by a fibrous pseudocapsule.

Rhabdomyomatous mesenchymal hamartoma demonstrates the haphazard interposition of variably sized fascicles or single fibers of mature striated muscle in the dermis and superficial subcutis.[72–74] The muscular bands mold themselves to cuta-

neous adnexae and may be associated with neural branches. A polypoid configuration is reproducible in these cases (Fig. 19-8).

The bases of the excrescences are narrower than their distal aspects, yielding a club-shaped image.

Benign Vascular (Endothelial) Neoplasms
Clinical Features

There are basically only two types of benign cutaneous vascular neoplasms—lymphangiomas and hemangiomas. The former have two potential clinical presentations. *Superficial circum-*

Figure 19-8. Unusual cutaneous hamartoma containing mature striated muscle.

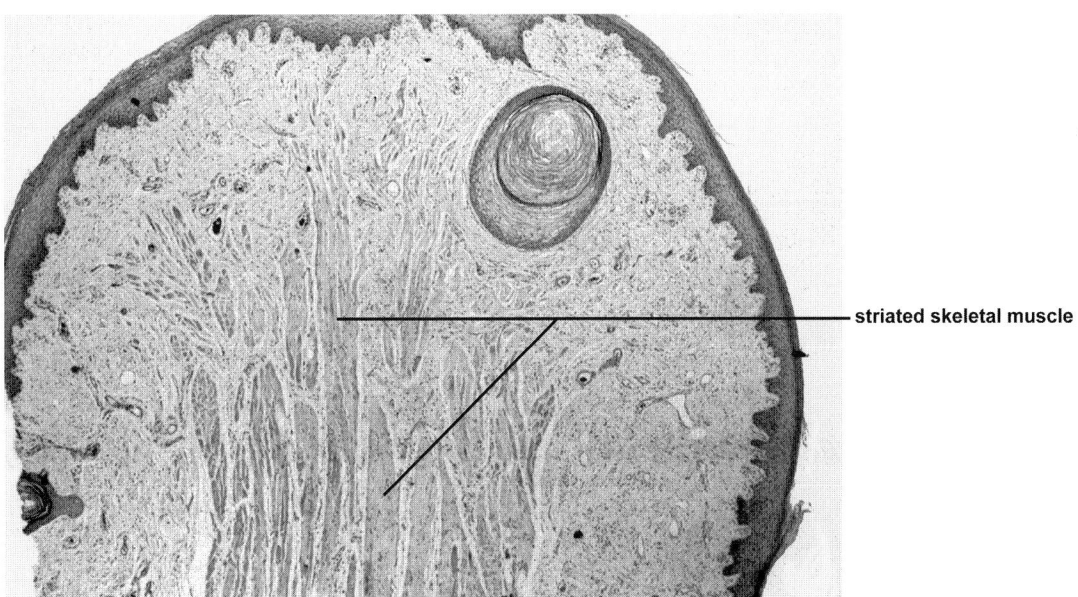

striated skeletal muscle

scribed lymphangiomas usually arise early in life, as multifocal papules or verrucoid lesions. *Deep lymphangiomas* may be seen at any age and take the form of large, ill-defined, fluctuant nodules or plaques. Both variants tend to affect the head and neck and the skin of the axillae, but other topographic sites may be involved as well.[75–78]

Hemangiomas may be observed throughout life and assume relatively uniform macroscopic characteristics.[79–81] They are blue-red, nonulcerated, relatively well-circumscribed, variably fluctuant masses that may be macular, plaque-like, or protuberant in nature and commonly blanch when manually compressed by the examiner. The sizes of hemangiomas vary considerably, from 1 to 2 mm to more than 20 cm in greatest dimension. Large areas of the skin surface may be affected by lesions that are part of the Sturge-Weber syndrome, and these also tend to be confined to one side of the body. Hemangiomas are commonly congenital proliferations, and, if so, they usually regress spontaneously with maturation of the host.[79,81] Patients with *Kimura's disease* (tentatively included as a form of cutaneous hemangioma) often have multifocal nodular and -violaceous lesions of the skin, peripheral eosinophilia, and enlargement of those lymph nodes draining the affected cutaneous area.[82] Another distinctive subtype, "*targetoid hemosiderotic*" *hemangioma*, is named for its characteristic clinical appearance, simulating that of an archery target at some stage of lesional evolution.[83]

Despite the fact that all cutaneous hemangiomas are benign, some variants—such as lobular capillary hemangioma and infiltrating hemangioma—may be floridly multifocal and difficult to approach surgically.[84] Recurrence of such lesions therefore does *not* necessarily indicate progression to a biologically aggressive neoplasm.

Histopathologic Features

Superficial circumscribed lymphangiomas are typified by a proliferation of small, thin-walled vessels in the superficial papillary dermis, lined by attenuated endothelial cells (Fig. 19-9). They have no discernible pericytic cuff and are filled with slightly eosinophilic luminal material. The overlying epidermis commonly forms "collarettes" around the lymphatic vascular channels, and acanthosis or hyperkeratosis also may be apparent. Accompanying inflammation in the surrounding corium is scant or absent.[78,85]

Deep lymphangiomas are composed of larger vascular spaces that are centered in the deep reticular dermis and subcutis, with no epidermal reaction to them. Luminal proteinaceous lymphatic fluid is abundant, and it characteristically assumes a "scalloped" appearance. Lesional endothelial cells are again flattened and inconspicuous.[75–77] Surrounding connective tissue is usually sclerotic; numerous lymphoid cells may be admixed with the lymphatic channels and are often present within them as well. Erythrocytes are scarce in both forms of cutaneous lymphangioma.

In the past few years, several microscopic variants of hemangioma of the skin have been recognized. These include the well-known capillary and cavernous subtypes—composed of small-bore and large ectatic vascular spaces, respectively—as well as

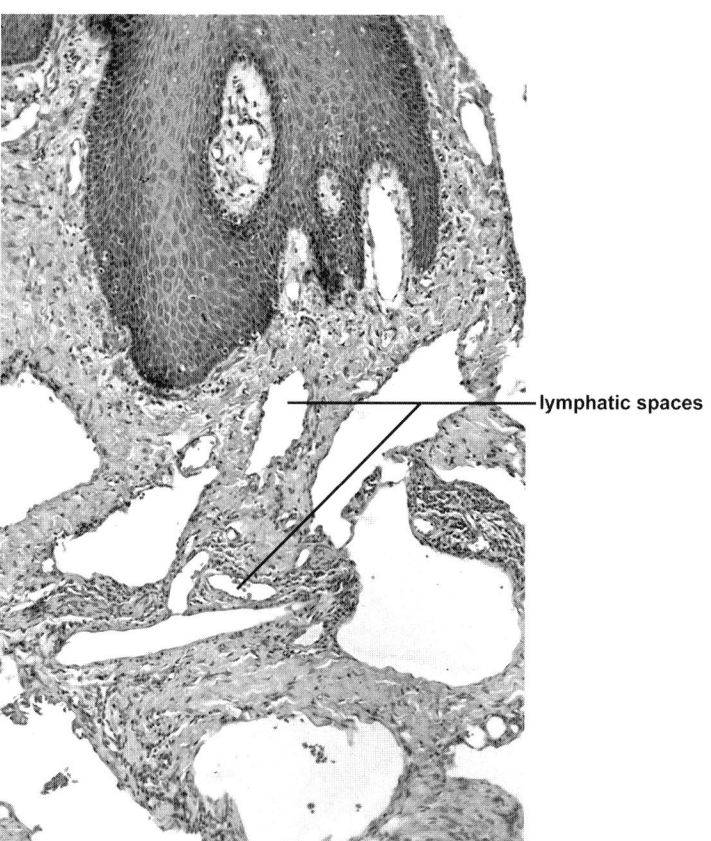

lymphatic spaces

Figure 19-9. The superficial lymphangiomyoma consists of multiple complex dilated vascular channels that often abut the superficial epidermis. In this example, there are numerous dilated vascular channels that do not contain blood. Vascular spaces containing blood would naturally be in the hemangioma category.

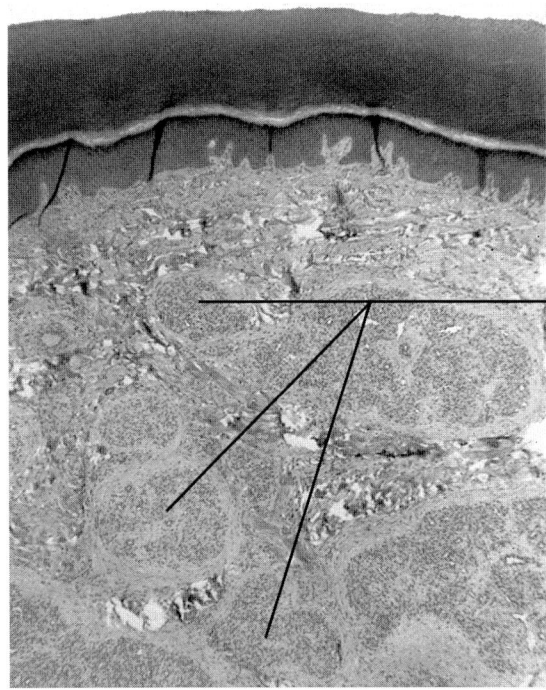

lobular groups
of capillaries

Figure 19-10. The characteristic feature of many hemangiomas such as this lobular capillary hemangioma is the presence of small capillary-sized vessels arranged in groups or lobules. Variable amounts of connective tissue separate the lobules. When these lesions form an exophytic mass with an ulcerated epidermal surface, the term used is *pyogenic granuloma*.

mixed capillary-cavernous/venous hemangiomas,[79] lobular capillary hemangiomas ("pyogenic granulomas"),[86] "cellular" capillary hemangiomas,[86] acquired tufted hemangiomas,[87] glomeruloid hemangiomas,[88] verrucous hemangiomas,[89] infiltrating hemangiomas,[90] targetoid hemangiomas,[83,91] epithelioid ("histiocytoid") hemangiomas,[92,93] and Kimura's tumor/disease.[82,93]

The basic structure of all of these proliferations is that of *organized formation of complete intercellular lumina*, mantled by pericytic cuffs of variable thickness and lined by bland endothelial cells with a spectrum of appearances.[94] Another feature common to all the hemangiomas (possibly excepting "infiltrating" and "targetoid" lesions) is a *lobular* configuration.[86,94] Discrete groups of lesional blood vessels and investing pericytes are separated from one another by fibrous stroma, and they contain a central "feeder" vessel in each lobule.[85] Indeed, the *lobular capillary hemangioma* is the prototypical example of this morphologic arrangement (Fig. 19-10). Although the latter tumor is most commonly superficial and polypoid, often with overlying ulceration, it also may be seen deep in the dermis or subcutis.[95] Lobular capillary hemangiomas that are traumatized may show regenerative nuclear atypia and mitotic activity in constituent endothelial cells.[85] Noticing that the lobular character of the tumor is retained in these circumstances should help to avoid erroneous interpretations.

"Cellular" capillary hemangioma is simply regarded as a variant form of lobular capillary hemangioma in which the boundaries between adjacent lobules are indistinct, and the lumina formed by constituent endothelial cells are extremely small. This lesion is synonymous with the "angioblastoma" of Nakagawa.[96] Another alternative designation, that of "juvenile hemangioendothelioma," is unacceptable for diagnostic use, because hemangioendotheliomas in general are regarded as potentially malignant neoplasms.

Verrucous hemangioma is a variant of cavernous hemangioma that is typified by overlying epidermal papillomatosis, parakeratosis, and hyperkeratosis.[89] Keratinocytic rete ridges extend downward in this tumor to "embrace" or surround lesional blood vessels, much in the same manner as that observed in angiokeratoma (see below).

Acquired tufted hemangioma is another subtype of lobular capillary hemangioma in which the lobules of tumor cells project into ectatic but pre-existing dermal veins and lymphatics.[87,97] This arrangement yields a low-power appearance that has been likened to "cannon balls in the dermis" by Wilson-Jones and Orkin[97] (Fig. 19-11). In light of this description, it is likely that some examples of "intravenous pyogenic granuloma" described by Cooper et al[98] would currently be regarded as acquired tufted hemangiomas.

Glomeruloid hemangioma is a newly described variant in which proliferating vascular channels take on the size of dermal venules and are grouped together in discrete clusters such that they passingly resemble glomeruli of the kidney on low-power microscopy.[99] They are associated with the *POEMS* syndrome, a constellation of disorders (*p*olyneuropathy, *o*rganomegaly, *e*ndocrinopathies, *m*onoclonal gammopathies, and *s*kin lesions) that is usually linked to an underlying lymphoproliferative disease or plasma cell dyscrasia.[88,99]

Infiltrating hemangioma is again composed of venule-sized channels, but this lesion differs from the others described thus far because it shows no circumscription. A disorganized proliferation of randomly arranged (but complete) luminal profiles is seen throughout the dermis and subcutis, and it may involve underlying fascia, muscle, viscera, and bones, justifying diagnostic use of the term *angiomatosis*.[90]

The *targetoid hemosiderotic hemangioma*, as well as another closely allied variant, *microvenular hemangioma*, are probably related to the infiltrating variant just cited.[83,91,100] Nonetheless,

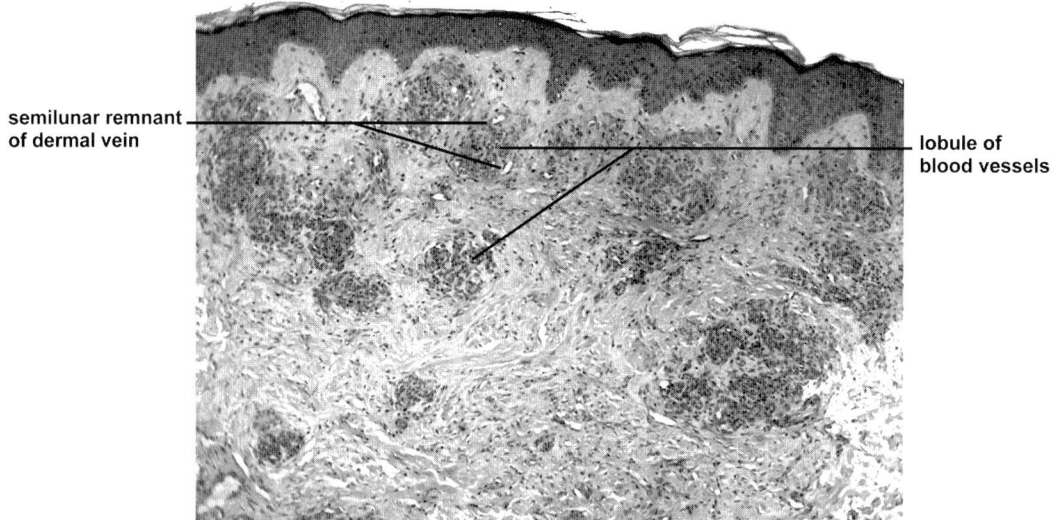

semilunar remnant of dermal vein

lobule of blood vessels

Figure 19-11. The tufted angioma has the histologic appearance of cannon balls in the dermis. In this angioma, the lobules of small blood vessels project into pre-existing ectatic dermal veins.

the first two of these lesions shows a greater penchant for formation of *in*complete and interanastomosing vascular spaces that "dissect" through dermal collagen and subcuticular tissue[83] (Fig. 19-12). Small papillary projections of bland endothelial cells also may project into the lumina of targetoid hemangiomas.[86,91] These histologic features often cause considerable concern regarding the potential diagnosis of a vascular sarcoma. Nonetheless, the advancing boundaries of targetoid hemangiomas are relatively well-defined (unlike those of endothelial malignancies), and an organized rim of dense hemosiderin deposition is often apparent peripherally.[91] Other lesions with closely similar microscopic features include the so-called benign lymphangioendothelioma[101] and angioreticulohistiocytoma.[102] Benign lymphangioendothelioma contains proteinaceous lymphatic fluid rather than luminal erythrocytes, lacks stromal hemosiderin deposits, has a more regimented superficial constituency by vertically aligned vascular spaces, and may be invested by lymphoid infiltrates. Angioreticulohistiocytoma

Figure 19-12. The targetoid hemangioma is often hemosiderotic. Histologically, this lesion forms vessels with incomplete anastomosing vascular spaces. It is important therefore to correlate the clinical presentation as well as the shape of the overall lesion. The microvenular hemangioma is also very similar to this lesion but occurs deeper in the dermis.

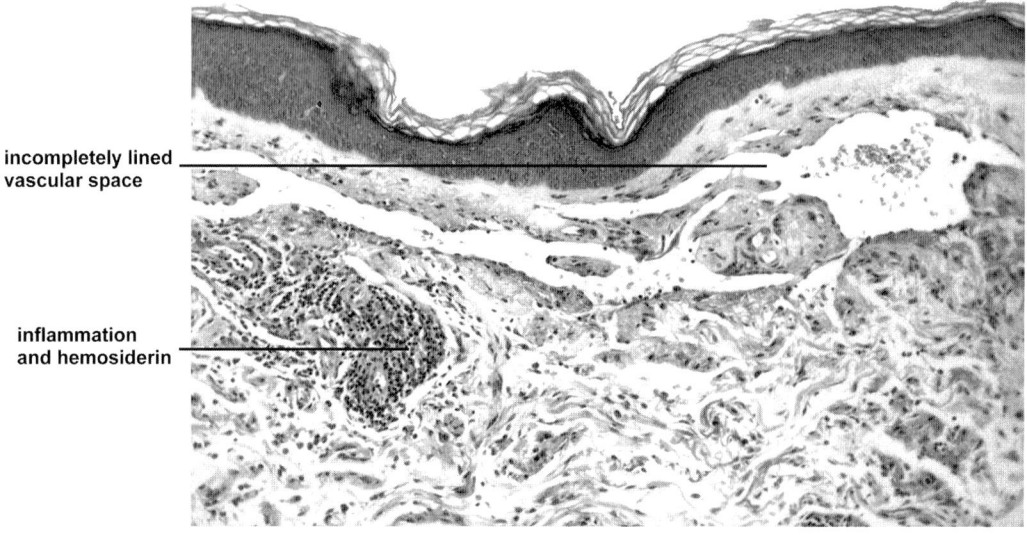

incompletely lined vascular space

inflammation and hemosiderin

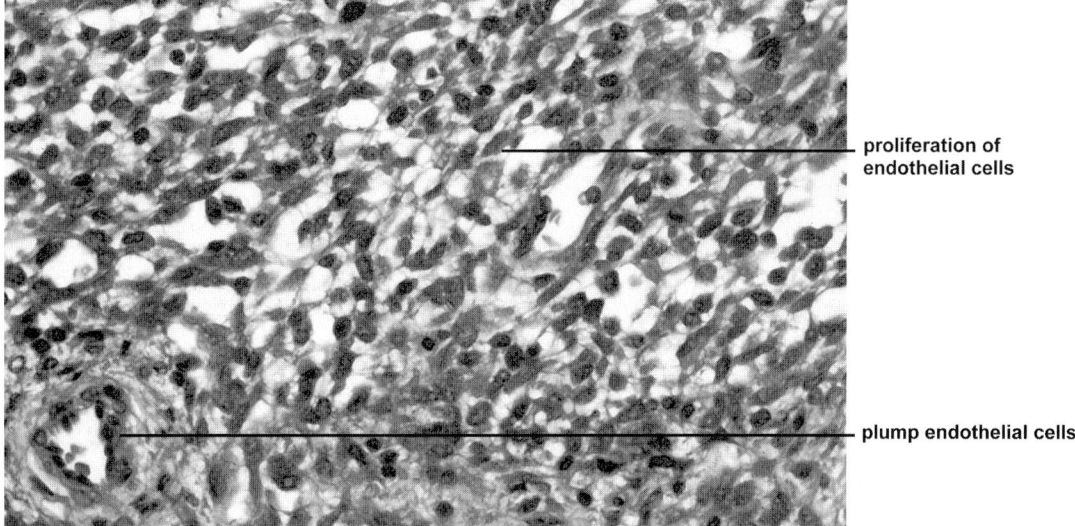

proliferation of
endothelial cells

plump endothelial cells

Figure 19-13. The epithelioid hemangioma is characterized by plump cuboidal endothelial cells that line constituent blood vessels. The lumina of the vascular spaces are often obscured because of the proliferation of the plump endothelial cells. Nuclei are enlarged and histiocytic-like, thus giving the origin for the alternate name of *histiocytoid hemangioma.*

contains multinucleated stromal cells that border vascular spaces and, in some foci, may appear to line them.

The lesion now known as *epithelioid hemangioma*[96] has been the subject of considerable terminologic debate in recent years. Alternative designations for this tumor include "angiolymphoid hyperplasia with eosinophilia"[103] and "histiocytoid" hemangioma.[95] The key feature of epithelioid hemangiomas is the plump, cuboidal appearance of the endothelial cells that line constituent blood vessels (Fig. 19-13). The latter channels have the dimensions of capillaries or venules, and their lumina are indistinct because of the space occupied by proliferating endothelia. Nuclear contours in the tumor cells are round or slightly indented, chromatin is dispersed, and nucleoli are indistinct.[93] These characteristics led Rosai et al[92] to focus on morphologic similarities between the nuclei of such neoplasms and those of histiocytes. Angiolymphoid hyperplasia with eosinophilia is nothing more than an inflamed version of epithelioid hemangioma, in which the stroma between constituent dermal blood vessels is rich in lymphocytes and eosinophils.[103]

Like other morphologic variants of hemangioma, a basically lobular substructure is observed in epithelioid hemangiomas as well. Nevertheless, a unique finding is their potential association with large arteries or veins in the skin such that the tumoral blood vessels appear to "spin off" of pre-existing vascular adventitia like a swarm of bees.

Considerable attention also has been given to the possible synonymity between epithelioid hemangioma and *Kimura's disease/tumor.*[82] However, points of convincing clinicopathologic dissimilarity do exist between these two neoplasms. Kimura's tumor features a striking stromal lymphoid infiltrate—complete with germinal centers—and is centered more deeply in the skin. Moreover, constituent vessels are more elongated than those of epithelioid hemangioma, and tumor cell nuclei do not have the complex contours of those in the latter lesion. Kimura's disease

often includes the presence of regional lymphadenopathy and eosinophilia in the peripheral blood, whereas epithelioid hemangiomas are unassociated with these findings.[93]

Benign Neural Tumors

Neuromas and Ganglioneuromas

Clinical Features

Two types of cutaneous neuroma are recognized at the present time—*post-traumatic neuroma*[104,105] and *palisading neuroma.*[106,107] Both of these variants present as small nodular tan-pink lesions; post-traumatic neuromas tend to affect the extremities (where mechanical injuries are most common),[105] whereas palisading neuromas occur almost exclusively on the face.[106] Both favor adult patients, with no predilection for gender.

Ganglioneuromas rarely arise in the skin,[108] but rather are typically found in modified mucosal surfaces such as the lips and genital skin. They are largely restricted to patients with the multiple endocrine neoplasia syndrome, type 2b (Gorlin syndrome)[109] in which medullary thyroid carcinoma, pheochromocytoma, parathyroid hyperplasia, and a marfanoid habitus are also seen. Mucosal ganglioneuromas are typically multiple and take the form of irregular nodules of variable size.[108] However, a case of solitary ganglioneuroma of the skin has been reported, under the rubric of "ganglion cell choristoma."[110]

Histopathologic Features

Post-traumatic neuromas are actually misnamed in that they do not represent truly neoplastic proliferations of peripheral nerves. They are the result of aberrant reinnervation after traumatic disruption of axons and consequent intraneurial scarring.[104] Accordingly, one observes relatively banal nerve bundles that are distorted by fibrous bands within them and surrounding them (Fig. 19-14). Regenerating axonal fibers may be "blocked" from

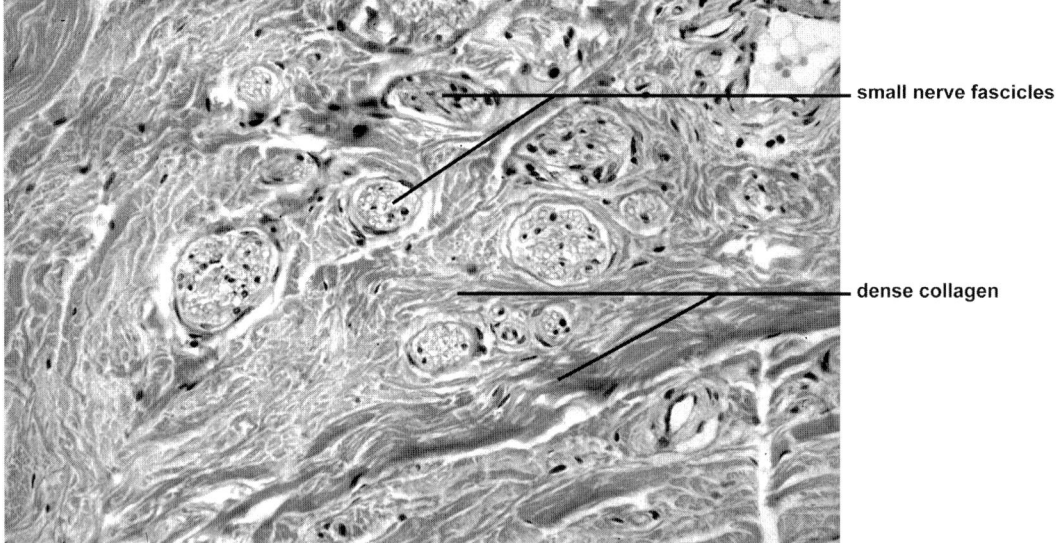

small nerve fascicles

dense collagen

Figure 19-14. The traumatic neuroma is characterized by small fascicles of peripheral nerve that have proliferated and are thus found in the dense fibrous stroma. Following transection, axons proliferate in an effort to find the Schwann cell sheath on the other side of the transection. If instead they project into adjacent connective tissue, a dense fibrosis results.

establishing continuity with distal portions of the Schwann sheath by such zones of fibrosis, yielding micronodular proliferations of axons and accompanying Schwann cells.[105] Adjacent blood vessels may contain organizing microthrombi.

Palisading neuromas, by contrast, are probably neoplasms. They are centered in the mid-dermis and show a thin peripheral fibrous capsule. Fascicles of bland, amitotic spindle cells are intertwined around one another, and tumor cell nuclei manifest a tendency to align themselves in registers or palisades within each fascicle[106,107] (Fig. 19-15). Nuclear contours are serpiginous or comma shaped, and the cytoplasm is slightly eosinophilic. However, it lacks the fibrillation that would be expected in a smooth muscle tumor, which represents the most likely histopathologic diagnostic alternative. Similarly, fascicles cut in cross section do not exhibit the zones of perinuclear cytoplasmic clarity that are seen in leiomyomas.

Ganglioneuromas differ only slightly from the description just given. The points of dissimilarity between these tumors and palisaded neuromas include a lack of encapsulation in ganglioneuromas and, more importantly, the presence of well-formed ganglion cells that are interspersed throughout.[108,110] The latter elements are variable in number, but they are easily recognized by their polyhedral shape, vesicular nuclei, and prominent nucleoli.

Neurofibromas

Clinical Features

Neurofibromas of the skin are not uncommon as sporadic neoplasms, in which case they are nondescript soft papules or nodules measuring up to 3 cm in greatest dimension. Any skin field may be affected by solitary neurofibromas (including modified mucosae), and they are likewise seen at all ages.[111,112]

Multiple neurofibromas—particularly if they are accompanied by café au lait lesions and are seen in patients under 10 years of age—strongly suggest a diagnosis of von Recklinghausen's disease.[113–115] The plexiform variant of these neoplasms, which is *pathognomonic* of von Recklinghausen's disease even if solitary,[113,116] is characterized by extension of the tumor into branches of a nerve or plexus. It can greatly distort the superficial soft tissue so that the affected skin acquires a pendulous appearance ("elephantiasis neuromatosa").[113] The cut surface of plexiform neurofibromas has been likened to a "bag of worms."

Histopathologic Features

Neurofibromas are paucicellular tumors with a bland cytologic appearance, serpiginous nucleocytoplasmic contours, and infiltrative, poorly delimited boundaries with surrounding dermis or soft tissue. These lesions are microscopically uniform throughout (Fig. 19-16) and may be restricted to the corium or extend deeply into the subcutis. Myxoid stromal change is relatively common, but a tendency toward nuclear palisading is generally not appreciated in neurofibromas. The tumor cells are arranged haphazardly, with entrapment of dermal collagen and appendages.[113] Intralesional mast cells are often numerous.

By contrast, *plexiform neurofibroma* has a distinctive configuration that recalls a distorted neural plexus. Irregular fascicles of proliferating but banal Schwann cells are separated from one another by myxofibrous stroma or adipose tissue in this neoplasm such that each grouping of spindle cells resembles a miniature nerve trunk (Fig. 19-17). Occasionally, melanin-containing cells or structures resembling meissnerian or pacinian corpuscles may punctuate these proliferations.[113,117] To reiterate, making the histologic interpretation of plexiform neurofibroma is tantamount to assigning a diagnosis of von Recklinghausen's disease to the pa-

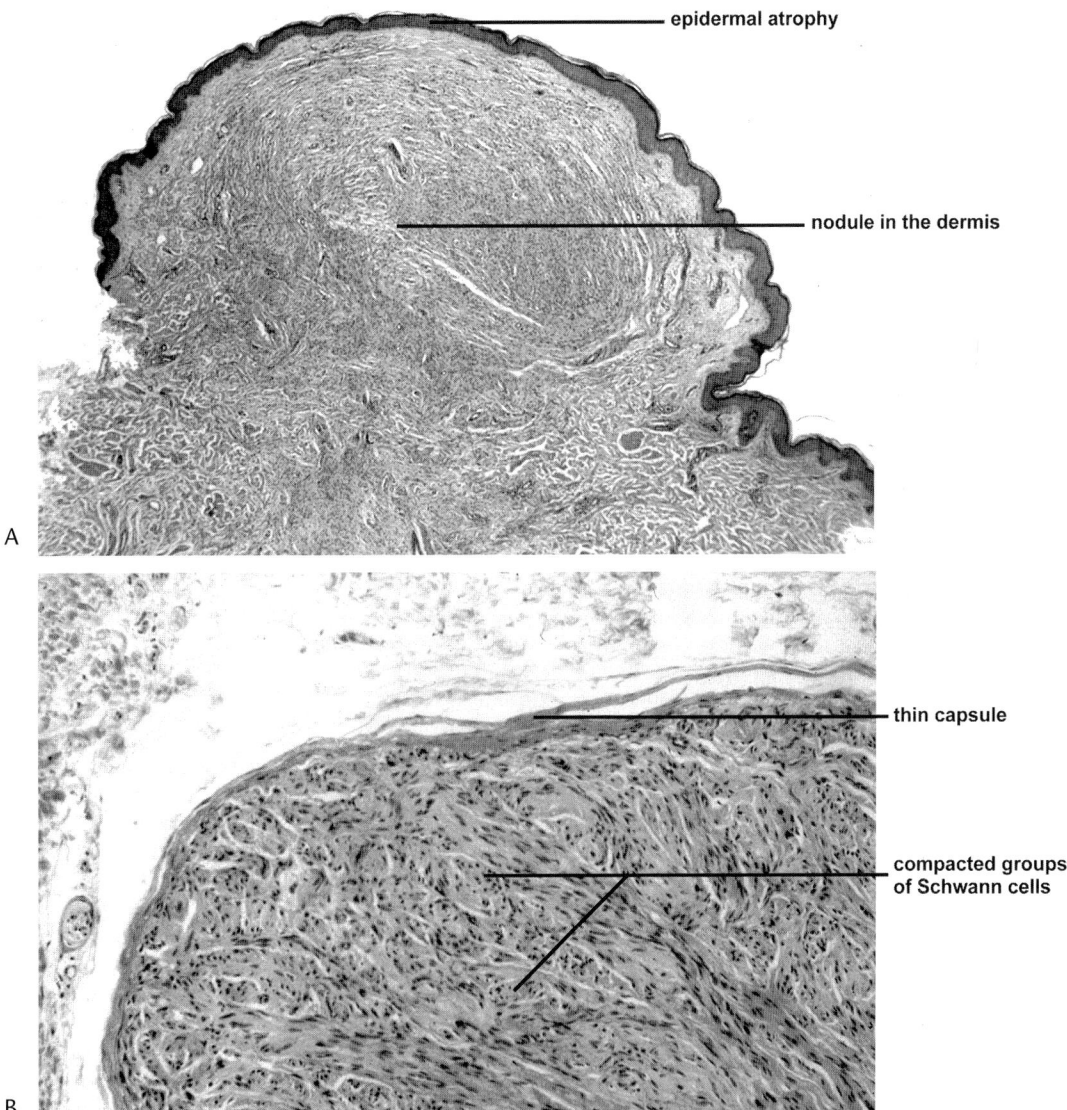

— epidermal atrophy

— nodule in the dermis

A

— thin capsule

— compacted groups
of Schwann cells

B

Figure 19-15. **(A)** A papule produced by a palisaded and encapsulated neuroma. The epidermis is slightly atrophic over the lesion. The lesion forms a distinct nodule in the dermis and is thinly to variably encapsulated. **(B)** Thin encapsulation of the palisaded encapsulated neuroma. Weak attempts at palisading or Verocay body formation are present. Silver staining would reveal fewer axons present. This is in contrast to the neurofibroma, which should contain fewer axons, and the schwannoma, which should never contain axons.

tient; hence, one should require that the above-cited microscopic features are all present before taking this step.

Mitotic activity, local hypercellularity, necrosis, and nuclear atypia are worrisome features in lesions thought to be neurofibromas. It is well-known that great difficulty may be encountered in distinguishing such neoplasms from selected malignant peripheral nerve sheath tumors (see below) of low histologic grade, particularly if they are several centimeters in size.[118] Therefore, reports of lesions with the alarming features just cited should make special note of them, and the preferred diagnostic terminology in such instances is "peripheral nerve sheath tumor of indeterminate biologic potential."

Another problem concerning neurofibromas is their distinction from ordinary but extensively "neurotized" melanocytic intradermal nevi. Serial sections are often required to search for small foci of residual melanocytes in the latter lesions, and it is admittedly impossible to make the distinction just cited in some cases.

Neurilemmomas (Schwannomas)

Clinical Features

Neurilemmomas (schwannomas) rarely occur in skin because they are lesions of deep nerve trunks. There is a potential association between cutaneous variants of the former neoplasms and

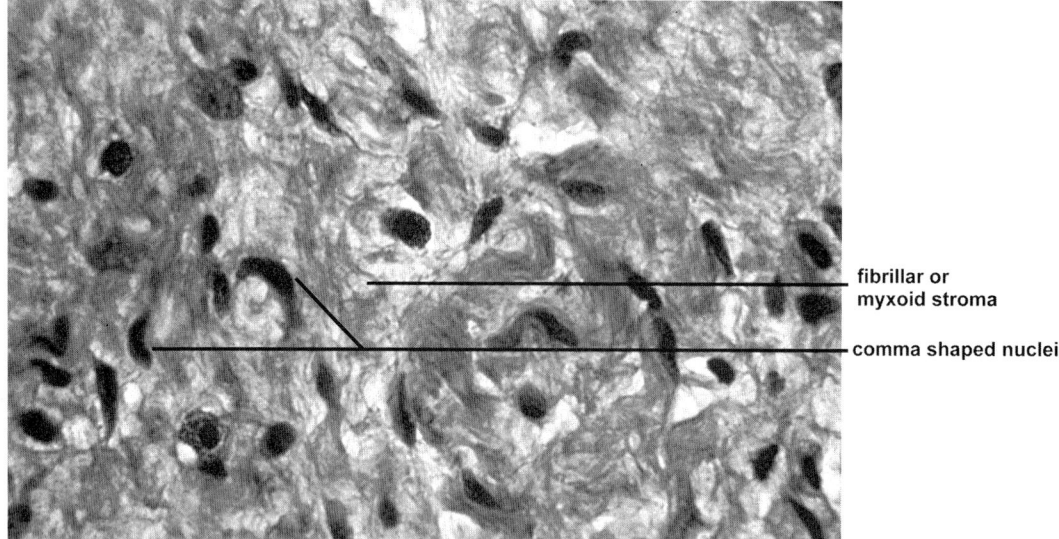

fibrillar or
myxoid stroma

comma shaped nuclei

Figure 19-16. The neurofibroma is composed of nuclei that are comma or S shaped. The intervening extracellular matrix is finely fibrillar. Mast cells are numerous.

von Recklinghausen's disease if the lesions are multifocal; this is a rare occurrence.[113]

Histopathologic Features

Neurilemmomas differ from neurofibromas in two respects. First, they demonstrate a biphasic cellular growth pattern. Second, they are often encapsulated and contain internal thick-walled stromal blood vessels.[112]

The two major microscopic patterns in neurilemmoma are known as the "Antoni A" (densely cellular) and "Antoni B" (paucicellular) configurations. These feature the presence of dense spindle cell foci with potential nuclear palisading (Verocay bodies) and myxoid or edematous, paucicellular areas composed of bland myxoid or stellate tumor cells[113,119] (Fig. 19-18). Intratumoral mast cells are again numerous. Nuclear characteristics are usually bland, although traumatized, long-standing superficial ("ancient") neurilemmomas may show nuclear enlargement and hyperchro-

Figure 19-17. The plexiform neurofibroma is simply a neurofibroma that involves a nerve plexus. Thus, the tumor infiltrates out all the branches of a nerve plexus. Therefore, when cut in cross section, multiple lobules of tumor are seen as shown here. It is written that one plexiform neurofibroma makes the diagnosis of von Recklinghausen's disease.

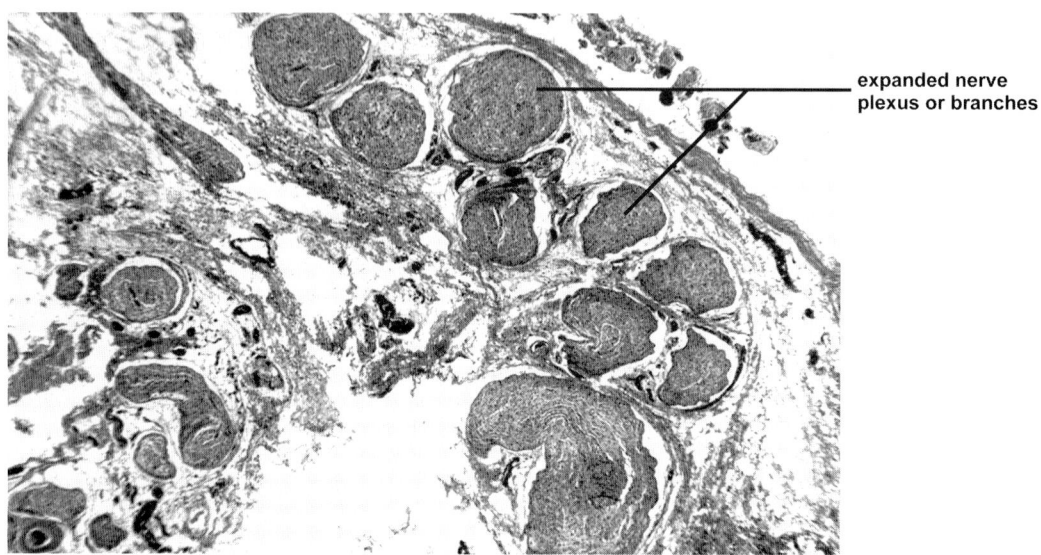

expanded nerve
plexus or branches

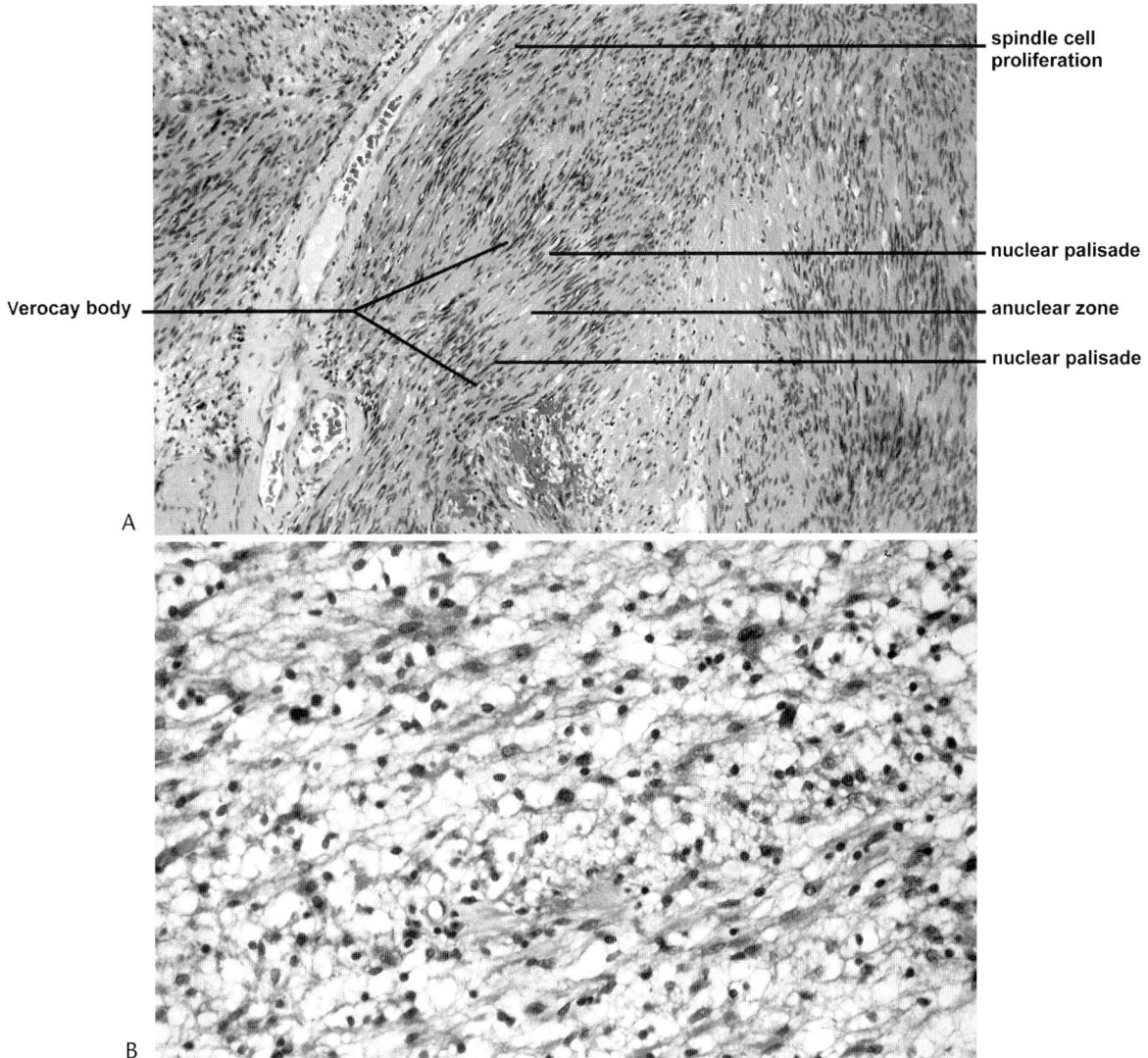

Figure 19-18. (**A**) Field of Antoni A type tissue in a schwannoma. Also noted are rows of dark-staining nuclei that bound anuclear regions (the Verocay body). (**B**) Antoni B type tissue. Antoni B tissue is not merely a degenerated product of Antoni A, since they both reproduce true in tissue culture. Mast cells are also found in Antoni B type tissue.

masia as secondary changes. Mitotic activity is scanty, but, unlike the case with neurofibroma, some division figures may be "tolerated" without alarm as long as a biphasic pattern is present.

Neurilemmoma is much more "versatile" than other peripheral nerve sheath tumors, with respect to its modes of microscopic differentiation. Variants of this neoplasm include one containing small groups of epithelium, with or without mucin production (*"glandular" neurilemmoma*)[120]; another showing an admixture of melaninized cells (*"melanotic" neurilemmoma*)[121,122]; a *plexiform* subtype in which the macroscopic appearance of the tumor simulates that of plexiform neurofibroma (but where linkage with von Recklinghausen's disease is lacking)[123,124]; a variant dominated by plump epithelioid tumor cells (*"epithelioid" neurilemmoma*)[125]; and a form in which *both* melaninization and psammomatous calcification are apparent (*"psammomatous-melanotic"*

neurilemmoma).[126] Some authors have used the term *cellular schwannoma* in describing some cutaneous tumors with extremely dense Antoni A areas. However, the latter designation is most properly applied to a restricted subset of neurilemmomas that occur in the deep soft tissues of the midline.[127] Hence, I do not endorse its application in the context of dermatopathology.

Neurothekeomas; Pacinian Neurofibroma; Dermal Nerve Sheath Myxoma

Clinical Features

"Neurothekeoma" is an unusual benign peripheral nerve sheath tumor that tends to arise in the skin of the head, neck, and arms in patients under 30 years of age. It presents as a nontender, soft,

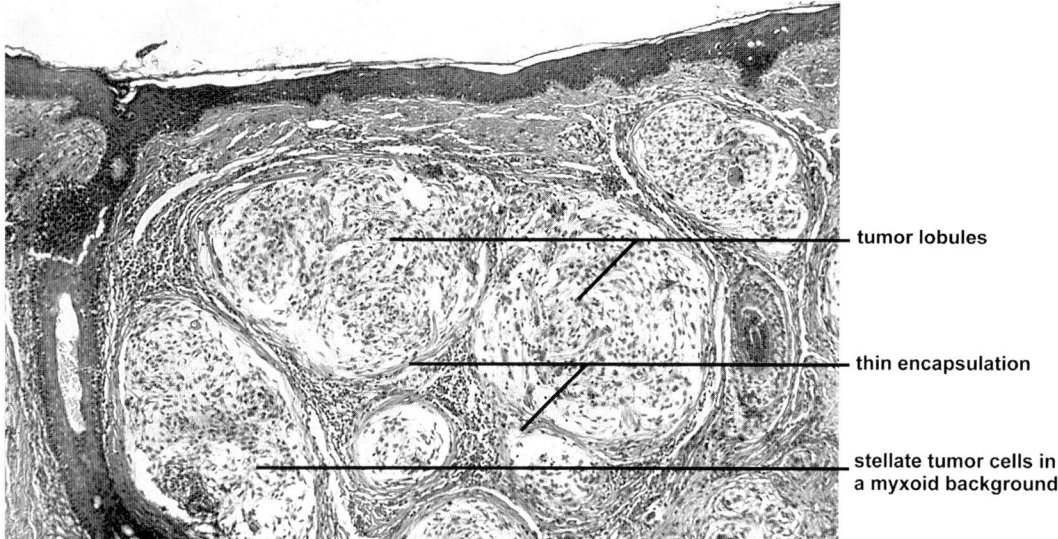

Figure 19-19. The neurothekeoma is characterized by a multilobulated and thinly encapsulated tumor in the dermis. In this example, the lobules are myxoid in character and are made up of the thin stellate tumor cells.

tan nodule measuring up to 3 cm. The cut surfaces of such lesions are often myxoid or "slimy."[113,128–130]

Histopathologic Features

Neurothekeomas are circumscribed neoplasms that are comprised of distinctive theques of spindled epithelioid or stellate cells in a lobular and concentric arrangement and with a generally bland cytologic appearance (Fig. 19-19). The background stroma is variably myxoid or myxofibrous, and the tumor is centered in the deep dermis or superficial subcutis. Limited mitotic activity may be observed but is of no prognostic consequence in neurothekeoma, and focal but modest nuclear hyperchromasia of epithelioid or multinucleated cells also may be evident in some cases.[128] Although the great majority of other benign peripheral nerve sheath tumors are immunoreactive for S-100 protein and the CD57 antigen, these markers are lacking in neurothekeomas.[131] Such results have prompted the suggestion that these neoplasms may pursue perineurial cell differentiation.

Recent reports have appeared on *cellular neurothekeoma*. This variant is more superficially located in the dermis and has a more vaguely theque-like growth pattern. Moreover, constituent cells may be polygonal, with "glassy" eosinophilic cytoplasm and nuclei that resemble those of ordinary nevocytes[132] (Fig. 19-20). Indeed, the major differential diagnostic problem in cases of cellular neurothekeoma lies in excluding epithelioid or Spitz nevi. Immunostains may contribute to resolving such uncertainties; the latter proliferations are uniformly positive for S-100 protein, whereas cellular neurothekeomas are not.[132]

Granular Cell Tumors

Clinical Features

Granular cell tumors are tan, dome-shaped nodules with smooth surfaces, measuring up to 3 cm in greatest dimension. They occur at all ages and all topographic locations, with no preference for either gender,[133] and may be multifocal.

Histopathologic Features

The hallmark of granular cell tumor is its composition by polyhedral cells with eccentric oval nuclei, dispersed nuclear chromatin, and overtly granular eosinophilic cytoplasm.[134] The neoplastic cells permeate the dermis irregularly, entrapping collagen bundles and cutaneous adnexae, and may extend into the superficial subcutis (Fig. 19-21). The low-power appearance of this lesion is circumscribed but not encapsulated.[135,136] Rare mitotic figures may be seen in benign granular cell tumors; however, atypical division figures, necrosis, vascular permeation, and overlying ulceration should prompt one to consider an alternative diagnosis[137] (see subsequent section on malignant peripheral nerve sheath tumors). Granular cell tumors (approximately 85%) show electron microscopic evidence of schwannian differentiation[138–140] and immunoreactivity for S-100 protein, CD57 antigen, and myelin basic protein.[138,139] Granular cell change may be a nonspecific degenerative alteration (reflecting an abundance of secondary cytoplasmic phagolysosomes) in neoplasms that are not neural in nature. For example, it has been reported in myogenous and epithelial proliferations as well.[138,141] Granular cell variants of other lesions do not show exceptional behavior when compared with their "conventional" forms.

Benign Tumors of Adipose Tissue

Lipomas

Clinical Features

Lipomas are almost ubiquitous in the adult population, and these "lumps" and "bumps" are generally part of the normal variation in human physiognomy that we have come to accept. Nonetheless, when they arise in cosmetically unacceptable locations or in patients who are naturally anxious about "growths," the dermatologist or surgeon provides the pathologist with examples to study histologically. On macroscopic grounds, lipomas are easily compressible, mobile, irregularly nodular lesions that may be located in the deep soft tissues or the subcutis and range in size from 2 to 10 cm.[142] The bright, fatty, yellow nature of such tumors on cut section is usually obvious.

Particular clinical variants of lipoma with which the dermatologist must be familiar include the "spindle cell,"[143] "pleomorphic,"[144] and vascular (angiolipomatous)[145] subtypes. The first of these is most often seen in elderly patients on the upper trunk, with men predominating. The base of the neck and the interscapular region are particularly common sites of origin for spindle cell lipomas.[146] These lesions are firmer and more fixed to surrounding tissue than the usual lipoma, and therefore may engender some concern. Pleomorphic lipomas likewise may have a firm consistency and are observed on the extremities or the head and neck.[147] Angiolipomas have a broader anatomic distribution, but are distinguished from other lipoma variants by their tendency to be painful when traumatized or palpated.[148]

Rare patients manifest the syndrome of familial lipomatosis, wherein hundreds of fatty lesions appear throughout adult life in all topographic sites.[149,150] Lipomas also may be components of Gardner syndrome (with familial adenomatous polyposis of the colon).[142]

Histopathologic Features

In their usual banal form, lipomas represent localized overgrowths of mature thinly encapsulated adipocytes. Internal stroma is delicate and inconspicuous, and there is no tendency for matrical sclerosis with increasing size.[150,151]

Spindle cell lipoma is a triphasic neoplasm in which lobules of mature fat cells are interposed with dense zones of bland spindle cell growth and other areas of prominent myxoid stromal change. In some cases, the latter two components may be dominant, leading to diagnostic consideration of a neural or fibroblastic proliferation. In rare examples, metaplastic osteoid or cartilage is seen in such tumors as well.[143,146] Another lesion that resembles spindle cell lipoma is the fibrous hamartoma of infancy.[48] However, these proliferations occur in mutually exclusive patient populations.

Pleomorphic lipoma differs from the usual type by its content of "floret" cells.[144,147] These are multinucleated and atypical but cytologically bland elements interspersed throughout the background population of mature adipocytes (Fig. 19-22). A modest increase in stromal fibrous tissue also may be apparent within such masses, recalling the image of well-differentiated sclerosing liposarcomas of deep soft tissue. Nonetheless, the overall configuration of the mass—including sharp circumscription, a superficial location, and a lack of mitotic activity and lipoblasts—serves to allay any concern over a diagnosis of malignancy.[147] As stated previously, liposarcoma virtually never arises in the subcutis.

Angiolipoma is typified by the proliferation of small groups of capillary- or venule-sized blood vessels within an otherwise typical lipoma.[145,148] The vascular clusters tend to be disposed toward the periphery of fat lobules and may also be associated with small collections of nondescript spindle cells[148] (Fig. 19–23). One form of this neoplasm features a prominent overgrowth of vascular elements containing fibrin microthrombi, such that they actually dominate the mass. Such tumors, known as "cellular" angiolipomas,[152] can be confused with angioleiomyomas and other lesions that are basically spindle cell proliferations. Nonetheless, the consistent presence of lobulated aggregates of fat cells, microthrombi in stromal blood vessels, and foci of myxoid stromal change serve to separate angiolipomas from the other possibilities.[153]

Figure 19-20. The cellular neurothekeoma is characterized by lobules composed of epithelioid cells, often with atypia or even mitoses. The silhouette of the lobular arrangement still exists and is the greatest aid to diagnosis.

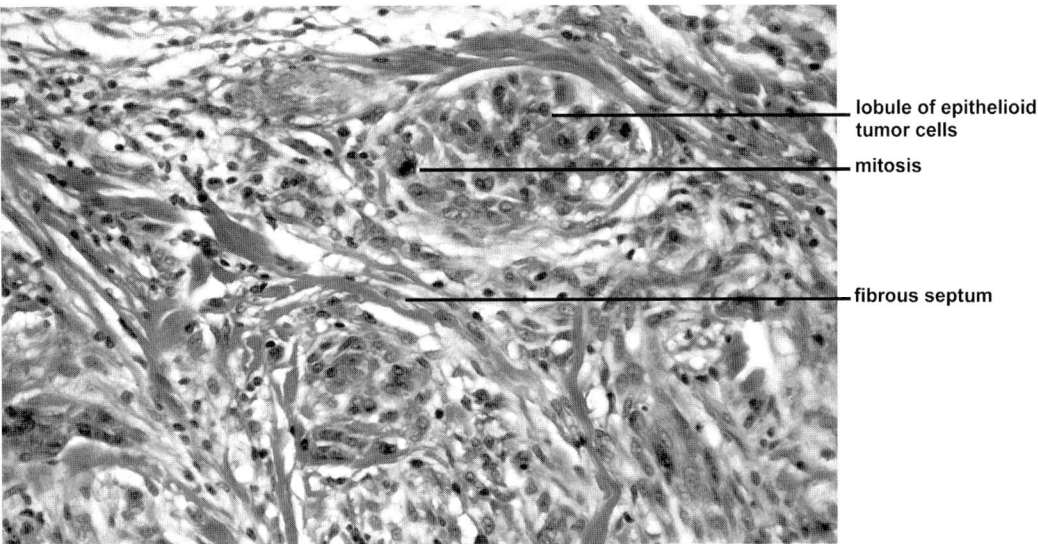

lobule of epithelioid tumor cells

mitosis

fibrous septum

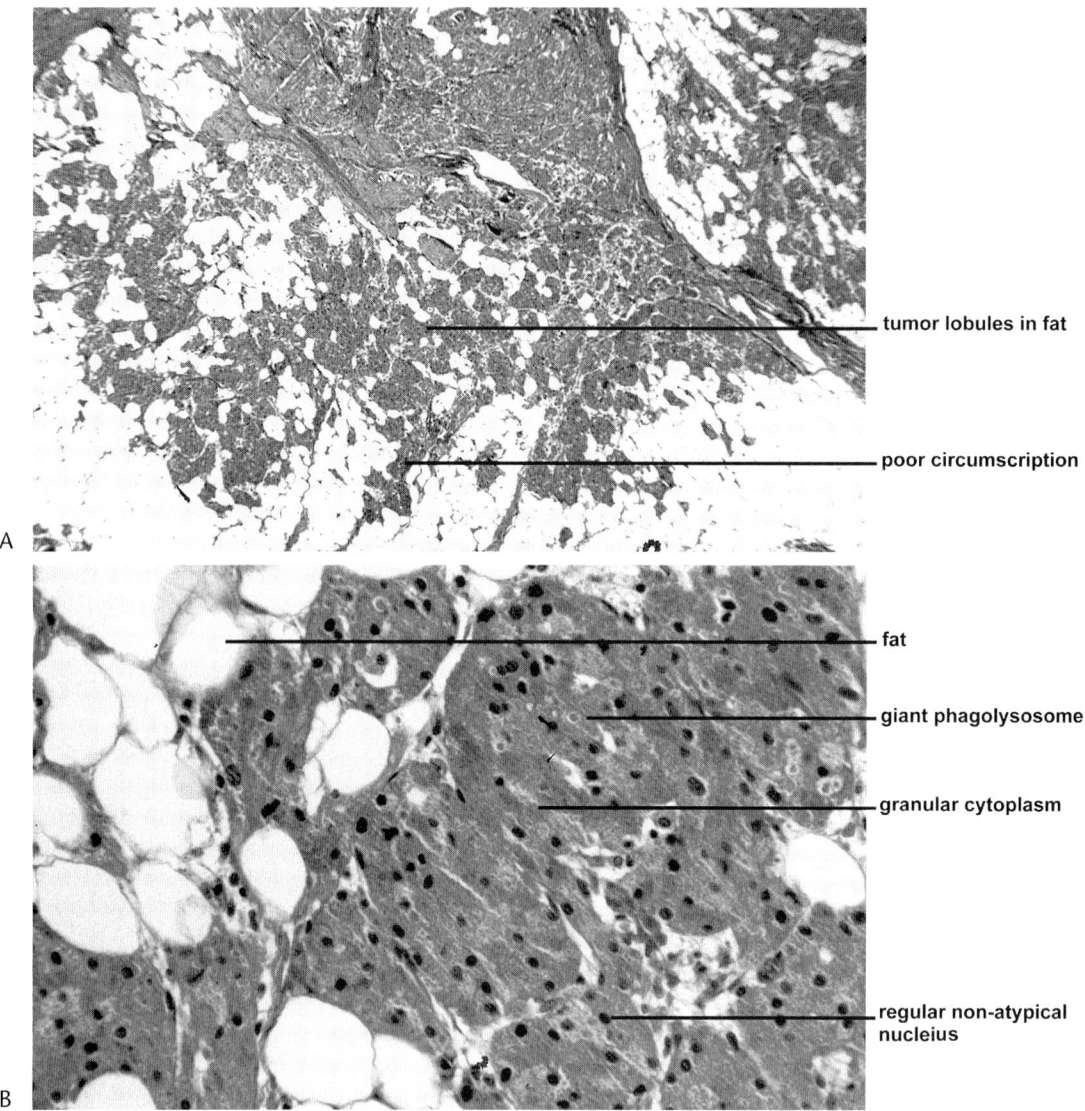

A

B

tumor lobules in fat

poor circumscription

fat

giant phagolysosome

granular cytoplasm

regular non-atypical nucleius

Figure 19-21. (**A**) The granular cell tumor can occur in any body site, including the brain. In this example occurring in adipose tissue, it is evident that the lesion is not compact or encapsulated. The finding is the same when it occurs in dense connective tissue. (**B**) Characteristic epithelioid cells with pink granular cytoplasm that have small, dark, nonatypical nuclei. The overall silhouette of a tumor with an indistinct outline should not make one worry about malignancy.

Lipoblastomas

Clinical Features

Lipoblastoma is confined to patients under 5 years of age and may occur singly or as part of a disseminated process ("lipoblastomatosis").[153–155] The great majority of these lesions are seen in the subcutis of the arms and legs as firm but compressible nodules of variable sizes. On cut section, they are well demarcated and have a variably white-yellow appearance.

Histopathologic Features

Lipoblastoma demonstrates a range of embryonic-type adipocytic differentiation. Accordingly, it contains a mixture of mature fat cells, bland stellate cells in a myxoid stroma, and lipoblasts with eccentric nuclei and monovacuolated cytoplasm.[25,154] The overall growth pattern is lobular, with aggregates of tumor cells separated from one another by delicate fibrovascular septa. Myxoid zones are often most prominent at the peripheries of the cellular lobules; areas of prominent stromal vascularity may be apparent within them, in likeness to those seen in angiolipomas.[25] Mitotic activity is typically absent but may be observed in some lipoblastomas.

Because of the presence of lipoblasts and myxoid foci, lipoblastoma has been confused in the past with myxoid liposarcoma. Nevertheless, it should be remembered that liposarcoma is vanishingly rare in early childhood,[153] and it virtually never arises in superficial soft tissue.

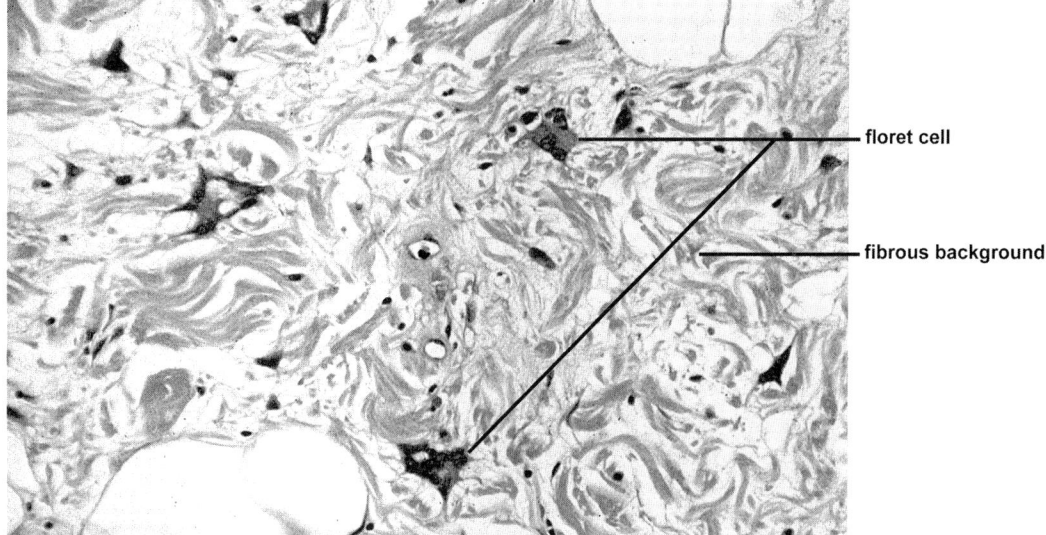

Figure 19-22. The pleomorphic lipoma is characterized by numerous floret cells. The floret cells are multinucleate giant cells with the nuclei arranged on the periphery. Some degree of inflammation is also often present. A fibrous background such as in the present example may be seen.

Hibernomas

Clinical Features

Hibernomas are exceedingly rare tumors that demonstrate differentiation toward brown (fetal) fat.[156,157] They may be observed in patients of all ages. The subcuticular soft tissues of the head and neck, upper trunk, and axillae are the favored sites of origin. The clinical appearance of such tumors is identical to that of conventional lipomas, but hibernomas are tan-brown rather than yellow on cut section.[156] One may regard them simply as "fetal lipomas" because of these attributes.

Histopathologic Features

The cells of hibernomas are multivacuolated with eosinophilic cytoplasm and internal lipofuscin granules (Fig. 19-24). These lesions are usually well circumscribed or encapsulated, lobulated, and devoid of mitoses.[156,157]

Figure 19-23. The angiolipoma is a very vascular lipoma that often contains fibrin thrombi in vascular lumina. As illustrated, rouleaux formations of erythrocytes are also often present.

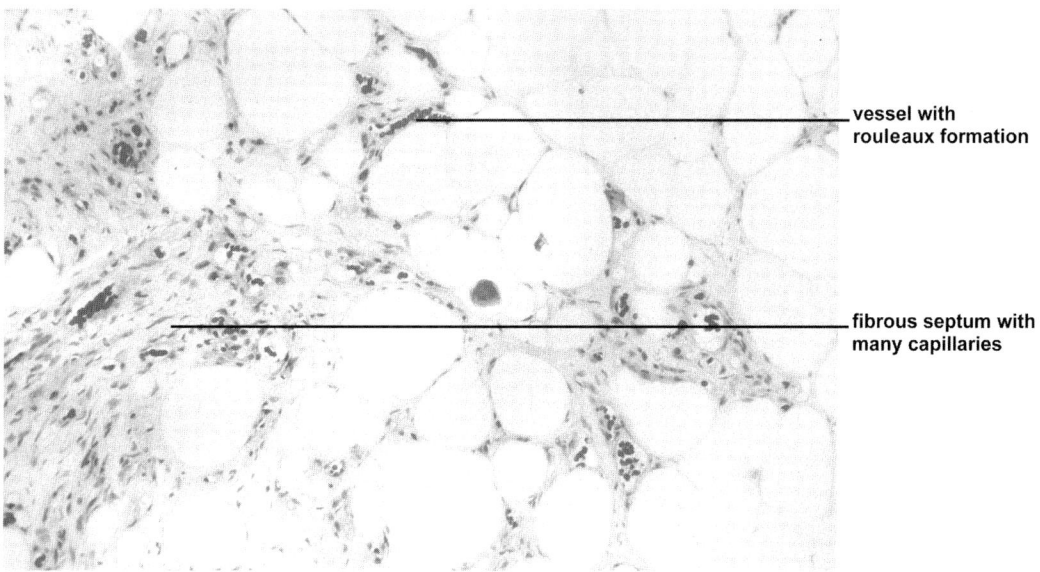

Figure 19-24.   The hibrinoma is a mass of fetal or brown fat. While occurring anywhere in a fetus, it is most commonly found in the scapular region in adult life. The finely vacuolated fat cells are characteristic of this lesion.

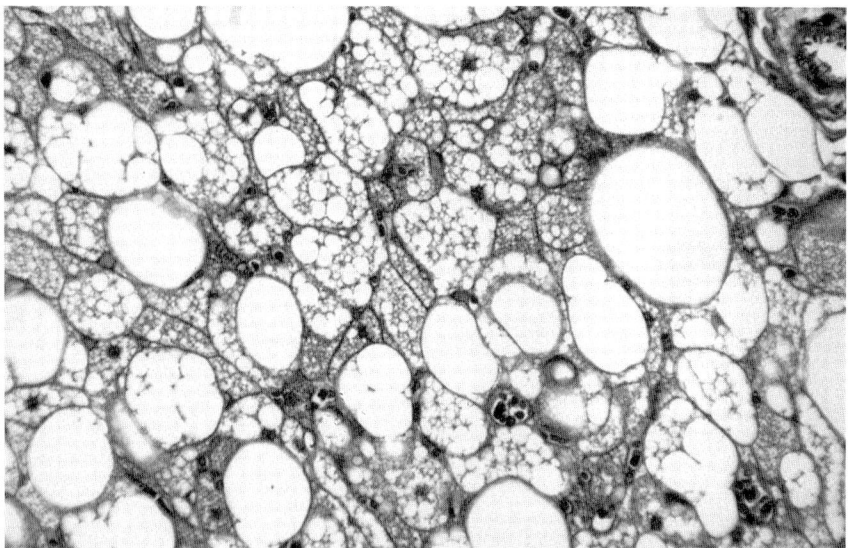

Benign "Fibrohistiocytic" Tumors

Dermatofibromas

Clinical Features

Dermatofibromas are frequently seen by all dermatologists, perhaps representing the most common mesenchymal tumors of the skin. These lesions are firm papules or nodules measuring less than 1 cm with slightly irregular borders; they may be multiple or familial; and they "dimple" when laterally compressed.[158–162] Any skin field may be affected, but the extremities are favored; patients are generally postpubertal.[159] Overlying epidermal hyperpigmentation is often present, and a diagnosis of melanoma may be considered by the clinician. Pseudoepitheliomatous hyperplasia over dermatofibromas may simulate basal cell carcinoma or squamous cell carcinoma microscopically.[163] Dermatofibroma may be the endpoint in a spectrum of maturation exhibited by benign fibrohistiocytic lesions of the skin. As such, it is closely related to juvenile xanthogranuloma, nodular histiocytoma, "fibrous histiocytoma," and "subepidermal fibroma" and probably represents a relatively mature member of this group that reflects a long period of clinical evolution.[164]

Histopathologic Features

Dermatofibromas are circumscribed lesions; they show a variably dense composition by compact spindle cells in the dermis, admixed with an abundantly collagenous matrix and scattered foamy histiocytes (Fig. 19-25). As in "fibrohistiocytic" tumors

Figure 19-25.   The dermatofibroma is a dermal-based proliferation of fibroblasts and histiocytic cells. In this example, as in many, there is hyperplasia of the overlying epidermis. There is commonly a spray-like extension of the tumor elements into the subcutis which does not portend a poor prognosis. Instead, such findings are to be expected.

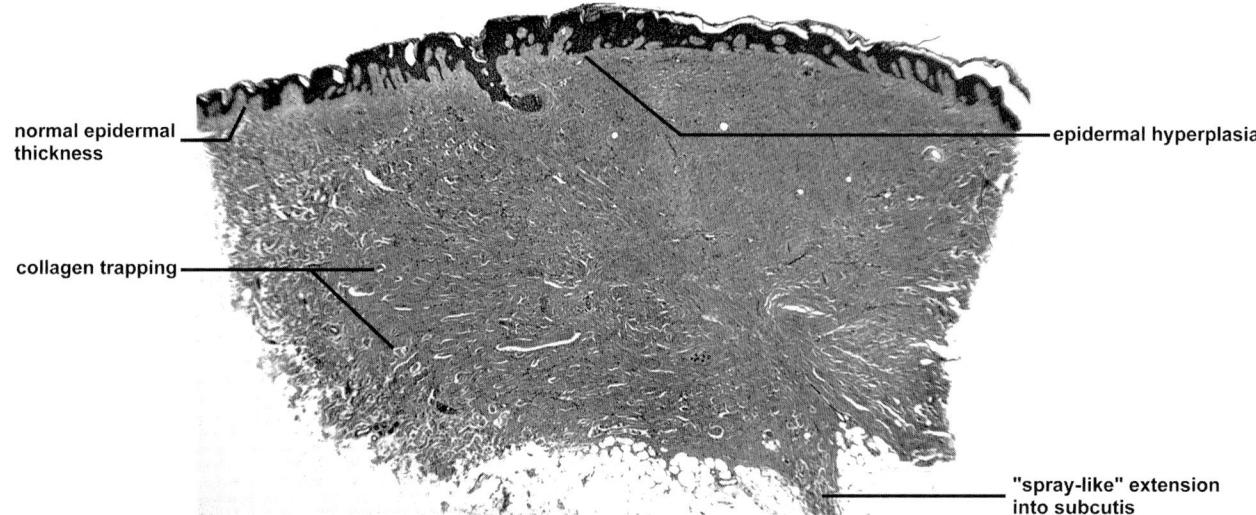

in general, a "storiform" pattern and cells of the Touton or floret types are often seen[162,165] (Fig. 19-26). Their peripheral aspects blend gradually with the surrounding connective tissue, often isolating rounded, sclerotic bundles of collagen (Fig. 19-27); when subcutaneous involvement is present, it is limited and confined to extension into interlobular fibrous septa of the hypodermis.[159,160,164,166] Stromal vascularity in this neoplasm is represented by delicately arborizing capillaries that may assume a "chicken-wire" configuration. Mitotic activity is variable, as is the presence of focal nuclear hyperchromasia and pleomorphism in proliferating cells. Extremes in the latter characteristics have resulted in such terms as *pleomorphic fibroma, atypi-*

cal fibrous histiocytoma, and *dermatofibroma with monster cells* in reference to variations in the general microscopic attributes of dermatofibromas.[165,167,168] There is no reliable evidence to suggest that these neoplasms ever undergo aggressive transformation.

One special subtype of dermatofibroma contains vascular lakes that are mantled by giant cells, fibroblasts, and macrophages, surrounded by zones of intratumoral hemorrhage and hemosiderin deposition. This lesion is known as *aneurysmal fibrous histiocytoma* (Fig. 19-28), which arises principally in middle-aged adults as a slowly growing papule or nodule with a long evolution.[169,170] Other variants of dermatofibroma

Figure 19-26. Dermatofibromas can have a variable cellular composition. They contain variable percentages of fibroblasts and histiocytic cells. Multinucleate cells may be present. (**A**) Near storiform pattern, which may be seen. (**B**) Xanthoma cells, which are also often found in a dermatofibroma. A variation in the cellular composition in these lesions indicates a benign tumor. This feature, as well as the overlying epidermal hyperplasia, are not features of dermatofibrosarcoma protuberans.

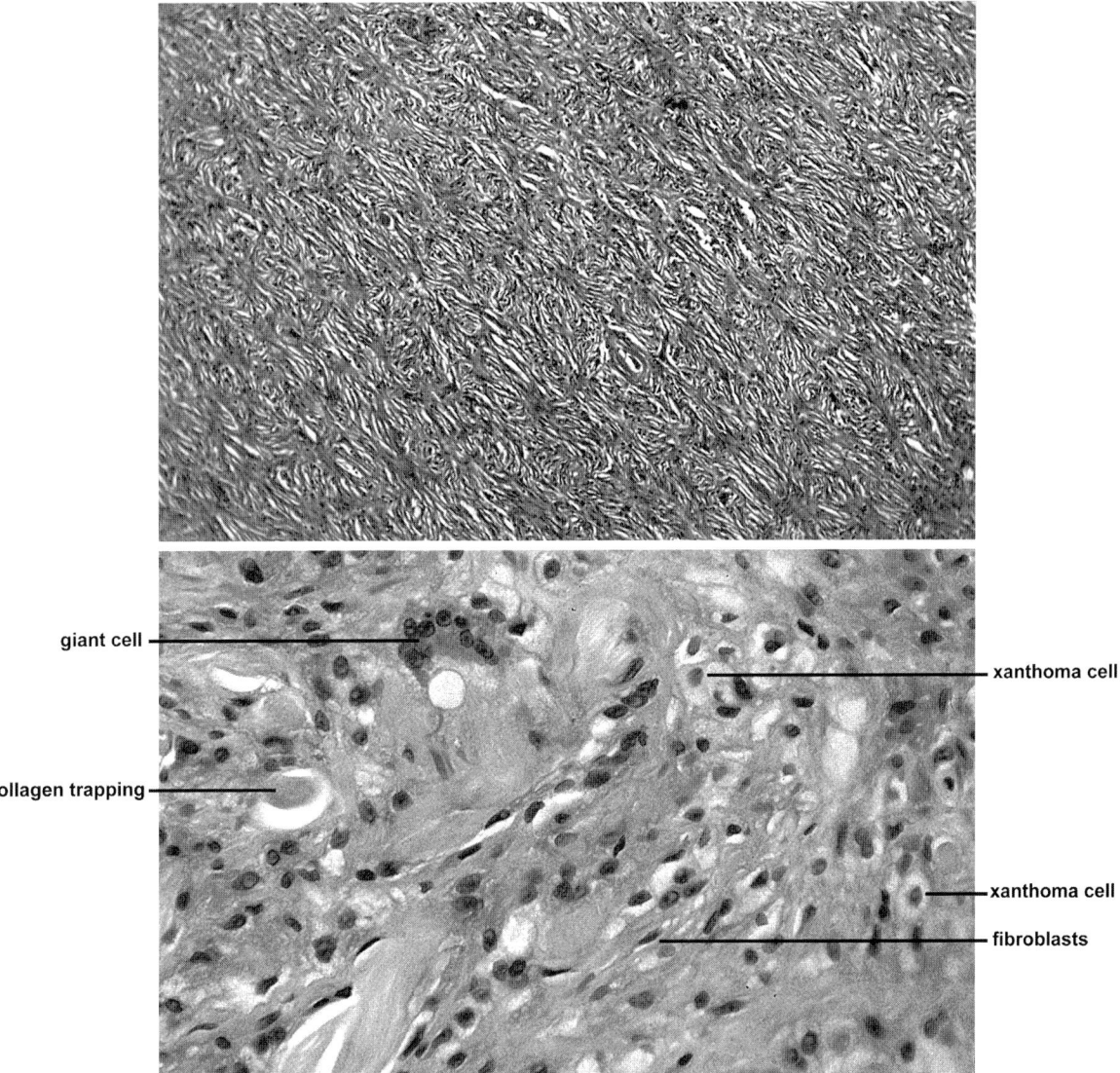

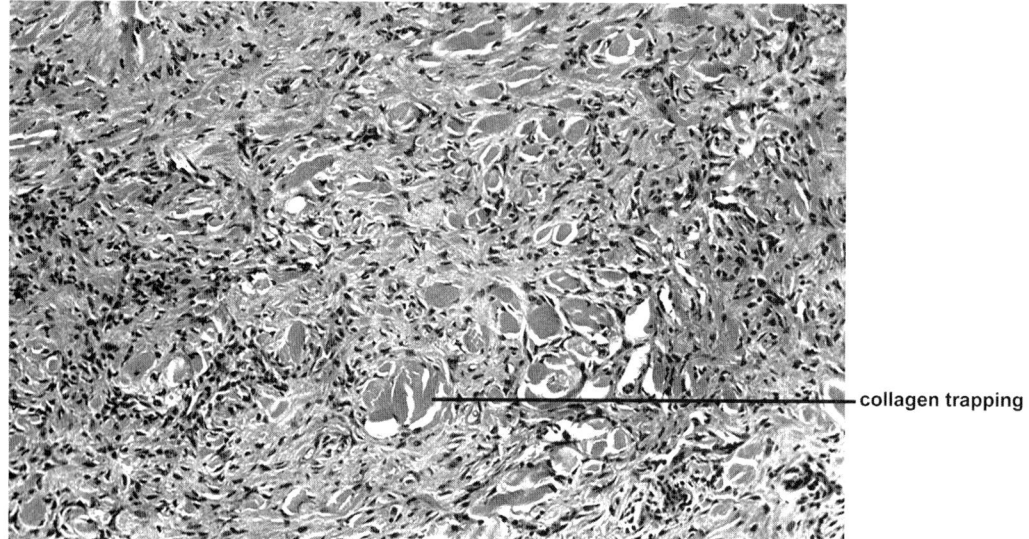

collagen trapping

Figure 19-27. The dermatofibroma characteristically has distinct boundaries. In this example taken from the lateral border of a dermatofibroma, collagen trapping is illustrated. The dermal collagen bundles are swollen, and there are retraction clefts between the distinct collagen bundles and the surrounding tumor elements. This is also not a feature of dermatofibrosarcoma protuberans.

include lesions with abundant reactive lymphoid infiltration; entrapped and proliferating epithelium; nuclear palisading; marked hemosiderosis; and divergent smooth muscular or granular cell components.[171–174]

Benign Recurring Fibrous Histiocytomas

Clinical Features

This tumor may occur at any age, with a wider topographic distribution than that of usual dermatofibromas. They are more deeply based in the dermis and subcutis and have a multinodular appearance. Recurrence after seemingly adequate excision is observed in up to 40% of cases. In light of all of these attributes, the terms *benign fibrous histiocytoma with potential for local recurrence* (BFHPR) or *atypical fibrous histiocytoma* have been appended to such proliferations.[175,176]

Histopathologic Features

In parallel with the aforementioned points of clinical dissimilarity between BFHPR and dermatofibroma, the microscopic appearances of these tumors are also reproducibly divergent. BFHPR is composed entirely of fusiform or stellate cells in short fascicles or storiform arrays, without any multinucleated elements or nuclear pleomorphism and only a few foam cells.[175] It shows a multinodular profile on low-power microscopy and often involves the subcutis, in contrast to the uninodular, irregularly expansile, and almost purely dermal nature of dermatofibroma.[176] Hyalinized, keloidal-type stromal collagen is commonly entrapped by the tumor cells in BFHPR, and a delicately branching vascular matrix is routinely apparent.[176] Mitotic activity can almost always be found, but pathologic division figures are absent.[175,176]

Giant Cell Tumors of Tendon Sheaths

Clinical Features

Giant cell tumors of tendon sheath (GCTTS) are confined to the distal extremities (particularly the digits) of adult patients. They present as slowly growing, nodular tan-pink masses that may restrict joint mobility and project into the skin in a protuberant fashion.[177–179] Synonyms for such lesions are *nodular tenosynovitis*[177] and *tendon sheath fibroma*.[180,181] Simple excision is usually curative, although examples of recurrence have indeed been reported.

Histopathologic Features

An admixture of plump fusiform cells, polygonal cells, foam cells, and osteoclast-like giant cells is observed in GCTTS, sometimes in equal proportions and otherwise with one or the other of these elements predominating[177–179] (Fig. 19-29). The stroma is characteristically rich in collagen, and connection to a tendon sheath or synovial membrane is obvious microscopically in a sizable number of cases. Collagenous stroma represents the predominant element in "tendon sheath fibromas."[180,181] Nuclei of the proliferating cells are bland, but mitotic activity may be brisk in some examples. The latter finding is of no clinical consequence.

Other Benign Neoplasms

Myxomas, Angiomyxomas, and Angiomyofibroblastomas

Myxomas of the skin are extremely uncommon, and most lesions labeled as such in the past represent dermal mucous cysts of the digits rather than actual neoplasms.[182] True myxomas are most often seen in patients who have the NAME syndrome

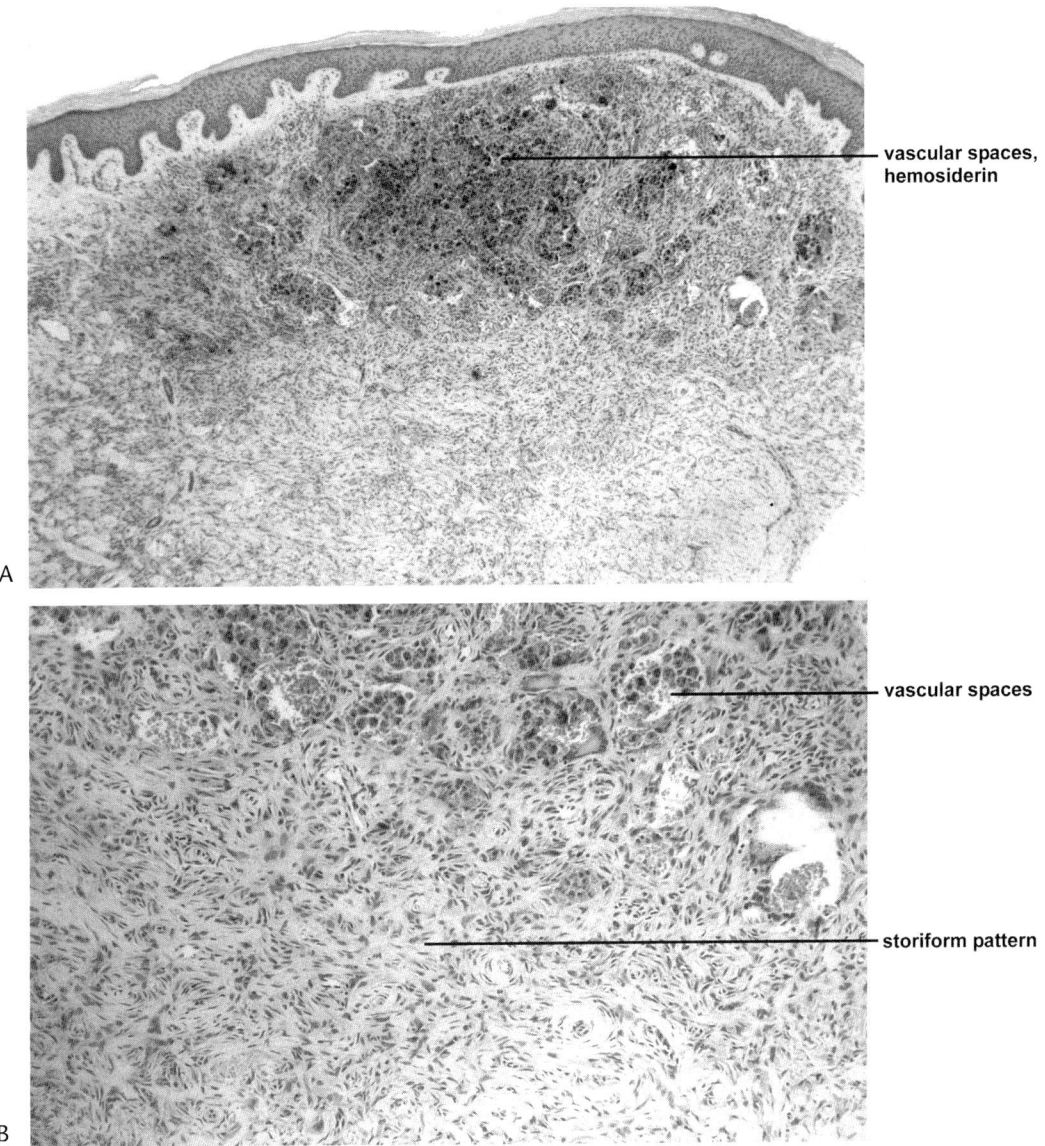

Figure 19-28. (**A**) Upper portion and epidermis in an aneurysmal type of dermatofibroma. The vascular lakes and hemosiderin pigmentation at the surface cause a distinct dark clinical presentation. (**B**) Deeper portion of the lesion and the vascular sclerosis that results as the lesion matures.

(*n*evi, *a*trial myxomas, *m*yxomas of skin and mammary glands, and *e*phelides). These individuals are adolescents and young adults who also manifest endocrine hyperactivity (particularly Cushing syndrome) as part of a complex disorder with autosomal dominant inheritance.[183]

Cutaneous myxomas in this setting are papules or nodules that average approximately 1 to 2 cm in maximal diameter, occurring on the face and trunk. The lesions are soft, compressible, and tan or pink. Although cutaneous tumors in the NAME syndrome represent only a cosmetic nuisance, they may be an invaluable clue to the existence of this complex. Such a realization may be life-saving for the patient, inasmuch as either the atrial myxomas or endocrinopathies that constitute additional parts of the syndrome may prove fatal if left untreated.[183]

Histologically, cutaneous myxomas are centered in the dermis or superficial subcutis. They are extremely paucicellular on low-power microscopy, appearing mainly as circumscribed, lightly basophilic "balls of mucus." Within the abundant myxoid stroma, one finds scant numbers of bland, fusiform, or stellate fibroblast-like cells that are widely separated and admixed with inconspicuous fibrovascular stromal elements. Occasional vacuolated polygonal cells may be apparent as well, potentially simulating adipocytes or lipoblasts. However, colloidal iron or Alcian blue stain shows that their cytoplasmic vacuoles contain stromal mucin rather than fat. Myxomas never demonstrate mitotic activity or nuclear atypia in the proliferating cells.[183]

*Angio*myxomas differ substantially from the clinicopathologic sketch just provided. They arise almost exclusively in the genital

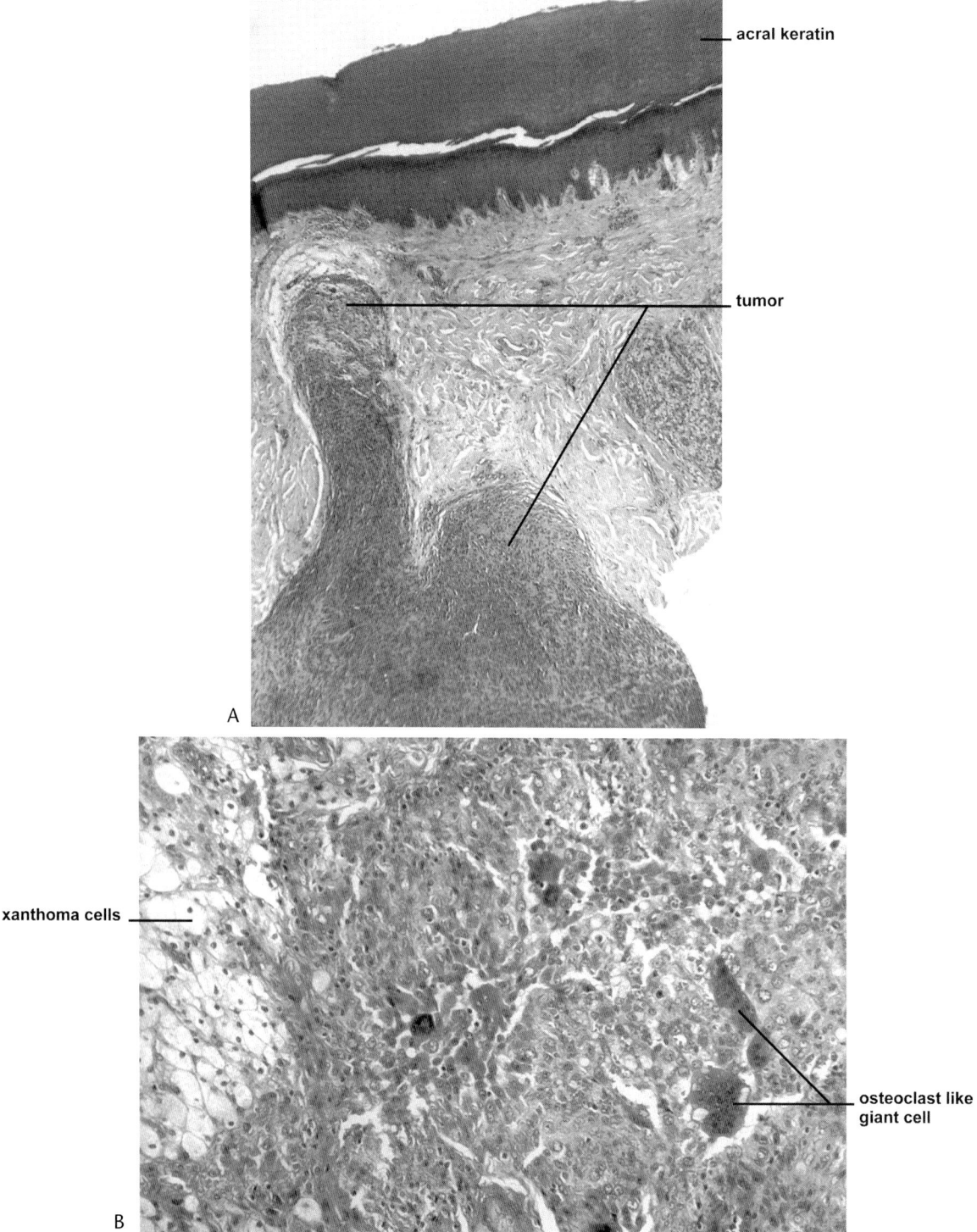

acral keratin

tumor

xanthoma cells

osteoclast like giant cell

A

B

Figure 19-29. **(A)** Giant cell tumor of tendon sheath with an irregular shape. The shape is irregular enough that a projection of tumor is nearly in contact with epidermis. This makes it easy for the dermatologist to biopsy with the usual punch. **(B)** Characteristic triphasic features of a giant cell tumor of tendon sheath. The characteristics are osteoclast-like giant cells, fibroblasts, and anthoma cells. Mitoses are rarely found.

skin and pelvic soft tissues of young adults, with a striking female predominance. Such lesions are nodular or plaque-like, often attain a size of 10 cm or more, and are ill defined microscopically.[184] There is no known association between angiomyxomas and the NAME syndrome. Moreover, the behavior of these tumors in pelvic or genital sites is potentially locally aggressive, with repeated recurrence and infiltrative growth into deep soft tissues being commonplace. The latter features account for the designation of "aggressive" angiomyxoma, which is often applied in such cases.[184]

The microscopic appearance of angiomyxoma is similar to that of cutaneous myxoma except for four important features. The former tumor is larger, more deeply seated, and more ill defined at its peripheries, often blending imperceptibly with surrounding connective tissue and subjacent striated muscles. In addition, stromal vascularity is prominent in angiomyxoma, being represented by a profusion of venule-sized blood vessels or dilated capillaries.[184] In other respects, the cytologic and architectural attributes of this neoplasm are virtually identical to those of myxoma.

Fletcher et al[185] have described a potential simulant of angiomyxoma that also occurs in the genital skin of young women. This nodular neoplasm, known as *angiomyofibroblastoma*, may clinically simulate a Bartholin's gland cyst or vulvar lipoma; it shows a sharply circumscribed image and a substantial degree of cellularity on scanning microscopy. The neoplasm is composed of narrow groupings of bland stellate, polygonal, and spindle cells set in a myxoid matrix, supported by a distinctive network of fibrovascular stroma that is rich in capillaries. Zones of relatively high cellularity alternate with hypodense foci in this lesion, but mitotic activity is limited and nuclear atypia are absent. Thick bundles of collagen often are entrapped within angiomyofibroblastomas, again in contrast to the appearance of angiomyxoma.[185]

Cutaneous Chondroma and Osteoma

Examples of *chondroma* and *osteoma* also have been reported as primary lesions of the skin and superficial soft tissues.[186–188] However, the true existence of these tumors, as distinct from unusual variants of cutaneous mixed tumor ("chondroid syringoma"), periosteal reactions in underlying bones involving the skin secondarily, and metaplastic changes in various other lesions,[189–192] may be questioned.

Biologically "Borderline" Cutaneous Mesenchymal Tumors

"Borderline" tumors may be defined as those that have a substantial tendency to recur—often with significant morbidity—and, in rare circumstances, metastasize to distant sites as well. In the skin, three particular classes of neoplasms include such lesions: endothelial proliferations, myogenous tumors, and others of a "fibrohistiocytic" character.

Borderline Endothelial Tumors

Papillary Endovascular Angioendotheliomas

Clinical Features. Papillary endovascular angioendotheliomas (PEA) were first described by Dabska[193] in 1969 and have subsequently become known by her name (i.e., Dabska's

tumor). They are apparently seen only in children and adolescents, as fluctuant, ill-defined reddish plaques or nodules that range in size up to 5 cm. A zone of dermal edema may surround such neoplasms.[193,194] "Metastases" of PEA to regional lymph nodes were reported in a seminal series of cases, but other authors have since suggested the alternative interpretation that the nodal implants actually represented tumor "satellites" as part of a field neoplasia phenomenon.[195] Nevertheless, PEA does have a marked propensity to recur locally after surgical excision, justifying its inclusion as a "borderline" proliferation.[193,196]

Histopathologic Features. The microscopic features of PEA are distinctive. As its name suggests, this tumor is confined to pre-existing vascular spaces in the curium, most of which have the properties of dilated lymphatic channels. Also in similarity to deep lymphangiomas of the skin, PEA features contiguous dermal fibrosis and intralesional aggregates of lymphocytes. The latter cells are also evident in intimate admixture with plump endothelial cell clusters inside the affected vessels.[85,193,196]

The papillae of PEA are composed of polyhedral cells with round nuclei, dispersed chromatin, and small nucleoli. As mentioned, mature lymphocytes commonly mantle the peripheral aspects of the papillary formations, and they contain internal, globular, intercellular deposits of eosinophilic basement membrane material. These inclusions may be labeled with the periodic acid–Schiff stain or with immunostains for laminin and collagen type IV.[85]

Adjacent blood vessels in PEA that do not contain papillae are nonetheless lined by atypical endothelial cells, with hyperchromatic nuclei. Small areas of racemose vascular proliferation also may be apparent in the dermis, as seen in well-differentiated angiosarcomas. Mitotic activity is present but limited.[85,193]

Epithelioid Hemangioendotheliomas

Clinical Features. Epithelioid hemangioendotheliomas (EH) are subcutaneous lesions that uncommonly involve the dermis. As such, they present as firm tan-pink nodules and plaques measuring several centimeters in maximum diameter. Adult patients are primarily affected, with a slight predilection for women. The trunk and extremities are the usual sites of origin.[85,197] Some patients with EH of the skin will concurrently have histologically identical tumors in the lung (which were known in the past as *intravascular bronchoalveolar tumors*) and the liver.[198] Under these conditions, it is impossible to determine whether the visceral and cutaneous lesions are independent primary neoplasms or whether they represent metastases of one another. EH recurs in up to 40% of cases, and approximately 15% metastasize to distant extracutaneous locations.[197,198]

Histopathologic Features. EH is typified by disorganized sheets and cords of large polyhedral tumor cells with amphophilic cytoplasm, prominent cytoplasmic vacuoles, and round but eccentric nuclei. Chromatin is vesicular, and small nucleoli are often seen.[197] The neoplastic cells make no attempt to form complete intercellular vascular lumina, as seen in epithelioid *hemangiomas*.[85] However, like the latter tumor, EH has a proclivity for growth around pre-existing large blood ves-

Figure 19-30. The leiomyosarcoma is characterized by atypical elongate spindle cells arranged in fascicles that intersect at acute angles. The cytoplasm has a characteristic eosinophilic appearance, similar to smooth muscle. Atypical mitoses were present in this example. Where the fascicles were cut in cross section, a clear halo appears around the nuclei.

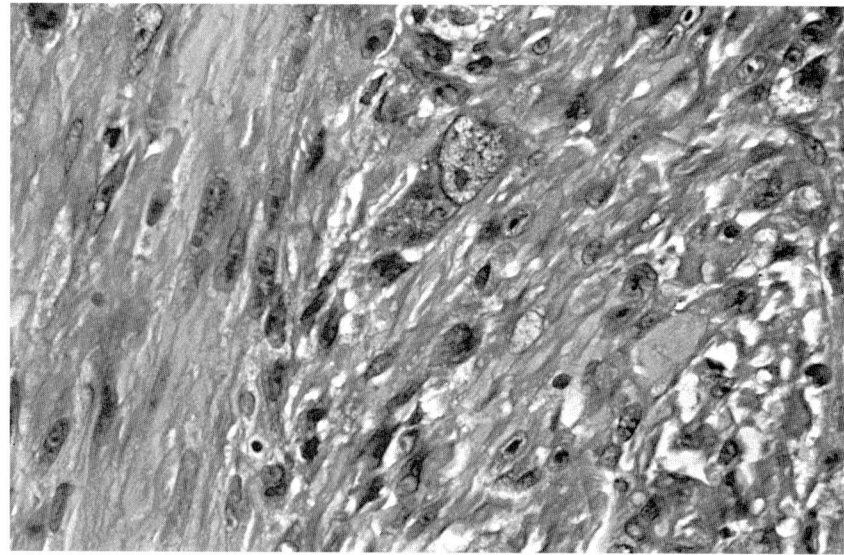

sels. Mitotic activity and necrosis may be apparent, but they are relatively inconspicuous when present. The background stroma is variably fibrous or myxoid in character.[198]

Two diagnostic errors are common in the evaluation of PEA. First, one may focus on the cord-like arrays of polygonal cells in some cases, leading to a misinterpretation of metastatic carcinoma. Second, those lesions with extensive cytoplasmic vacuolization may erroneously be labeled as adipocytic in nature. The application of electron microscopy or immunohistochemical studies for epithelial and endothelial determinants (see above) is useful in resolving such uncertainties.[85]

Spindle Cell Hemangioendothelioma

Clinical Features. Spindle cell hemangioendothelioma (SCH) is a relatively recently described tumorous entity that is seemingly confined to the skin and subcutis.[199,200] It has a long period of evolution—up to 30 years—and therefore usually presents in young adulthood.[199] This neoplasm has a marked tendency for multifocality and a predilection for the skin of the extremities.[200] It also may arise in the setting of Mafucci syndrome in which multiple enchondromas of bone are also observed.[199,200]

SCH is a multinodular, red-violet, fluctuant lesion that can attain a size of several centimeters. Its borderline status stems from the fact that local recurrence after surgical excision is a common event, being seen in up to 70% of cases.[199] Only one documented instance of distant metastasis has been reported to date, and this case was unusual in that the patient had received radiation.[199] A controversy surrounding this neoplasm centers on whether it is, indeed, a neoplasm. Some authors prefer the view that SCH represents a reactive endothelial proliferation.[201,202]

Histopathologic Features. SCH has a distinctive microscopic appearance that represents an "amalgamation" of the attributes of cavernous hemangioma and Kaposi's sarcoma.[85,199,200] One observes an intimate admixture of large, ectatic vascular spaces in the dermis—which often contain luminal thrombi and may harbor calcifications as well—with spindle cell foci showing extravasation of erythrocytes and intracytoplasmic vacuoles. The

latter finding is shared with *epithelioid* hemangioendothelioma, as described above. Nuclei of the tumor cells in both components of SCH are relatively bland, and mitotic activity is limited. The peripheral borders of the proliferation are poorly defined, and small "satellite" lesions may be observed within several millimeters on either side of the main mass.[200] Permeation into the subcutis or deeper soft tissues is relatively common. Small areas featuring racemose, interanastomosing, "dissecting" vascular channels may be noted as well.

Borderline Myogenous Tumors

Dermal Leiomyosarcoma

Clinical Features. Superficial (dermal) leiomyosarcomas (DLMS) are relatively uncommon lesions, accounting for less than 5% of all malignant mesenchymal tumors.[137,203–205] Patients with these neoplasms are adults with a mean age of 50 years. Males predominate by a ratio of 2:1.[204] Favored locations for DLMS are the proximal extremities, particularly on the dorsal surfaces. The evolution of this tumor is slow, and most have been present for years before excision. Placement of DLMS in the "borderline" category is a reflection of its clinical behavior; this lesion recurs in 30% to 40% of cases, but metastasis is exceedingly rare.[137,203,206]

Histopathologic Features. DLMS is thought to demonstrate differentiation toward pilar musculature.[206] It is composed of intertwined fascicles of fusiform cells, like leiomyoma of the skin. Also similar to the latter neoplasm, nuclei in DLMS are blunt ended and cytoplasm is eosinophilic and fibrillar.[137] Pertinent differences between benign and borderline cutaneous smooth muscle tumors include nuclear detail in these two groups of neoplasms, as well as relative mitotic activity. The cells of leiomyomas have dispersed chromatin and physiologic nucleocytoplasmic ratios, whereas those of DLMS show enlarged nuclei with coarse chromatin and discernible nucleoli. Mitotic activity is absent in the former of these tumors, but DLMS regularly demonstrates its presence (Fig. 19-30). A rarely seen variant of cutaneous leiomyosarcoma is composed partially or wholly of granular cells,[141] potentially causing confusion with neural granular cell tumor.

There is no "maximum level" of mitotic activity above which a diagnosis of DLMS should be made, in contradistinction to the guidelines governing the classification of *visceral* smooth muscle tumors. In fact, the observation of *any* mitoses in cutaneous lesions of this type should raise considerable doubt over a benign interpretation.[206]

Superficial Hemangiopericytoma

Clinical Features. Hemangiopericytoma (HPC) only uncommonly arises in the subcutis, and most examples of this tumor are situated in the deep soft tissues.[66,207] Bona fide examples of subcuticular HPC are nodular, firm, reddish lesions that may attain a maximum size of 5 to 6 cm. They may be slightly tender

to palpation, in likeness to other smooth muscle tumors.[208] Adults are affected almost exclusively, with a peak incidence during middle life, and the extremities are the favored sites of origin for these neoplasms. Biologically, HPC of the subcutis has the potential to recur in up to 50% of cases. Examples that metastasize distantly are rare (less than 1%).[66]

Histopathologic Features. HPC is a cytologically monotonous, unencapsulated neoplasm that is composed of bluntly fusiform or polyhedral cells. These are arranged in large clusters or sheets, punctuated by numerous blood vessels with the caliber of venules or capillaries (Fig. 19-31). Vascular lumina in most examples focally demonstrate a "staghorn" configuration, branching like the antlers of a deer.[207] It should be noted that this histologic finding is not the sole criterion for the diagnosis of HPC; staghorn vessels also may be observed in tumors of epi-

Figure 19-31. (A) Hemangiopericytoma with apparently distinct borders. These can be found almost exclusively in the dermis and subcutis. (B) Prominent vascular channels that exist in a staghorn pattern. In the clearly benign form, mitoses are fewer than 4/10 hpf.

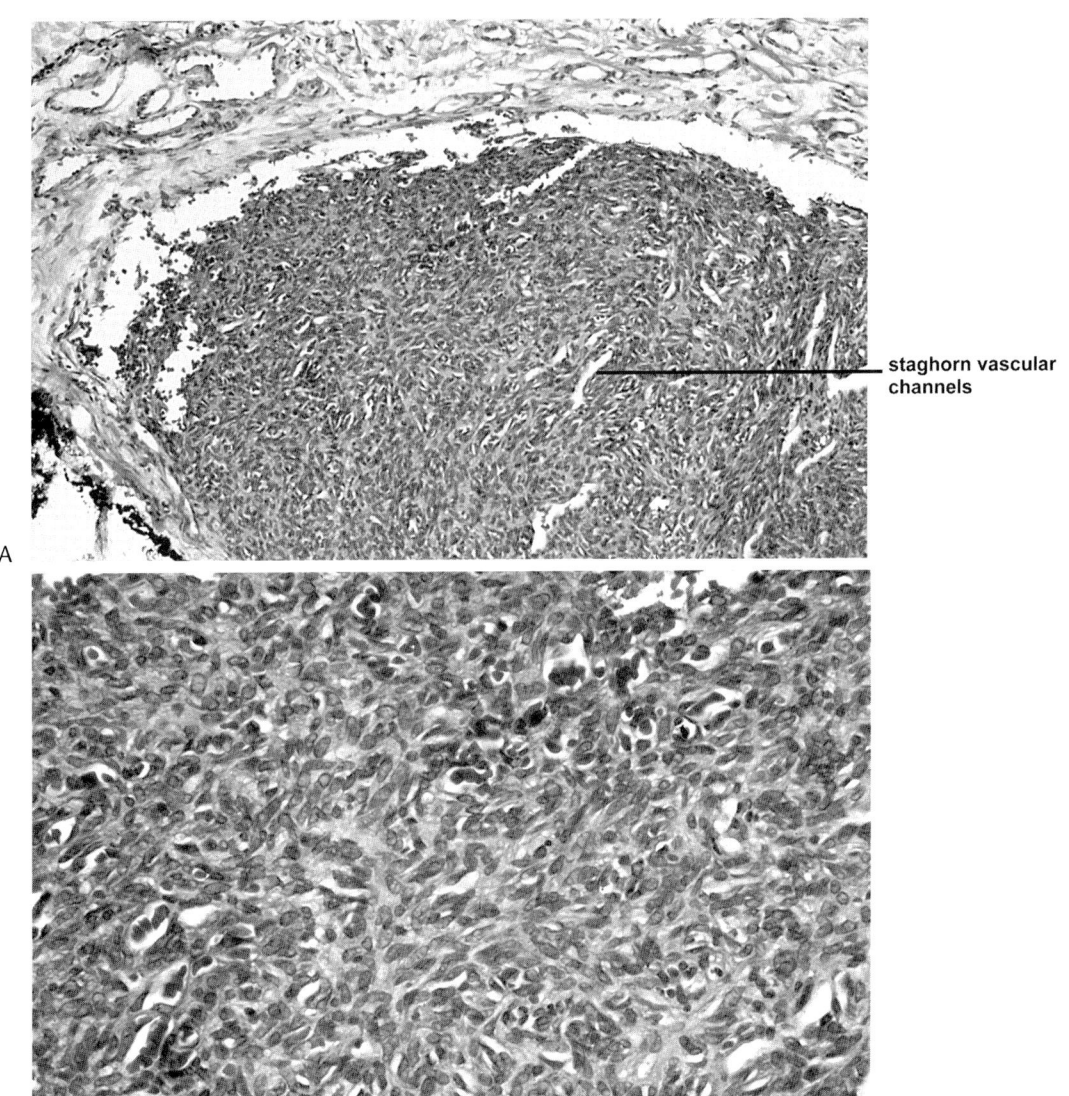

staghorn vascular channels

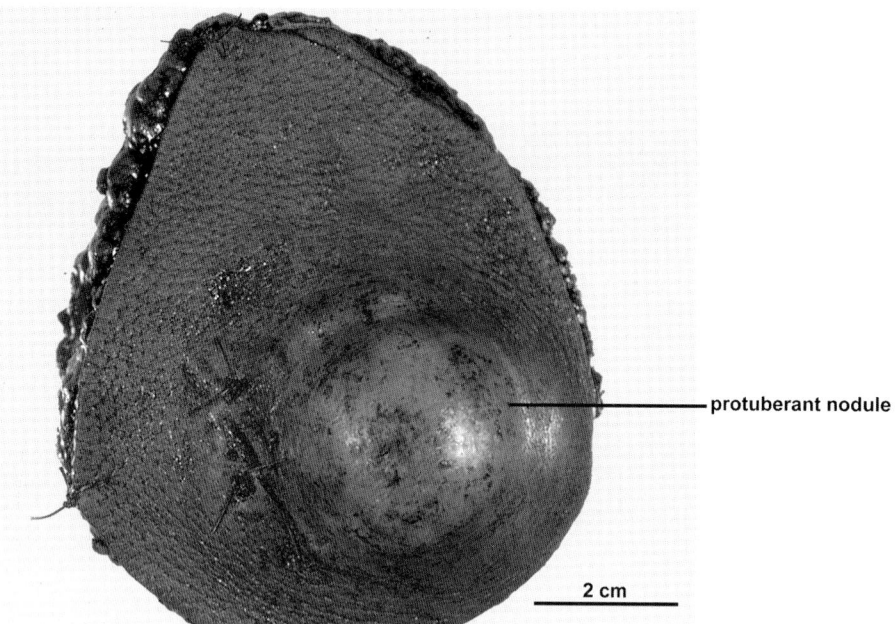

protuberant nodule

2 cm

Figure 19-32. This gross example of a dermatofibrosarcoma protuberans displays the origin of the name. It characteristically forms a nodule that is raised above the skin surface late in the course.

thelial, cartilaginous, and leiomyomatous or leiomyosarcomatous natures.[137]

Nuclear chromatin in the tumor cells of HPC is compact and hyperchromatic; accordingly, nucleoli are difficult to discern. Cytoplasm is modest in amount and amphophilic.

Several microscopic features are worrisome in regard to the potential for superficial HPC to recur or metastasize. These include a mitotic count of 4 or more per 10 high power ($\times$ 40) fields, spontaneous necrosis, and focally marked nuclear pleomorphism and atypia.[66] If such findings are observed, a note should be made in the pathology report that the neoplasm may have the ability to spread distantly, and close follow-up should be urged.

Differential diagnosis between HPC and lesions *simulating* it may be extremely difficult (if not impossible) on conventional microscopy. Immunostains are useful in this regard. Although it putatively shows modified myogenous differentiation, HPC is reactive only for vimentin and does not express actin isoforms or desmin, in contrast to leiomyoma and leiomyosarcoma. It similarly lacks epithelial markers, unlike carcinomas and sarcomas that represent histologic mimics of HPC.[209]

Borderline "Fibrohistiocytic" Neoplasms

Dermatofibrosarcoma Protuberans

Clinical Features. Dermatofibrosarcoma protuberans (DFSP) is typically a slowly growing, firm, reddish plaque or nodule that tends to arise on the proximal extremities and trunk.[137] Most patients are adults,[210] but cases in children also have been well documented.[211] The overlying skin may be attenuated or ulcerated.[210–214]

DFSP shows a reproducible tendency to recur after simple surgical excision and does so in approximately 50% of cases. With repeated regrowth of this tumor, it may assume a multinodular appearance, and the development of regional satellite lesions is also possible.[137] The latter eventuality is worrisome, because metastasizing variants of this tumor have usually recurred many times before distant spread occurs[212]; the disease-free interval between successive recurrences typically shortens each time.

Histopathologic Features. As its name implies, DFSP is a tumor that by definition protrudes above the surface of the contiguous, uninvolved skin (Fig. 19-32). Accordingly, neoplastic cells are typically seen throughout the dermis, and many lesions lack a grenz zone. DFSP is the archetypal storiform lesion in which short spindle cells are arranged in a "pinwheel" fashion throughout the mass[210] (Fig. 19-33). Nuclei show only modest pleomorphism and dispersed chromatin, and mitoses are generally scarce. The giant cells that are so common in benign cutaneous fibrohistiocytic neoplasms are absent in DFSP[137]; hence, observation of such elements should lead the pathologist to another diagnostic interpretation.

In its deep aspects, DFSP tends to infiltrate the subcuticular fat in a permeative fashion (Fig. 19-34) rather than using interlobular fibrous septa as scaffolds for downward growth as seen in unusually large dermatofibromas.[166] A time-honored adage for some dermatopathologists has been that DFSP and dermatofibroma differ only in their vertical extent of growth.[166] However, careful scrutiny of each neoplasm shows additional points of dissimilarity. The abundant collagenous stroma, xanthoma cells, and multinucleated giant cells of dermatofibroma are not seen in DFSP; conversely, storiform growth is much more pronounced in the latter tumor. The DFSP tends to infiltrate the subcutis in planes parallel to the epidermis, whereas the dermatofibroma produces short radiating extensions. Both lesions may induce hyperpigmentation and acanthosis in the overlying epidermis, but true epidermal hyperplasia is seen only in the dermatofibroma.[166,176,213]

Several microscopic variants of DFSP are now recognized. The *myxoid* subtype demonstrates a stromal mucin-rich matrix in which small capillaries are regularly interspersed; storiform growth is only vaguely represented in this lesion.[215] *Pigmented* DFSP is also known as the "Bednar tumor." It is virtually identical to conventional dermatofibrosarcoma except that pigmented stellate and spindle cells are regularly interspersed throughout the mass.[216] These have been shown convincingly to contain melanin, and I have seen examples of Bednar tumor that were misdiagnosed as melanomas as a consequence of this finding.

Other variants of DFSP show a partial composition by granular cells, or densely cellular, *fibrosarcoma-like* zones, in which the degree of nuclear atypia and mitotic activity is greater and a "herringbone" pattern of cell growth is observed[217–219] (Fig. 19-35). Lastly, evolution of DFSP into a high-grade pleomorphic tumor (with the features of malignant fibrous histiocytoma) has been reported.[220,221] I consider the latter form to represent *dedifferentiated* DFSP. It is tempting to speculate that metastasis of dermatofibrosarcomas will not occur until dedifferentiation supervenes, but I know of no systematic evaluation of this premise in the literature. A study by Connelly and Evans[219] failed to document an association of this type between fibrosarcoma-like growth in DFSP and heightened aggressiveness.

Some may consider the distinction between BFHPR (see above) and DFSP to represent a fine point of academia. I do not share this view because of differences in histology[179] and the documented metastatic potential of some recurring dermatofibrosarcomas.[137] To reiterate, distant spread has never been reported with reference to BFHPR.[175,176]

Giant Cell Fibroblastoma

Clinical Features. In 1983, Shmookler and Enzinger[222] reported a peculiar tumor of childhood that they designated as *giant cell fibroblastoma* (GCF). Patients with this lesion are less than 20 years old, and it typically takes the form of an ill-defined skin-colored nodule on the trunk or extremities. The cut surfaces of GCF are commonly described as "gelatinous."[223–226]

GCF recurs in up to 50% of cases after excision; however, there have been no examples of distant metastases to date.[223,226] This neoplasm is grouped with the fibrohistiocytic proliferations because of the observation that *recurrent* GCF may be indistinguishable from DFSP (in either classic or variant forms) microscopically[223]; moreover, de novo DFSP may contain GCF-like foci.[227]

Histopathologic Features. A biphasic pattern of growth typifies GCF. Superficial elements of the neoplasm in the papillary and reticular dermis are represented by bland stellate cells that are set in a fibromxyoid stroma, punctuated by floret-type multinucleated giant cells.[223] Deeper components assume an "angiectoid" appearance in which interconnecting pseudovascular spaces are observed. The latter channels are lined in part by floret cells and do not contain erythrocytes.[225] Peripheral aspects of the proliferation blend with the surrounding dermis, but the deep interface with subjacent subcutaneous fat is usually more distinct. Mitotic figures are rare in GCF, and storiform growth is lacking in de novo examples.

As cited above, *recurrent* lesions may retain the histologic profile just described, or they may acquire nearly all of the microscopic features of conventional DFSP. A case of GCF that regrew as a Bednar tumor has been documented.[228]

Differential diagnosis primarily centers on angiosarcoma and rudimentary meningocele (see below). These lesions are easily excluded from consideration by attention to clinical data alone, because angiosarcoma virtually never occurs in children or ado-

Figure 19-33. The most common architectural pattern of a dermatofibrosarcoma protuberans is that of a storiform arrangement of short fibroblastic cells. Only a single cell type is present. The multiform composition of the benign dermatofibroma is not seen.

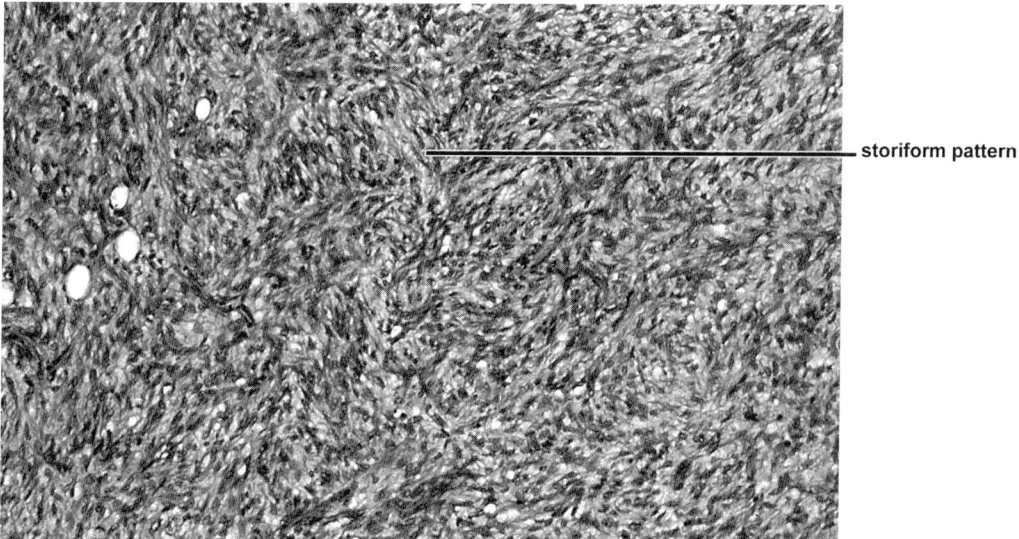

storiform pattern

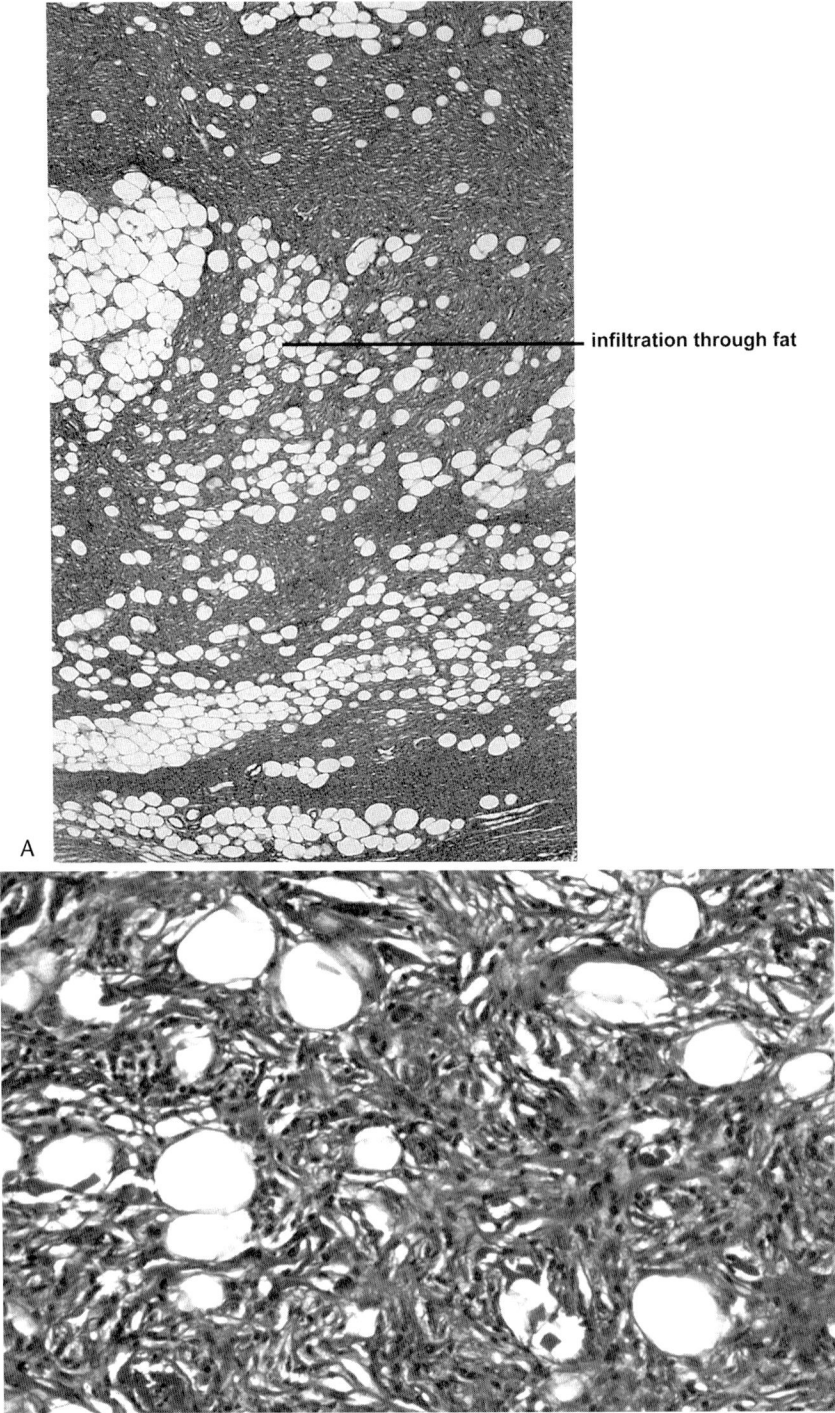

infiltration through fat

Figure 19-34. (**A**) Whereas a dermatofibroma is dermal based, the dermatofibrosarcoma protuberans (DFSP) is based in the deep dermis and subcutis. In this example, it is noted that the tumor infiltrates deeply into adipose tissue. Not only does it infiltrate into adipose tissue, but it does so in a vertical as well as a horizontal pattern. It has been written that the parallel planes of infiltration are characteristic of a DFSP. (**B**) Characteristics of the storiform pattern in the infiltrated adipose tissue.

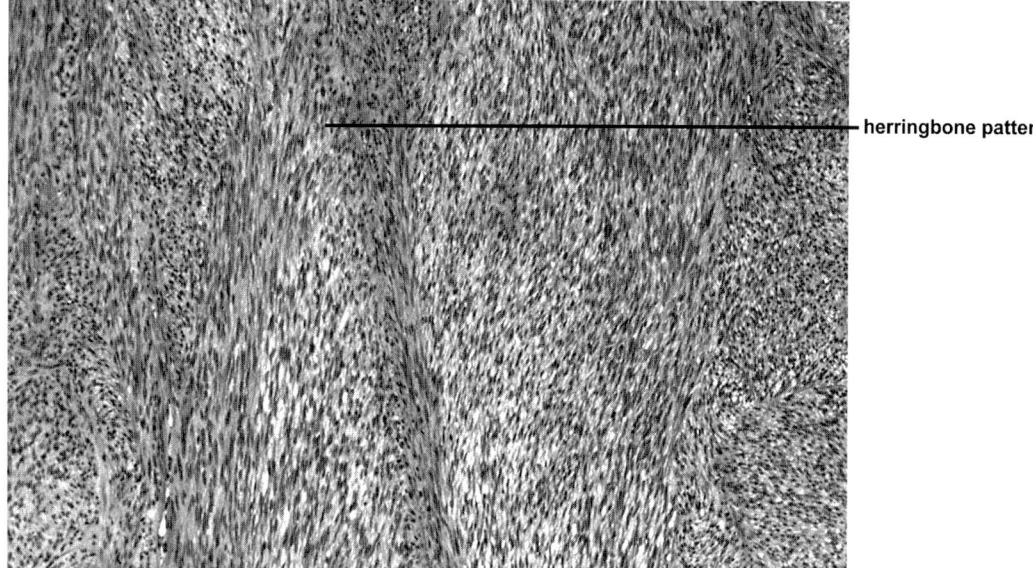

herringbone pattern

Figure 19-35. The dermatofibrosarcoma protuberans may eventuate in a fibrosarcomatous pattern. Successive recurrences have been reported to be associated with this pattern as well as with ultimate metastasis.

lescents, and rudimentary meningocele does not affect the trunk or extremities.[229]

Plexiform Fibrous Histiocytomas

Clinical Features. Plexiform fibrous histiocytoma (PFH) was first described by Enzinger and Zhang[230] in 1988. In that series, 65 patients were described, all of whom were children, adolescents, or young adults. They had nodular lesions that most often arose in the subcutaneous tissues of the extremities and that measured up to several centimeters at diagnosis. There were no particularly distinguishing macroscopic characteristics of such tumors.

Since that time, several other examples of PFH have been documented.[231] It has become increasingly clear that this neoplasm has a marked proclivity for local recurrence (in up to 67% of cases), but there have been only two instances of metastasis to regional lymph nodes. No patient with PFH has died of the tumor.[232,233]

Histopathologic Features. On low-power microscopy, PFH has an appearance close to that of plexiform neural tumors and causes differential diagnostic difficulty with regard to the latter neoplasms. One observes fascicles of spindle cells in the corium and subcutis, separated from one another by unremarkable dermal fibrous or subcuticular adipose tissue. The aggregates of tumor cells are arranged in such a manner that they recapitulate the image of a miniature nerve plexus.[230]

However, closer inspection shows several points of difference between PFH and peripheral nerve sheath neoplasms. The former lesion is composed of relatively nondescript spindle cells with enlarged, minimally pleomorphic, slightly hyperchromatic nuclei and notable mitotic activity. Focal storiform growth within each fascicle is often seen, and the tumor cells also may mantle small pseudovascular spaces or myxoid foci. A key finding is the presence of osteoclast-like giant cells, which

are interspersed among the fusiform elements.[230,231] These are essentially never observed in nerve sheath tumors.

The margins of PFH are indistinct, and one cannot always be certain that the lesion has been excised completely in limited resection specimens. This feature probably contributes to the high incidence of local recurrence reported in most series.

Angiomatoid Malignant Fibrous Histiocytoma

Clinical Features. Among all superficial mesenchymal neoplasms, the angiomatoid malignant fibrous histiocytoma (AMFH) is unusual in many respects. Patients tend to be adolescents—with a mean age of 17 years—but occasional examples also arise in elderly adults.[232–234] The extremities, trunk, and head and neck are the preferred sites of origin for AMFH, the sizes of which range from 0.5 to 12 cm. On cut section, the tumor has an obviously cystic and hemorrhagic quality and is composed of dense white-gray tissue.[233]

Most notably, this lesion may be associated with systemic symptoms and signs, including hypochromic-microcytic anemia, extreme fatigue, weight loss, and fever, even though the tumor mass may be relatively small and localized. All these problems resolve after resection of the neoplasm.[234]

Costa and Weiss[233] have evaluated 108 examples of AMFH, observing 4.7% metastases in local recurrence in 12% of cases and death in one patient. Hence, it would appear that a biologically "borderline" status is appropriate for this neoplasm.

Histopathologic Features. The three basic microscopic constituents of AMFH are (1) solid sheets of spindled or bluntly fusiform tumor cells, focally assuming a storiform growth pattern; (2) central erythrocytic pools that are not mantled by endothelial cells; and (3) surrounding lymphoid inflammation (often with germinal center formation) with or without a fibrous pseudocapsule[232–234] (Fig. 19-36).

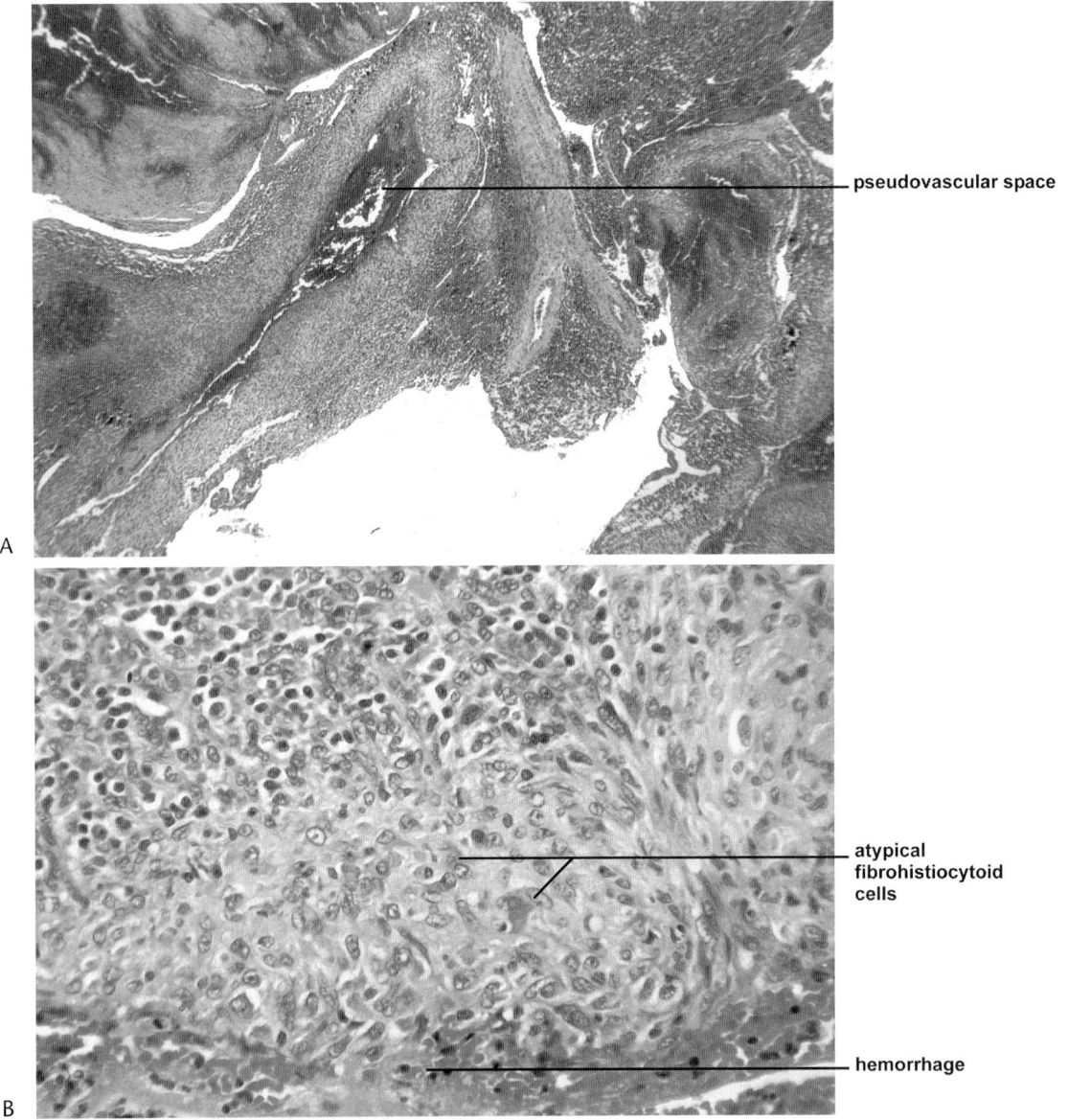

Figure 19-36. (A) Low-power pattern of pseudovascular spaces found in an angiomatoid malignant fibrous histiocytoma. (B) Edge of one of the pseudovascular spaces. Adjacent to the hemorrhage and necrosis are the features of atypical cells of a malignant fibrous histiocytoma. Giant cells as well as elongate fibroblast forms are noted.

The degree of nuclear atypia in the cells of AMFH is modest; chromatin is vesicular, with small nucleoli and mitotic activity. Scattered pleomorphic giant cells may be dispersed throughout the neoplastic population in some cases; myxoid stromal change and deposition of hemosiderin also may be seen.[234]

An important diagnostic error in reference to AMFH is to mistake the tumor for an organizing hematoma. It should be remembered that broad, compact sheets of spindle cells are never observed in the latter lesion, as regularly seen in AMFH. Negative results of immunostains for endothelial markers also assist in excluding true vascular neoplasms.

Overtly Malignant Neoplasms

Those mesenchymal neoplasms that demonstrate a reproducible tendency for recurrence *and* distant metastasis are rightly considered to be overtly malignant. These tumors manifest a variety of cellular lineages, as detailed below. As mentioned at the outset of this chapter, they are grouped together by generic histologic appearance because many malignant lesions have the capacity to manifest an undifferentiated image on conventional microscopy. Accordingly, differential diagnostic considerations are broader and receive more attention than those presented above.

Small Cell Neoplasms

Peripheral Neuroepithelioma/Extraskeletal Ewing's Sarcoma

Clinical Features. Peripheral neuroepithelioma[235] (PNE; also known as *primitive neuroectodermal tumor*[236,237]) is considered to be closely allied, if not identical, to *extraskeletal Ewing's sarcoma*.[238–240] Both lesions are rare in the superficial subcutis and dermis, where they present as nodular, red-violet, ill-defined tumefactions.[235,238,239] Patients with PNE are usually children, adolescents, or young adults, but older individuals are occasionally affected as well. The neoplasms may attain a maximum dimension of 10 cm and are rapidly growing. The trunk and extremities are favored locations for PNE.[235] Even with prompt diagnosis and therapy, PNE has a 5-year mortality rate of approximately 50%; distant metastases to lungs, liver, bones, and brain are common.[241]

Histopathologic Features. PNE represents one of the quintessential small round cell tumors. One observes sheets, vague nests, and occasional cords of closely apposed monomorphic neoplastic cells that are approximately twice to three times the size of mature lymphocytes (Fig. 19-37). Tumor cells are often embedded in a fine fibrillar background. These aggregates are separated from one another by a delicate but complex fibrovascular stromal network. Mitotic activity is variable but may be surprisingly sparse; similarly, cellular apoptosis and regional necrosis may or may not be present.[242] The nuclear detail of PNE is the most helpful clue to its recognition. Chromatin is typically evenly distributed, and nucleoli, if present, are small. Cytoplasm is modest in amount and amphophilic.[235]

A minority of PNE cases will exhibit the presence of intercellular rosettes, betraying the primitive neural nature of this neoplasm.[235] However, the fibrillary intercellular meshwork seen in many examples of metastatic *neuroblastoma*—an important differential diagnostic alternative—is lacking in PNE.[242] Similarly, focal nuclear pleomorphism and multinucleation are uniformly absent in contrast to the characteristics of small round cell (embryonal or alveolar) *rhabdomyosarcoma*. *Merkel cell carcinoma* also enters into diagnostic consideration in this context, because the latter tumor may arise deep in the skin without any intervening dermal component. Because it is somewhat related to PNE in terms of cellular differentiation, electron microscopy or immunohistology is often necessary to distinguish between these lesions.[243] Discriminating results of such analyses (as applied to small round cell tumors in general) are outlined in Table 19-2.

Finally, *malignant lymphoma* of the subcutis may simulate any of the other small cell neoplasms, including PNE.[243] The nuclei of lymphoid cells differ from those of other alternatives, because they are more irregular in contour and have a greater tendency to overlap one another. The most certain indicator of hematopoietic differentiation is the CD45 immunostain.[244]

Metastatic Neuroblastoma

Clinical Features. Neuroblastomas involve the skin only in stage IV or IVs disease, and the great majority are therefore seen in infants. These tumors are multiple and present as blue-violet cutaneous nodules and papules (potentially in any skin field) in contrast to the clinical appearance of other small round cell tumors.[245]

Histopathologic Features. The neurofibrillary matrical background (Fig. 19-38) of neuroblastoma was mentioned above in reference to the differential diagnosis of PNE. This attribute is the most useful discriminant between the two lesions

Figure 19-37. The peripheral neuroepithelioma is a small round cell tumor. The tumor cells are arranged in vague nests and sheets and embedded in a vague finely fibrillar background. Apoptosis and mitotic activity are variable. The tumors are similar to neuroblastoma but possess less extracellular neurofibrillary matrix than a neuroblastoma.

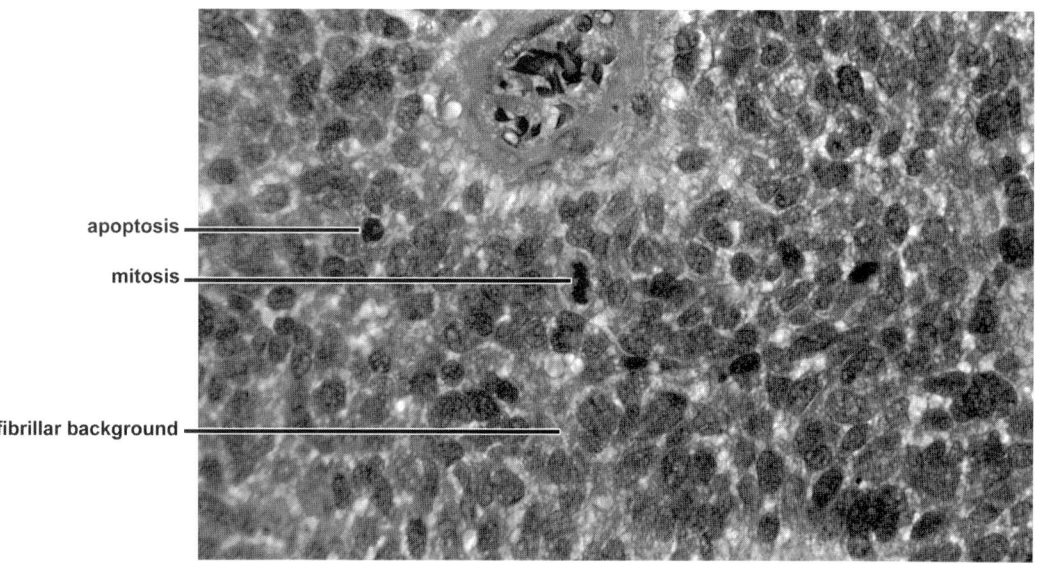

Table 19-2. Specialized Features of Malignant Cutaneous Small Round Cell Neoplasms

Tumor Type	Electron Microscopy					Immunohistochemistry				
	ICJ	FIL	NSG	MTL	GLY	BL	KER	DES	SYN/LEU7	LCA
Ewing's sarcoma/peripheral neuroepithelioma	+	0	±	±	±	±	0	0	±	0
Rhabdomyosarcoma	0	+	0	0	+	+	0	+	0	0
Neuroendocrine carcinoma	+	+	+	0	±	±	+	0	+	0
Metastatic neuroblastoma	±	±	±	+ +	0	0	0	0	+ +	0
Malignant lymphoma	0	0	0	0	0	0	0	0	0	+ +

Abbreviations: ICJ, intercellular junctional complexes; FIL, cytoplasmic microfilaments; NSG, neurosecretory granules; MTL, microtubules; GLY, cytoplasmic glycogen; BL, pericellular basal lamina; KER, keratin; DES, desmin; SYN, synaptophysin; LCA, leukocyte common antigen (CD45).

on conventional microscopy, because they are otherwise closely similar histologically. In difficult cases involving solitary metastases of "undifferentiated" neuroblastoma, electron microscopy and immunohistology are capable of providing a final interpretation[243] (Table 19-2).

Rhabdomyosarcoma

Clinical Features. Rhabdomyosarcoma is an extremely rare primary cutaneous neoplasm. Indeed, only a few cases exclusive to skin have been well documented.[246,247] It arises primarily in the head and neck of children who have a rapidly growing red-violet nodular mass.[247] Rhabdomyosarcoma is an aggressive, often lethal neoplasm that usually metastasizes distantly; thus, rapid diagnosis and polychemotherapy are necessary to any chance of cure.

Histopathologic Features. Although rhabdomyosarcoma is generically classified as a small round cell tumor, there are three subtypes. *Embryonal rhabdomyosarcoma* is composed of small cells with eosinophilic cytoplasm arranged in sheets. Foci of myxoid stromal change may be present. *Alveolar rhabdomyosarcoma* exhibits small cells with eosinophilic cytoplasm arranged in a distinctive alveolar pattern. Tumor cell dyscohesion yields irregular clefts and acinus-like structures (Fig. 19-39). Mitotic activity is usually brisk in all forms of rhabdomyosarcoma, and individual cell necrosis is a common finding as well. Although *pleomorphic* and *spindle cell* variants of the neoplasm have been described in deep soft tissue sites, they are unknown as primary cutaneous lesions.[247,248]

Differential diagnosis with other small round cell neoplasms is largely as described above in reference to PNE. Discriminating features of rhabdomyosarcoma include the ultrastructural presence of cytoplasmic thick and thin filaments that aggregate into primitive

Figure 19-38. The metastatic neuroblastoma has similarities to the peripheral neuroepithelioma. The chromatin pattern noted in this example of neuroblastoma is much more dense than in peripheral neuroepithelioma. Significant in the diagnosis of neuroblastoma is the presence of cells that possess small, triangular portions of cytoplasm. This is indicative of neuronal differentiation. Rosettes may also be found.

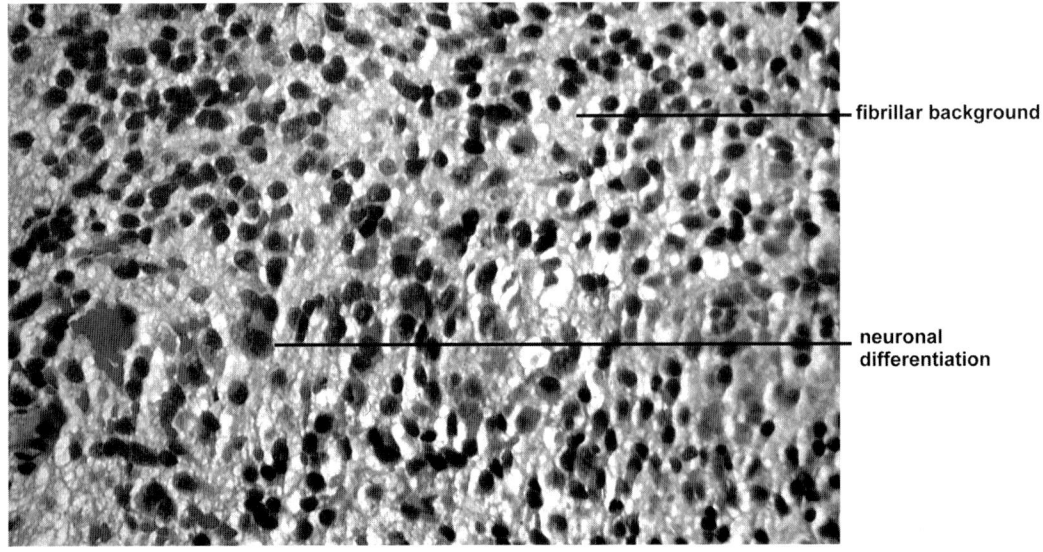

fibrillar background

neuronal differentiation

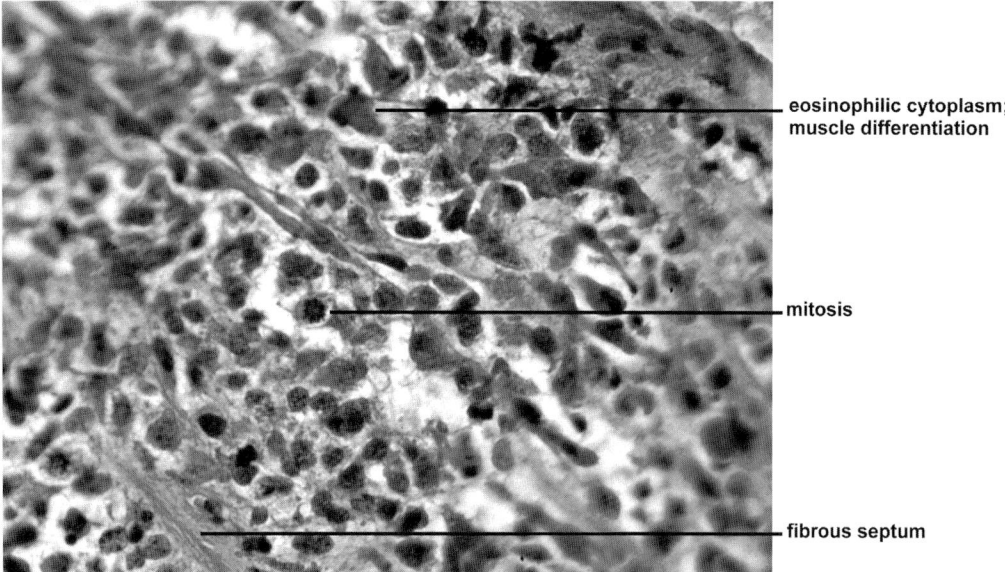

eosinophilic cytoplasm; muscle differentiation

mitosis

fibrous septum

Figure 19-39.   The alveolar rhabdomyosarcoma is another form of small round cell tumor. The example shown is an alveolar rhabdomyosarcoma in which spaces are lined by small tumor cells in an alveolar pattern. The small tumor cells possess small quantities of eosinophilic cytoplasm that mark for muscle determinants.

sarcomeres; immunohistologic reactivity for desmin and muscle-specific actin is of great diagnostic assistance [243,247] (Table 19-2).

In the differential diagnosis is the lesion known as *malignant Triton tumor*, a malignant peripheral nerve sheath (schwannian) sarcoma with divergent rhabdomyosarcomatous differentiation.[249,250] This lesion is seen principally in adults.

Spindle Cell Neoplasms

Subcuticular Leiomyosarcoma

Clinical Features.   The clinical features of subcutaneous leiomyosarcoma are identical to those of its dermal variant (see above) except that the former lesion tends to be larger and, ob-

viously, more deeply seated.[204–206] It recurs approximately twice as often as DLMS does, and distant metastases to the lungs, other soft tissue sites, and the liver are observed in 30% to 40% of cases.[137]

Histopathologic Features.   Subcutaneous leiomyosarcoma is similar microscopically to DLMS, but demonstrates a greater degree of cellular pleomorphism, nuclear atypia, and mitotic activity (Fig. 19-40). Fascicles of fusiform cells in this tumor extend deeply into the adipose tissue and often involve underlying fascia and striated muscle as well.[204,205] Prominent stromal vascularity is also more common in the subcutaneous variant of leiomyosarcoma, yielding the designations of *angioleiomyosar-*

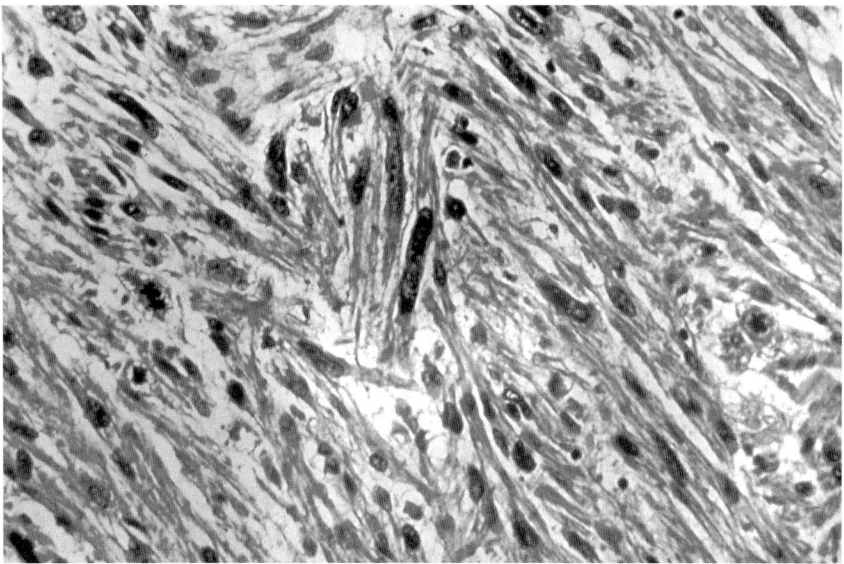

Figure 19-40.   The deep leiomyosarcoma. Similar to the dermal leiomyosarcoma is a spindle cell malignant neoplasm. This example displays very pleomorphic spindle cells arranged in short fascicles that intersect at acute angles. Foci of necrosis were prominent within the tumor.

Figure 19-41. The malignant peripheral nerve sheath tumor is a sarcoma that arises from nerve sheath. It may arise from neurilemmoma, neurofibroma, or be malignant de novo. This example is characterized by atypical spindle cells with small foci of necrosis. The nuclei maintain a near palisaded pattern. The nuclei are also short and maintain comma or S shapes.

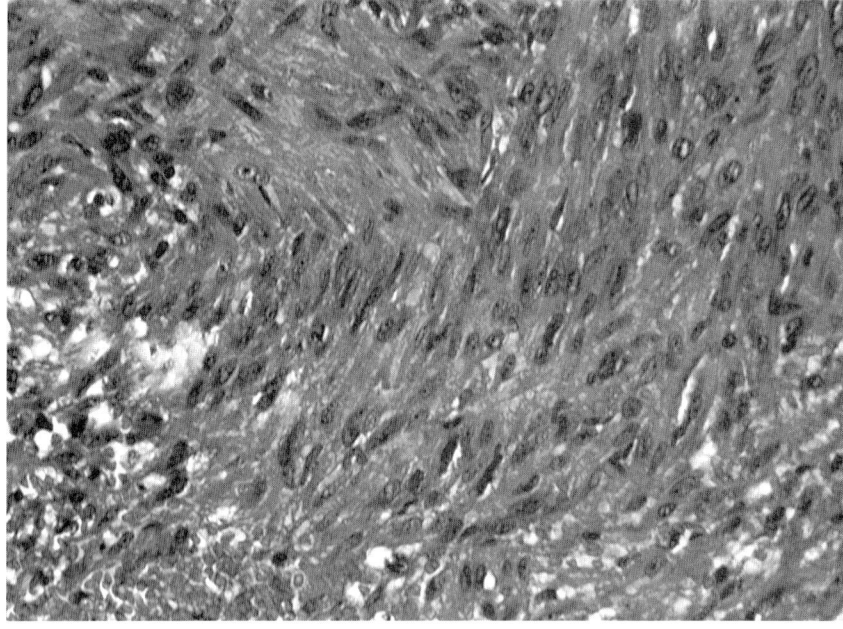

coma or *vascular leiomyosarcoma*. In fact, based on the results of immunohistologic analysis showing frequent reactivity for the CD57 antigen (a potential marker of vascular medial smooth muscle) in subcutaneous leiomyosarcoma, a proposal has been made that this subtype pursues specialized vascular myogenous differentiation.[209]

Malignant Peripheral Nerve Sheath Tumors

Clinical Features. Outside the setting of von Recklinghausen's disease, the existence of cutaneous malignant peripheral nerve sheath tumors (MPNST) has been questioned in the past. It is well recognized that approximately 1% to 3% of patients with von Recklinghausen's disease—both children and adults—will develop malignant transformation in superficial neurofibromas, in which cases the latter lesions rapidly expand in size and often become painful.[251]

Sporadic cutaneous MPNST have been increasingly accepted as bona fide entities over the past few years. These lesions are nodules or plaques with variable growth rates, and they have a propensity to arise on the trunk or extremities of adults.[252,253] Ulceration may supervene, and local paresthesias or dysesthesias are sometimes observed if the masses are associated with major nerves.

The behavior of MPNST is generally predicated on its size, location, and surgical resectability. However, tumors arising in the skin more often demonstrate local recurrence (in approximately 80% of cases) than distant metastasis (15% to 20%).[253]

Histopathologic Features. The microscopic features of MPNST are variable; indeed, this neoplasm is one of the great "chameleons" of pathology. In most cases, one observes a modestly pleomorphic proliferation of spindle cells in the dermis and subcutis in which cellularity is highly variable from region to region. Most have "wavy" or serpiginous nuclei[252,253] (Fig. 19-41). The tumors cells are randomly arranged or configured

in acute angle intersecting fascicles (the so-called herringbone growth pattern) (Fig. 19-42). Myxoid stromal change is evident in approximately one-third of all cases, and a focal storiform arrangement of tumor cells is often observed.[253]

These lesions entrap cutaneous appendages rather than destroying them, but the peripheral margins of growth are indistinct. Permeation into the subcutis and underlying soft tissue is common. Nuclear atypia are modest to moderate, and mitotic activity is present but not striking.

Occasional examples of cutaneous MPNST—particularly those occurring in patients with von Reckinghausen's disease—manifest divergent mesenchymal differentiation. Tumors showing foci of rhabdomyosarcomatous elements are known as *malignant Triton tumors*[249] (Fig.19-43). Although de novo rhabdomyosarcoma is a highly aggressive neoplasm, Triton tumors are no different biologically from conventional MPNST. Other divergent elements that have been reported in such lesions include osteosarcoma, pigmented malignant melanoma (*melanotic MPNST*), chondrosarcoma, adenocarcinoma (*glandular MPNST*), and angiosarcoma.[253,254] Electron microscopic evaluation demonstrates elongated, overlapping cytoplasmic processes in the spindle cells of MPNST with focal pericellular basal lamina and primitive appositional plaques.[137]

Immunohistologic studies show reactivity for S-100 protein in approximately 50% of cases, CD57 in 33%, and myelin basic protein in 15% to 20%.[255] When used as a panel, one or more of these markers is present in 70% of all lesions. Divergent tumors also may express desmin or muscle-specific actin, keratin, or von Willebrand factor and the CD31 or CD34 antigens. In light of this heterogeneity in the immunophenotype of MPNST, it may be safely said that ultrastructural assessments are usually more definitive in resolving diagnostic difficulties.[8]

Differential diagnosis includes leiomyosarcoma, spindle cell squamous carcinoma, DFSP, atypical fibroxanthoma, and desmoplastic or neurotropic melanoma.[252] All but the last of these possibilities are adequately distinguished from MPNST

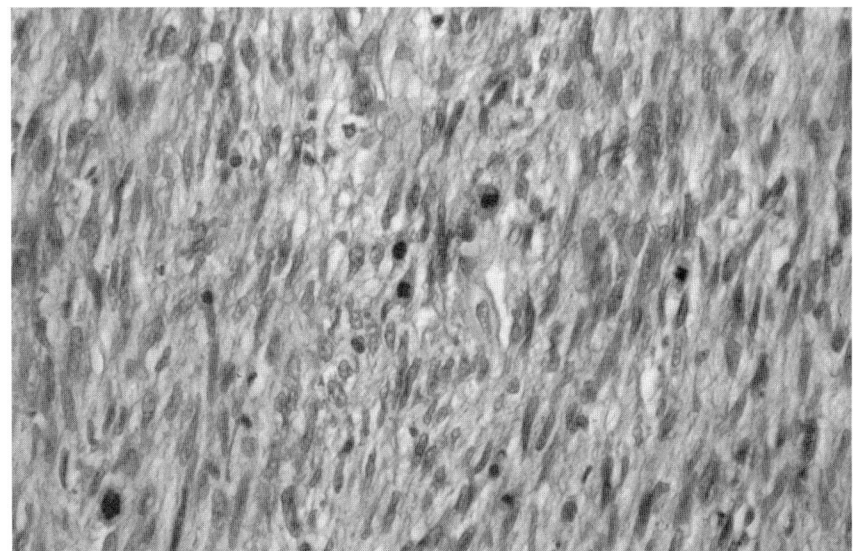

Figure 19-42. The tumor may also display a sarcomatous, herringbone pattern with numerous mitoses. The mitotic rate in a malignant peripheral nerve sheath tumor may be as low as 2/20 hpf.

by electron microscopy and immunohistology [137] (Table 19-3). It must be acknowledged that neuroid spindle cell melanomas and true nerve sheath tumors share many points of synonymity.[256] Ultrastructural features of the two groups are virtually identical inasmuch as spindle cell melanomas often lose their synthesis of cytoplasmic premelanosomes.[257] Similarly, the HMB-45 antigen, a specific determinant of melanocytic cells, is absent in almost all neuroid melanomas and is not seen in MPNST.[258] Thus, one may not be able to make this distinction with certainty in the absence of a concurrent or previous intraepidermal melanocytic proliferation at the same anatomic site. Separation of the two tumors may not be *necessary* because of similarities in their biologic potential and behavior.[256]

Kaposi's Sarcoma

Clinical Features.   The clinical characteristics of Kaposi's sarcoma (KS) are familiar to most physicians because of the tremendous increase in its incidence occasioned by the AIDS epidemic in the 1980s. Prior to that time, KS was a relatively rarely encountered lesion outside of the Mediterranean Basin and Africa.[259]

This neoplasm occurs in four well-defined clinical settings.[259–261] *Classic* KS is a disease that predominantly affects elderly men of Middle-Eastern or Italian heritage and that manifests as multiple, coalescent, red-brown macules and plaques on the distal lower extremities. A subset of patients has lesions that resemble deep lymphangiomas, accompanied by lym-

Figure 19-43.   The malignant Triton tumor is a malignant peripheral nerve sheath tumor that contains a component of striated muscle. Other divergent elements can be found in these tumors such as malignant melanoma, osteosarcoma, chondrosarcoma, adenocarcinoma, and angiosarcoma.

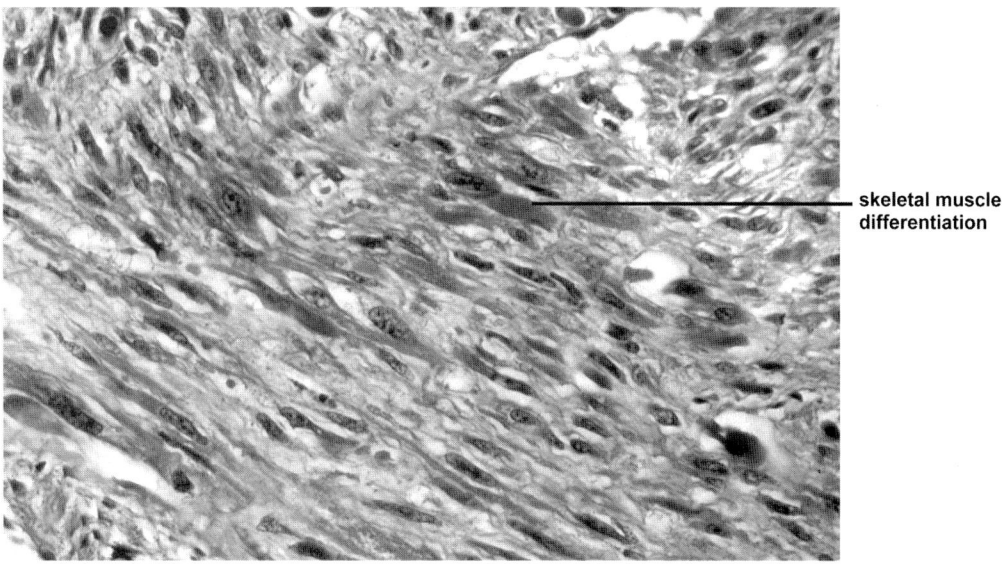

skeletal muscle differentiation

Table 19-3. Specialized Pathologic Features of Malignant Cutaneous Spindle Cell Tumors

Tumor	Electron Microscopy			Immunohistochemistry						
	ICJ	WPB	ECP	FDBC	KER	VIM	S-100	LEU7	DES	CD31/UEL
Leiomyosarcoma	0	0	0	+	0	±	±	±	+	0
MPNST	0	0	+	0	0	+	±	±	0	0
Spindle cell angiosarcoma	±	±	0	0	0	+	0	0	0	+
Spindle cell squamous carcinoma	+	0	0	0	+	±	0	0	0	0
Spindle cell malignant melanoma	0	0	±	0	0	+	+	±	0	0
Kaposi's sarcoma	0	0	0	±	0	+	0	0	0	0

Abbreviations: ICJ, intercellular junctional complexes; ECP, elongated cytoplasmic processes; KER, keratin; S-100, S-100 protein; UEL, *Ulex europaeus* I lectin binding; WPB, Weibel-Palade bodies; FDBC, filament-dense body complexes; VIM, vimentin; DES, desmin; MPNST, malignant peripheral nerve sheath tumor.

phedema of the extremities. Nodular, sometimes ulcerated tumors of the skin and viscera eventually supervene in this variant, but only after a prolonged period of time. African KS is seen in young black patients from restricted portions of the African continent. Women are almost as frequently afflicted as men, and their mean age is less than that of classic KS patients by two to three decades. The disorder is more rapidly progressive in African KS, with relatively early appearance of nodular lesions and involvement of lymph nodes and internal organs. *KS associated with iatrogenic immunosuppression* shares clinical features with both the classic and African subtypes and primarily affects recipients of allogeneic organ transplants. AIDS-related KS is precipitated by infection with the HIV. At the outset of the AIDS pandemic, it was first noted in young homosexual men,[262] with lesser numbers of cases in intravenous drug abusers and recipients of infected blood products.

Although the other manifestations of AIDS have become more evenly distributed among all infected patient populations, KS has remained largely confined to gay males. In fact, its incidence has already begun to decline, even though the number of HIV-infected individuals continues to rise on a worldwide scale. The reasons for these epidemiologic peculiarities are unknown at the present time.[263]

AIDS-related KS has a deceptively innocuous appearance at its onset, taking the form of ill-defined macular "patches" that often resemble ecchymoses.[256,264] In contrast to the topographic confinement of the classic variant, KS in AIDS patients may affect virtually any skin field and also is seen in the mucosa.[262] Visceral involvement also appears rapidly, in likeness to that in the African form. KS has been associated with HLA-DR5 and cytomegalovirus infection.[265–267] The tumor has been considered an altered tissue response and a true neoplasm.[268,269] It may be a tumor of endothelial or myogenic cells.[270,271]

Clinically, "early" KS most often takes a macular or "patch" form.[264] Microscopically, this variant is extremely subtle. One sees only a limited proliferation of small, attenuated, interanastomosing but bland blood vessels in the periappendageal reticular corium, together with an excess of nondescript spindle cells throughout the dermal connective tissue (Fig. 19-44). In addition, small pre-existing blood vessels are often invested by a lymphoplasmacytic infiltrate. The "promontory" sign, wherein

neovascular channels are formed around native vessels—yielding profiles that simulate the promontory of a cliff—is a helpful diagnostic finding[85,260,264] (Fig. 19-45). Small groupings of venule-like blood vessels are also interspersed randomly throughout the dermis in some cases, and extravasated erythrocytes are inconspicuous if present at all.[260] McNutt et al[272] have also called attention to the fact that endothelial cells within "new" (neoplastic) blood vessels of KS are often apoptotic in the patch stage. This observation is unique and would not be expected in benign vascular proliferations.

"Plaque"-stage KS features the appearance of more organized aggregates of spindle cells, forming small fascicles in admixture with capillary-sized neovascular channels, extravasated erythrocytes, hemosiderin, and stromal hemosiderin granules[85,259,260,273] (Fig. 19-46). The groupings of neoplastic cells are most often diffusely dispersed throughout the dermis, but they sometimes assume a pseudolobular configuration.[260] Another useful diagnostic clue that appears at this phase of tumor evolution is the presence of hyaline globules in the neoplastic endothelial cells. These represent phagocytosed erythrocytes, as documented by the peroxidase reaction, and they also may be stained with the periodic acid–Schiff–diastase method.[259] Hyaline globules are not sufficient unto themselves for a diagnosis of KS, because they can rarely be seen in non-neoplastic vascular proliferations of the skin.[260,273] However, they are helpful when interpreted in the proper context. Finally, small papillary projections of tumor cells may be observed within ectatic neovascular spaces in this stage of KS, together with racemose, "dissecting" luminal profiles throughout the dermis.[273]

The truly spindle cell stage of KS is its "nodular" phase, where fusiform elements compose the bulk of the proliferating cell population. Their nuclei are only modestly hyperchromatic, with indistinct nucleoli, and cytoplasm is scant and amphophilic. A notable diagnostic feature is the presence of cytoplasmic vacuoles in the spindle cells (Fig. 19-47), probably representing a primitive attempt at vascular lumen formation.[274] Another helpful microscopic finding is that the fusiform cells of KS appear to "spare" dermal zones that surround pre-existing vessels, leaving hypocellular cuffs around the latter struc-

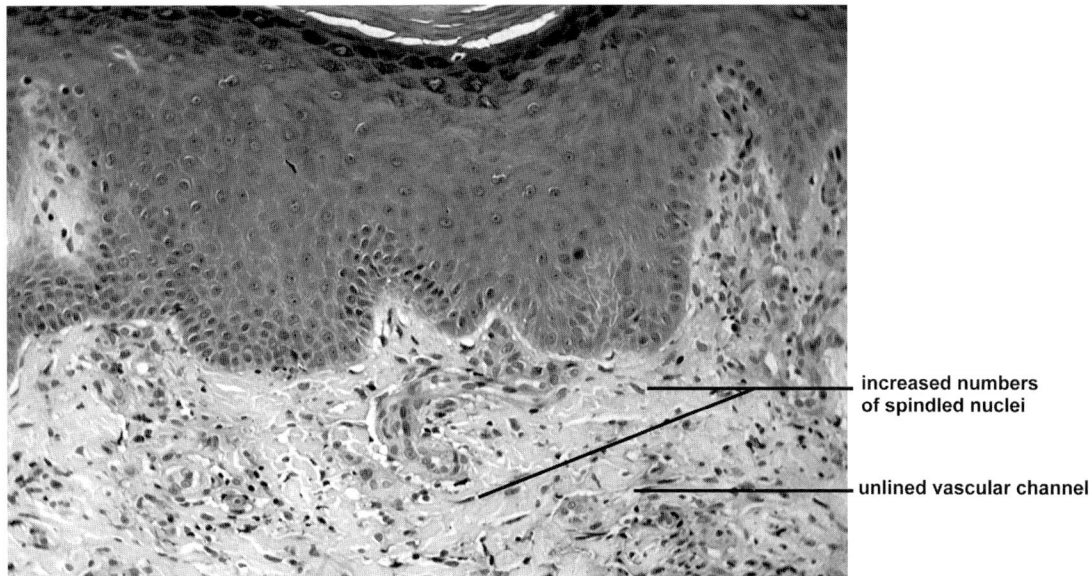

increased numbers
of spindled nuclei

unlined vascular channel

Figure 19-44. Early Kaposi's sarcoma is characterized by a proliferation of small attenuated anastomosing bland blood vessels in the dermis. Small numbers of spindle cells are also present and can be seen as increased numbers of nuclei between the collagen bundles.

tures.[275] Extravasated erythrocytes and stromal hemosiderin deposition are maximal in scope in the nodular stage of KS, and hyaline globules often are numerous in the neoplastic cells.

Differential diagnosis includes leiomyosarcoma, spindle cell melanoma, spindle cell squamous carcinoma, MPNST, and spindle cell angiosarcoma. All but the last of these possibilities are easily excluded by attention to histologic detail or application of immunostains.[260,273,274]

Spindle cell angiosarcoma is a rare lesion, the microscopic attributes of which are nearly identical to those of nodular KS.[85,274] Nevertheless, the clinical features of the two conditions usually differ substantially. Spindle cell angiosarcoma also exhibits a much higher degree of nuclear atypia and mitotic activity. Moreover, immunostains for *Ulex europaeus*, CD31, and CD34 are typically positive in spindle cell angiosarcoma but not in spindle cell KS[259] (Table 19-3).

Figure 19-45. The promontory sign consists of neovascular proliferations that form around pre-existing vessels. This is a helpful, but not absolutely diagnostic, feature.

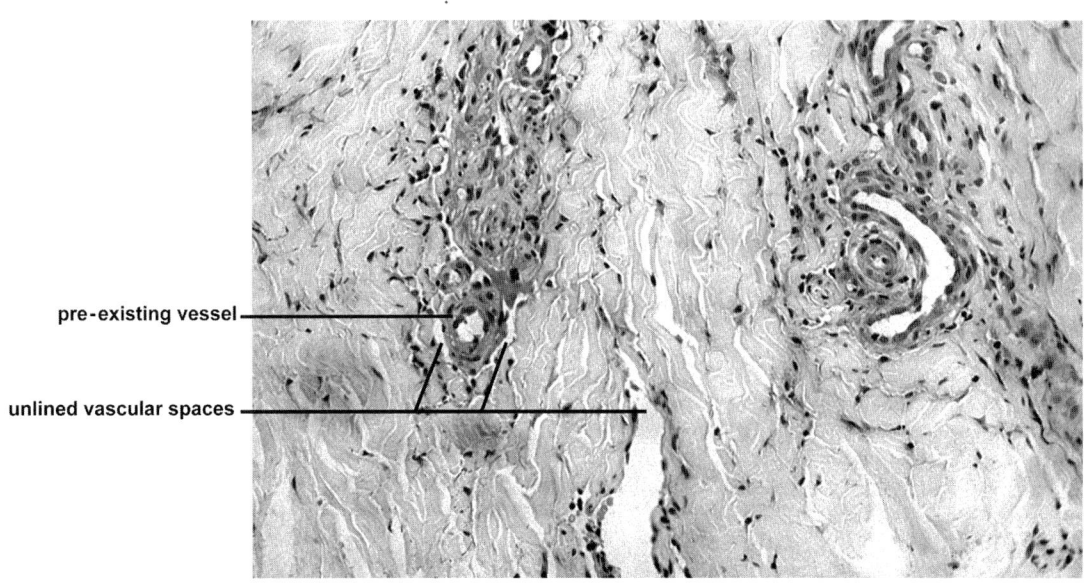

pre-existing vessel

unlined vascular spaces

Figure 19-46. The plaque stage features increased quantities of spindle cells and irregular capillaries. Between the spindle cells there are nonendothelial lined spaces that contain erythrocytes. Hemosiderin is present throughout.

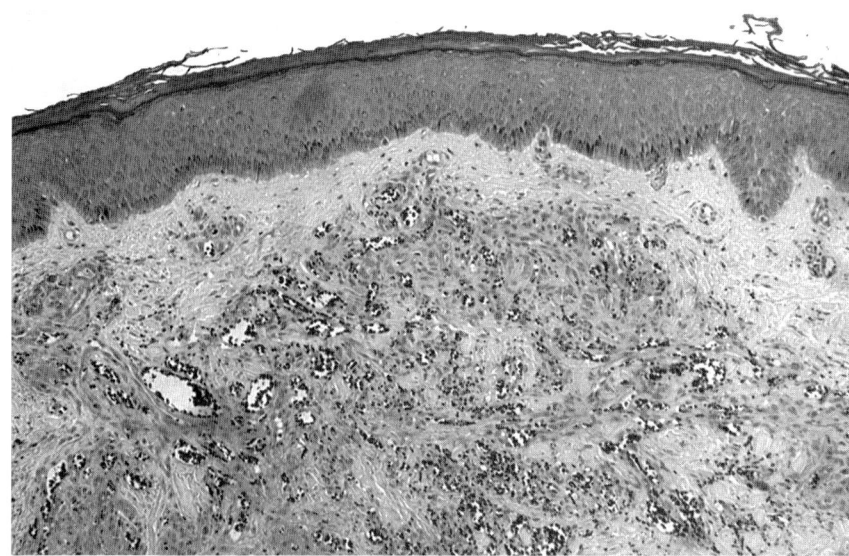

Epithelioid (Polygonal Cell) Neoplasms

Epithelioid Sarcoma

Clinical Features. Epithelioid sarcoma (ES) was first described by Enzinger[276] in 1970 as a neoplasm of the superficial soft tissues that could be confused with metastatic carcinoma or necrobiotic granuloma. It principally affects the extremities of adolescents and young adults, taking the forms of a nodular, plaque-like, or chronic ulcerative lesion ranging up to 5 cm in size.[277–281] ES also may rarely affect elderly patients.[279] This tumor may be clinically misdiagnosed as an ulcerative granuloma, deep granuloma annulare, or a rheumatoid lesion.

This neoplasm spreads along fascial planes, ligaments, and tendon sheaths.[276,277] Therefore, it is difficult to eradicate surgically without recourse to wide excision or amputation. The clinical evolution of ES is prolonged, spanning many years before and after diagnosis. Most patients ultimately develop distant metastases and succumb to the tumor.[277] Relatively favorable prognostic features include a short period of growth before diagnosis; small lesional size; and complete resectability.[277]

Histopathologic Features. ES is the prototypic epithelioid cell malignancy of the dermis and superficial soft tissues (see Fig. 19–48). Tumor cells are plump or slightly spindle shaped, with round or oval central nuclei and a moderate amount of amphophilic or eosinophilic cytoplasm.[276] They often surround a central area of necrosis or collagenous necrobiosis, mimicking a palisading granuloma, and this resemblance is further heightened by the fact that nuclear atypia are modest in many instances[276,278,279] (Fig. 19-48). Careful scrutiny will usually reveal mitotic activity and peripheral infiltration of adjacent soft tissue. Alternatively, the neoplastic cells may be grouped into tight clusters, separated from one another by collagenous stroma. This pattern may simulate metastatic carcinoma or melanoma.[280] However, glandular lumina, squamous eddies, and melanin pigment are not observed in ES.

Figure 19-47. The tumor stage of Kaposi's sarcoma consists of dense masses of atypical spindle cells separated by erythrocyte-containing channels. The channels are not lined by endothelial cells. The nonendothelial cell–lined slit containing erythrocytes is a recurring element in Kaposi's sarcoma.

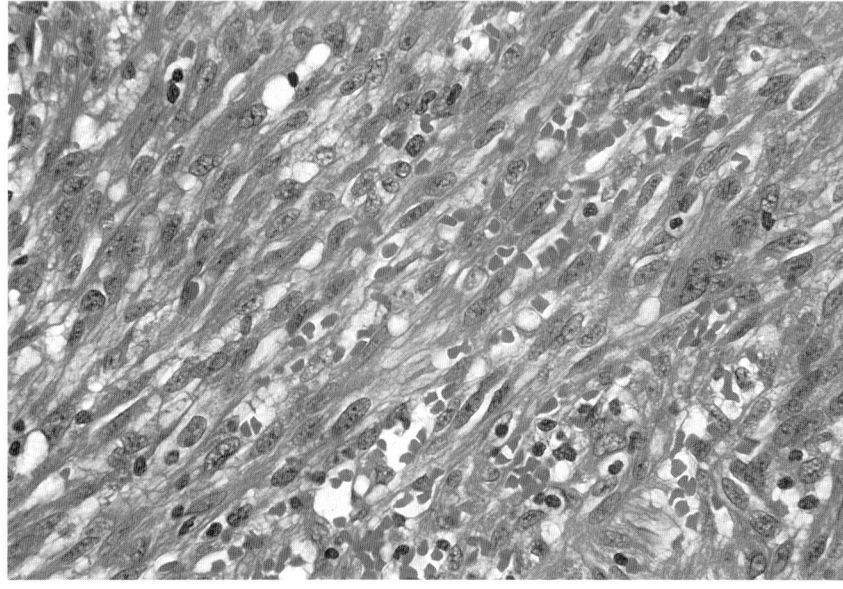

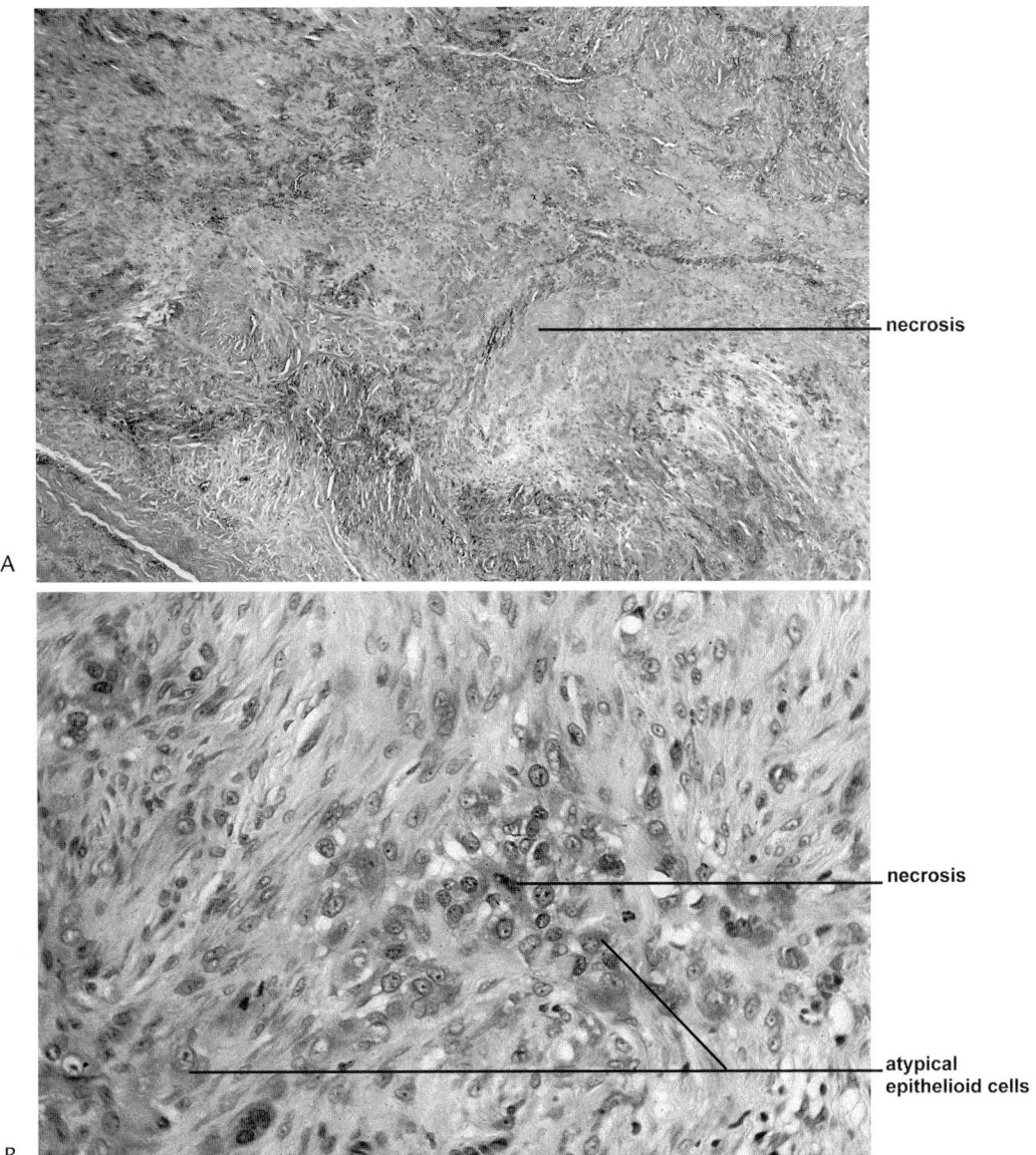

Figure 19-48. (**A**) Low-power view of epithelioid sarcoma. At low power it has the superficial appearance of a granulomatous reaction. Necrosis is often present, adding to that similarity. (**B**) Careful scrutiny will reveal the atypical epithelioid cells. The neoplastic cells may be grouped in small clusters or may be widely separated. If numerous, the pattern can mimic metastatic carcinoma or melanoma. Melanin is never observed.

Distinction from necrobiotic granuloma is facilitated by application of immunostains to keratin and CD45 antigen. ES is an unusual primary soft tissue tumor in that it regularly exhibits keratin expression, along with nonreactivity for CD45. By contrast, the constituent cells of granulomas are keratin negative and CD45 positive.[282]

Clear Cell Sarcoma (Melanoma of Soft Parts)

Clinical Features. Clear cell sarcoma is a soft tissue tumor with an intimate association with fasciae, ligaments, and tendons.[283] It occurs primarily on the extremities of young adults.[284] This tumor is more deeply seated than ES, however, and it therefore typically presents as a nodular, nonulcerated mass. Depending on whether it is distally or proximally located on the arms or legs, the size of clear cell sarcoma varies considerably at diagnosis.[285]

The course of clear cell sarcoma is slow, despite the fact that it has been shown to demonstrate melanocytic differentiation.[286–289] Despite the subcuticular (or deeper) location, metastasis and mortality are, as in ES cases, often seen only after long follow-up periods.[290] A conventional cutaneous melanoma of similar size and depth would certainly be expected to behave more aggressively than this, and the reasons for such disparities are unknown. Radical surgical excision is recommended in the treatment of clear cell sarcoma.[284,290]

Histopathologic Features. Clear cell sarcoma is composed of polyhedral to slightly spindled plump cells, with variably lucent or lightly eosinophilic cytoplasm (Fig. 19-49). Cellular growth may be clustered, fascicular, or sheet-like, and small foci of spontaneous necrosis are frequently seen.[283,285] Nuclei are round, with vesicular chromatin and prominent nucleoli. As in cutaneous melanomas, intranuclear invaginations of cytoplasm are common.[284] Mitotic activity is variable but always present.

Cytoplasmic melanin is visible by conventional microscopy or silver-impregnation histochemistry in approximately 30% to 40% of cases.[289] This pigment is usually widely dispersed and never attains the density seen in cutaneous melanocytic neoplasms. Immunohistochemical analysis shows consistent reactivity for vimentin, S-100 protein, and the HMB-45 antigen in clear cell sarcoma. This profile is identical to that seen in melanoma, but is not recapitulated by any other primary epithelioid tumor of the skin.[8,291]

The differential diagnosis of clear cell sarcoma includes epithelioid sarcoma, metastatic carcinoma, metastatic melanoma, and epithelioid malignant peripheral nerve sheath tumor (see below).[291] Immunohistologic assessments are the surest means of excluding most of these possibilities (Table 19-4). Metastatic

Figure 19-49. **(A)** Clear cell sarcoma with arrangement of cells in large lobules and sheets. Pigment is not identified. Small foci of hemorrhage are present. **(B)** Characteristic cells that have a vague resemblance to nevocytes. Central nucleoli and intranuclear pseudoinclusions can be found. The tumors are consistently HMB-45 and S-100 positive.

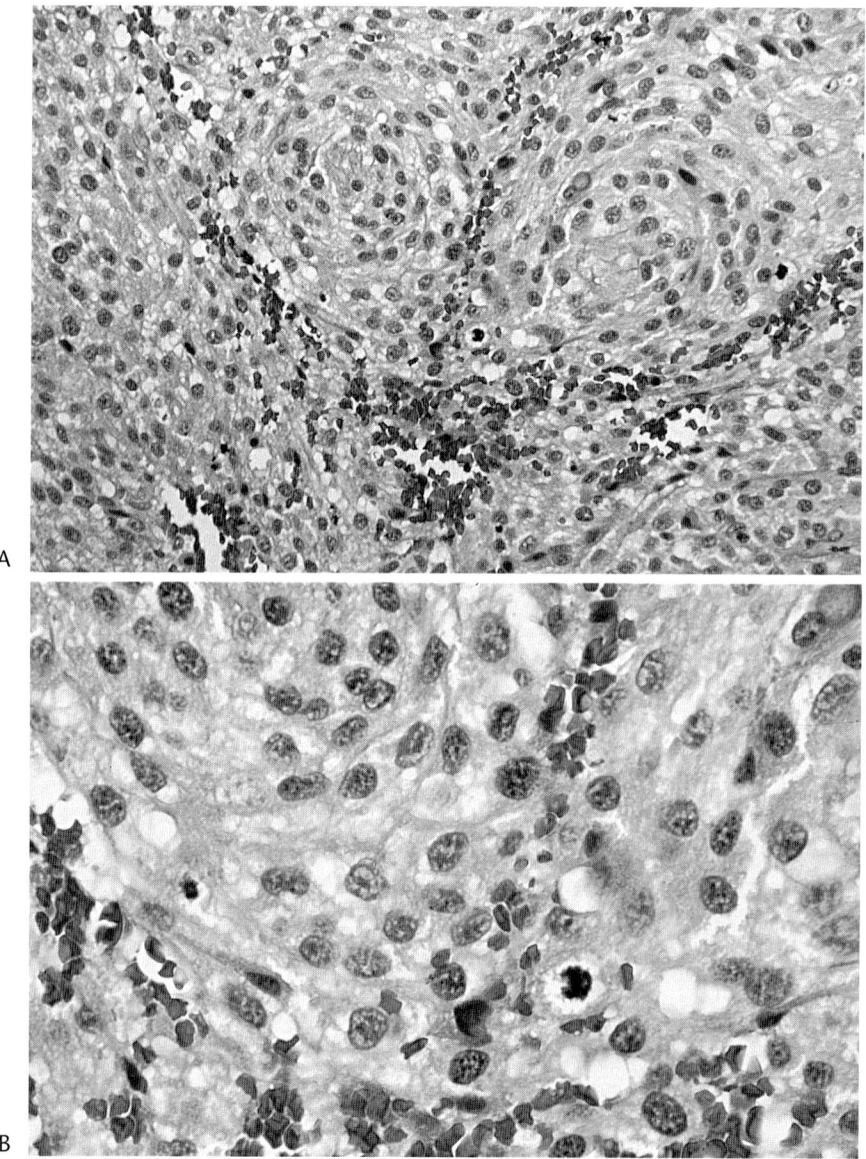

Table 19-4. Specialized Pathologic Features of Malignant Cutaneous Epithelioid Tumors

Tumor	Electron Microscopy				Immunohistochemistry							
	ICJ	PRML	WPB	ECP	FDBC	KER	VIM	S-100	HMB	LEU7	SMA	CD31
Epithelioid sarcoma	±	0	0	0	0	+	+	±	0	0	0	0
Clear cell sarcoma	±	±	0	0	0	0	+	+	+	0	0	0
Epithelioid angiosarcoma	±	0	±	0	0	0	+	0	0	0	0	+
Epithelioid MPNST and MGCTS	±	0	0	±	0	0	+	±	0	±	0	0
Epithelioid leiomyosarcoma	±	0	0	0	+	0	±	0	0	±	+	0
Malignant rhabdoid tumor	±	0	0	0	0	±	+	±	0	0	0	0
Metastatic carcinomas	+	0	0	0	0	+	±	±	0	±	0	0

Abbreviations: ICJ, intercellular junctional complexes; WPB, Weibel-Palade bodies; FDBC, filament-dense body complexes; VIM, vimentin; HMB, HMB-45 antigen; CD31, CD31 antigen; MGCTS, malignant granular cell tumor of the skin; PRML, premelanosomes; ECP, elongated cytoplasmic processes; KER, keratin; S-100, S-100 protein; SMA, smooth muscle actin; MPNST, malignant peripheral nerve sheath tumor.

melanoma, by contrast, differs microscopically from clear cell sarcoma only in its peripheral pattern of growth. When they are seen as secondary implants in soft tissue, nodules of melanoma have sharply circumscribed borders; by contrast, clear cell sarcoma infiltrates irregularly into the surrounding connective tissue.[289]

Epithelioid Leiomyosarcoma

Clinical Features. There are no appreciable differences in the clinical presentation or behavior of epithelioid cutaneous leiomyosarcoma compared with the usual histologic forms of this neoplasm.[206]

Histopathologic Features. Epithelioid leiomyosarcoma is composed predominantly of polygonal cells arranged in sheets or clusters. Nuclei are vesicular with variably prominent nucleoli, and the cytoplasm is lightly eosinophilic and homogeneous. Mitotic activity is routinely observed.[292] Epithelioid leiomyosarcoma provides few histologic clues to its myogenous nature. This is appreciated only by electron microscopy—showing pinocytosis, plasmalemma-associated dense plaques, cytoplasmic microfilaments and dense bodies, and pericellular basal lamina—or immunohistologic studies demonstrating reactivity for desmin and muscle-specific actin.[8]

Differential diagnosis includes virtually all other epithelioid malignancies of the skin.[291] The distinguishing characteristics of these lesions are outlined in Table 19-4.

Epithelioid Malignant Peripheral Nerve Sheath Tumors

Clinical Features. The clinical features of epithelioid malignant peripheral nerve sheath tumors (MPNST) are identical to those of the spindle cell form of this tumor, and the reader is referred back to the discussion of the latter variant for details.

Histopathologic Features. Epithelioid MPNST is greatly dissimilar to spindle cell nerve sheath sarcomas in that it is composed solely of polyhedral cells that are arranged in cords, clusters, and sheets, often separated by myxoid or mucinous stromal material. Nuclei are vesicular with prominent nucleoli, mitotic activity is brisk, and cytoplasm is amphophilic or eosinophilic[293,294] (Fig. 19-50). Identification of this tumor in distinction to other epithelioid sarcomas is aided in some cases by an obvious association with a large cutaneous or subcutaneous nerve. It can be *complicated* by the fact that epithelioid MPNST may rarely show melanin production in mimicry of melanotic neurilemmomas or melanomas.

The latter eventuality may produce great consternation in the differential diagnosis with metastatic melanoma (particularly with its "myxoid" variant[295]) or with clear cell sarcoma. This problem is solved only with electron microscopy or immunohistology. The first of these studies shows the generic ultrastructural features of MPNST (see above), but may indeed demonstrate premelanosomes in the pigmented elements. Immunohistologically, HMB-45 is not observed in epithelioid MPNST, as expected in truly melanocytic neoplasms.[8]

Malignant Granular Cell Tumors

Clinical Features. Malignant cutaneous granular cell tumors (MGCT) are exceedingly rare, and less than 30 examples have been documented.[296–299] They have an average size of 4 cm and are seemingly restricted to adult patients, with a female predominance.[137] Although any anatomic location may be the site of origin for MGCT of the skin, most have occurred on the proximal extremities or trunk as subcuticular nodules or ill-defined plaques. Recurrence after adequate surgical excision is the usual indicator that a granular cell tumor is other than benign as usual.[141] Metastases of MGCT have been seen in over 50% of

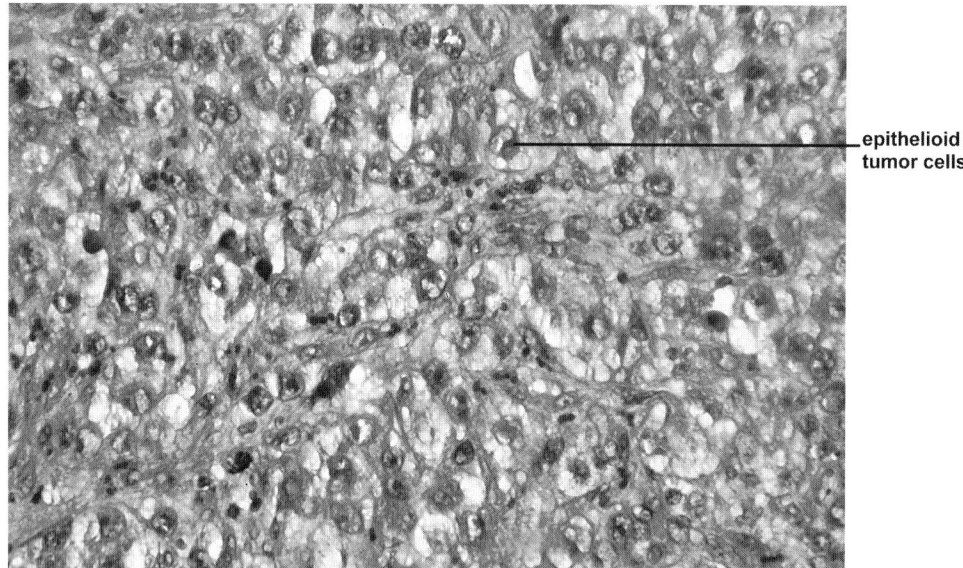

epithelioid
tumor cells

Figure 19-50. The malignant epithelioid schwannoma of the dermis or the epithelioid malignant peripheral nerve sheath tumor is a very rare lesion. This example arose in the superficial dermis of the great toe. Large epithelioid cells are present in small and large groups separated by fibrovascular stroma. Mitoses were prominent in some areas. The lesion was S-100 positive but HMB-45 negative. There was no indication of melanosomes or premelanosomes by electron microscopy.

reported cases, involving the regional lymph nodes, lungs, liver, bones, and brain (Fig. 19-51). Mortality approximates 80%.[137]

Histopathologic Features. The microscopic features of MGCT are closely similar to those of its benign counterpart. However, histologic signs of malignancy in such lesions include broad zones of spontaneous necrosis, obvious invasion of stromal blood vessels, and numerous mitotic figures with atypical forms.[137]

Although most MGCT, like their benign counterparts, demonstrate a schwannian phenotype by electron microscopy and immunohistologic analysis,[299] a subset of granular cell tumors exists that is microscopically atypical and that has an "uncommitted" immunophenotype.[141] These lesions are usually polypoid, with a maximum size of 2 cm or less. They may recur, but metastasis is unreported to date.

The differential diagnosis of MGCT of the skin includes other primary cutaneous neoplasms and also metastatic tumors with a granular cell appearance. Leiomyosarcoma of the skin may have a predominantly granular cell phenotype, as rarely may basal cell carcinoma.[141] Likewise, selected examples of metastatic renal cell carcinoma or mammary adenocarcinoma with granular cell change may simulate the appearance of primary MGCT of the skin.[300] Distinguishing characteristics of these lesions are outlined in Table 19-5.

Malignant Rhabdoid Tumor of the Skin

Clinical Features. Malignant rhabdoid tumor of the skin is another rare lesion that occurs in dermis or subcutis.[301,302] Typical macroscopic features are uncertain at this time. Those examples that have been documented to date have taken the form of ill-defined nodules in the scalp or genital skin of adults, measuring several centimeters in greatest dimension. This neoplasm is extremely aggressive, fast growing, and often metastasizes widely. These features characterize the behavior of rhabdoid tumors of the viscera, which have been documented in the kidney, liver, uterus, oral cavity, urinary bladder, deep soft tissues, heart, and central nervous system.[303]

Histopathologic Features. Malignant rhabdoid tumors are characterized by sheets and clusters of neoplastic cells. Nuclei are oval or round with dense chromatin and prominent nucleoli. Amphophilic or eosinophilic cytoplasm contains a characteristic eosinophilic, homogeneous fibrillar material that displaces the nucleus to one side[303] (Fig. 19-52). Cutaneous appendages are effaced, and the lesions permeate surrounding connective tissue.[301,302] Mitotic activity is abundant in rhabdoid tumors, and atypical division figures are common.

Ultrastructurally, malignant rhabdoid tumors show perinuclear aggregates of whorled intermediate filaments, corresponding to the "hyaline masses" seen at a light microscopic level.[303] Intercellular junctional complexes may be present as well. Immunopathologic characteristics of these neoplasms have varied considerably, according to their topographic origins. In the skin, reactivity with antibodies to keratin, epithelial membrane antigen, vimentin, and carcinoembryonic antigen has been documented.[301,302] In other anatomic locations, malignant rhabdoid tumors may also express glial fibrillary acidic protein, S-100 protein, desmin, and muscle-specific actin. These attributes have led some authors to conclude that rhabdoid tumors do not represent a specific tumor. Instead, they propose that the rhabdoid phenotype is a common morphologic pathway assumed by poorly differentiated aggressive

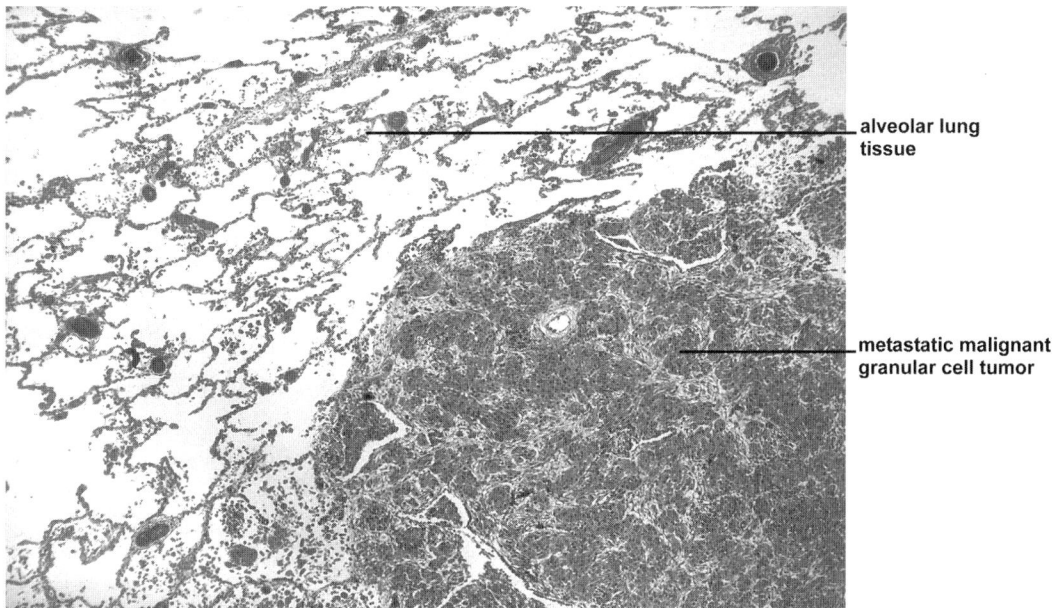

Figure 19-51. Malignant granular cell tumors are rare. This particular example metastasized to the lungs. Note the relatively small size of tumor nuclei. Nonetheless, tumor nuclei in this example are larger than standard size for granular cell tumor.

tumors.[303,304] Indeed, in particular reference to the skin, it should also be remembered that malignant melanoma is also capable of assuming a "rhabdoid" appearance in primary or metastatic lesions.[305] Thus, an unqualified diagnosis of malignant rhabdoid tumor of the skin must follow the exclusion of melanocytic differentiation through appropriate special studies.

Angiosarcoma

Clinical Features. Angiosarcoma of the skin is characteristically seen in one of several well-defined clinical contexts. These encompass idiopathic proliferations on the scalp or face of elderly patients; occurrence in a field of prior therapeutic irradiation after a "lag" period of 5 or more years; and development in

Table 19-5. Differential Diagnosis of Malignant Cutaneous Tumors With a Predominantly Granular Cell Microscopic Appearance

Tumor	Electron Microscopy			Immunohistochemistry								
	ICLF	ICJ	TF	FDBC	KER	EMA	VIM	SMA	GCP	S-100	ERP	CD31
PMGCTS	0	0	0	0	0	0	+	0	0	±	0	0
Metastatic breast carcinoma	±	+	0	0	+	+	±	0	±	±	±	0
Metastatic renal cell carcinoma	±	+	0	0	+	+	±	0	0	0	0	0
Granular cell leiomyosarcoma	0	0	0	+	0	0	±	+	0	±	0	0
Granular cell basal cell carcinoma	0	+	+	0	+	0	0	0	0	0	0	0
Granular cell angiosarcoma	0	±	0	0	0	0	+	0	0	0	0	+

Abbreviations: ICLF, intracellular lumen formation; TF, tonofilaments; KER, keratin; VIM, vimentin; GCP, gross cystic disease fluid protein-15; ERP, estrogen receptor protein; ICJ, intercellular junctional complexes; FDBC, filament-dense body complexes; EMA, epithelial membrane antigen; SMA, smooth muscle actin; S-100, S-100 protein; CD31, CD31 antigen.

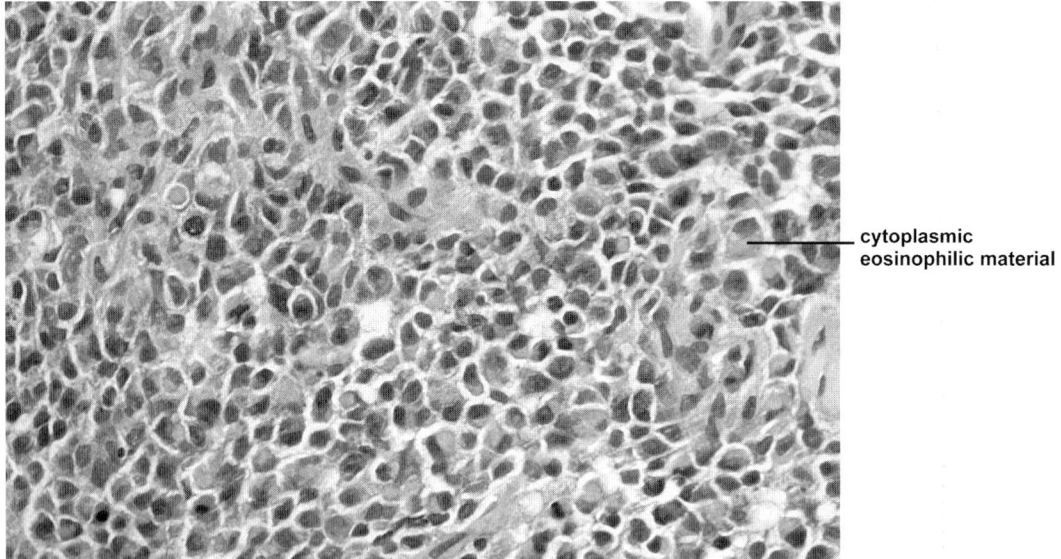

cytoplasmic eosinophilic material

Figure 19-52. The malignant rhabdoid tumor, wherever it occurs, is characterized by partially necrotic sheets of malignant cells. The nuclei are oval and pushed to one side by an intracytoplasmic whorl of eosinophilic fibrillar material. The tumors are highly malignant and spread rapidly. Mitotic activity is high.

an area of chronic cutaneous lymphedema (the so-called Stewart-Treves syndrome).[306] A small minority of tumors do arise outside of the situations just cited as lesions of the extremities or trunk in individuals with no apparent predisposing conditions.

Angiosarcomas likewise show a variety of macroscopic presentations. They may be large, multinodular, ill-defined, violaceous, bloody, and sometimes ulcerated masses; vague ecchymosis-like macular lesions; ligneous, "brawny" alterations in the skin that simulate erysipelas; and multifocal, seemingly discrete bluish-red nodules that imitate cavernous hemangiomas.[85]

The behavior of angiosarcoma is uniformly aggressive. Those patients whose neoplasms are less than 10 cm in maximum dimension may benefit from radical surgical excision and postoperative irradiation, but almost all affected individuals will eventually die of unmanageable local tumor growth or distant metastases.[307]

Histopathologic Features. In the classic form, angiosarcoma is a disorganized proliferation of polyhedral atypical endothelial cells with hyperchromatic nuclei and scant amphophilic cytoplasm. The tumor cells form racemose, interconnecting, "sieve-like" vascular channels in the skin that "dissect" through dermal collagen and deeper tissues and contain luminal red blood cells.[308-311] Cutaneous appendages are entrapped or destroyed by the proliferation; hemosiderin and chronic inflammatory cells may be interspersed throughout the lesion. Large tumors may ulcerate the overlying epidermis multifocally. Micropapillae of neoplastic cells frequently project into the neovascular channels of angiosarcomas, and the supporting (stromal) blood vessels also may show nuclear atypia in endothelial cells (Fig. 19-53). Mitotic activity is variable but always present. Necrosis may or may not be observed.[309,311]

Several well-documented microscopic variants of angiosarcoma have been recognized. These include the spindle cell subtype (as described above),[85,274] a solid "epithelioid" form,[312]

"minimal-deviation" (hemangioma-like) angiosarcoma,[313] a granular cell variant,[314] and a pleomorphic subtype with the potential to simulate atypical fibroxanthoma or malignant fibrous histiocytoma[306] (see below). Akiyama et al[315] also have reported two cases in which benign melanocytes and melanophages were intermixed with the neoplastic endothelial cells in the dermis.

Epithelioid angiosarcoma is composed entirely or predominantly of plump polyhedral cells that imitate true epithelia.[274,312] These occupy much of the lumen in vascular spaces formed by such lesions, and therefore the latter channels often contain few discernible erythrocytes and are not readily recognized as endothelial in nature.

Simulants of spindle cell angiosarcoma are discussed above in connection with KS. Epithelioid vascular tumors may simulate true epithelial neoplasms (particularly "pseudovascular" or "angiomatoid" squamous carcinomas,[316] melanoma and clear cell sarcoma, epithelioid sarcoma, epithelioid leiomyosarcoma, and large cell lymphoma.[85] Pleomorphic variants of angiosarcoma can be confused with atypical fibroxanthoma, primary or metastatic undifferentiated carcinomas, melanoma, and malignant fibrous histiocytoma.[85] Immunohistologic analysis is the most useful diagnostic tool. Endothelial tumors are reactive for vimentin, von Willebrand factor, CD31 and CD34 antigens, and *Ulex europaeus* I agglutinin receptors; they lack cytokeratin, epithelial membrane antigen, desmin, muscle-specific actin, and S-100 protein, as seen in the alternatives just cited[317] (Table 19-4).

Pleomorphic Malignant Mesenchymal Tumors of the Skin

Atypical Fibroxanthoma

Clinical Features. Atypical fibroxanthoma (AFX) of the skin was recognized by Helwig[318] in 1963. It is seen principally in the sun-exposed skin of elderly patients, although 25% arise in

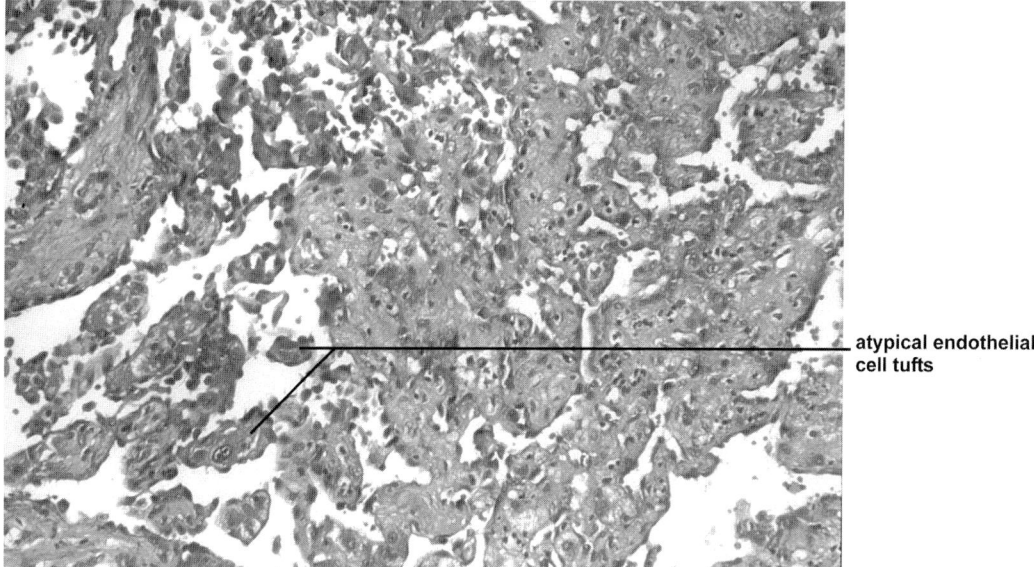

atypical endothelial
cell tufts

Figure 19-53. The typical angiosarcoma displays both spindled and papillary areas. In this central portion of the tumor there is a papillary area characterized by endothelial tufts that project into irregular vascular lumina.

areas of the trunk or extremities that are covered by clothing.[137] The ears, nose, and cheeks are the most frequent sites of origin. There is a male predominance, with a gender ratio of 2:1. Examples of AFX have been reported after previous therapeutic irradiation to the affected skin field.[319] In all cases, it is a nodular, protuberant, red-pink lesion with an average size of 2 cm and potential ulceration.[319–321]

Even though it was initially considered to be a "pseudosarcoma" of the skin, it is now apparent that AFX is a true neoplasm. Examples with repeated recurrence have been documented, as well as others that have metastasized to distant sites.[322] Metastasis is rare, and most AFX are cured by adequate surgical excision.[137] It may therefore be argued that discussion of this tumor would have been more appropriate in the section on borderline cutaneous neoplasms. Nevertheless, because of its many similarities to malignant fibrous histiocytoma, AFX is included in this category.

Histopathologic Features. AFX is a dermally centered proliferation that usually abuts the epidermal basement membrane or is separated from it by only a narrow grenz zone[318] (Fig. 19-54). The lesion typically extends downward into the superficial subcutis or deeper; its peripheral borders are indistinct. Surrounding dermal actinic elastosis is usually striking.[319–321] The tumor cells are spindle shaped, stellate, or multinucleated and pleomorphic, with hyperchromatic or vesicular chromatin, prominent nucleoli, and amphophilic cytoplasm (Fig. 19-55). They are arranged haphazardly or in vaguely storiform or fascicular configurations. Mitotic activity is always brisk with atypical division figures.[137] Small areas of spontaneous necrosis are observed in approximately 50% of cases, and foamy histiocytes may be admixed with the tumor cells surrounding these foci. Rare examples of AFX have been reported in which "divergent" mesenchymal differentiation was apparent.[323,324]

Helwig and May[322] have shown that deep invasion by AFX into the subcutaneous fat or obvious permeation of blood vessels by the tumor are associated with potential for recurrence and metastasis.[322] Thus, lesions showing these attributes should be excised widely, with close patient monitoring thereafter.

Differential diagnosis of AFX is principally centered on the exclusion of two other tumors that may imitate this lesion to perfection: pleomorphic and spindle cell ("sarcomatoid") squamous carcinoma of the skin[325] and sarcomatoid malignant melanoma.[326] The presence of small foci with overt squamous differentiation or pigmentation in the latter neoplasms sometimes allows for their recognition by conventional microscopy. Most pathologists make the distinction between the three types through the application of immunohistologic stains. Keratin reactivity separates squamous carcinomas from the other two possibilities, and a similar association exists between sarcomatoid malignant melanoma and positivity for S-100 protein. AFX lacks both of these markers. All three neoplasms consistently express vimentin.[14,327]

Superficial Malignant Fibrous Histiocytoma

Clinical Features. That malignant fibrous histiocytoma (MFH) is most often a sarcoma of the deep soft tissues is reflected by the fact that only 25% involve the subcutis through primary growth or upward extension from an underlying lesion.[137,328] Overall, MFH is a neoplasm of adults, with a peak incidence in the seventh decade of life and a relatively equal distribution between the genders. Most superficial examples occur on the proximal extremities, although other anatomic locations have been affected. The average size of such tumors is 4 to 5 cm.[137]

Enzinger[329] has offered the opinion that the differences between the biologic potentials of AFX and MFH are solely determined by relative tumor size and depth of origin. Lesions that

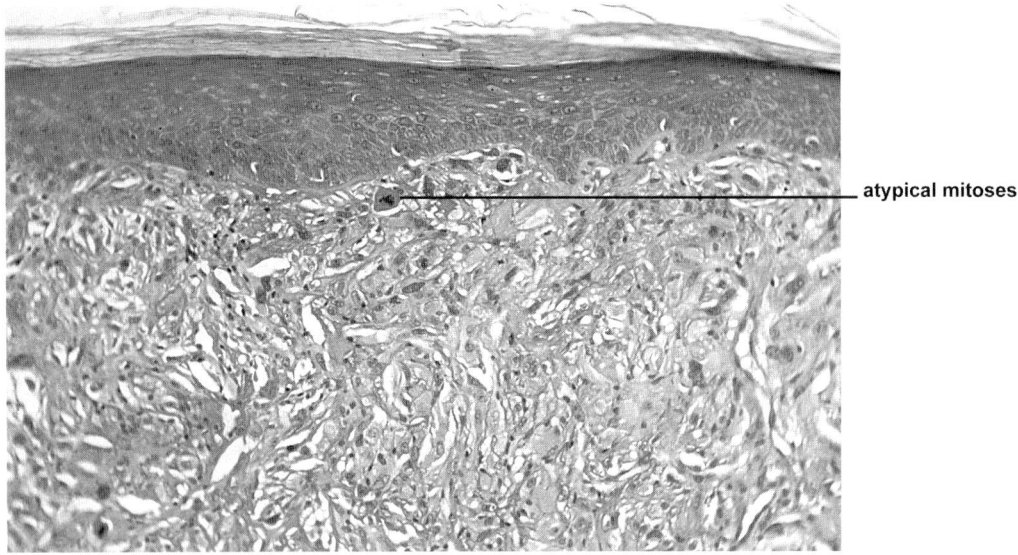

Figure 19-54. The atypical fibroxanthoma characteristically abuts the epidermis or displays a thin grenz zone. The architecture is often storiform, as here, or elongate in a spindle pattern. Bizarre cellular elements are often present. The mitotic rate is high.

are small and superficially located infrequently recur or metastasize, probably because they are diagnosed at an early stage of evolution. By contrast, MFH of the subcutis and superficial soft tissues recurs in 30% of cases and spreads distantly in 10%.[137] Accordingly, all neoplasms in this generic category should be thoroughly excised surgically.

Histopathologic Features. The microscopic attributes of superficial MFH mirror those of its more deeply seated counterparts, and they are virtually identical to the histologic characteristics of AFX (see above). Malignant fibrous histiocytomas in general have been subdivided into *spindle cell/pleomorphic, myxoid, "monomorphic-histiocytic," inflammatory,* and giant cell histologic variants.[328]

Figure 19-55. The atypical fibroxanthoma displays bizarre cellular elements as well as pleomorphic giant cells. Mitoses are frequent. The overall architecture is identical to that of the storiform/pleomorphic malignant fibrous histiocytoma. The atypical fibroxanthoma is, however, the same tumor that occurs in the superficial dermis. The prognosis changes significantly if the tumor reaches the subcutis.

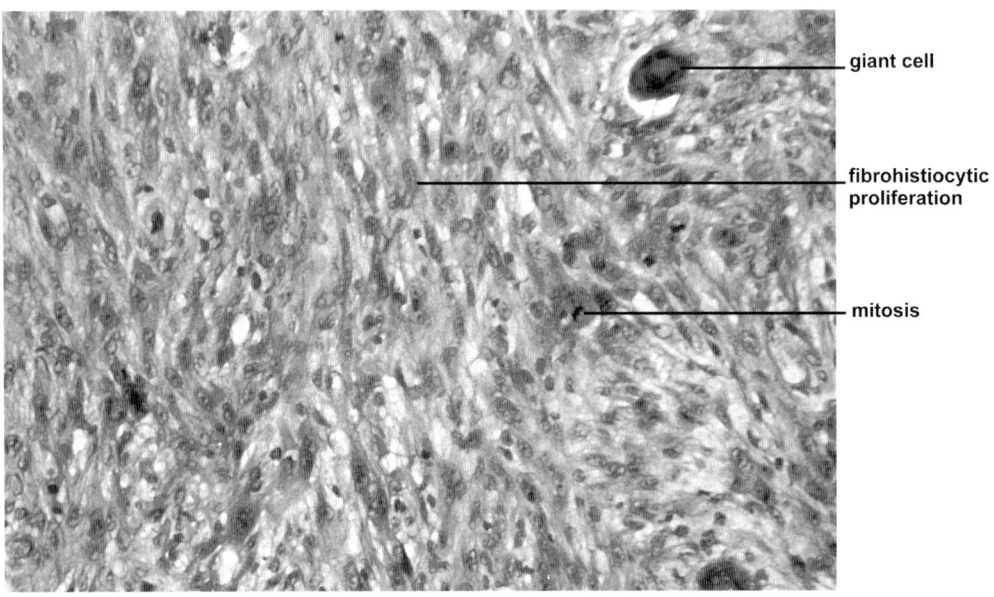

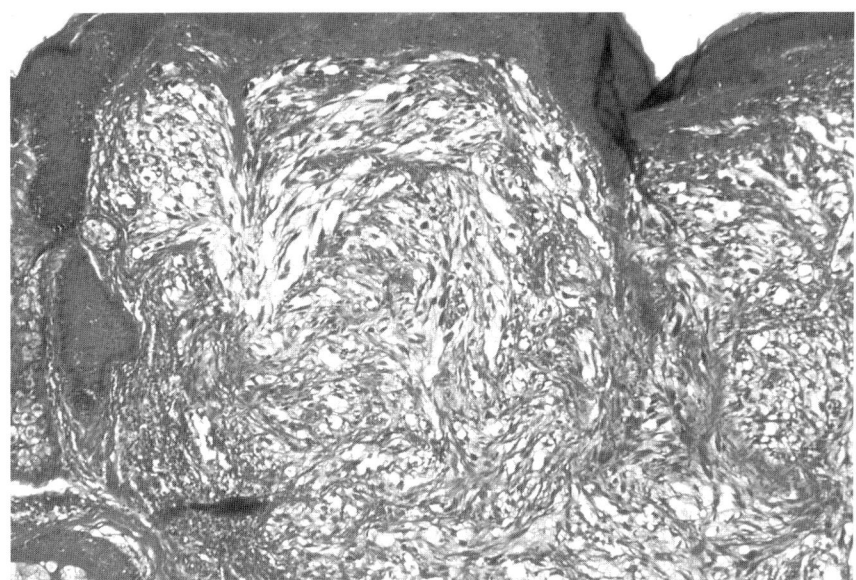

Figure 19-56. The myxoid malignant fibrous histiocytoma or atypical fibroxanthoma displays a faint storiform, spindle cell pattern in a myxoid background. In this example, the tumor abuts the epidermis.

Only the myxoid subtype (Fig. 19-56) is different biologically in that it has a lower incidence of recurrence and distant metastasis.[330]

In likeness to cases of AFX, the differential diagnosis of superficial MFH includes metastatic anaplastic carcinoma and melanoma (Fig. 19-57). In addition, one must consider "dedifferentiated" examples of deep soft tissue sarcomas that may involve the subcutis secondarily. The latter include synovial sarcoma, liposarcoma, leiomyosarcoma, rhabdomyosarcoma, and MPNST.[331] Either electron microscopy or immunohistochemistry can be employed to distinguish these neoplasms from one another[8] (Table 19-6).

Primary Cutaneous "Osteosarcoma"

Clinical Features. Three cases of putatively primary osteosarcoma of the skin and subcutis have been documented.[332,333] These presented as hard nodular masses in adult patients. No follow up was reported, and no meaningful statements can be made on their biologic behavior.

Histopathologic Features. Cutaneous "osteosarcoma" was described as a pleomorphic dermal or subcuticular proliferation of atypical cells with fusiform, stellate, and pleomorphic shapes mixed with osteoclast-like giant cells. Chondroid and delicate osteoid matrix surrounded the tumor cells. Mitotic activity was brisk, and necrosis was apparent.[332,333]

Osteosarcoma cutis is tenable on conceptual grounds. Other malignant mesenchymal tumors may demonstrate divergent osteochondroid matrix formation, with or without osteoclast-like giant cells. These include AFX, melanoma, and MPNST.[254,324,326] Ultrastructural studies and immunohistologic stains for keratin are also mandatory in this context, because spindle cell carcinoma is capable of exhibiting osteoid

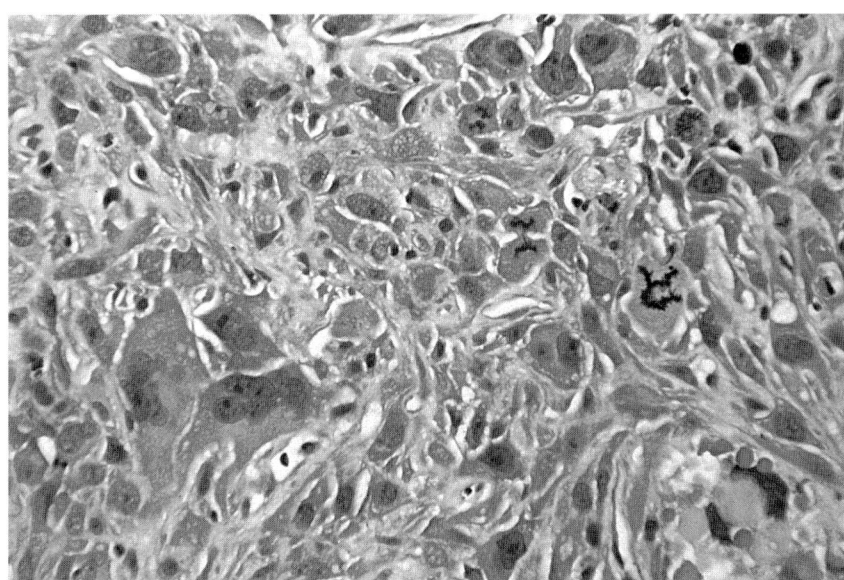

Figure 19-57. The typical giant cell/pleomorphic malignant fibrous histiocytoma shows a predominance of large giant cell forms. Very pleomorphic epithelioid cells are frequently present that can mimic very poorly differentiated carcinomas and melanomas. Many believe that the malignant fibrous histiocytoma is a differentiated end product that can originate from carcinomas as well as sarcomas.

Table 19-6. Specialized Pathologic Features of Pleomorphic Malignant Cutaneous Tumors

Tumor	Electron Microscopy			Immunohistochemistry						
	ICJ	PRML	FDBC	ECP	KER	VIM	EMA	S-100	LEU7	HMB
Atypical fibroxanthoma/malignant fibrous histiocytoma	0	0	0	0	0	+	0	0	0	0
Pleomorphic squamous cell carcinoma	+	0	0	0	+	±	±	0	0	0
Pleomorphic malignant melanoma	±	+	0	0	0	+	0	+	±	+
Dedifferentiated sarcomas (see text)	±	0	±	±	±	+	±	±	±	0
Osteosarcoma[a]	0	0	0	0	0	+	0	0	0	0

[a] Light microscopic demonstration of diffuse osteoid formation distinguishes osteosarcoma from atypical fibroxanthoma and malignant fibrous histiocytoma.

Abbreviations: ICJ, intercellular junctional complexes; FDBC, filament-dense body complexes; KER, keratin; EMA, epithelial membrane antigen; LEU7, Leu 7 antigen; PRML, premelanosomes; ECP, elongated cytoplasmic processes; VIM, vimentin; S-100, S-100 protein; HMB, HMB-45 antigen.

formation and may show no overtly epithelial foci on conventional microscopy.[334]

Myxoid Malignant Neoplasms of the Skin

Subcutaneous Myxopapillary Ependymoma

Clinical Features. Myxopapillary ependymoma (ME) is a neoplasm that is usually observed at the inferior end of the spinal cord, the cauda equina, and filum terminale. This tumor may rarely arise outside of the meninges in the subcutis in the sacrococcygeal region.[335,336] Primary subcuticular ME affects children and adults alike, with a median age of 17 years at presentation. These individuals complain of slowly growing, nodular, firm masses in the "pilonidal" area of the intergluteal cleft; the lesions may occasionally be painful, and they range from 1 to 12 cm in greatest dimension.[336]

Even with adequate excision, ME of the skin recur locally in 15% of cases. In addition, the tumor metastasizes distantly (to lymph nodes and lungs) in up to 20% of patients and may prove fatal after a protracted period of follow up.[336]

Histopathologic Features. ME is a microscopically distinctive lobulated proliferation that demonstrates the formation of broad papillae set in a basophilic, myxoid, focally microcystic stroma. Its peripheral aspect is infiltrative superficially or may be partially encapsulated.

Differential diagnosis of ME includes benign ependymal rests of the sacrococcygeal region,[337] chordomas involving the skin secondarily,[338] and overgrowth of a sacrococcygeal teratoma by yolk sac carcinoma.[339] The first of these possibilities demonstrates essential microscopic identity to ME except that only minute foci of ependymal tissue are observed (with an aggregate size of less than 0.5 cm), and a mass lesion is never present clinically in cases of ependymal rests.[337] Chordomas do not contain papillary structures and are instead composed of cords

and clusters of vacuolated polyhedral cells in a myxoid stroma.[338] They are immunoreactive for keratin but not glial fibrillary acidic protein,[8] whereas ME shows the converse of this profile.[336] Teratoma-related yolk sac carcinomas are confined to infants. Although these neoplasms may exhibit micropapillae and structures passingly resembling pseudorosettes ("Schiller-Duvall bodies"), the myxoid stroma of ME is absent in yolk sac tumors.[339] Moreover, the latter lesions are again reactive for keratin polypeptides but lack glial proteins.

Non-Neoplastic Cutaneous Mesenchymal Proliferations

There are several reactive proliferations of mesenchymal cells in the skin and subcutis that may cause diagnostic consternation or be confused with true neoplasms. These are outlined in the following sections.

Elastofibroma Dorsi

Elastofibroma dorsi is a peculiar reaction to injury seen in the superficial soft tissues of the upper trunk, particularly those under and near the scapulae. Patients with this condition are typically middle-aged males, most of whom have worked in trades requiring heavy manual labor.[340,341] The lesion presents as an ill-defined, 2- to 3-cm nodule or plaque, which is often painful upon motion of the upper trunk or the shoulders. It also may be tender to palpation.

Microscopically, elastofibroma dorsi basically represents a sclerosing proliferation of fibroblasts in the connective tissue of the lower dermis and subcutis. It may simply have the appearance of an organized scar on conventional microscopy, but close inspection will often disclose lightly bluish discoloration and fragmentation of "collagen" fibers in the lesion.[342] When elastic tissue stains are applied, these foci are seen to contain pathognomonic abundant but abnormal elastic fibers that are often bulbous, sharply truncated, or convoluted.[341]

Nodular Fasciitis

Nodular fasciitis represents an idiosyncratic response to minor injury that is seen in the superficial soft tissues, primarily those of the distal extremities in children, adolescents, and young adults.[343] It also has been observed in other locations, including the oral cavity, salivary glands, and deep soft tissues. It may rarely occur in elderly individuals as well.[344] The typical clinical history is that of a very rapidly evolving mass that is slightly tender. The patient may or may not remember an episode of trauma to the area, because in some cases this is so minor that it escapes notice.[342] Differences in the clinical presentation of several clinical variants of the process are also determined by the *site* of the proliferation. Hence, *cranial fasciitis*, *intravascular fasciitis*, and *parosteal fasciitis*[345–347] may all be regarded as variations of the same pathologic entity.

Microscopically, nodular fasciitis is typified by a loosely fascicular, disorganized, or storiform proliferation of cytologically bland fibroblasts and myofibroblasts; these contain ample amphophilic cytoplasm and oval nuclei with dispersed chromatin. The cells are separated from one another by variably edematous stroma with a myxoid aura, and acute and chronic inflammatory cells are often interspersed throughout[342] (Figs. 19-58 and 19-59). The proliferation resembles a "tissue culture" appearance because of its dyscohesive cellular nature.[343] Supporting blood vessels are numerous, thin walled, and capillary sized, and zones of spontaneous erythrocytic extravasation are numerous.[344] Foci of "keloidal"-type matrical collagen are often seen in these lesions as well.

Small nucleoli may be seen in the proliferating cells of nodular fasciitis, and mitotic activity is characteristically brisk.[343–348] The latter features largely account for the histopathologic confusion of this lesion with true sarcomas (primarily leiomyosarcoma or MFH). Nonetheless, the latter neoplasms are cytologically atypical, uncommonly contain inflammatory cells, and virtually never show prominent stromal erythrocyte extravasation or tissue culture appearance as seen in nodular fasciitis.

Attention to these distinguishing microscopic features and characteristic clinical information will allow for the confident recognition of nodular fasciitis in the vast majority of cases. It may then be excised conservatively, and the patient may be reassured as to the reactive nature of the proliferation.

However, examples of nodular fasciitis do exist wherein organization (maturation) of the lesion obscures many of its salient features and heightens a similarity to a true mesenchymal neoplasm. In these instances, it may truthfully be impossible to exclude the possibility of a low-grade sarcoma. Immunohistochemical analysis is of no assistance, because the myofibroblasts in nodular fasciitis share many points of antigenic similarity with tumor cells in leiomyosarcoma (including reactivity for smooth-muscle actin, desmin, and vimentin). A practical solution to this dilemma is to recommend complete but conservative excision, with subsequent follow up of the patient. Nodular fasciitis essentially never recurs, and lesional regrowth should be considered tantamount to an exclusion of this diagnosis.[348] In the circumstances just enumerated, the pathologic interpretation of "myofibroblastic proliferation of uncertain biologic potential" is a prudent one.

Keloids and Hypertrophic Scars

Some individuals react to trauma idiosyncratically by the formation of other lesions that differ from nodular fasciitis. These are known as *keloids* and *hypertrophic scars*, and they are most often seen in nonwhite patients.[349] Minor abrasions, punctures, or lacerations may serve as the impetus for development of these proliferations, as may prior surgical procedures.[350] Clinically, one observes hard, variably sized nodules and plaques that attenuate the overlying epidermis and have a shiny red-pink appearance.[351]

The histologic appearance of hypertrophic scars and keloids is that of a continuum, wherein there are dense aggregates of dermal fibroblasts and the collagenous matrix they produce (Fig. 19-60 and 19-61). Cutaneous appendages and overlying

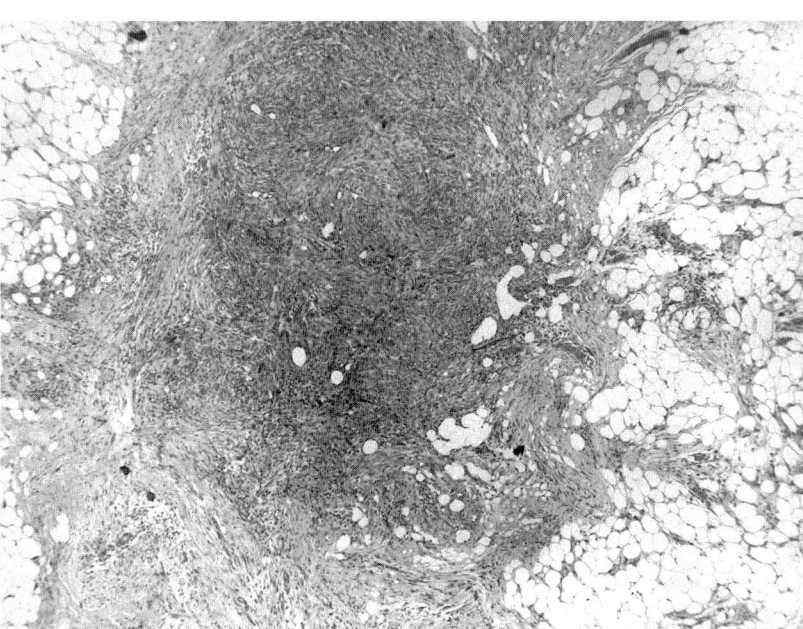

Figure 19-58. Nodular fasciitis is actually a reaction, probably to injury. It is a sharply demarcated proliferation of fibroblastic cells, some endothelial cells, and scattered lymphocytes as noted here. The distinct border with adjacent adipose tissue is noted, but the overall configuration is that of a stellate scar.

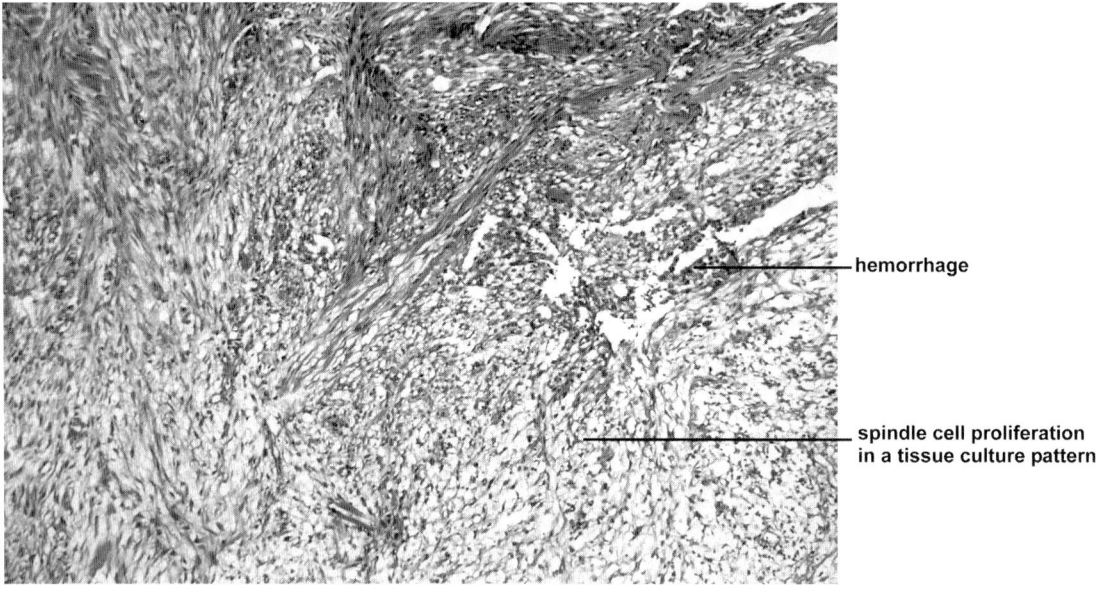

hemorrhage

spindle cell proliferation
in a tissue culture pattern

Figure 19-60. The hypertrophic scar is characterized by ba-sophilic fibroblasts that replace all normal structures where the lesion occurs. Elongate capillaries in the proliferating fibroblasts are often oriented perpendicular to the overlying epidermis.

Figure 19-61. The keloid is very similar to the hypertrophic scar but is characterized specifically by the presence of large, broad, eosinophilic collagen bands. These keloidal bands increase in number as the lesion ages.

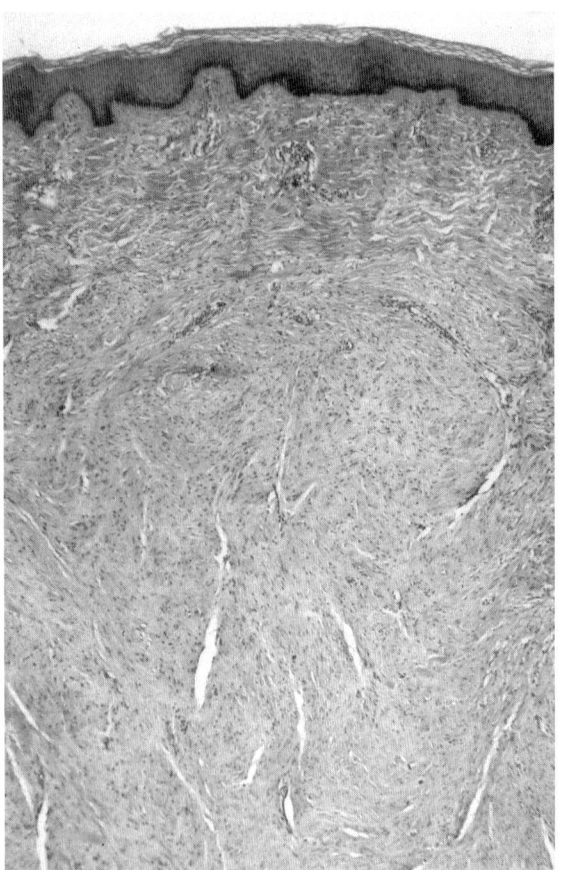

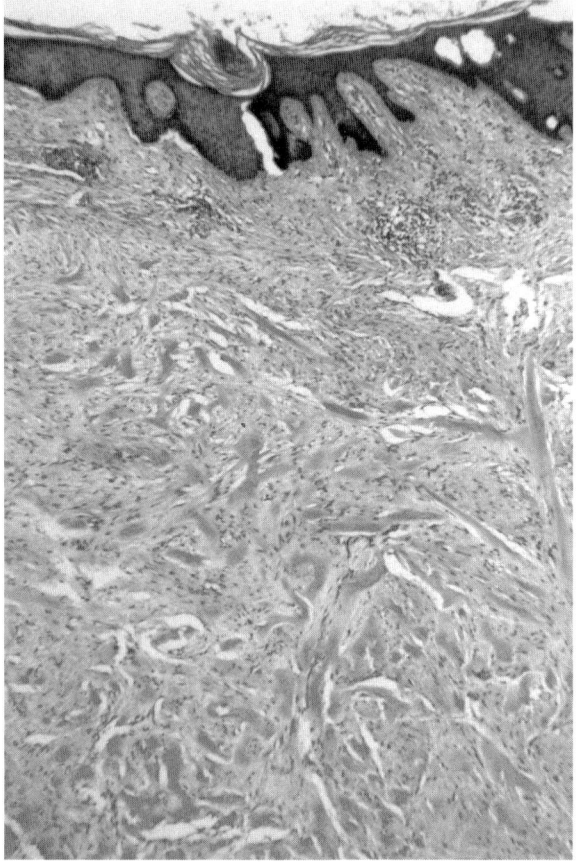

Figure 19-59. The fibroblastic cells of nodular fasciitis are elongate and are separated from one another in a tissue culture pattern. There are also extravasated erythrocytes and lymphocytes. Mild nuclear atypia as well as atypical mitoses may be present, but the overall pattern must be used for diagnosis.

rete ridges are usually effaced, and there is commonly a peripheral zone of capillary proliferation and scant chronic inflammation at the border of the lesion.[349] As hypertrophic scars mature, their high level of cellularity gives way to the accumulation of hyalinized, brightly eosinophilic collagen that is arranged haphazardly in broad bands in the dermis and superficial subcutis. The latter stage typifies the fully formed keloid.[350]

Inflammatory Pseudotumors of the Skin

Several examples of an unusual dermal proliferation designated as "inflammatory pseudotumor of the skin" (IPS) have been described.[352] Patients were all adults, who presented with nodular, nontender, skin-colored or pink tumefactions on the neck or extremities. There was no history of trauma or other possibly predisposing conditions, and the lesional sizes ranged from 0.8 to 1.3 cm.

Microscopically, pseudoencapsulated uninodular proliferations of bland fibroblasts and stromal venule- or capillary-sized blood vessels were apparent in the deep dermis and subcutis, admixed with abundant mature collagen fibers. Numerous lymphocytes and plasma cells were interspersed throughout, with lesser numbers of neutrophils and eosinophils. In 50% of cases, well-formed germinal centers were evident at the lesional peripheries.[352] Many of the supporting blood vessels in IPS showed a concentric adventitial cuff of hyalinized collagen, yielding a "targetoid" configuration. Immunostaining for S-100 protein demonstrated many intralesional Langerhans cells as well.

The major differential diagnostic considerations in IPS cases include nodular fasciitis, angiolymphoid hyperplasia with eosinophilia, Kimura's disease, and lymphocyte-rich dermatofibromas. The unique conjunction of compactly proliferating fibroblasts and well-organized lymphoplasmacytic infiltrates serves to distinguish inflammatory pseudotumors from these other entities, described above.

Mesenchymal "Nevi" (Hamartomas)

Patients with *tuberous sclerosis* (Bourneville's disease) may develop angiofibromas, hypopigmented macules, or connective tissue nevi of the skin. The last of these lesions, also known as *shagreen patches*, most often are observed in the lumbosacral region as elevated, rough papules and plaques. On microscopic examination, one sees either densely aggregated bundles of somewhat hyalinized collagen in the dermis, mimicking morphea, or tumefactive fascicles of normal collagen fibers that are bordered by fragmented elastic fibers in these connective tissue nevi.[353] Identical collagenous malformations may be observed occasionally in patients who do *not* have a familial history of tuberous sclerosis and who lack other signs of the disorder themselves. A closely related lesion is the *juvenile (isolated) elastoma*, which is composed of a circumscribed, tangled proliferation of relatively normal elastic fibers in the dermis.[353,354]

Still other connective tissue nevi exist that feature localized accumulations of dense dermal collagen fibers and fragmented or deficient elastic fibers.[353,355] When seen in association with roentgenographic densities in multiple bones (osteopoikilosis), they may constitute a part of the autosomal dominant *Buschke-Ollendorff syndrome* (dermatofibrosis lenticularis disseminata).[356] In other patients, similar lesions may arise sporadically in the pectoral skin and be unrelated to bony abnormalities. In the latter setting, such malformations are called *mesenchymal nevi of the Lewandowsky type*.[357] Histologically analogous lesions of the trunk and extremities that *lack* elastic fibers altogether (*collagenomas*) also occur in either sporadic[353] or familial (autosomal dominant[358]) forms and show no well-documented association with other cutaneous or visceral abnormalities.

Another heritable condition — *Cowden's disease* (an autosomal dominant syndrome typified by facial trichilemmomatous follicular hamartomas, hamartomatous or ganglioneuromatous intestinal polyposis, oral papillomatosis, and an increased risk of visceral carcinomas[359,360])—is also associated with peculiar hamartomatous fibrous cutaneous proliferations. They have been termed *storiform collagenoma* or *sclerotic fibroma*,[361] and present as nondescript, firm, single or grouped nodules or papules, usually in the facial skin (Fig. 19-62). Multifocality constitutes strong evidence favoring the presence of the syndromic complex.[361] This dermal lesion is sharply circumscribed histologically; it is characterized by hyalinized hypocellular fascicles of collagen that "spin" around one another like the blades of a child's pinwheel. In likeness to the shagreen patch, isolated storiform collagenoma may also occur in patients with no familial or personal evidence of syndromic disease.[362]

Common *acrochordons* ("skin tags") are almost ubiquitous mesenchymal nevi that may affect any skin field at any age; they are soft, polypoid, papillomatous lesions with a narrow stalk.[363] Some acrochordons undoubtedly represent intradermal melanocytic nevi that are undergoing resolution by extrusion, as supported by the occasional observation of small nests of nevocytes in these proliferations. Others may be regressing seborrheic keratoses. However, the usual case shows only a bland fibrovascular connective tissue core that is mantled by slightly papillomatous epidermis.[364]

Nevus lipomatosus is another cutaneous mesenchymal malformation that is commonly congenital in nature.[365] This condition most often presents as multiple soft yellow-tan papules or nodules in the skin of the buttock, trunk, or extremities, and these lesions may coalesce to form irregular plaques. Rarely, infants have disseminated nevus lipomatosus and extensively folded skin ("Michelin tire baby syndrome").[366] Isolated lesions also may be observed in children and adults, and these are nearly impossible to separate clinically from acrochordons.

The primary microscopic attribute of nevus lipomatosus is the presence of small groups of mature adipocytes at all levels of the dermis, particularly centered around adnexae and blood vessels. Accordingly, the junction between the corium and subcutis is often blurred.[367]

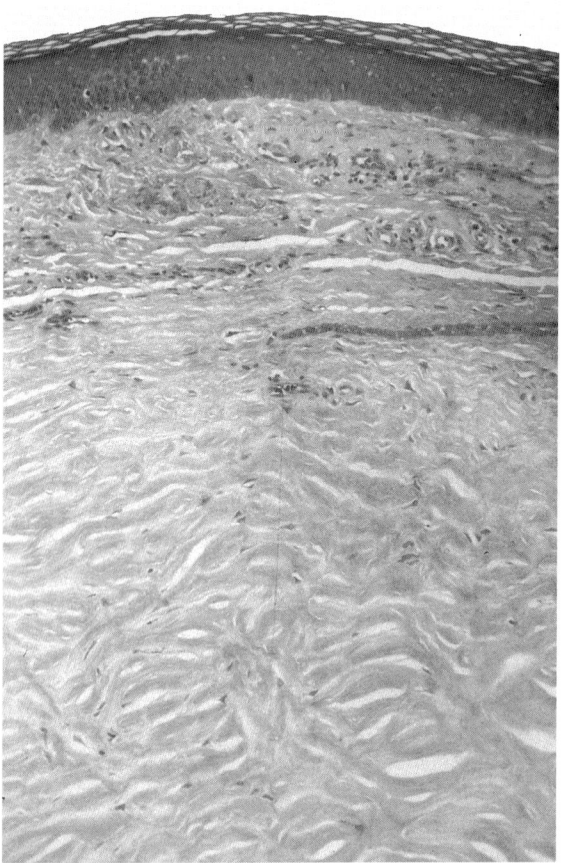

Figure 19-62. The circumscribed collagenoma is a characteristic dermal lesion. It is a distinct nodule characterized by concentric collagen bands with few intervening fibroblastic nuclei.

Smooth muscle hamartomas are thought to be malformations of the arrectores pilorum.[59,368] Because leiomyomatous hamartomas are intimately related to *Becker's nevi* and probably constitute another point on the same clinicopathologic spectrum with the latter lesions,[369] these two proliferations are herein considered as one entity and termed *smooth muscle malformations* (SMMF). The trunk and the extremities are the most common sites of origin for such nevi, and they are principally seen in children as congenital proliferations.[59,365] The lesions are firm macules or plaques that may attain a size of up to 10 cm, with or without hyperpigmentation or coarse hypertrichosis. Slight abrasion of these hamartomas often causes them to contract (pseudourtication).

Microscopically, the salient components of SMMF are disordered fascicles of morphologically normal smooth muscle fibers that are often centered on hair follicles in the papillary and reticular dermis (Fig. 19-63). Melanocytic hyperplasia is often evident in the basal layer of the epidermis, and acanthosis also may be apparent.[59,365] Individual hairs within the lesional area sometimes show abnormally thick contours or are otherwise distorted. It may be difficult for the histologist to separate some SMMF from true leiomyomas of the skin, and accurate clinical information is vital in these instances.

One vascular connective tissue nevus, *nevus flammeus* (port wine stain), is relatively common in the general population, but it is most well known for its association with other pathologic elements of *Sturge-Weber* or *Klippel-Trenaunay-Weber* syndrome.[85,370,371] Clinically, nevus flammeus takes the form of a variably prominent red-violet patch or plaque that is usually confined to one side of the body. It may be relatively inconspicuous or involve a large portion of the skin surface; the latter eventuality is most often observed in syndromic rather than sporadic cases.[372]

The histologic appearance of this lesion is that of dermal telangiectasia rather than a true hemangioma. Dilated vascular spaces of varying sizes are dispersed throughout the corium, separated by relatively normal connective tissue and cutaneous appendages.[370] With advancing age of the patient, the telangiectatic vessels may increase in caliber so that they resemble large veins. In children, this vascular malformation may be subtle, being composed of attenuated capillaries in the superficial dermis.[373]

Cutaneous telangiectasias are also part of the *Osler-Weber-Rendu syndrome*, in association with vascular abnormalities of the mucosae, ears, and nail beds. This autosomal dominant complex presents itself in adolescence or young adulthood as a generalized profusion of tiny macular or papular red lesions. Hemorrhage from the nose and gut is potentially life threatening in the Osler-Weber-Rendu syndrome. The microscopic characteristics of the disease are analogous to those of early-stage nevus flammeus, being represented by numerous small-caliber, thin-walled blood vessels that are randomly distributed throughout the corium or the submucosa of the oral cavity.[374–376]

Tumefactive Non-Neoplastic Vascular Proliferations

Lesions that Simulate Kaposi's Sarcoma

As a by-product of the AIDS pandemic and consequently increased interest in vascular lesions of the skin, several non-neoplastic proliferations have been identified that may simulate KS. These include "acroangiodermatitis," proliferating dermal scars, and reactions to application of Monsel solution.

Acroangiodermatitis (AAD) is a proliferative reaction to dermal erythrocyte extravasation that occurs in the setting of severe venous stasis in the lower extremities due to venous valvular insufficiency. Clinically, it is therefore seen in patients with severe venous varicosities of the legs, who tend to be elderly.[377] The lesions of AAD are typically slowly evolving, brawny, red-brown macules, papules, or plaques, but they also may assume a more violaceous nodular character in some instances. Depending on the symmetry or asymmetry of the venous insufficiency, one or both legs may be affected. The areas of skin surrounding the lateral malleoli and dorsal surfaces of the feet are primarily involved by this process.

Patients with classic KS do not tend to have venous stasis of the legs, except by serendipity.[261] Thus, physical examination and careful history taking regarding the course and pace of the eruption will usually permit a diagnosis of AAD to be made solely on clinical grounds.

In those cases where these features are indeterminate, biopsy may be useful. AAD shows a lobular pattern of capillary and venular proliferation in the dermis, particularly in its superficial aspect. There is no proclivity for new vessels to cluster around old ones (i.e., the "promontory sign" is lacking in AAD); there is no interstitial dermal hypercellularity; and the degree of lesional hemosiderin deposition greatly outstrips the extent of visible red cell extravasation in this condition. The latter microscopic features differ markedly from those seen in KS.

Not uncommonly, biopsies of *proliferating scars* (following episodes of injury that the patient may not remember) are performed under the impression that these lesions represent cutaneous neoplasms. The resulting histologic profile is essentially that of organizing granulation tissue, featuring a regimented proliferation of capillaries and venules that are typically oriented vertically within the dermis.[273] Proliferation of intervening fibroblasts and myofibroblasts is frequent, with variable edema or dense collagen deposition in the surrounding dermal stroma. If the scar has been traumatized, red cell leakage and hemosiderin deposition may again be observed. Nonetheless, the overall image of this lesion is only superficially like that of KS, and diagnostic separation of the two conditions is typically straightforward.

The characteristics of *reactions to the application of Monsel solution* (a surgical styptic) are also closely similar to those of proliferating scars. Because this pharmaceutical includes iron salts, large irregular or rhomboidal clusters of iron pigment are also observed in tissue reactions to Monsel solution[378] (Fig. 19-64).

An extremely interesting condition that has been recognized for only a few years is that known as *bacillary (epithelioid) angiomatosis*.[379] It is observed in patients who are infected with HIV, leading to particular concern that they have KS. Red-violet cutaneous nodules and plaques of variable sizes are seen in this disorder, without topographic predilections. The viscera also may be involved, heightening the mimicry of KS.[380]

Nevertheless, the histologic features of bacillary angiomatosis differ substantially from those of KS and are instead more similar to those of epithelioid hemangioma. Organized sheets or clusters of completely formed vascular channels are observed in the dermis, with indistinctly lobular profiles; an epidermal collarette is rather frequently seen at the lateral borders of the proliferation (Fig. 19-65). Constituent endothelial cells are plump with abundant cytoplasm and bland nuclear features, although mitotic activity and limited foci of necrosis may be apparent.[379] Intralesional neutrophilia is a distinctive finding.[260] Close examination of the cells shows granular cytoplasmic inclusions that represent clusters of bacilliform organisms.[379] These have been shown to bear a taxonomic relationship to the cat-scratch agent, and they may be highlighted with the Warthin-Starry stain.[379,381] Virtually identical cutaneous lesions are also seen in association with infection by another bacillus, *Bartonella*, in South American patients with *Carrion's disease (verruga peruana)*.[382,383]

Treatment of bacillary angiomatosis with appropriate antibiotics results in resolution of the disease.[381] Thus, pathologic confusion of this process with KS is a particularly egregious error.

A related but histologically dissimilar cutaneous proliferation is seen in patients with AIDS who are infected with atypical mycobacteria. In this context, spindle cell lesions of the skin may be observed that emulate nodular KS.[384] They are composed of dermal fibroblast-like cells arranged in whorling fascicles, admixed with bands of sclerotic collagen, lymphocytes, and plasma cells. Careful scrutiny of the cytoplasm in the fusiform elements reveals granular inclusions that represent clumps of mycobacteria. These may be further delineated with Ziehl-Neelsen or Fite stains.[384] Appropriate antibiotic treatment of such *spindle cell reactions to mycobacteria* results in only variable resolution of the lesions, but they clearly should not be confused with KS.

Potential Simulators of Angiosarcoma

There are two non-neoplastic cutaneous proliferations that may be mistaken for angiosarcoma by the unwary pathologist. These include *papillary intravascular endothelial hyperplasia* (PIEH; "Masson's vegetant intravascular hemangioendothelio-

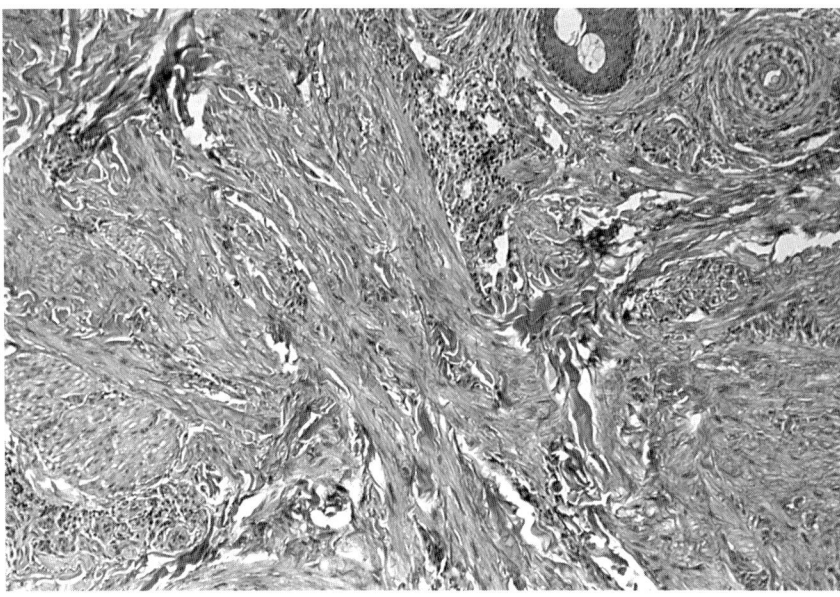

Figure 19-63. Smooth muscle hamartomas of the skin are very similar to leiomyomas except that the smooth muscle proliferations are very irregular, rather than nodular or ovoid. They are often associated with dermal appendages.

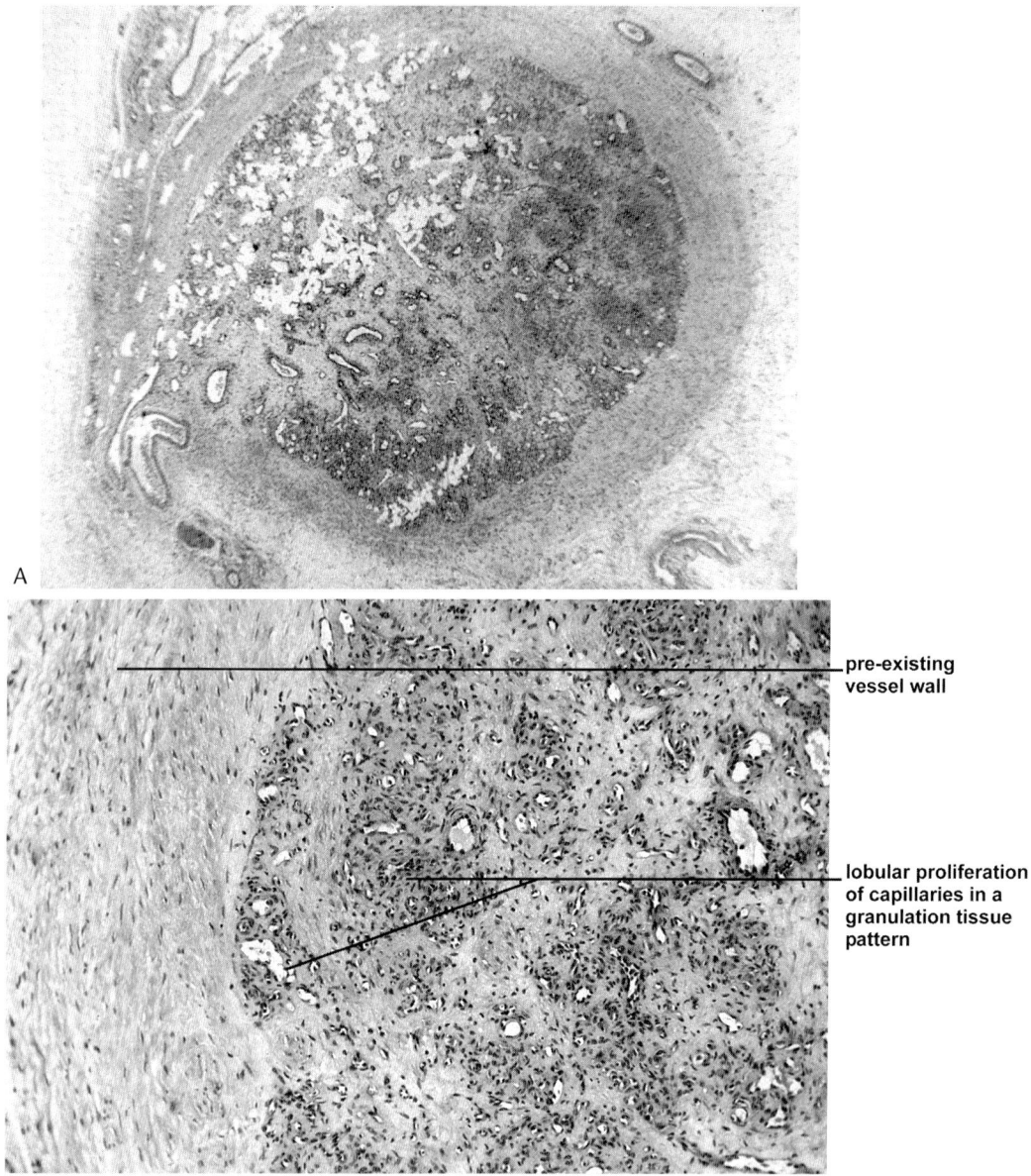

Figure 19-66.   *Intravascular pyogenic granuloma* is the term most defining of this lesion. **(A)** Low-power view in which granulation tissue fills the lumen of a thrombosed vessel. Similar proliferations can occur in venous lakes as well as in pre-existing hemangiomas. The occurrence in a pre-existing hemangioma can make the diagnosis more difficult. **(B)** Granulation tissue in a lobular pattern similar to a pyogenic granuloma. Note the wall of the pre-existing vessel on the left side of the field.

ma").[385,386] PIEH is seen as a consequence of trauma and thrombosis within pre-existing hematomas, hemangiomas, varices, or otherwise-dilated blood vessels, usually on the distal extremities.[385]

Microscopic examination of PIEH shows a racemose proliferation of bland endothelial cells that mantles hyalinized pseudopapillary cores of organized fibrinous thrombotic material.[386,387] Low-power assessment clearly demonstrates sharp confinement of the lesion to the lumen of a thrombosed hematoma or a large vein or artery (Fig. 19–66). The latter point

is crucial to correct interpretation, because the *internal* aspects of PIEH may otherwise easily be mistaken for those of a low-grade angiosarcoma.[386]

Angiokeratomas

Angiokeratomas are seen in two clinical settings, as isolated, sporadic, papulonodular, red-violet lesions or as multiple papules that tend to affect the genital skin and lower extremities in patients with *Fabry's disease* (angiokeratomatosis corporis diffusum universale—an X-linked recessive deficiency of tri-hexosylceramide α-galactosidase that results in degeneration of the nervous system and renal insufficiency). Syndromic abnormalities tend to present themselves in adolescence or early adulthood, whereas isolated angiokeratoma is potentially seen in individuals of all ages.[387–390]

Histologically, there is no difference in the light microscopic appearance of isolated and Fabry's angiokeratomas. They represent blood lakes in the upper dermis that are surrounded by complete collarettes of epidermis, with slight overlying hyperkeratosis and papillomatosis (Fig. 19-67). A resemblance to verrucous hemangioma therefore exists, but the latter proliferation differs in that it affects the deep reticular dermis as well. Syndromic angiokeratomas may be distinguished from sporadic examples by electron microscopy. Ultrastructural analysis shows lamellated intralysosomal "myelin figures" in lesional endothelial cells, pericytes, and fibroblastic stromal cells of the dermis in patients with Fabry's disease, but not in those with sporadic angiokeratoma.

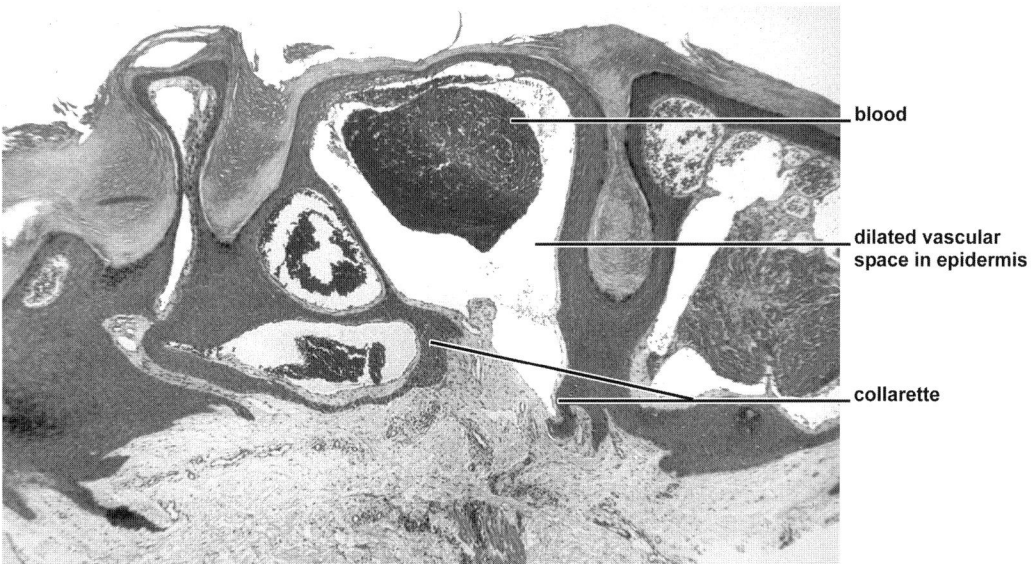

Figure 19-67. The angiokeratoma is characterized by dilated vascular channels that are projected into the epidermis. The surrounding epidermis forms collarettes. The vessels contain blood and often thrombus. The overall appearance, without the blood, is nearly identical to lymphangioma.

blood

dilated vascular space in epidermis

collarette

REFERENCES

1. Dehner LP: Pediatric Surgical Pathology. 2nd Ed. Williams & Wilkins, Baltimore, 1987
2. Lendrum AC: Painful tumours of the skin. Ann R Coll Surg Engl 1:62, 1947
3. Laskin WB, Silverman TA, Enzinger FM: Postradiation soft tissue sarcomas. Cancer 62:2330, 1988
4. Ducatman BS, Scheithauer BW: Postirradiation neurofibrosarcoma. Cancer 51:1028, 1983
5. Goette DK, Detlefs RL: Postirradiation angiosarcoma. J Am Acad Dermatol 12:922, 1985
6. Muggia FM, Lonberg M: Kaposi's sarcoma and AIDS. Med Clin North Am 70:109, 1986
7. Ghadially FN: Diagnostic Electron Microscopy of Tumours. 2nd Ed. Butterworths, London, 1985
8. Wick MR, Swanson PE, Manivel JC: Immunohistochemical analysis of soft tissue sarcomas: comparisons with electron microscopy. Appl Pathol 6:169, 1988
9. Carstens PHB: The Weibel-Palade body in the diagnosis of endothelial tumors. Ultrastruct Pathol 2:315, 1981
10. Llombart-Bosch A, Peydro-Olaya A, Pellin A: Ultrastructure of vascular neoplasms. Pathol Res Pract 174:1, 1982
11. Ordonez NG, Batsakis JG: Comparison of *Ulex europaeus* I lectin and factor VIII-related antigen in vascular lesions. Arch Pathol Lab Med 108:129, 1984
12. Traweek ST, Kandalaft PL, Mehta P, Battifora H: The human hematopoietic progenitor cell antigen (CD34) in vascular neoplasia. Am J Clin Pathol 96:25, 1991
13. Battifora H: Assessment of antigen damage in immunohistochemistry: the vimentin internal control. Am J Clin Pathol 96:669, 1991
14. Wick MR, Kaye VN: The role of diagnostic immunohistochemistry in dermatology. Semin Dermatol 5:346, 1986
15. Graham JH, Sanders JB, Johnson WC, Helwig EB: Fibrous papule of the nose: a clinicopathological study. J Invest Dermatol 45:194, 1965
16. Rosen LB, Suster S: Fibrous papules: a light microscopic and immunohistochemical study. Am J Dermatopathol 10:109, 1988
17. Saylan T, Marks R, Wilson-Jones E: Fibrous papule of the nose. Br J Dermatol 85:111, 1971
18. Zackheim MS, Pinkus H: Perifollicular fibromas. Arch Dermatol 82:913, 1960

19. Guitart J, Bergfeld WF, Tuthill RJ: Fibrous papule of the nose with granular cells: two cases. J Cutan Pathol 18:284, 1991

20. McGibbon DH, Wilson-Jones E: Fibrous papule of the face (nose): fibrosing melanocytic nevus. Am J Dermatopathol 1:345, 1979

21. Cerio R, Rao BK, Spaull J, Wilson-Jones E: An immunohistochemical study of fibrous papule of the nose: 25 cases. J Cutan Pathol 16:194, 1989

22. Chung EB, Enzinger FM: Infantile myofibromatosis. Cancer 48:1807, 1981

23. Allen PW: The fibromatoses: a clinicopathologic classification based on 140 cases (part I). Am J Surg Pathol 1:255, 1977

24. Allen PW: The fibromatoses: a clinicopathologic classification based on 140 cases (part II). Am J Surg Pathol 1:305, 1977

25. Coffin CM, Dehner LP: Soft tissue tumors in the first year of life: a report of 190 cases. Pediatr Pathol 10:509, 1990

26. Shapiro L: Infantile digital fibromatosis and aponeurotic fibroma. Arch Dermatol 99:37, 1969

27. Dabney KW, MacEwen GD, David NE: Recurring digital fibrous tumor of childhood. J Pediatr Orthop 6:612, 1986

28. Mehregan AH, Nabai H, Matthews JE: Recurring digital fibrous tumor of childhood. Arch Dermatol 106:375, 1972

29. Allen PW, Enzinger FM: Juvenile aponeurotic fibroma. Cancer 26:857, 1970

30. Goldman RL: The cartilage analogue of fibromatosis (aponeurotic fibroma): further observations based on 7 new cases. Cancer 26:1325, 1970

31. Fayad MN, Tacoub A, Salman S et al: Juvenile hyalin fibromatosis: two new patients and review of the literature. Am J Med Genet 26:123, 1987

32. Ramberger K, Krieg T, Kunze D et al: Fibromatosis hyalinica multiplex (juvenile hyalin fibromatosis). Cancer 56:614, 1985

33. Taylor LJ: Musculoaponeurotic fibromatosis: a report of 28 cases and review of the literature. Clin Orthop Rel Res 224:294, 1987

34. Ayala AG, Ro JY, Goepfert H et al: Desmoid fibromatosis: a clinicopathologic study of 25 children. Semin Diagn Pathol 3:138, 1986

35. Sundaram M, Duffrin H, McGuire MH, Vas W: Synchronous multicentric desmoid tumors (aggressive fibromatosis) of the extremities. Skel Radiol 17:16, 1988

36. Posner MC, Shiu MH, Newsome JL et al: The desmoid tumor: not a benign disease. Arch Surg 124:191, 1989

37. Daimaru Y, Hashimoto H, Enjoji M: Myofibromatosis in adults (adult counterpart of infantile myofibromatosis). Am J Surg Pathol 13:859, 1989

38. Smith KJ, Skelton HG, Barnett TL et al: Cutaneous myofibroma. Mod Pathol 2:603, 1989

39. Hogan SF, Salassa JR: Recurrent adult myofibromatosis: a case report. Am J Clin Pathol 97:810, 1992

40. Kamino H, Reddy VB, Gero M, Greco MA: Dermatomyofibroma. J Cutan Pathol 19:85, 1992

41. Larsen D, Posche L: Dupuytren's contracture, with special reference to pathology. J Bone Joint Surg 40A:773, 1958

42. Aviles E, Arlen M, Miller T: Plantar fibromatosis. Surgery 69:117, 1971

43. Briselli MF, Soule EH, Gilchrist GS: Congenital fibromatosis: report of 18 cases of solitary and 4 cases of multiple tumors. Mayo Clin Proc 55:554, 1980

44. Seibert JJ, Seibert RW, Weisenburger DS et al: Multiple congenital hemangiopericytomas of head and neck. Laryngoscope 88:1006, 1978

45. Yokoyama R, Tsuneyoshi M, Enjoji M et al: Extra-abdominal desmoid tumors: correlations between histologic features and biologic behavior. Surg Pathol 2:29, 1989

46. Bhawan J, Bacchetta C, Joris I, Majno G: A myofibroblastic tumor—infantile digital fibroma. Am J Pathol 94:19, 1979

47. Choi KC, Hashimoto K, Setoyama M et al: Infantile digital fibromatosis: immunohistochemical and immunoelectron microscopic studies. J Cutan Pathol 17:225, 1990

48. Paller AS, Gonzalez-Crussi F, Sherman JO: Fibrous hamartoma of infancy: eight additional cases and a review of the literature. Arch Dermatol 125:88, 1989

49. Montgomery H, Winkelmann RK: Smooth-muscle tumors of the skin. Arch Dermatol 79:32, 1959

50. Fox SR: Leiomyomatosis cutis. N Engl J Med 263:1248, 1960

51. Kloepfer HW, Krafchuk J, Derbes V et al: Hereditary multiple leiomyomas of the skin. Am J Hum Genet 10:48, 1958

52. Thompson JA: Therapy of painful cutaneous leiomyomas. J Am Acad Dermatol 13:865, 1985

53. Fisher WC, Helwig EB: Leiomyomas of the skin. Arch Dermatol 88:510, 1963

54. Headington JT, Beals TF, Niederhuber JE: Primary leiomyosarcoma of the skin: a report and critical appraisal. J Cutan Pathol 4:308, 1977

55. Magner D, Hill DP: Encapsulated angiomyoma of the skin and subcutaneous tissue. Am J Clin Pathol 35:137, 1961

56. MacDonald DM, Sanderson RV: Angioleiomyoma of the skin. Br J Dermatol 91:161, 1974

57. Hachisuga T, Hashimoto H, Enjoji M: Angioleiomyoma: a clinicopathologic reappraisal of 562 cases. Cancer 54:126, 1984

58. Berger TG, Levin MW: Congenital smooth muscle hamartoma. J Am Acad Dermatol 11:709, 1984

59. Tsambaos D, Orfanos CE: Cutaneous smooth muscle hamartoma. J Cutan Pathol 9:33, 1982

60. Girard C, Graham JH, Johnson WC: Arteriovenous hemangioma (arteriovenous shunt): a clinicopathological and histochemical study. J Cutan Pathol 1:73, 1974

61. Carapeto FJ, Garcia-Perez A, Winkelmann RK: Acral arteriovenous tumor. Acta Dermatol Venereol 57:155, 1977

62. Connelly MG, Winkelmann RK: Acral arteriovenous tumor: a clinicopathologic review. Am J Surg Pathol 9:15, 1985

63. Shugart RR, Soule EH, Johnson EW: Glomus tumors. Surg Gynecol Obstet 117:334, 1963

64. Conant MA, Wiesenfeld SL: Multiple glomus tumors of the skin. Arch Dermatol 103:481, 1971

65. Kaye VN, Dehner LP: Cutaneous glomus tumor. Am J Dermatopathol 13:2, 1991

66. Enzinger FM, Smith BH: Hemangiopericytoma: an analysis of 106 cases. Hum Pathol 7:61, 1976

67. Czernobilsky B, Cornog JL Jr, Enterline HT: Rhabdomy-

oma: report of cases with ultrastructural and histochemical studies. Am J Clin Pathol 49:782, 1968

68. Hajdu SI: Pathology of Soft Tissue Tumors. Lea & Febiger, Philadelphia, 1979

69. Dehner LP, Enzinger FM, Font RL: Fetal rhabdomyoma: an analysis of nine cases. Cancer 30:160, 1972

70. Dehner LP: Juvenile rhabdomyoma. Pediatr Pathol (in press)

71. Sangueza O, Sangueza P, Jordan J, White CR Jr: Rhabdomyoma of the tongue. Am J Dermatopathol 12:492, 1990

72. Sahn EE, Garen PD, Pai GS et al: Multiple rhabdomyomatous mesenchymal hamartomas of skin. Am J Dermatopathol 12:485, 1990

73. Mills AE: Rhabdomyomatous mesenchymal hamartoma of skin. Am J Dermatopathol 11:58, 1989

74. Ashfaq R, Timmons CF: Rhabdomyomatous mesenchymal hamartoma of skin. Pediatr Pathol 12:731, 1992

75. Flanagan BP, Helwig EB: Cutaneous lymphangioma. Arch Dermatol 113:24, 1977

76. Fisher I, Orkin M: Acquired lymphangioma (lymphangiectasis). Arch Dermatol 101:230, 1970

77. Peachy RO, Limm CC, Whimster IW: Lymphangioma of skin: a review of 65 cases. Br J Dermatol 83:519, 1970

78. Whimster IW: The pathology of lymphangioma circumscriptum. Br J Dermatol 10:35, 1974

79. Margileth AM: Cutaneous vascular tumors. Med Probl Pediatr 17:101, 1975

80. Donsky HJ: Vascular tumors of the skin. Can Med Assoc J 99:993, 1968

81. Simpson JR: Natural history of cavernous hemangiomata. Lancet 2:1057, 1959

82. Iizuka S: Eosinophilic lymphadenitis and granulomatosis: Kimura's disease. Nihon Univ Med J 18:900, 1959

83. Santa Cruz DJ, Aronberg J: Targetoid hemosiderotic hemangioma. J Am Acad Dermatol 19:550, 1988

84. Dekaminsky AR, Otero AC, Kaminsky CA et al: Multiple disseminated pyogenic granulomas. Br J Dermatol 98:461, 1978

85. Wick MR, Manivel JC: Vascular neoplasms of the skin: a current perspective. Adv Dermatol 4:185, 1989

86. Mills SE, Cooper PH, Fechner RE: Lobular capillary hemangioma: the underlying lesion of pyogenic granuloma. Am J Surg Pathol 4:471, 1980

87. Padilla RS, Orkin M, Rosai J: Acquired "tufted" hemangioma (progressive capillary hemangioma). Am J Dermatopathol 9:292, 1987

88. Bardwick PA, Zvaifler NJ, Gill GN et al: Plasma cell dyscrasia with polyneuropathy, organomegaly, endocrinopathy, M Protein, and skin changes: The POEMS syndrome. Medicine (Baltimore) 59:311, 1980

89. Imperial R, Helwig EB: Verrucous hemangioma: a clinicopathologic study of 21 cases. Arch Dermatol 96:247, 1967

90. Rao VK, Weiss SW: Angiomatosis of soft tissue: an analysis of the histologic features and clinical outcome in 51 cases. Am J Surg Pathol 16:764, 1992

91. Rapini RP, Golitz LE: Targetoid hemosiderotic hemangioma. J Cutan Pathol 17:233, 1990

92. Rosai J, Gold J, Landy R: The histiocytoid hemangiomas:

a unifying concept embracing several previously described entities of skin, soft tissue, large vessels, bone, and heart. Hum Pathol 10:707, 1979

93. Urabe A, Tsuneyoshi M, Enjoji M: Epithelioid hemangioma versus Kimura's disease: a comparative clinicopathologic study. Am J Surg Pathol 11:758, 1987

94. Nichols GE, Gaffey MJ, Mills SE, Weiss LM: Lobular capillary hemangioma: an immunohistochemical study including steroid hormone receptor status. Am J Clin Pathol 97:770, 1992

95. Cooper PH, Mills SE: Subcutaneous granuloma pyogenicum: lobular capillary hemangioma. Arch Dermatol 118:30, 1982

96. Satomi I, Tanaka Y, Murata J et al: A case of angioblastoma (Nakagawa). Rinsho Dermatol 23:703, 1981

97. Wilson-Jones E, Orkin M: Tufted angioma (angioblastoma): a benign progressive angioma, not to be confused with Kaposi's sarcoma or low-grade angiosarcoma. J Am Acad Dermatol 20:214, 1989

98. Cooper PH, McAllister HA, Helwig EB: Intravenous pyogenic granuloma: a study of 18 cases. Am J Surg Pathol 3:221, 1979

99. Chan JKC, Fletcher CDM, Hicklin GA, Rosai J: Glomeruloid hemangioma: a distinctive cutaneous lesion of multicentric Castleman's disease associated with POEMS syndrome. Am J Surg Pathol 14:1036, 1990

100. Hunt SJ, Santa Cruz DJ, Barr RJ: Microvenular hemangioma. J Cutan Pathol 18:235, 1991

101. Wilson-Jones E, Winkelmann RK, Zachary CB, Reda AM: Benign lymphangioendothelioma. J Am Acad Dermatol 23:229, 1990

102. Wilson-Jones E, Cerio R, Smith NP: Multinucleate cell angiohistiocytoma: an acquired vascular anomaly to be distinguished from Kaposi's sarcoma. Br J Dermatol 122:651, 1990

103. Mehregan AH, Shapiro L: Angiolymphoid hyperplasia with eosinophilia. Arch Dermatol 103:50, 1971

104. Reed RJ, Bliss BO: Morton's neuroma: regressive and productive intermetatarsal elastofibrositis. Arch Pathol 95:123, 1973

105. Scotti TM: The lesion of Morton's metatarsalgia (Morton's toe). Arch Pathol 63:91, 1957

106. Reed RJ, Fine RM, Meltzer HD: Palisaded encapsulated neuromas of the skin. Arch Dermatol 106:865, 1972

107. Dover JS, From L, Lewis A: Clinicopathologic findings in palisaded encapsulated neuromas. J Cutan Pathol 13:77, 1986

108. Geffner RE: Ganglioneuroma of the skin. Arch Dermatol 122:377, 1986

109. Carney JA, Sizemore GW, Lovestedt SA: Mucosal ganglioneuromatosis, medullary thyroid carcinoma, and pheochromocytoma: multiple endocrine neoplasia, type 2b. Oral Surg 41:739, 1976

110. Rios JJ, Siaz-Cano SJ, Rivera-Hueto F, Willar JL: Cutaneous ganglion cell choristoma. J Cutan Pathol 18:469, 1991

111. Oshman RG, Phelps RG, Kantor I: A solitary neurofibroma on the finger. Arch Dermatol 122:1185, 1988

112. Stout AP: Neurofibroma and neurilemoma. Clin Proc 5:1, 1946

113. Harkin JC, Reed RJ: Tumors of the peripheral nervous system. p. 29. In Atlas of Tumor Pathology (Series 2, Fascicle 3). Armed Forces Institute of Pathology, Washington, DC, 1969

114. McCarroll HR: Clinical manifestations of congenital neurofibromatosis. J Bone Joint Surg 32A:601, 1950

115. Preston FW, Walsh WS, Clarke TH: Cutaneous neurofibromatosis (von Recklinghausen's disease): clinical manifestations and incidence of sarcoma in 61 male patients. Arch Surg 64:813, 1952

116. Ross DE: Skin manifestations of von Recklinghausen's disease and associated tumors (neurofibromatosis). Am Surg 31:729, 1965

117. Saxen E: Tumours of tactile end-organs. Acta Pathol Microbiol Scand 25:66, 1948

118. Daimaru Y, Hashimoto H, Enjoji M: Malignant peripheral nerve sheath tumors (malignant schwannomas). Am J Surg Pathol 9:434, 1985

119. Saxen E: Tumors of the sheaths of the peripheral nerves (studies on their structure). Acta Pathol Microbiol Scand, suppl. 79:1, 1948

120. Woodruff JM: Peripheral nerve tumors showing glandular differentiation (glandular schwannomas). Cancer 37:2399, 1976

121. Font RL, Truong LD: Melanotic schwannoma of soft tissues. Am J Surg Pathol 8:129, 1984

122. Mennemeyer RP, Hammar SP, Titus JS et al: Melanotic schwannoma. Am J Surg Pathol 3:3, 1979

123. Fletcher CDM: Benign plexiform (multinodular) schwannoma: a rare tumor unassociated with neurofibromatosis. Histopathology 10:971, 1986

124. Iwashita T, Enjoji M: Plexiform neurilemmoma. Virchows Arch A 411:305, 1987

125. Taxy JB, Battifora H: Epithelioid schwannoma: diagnosis by electron microscopy. Ultrastruct Pathol 2:19, 1981

126. Carney JA: Psammomatous melanotic schwannoma. Am J Surg Pathol 14:206, 1990

127. Fletcher CDM, Davies SE, McKee PH: Cellular schwannoma: a distinct pseudosarcomatous entity. Histopathology 11:21, 1987

128. Gallager RL, Helwig EB: Neurothekeoma: a benign cutaneous tumor of neural origin. Am J Clin Pathol 74:759, 1980

129. MacDonald DM, Wilson-Jones E: Pacinian neurofibroma. Histopathology 1:247, 1977

130. Fletcher CDM, Chan JKC, McKee PH: Dermal nerve sheath myxoma: a study of 3 cases. Histopathology 10:135, 1986

131. Aronson PJ, Fretzin DF, Potter BS: Neurothekeoma of Gallager and Helwig (dermal nerve sheath myxoma variant): report of a case with electron microscopic and immunohistochemical studies. J Cutan Pathol 12:506, 1985

132. Barnhill RL, Mihm MC Jr: Cellular neurothekeoma: a distinctive variant of neurothekeoma mimicking nevomelanocytic tumors. Am J Surg Pathol 14:113, 1990

133. Lack EE, Worsham GF, Callihan MD et al: Granular cell tumor: a clinicopathologic study of 110 patients. J Surg Oncol 13:301, 1980

134. Sobel HJ, Churg J: Granular cells and granular cell lesions. Arch Pathol 77:132, 1964

135. Sobel HJ, Marquet E: Granular cells and granular cell lesions. Pathol Annu 9:43, 1974

136. Apisarnthanarax P: Granular cell tumor: an analysis of 16 cases and review of the literature. J Am Acad Dermatol 5:171, 1981

137. Manivel JC, Dehner LP, Wick MR: Nonvascular sarcomas of the skin. p. 211. In Wick MR (ed): Pathology of Unusual Malignant Cutaneous Tumors. Marcel Dekker, New York, 1985

138. Abenoza P, Sibley RK: Granular cell myoblastoma and schwannoma: a fine structural and immunohistochemical study. Ultrastruct Pathol 11:19, 1987

139. Penneys NS, Adachi K, Ziegels-Weissman J, Nadji M: Granular cell tumors of the skin contain myelin basic protein. Arch Pathol Lab Med 107:302, 1983

140. Sobel HJ, Schwartz R, Marquet E: Light and electron microscopic study of the origin of granular cell myoblastoma. J Pathol 109:101, 1973

141. LeBoit PE, Barr RJ, Burall S et al: Primitive polypoid granular cell tumor and other cutaneous granular cell neoplasms of apparent non-neural origin. Am J Surg Pathol 15:48, 1991

142. Arnold HL, Odom RB, James WD (eds): Andrews' Diseases of the Skin: Clinical Dermatology. 8th Ed. WB Saunders, Philadelphia, 1990

143. Fletcher CDM, Martin-Bates E: Spindle-cell lipoma: a clinicopathological study with some original observations. Histopathology 11:803, 1987

144. Griffin TD, Goldstein J, Johnson WC: Pleomorphic lipoma. J Cutan Pathol 19:330, 1992

145. Dixon AY, McGregor DH, Lee SH: Angiolipomas: an ultrastructural and clinicopathologic study. Hum Pathol 12:739, 1981

146. Enzinger FM, Harvey DJ: Spindle-cell lipoma. Cancer 36:1852, 1975

147. Shmookler BM, Enzinger FM: Pleomorphic lipoma: a benign tumor simulating liposarcoma. A clinicopathologic analysis of 48 cases. Cancer 47:126, 1981

148. Howard WR, Helwig EB: Angiolipoma. Arch Dermatol 82:924, 1960

149. Kurzweg FT, Spencer R: Familial multiple lipomatosis. Am J Surg 82:762, 1951

150. Osment LS: Cutaneous lipomas and lipomatosis. Surg Gynecol Obstet 127:129, 1968

151. Sahl WJ Jr: Mobile encapsulated lipomas. Arch Dermatol 114:1684, 1978

152. Hunt SJ, Santa Cruz DJ, Barr RJ: Cellular angiolipoma. Am J Surg Pathol 14:75, 1990

153. Kauffman SL, Stout AP: Lipoblastic tumors of children. Cancer 12:912, 1959

154. Chung EB, Enzinger FM: Benign lipoblastomatosis: an analysis of 35 cases. Cancer 32:482, 1973

155. Mahour GH, Bryan BJ, Isaacs H Jr: Lipoblastoma and lipoblastomatosis: a report of six cases. Surgery 104:577, 1988

156. Rigor VU, Goldstone SE: Hibernoma: a case report and discussion of a rare tumor. Cancer 57:2207, 1986

157. Dardick I: Hibernoma: a possible model of brown fat histogenesis. Hum Pathol 9:321, 1978

158. Fitzpatrick TB, Gilchrist BA: Dimple sign to differentiate

benign from malignant cutaneous lesions. N Engl J Med 296:1518, 1977

159. Gonzalez S, Duarte I: Benign fibrous histiocytoma of the skin: a morphologic study of 290 cases. Pathol Res Pract 174:379, 1982

160. Niemi KM: The benign fibrohistiocytic tumors of the skin. Acta Dermatol Venereol, suppl. 50:1, 1970

161. Baraf CS, Shapiro L: Multiple histiocytomas. Arch Dermatol 101:588, 1970

162. Roberts JT, Byrne EH, Rosenthal D: Familial variant of dermatofibroma with malignancy in the proband. Arch Dermatol 117:12, 1981

163. Schoenfeld RJ: Epidermal proliferations overlying histiocytomas. Arch Dermatol 90:266, 1964

164. Marrogi AJ, Dehner LP, Coffin CM, Wick MR: Benign cutaneous histiocytic tumors in childhood and adolescence, excluding Langerhans' cell proliferations: a clinicopathologic and immunohistochemical analysis. Am J Dermatopathol 14:8, 1992

165. Leyva WH, Santa Cruz DJ: Atypical cutaneous fibrous histiocytoma. Am J Dermatopathol 8:467, 1986

166. Kamino H, Jacobson M: Dermatofibroma extending into the subcutaneous tissue: differential diagnosis from dermatofibrosarcoma protuberans. Am J Surg Pathol 14:1156, 1990

167. Fukamizu H, Oku T, Inoue K et al: Atypical (pseudosarcomatous) cutaneous histiocytoma. J Cutan Pathol 10:327, 1983

168. Tamada S, Ackerman AB: Dermatofibroma with monster cells. Am J Dermatopathol 9:380, 1987

169. Santa Cruz DJ, Kyriakos M: Aneurysmal (angiomatoid) fibrous histiocytoma of the skin. Cancer 47:2053, 1981

170. Sood U, Mehregan AH: Aneurysmal (angiomatoid) fibrous histiocytoma. J Cutan Pathol 12:157, 1985

171. Barker SM, Winkelmann RK: Inflammatory lymphadenoid reactions with dermatofibroma/histiocytoma. J Cutan Pathol 13:222, 1986

172. Goette DK, Helwig EB: Basal cell carcinomas and basal cell carcinoma-like changes overlying dermatofibromas. Arch Dermatol 111:589, 1975

173. Schwob VS, Santa Cruz DJ: Palisading cutaneous fibrous histiocytoma. J Cutan Pathol 13:403, 1986

174. Bernstein JC: Hemosiderin histiocytoma of the skin. Arch Dermatol 40:390, 1939

175. Franquemont DW, Cooper PH, Shmookler BM, Wick MR: Benign fibrous histiocytoma of the skin with potential for local recurrence. Mod Pathol 3:158, 1990

176. Marrogi AJ, Dehner LP, Coffin CM, Wick MR: Atypical fibrous histiocytoma of the skin in childhood and adolescence. J Cutan Pathol 19:268, 1992

177. Jones FE, Soule EH, Coventry MB: Fibrous histiocytoma of synovium (giant cell tumor of tendon sheath pigmented nodular synovitis): a study of 118 cases. J Bone Joint Surg 51A:76, 1969

178. Phalen GS, McCormack LJ, Gazale WJ: Giant cell tumor of tendon sheath (benign synovioma) in the hand: evaluation of 56 cases. Clin Orthop 15:140, 1959

179. King DT, Millman AJ, Gurevitch AW et al: Giant cell tumor of the tendon sheath involving skin. Arch Dermatol 114:944, 1978

180. Chung EB, Enzinger FM: Fibroma of tendon sheath. Cancer 44:1945, 1979

181. Humphreys S, McKee PH, Fletcher CDM: Fibroma of tendon sheath: a clinicopathologic study. J Cutan Pathol 13:331, 1986

182. Johnson WC, Graham JH, Helwig EB: Cutaneous myxoid cyst. JAMA 191:15, 1965

183. Carney JA, Gordon H, Carpenter PC et al: The complex of myxomas, spotty pigmentation, and endocrine overactivity. Medicine (Baltimore) 64:270, 1985

184. Steeper TA, Rosai J: Aggressive angiomyxoma of the female pelvis and perineum. Am J Surg Pathol 7:463, 1983

185. Fletcher CDM, Tsang WYW, Fisher C et al: Angiomyofibroblastoma of the vulva. Am J Surg Pathol 16:373, 1992

186. Dahlin DC, Salvador AH: Cartilaginous tumors of the soft tissues of the hands and feet. Mayo Clin Proc 49:721, 1974

187. Holmes HS, Bovenmeyer DA: Cutaneous cartilaginous tumor. Arch Dermatol 112:839, 1976

188. Burgdorf WHC, Nasemann T: Cutaneous osteoma: a clinical and histopathological review. Arch Dermatol Res 260:121, 1977

189. Collina G, Annessi G, DiGregorio C: Cellular blue nevus associated with osteoma cutis. Histopathology 19:473, 1991

190. Hirsh P, Helwig EB: Chondroid syringoma: mixed tumor of the skin of salivary gland type. Arch Dermatol 84:835, 1961

191. Dupree WB, Enzinger FM: Fibro-osseous pseudotumor of the digits. Cancer 58:2103, 1986

192. Bowyer SL, Blane CE, Sullivan DB et al: Childhood dermatomyositis: factors predicting functional outcome and development of dystrophic calcification. J Pediatr 103:882, 1983

193. Dabska M: Malignant endovascular papillary angioendothelioma of the skin in childhood: clinicopathologic study of 6 cases. Cancer 24:503, 1969

194. DeDulanto F, Armijo-Moreno M: Malignant endovascular papillary hemangioendothelioma of the skin: the nosological situation. Acta Dermatol Venereol 53:403, 1973

195. Manivel JC, Wick MR, Swanson PE et al: Endovascular papillary angioendothelioma of childhood: a vascular tumor possibly characterized by "high" endothelial differentiation. Hum Pathol 17:1240, 1986

196. Patterson K, Chandler RS: Malignant endovascular papillary angioendothelioma: cutaneous borderline tumor. Arch Pathol Lab Med 109:671, 1985

197. Weiss SW, Enzinger FM: Epithelioid hemangioendothelioma: a vascular tumor often mistaken for a carcinoma. Cancer 50:970, 1982

198. Weiss SW, Ishak KG, Dail DH et al: Epithelioid hemangioendothelioma and related lesions. Semin Diagn Pathol 3:259, 1986

199. Weiss SW, Enzinger FM: Spindle-cell hemangioendothelioma. Am J Surg Pathol 10:521, 1986

200. Scott GA, Rosai J: Spindle-cell hemangioendothelioma. Am J Dermatopathol 10:281, 1988

201. Fletcher CDM, Beham A, Schmid C: Spindle-cell hemangioendothelioma: a clinicopathological and immunohistochemical study indicative of a non-neoplastic lesion. Histopathology 18:291, 1991

202. Imayama S, Murakamai Y, Hashimoto H, Hori Y: Spindle-cell hemangioendothelioma exhibits the ultrastructural features of reactive vascular proliferation rather than of angiosarcoma. Am J Clin Pathol 97:279, 1992

203. Wolff M, Rothenberg D: Dermal leiomyosarcoma: a misnomer? Prog Surg Pathol 7:147, 1986

204. Dahl I, Angervall L: Cutaneous and subcutaneous leiomyosarcoma: a clinicopathologic study of 47 patients. Pathol Eur 9:307, 1974

205. Fields JP, Helwig EB: Leiomyosarcoma of the skin and subcutaneous tissue. Cancer 47:156, 1981

206. Swanson PE, Stanley MW, Scheithauer BW, Wick MR: Primary cutaneous leiomyosarcoma. J Cutan Pathol 15:129, 1988

207. Stout AP, Murray MR: Hemangiopericytoma. Am J Surg 116:26, 1942

208. Saunders TS, Fitzpatrick TB: Multiple hemangiopericytomas: their distinction from glomangiomas (glomus tumors). Arch Dermatol 76:731, 1957

209. D'Amore ESG, Manivel JC, Sung JH: Soft tissue and meningeal hemangiopericytomas: an immunohistochemical and ultrastructural study. Hum Pathol 21:414, 1990

210. Burkhardt BR, Soule EH, Winkelmann RK, Ivins JC: Dermatofibrosarcoma protuberans: a study of fifty-six cases. Am J Surg 111:638, 1966

211. McKee PH, Fletcher CDM: Dermatofibrosarcoma protuberans presenting in infancy and childhood. J Cutan Pathol 18:241, 1991

212. McPeak CJ, Cruz T, Nicastri AD: Dermatofibrosarcoma: an analysis of 86 cases—five with metastases. Ann Surg 166:803, 1967

213. Taylor HB, Helwig EB: Dermatofibrosarcoma protuberans: a study of 115 cases. Cancer 15:717, 1962

214. Fletcher CDM, Evans BJ, Macartney JC et al: Dermatofibrosarcoma protuberans: a clinicopathological and immunohistochemical study with a review of the literature. Histopathology 9:921, 1985

215. Frierson HF Jr, Cooper PH: Myxoid variant of dermatofibrosarcoma protuberans. Am J Surg Pathol 7:445, 1983

216. Dupree WB, Langloss JM, Weiss SW: Pigmented dermatofibrosarcoma protuberans (Bednar tumor): a pathologic, ultrastructural, and immunohistochemical study. Am J Surg Pathol 9:630, 1985

217. Wrotnowski U, Cooper PH, Shmookler BM: Fibrosarcomatous change in dermatofibrosarcoma protuberans. Am J Surg Pathol 12:287, 1988

218. Ding J, Hashimoto H, Enjoji M: Dermatofibrosarcoma protuberans with fibrosarcomatous areas: a clinicopathologic study of nine cases and a comparison with allied tumors. Cancer 64:721, 1989

219. Connelly JH, Evans HL: Dermatofibrosarcoma protuberans: a clinicopathologic review with emphasis on fibrosarcomatous areas. Am J Surg Pathol 16:921, 1992

220. Volpe R, Carbone A: Dermatofibrosarcoma protuberans metastatic to lymph nodes and showing a dominant histiocytic component. Am J Dermatopathol 5:327, 1983

221. O'Dowd J, Laidler P: Progression of dermatofibrosarcoma protuberans to malignant fibrous histiocytoma: report of a case with implications for tumor histogenesis. Hum Pathol 19:368, 1988

222. Shmookler BM, Enzinger FM: Giant cell fibroblastoma: a peculiar childhood tumor, abstracted. Lab Invest 46:7A, 1983

223. Shmookler BM, Enzinger FM, Weiss SW: Giant cell fibroblastoma. Cancer 64:2154, 1989

224. Abdul-Karim W, Evans HL, Silva EG: Giant cell fibroblastoma: a report of three cases. Am J Clin Pathol 83:165, 1985

225. Dymock RB, Allen PW, Stirling JW et al: Giant cell fibroblastoma: a distinctive recurrent tumor of childhood. Am J Surg Pathol 11:263, 1987

226. Fletcher CDM: Giant cell fibroblastoma of soft tissue: a clinicopathological and immunohistochemical study. Histopathology 13:499, 1988

227. Beham A, Fletcher CDM: Dermatofibrosarcoma protuberans resembling giant cell fibroblastoma: report of two cases. Histopathology 17:165, 1990

228. DeChadarevian JP, Coppola D, Billmire DF: Bednar tumor pattern in recurring giant cell fibroblastoma. Am J Clin Pathol 100:164, 1993

229. Marrogi AJ, Swanson PE, Kyriakos M et al: Rudimentary meningocele: clinicopathologic features and differential diagnosis. J Cutan Pathol 18:178, 1991

230. Enzinger FM, Zhang R: Plexiform fibrohistiocytic tumor presenting in children and young adults: an analysis of 65 cases. Am J Surg Pathol 12:818, 1988

231. Hollowood K, Holley MP, Fletcher CDM: Plexiform fibrohistiocytic tumour: clinicopathological, immunohistochemical, and ultrastructural analysis in favor of a myofibroblastic lesion. Histopathology 19:503, 1991

232. Kay S: Angiomatoid malignant fibrous histiocytoma: report of two cases with ultrastructural observations of one case. Arch Pathol Lab Med 109:934, 1985

233. Costa MJ, Weiss SW: Angiomatoid malignant fibrous histiocytoma: a followup study of 108 cases with evaluation of possible histologic predictors of outcome. Am J Surg Pathol 14:1126, 1990

234. Enzinger FM: Angiomatoid malignant fibrous histiocytoma: a distinct fibrohistiocytic tumor of children and young adults, simulating a vascular neoplasm. Cancer 44:2146, 1979

235. Hashimoto H, Enjoji M, Nakajima T et al: Malignant neuroepithelioma (peripheral neuroblastoma): a clinicopathologic study of 15 cases. Am J Surg Pathol 7:309, 1983

236. Dehner LP: Peripheral and central neuroectodermal tumors: a nosologic concept seeking a consensus. Arch Pathol Lab Med 110:997, 1986

237. Jacinto CM, Grant-Kels JM, Knibbs DR et al: Malignant peripheral neuroectodermal tumor presenting as a scalp nodule. Am J Dermatopathol 13:63, 1991

238. Patterson JW, Maygarden SJ: Extraskeletal Ewing's sarcoma with cutaneous involvement. J Cutan Pathol 13:46, 1986

239. Peters MS, Reiman HM Jr, Muller SA: Cutaneous extraskeletal Ewing's sarcoma. J Cutan Pathol 12:476, 1985

240. Mierau GW: Extraskeletal Ewing's sarcoma (peripheral neuroepithelioma). Ultrastruct Pathol 9:91, 1985

241. Jurgens H, Bier V, Harms D et al: Malignant peripheral neuroectodermal tumors. Cancer 61:349, 1988

242. Triche TJ, Askin F: Neuroblastoma and the differential di-

agnosis of small-, round-, blue-cell tumors. Hum Pathol 14:569, 1983

243. Wick MR, Scheithauer BW: Primary neuroendocrine carcinoma of the skin. p. 107. In Wick MR (ed): Pathology of Unusual Malignant Cutaneous Tumors. Marcel Dekker, New York, 1985

244. Michels S, Swanson PE, Frizzera G et al: Immunostaining for leukocyte common antigen using an amplified avidin-biotin-peroxidase complex method and paraffin sections. Arch Pathol Lab Med 111:1035, 1987

245. Shapiro L: Neuroblastoma with multiple cutaneous metastases. Arch Dermatol 99:502, 1969

246. Wiss K, Solomon AR, Raimer SS et al: Rhabdomyosarcoma presenting as a cutaneous nodule. Arch Dermatol 124:1687, 1988

247. Chang Y, Dehner LP, Egbert B: Primary cutaneous rhabdomyosarcoma. Am J Surg Pathol 14:977, 1990

248. Agamanolis DP, Dasu S, Krill CE: Tumors of skeletal muscle. Hum Pathol 17:778, 1986

249. Kiryu H, Urabe H: Malignant Triton tumor. Am J Dermatopathol 14:255, 1992

250. Daimaru Y, Hashimoto H, Enjoji M: Malignant "Triton" tumors: a clinicopathologic and immunohistochemical study of nine cases. Hum Pathol 15:768, 1984

251. D'Agostino AN, Soule EH, Miller RH: Sarcomas of the peripheral nerves and somatic soft tissues associated with multiple neurofibromatosis (von Recklinghausen's disease). Cancer 16:1015, 1963

252. George E, Swanson PE, Wick MR: Malignant peripheral nerve sheath tumors of the skin. Am J Dermatopathol 11:213, 1989

253. Dabski C, Reiman HM Jr, Muller SA: Neurofibrosarcoma of skin and subcutaneous tissues. Mayo Clin Proc 65:164, 1990

254. Ducatman BS, Scheithauer BW, Piepgras DG et al: Malignant peripheral nerve sheath tumors: a clinicopathologic study of 120 cases. Cancer 57:2006, 1986

255. Wick MR, Swanson PE, Scheithauer BW, Manivel JC: Malignant peripheral nerve sheath tumor: an immunohistochemical study of 62 cases. Am J Clin Pathol 87:425, 1987

256. Wick MR: Malignant peripheral nerve sheath tumors of the skin. Mayo Clin Proc 65:279, 1990

257. DiMaio SM, Mackay B, Smith JL et al: Neurosarcomatous transformation in malignant melanoma: an ultrastructural study. Cancer 50:2345, 1982

258. Gown AM, Vogel AM, Hoak D et al: Monoclonal antibodies specific for melanocytic tumors distinguish subpopulations of melanocytes. Am J Pathol 123:195, 1986

259. Wick MR: Kaposi's sarcoma unrelated to the acquired immunodeficiency syndrome. Curr Opin Oncol 3:377, 1991

260. Chor PJ, Santa Cruz DJ: Kaposi's sarcoma: a clinicopathologic review and differential diagnosis. J Cutan Pathol 19:6, 1992

261. Gottlieb GJ, Ackerman AB (eds): Kaposi's Sarcoma: a Text and Atlas. Lea & Febiger, Philadelphia, 1988

262. Gottlieb GJ, Ackerman AB: Kaposi's sarcoma: an extensively disseminated form in young homosexual men. Hum Pathol 13:882, 1982

263. Jaffe HW: Acquired immune deficiency syndrome: epi-

demiologic features. J Am Acad Dermatol 22:1167, 1990

264. Ackerman AB: The patch stage of Kaposi's sarcoma. Am J Dermatopathol 1:165, 1979

265. Pollack MS, Safai B, Myskowski PL et al: Frequencies of HLA and Gm immunogenetic markers in Kaposi's sarcoma. Tissue Antigens 21:1, 1983

266. Boldogh I, Beth E, Huang ES et al: Kaposi's sarcoma: IV. Detection of CMV-DNA, CMV-RNA, and CMNA in tumor biopsies. Int J Cancer 28:469, 1981

267. Fenoglio CM, Oster M, LoGerfo P et al: Kaposi's sarcoma following chemotherapy for testicular cancer in a homosexual man: demonstration of cytomegalovirus DNA in sarcoma cells. Hum Pathol 13:955, 1982

268. Costa J, Rabson AS: Generalized Kaposi's sarcoma is not a neoplasm. Lancet 1:58, 1983

269. Delli-Bovi P, Basilico C: Isolation of a rearranged human transforming gene following transfection of Kaposi's sarcoma DNA. Proc Natl Acad Sci USA 84:5660, 1987

270. Beckstead JH, Wood GS, Fletcher V: Evidence for the origin of Kaposi's sarcoma from lymphatic endothelium. Am J Pathol 119:294, 1985

271. Harrison AC, Kahn LB: Myogenic cells in Kaposi's sarcoma: an ultrastructural study. J Pathol 124:157, 1978

272. McNutt NS, Fletcher V, Conant MA: Early lesions of Kaposi's sarcoma in homosexual men: an ultrastructural comparison with other vascular proliferations in skin. Am J Dermatopathol 3:62, 1983

273. Blumenfeld W, Egbert BM, Sagebiel RW: Differential diagnosis of Kaposi's sarcoma. Arch Pathol Lab Med 109:123, 1985

274. Snover DC, Rosai J: Vascular sarcomas of the skin. p. 181. In Wick MR (ed): Pathology of Unusual Malignant Cutaneous Tumors. Marcel Dekker, New York, 1985

275. Templeton AC: Kaposi's sarcoma. Pathol Annu 17:315, 1981

276. Enzinger FM: Epithelioid sarcoma: a sarcoma simulating a granuloma or a carcinoma. Cancer 26:1029, 1970

277. Chase DR, Enzinger FM: Epithelioid sarcoma: prognostic factors and treatment. Am J Surg Pathol 9:241, 1985

278. Heenan PJ, Quirk CJ, Papadimitriou JM: Epithelioid sarcoma: a diagnostic problem. Am J Dermatopathol 8:95, 1986

279. Shmookler BM, Gunther SF: Superficial epithelioid sarcoma: a clinical and histologic simulant of benign cutaneous disease. J Am Acad Dermatol 14:893, 1986

280. Schmidt D, Harms D: Epithelioid sarcoma in children and adolescents: an immunohistochemical study. Virchows Arch A 410:423, 1987

281. Weissman D, Amenta PS, Kantor GR: Vulvar epithelioid sarcoma metastatic to the scalp. Am J Dermatopathol 12:462, 1990

282. Manivel JC, Wick MR, Dehner LP, Sibley RK: Epithelioid sarcoma: an immunohistochemical study. Am J Clin Pathol 87:310, 1987

283. Enzinger FM: Clear cell sarcoma of tendons and aponeuroses: an analysis of 21 cases. Cancer 18:1164, 1965

284. Eckardt JJ, Pritchard DJ, Soule EH: Clear cell sarcoma: a clinicopathologic study of 27 cases. Cancer 52:1482, 1983

285. Pavlidis NA, Fisher C, Wiltshaw E: Clear cell sarcoma of tendons and aponeuroses: a clinicopathologic study. Cancer 54:1412, 1984

286. Bearman RM, Noe J, Kempson RL: Clear cell sarcoma with melanin pigment. Cancer 36:977, 1975
287. Boudreaux D, Waisman J: Clear cell sarcoma with melanogenesis. Cancer 41:1387, 1978
288. Ekfors TO, Rantakokko V: Clear cell sarcoma of tendons and aponeuroses: malignant melanoma of soft tissues? Report of 4 cases. Pathol Res Pract 165:422, 1979
289. Chung EB, Enzinger FM: Malignant melanoma of soft parts. Am J Surg Pathol 7:405, 1983
290. Sara AS, Evans HL, Benjamin RS: Malignant melanoma of soft parts (clear cell sarcoma): a study of 17 cases with emphasis on prognostic factors. Cancer 65:367, 1990
291. Swanson PE, Wick MR: Clear cell sarcoma: an immunohistochemical analysis of six cases and comparison with other epithelioid neoplasms of soft tissue. Arch Pathol Lab Med 113:55, 1989
292. Rachman R, Meranze DR, Zibelman CS et al: Malignant leiomyoblastoma. Am J Clin Pathol 49:556, 1968
293. DiCarlo EF, Woodruff JM, Bansal M, Erlandson RA: The purely epithelioid malignant peripheral nerve sheath tumor. Am J Surg Pathol 10:478, 1986
294. Morgan KG, Gray C: Malignant epithelioid schwannoma of superficial soft tissue? A case report with immunohistology and electron microscopy. Histopathology 9:765, 1985
295. Bhuta S, Mirra JM, Cochran AJ: Myxoid malignant melanoma. Am J Surg Pathol 10:203, 1986
296. Cadotte M: Malignant granular cell myoblastoma. Cancer 33:1417, 1974
297. Al-Sarraf M, Loud A, Vaitkevicius V: Malignant granular cell tumor. Arch Pathol 91:550, 1971
298. MacKenzie DH: Malignant granular cell myoblastoma. J Clin Pathol 20:739, 1967
299. Shimamura K, Osamura RY, Ueyama Y et al: Malignant granular cell tumor of the right sciatic nerve. Cancer 53:524, 1984
300. Franzblau MJ, Manwaring J, Plumhof C et al: Metastatic breast carcinoma mimicking granular cell tumor. J Cutan Pathol 16:218, 1989
301. Dabbs DJ, Park HK: Malignant rhabdoid skin tumor: an uncommon primary skin neoplasm. J Cutan Pathol 15:109, 1988
302. Perrone T, Swanson PE, Twiggs L et al: Malignant rhabdoid tumor of the vulva. Am J Surg Pathol 13:848, 1989
303. Tsokos M, Kouraklis G, Chandra RS et al: Malignant rhabdoid tumor of the kidney and soft tissues: evidence for a diverse morphological and immunocytochemical phenotype. Arch Pathol Lab Med 113:115, 1989
304. Weeks DA, Beckwith B, Mierau GW: Rhabdoid tumor: an entity or a phenotype? Arch Pathol Lab Med 113:113, 1989
305. Chang ES, Dehner LP, Wick MR: Metastatic melanoma with "rhabdoid" differentiation, abstract. Lab Invest 66:31A, 1992
306. Cooper PH: Angiosarcomas of the skin. Semin Diagn Pathol 4:2, 1987
307. Holden CA, Spittle MF, Wilson-Jones E: Angiosarcoma of the face and scalp: prognosis and treatment. Cancer 59:1046, 1987
308. Wilson-Jones E: Malignant angioendothelioma of the skin. Br J Dermatol 76:21, 1964
309. Girard C, Johnson WC, Graham JH: Cutaneous angiosarcoma. Cancer 26:868, 1970
310. Hodgkinson DJ, Soule EH, Woods JE: Cutaneous angiosarcoma of the head and neck. Cancer 44:1106, 1979
311. Maddox JC, Evans HL: Angiosarcoma of skin and soft tissue: a study of forty-four cases. Cancer 48:1907, 1981
312. Perez-Atayde AR, Achenback H, Lack EE: High-grade epithelioid angiosarcoma of the scalp: an immunohistochemical and ultrastructural study. Am J Dermatopathol 8:411, 1986
313. Miyachi Y, Imamura S: Very low-grade angiosarcoma. Dermatologica 162:206, 1981
314. McWilliam LJ, Harris M: Granular cell angiosarcoma of the skin: histology, electron microscopy, and immunohistochemistry of a newly recognized tumor. Histopathology 9:1205, 1985
315. Akiyama M, Naka W, Harada T, Nishikawa T: Angiosarcoma with dermal melanocytosis. J Cutan Pathol 16:149, 1989
316. Nappi O, Wick MR, Pettinato G et al: Pseudovascular adenoid squamous cell carcinoma of the skin: a neoplasm that may be mistaken for angiosarcoma. Am J Surg Pathol 16:429, 1992
317. Swanson PE, Wick MR: Immunohistochemical evaluation of cutaneous vascular neoplasms. Clin Dermatol 9:243, 1991
318. Helwig EB: Atypical fibroxanthoma. Texas J Med 59:664, 1963
319. Fretzin DF, Helwig EB: Atypical fibroxanthoma of the skin: a clinicopathologic study of 140 cases. Cancer 31:1541, 1973
320. Alguacil-Garcia A, Unni KK, Goellner JR: Atypical fibroxanthoma of the skin. Cancer 40:1471, 1977
321. Dahl I: Atypical fibroxanthoma of the skin: a clinicopathological study of 57 cases. Acta Pathol Microbiol Scand 84:183, 1976
322. Helwig EB, May D: Atypical fibroxanthoma of the skin with metastasis. Cancer 57:368, 1986
323. Jacobs DS, Edwards WD, Ye RC: Metastatic atypical fibroxanthoma of skin. Cancer 35:457, 1975
324. Wilson PR, Strutton GM, Stewart MR: Atypical fibroxanthoma: two unusual variants. J Cutan Pathol 16:93, 1989
325. Evans HL, Smith JL: Spindle-cell squamous carcinomas and sarcoma-like tumors of the skin: a comparative study of 38 cases. Cancer 45:2687, 1980
326. Nakhleh RE, Wick MR, Rocamora A et al: Morphologic diversity in malignant melanomas. Am J Clin Pathol 93:731, 1990
327. Ma CK, Zarbo RJ, Gown AM: Immunohistochemical characterization of atypical fibroxanthoma and dermatofibrosarcoma protuberans. Am J Clin Pathol 97:487, 1992
328. Weiss SW, Enzinger FM: Malignant fibrous histiocytomas: an analysis of 200 cases. Cancer 39:1672, 1977
329. Enzinger FM: Atypical fibroxanthoma and malignant fibrous histiocytoma. Am J Dermatopathol 1:185, 1979
330. Weiss SW, Enzinger FM: Myxoid variant of malignant fibrous histiocytoma. Cancer 39:1672, 1977
331. Brooks JJ: The significance of double phenotypic patterns and markers in human sarcomas. Am J Pathol 125:113, 1986

332. Chung EB, Enzinger FM: Extraskeletal osteosarcoma. Cancer 60:1132, 1987

333. Kuo TT: Primary osteosarcoma of the skin. J Cutan Pathol 19:151, 1992

334. Feldman PS, Barr RJ: Ultrastructure of spindle-cell squamous carcinoma. J Cutan Pathol 3:17, 1976

335. Chou S, Soucy P, Carpenter B: Extraspinal ependymoma. J Pediatr Surg 22:802, 1987

336. Helwig EB, Stern JB: Subcutaneous sacrococcygeal myxopapillary ependymoma: a clinicopathologic study of 32 cases. Am J Clin Pathol 81:156, 1984

337. Pulitzer DR, Martin PC, Collins PC, Ralph DR: Subcutaneous sacrococcygeal ("myxopapillary") ependymal rests. Am J Surg Pathol 12:672, 1988

338. Chambers CW, Schwinn CP: Chordoma: a clinicopathologic study of metastasis. Am J Clin Pathol 72:765, 1979

339. Bale PM, Painter DM, Cohen D: Teratomas in childhood. Pathology 7:209, 1975

340. Dixon AY, Lee SH: An ultrastructural study of elastofibromas. Hum Pathol 11:257, 1980

341. Gartmann H, Groth W, Kuhn A: Elastofibroma dorsi. Z Hautkr 63:525, 1988

342. Shimizu S, Hashimoto H, Enjoji M: Nodular fasciitis: an analysis of 250 patients. Pathology 16:161, 1984

343. Price EB Jr, Silliphant WM, Shuman R: Nodular fasciitis: a clinicopathologic analysis of 65 cases. Am J Clin Pathol 35:122, 1961

344. Meister P, Buckmann FW, Konrad EA: Nodular fasciitis: an analysis of 250 patients. Pathology 16:161, 1984

345. Lauer DH, Enzinger FM: Cranial fasciitis of childhood. Cancer 45:401, 1980

346. Patchefsky AS, Enzinger FM: Intravascular fasciitis. Am J Surg Pathol 5:29, 1981

347. Hutter RV, Foote FW, Francis KC et al: Parosteal fasciitis. Am J Surg 104:800, 1962

348. Bernstein KE, Lattes R: Nodular (pseudosarcomatous) fasciitis: a nonrecurrent lesion. Clinicopathologic study of 134 cases. Cancer 49:1668, 1982

349. Murray JC, Pollack SV, Pinnell SR: Keloids and hypertrophic scars. Clin Dermatol 2:121, 1984

350. Ketchum LD, Cohen IK, Masters FW: Hypertrophic scars and keloids: a collective review. Plast Reconstr Surg 53:140, 1974

351. Murray JC, Pollack SV, Pinnell SR: Keloids: a review. J Am Acad Dermatol 4:461, 1981

352. Hurt MA, Santa Cruz DJ: Cutaneous inflammatory pseudotumor. Am J Surg Pathol 14:764, 1988

353. Uitto J, Santa Cruz DJ, Eizen AZ: Connective tissue nevi of the skin. J Am Acad Dermatol 3:441, 1980

354. Weidman FD, Anderson NP, Ayres S: Juvenile elastoma. Arch Dermatol Syphilol 28:182, 1933

355. Sosis AC, Johnson WC: Connective tissue nevus. Dermatologica 144:57, 1972

356. Cole GW, Barr RJ: An elastic tissue defect in dermatofibrosis lenticularis disseminata (the Buschke-Ollendorff syndrome). Br J Dermatol 118:44, 1982

357. Lewandowsky F: Naevus elasticus regionis mammariae. Arch Klin Exp Dermatol 90:131, 1921

358. Henderson RR, Wheeler CE Jr, Abele DC: Familial cutaneous collagenoma: report of cases. Arch Dermatol 98:23, 1968

359. Brownstein MH, Mehregan AH, Bikowski JB et al: The dermatopathology of Cowden's syndrome. Br J Dermatol 100:667, 1979

360. Brownstein MH, Wolf M, Bikowski JB: Cowden's disease: a cutaneous marker of breast cancer. Cancer 41:2393, 1978

361. Requena L, Gutierrez J, Sanchez-Yus E: Multiple sclerotic fibromas of the skin: a cutaneous marker of Cowden's disease. J Cutan Pathol 19:346, 1991

362. Metcalf JS, Maize JC, LeBoit PE: Circumscribed storiform collagenoma (sclerotic fibroma). Am J Dermatopathol 13:122, 1992

363. Templeton HJ: Cutaneous tags of the neck. Arch Dermatol 33:495, 1933

364. Stegmaier OC: Natural regression of the melanocytic nevus. J Invest Dermatol 32:413, 1959

365. Slifman NR, Harrist TJ, Rhodes AR: Congenital arrector pili hamartoma. Arch Dermatol 121:1034, 1985

366. Burgdorf WHC, Doran CK, Worret WI: Folded skin with scarring. Michelin tire baby syndrome. J Am Acad Dermatol 7:90, 1982

367. Mehregan AH, Tarafogli VL, Ghandchi A: Nevus lipomatosus cutaneus superficialis (Hoffman-Zurhelle). J Cutan Pathol 2:307, 1975

368. Stokes JH: Nevus pilaris with hyperplasia of non-striated muscle. Arch Dermatol Syphilol 7:481, 1923

369. Urbanek RW, Johnson WC: Smooth muscle hamartoma associated with Becker's nevus. Arch Dermatol 114:104, 1978

370. Lindenhauer SM: The Klippel-Trenaunay syndrome: varicosities, hypertrophy and hemangioma with no arteriovenous fistula. Ann Surg 162:303, 1965

371. Bluefarb SM: Sturge-Weber syndrome. Arch Dermatol Syphilol 59:531, 1949

372. Barsky SH, Rosen S, Geer DE et al: The nature and evolution of port-wine stains. J Invest Dermatol 74:154, 1980

373. Bowers RE, Graham EA, Tomlinson KA: The natural history of the strawberry nevus. Arch Dermatol 82:667, 1960

374. Chandler D: Pulmonary and cerebral arteriovenous fistula with Oster's disease. Arch Intern Med 116:277, 1965

375. Smith CR Jr, Bartholomew LG, Cain JG: Hereditary hemorrhagic telangiectasia and gastrointestinal hemorrhage. Gastroenterology 44:1, 1963

376. Waller JD, Greenberg JH, Lewis CW: Hereditary hemorrhagic telangiectasia with cerebrovascular malformations. Arch Dermatol 112:49, 1976

377. Mali JWH, Kuiper JP, Hamers AA: Acroangiodermatitis of the foot. Arch Dermatol 92:515, 1965

378. Wood C, Severin GL: Unusual histiocytic reaction to Monsel's solution. Am J Dermatol 2:261, 1980

379. Tsang WYW, Chan JKC: Bacillary angiomatosis. A "new" disease with a broadening clinicopathologic spectrum. Histol Histopathol 7:143, 1992

380. Steeper TA, Rosenstein H, Weiser J et al: Bacillary epithelioid angiomatosis involving the liver, spleen, and skin in an AIDS patient with concurrent Kaposi's sarcoma. Am J Clin Pathol 97:713, 1992

381. Bachelez H, Oskenhendler E, Lebbe C et al: Bacillary angiomatosis in HIV-infected patients: report of three cases with different clinical courses and identification of

Rochalimaea quintana as the aetiological agent. Br J Dermatol 133:983, 1995

382. Arias-Stella J, Lieberman PH, Erlandson RA et al: Histology, immunohistochemistry, and ultrastructure of the verruga in Carrion's disease. Am J Surg Pathol 10:595, 1986

383. Arias-Stella J, Lieberman PH, Garcia-Caceres U et al: Verruga peruana mimicking malignant neoplasms. Am J Dermatol 9:279, 1987

384. Reed J, Brigati D, Flynn S et al: Immunocytochemical identification of *Rochalimaea henselae* in bacillary (epithelioid) angiomatosis, parenchymal bacillary peliosis, and persistent fever with bacteremia. Am J Surg 16:650, 1992

385. Rosai J, Akerman LR: Intravascular atypical vascular proliferation. Arch Dermatol 109:714, 1974

386. Reed CN, Cooper PH, Swerlick RA: Intravascular papillary endothelial hyperplasia. Multiple lesions simulating Kaposi's sarcoma. J Am Acad Dermatol 10:110, 1984

387. Bruce DH: Angiokeratoma circumscriptum and angiokeratoma scroti. Arch Dermatol 81:388, 1960

388. Haye KR, Rebello DJA: Angiokeratoma of Mibelli. Acta Derm Venereol (Stockh) 41:56, 1961

389. Johnson WC: Pathology of cutaneous vascular tumors, review. Int J Dermatol 15:239, 1976

390. Goldman L, Gibson SH, Richfield DF: Thrombotic angiokeratoma circumscriptum simulating melanoma. Arch Dermatol 117:138, 1981

20

NEOPLASMS OF MELANOCYTES

GENERAL CONSIDERATIONS

Terminology

Because many of the controversies regarding melanocytic neoplasms have revolved around the terms used to describe them, we first briefly review the most salient of these.

Melanocytes are cells that migrate from the neural crest to the skin during embryogenesis and have the capacity to synthesize the pigment melanin. In normal skin, they reside in the basal layer of the epidermis and in the bulbs of hair follicles.

Nevus cells are the constituents of benign neoplasms of melanocytes. Because the term *nevus* in its strict sense means a malformation, the term *nevus cell*, although widely understood, is poor and should be avoided; *melanocyte* is preferable. Pierre Masson[1] believed that the junctional cells of a compound nevus derived from epidermal melanocytes and the dermal component from the Schwann cells of nerves. He termed these dermal constituents *nevus cells*. It later became convention to refer to the intradermal melanocytes of a compound nevus as *nevus cells* and the intraepidermal portion as *melanocytes*. Because there is no credence given currently to the belief that epidermal and dermal components of a compound nevus have separate derivations, there seems little point in preserving this distinction.

While the term *dysplasia* in its original sense means a malformation, this meaning has been displaced by its recent usage as a synonym for *cytologic atypia* and, when modified by a cellular lineage (i.e., melanocytic dysplasia), to refer to neoplasms that are at a partially transformed, intermediate stage between benign and malignant. Because the term *dysplastic nevus* has been so widely used, we consider it herein as synonymous for the flat, acquired melanocytic nevus found most often on the trunk, also known as *Clark nevus*.

Melanoma and *malignant melanoma* are synonymous. We use the term *melanoma in situ* to refer to malignant melanoma when it is still at an intraepithelial stage in its development, recognizing that it is, at that stage, incapable of metastasis. *Atypical melanocytic hyperplasia, pagetoid melanocytic proliferation*, and a variety of other terms have been used to describe

similar neoplasms in a way that conveys uncertainty as to the nature of the proliferation. In our opinion, *hyperplasias* are proliferations of cells that are incited by a stimulus, but cease to grow, and ultimately involute once that stimulus is removed. Hyperplasia of melanocytes does occur, but in very few settings, such as in pigmented basal cell and squamous cell carcinomas and in phytophotodermatitis.

Much of the literature regarding the biology of malignant melanoma is muddled by indiscriminant use of the term *recurrent melanoma* to refer both to cases in which the primary neoplasm was not excised, and persisted (i.e., recurred clinically) at the site of the biopsy, and to cases in which satellite or distant metastases occurred. *Persistent melanoma* seems to be preferable to describe incompletely excised neoplasms that regrew in contiguity with surgical scars, and satellite or distant metastases should be specified as such. Sometimes it is difficult to tell whether a patient has persistent or locally metastatic melanoma. In such cases the sectioning diagram and microscopic slides from the initial excisional specimen should be reviewed to determine whether an extension of the neoplasm to surgical margins could have been missed.

Biopsy Technique

Although this is a textbook of dermatopathology and not of clinical dermatology or dermatologic surgery, it is appropriate to comment on proper biopsy technique for the evaluation of melanocytic neoplasms. Dermatopathologists are often asked about biopsy technique by clinical colleagues and are in an excellent position to comment on many aspects of it, as the adequacy and accuracy of histopathologic examination depends on one's ability to evaluate many criteria that can be compromised by faulty sampling. Dermatopathologists also receive re-excision specimens in cases in which malignant melanoma has been diagnosed or suspected or in which it could not be excluded and so have developed a wealth of experience to draw on.

Shave biopsy can be an appropriate technique to remove melanocytic neoplasms in several settings. Melanocytic nevi that are removed for cosmetic reasons are often best subjected to this technique. If shave biopsies are to be performed on lesions suspected of being dysplastic or Clark nevi, the shave should begin and end several millimeters beyond the borders of the pigmented lesion, as melanocytes can extend within the epidermis and sometimes within the papillary dermis without producing clinical pigmentation. If this is not done, the degree of lateral circumscription of the lesion cannot be evaluated. Scoring the skin with the scalpel blade before performing the shave to ensure adequate clearance can be helpful. Placing the shaved specimen on a piece of cardboard prior to fixation in formalin can prevent its curling and the confusing histopathologic picture from tangential sectioning that can result. While the edges of the specimen should be thin, all too often shave biopsy specimens are transected within the papillary dermis, making maturation of melanocytes impossible to evaluate.

Punch biopsy is rarely appropriate for melanocytic neoplasms. Punches taken from pigmented patches can provide a clue as to the findings in the remainder of the lesion, and punch excisions (in which the circumference of the punch is larger than that of the neoplasm by a millimeter or more) are appropriate uses. Punch biopsies of suspected malignant melanomas that are taken through the thickest portion of the neoplasm can disrupt the neoplastic cells, driving them deeper into the dermis,[2] and, if the punch does not extend beneath the deepest cells, it can compromise the accurate measurement of thickness.

Incisional biopsies taken with a scalpel in such a way as to provide some information regarding circumscription, symmetry, and maturation can be appropriate when an *excisional biopsy* would be too difficult because of the location of the lesion, its size, or the condition of the patient. Excisional biopsies are optimal for the pathologic evaluation of most melanocytic neoplasms, should extend into the subcutaneous fat, and result in histopathologic clearance of the lateral margins of the neoplasm (clinical margins of 1 to 2 mm). The majority of malignant melanomas sampled by excisional biopsy with even minimally clear margins will not persist at the sites of those biopsies, even if the histopathologic diagnosis is missed.

Approach to Histopathologic Diagnosis

The salient question in the evaluation of many melanocytic neoplasms is whether the correct diagnosis is malignant melanoma. While there is no histopathologic feature whose presence or absence is completely specific or sensitive for the diagnosis of malignant melanoma, there are generic criteria that can be applied to the examination of most melanocytic neoplasms if the exceptions to these criteria are kept in mind. Many of these criteria are reiterated throughout this chapter.

The *shape* or *silhouette* of a melanocytic neoplasm is an important feature to evaluate. Most congenital or acquired melanocytic nevi are horizontally oriented with respect to the surface of the skin, as are most malignant melanomas. Blue nevi and cutaneous metastases of malignant melanoma are often taller than they are broad and hence appear vertically oriented with respect to the skin surface. Rarely, primary malignant melanomas that extend deeply along a hair follicle will be vertically oriented.

The *size* of a melanocytic neoplasm is relevant because only a few benign melanocytic neoplasms grow to become larger than 1 cm: congenital melanocytic nevi, some Spitz or blue nevi, and rare dysplastic or Clark nevi can. A *growth pattern appropriate for size* is important. Most malignant melanomas begin as proliferations of melanocytes as single cells at the dermoepidermal junction, as do most acquired melanocytic nevi. Acquired melanocytic nevi rapidly evolve into nested proliferations so that if a junctional neoplasm consists largely of nested cells when it is still quite small (less than 3 mm) it is unlikely to be a malignant melanoma.

The *symmetry* of a melanocytic neoplasm around a central axis is an important feature, as many malignant melanomas are asymmetric (perhaps due to the evolution of new clones of cells with different growth rates and other characteristics). Symmetry of overall configuration (silhouette), size of nests, cytologic features, pigmentation, and inflammatory infiltrates should all be examined because each of these alone can be the only clue to the diagnosis of malignant melanoma at scanning magnification. Benign melanocytic neoplasms that are typically asymmetric include some blue nevi, most combined nevi, and some dysplastic or Clark nevi.

Poor *lateral circumscription* is a clue to the diagnosis of malignant melanoma clinically, and its histopathologic correlate is the extension of single melanocytes beyond the lateralmost junctional nest within the epidermis. A feature that especially favors malignant melanoma is the presence of single melanocytes at the advancing edge of the neoplasm, above the basal layer of the epidermis. Some lesions that are poorly circumscribed clinically feature junctional nests that are distributed at irregular intervals lateral to central, compound component. Some simple lentigines, lentiginous junctional or compound nevi, nevi on acral surfaces, and some dysplastic or Clark nevi have single melanocytes that are lateral to the most lateral junctional nest, as do many malignant melanomas.

The balance between junctional melanocytes arranged as *single cells* and in *nests* can be a useful diagnostic feature. In many malignant melanomas, there are areas in which single melanocytes predominate along the dermoepidermal junction. Simple lentigines, lentiginous junctional and compound nevi, some dysplastic or Clark nevi, and some congenital melanocytic nevi also have mostly single melanocytes in their junctional components. In such cases, the single melanocytes are usually distributed evenly throughout the neoplasm as opposed to malignant melanoma, in which they are irregularly scattered.

Upward migration of melanocytes within the epidermis, or within the epithelium of hair follicles or sweat ducts, is often seen in malignant melanoma. As melanocytes migrate from the neural crest to the basal layer of the epidermis in embryonic life, their further migration within epithelia in malignant melanoma may be a reversion to a primitive behavior. Upward scatter, or pagetoid upward migration of melanocytes, also occurs outside the setting of malignant melanoma in some congenital melanocytic nevi biopsied in the first months of life, in junctional or compound nevi that have been traumatized, in many melanocytic nevi on acral skin and in the epithelium of nailbeds, in junctional or compound Spitz nevi, especially in children and in teenagers, and in melanocytic nevi that persist despite attempts to remove them, especially by shave biopsy.

Mitotic figures are present in dermal melanocytes in many malignant melanomas, and their number may have a bearing on the patient's prognosis. Mitoses can also be detected in the uppermost cells of Spitz nevi (and sometimes in cells deep within the neoplasm, especially in young children). Mitotic figures have been documented in melanocytes in the superficial dermis in compound and in intradermal nevi.[3] The "cellular" variants of blue nevi can also contain mitotic figures, but atypical mitoses have not been reported in cellular blue nevi.[4]

Maturation of melanocytes refers to the diminution in the sizes of nests, cells, nuclei, and nucleoli in the deep portions of some melanocytic neoplasms. These morphologic changes are accompanied by a decrease in melanin and in the enzymes that help to synthesize it and by diminished numbers of cycling cells. Maturation is evident in benign neoplasms that begin as proliferations of cells at the dermoepidermal junction, such as compound and intradermal nevi, including Spitz nevi, and also in some that do not, such as congenital nevi. While occasional primary lesions of malignant melanoma show some features of maturation, many epidermotropic metastases of malignant melanoma have melanocytes at their bases that are much smaller than those in the superficial part of the metastasis.[5] Maturation is not evident at all in blue nevi of all types and in portions of combined nevi that resemble blue nevi. Melanocytic neoplasms that are entirely intraepidermal cannot, of course, show maturation.

Perineural invasion is present in some malignant melanomas, particularly those in which the dermal component consists mainly of spindled cells. Such melanomas often arise in the sun-damaged skin of the head and neck (so-called lentigo maligna melanoma) or on the skin of the hands and feet (so-called acral lentiginous melanoma), but occasionally arise on the skin of the trunk. Melanocytes are evident around and within small cutaneous nerves in many congenital nevi, and perineural melanocytes have been described in Spitz nevi.[6]

Lymphatic invasion by a melanocytic neoplasm is likewise not pathognomonic of malignant melanoma. To be an authentic example of lymphatic invasion, melanocytes should either appear to be attached to lymphatic endothelial cells or be enmeshed in fibrin or both. Lymphatic invasion is often simulated by retraction artifact in many forms of melanocytic nevi in which a cleft surrounds a nest of melanocytes, separating them from a thin rim of compressed fibroblasts. Small nests of melanocytes in a subendothelial location in the dermis of congenital and acquired nevi can be misinterpreted as representing lymphatic invasion. True lymphatic invasion occurs in some Spitz nevi.[7]

The most objective way to arrive at a diagnosis of a melanocytic neoplasm is to examine its histopathology without benefit of clinical information, arrive at an impression, and then revise those findings, if necessary, following review of the clinical setting. There are some important clinical features that should be kept in mind as part of the general approach outlined herein. The *age of the patient* is highly relevant. Malignant melanoma can arise in congenital nevi in children, but melanoma arising de novo is rare before puberty. Therefore, the histopathologic features of a *lesion* should be compelling before a diagnosis of malignant melanoma is made in a child. Conversely, new (junctional) melanocytic nevi uncommonly arise in patients in their seventh and eighth decades, and a junctional or intraepidermal melanocytic neoplasm in an older patient should have compelling features of benignity before the diagnosis of melanoma in situ is discarded. The *site* that a neoplasm occurs at is likewise important. Acquired melanocytic nevi show regional variation in their histopathologic appearances. Junctional and compound nevi on acral skin feature upward migration of single melanocytes within the epidermis, and nevi on or near genital skin can show lateral confluence of junctional nests. Both signs in other contexts would raise the possibility of malignant melanoma. The *size of the lesion as described clinically* can be a crucial piece of information; all too often small, partial biopsies of large lesions are performed, without informing the dermatopathologist. A 2 mm punch biopsy that appears to show a banal compound melanocytic nevus has different implications when it represents the entirety of a lesion in a 28-year-old person and when it is a sample from a 2.8 cm lesion in a 74-year-old person.

LENTIGO SIMPLEX AND LENTIGINOUS NEVI

A lentigo simplex is a small, pigmented macule produced by an increased number of single melanocytes situated along the dermoepidermal junction. Most lentigines remain stable, but some evolve into a junctional or compound melanocytic nevus. In lentiginous compound nevi the epidermal features are those of a simple lentigo, but there are also melanocytes in the papillary dermis.

Clinical Features

Most simple lentigines and lentiginous compound nevi are small (less than 4 mm in diameter) and dark brown with sharply defined borders that can be rounded or jagged. A reticulated network of pigment may be visible on close examination, especially when the skin is stretched. Simple lentigines mainly occur on the extremities and seem to be more numerous in sun-exposed skin. Some lesions with the clinical and histopathologic features of simple lentigines that occurred in sun-exposed skin have been termed *reticulated black solar lentigo* or *ink spot lentigo*.[8] The presence of numerous simple lentigines can be a marker of Carney's complex, in which atrial myxomas are the most dire feature, and it can also be a feature of xeroderma pigmentosum. Numerous simple lentigines have been produced in patients with psoriasis by treatment with psoralens and ultraviolet light A; these are known as *PUVA lentigines*. Hyperpigmented macules that are clinically similar to simple lentigines occur on the lips and are known as *labial melanotic macules*. Similar lesions are found on the lips of patients with Peutz-Jeghers syndrome. Larger pigmented patches, often irregular in shape, can occur on genital skin and have been described under the names *benign genital melanosis* and *vulvar melanosis*.[9] These conditions are not forms of simple lentigo, as there is no substantial increase in the number of melanocytes in the basal layer.

Histopathologic Features

Simple lentigines are characterized by their small size and sharp lateral circumscription. The rete ridges are slender, elongated, bulbous, and sometimes club shaped. Single melanocytes are present in increased numbers along the sides and bases of the ridges. The basal layer of the epidermis is usually hyperpigmented. The cornified layer above a simple lentigo is often compact or laminated and may contain flecks of pigment, simulating parakeratosis. The papillary dermis often shows delicate fibroplasia, melanophages, and a sparse lymphocytic infiltrate (Fig. 20-1).

There are several variable features in simple lentigines. When serially sectioned, almost all display at least a few small nests of melanocytes at the dermoepidermal junction; perhaps these lesions might better be called *small lentiginous nevi*.[10] Giant melanosomes can be seen within the cytoplasms of junctional melanocytes. The rete ridges of some simple lentigines are connected at their bases. Some lentigines have horizontally oriented, thickened collagen bundles (lamellar fibroplasia) in the papillary dermis. Clusters of melanocytes with small, round nuclei may be present in the papillary dermis, in which event the lesion may be termed a *lentiginous compound nevus* (Fig. 20-2). Rarely, sporadic, simple lentigines can have large melanocytes, and cytologically atypical melanocytes have been reported in PUVA-induced lentigines[11] and in lentigines in patients with xeroderma pigmentosum.[12]

In labial lentigines, both of the sporadic type and in patients with the Peutz-Jeghers syndrome and in genital melanosis, there is basilar hyperpigmentation without a discernible increase in the number or size of melanocytes.

Clinicopathologic Correlation

The intense pigmentation seen in simple lentigines and lentiginous compound nevi is the result of a marked increase in the melanin content of the basal epidermis, the cornified layer, and the papillary dermis. The reticular pigment network seen on close clinical examination derives from hyperpigmented rete ridges that branch radially from the center of the lesion. It is impossible to discern whether a lesion is a lentigo simplex or a lentiginous compound nevus clinically, as the dermal component in the latter is too scanty to result in elevation of the surface of the lesion.

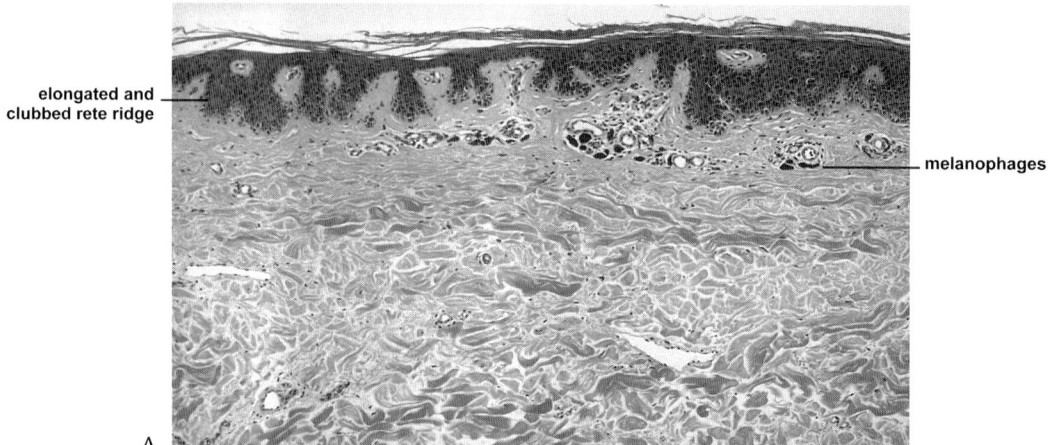

Figure 20-1. Simple lentigo. There are increased numbers of single melanocytes along the sides and bases of elongated rete ridges (**A**). The papillary dermis contains infiltrates of lymphocytes and melanophages (**B**), and there is hyperpigmentation of both the basal and cornified layers (**C**). *Continued.*

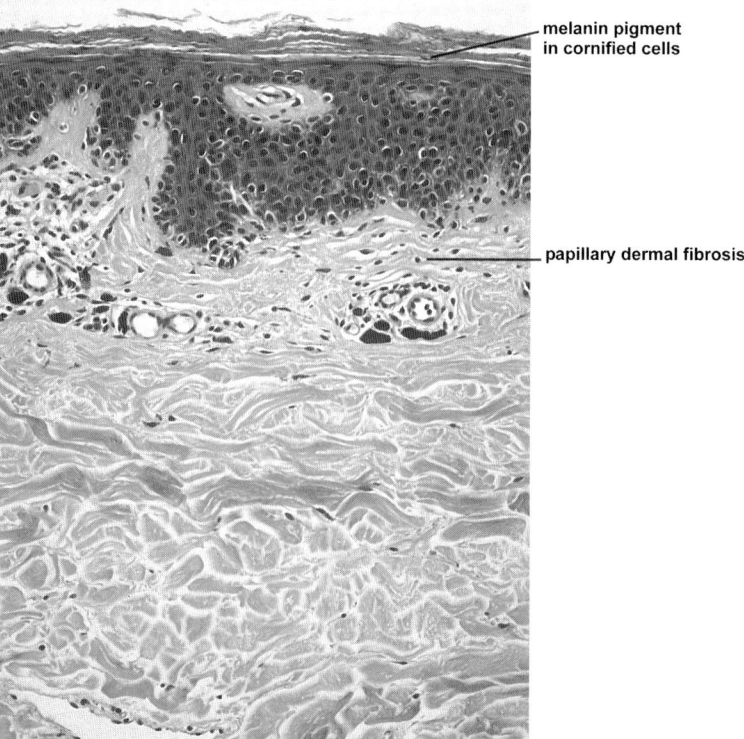

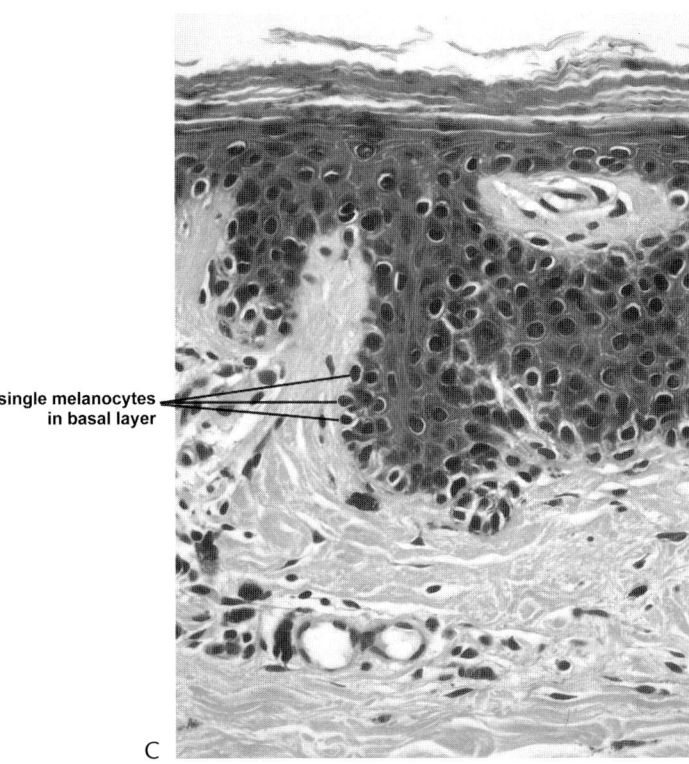

Figure 20-1. *Continued.* There is hyperpigmentation of both the basal and cornified layers **(C)**.

single melanocytes in basal layer

C

Differential Diagnosis

Simple lentigines are often confused with solar lentigines in part because the two conditions have been confounded in the literature.[13] Solar lentigines are broad, flat, light brown macules with waxy surfaces. They are proliferations of pigmented keratinocytes in which melanocytes produce abundant pigment. Although this type of lentigo is usually stable, it may evolve into

a reticulated seborrheic keratosis. Unlike simple lentigines the number of melanocytes is not discernibly increased. The rete ridges of solar lentigines are broader and more bulbous than those of simple lentigines, and the cornified layer usually contains less pigment. By definition, solar lentigines occur in sun-damaged skin, and the basophilic fibers of solar elastosis are present in the subjacent reticular dermis.

As almost all simple lentigines contain a few junctional nests

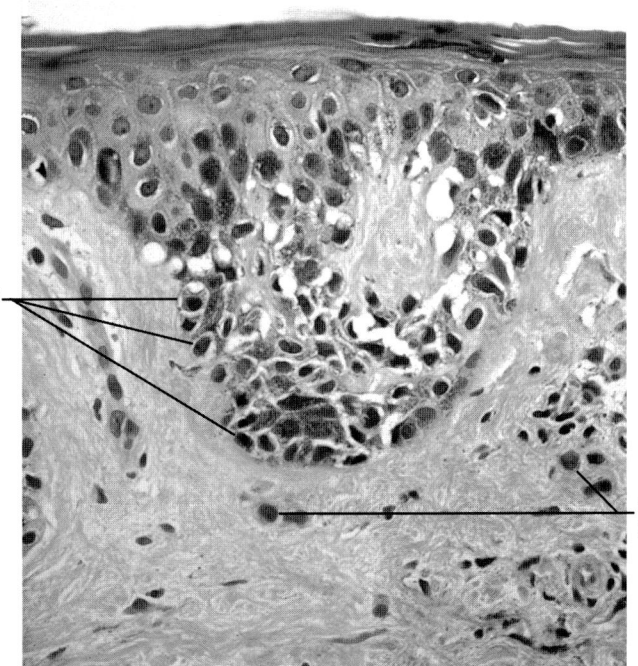

single melanocyte in basal layer

melanocytes in papillary dermis

Figure 20-2. A lentiginous compound nevus. In addition to the features seen in a simple lentigo, there are small round melanocytes in the papillary dermis. Because the clinical findings in this type of lesion are determined by the amount and distribution of melanin, lentiginous compound nevi are indistinguishable from simple lentigines clinically.

on serial sectioning, the dividing line between a simple lentigo and a junctional nevus is arbitrary. If most of a lesion resembles a simple lentigo, but a few junctional nests are present, the lesion can be termed a *lentiginous junctional nevus*. Some simple lentigines or lentiginous junctional or compound nevi can have features seen in dysplastic or Clark nevi such as lamellar fibroplasia and fusion of bases of adjacent rete ridges. It seems likely that there is a continuum between simple lentigines and these nevi, and it seems pointless to agonize over their differential diagnosis, as the clinical import of a single, presumably small dysplastic nevus is minimal.

Simple lentigines differ from labial melanotic macules and genital melanosis in that the number of basilar melanocytes is noticeably increased. Labial melanotic macules in turn need to be distinguished from another form of mucosal pigmentation known as *melanoacanthoma*.[14] Melanoacanthoma of the oral cavity (the term *melanoacanthoma* has also been used to describe a type of seborrheic keratosis that has numerous dendritic melanocytes) seems to be a hyperpigmented inflammatory process. Microscopically, it features spongiosis, epithelial hyperplasia, and hyperplasia of dendritic melanocytes that are present above the basal layer.

Lentigo maligna is a term sometimes used for malignant melanoma in situ arising in sun-damaged skin, usually of the head or neck. This condition is usually easily differentiated from simple lentigo both clinically and pathologically. The use of the term *lentigo* in both conditions has given rise to the misconception that they are related. Clinically the form of malignant melanoma in situ termed *lentigo maligna* is a large and poorly circumscribed patch with variable pigmentation, in contrast to the small, sharply circumscribed, and darkly but evenly pigmented simple lentigo. Histologically, in both melanoma in situ of the lentigo maligna type and simple lentigo there are increased numbers of single melanocytes at the dermoepidermal junction. In melanoma in situ they are randomly distributed, while in simple lentigines melanocytes are increased along the sides and bases of rete ridges and are absent or fewer in the basal layer above dermal papillae (sometimes termed the *inter-retial epidermis*). The rete ridge pattern in melanoma in situ of the lentigo maligna type is usually diminished, while in a simple lentigo it is accentuated. Only in the most advanced portion of many examples of this type of melanoma in situ will there be elongated rete; generally, such areas will also show nests of melanocytes, some upwardly migrating cells, and lymphocytic infiltrates in the subjacent dermis.

Pathophysiology

The formation of simple lentigines appears to be under genetic control. They are markedly increased in patients with familial melanoma and numerous large irregular nevi, and in patients with Carney's complex, Peutz-Jeghers syndrome, and xeroderma pigmentosum.

ACQUIRED JUNCTIONAL, COMPOUND, AND INTRADERMAL NEVI

Nevus, used in a generic sense, denotes any congenital malformation of the skin. When used in an unqualified manner, or in reference to melanocytes, it describes a benign neoplasm that can be acquired or congenital. Melanocytic nevi, whether acquired or congenital, are junctional, compound, or intradermal, depending on the distribution of their cells. Junctional nevi have nests of melanocytes and often individual melanocytes at the dermoepidermal junction. In compound nevi there are melanocytes in the dermis in addition to those at the junction. Intradermal nevi usually have a few small residual nests of melanocytes at the dermoepidermal junction. The intradermal cells of a melanocytic nevus are often referred to as *nevus cells* (as distinct from *melanocytes*), a term that derived from the belief of early twentieth century pathologists that some of these cells were derived from Schwann cells of dermal nerves rather than from junctional melanocytes.

If an acquired nevus is composed of large spindle or ovoid melanocytes it is a Spitz nevus; if it is wholly dermal and composed in part of pigmented, dendritic melanocytes or nests of ovoid melanocytes it is a blue nevus. If neither of these cell types is present, the lesion is an "ordinary" acquired nevus, an unsatisfactory term that blurs the differences between several types of acquired nevus.

Clinical Features

Some generalizations can be made about the diversity of the clinical appearance of "ordinary" acquired nevi. Most acquired nevi are small, usually less than 4 mm in diameter, but they can be up to several centimeters in diameter. They may be flat, dome shaped, papillated, or occur as a sessile polyp. Their pigmentation ranges from skin colored to dark brown and is usually evenly or uniformly distributed. Acquired nevi usually are sharply demarcated from the surrounding skin.

Regional variation in the appearance of melanocytic nevi is evident clinically and histologically. Small acquired melanocytic nevi on the face are generally round, small, and slightly domed. Acquired compound melanocytic nevi on the trunk often exceed 4 mm in diameter, are irregularly ovoid in shape, and have a small papular component centrally. Some of these nevi (so-called dysplastic or Clark nevi) may be poorly circumscribed and asymmetric and have hues of pink, tan, and brown (i.e., clinical features that raise the possibility of malignant melanoma). A ring of erythema is often seen at their periphery. Some patients have dozens of such nevi, some of them exceptionally large, as well as nevi of other types. These patients sometimes have relatives who have similar numbers of nevi and melanoma, the so-called dysplastic nevus syndrome. Melanocytic nevi on acral skin are usually intensely pigmented with reticulated borders and stippled pigment. Terminal hairs can occur in acquired nevi but are more often present in congenital nevi.

As a melanocytic nevus ages and evolves from the junctional to the intradermal stage, its pigmentation diminishes. Junctional lesions tend to be flat; compound and early intradermal ones are elevated; and late, intradermal, melanocytic nevi can recede and become inconspicuous.[15] Rarely, intradermal nevi become bulky, exophytic, lobulated masses.[16]

Because of their evolution, junctional melanocytic nevi tend to occur in children and adolescents; intradermal nevi tend to affect adults. However, a broad age range exists for all stages of this common neoplasm. A rare form of compound nevus usually seen in children has a target-like configuration and is called *Cockarde nevus*.[17]

Histopathologic Features

Junctional Nevi

In junctional melanocytic nevi there are both nests of melanocytes and increased individual melanocytes at the dermoepidermal junction. Junctional nests often protrude slightly into the papillary dermis. The melanocytes within a junctional nest can appear either tightly or loosely packed. Most junctional nests in acquired nevi are discrete and round or ovoid. They are generally situated along or at the base of rete ridges rather than directly above dermal papillae. The rete ridges are often elongated and can connect at their bases. The solitary melanocytes that accompany melanocytic nests in benign acquired nevi are also situated along rete ridges and do not extend much beyond the lateralmost nests of a junctional nevus.

The cytologic features of melanocytes in "ordinary" junctional nevi vary. In general, cytoplasm is inconspicuous, and fixation results in its contraction around the nucleus; only remnants of dendritic processes are seen. The nuclei of melanocytes in a junctional nevus are usually smaller than those of adjacent keratinocytes. In "ordinary" junctional nevi there are small nucleoli, which usually are blue in properly balanced, hematoxylin and eosin-stained sections. The amount of pigment can vary in the cells in a junctional nest, but usually is uniform from nest to nest within a nevus. Giant melanosomes are sometimes seen in junctional nevi (Fig. 20-3).

Exceptions to these prototypic cytologic features are frequent. Dendritic processes may be conspicuous in junctional melanocytic nevi in dark-skinned persons. In junctional melanocytic nevi in some children, adolescents, and, less commonly, in some adults there may be abundant cytoplasm and fine melanin granules, resulting in an "epithelioid" or "pagetoid" appearance. The nuclei of cells of this type are uniformly small and have tiny nucleoli. Powdery-appearing melanin can be transferred to keratinocytes and make the cytoplasm of some keratinocytes similar in appearance. These cells can nonetheless be recognized as keratinocytes by the presence of a distinct cell membrane and intercellular bridges. Melanocytic giant cells with eosinophilic cytoplasm, a scalloped border, and numerous small, round nuclei are present in some junctional nevi and in the junctional component of some compound nevi. As in simple lentigines, the papillary dermis can contain a sparse lymphocytic infiltrate, fibroplasia, and melanophages.

In most junctional nevi there are few, if any, melanocytes in the upper spinous, granular, or cornified layers. Exceptions include junctional nevi that have been irritated or traumatized and junctional nevi on acral skin, especially that of the palms, soles, nailbeds, elbows, or knees.[18] In traumatized nevi and in acral nevi there may be individual melanocytes or small melanocytic nests scattered throughout all levels of the epidermis, but this upward scatter does not usually extend laterally much beyond the last junctional nest on either side of the lesion (i.e., lateral confinement is present; Fig. 20-4). Evidence that a nevus has been traumatized may include scale-crusts, the presence of erosion or ulceration of the epidermis, and subepidermal fibrin deposition or hemorrhage. Upward migration of melanocytes in acral nevi may be due to the constant friction or pressure to which those sites are subjected.

Some broad junctional nevi, especially on the trunk, can have features of so-called dysplastic or Clark nevi, such as bridging of adjacent rete ridges by nests of melanocytes, lamellar or concentric fibroplasia of the papillary dermis, and moderately dense lymphocytic infiltrates. These nevi are identical to their compound counterparts except for the presence of melanocytes in the papillary dermis in the latter.

Compound Nevi

The fate of most junctional nevi is to become compound, probably by stimulating the production of extracellular matrix that surrounds the junctional nests. As melanocytes become incorporated into the adventitial dermis they begin to mature. The more deeply situated and, presumably, older aggregates of melanocytes become smaller. The size of melanocytes that comprise these aggregates and the size of their nuclei diminish. Pigmentation diminishes with maturation. Nucleoli are barely perceptible in the deepest dermal cells of most compound nevi. In many older compound and intradermal nevi there are further involutional changes, such as neurotization, fibrosis, and fatty change.

Compound nevi have diverse histologic appearances. Lentiginous compound nevi, in which single melanocytes rather than nests of melanocytes are the predominant population at the dermoepidermal junction, have epidermal features indistinguishable from those of a simple lentigo and compact clusters of small, round melanocytes in the papillary dermis. The epidermis above compound nevi can be variably pigmented. Although most compound nevi induce some epidermal hyperplasia, some can evoke a striking elongation and interanastomosis of rete ridges with hyperkeratosis that simulates a seborrheic keratosis clinically and histologically. The papillary dermis in most compound nevi is thickened and elevates the surface of the lesion.

Many compound nevi, especially on the trunk or proximal extremities, involve only the dermoepidermal junction and papillary dermis. In these superficial acquired compound nevi there are often junctional nests of melanocytes with an abundant, pale-staining cytoplasm. These nests extend laterally beyond the dermal component. Adjacent rete may appear to be bridged by nests of horizontally oriented melanocytes with an ovoid or spindled nucleus. Slight vascular ectasia, a sparse or moderately dense lymphocytic infiltrate, and horizontally oriented fibrosis (lamellar fibroplasia) of the papillary dermis further typify the changes at the periphery of this type of compound nevus. Sometimes melanocytes with cytologic features indistinguishable from their junctional counterpart are evident in the dermis in areas of fibroplasia. Only exceptionally are the melanocytes markedly atypical by standard cytopathologic criteria or there is a dense lymphocytic infiltrate (Fig. 20-5).

This "atypical" compound nevus with melanocytic "dysplasia" has provoked great controversy. In 1978, Clark and co-workers[19] described two kindreds with numerous family members who had malignant melanoma and many large, clinically atypical nevi that had unusual histologic features. Later, Clark and co-workers[20] termed these histologic changes *melanocytic dysplasia* and referred to the lesions as *dysplastic nevi*. They held it requisite that such lesions contain at least a proportion of cells whose cytologic atypia is easily identifiable. The identification of a histologically dysplastic nevus in a patient without a family history of melanoma nonetheless indicates an increased lifetime risk of melanoma according to these workers.[21]

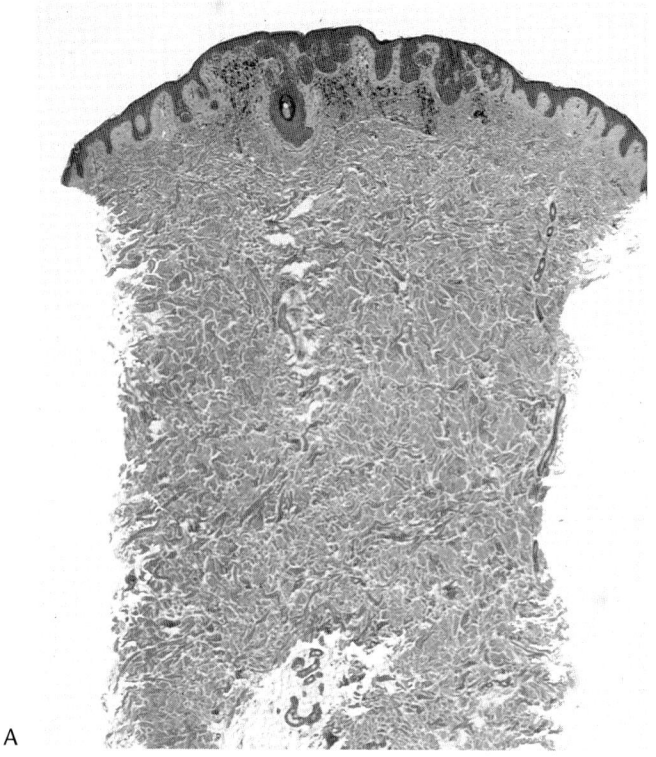

A

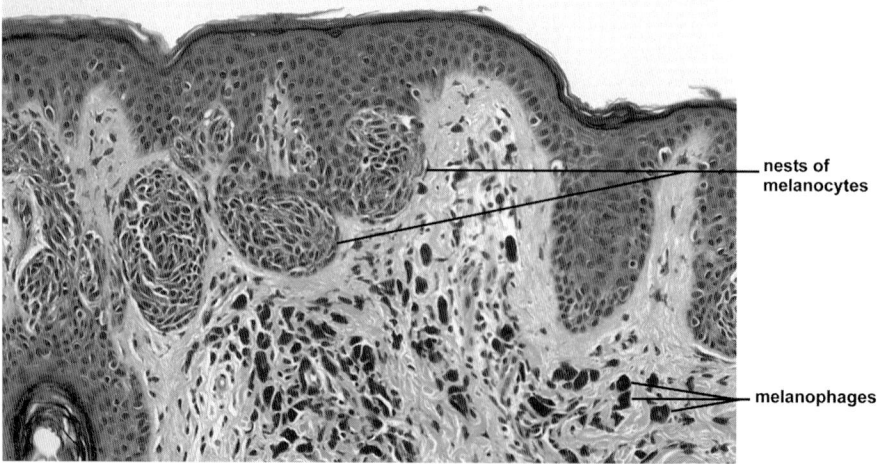

B

nests of
melanocytes

melanophages

Figure 20-3. A junctional melanocytic nevus. Note the sharply circumscribed, slightly elevated area on the surface of this punch biopsy specimen
(**A**). There are well-circumscribed, rounded nests of melanocytes at the
bases of rete ridges (**B**).

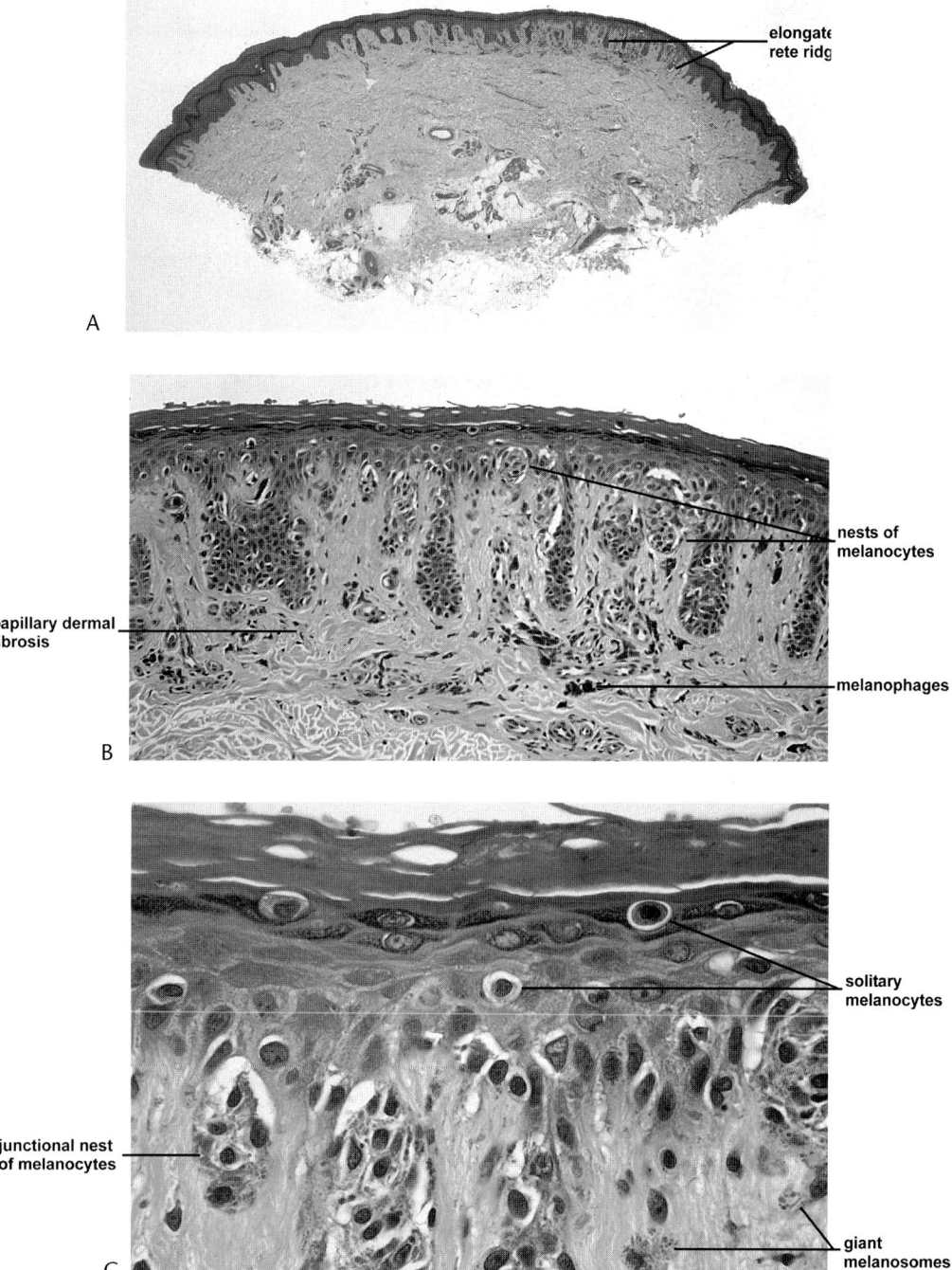

Figure 20-4. A junctional melanocytic nevus on acral skin. In this nevus from the dorsal hand, the altered rete ridge pattern is discernible at scanning magnification **(A)**. There are both nested and single melanocytes along the junction, with the largest nests being roughly equal in size **(B)**. In nevi on the hands, feet, elbows and knees, the scatter of solitary melanocytes above the junction does not indicate melanoma **(C)**. The reason for the upward scatter of single cells in this setting is unknown.

In a series of papers Ackerman and Mihara[22] and Ackerman[23] attempted to demonstrate that the type of nevus described by Clark's group is relatively common, that the implication of these histologic features is minimal, and that the terminology that has been applied to them is inappropriate. These arguments were advanced by several population-based studies in which nevi with "dysplastic" features had an estimated prevalence of 80% in the white population.[24] In addition, histologic "dyspla-sia" was found to be common in clinically ordinary nevi.[25] It seems clear that such features as extension of junctional nests beyond the dermal component, bridging of adjacent rete ridges, fibroplasia of the papillary dermis, and slight variability in the size and shape of junctional melanocytic nuclei are not proof that a melanocytic nevus is about to turn into a melanoma; whether these findings in any way mark nevi that are partially transformed (i.e., have undergone genetic alterations that are in-

Figure 20-5. A compound melanocytic nevus, Clark or dysplastic type. At scanning magnification, the neoplasm is barely elevated with respect to the surrounding skin (**A**). Junctional nests extend to one side of the dermal component (**B**). In the center of the lesion, there are small round melanocytes clustered in the papillary dermis (**C**). *Continued.*

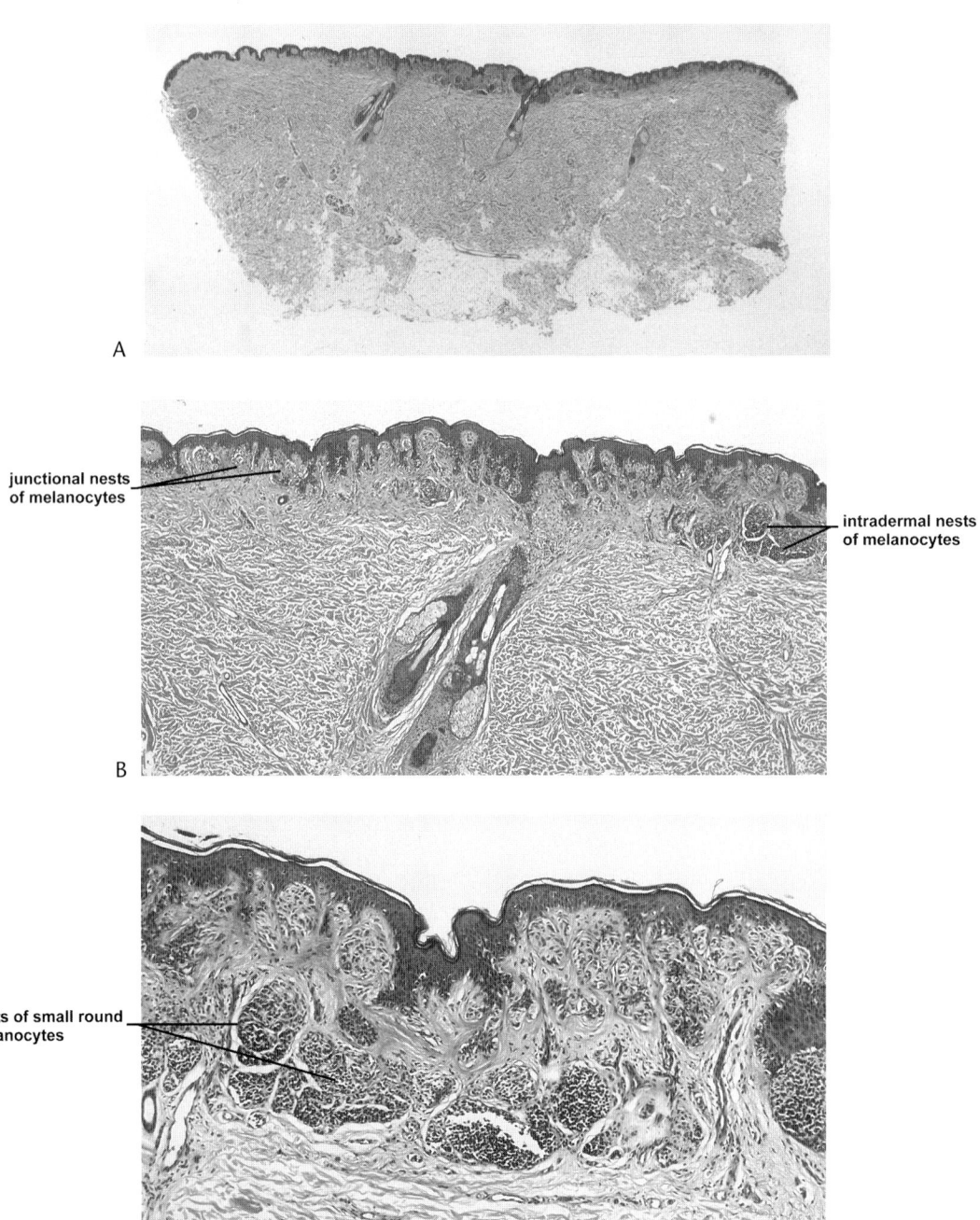

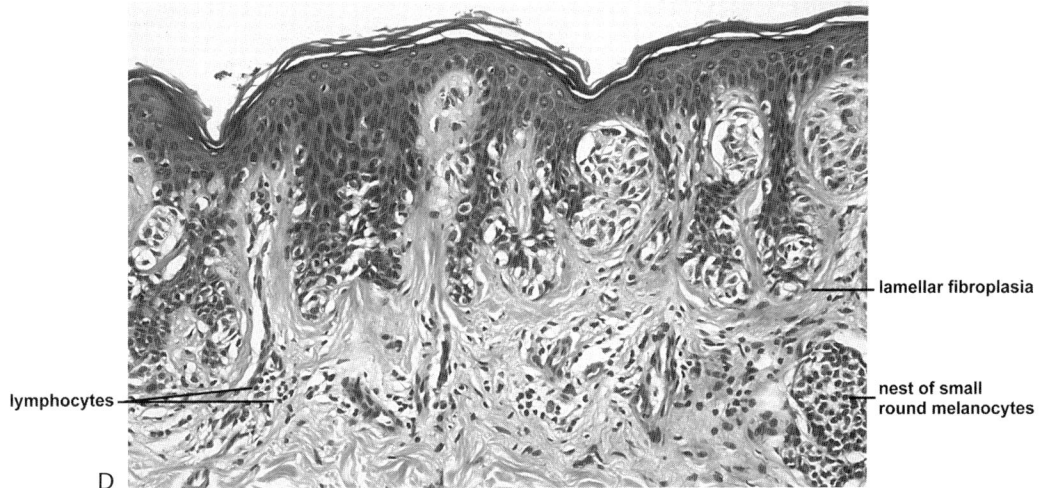

lamellar fibroplasia

nest of small
round melanocytes

lymphocytes

D

Figure 20-5. *Continued.* Junctional nests are situated near the bases of branching rete ridges, above lamellar fibroplasia, with sparse infiltrates of lymphocytes and melanophages **(D).**

termediate between "banal" nevi and melanoma) is yet to be proven.

There is however, a consensus that when many atypical nevi occur in a person with a family history of melanoma whose family members with melanoma *also* have numerous and/or large acquired nevi, that person has a lifetime risk of developing malignant melanoma that approaches 100%.[26] The judgement that a patient fits into this category should be made clinically and not by microscopic examination of a single lesion.

The best designation for these nevi and for the familial condition in which many of them are seen in a patient with malignant melanoma is not yet clear. Clark and Ackerman[27] suggested the term *compound nevus showing dysplasia of the type seen in the dysplastic nevus syndrome*, but insisted that this term should not be applied unless easily identifiable cytologic atypia is present. Sagebiel et al[28] advocated the term *low grade melanocytic dysplasia* for compound nevi in which junctional nests extend beyond the dermal component and bridging, fibroplasia, and lymphocytic infiltrates are present and *severe dysplasia* for those rare examples in which some melanocytes at the dermoepidermal junction or within the papillary dermis have

large, atypical nuclei. Ackerman and Magana-Garcia[29] recognized the distinctive low-power pattern of these nevi, for which they proposed the name *Clark nevus*. In 1992, a consensus conference of the National Institutes of Health recommended that the term *dysplastic nevus* be abandoned and that these lesions be referred to histologically as *nevus with atypical cytological and/or architectural features* and clinically as *atypical moles*.[30]

The behavior of these nevi is less controversial. Most persist, but some involute. Involution can be inferred by the presence of epidermal and papillary dermal alterations in the absence of melanocytes in either a part or throughout a lesion. Typically, there is lamellar or concentric fibroplasia and elongated rete devoid of junctional nests that flank a collection of mature nevus cells in the papillary dermis (Fig. 20-6). Sometimes, only a few melanocytes persist in the papillary dermis. Only rarely do socalled dysplastic or Clark nevi give rise to malignant melanoma, although they may do so more commonly than other types of compound nevi.[31] Upward scatter of atypical melanocytes within the epidermis, especially on one edge of the lesion, can herald the evolution of malignant melanoma in situ in such a nevus.

Figure 20-6. A Clark nevus that has largely involuted. The altered epidermis and papillary dermis remain, despite the near absence of melanocytes. This eventuation is by far the most common fate of Clark or dysplastic nevi.

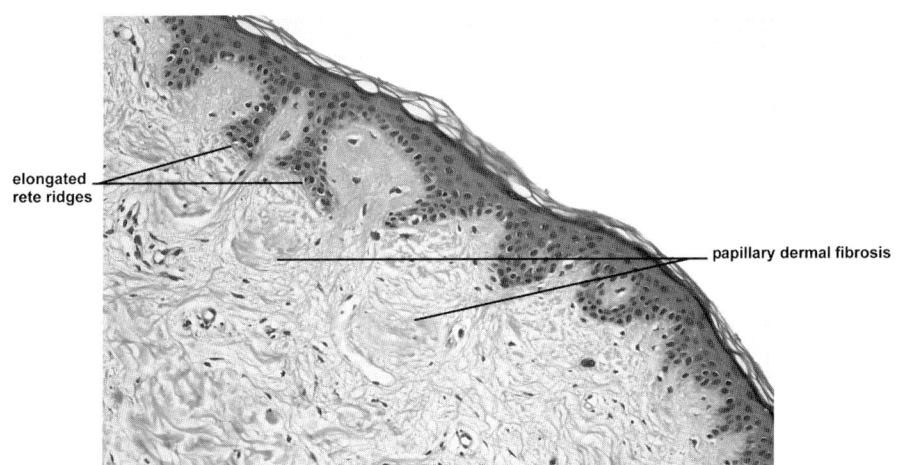

elongated
rete ridges

papillary dermal fibrosis

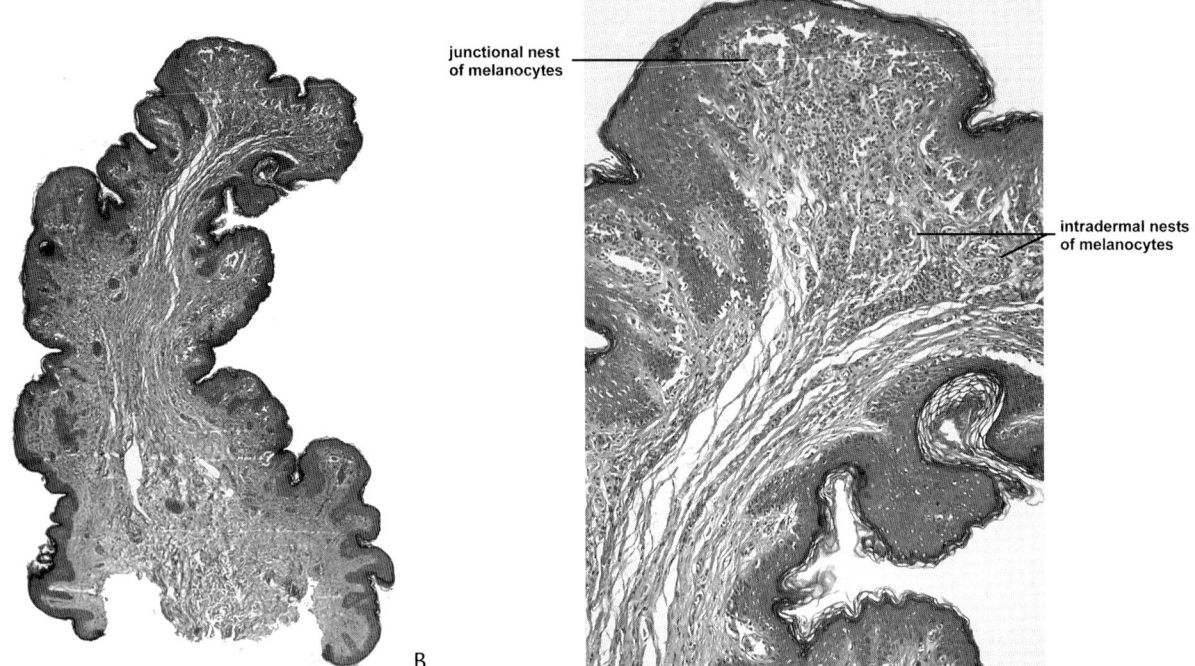

junctional nest
of melanocytes

intradermal nests
of melanocytes

A

B

Figure 20-7. A polypoid melanocytic nevus. This type of nevus often occurs in the same flexural areas as do skin tags and shares their shape **(A)**. Melanocytes are present both at the junction and in the dermis of this compound example **(B)**. There are small junctional nests and clusters of mature appearing cells in the dermis **(C)**.

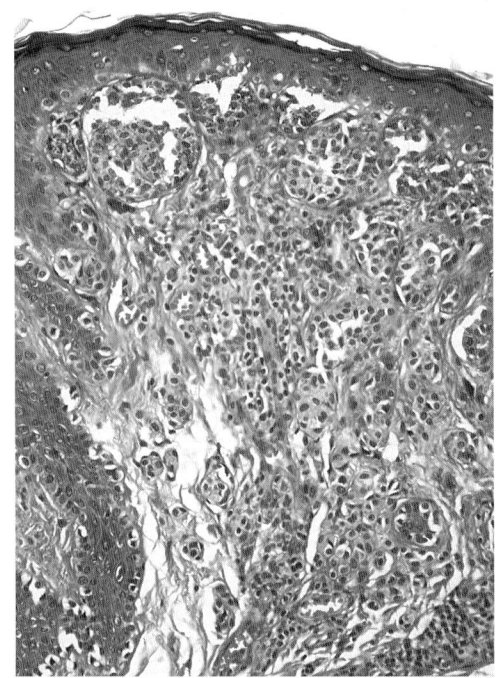

C

Some compound nevi in flexural areas such as the axillae and groins may develop small sac-like growths that resemble skin tags or acrochordons (Fig. 20-7). In most of these compound nevi, junctional nests do not extend much beyond the protuberant compound portion, but on occasion there will be lateral extension of junctional nests, bridging, and fibroplasia similar to those seen in dysplastic or Clark nevi. If the specimen includes reticular dermis, melanocytes can lie as strands between collagen bundles or can be clustered periappendageally, features seen in congenital nevi.

Small, acquired compound nevi on the face have an inverted wedge shape whose apex lies in the deep reticular dermis.[29] Periappendageal clustering of melanocytes is prominent and may be caused by a regional difference in the interaction between facial mesenchyme and melanocytes. The presence of melanocytes in and around pilosebaceous structures is frequently associated with the congenital origin of nevi when it occurs at other body sites, but this relationship may not hold true for nevi on the head or neck or, as mentioned above, for skin tag-like nevi (Fig. 20-8). Nevi in the beard area of men often have superficial areas of fibrosis from traumatization during shaving.

Compound nevi located along the milk line, especially those from the axillae, breasts, and groins, often have some features that may be seen in malignant melanomas (i.e., confluence of large junctional nests that contain melanocytes with abundant pale cytoplasm, some large nuclei, and necrotic melanocytes). Rarely, upward migration of single melanocytes is evident. Several studies have found that these changes do not imply malignant transformation.[18,32] Even proponents of the theory that single "dysplastic" nevi are markers of an increased lifetime risk of

malignant melanoma do not regard milk-line nevi as such a marker.

Compound nevi on acral skin can display the same upward scatter of single melanocytes as junctional nevi do at these sites. The dermal portion often has clusters of small round nevus cells around eccrine ducts. Lamellar fibroplasia is rare in compound nevi of the palms and soles.

Aside from halo reactions, there are two secondary inflammatory changes that occur with some frequency in compound

Figure 20-8. A wedge-shaped melanocytic nevus on the face. These lesions share a periadnexal distribution of melanocytes with congenital nevi, and many of them may in fact be tardive congenital nevi, i.e., nevi in which melanocytes arrived in the dermis because of faulty migration before birth, but became evident clinically only after birth. *Continued.*

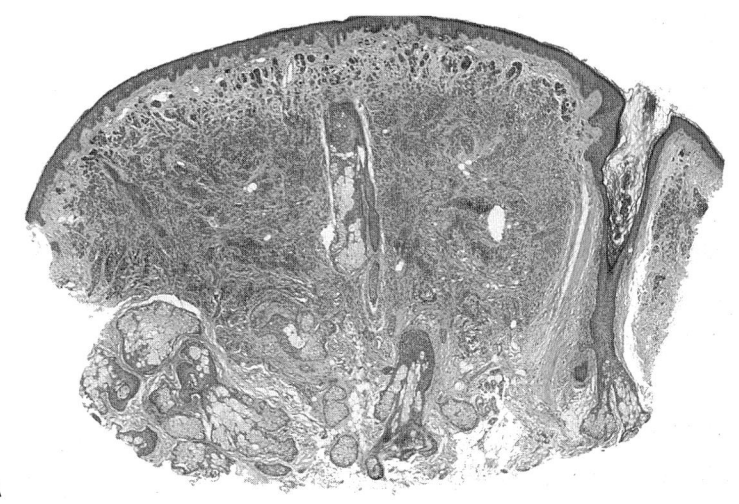

A

nests of melanocytes
in papillary dermis

melanocytes diffusely distributed
among collagen bundles of
reticular dermis

B

Figure 20-8. *Continued.*

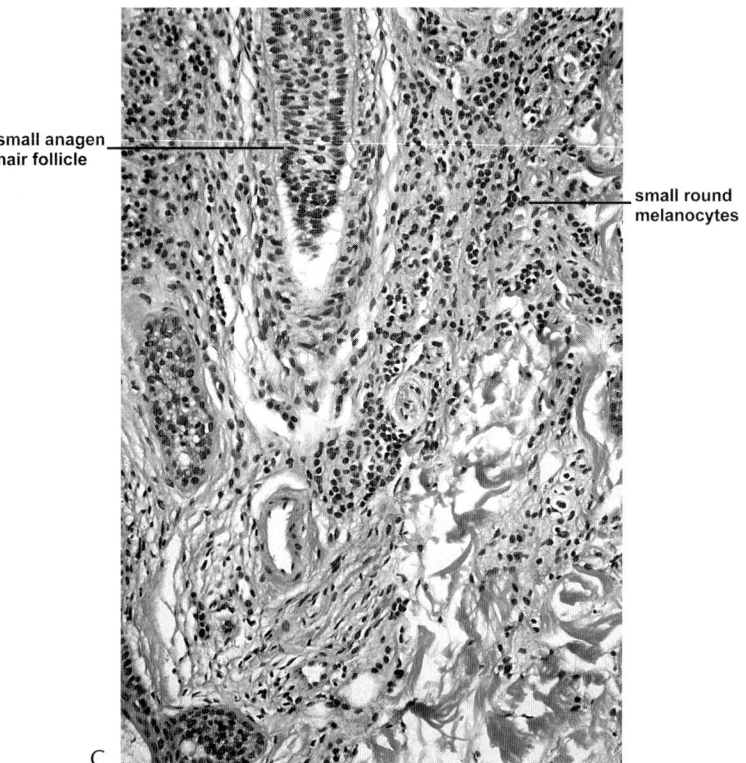

small anagen hair follicle

small round melanocytes

C

nevi. Hair follicles whose infundibula are constricted by the growth of a nevus can become cystic and rupture with suppurative and granulomatous dermatitis as a result. A compound nevus can also endogenously evoke spongiotic dermatitis, a change referred to as *halo eczema* or *Meyerson nevus*.[33] In some examples, the spongiotic changes are so prominent that level sections are required to demonstrate melanocytes.

Intradermal Nevi

Intradermal nevi are the end-stages of junctional and compound nevi, although many compound nevi remain stable during a person's lifetime. Junctional nests are still present in the majority of intradermal nevi, but serial sections are necessary to demonstrate their presence. The configuration of an intradermal nevus depends on the type of compound nevus that preceded it. The wedge-shaped compound nevi that are often found on the face, the polypoid nevi frequent in intertriginous areas, and "dysplastic" nevi all usually maintain their outlines even in their intradermal end-stage. Some intradermal nevi do not have distinctive shapes, and the types of compound nevi that preceded them cannot be discerned.

Regardless of the type of compound nevus from which they arose, intradermal nevi have many features in common that relate to their senescence. Maturation in nevi is evident as a decrease in the cellular and nuclear size of melanocytes with increased depth in a nevus. It is accompanied by loss of pigmentation in melanocytes in lesions whose upper portions were pigmented. In many very old nevi, further senescent changes can occur (Fig. 20-9). Melanocytes can come to resemble Schwann cells by virtue of S-shaped spindled nuclei and fibrillar or mucinous stroma replete with mast cells. Mucin can accumulate interstitially, a common finding in all neural

crest–derived proliferations. Neurotized nevus cells may aggregate to form so-called tactoid bodies or pseudomeissnerian corpuscles, ovoid structures whose nuclei are palisaded on opposite sides. Senescent nevi can also involute by developing areas of fibrosis or by replacing melanocytes with adipocytes. Adipocytes are not found in nevi from children, arguing against their presence due to malformation similar to that in nevus lipomatosis. Minute spicules of bone have been found in some old nevi, as have the rounded concretions known as *psammoma bodies.*

Clinicopathologic Correlation

The degree of pigmentation of melanocytes in a nevus diminishes as it matures from the junctional through the compound to the intradermal stage. Pigmented melanocytes are usually present only at the dermoepidermal junction or within the superficial dermis. The borders of melanocytic nevi are clinically circumscribed to the degree that junctional nests come to an abrupt end histologically. If single neoplastic melanocytes extend beyond the nests laterally, or if the distances between melanocytic nests that extend laterally beyond the dermal component are unequal, or if both junctional nests and dermal nevus cells are not homogeneously dispersed at the edge of a nevus, it will be poorly circumscribed clinically. Some melanocytic nevi have notched borders due to perifollicular hypopigmentation.

Superficial acquired nevi of the type termed a *dysplastic* or *Clark* nevus have architectural features that closely correspond to their clinical appearance. The macular peripheries of these nevi are areas that are predominantly junctional histologically. The erythematous halo that surrounds many of these lesions is produced by ectatic venules and a perivascular lymphocytic infiltrate. The central papule, if present, corresponds to an area in

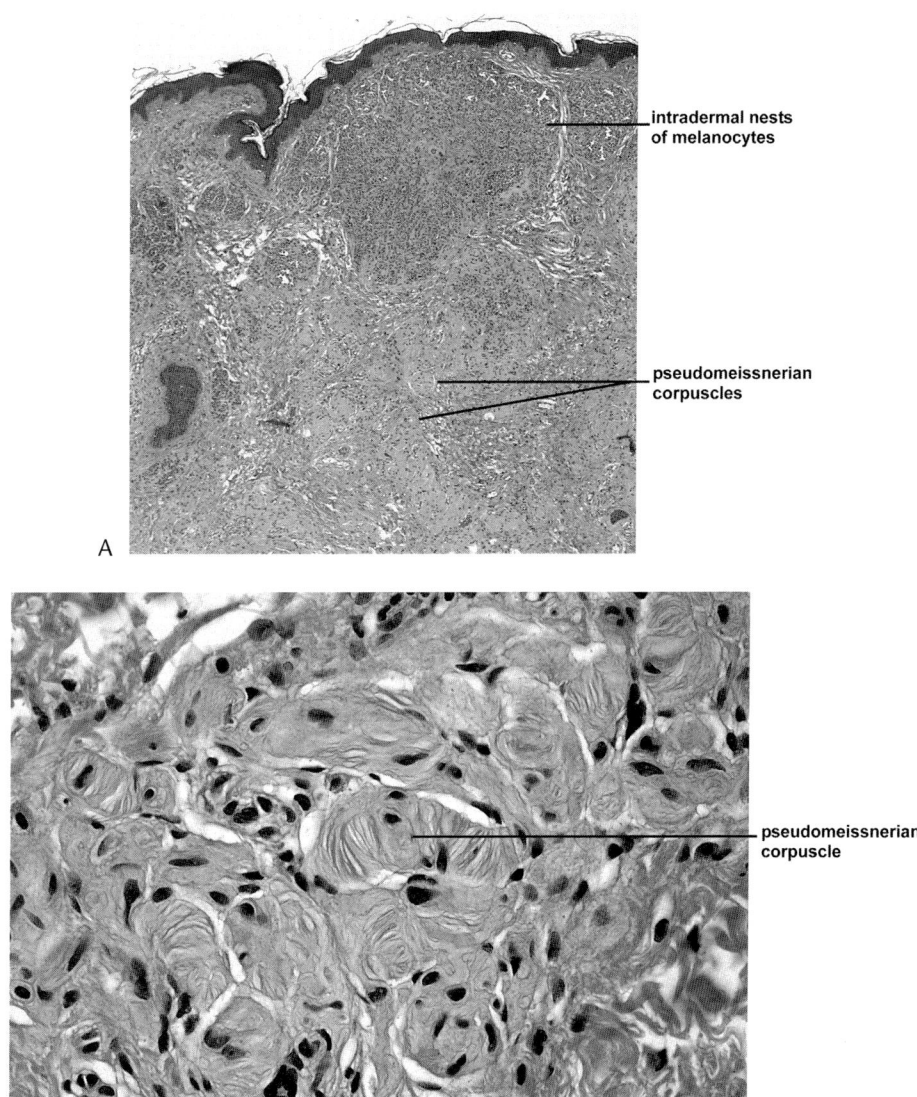

A

intradermal nests of melanocytes

pseudomeissnerian corpuscles

B

pseudomeissnerian corpuscle

Figure 20-9. An intradermal nevus with neurotization. Neurotization is the tendency of melanocytes in some nevi to adapt some of the phenotypic characteristics of Schwann cells, i.e., a spindle-shaped elaboration of basement membrane material, and the formation of structures resembling Meissner's corpuscles. Neurotization is often evident at scanning magnification as a pale zone in the deep portion of a predominately intradermal nevus **(A)**. Pseudomeissnerian corpuscles are formed by spindled melanocytes that elaborate laminated basement membrane material to form ovoid masses **(B)**.

which the lesion is compound. The targetoid configuration seen clinically in Cockarde nevi is most often due to a central compound nevus surrounded by a ring of junctional nests.[17]

Lobulated intradermal nevi, paradoxically, are large, even though their composition suggests involutional change, as neurotization and clusters of lipocytes are prominent.[15]

Inflammatory changes in nevi alter their appearance. In nevi that cause cystic dilation and rupture of underlying hair follicles, a red, scaly papule can arise, raising the specter of a "changing mole" clinically. In nevi with spongiotic dermatitis (halo eczema or Meyerson nevus) pre-existent nevi become red and scaly. The inflammatory changes regress without involution of the nevus as they do in halo reactions. Unlike halo nevi,

the lymphocytic infiltrates in nevi with spongiotic dermatitis do not disrupt melanocytic nests but, rather, are randomly distributed.

Differential Diagnosis

Melanocytic nevi at every stage of development can almost always be distinguished from malignant melanoma. Junctional nevi are generally small, well-circumscribed lesions in which melanocytes in nests outnumber those scattered singly. Individual melanocytes in junctional nevi are seen in the basal layer of the epidermis unless the lesion has been irritated or is on acral skin. Junctional nevi are generally symmetric in that the surface configuration, size of nests, distribution of cells, pigment, and lymphocytic host response on one side of a lesion generally resemble those seen on the other. In contrast, melanoma in situ can be asymmetric in respect to these features and have areas in which melanocytes disposed as individual cells outnumber nests. An exception to this contrast in appearances is the simple lentigo in which single melanocytes form the bulk of the lesion. In simple lentigines, however, single melanocytes are mostly arrayed along the sides and bases or rete ridges and are not as numerous in the basal layer of the epidermis in between the rete. Nests of malignant melanoma in situ can be large, irregular in shape, and appear to be laterally confluent with neighboring nests. Pigment, distribution and cytologic features of melanocytes, and the density of the lymphocytic infiltrate in the underlying dermis can each be asymmetric in malignant melanoma in situ. Circumscription is another diagnostic aid. Junctional nevi are generally sharply circumscribed laterally. Malignant melanoma in situ may display poor lateral circumscription, ending with an irregular trailing off of single melanocytes. Especially useful for the diagnosis of melanoma in situ is the finding of single melanocytes situated above the basal layer lateral to the lateralmost junctional nest, except in acral nevi, in which they can extend slightly lateral to the last nest. In some "dysplastic" nevi single melanocytes lie lateral to the lateralmost nest, but are usually distributed evenly throughout the lesion.

Compound nevi can be distinguished from malignant melanoma in situ by examining their intraepidermal portion for the above changes and their dermal component for symmetry and evidence of maturation. Maturation should be relatively even throughout a compound or intradermal nevus. Occasionally in "dysplastic" or Clark nevi there are large melanocytes within areas of fibrosis in the papillary dermis, but the large cells are usually singly dispersed or in nests that also include smaller melanocytes, indicating that they are not proliferating in an uncontrolled fashion. Mitotic figures are occasionally found in the superficialmost dermal melanocytes of a compound nevus and by themselves do not constitute evidence of malignancy.[3] Mitotic figures in the intraepidermal portion of compound nevi can be discounted because it is difficult to be sure that they are in melanocytes rather than in keratinocytes and because cellular proliferation in the junctional zone of a nevus is a normal finding. Mitotic figures within cytologically atypical melanocytes, a dense lymphocytic infiltrate, and an asymmetric arrangement of dermal melanocytes are often present in malignant melanoma. Asymmetry can, of course, be found in combined nevi, which are a composite of two different types of melanocytes.

Intradermal nevi sometimes simulate malignant melanoma, or vice versa. A malignant melanoma whose superficial portion has been traumatized may lack an in situ component and resemble an intradermal nevus. When the cells of such a melanoma are small, a misdiagnosis can easily be made. Melanocytes in the upper portion of an intradermal nevus that are arranged in sheets rather than as discrete nests and mitotic figures in melanocytes may be clues to the correct diagnosis. In most intradermal nevi, the size and shape of melanocytic aggregates will be relatively even at each depth in the dermis. In malignant melanoma simulating an intradermal nevus, aggregates at the same level of the dermis can have a markedly disparate size, shape, cytologic appearance, or pigmentation.

In some intradermal nevi, especially on the face, prominent single melanocytes in the basal layer of the epidermis overlie the central portion of the neoplasm (Fig. 20-10). Especially in shave biopsy specimens, these cells can raise the possibility of malignant melanoma in situ. Clues that prominent single melanocytes represent an intradermal nevus rather than a melanoma in situ include their distribution as scattered cells with intervening keratinocytes, retracted cytoplasm with surrounding clefts, and the absence of either upward migration or extension beyond or even to the lateral borders of the dermal component. Lymphocytic infiltrates beneath the epidermis of an intraepidermal nevus in which there are pronounced single melanocytes favors melanoma in situ.

Intradermal nevi that are largely neurotized can be indistinguishable from a neurofibroma histologically if residual, small, round nevus cells are not present. The immunohistochemical demonstration of factor XIIIa–containing dendritic cells and myelin basic protein in neurofibromas but not in neurotized nevi differentiate these two benign lesions.[34] As this differential diagnosis is seldom important in the management of patients, immunohistochemical studies to distinguish these lesions are largely a research tool.

Pathophysiology

The capacity to synthesize melanin is gradually lost as cells descend from the dermoepidermal junction into the papillary and reticular dermis. Mitotic activity also diminishes but does not cease entirely. Studies using thymidine labeling and immunoperoxidase staining with Ki-67, which labels a nuclear protein expressed in actively cycling cells, indicate that dermal melanocytes are also proliferating, albeit at a slower rate than their junctional counterparts.[35,36] Because errors in genomic replication may be among the causes of cancer, the relatively higher mitotic rate in the superficial portions of melanocytic nevi may account for the fact that almost all malignant melanomas that arise in association with nevi appear to begin at the junction.

The process of maturation may not be aptly named, as mature melanocytes are dendritic and produce pigment. In view of cellular and nuclear shrinkage and loss of organelles, *atrophy* better describes the changes seen in melanocytes deep in the dermis.[37]

HALO REACTIONS IN MELANOCYTIC NEVI

Halo nevi are not a separate type of nevus in the way that blue nevi and Spitz nevi are. Rather, they are melanocytic nevi, usually acquired and of the "ordinary" compound type (i.e., nevi composed of small round cells), that have provoked a dense lymphocytic infiltrate that permeates them and results in destruction of neoplastic melanocytes and non-neoplastic basilar melanocytes and keratinocytes in the surrounding dermis, producing a ring of depigmentation.

The term *halo reaction* describes a dense, permeative lymphocytic infiltrate in a nevus regardless of whether a clinical halo occurs.

Clinical Features

Halo nevi occur most frequently in children and adolescents and are rare after age 50.[38] Frequently, several halo nevi occur simultaneously. Depigmented halos have also been described around congenital melanocytic nevi, blue nevi, and malignant

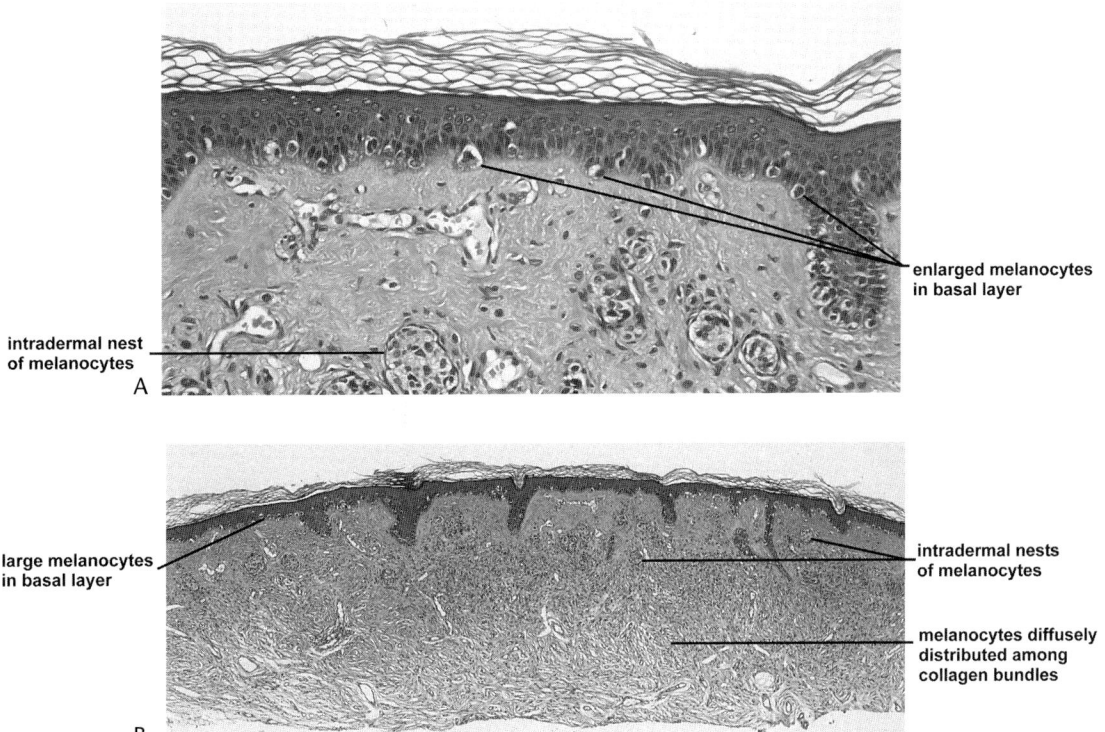

intradermal nest of melanocytes

A

enlarged melanocytes in basal layer

large melanocytes in basal layer

intradermal nests of melanocytes

melanocytes diffusely distributed among collagen bundles

B

Figure 20-10. A predominantly intradermal nevus on the face with prominent junctional melanocytes. Superficial shave biopsy specimens, or examination at high magnification without attention to the overall pattern of the lesion can lead to its misdiagnosis as melanoma in situ (**A**). The enlarged single melanocytes are present only directly above the dermal component, and only rare cells are present above the dermoepidermal junction (**B**).

melanomas. In some patients with malignant melanoma they have heralded the onset of a halo reaction in benign nevi.

The depigmented halos are symmetrically disposed around the central nevus, which, most often, is a red-brown or red papule. Nevi with a halo reaction histologically, but no halo clinically, are often erythematous.

Histopathologic Features

Most halo nevi have the overall features of a so-called dysplastic or Clark nevus, namely, melanocytes that are limited to the junctional zone and papillary dermis, arranged in nests along the dermoepidermal junction that exceed the dermal component in lateral span, and nests of melanocytes that bridge adjacent rete. The dermal portions of halo nevi are largely obscured by a dense, lymphocytic infiltrate that extends up to the dermoepidermal junction usually in both the center and periphery of the lesion. Melanocytes with karyorrhectic nuclei and, later, disruption of junctional nests of melanocytes by lymphocytes and necrosis of basilar keratinocytes and melanocytes are features of halo nevi. As melanocytes die, the papillary dermis becomes more visible and is often edematous and thickened by thin, delicate-appearing collagen bundles (Fig. 20-11).

The epidermis flanking the nevus shows loss of basilar melanocytes, scattered necrotic keratinocytes, infiltration by lymphocytes, and depigmentation. The latter can be detected by

the Fontana-Masson stain. Spitz nevi can develop halo reactions, and even when their melanocytic population entirely disappears they can be recognized for what they are by epidermal hyperplasia, compact hyperkeratosis, and Kamino bodies.

In some halo nevi, melanocytes with large monomorphous nuclei occur in the upper part of the dermis. The large nuclei of melanocytes in halo nevi are vesicular, with delicate nuclear membranes, and usually contain small nucleoli. These cells mature with descent.

Clinicopathologic Correlation

Depigmentation of the epidermis around a halo nevus is caused by T lymphocytes that have a cytotoxic effect on non-neoplastic basilar melanocytes. Even if these melanocytes do not die, their ability to synthesize pigment is impaired.

Differential Diagnosis

Melanomas with a dense, permeative, lymphocytic infiltrate are larger and more asymmetric than halo nevi. Mitotic figures can be seen in lymphocytes in halo nevi but are rare in melanocytes. Pagetoid intraepidermal spread of melanocytes is not a feature of halo nevi.

Some halo nevi have such dense lymphocytic infiltrates that they can be confused with cutaneous lymphoid hyperplasia or

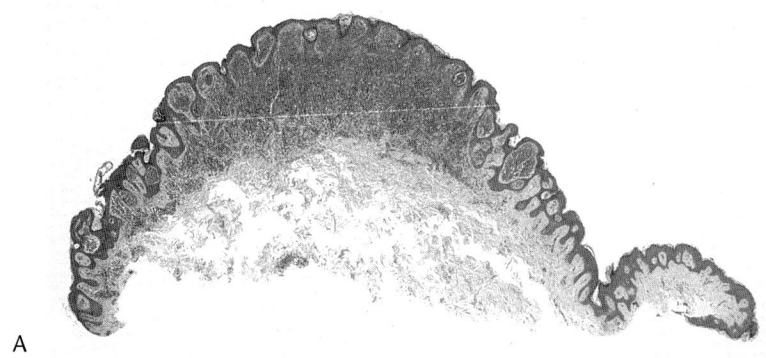

A

Figure 20-11. A Clark or dysplastic nevus with a halo reaction. At scanning magnification, the neoplasm and the reaction to it are present within the junctional zone and papillary dermis **(A)**. In the center of the lesion, melanocytes are obscured by dense infiltrates of lymphocytes, which ascend to the junction **(B)**. *Continued.*

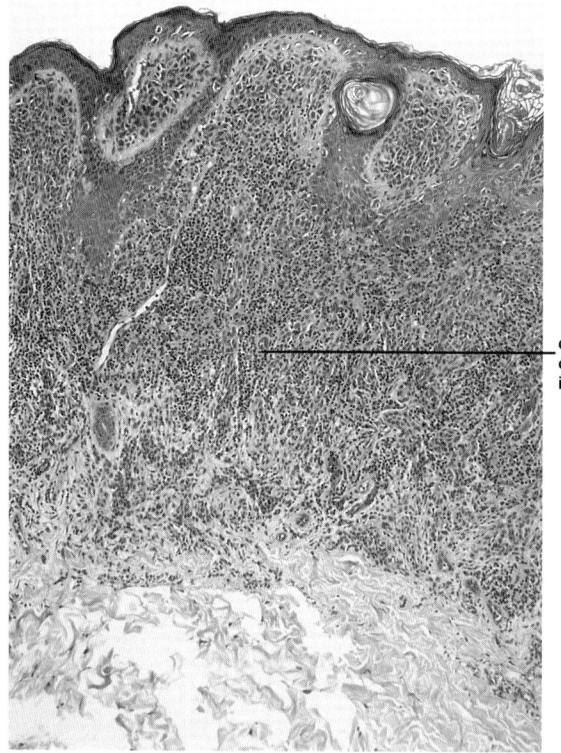

dense diffuse infiltrate of lymphocytes among intradermal melanocytes

B

lymphoma. Careful examination usually reveals a slight difference in nuclear size and cytologic features between the residual melanocytes and the infiltrating lymphocytes. In difficult cases, immunoperoxidase staining with antisera to S-100 protein can help demonstrate the melanocytic component.[39]

Both halo nevi and melanomas undergoing regression have areas in which melanocytes are diminished in number, in conjunction with dense lymphocytic infiltrates. In small, partial biopsy specimens it may be difficult or impossible to tell these two processes apart. Halo nevi tend to have the architectural features of dysplastic or Clark nevus and as such are well circumscribed and have elongated rete that are fused at their bases, sometimes even despite the absence of melanocytes. Pagetoid spread of melanocytes within the epidermis is not a feature of halo nevi, but can be detected in specimens of regressing or partially regressed melanoma. While confluence of junctional nests, and sometimes of nests of melanocytes in the superficial dermis, is evident in many halo nevi, large nodules of melanocytes are not present deep in the proliferation as they can be in

melanomas. If melanocytes are no longer present, the differential diagnosis between regressed melanoma and the remains of a halo nevus becomes even more difficult. There tend to be more numerous melanophages in regressed melanoma than in involuted halo nevi, with more complete diminution of the rete ridge pattern.

On occasion, halo nevi contain some dermal melanocytes that have a strikingly atypical nucleus. These atypical melanocytes do not form nests or sheets as they do in malignant melanoma but occur as single cells against a background of smaller ones with more banal appearance.

Pathophysiology

Circulating antibodies that reacted with the cytoplasm of the cells of malignant melanoma were detected in a patient with halo nevi.[40] A serologic factor would help explain why several halo nevi can occur in the same patient. Alternatively, the reaction could be entirely the result of cellular immunity and the antibody

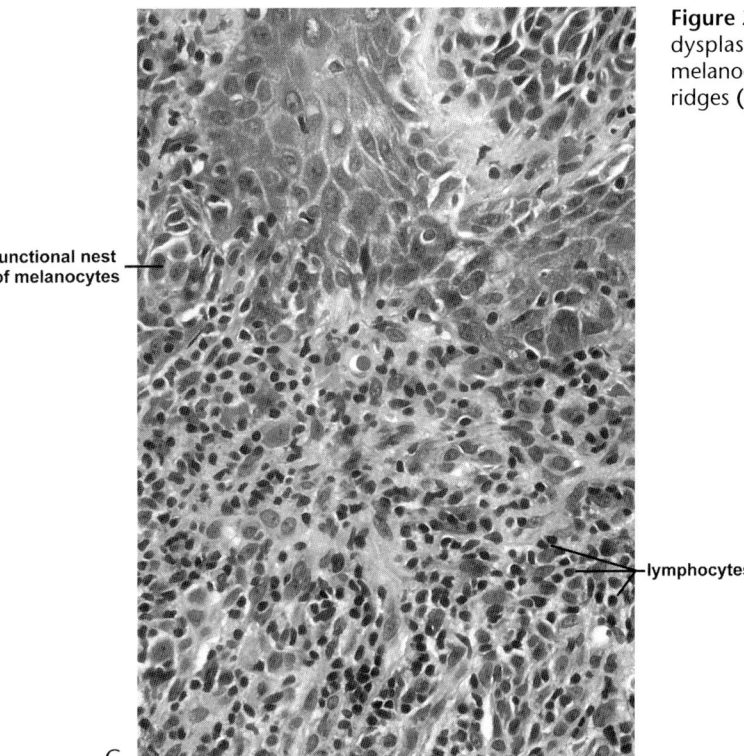

junctional nest of melanocytes

lymphocytes

C

Figure 20-11. *Continued.* The residual structure of this Clark or dysplastic nevus is evident as small clusters of junctional melanocytes, some of which bridge the bases of adjacent rete ridges (**C**).

to melanoma cell cytoplasm the result of cytotoxic damage unmasking an antigen. As in vitiligo, Langerhans cells persist in depigmented areas and migrate into the basal layer of the epidermis.

CONGENITAL MELANOCYTIC NEVI

Congenital melanocytic nevi are benign neoplasms of melanocytes that are evident clinically at or shortly after birth. Some lesions may be present at birth but only become visible when they acquire pigmentation thereafter. Estimates of the incidence of congenital nevi vary from less than 1% to 2.5% of newborn infants. Nevus spilus, or speckled lentiginous nevus, is a congenital nevus that features small dark macules or papules within a pigmented patch. Although blue nevi include forms that are doubtless congenital, and some blue nevi share a periappendageal distribution of melanocytes with congenital nevi, they are discussed separately.

Clinical Features

Congenital melanocytic nevi may be arbitrarily considered as small, large (or intermediate), and giant. Various authors have defined the large congenital nevi as more than 1.5 cm in diameter[41] or larger than a palm.[42] Giant congenital nevi have been defined as more than 20 cm in diameter or too large to excise and close without skin grafting. One commonly used classification considers nevi less than 1.5 cm as small, 1.5 to 20 cm as intermediate, and more than 20 cm as large.[43]

The color of a congenital nevus can range from tan to brown or dark brown; various hues can be present in the same lesion. Because the outline of a lesion can be irregular, small congenital nevi are often mistaken clinically for a dysplastic or Clark

nevus. The surface of a congenital nevus can be smooth or papillated, and terminal hairs can be present, especially in a so-called giant hairy nevus. The belief that the presence of terminal hairs indicates that a melanocytic lesion is benign is archaic and untrue. Some congenital nevi involving the scalp have a cerebriform appearance.[16] Speckled lentiginous nevi consist of a light brown patch within which are darker brown macules or papules. The condition can have a dermatomal distribution, and such lesions are called *zosteriform lentiginous nevus.*[44]

Histopathologic Features

Some histopathologic features are characteristic of congenital melanocytic nevi, but few are specific. The diagnosis of congenital melanocytic nevus is usually based on a lesion's clinical appearance or by history. It is nonetheless important for a dermatopathologist to be able to recognize a congenital nevus because exceptional changes occur in them that can be confusing.

Nearly all congenital melanocytic nevi are biopsied at a stage when they are compound or mostly intradermal. Rarely, congenital nevi in infants can be junctional, as can ones situated on the acral skin of small children.

In the superficial pattern of congenital melanocytic nevi biopsied at its compound stage there is often a band of melanocytes in the papillary dermis that extends into the perifollicular adventitial dermis.[45] Melanocytes can be arranged in strands between reticular dermal collagen bundles. Small, mature-appearing cells are present in and around eccrine ducts, arrector pili muscles, hair follicles, and venules. The presence of melanocytes within rather than around such structures appears to be a more specific sign of congenital origin, but melanocytes have even been found within hair follicle epithelium, eccrine ducts in the deep reticular dermis, and blood vessels in nevi that appeared during early childhood.[46] Adnexocentric distribution is probably the least reliable indicator of a true congenital origin of these features. The lack of a rigid histologic dividing line between small congenital nevi and nevi that appear during early childhood makes sense, as nevi evolve throughout life, and it would be surprising for parturition to end the development of these lesions (Fig. 20-12).

In some superficial congenital nevi compact aggregates of melanocytes bulge into lymphatic spaces. Penetration of these cells into lymphatic channels could give rise to the subcapsular collections of melanocytes sometimes seen in lymph nodes.

In the deep pattern of congenital nevus, generally seen in so-called giant or garment-sized lesions, melanocytes permeate the deep reticular dermis and extend into the septa of the subcutaneous fat.[47] The features noted above as characteristic of superficial congenital nevi may or may not be present (Fig. 20-13).

Unusual features seen in the dermis in congenital nevi include scattered dendritic melanocytes and melanophages, areas of Schwannian differentiation, balloon cells, areas resembling neurofibroma, foci of cartilaginous differentiation, and numerous multinucleated melanocytes with wreath-like configurations resembling juvenile xanthogranuloma. All of these findings are more often seen in deep than in superficial lesions.

Figure 20-12. A superficial congenital melanocytic nevus. At scanning magnification, melanocytes are arranged in a patchy fashion in the dermis, clustered around vessels and other adnexa **(A).** The dermal component is separated from the junction by a broad zone of uninvolved papillary dermis. Note a group of melanocytes around an eccrine duct **(B).** *Continued.*

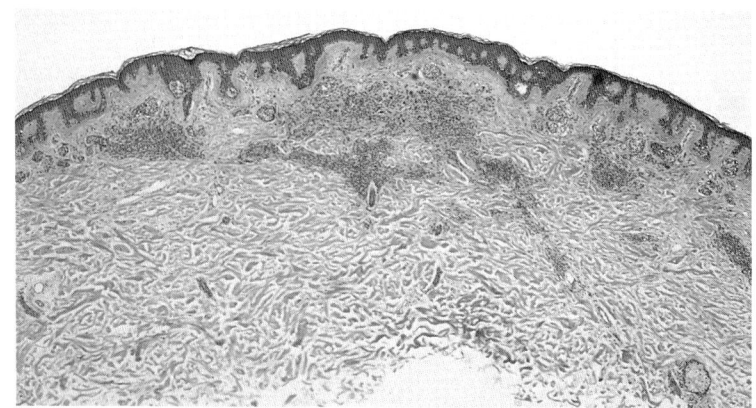

A

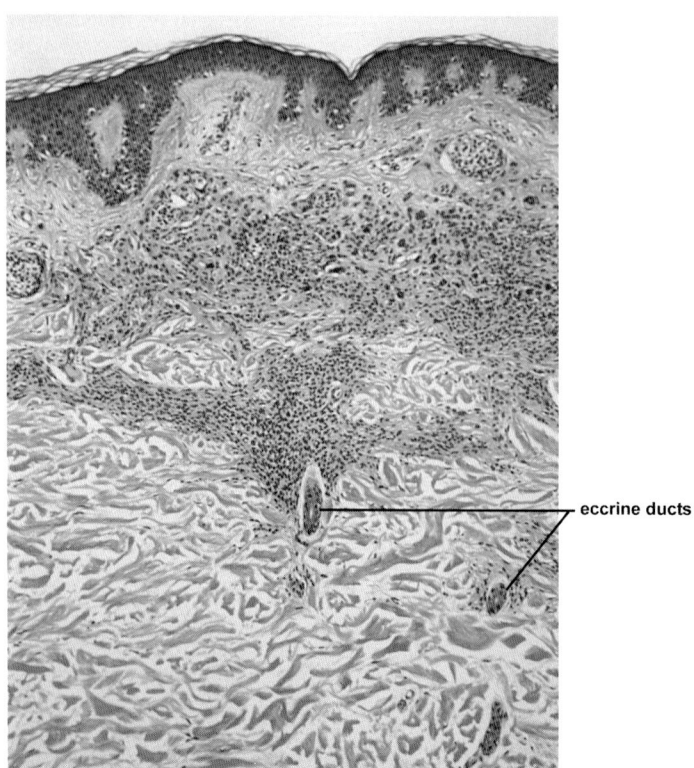

eccrine ducts

B

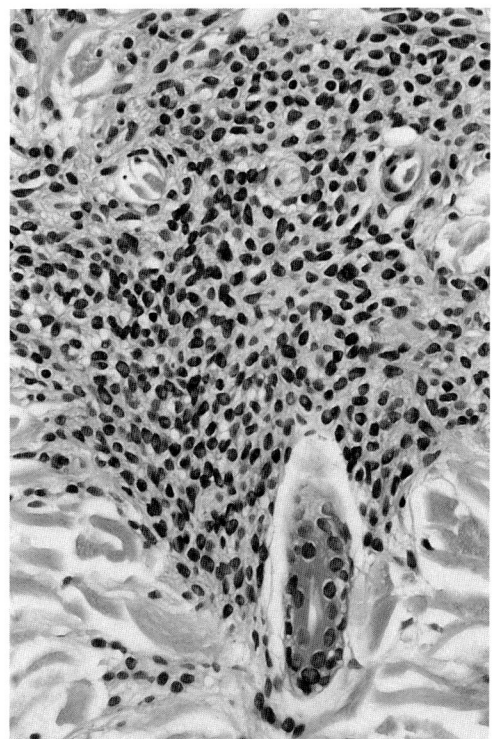

C

Figure 20-12. *Continued.* The melanocytes adjacent to the duct are arranged as strands between reticular dermal collagen bundles **(C)**. Prominent melanocytes, mostly arranged singly but also as small nests, are present at the junction. In congenital nevi, the wide gap between the junctional and dermal components suggests that melanocytes arrived at those sites separately, rather than first appearing at the junction and descending into the dermis **(D)**.

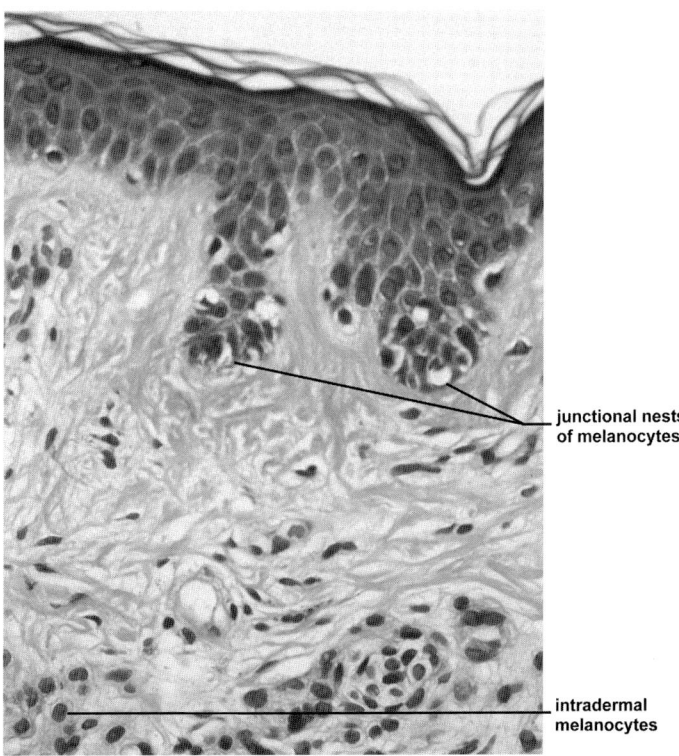

junctional nests of melanocytes

intradermal melanocytes

D

The junctional component of compound, congenital nevi is often lentiginous (i.e., along with basilar hyperpigmentation, there are elongated rete ridges, and areas in which solitary melanocytes outnumber those in nests). This lentiginous junctional component often extends laterally beyond the dermal component of superficial congenital nevi.

Several unusual histologic findings in congenital melanocytic nevi may simulate malignant melanoma. In some congenital nevi biopsied shortly after birth, and even in some in older infants, there may be pagetoid upward migration of small melanocytic nests and of individual melanocytes (Fig. 20-14). The nuclei of these melanocytes are quite uniform, in contrast to the pleomorphism usually present in the intraepidermal portion of malignant melanoma. Their cytoplasms are abundant, pale, finely vacuolated, and contain powdery melanin and may resemble balloon cells.[48] Papules or nodules may arise in congenital nevi that contain sheets of melanocytes that may contain a few cells in mitosis. Nodular melanocytic proliferation within a congenital nevus differs from a nodule of malignant melanoma arising in congenital nevi in that the nodules are small (less than 1 cm), melanocyte nuclei are uniform in size, necrotic cells are rare, and lymphocytic infiltrates are absent; maturation of melanocytes is evident in the deepest cells of the nodule (Fig. 20-15).

Figure 20-13. The deep form of congenital melanocytic nevus (**A**). The lesion has a mamillated surface, a cellular superficial portion, and a sparsely cellular deep component that extends into subcutaneous septa (**B**). *Continued.*

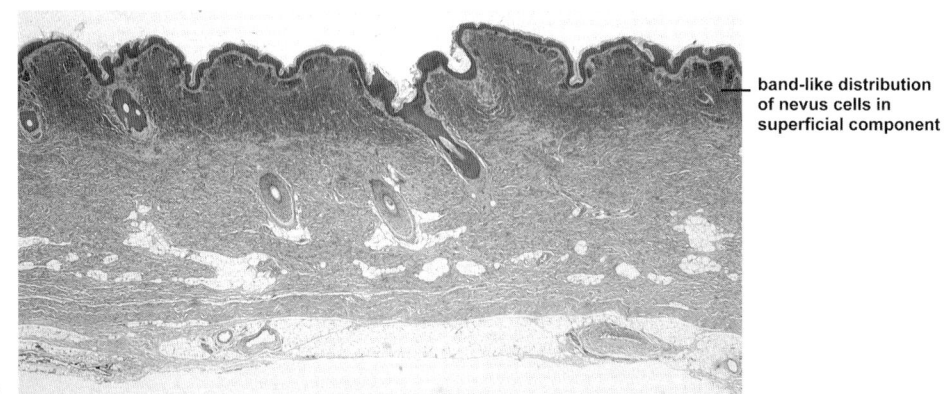

band-like distribution of nevus cells in superficial component

A

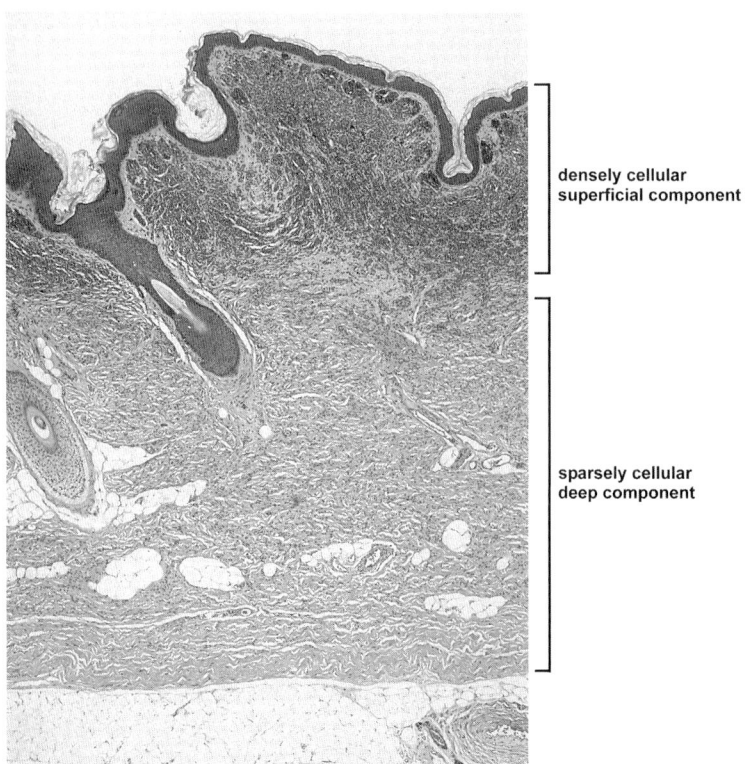

densely cellular superficial component

sparsely cellular deep component

B

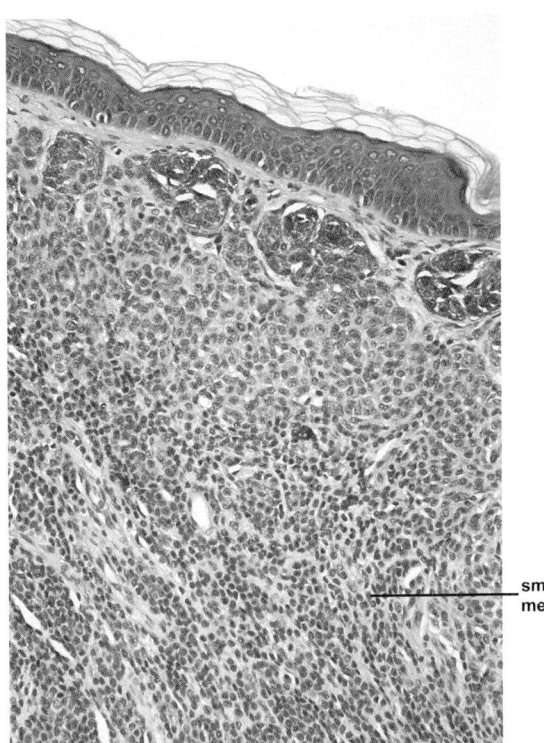

small, round
melanocytes

C

Figure 20-13. *Continued.* The superficial component contains melanocytes with scant cytoplasm and round nuclei **(C)**. The deep component has small spindled cells that could easily be mistaken for fibroblasts. In some cases, the deepest cells lie in fascia or even in skeletal muscle **(D)**.

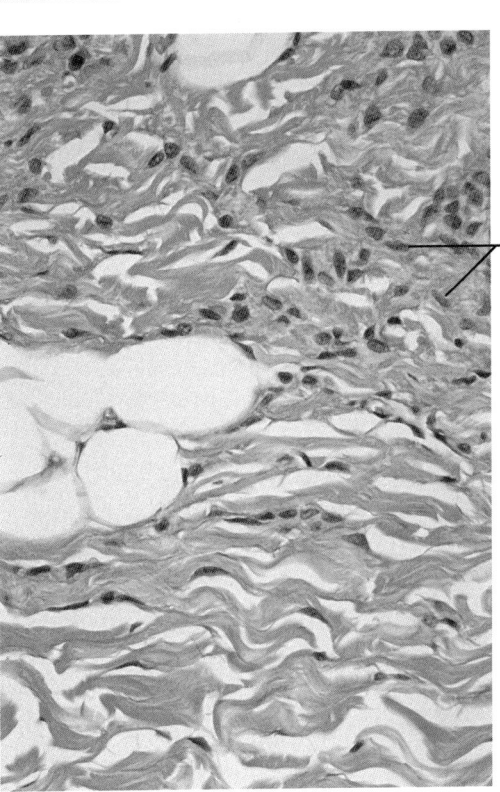

spindle shaped
melanocytes

D

Other unusual neoplasms have arisen within large congenital nevi.[49] Some of these have appeared to be malignant histologically but have not metastasized. These have included proliferations of spindled cells with frequent mitoses, rhabdomyoblasts, lipoblasts, and pseudo-Meissnerian corpuscles, as well as proliferations resembling neuroblastoma that matured via the formation of ganglion-like cells. Melanoma, proven by distant metastasis, can also present in unusual ways when it occurs within a giant congenital nevus. Melanomas arising in giant congenital nevi during childhood can begin in the dermis and often are characterized by cells that are round and have hyperchromatic nuclei with scant cytoplasm. Melanomas arising in congenital nevi during later life generally have a more conventional appearance and begin at the dermoepidermal junction.

In speckled (nevus spilus) or zosteriform lentiginous nevi the pigmented patch shows basilar hyperpigmentation, and the darker macules or papules have an epidermis with changes similar to those of a simple lentigo, with small round melanocytes in the subjacent dermis, clustered around eccrine ducts and hair follicles.[44]

Clinicopathologic Correlation

The range of colors in congenital melanocytic nevi depends in large part on the amount of melanin in the basal layer of the epidermis. In papillated congenital melanocytic nevi the epidermis is often hyperplastic. Interanastomosing rete ridges may enclose small horn pseudocysts, simulating a seborrheic keratosis. In older congenital nevi there is generally diminished pigmentation, corresponding to involution of the junctional component.

Figure 20-14. Pagetoid scatter of melanocytes in a congenital nevus biopsied shortly after birth. Note that hair follicles are closely spaced, an indication that the specimen is from a child **(A)**. A nest of small melanocytes is present within follicular epithelium. The epidermal zone in which pagetoid upward migration of melanocytes is present can only be discerned at this magnification by the finding of many melanophages in the dermis **(B)** *Continued.*

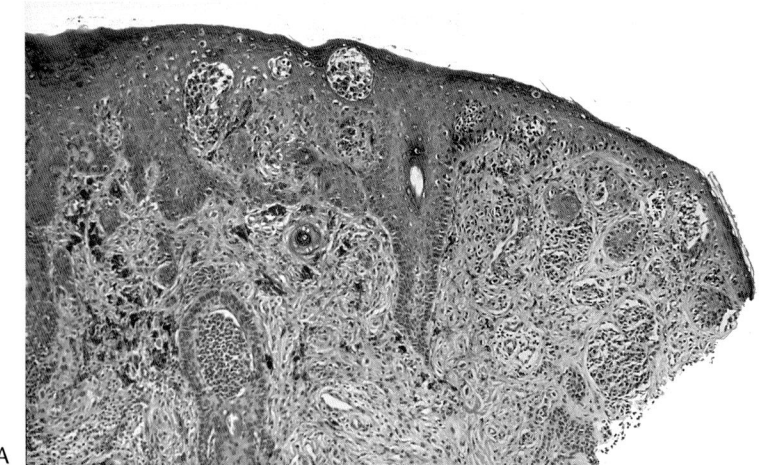

A

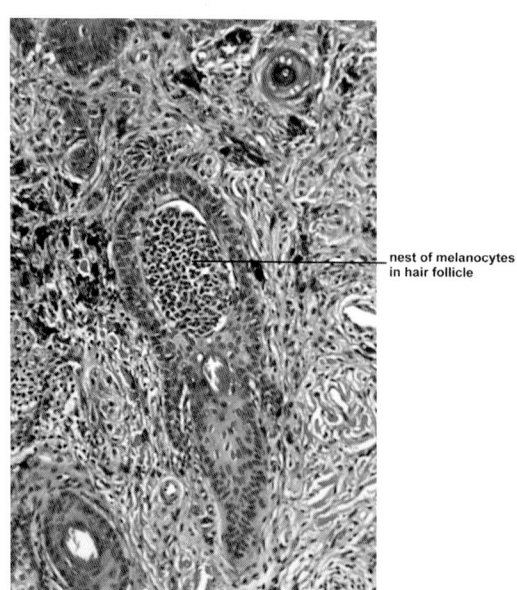

nest of melanocytes
in hair follicle

B

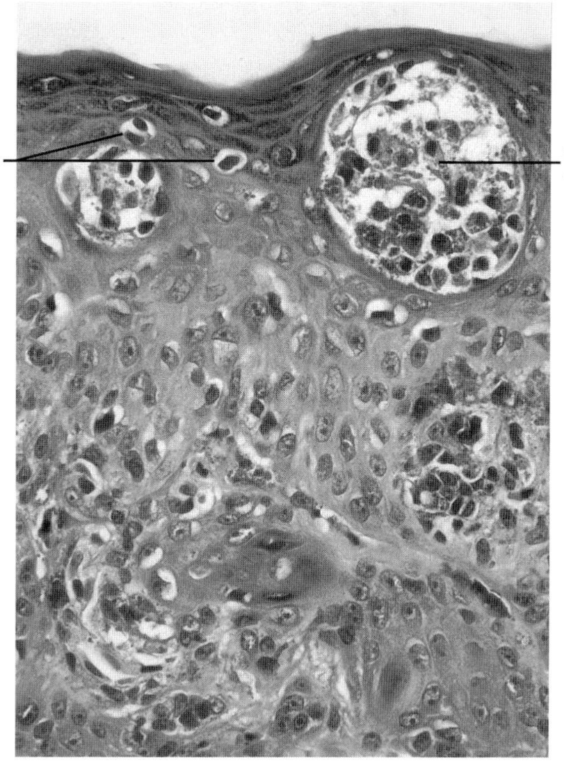

small cluster of two melanocytes and solitary melanocyte in upper level of epidermis

transepidermal migration of nest of melanocytes

Figure 20-14. *Continued.* In addition to nests at the junction, there are many individual melanocytes distributed in the suprabasilar epidermis and within hair follicle epithelium (**C**).

The various proliferations that arise in congenital nevi and simulate melanoma are usually evident clinically. A pagetoid melanocytic proliferation confined to the epidermis appears as a flat, dark brown area. A benign nodular melanocytic proliferation in a congenital nevus usually appears clinically as a dark brown to black, raised, smooth-surfaced lesion up to several centimeters in diameter. Malignant melanoma and other neoplasms arising in congenital nevi can present as large masses that sometimes ulcerate.

Differential Diagnosis

As there is no one feature that separates superficial congenital nevi from their acquired counterparts, the most common, but largely inconsequential, differential diagnosis of these lesions is with acquired nevi. When there is no clear history that a lesion was present at birth, it may be best to designate it as a nevus of the congenital type or as one with a congenital pattern. Breadth (especially greater than 1 cm), melanocytes within appendages or bulging into lymphatic spaces, or a pronounced perivascular distribution of melanocytes indicates that the nevus arose in utero or during early childhood.

Some small congenital nevi with a superficial histologic pattern have both clinical and pathologic features in common with dysplastic or Clark nevi. These small congenital nevi can have irregular pigmentation, a papular center, and a macular periphery. Junctional nests extend beyond the dermal component in

many such small, compound, congenital nevi. The proponents of the position that dysplastic nevi are uncommon lesions when precisely defined hold that the frequent changes seen at the "shoulders" of congenital nevi usually do not qualify as "melanocytic dysplasia" because lamellar fibroplasia, a lymphocytic infiltrate, and melanocytes with easily discernible nuclear atypia are not present.[50]

The various stimulants of melanoma that arise in congenital nevi can usually be differentiated from the rare cases in which melanoma does occur. The superficial spreading type of malignant melanoma shows greater nuclear pleomorphism than does its pagetoid simulant, and a lymphocytic host response is often present. A melanoma arising in the dermal portion of a congenital nevus is often composed of cells with a scant cytoplasm and a hyperchromatic nucleus and is also associated with a lymphocytic host response.

Pathophysiology

The risk of melanoma is greatest for giant congenital nevi, intermediate in large congenital nevi, and least in small ones. This is not accounted for by any finding aside from the number of melanocytes. Whether small congenital nevi should be removed prophylactically is a hotly debated topic.[51] The recent demonstration of a cellular population with an abnormal DNA content in histologically benign congenital nevi is of interest in this regard.[52]

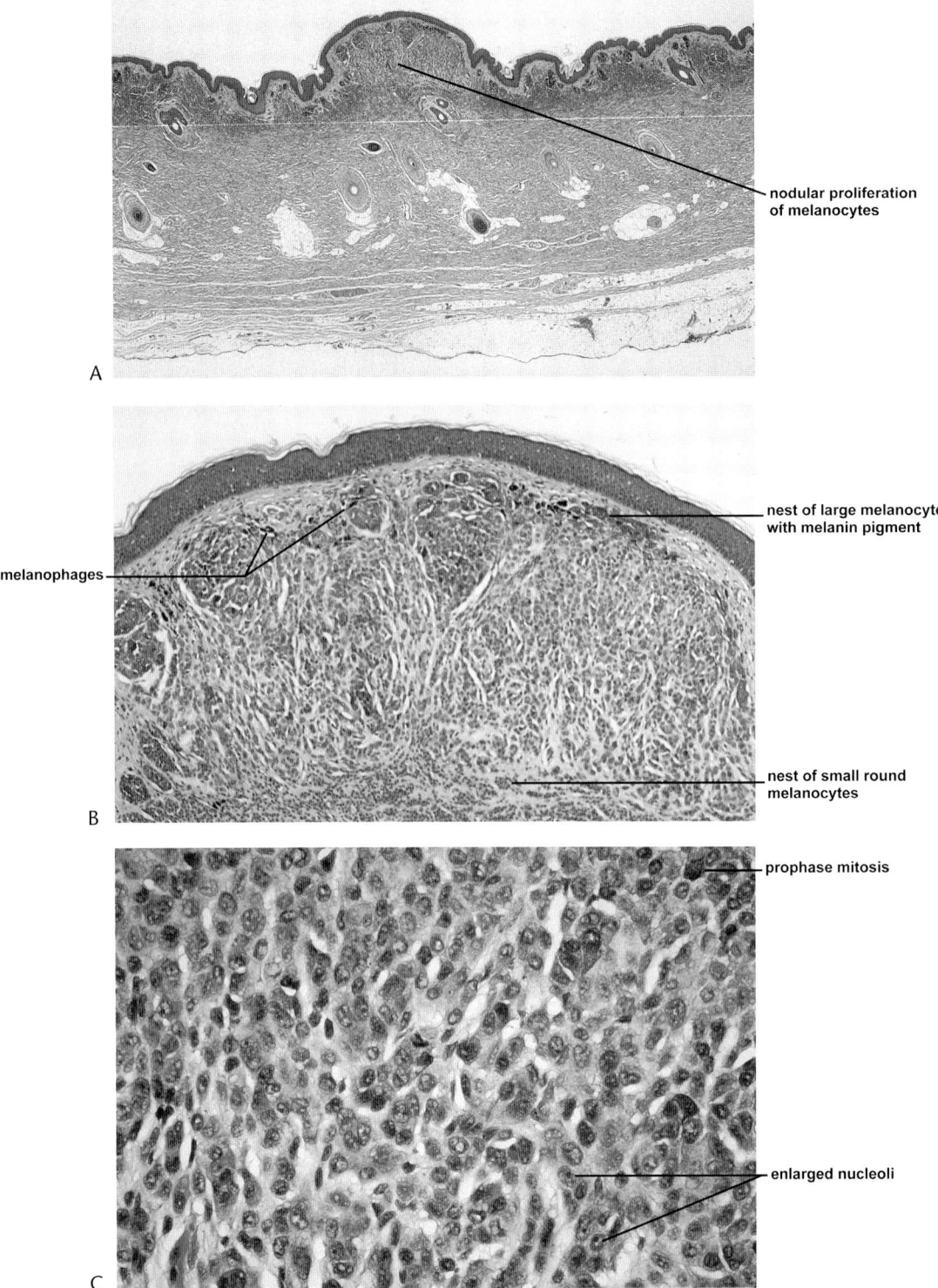

Figure 20-15. A nodular proliferation of melanocytes in the dermal portion of a congenital nevus. Some benign proliferations of melanocytes in large congenital nevi occur in the superficial portion of the lesion, resulting in a papule within the plaque formed by the nevus. The proliferation results in a zone in which melanocytes are more compactly arranged **(A)**. The nuclei of melanocytes in this area are larger than those in the remainder of the lesion. Note the superficial distribution of pigment in an umbrella-like pattern **(B)**. Occasional mitotic figures are present in melanocytes in the compactly arranged zone. **(C)**. *Continued.*

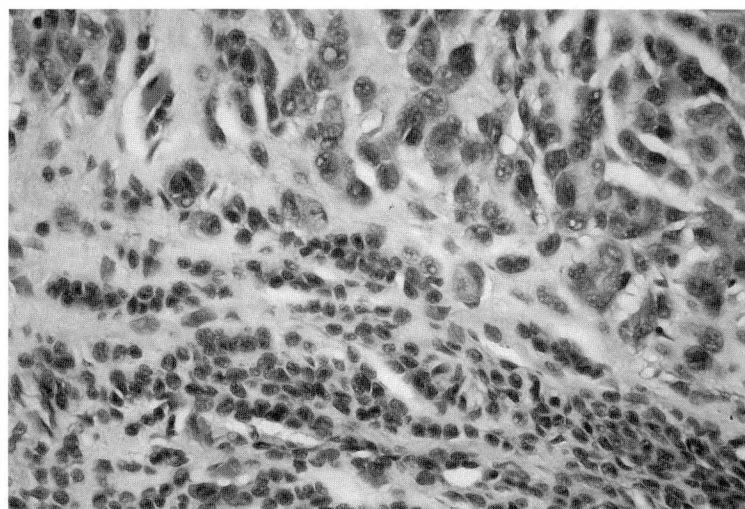

Figure 20-15. *Continued.* The melanocytes at the base of the papule have far smaller nuclei (**D**).

D

The origin of the features that simulate melanoma in congenital nevi is obscure. As a pagetoid proliferation is most common in infants, it has been suggested that it may be stimulated by maternal estrogens. Estrogen and progesterone receptors have been identified in congenital nevi, as well as "dysplastic" nevi and melanoma, but are not detected in banal intradermal nevi.[53]

SPITZ NEVUS

Spitz nevus, also known as a *spindle* or *epithelioid cell* nevus, is a benign neoplasm composed of large melanocytes that begin as junctional proliferations and may evolve into compound and, later, intradermal lesions. The term *juvenile melanoma*, which was originally used by Spitz to describe these neoplasms, has been abandoned.

Clinical Features

Spitz nevi can occur from birth to late adulthood, but most commonly occur before age 30. They are rapidly growing when they first appear, but later become stable.

The clinical appearance of Spitz nevus is diverse. Most are less than 1 cm in diameter, but exceptional lesions range up to 2 cm. Regardless of their size, radial symmetry and sharp lateral circumscription are clinically characteristic. Pigmentation is uniform within a given lesion. Many Spitz nevi in infants and children have little pigmentation and resemble a hemangioma. Others are tan or brown. The junctional or superficial compound variant of Spitz nevus (pigmented spindle cell nevus) often is dark brown.

A rare condition is agminated Spitz nevi in which several lesions occur in a circumscribed area of skin, sometimes on a hyperpigmented or hypopigmented patch. Some agminated Spitz nevi are present at birth. In another rare and frightening presentation, many Spitz nevi may "erupt" at separate sites or in a circumscribed area.[54]

Histopathologic Features

The earliest recognizable junctional Spitz nevus begins as a proliferation of large, single melanocytes at the dermoepidermal junction (Fig. 20-16). Reliable criteria do not exist to separate all of the earliest Spitz nevi from early lesions of malignant melanoma in situ. The earliest examples of Spitz nevus that are recognizable as such have cells that are often vertically oriented with large vesicular nuclei, abundant eosinophilic cytoplasm, multinucleated melanocytes, and clefts around the peripheries of melanocytes. Even at this embryonic stage, the epidermal changes that are so characteristically associated with Spitz nevus, such as hyperplasia of the spinous and granular layers, and compact hyperkeratosis first appear.

As junctional Spitz nevi develop further, nests of large melanocytes develop at the dermoepidermal junction[55] (Fig. 20-17). Within a given lesion, these nests are relatively uniform in size and are most often round. Clefts are frequently present between the junctional nests of Spitz nevus and the adjacent epidermis and separate the cells that comprise these nests. The junctional nests are often composed of elongated cells that are vertically oriented. As junctional Spitz nevi develop, the epidermis becomes more hyperplastic and hyperkeratotic.

Another finding in the epidermis of some junctional and compound Spitz nevi are Kamino bodies, which are a homogeneous-appearing dull pink in hematoxylin and eosin-stained sections, and they stain similarly to collagen with trichrome methods[56] (Fig. 20-18). Kamino bodies have a rounded or lobulated shape and may range in size from 10 to 110 μ in diameter, depending on whether they occur singly or in clumps. Kamino bodies appear to consist of basement membrane material and fibronectin, with an uncertain component of necrotic melanocytes and keratinocytes according to ultrastructural and immunohistochemical studies.[57] They stain with periodic acid–Schiff, and the staining is resistant to digestion with diastase. In trichrome stains, Kamino bodies stain the same color as subjacent dermal collagen.

The cytologic features of melanocytes in Spitz nevi are highly variable. Cytoplasm is always abundant, is usually densely eosinophilic; rarely it is finely vacuolated. Melanin can be abundant in the cells of a Spitz nevus in a dark-skinned person and in those of some junctional or superficial compound lesions in fair-skinned persons. A variant of Spitz nevus in which abundant melanin is present and in which the melanocytes are spindled has been termed *pigmented spindle cell nevus.*[58] Some

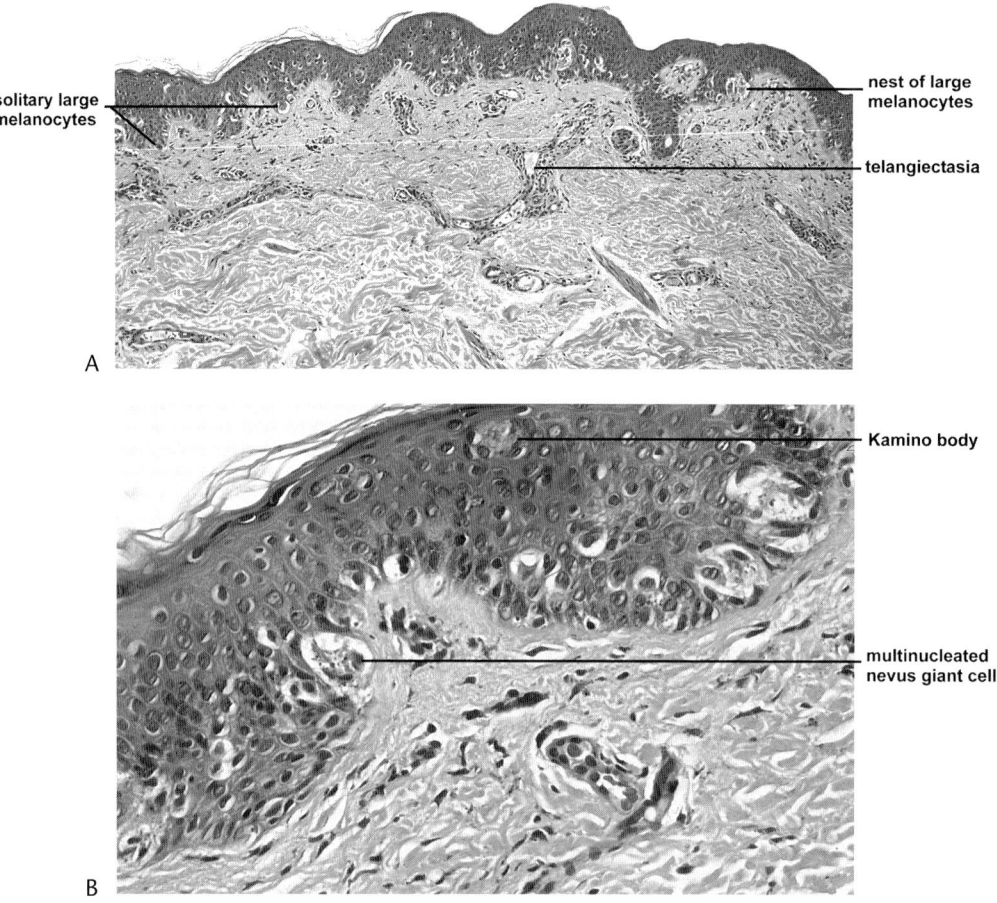

solitary large melanocytes

nest of large melanocytes

telangiectasia

A

Kamino body

multinucleated nevus giant cell

B

Figure 20-16. An evolving junctional Spitz nevus. At this incipient stage, solitary melanocytes outnumber those in nests **(A).** Some melanocytes are multinucleated, and a small Kamino body is present **(B).**

authors hold that this lesion, while related to Spitz nevus, is a separate entity whose evolution is different (Fig. 20-19).

The nuclear features of Spitz nevi have long been of interest, as it was their large size that led the pathologist Sophie Spitz to think that these lesions were a variant of malignant melanoma that occurred in childhood.[59] The nuclei of Spitz nevus are generally large and vesicular and round to ovoid. Although most Spitz nevi have small nucleoli, exceptional cases with large, eosinophilic nucleoli occur. It is rare to see diffusely hyperchromatic nuclei in Spitz nevus, and it is also unusual to find markedly irregular clumping of chromatin along the nuclear membrane. When cells with marked cytologic atypia occur, they are usually scattered among other cells that have a more banal appearance. Large eosinophilic inclusions (or pseudoinclusions) are sometimes evident in the nuclei of Spitz nevus and are thought to derive from cytoplasmic invaginations into the nucleus, cut in cross-section. Incorporation of these invaginations into the nucleus through apparent dissolution of the nuclear membrane has been observed by electron microscopy.[60]

Compound Spitz nevi show all of the superficial changes mentioned above and also have nests of melanocytes within the dermis (Fig. 20-20). The silhouette of a compound Spitz nevus often has an inverted wedge shape whose apex lies within the

deep reticular dermis or subcutis. The dermal cells are larger than the dermal melanocytes of ordinary compound nevi and are separated from each other by clefts. Generally, compound Spitz nevi are symmetric, sharply circumscribed, show maturation of the dermal component with descent, and lack significant upward migration within the epidermis. Spitz nevi in children often have edematous stroma and prominent telangiectatic vessels. Many of these features are examined in greater detail in the section on differential diagnosis.

Intradermal Spitz nevi are also inverted wedge-shaped lesions. The epidermis overlying an intradermal Spitz nevus sometimes loses many of the distinctive findings present in junctional or compound lesions. The dermis contains small nests or short fascicles of ovoid or spindled melanocytes. The size of these aggregates diminishes in the lower portion of lesions in which single melanocytes may be dispersed between collagen bundles. As an intradermal Spitz nevus ages, its cellularity may become scant. The stroma of an intradermal Spitz nevus is often sclerotic, hence the term *desmoplastic nevus* that has been applied to these lesions.[61] Symmetry, sharp lateral circumscription, maturation, and scarcity of mitoses in the deep portion of the lesion are all features of an intradermal Spitz nevus (Fig. 20-21).

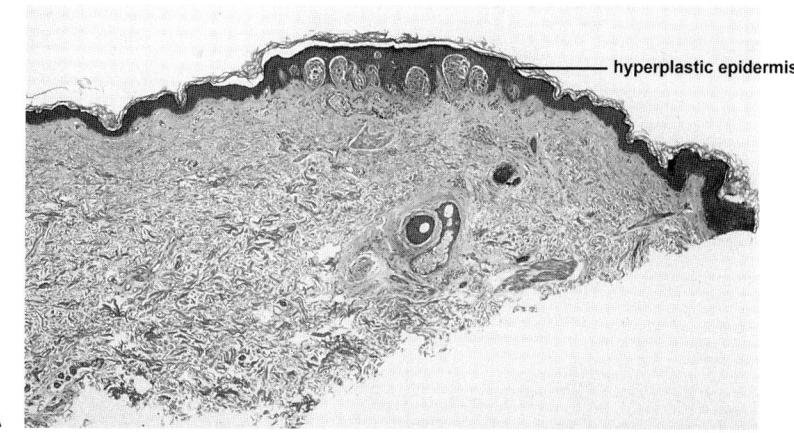

hyperplastic epidermis

A

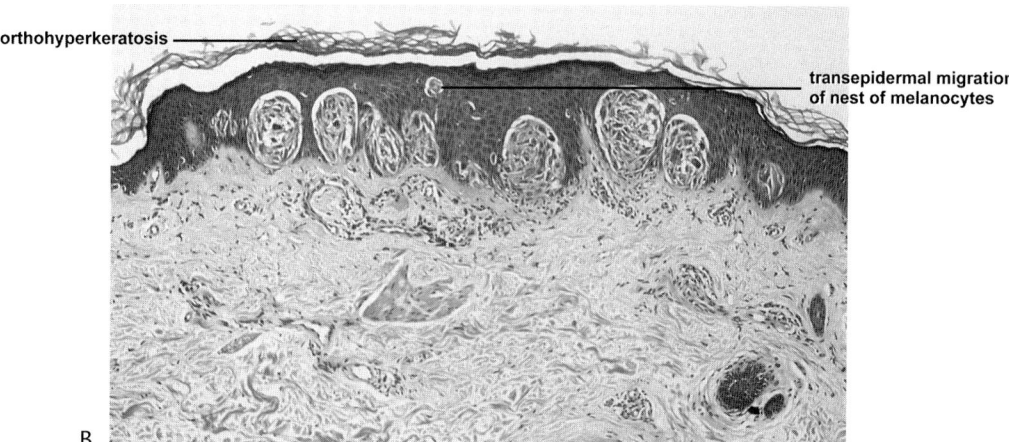

orthohyperkeratosis

transepidermal migration
of nest of melanocytes

B

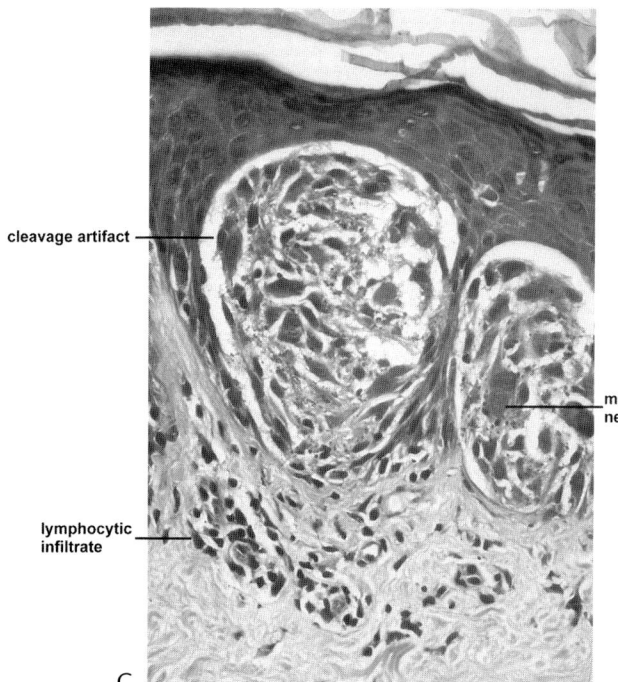

cleavage artifact

multinucleated
nevus giant cell

lymphocytic
infiltrate

C

Figure 20-17. A junctional Spitz nevus at a stage in which nests predominate over solitary cells. The lesion is very well circumscribed **(A)**. The epidermis overlying the junctional nests is irregularly hyperplastic, with slight compact hyperkeratosis. Note that the nests of melanocytes are similar in shape and are discrete **(B)**. Prominent clefts separate melanocytes of this Spitz nevus from each other and from the epidermis **(C)**.

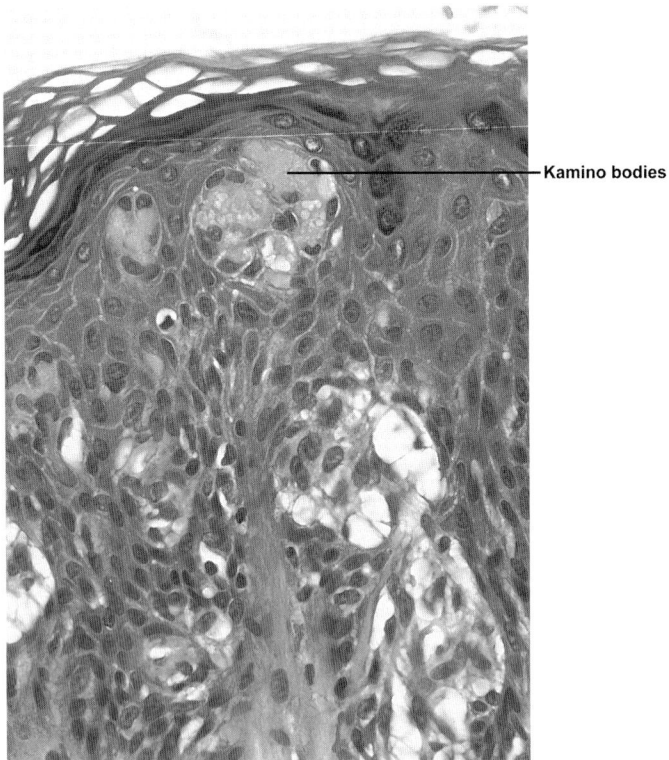

Kamino bodies

Figure 20-18. Kamino bodies in a Spitz nevus. Kamino bodies are a dull pink in hematoxylin and eosin–stained sections. They have polycyclic outlines, are surrounded by crescentically shaped keratinocytes, and sometimes have melanin inside them. They appear to be composed mainly of basement membrane material and extracellular substances such as fibronectin rather than effete cells.

Clinicopathologic Correlation

The red, smooth-surfaced papular Spitz nevus that occurs most often in children is sometimes mistaken for a hemangioma clinically. Histologically, the latter lacks melanin, is markedly edematous, and contains ectatic capillaries.

The sharply circumscribed, relatively flat, darkly pigmented variant of a Spitz nevus, seen most often in young adults, has been termed *pigmented spindle cell nevus.* Histologically, the lesions are junctional or compound. If compound, they are often limited to the papillary dermis. The melanocytes are by definition largely spindled and pigmented, although epithelioid melanocytes are also present in small numbers. The intensity of clinical pigmentation seems to correlate with the amount of melanoma in the epidermis. Lesions that are nearly black clinically often have melanin in the cornified layer microscopically. Some pigmented spindle cells variants of Spitz nevus have architectural similarities to so-called dysplastic, or Clark, nevi in that junctional nests extend beyond the dermal component, and the spindled cells that comprise them are horizontally oriented.

The intradermal Spitz nevus lacks pigment histologically and is markedly fibrotic. Because it appears as a hard, tan, flat to gently domed papule, it often resembles dermatofibroma clinically.

Differential Diagnosis and Pitfalls

The differential diagnosis of Spitz nevus versus melanoma is among the most difficult and hazardous in dermatopathology. It largely turns on rigorous application of the generic criteria outlined in the introduction to this chapter, buttressed by some specific ones.

The size of a melanocytic neoplasm, when correlated with its features, provides valuable information. Because Spitz nevi can range up to 2 cm in diameter, a mere measurement alone is not discriminatory. Spitz nevi begin as proliferations of single melanocytes, but rapidly evolve into nested growths. By the time that a Spitz nevus is 3 mm in diameter, its cells are mostly arranged in nests, while in most malignant melanomas of comparable size single melanocytes are still the predominant population.

Symmetry is most useful in the differential diagnosis of Spitz nevus versus malignant melanoma. Treacherously, both neoplasms can have identically symmetric silhouettes as discerned

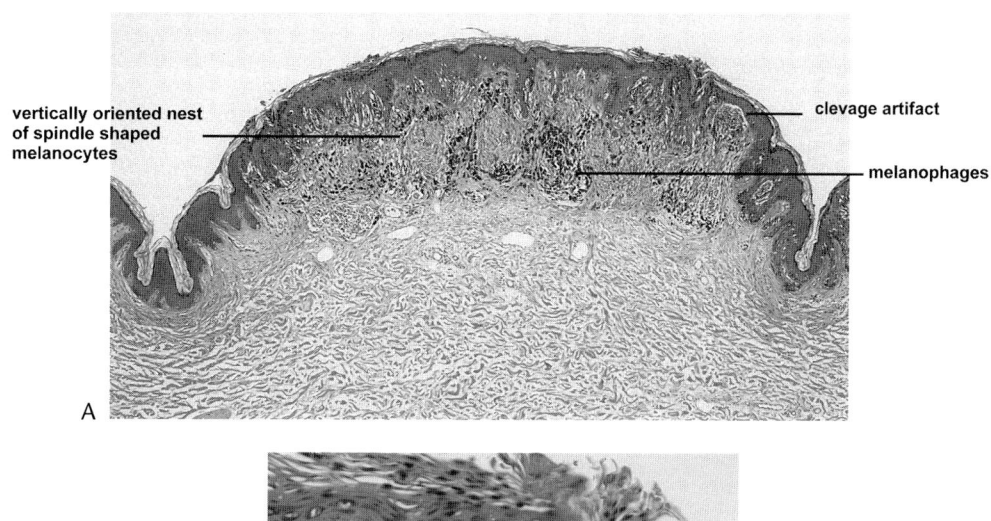

vertically oriented nest of spindle shaped melanocytes

clevage artifact

melanophages

A

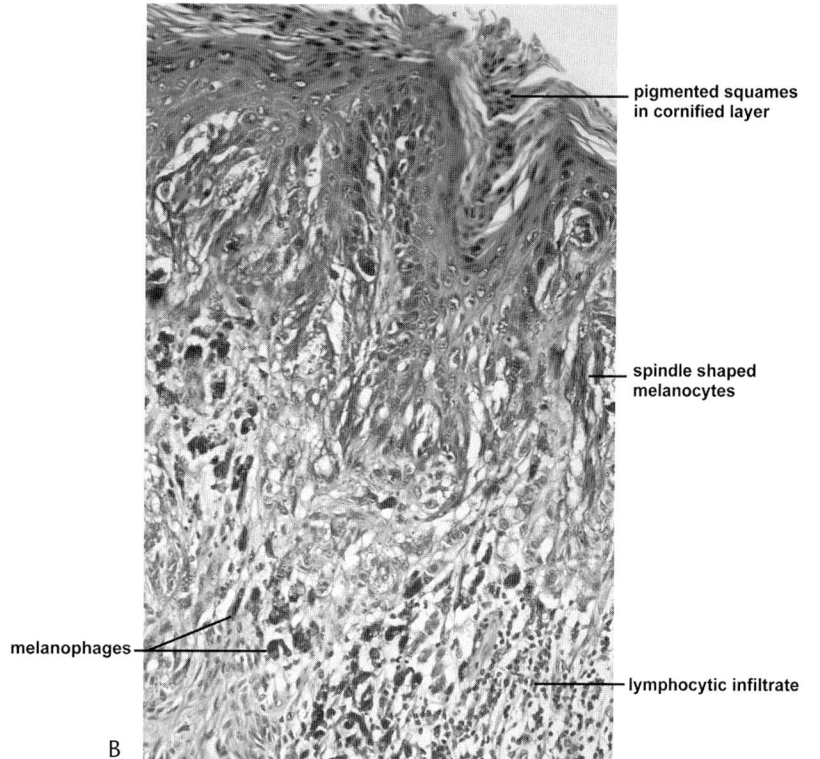

pigmented squames in cornified layer

spindle shaped melanocytes

melanophages

lymphocytic infiltrate

B

Figure 20-19. The pigmented spindle cell variant of Spitz nevus, also called pigmented spindle cell nevus of Reed. There is typically a small, symmetric and dome-shaped contour **(A)**. Spindled and pigmented melanocytes are present beneath an irregularly hyperplastic epidermis, with abundant melanin in the cornified layer **(B)**. *Continued.*

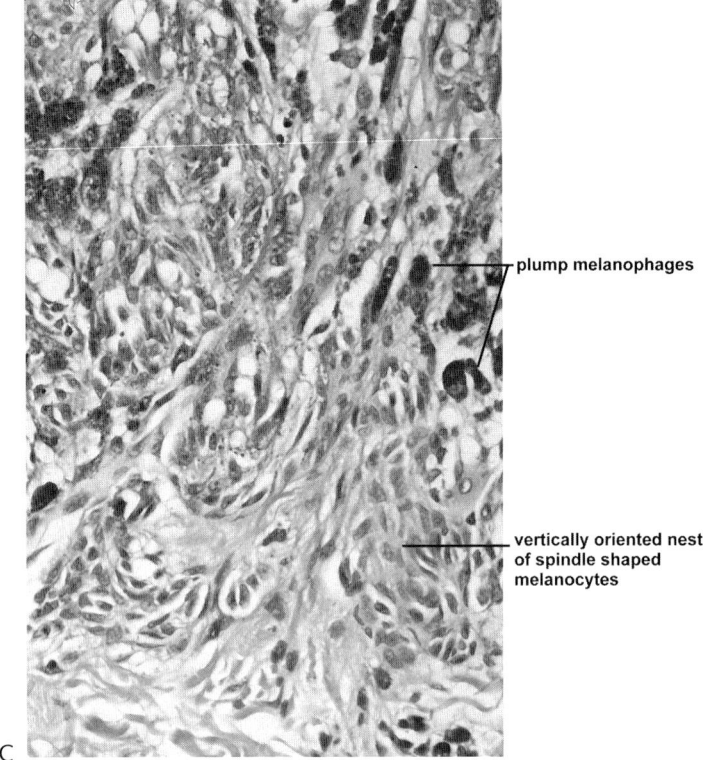

plump melanophages

vertically oriented nest of spindle shaped melanocytes

C

Figure 20-19. *Continued.* The spindled melano-cytes are accompanied by melanophages (**C**).

at scanning magnification. The evaluation of symmetry should therefore include comparisons of the epidermal changes, the size of junctional nests and cytologic features of the cells that compose them, pigmentation of melanocytes and numbers of melanophages, and the sizes and cytologic features of dermal melanocytes at each depth in the dermis. For example, the sil-houette of a melanocytic neoplasm can be symmetric, but if the nests of melanocytes at any given level of the dermis differ sig-nificantly in size or in their cytology, the diagnosis of malignant melanoma should be seriously considered.

Intraepidermal spread of melanocytes often occurs in Spitz nevi, and its presence per se should not result in a reflexive di-agnosis of malignant melanoma (Fig. 20-22). The extrusion of nests of melanocytes into the cornified layer is a common oc-currence in Spitz nevi. Single melanocytes can also ascend into the spinous, granular, and cornified layers in Spitz nevi. A key feature is that melanocytes arranged in nests outnumber those distributed singly, while the converse is often the case in melanoma. Single melanocytes are usually found in the centers of Spitz nevi, while they are randomly and homogeneously dis-tributed in melanoma. Spread of melanocytes above the basal layer of the epidermis tends to be most common in Spitz nevi in children and to diminish in frequency with age.[62]

Lateral circumscription is usually sharp except in the very earliest stages of Spitz nevus, in which rare melanocytes can be present lateral to the most outlying junctional nest.

Maturation, like symmetry, should be evaluated in a multi-

factorial fashion. Nests of melanocytes in Spitz nevi tend to di-minish in size with their descent into the dermis, and in fully de-veloped Spitz nevi the deepest cells are scattered individually. The cytoplasms of melanocytes in Spitz nevi are abundant in the superficial part of the lesion and, in most examples, become scanter in the deep part of the lesion. The nuclei of Spitz nevi likewise become smaller as cells descend, and their nucleoli be-come smaller. While some cells with large and sometimes eosinophilic nucleoli can be present in the upper part of Spitz nevi, only in rare examples are equally large nuclei seen at the base of a lesion. Maturation involves loss of the ability to repli-cate as cells descend, and it is rare to see mitotic figures in the deep part of a Spitz nevus. Some Spitz nevi are deeply pig-mented, but pigmentation of cells in the reticular dermis is rare in Spitz nevi in whites. Pigment was found in the deep part of two of three melanomas that resembled Spitz nevi in one se-ries.[63] Despite all of the modes by which the cells of Spitz nevi can mature, some examples are frustratingly devoid of signs of maturation yet in other respects fulfill every clinical and histopathologic criteria for Spitz nevus.

Some features that would intuitively point to the diagnosis of malignant melanoma rather than Spitz nevus, such as lymphatic and perineural invasion, can be seen in both conditions.[6,7,64]

The age of a patient should only be used as a last resort in making or not making a diagnosis of Spitz nevus, but can be of great help in avoiding an erroneous diagnosis. Because Spitz nevi begin as junctional neoplasms, develop into compound

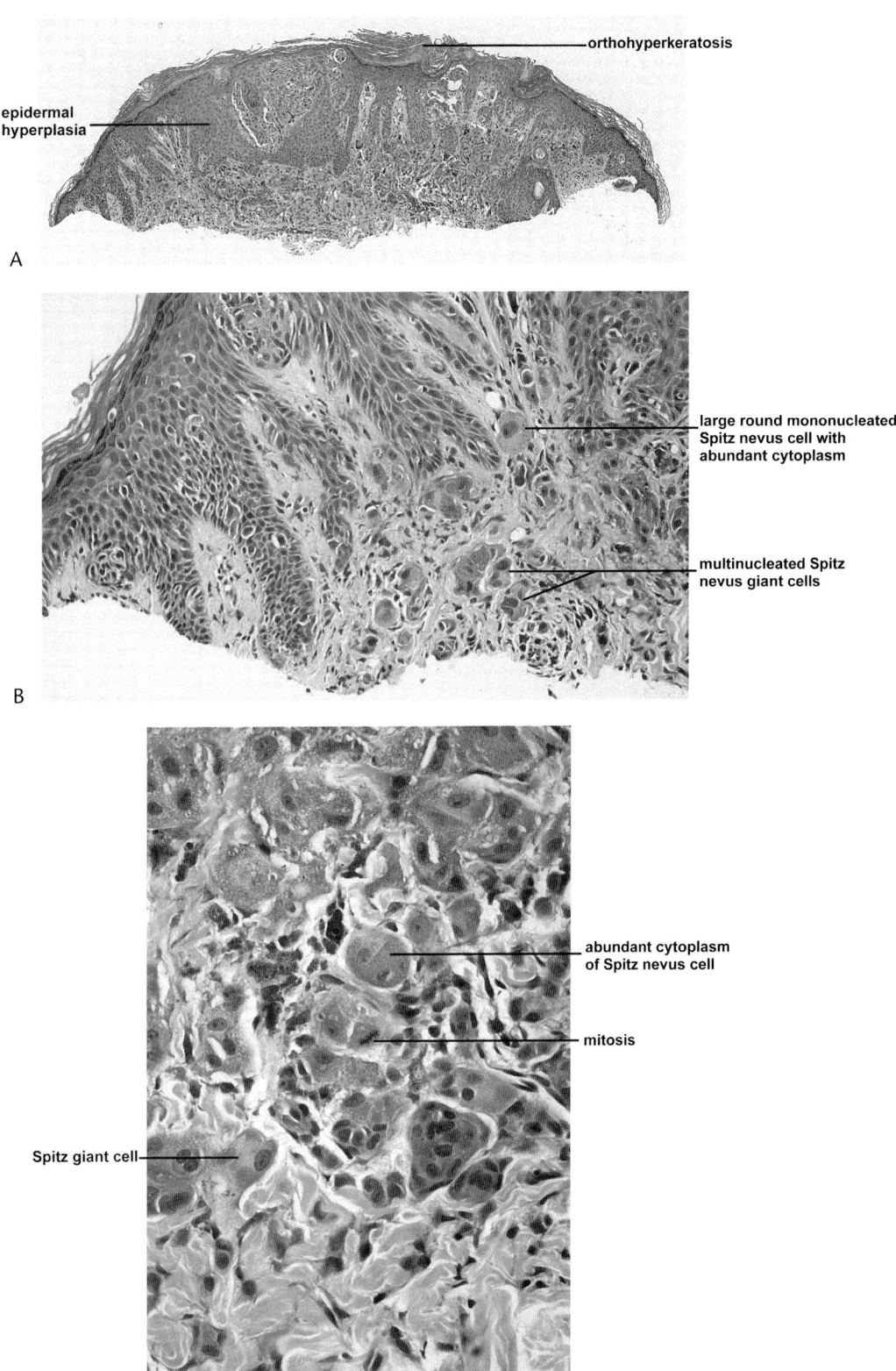

Figure 20-20. A compound Spitz nevus. The lesion has a domed shape, and is covered by a hyperplastic epidermis **(A)**. Strikingly enlarged melanocytes are present in a nested pattern at the junction, and as clusters in the superficial dermis **(B)**. Beneath the dermal nests are single, much smaller melanocytes that have insinuated themselves between collagen bundles **(C)**. Diminution of the size of nests with descent, accompanied by dispersion from nests to single cells at the base of the lesion are important features that favor Spitz nevus over melanoma in the context of a proliferation of large melanocytes.

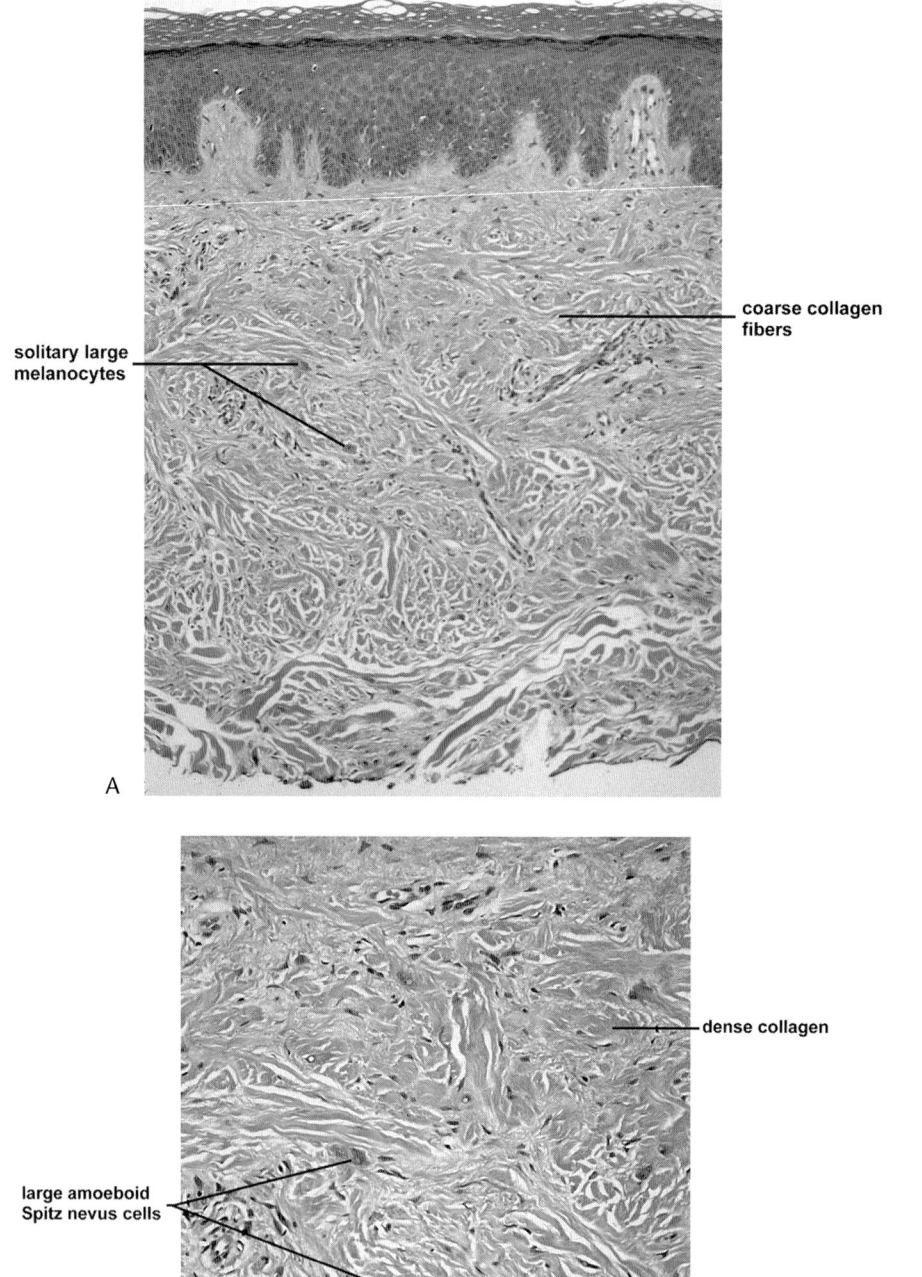

coarse collagen fibers

solitary large melanocytes

A

dense collagen

large amoeboid Spitz nevus cells

more deeply situated melanocytes have smaller nuclei and less cytoplasm

B

Figure 20-21. Desmoplastic Spitz nevus. In older, intradermal Spitz nevi, the neoplasm can consist entirely of single melanocytes disposed between thickened collagen bundles **(A)**. The abundant cytoplasm and large nuclei of the cells renders them visable even at intermediate magnification **(B)**. *Continued.*

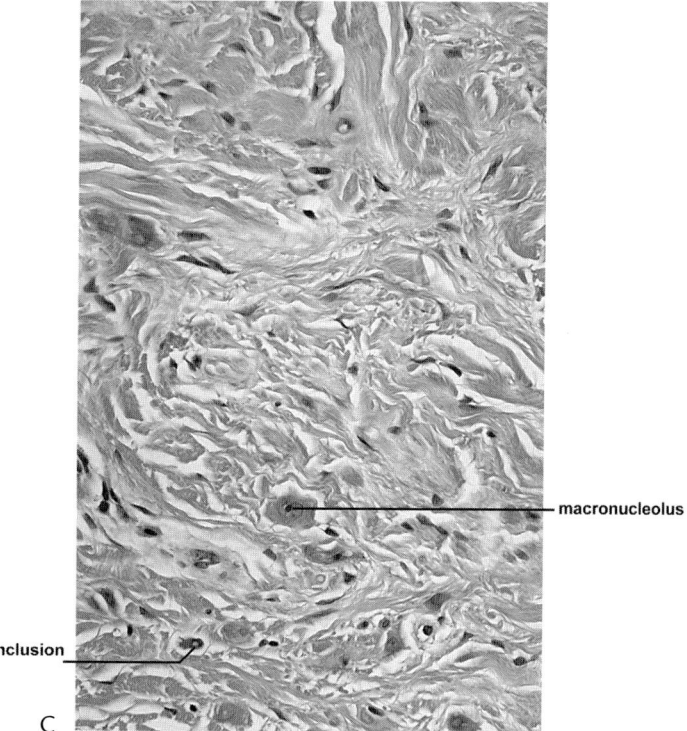

macronucleolus

nuclear pseudoinclusion
of cytoplasm

C

Figure 20-21. *Continued.* Note the ameboid shapes of the melanocytes, and their distribution as solitary cells (**C**). In desmoplastic melanoma, copious cytoplasm is exceptional, and aggregates of cells are often seen even at the base of a lesion.

ones, and eventuate as intradermal neoplasms, it is rare to find junctional Spitz nevi after age 40 or compound lesions after age 60. Conversely, most desmoplastic Spitz nevi are found in adults, although rare lesions play out their entire sagas in the first decade of life. Melanomas arise in congenital nevi in children, but seldom de novo. Unusual Spitz nevi are far more common than are malignant melanomas in children.

There are certainly malignant melanomas that have many features in common with Spitz nevi. These have been termed *spitzoid melanoma*. A recently published concept is that some Spitz nevus–like neoplasms have the capacity to spread to local lymph nodes but not beyond. Such cases have been termed *malignant Spitz nevi*.[65] The ultimate biologic behavior of such lesions awaits clarification, and it is unclear as to whether these neoplasms are a mixture of unusual Spitz nevi and melanomas or whether they truly are a discrete group of cases with limited metastatic potential. Features said to be characteristic of this entity include vertical orientation, extension into the subcutis with blunt borders, infiltrates of plasma cells, and ulceration.

Adjunctive techniques have to date had limited value in solving this difficult differential diagnosis. Immunophenotypic studies have not discriminated between Spitz nevus and melanoma. The cells of both stain positively for S-100 protein and the "melanoma marker" HMB-45 by the immunoperoxidase method. HMB-45 is actually a reasonably specific marker of melanocytic lineage and, with the exception of a few instances, should not be used in discriminating benign from ma-

lignant melanocytic neoplasms. Image analysis and flow cytometry have shown that cells with abnormal DNA content occur in Spitz nevi as they occur in malignant melanoma, although diploid cells predominate at the bases of Spitz nevi.[66]

While the differential diagnosis of Spitz nevus versus melanoma remains difficult, the criteria for telling these two neoplasms apart have been greatly refined over the last two decades. In our opinion, it would be a mistake to consider the two conditions to be on a spectrum. As the techniques of molecular biology find application in the study of melanocytic neoplasms, it is likely that clear-cut differences will be found that mirror the sharp distinction in the biologic behavior of these two neoplasms.

NEVUS OF OTA, NEVUS FUSCO-CAERULEUS ZYGOMATICUS, NEVUS OF ITO, AND MONGOLIAN SPOT

These conditions present as pigmented patches and are produced by sparsely distributed dendritic melanocytes, free melanin, and melanophages within the reticular dermis or submucosa. They can be regarded as variants of blue nevus, which in turn can be viewed as a form of congenital nevus. Because they are so alike and different from other blue nevi we have chosen to consider them separately.

Nevus of Ota occurs on the face and is localized to the distribution of the trigeminal nerve. Nevus fusco-caeruleus zygomaticus is also situated on the face, but differs from nevus of

Ota in that it is not a pigmented patch, but rather is a smaller speckled area that is bilateral and symmetric, with onset between 8 and 60 years. It is seen in Asians, and in a Chinese population it was much more common than nevus of Ota.[67] Nevus of Ito affects the area supplied by a nerve other than trigeminal, most often on the upper back or shoulder area. Mongolian spots are usually located on the sacral areas of infants, are often present at birth, and fade after a few months, but in rare cases persist into adulthood. Some consider these conditions to be variants of blue nevi.

Clinical Features

These conditions present as dusky blue-gray patches that have indistinct borders and do not change the surface contour of the overlying skin. Nevus of Ota may affect the nasopharyngeal, ocular, and auricular mucosae. Several central nervous system defects have been described in patients with nevus of Ota. Malignant melanoma has been reported to arise in nevus of Ota and nevus of Ito but not yet in nevus fusco-caeruleus zygomaticus or in mongolian spots.

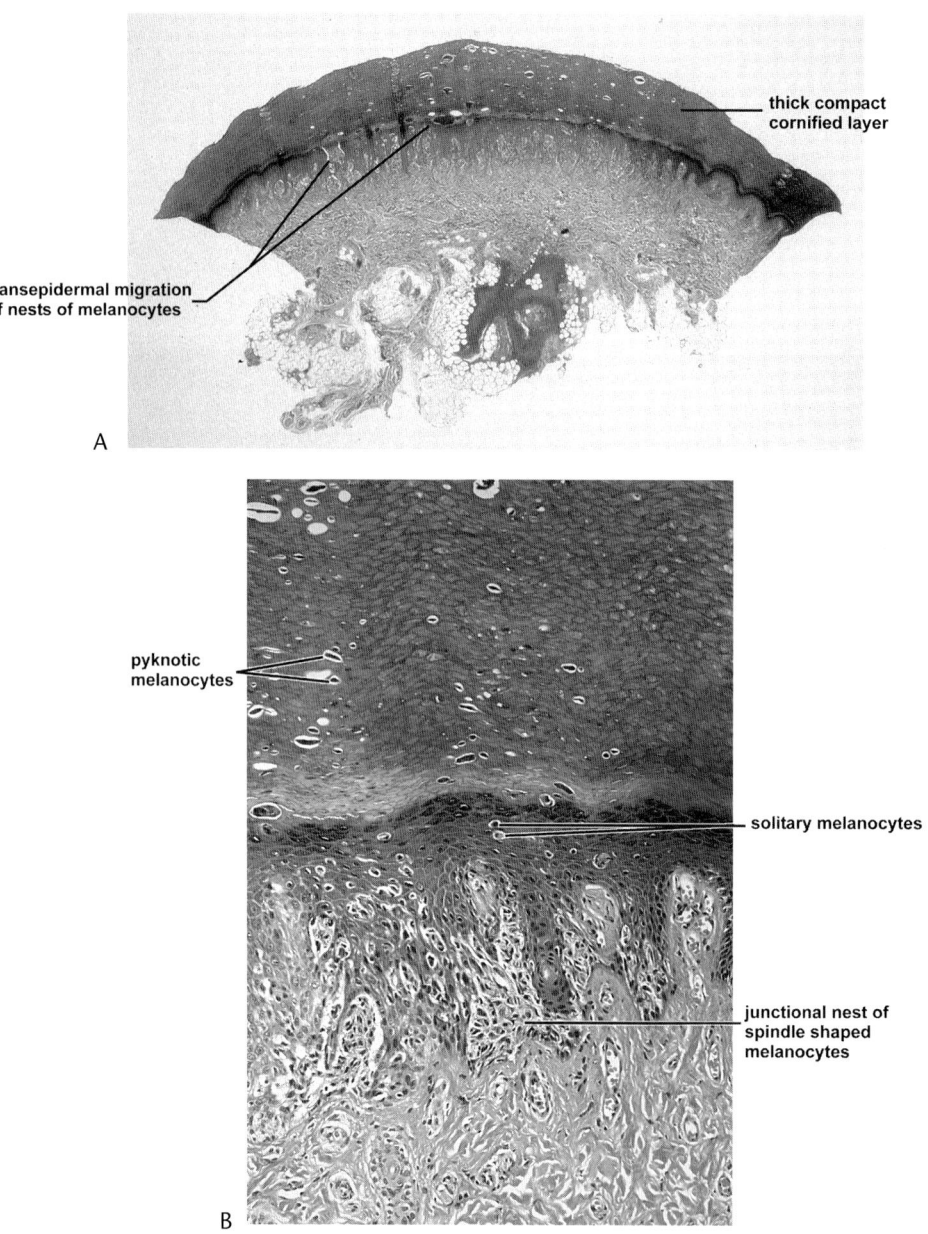

Figure 20-22. Pagetoid scatter of melanocytes in a Spitz nevus. This phenomenon does not necessarily indicate melanoma, because it can be seen to a limited extent in the centers of some otherwise unremarkable lesions. It is also common in traumatized Spitz nevi, Spitz nevi that persist following partial biopsy, and Spitz nevi on acral sites (seen here). Note the small size, dome shape, and characteristic epidermal changes in this lesion from a 2-year-old child (**A**). Distinct nests with peripheral clefts are present at the junction (**B**). *Continued.*

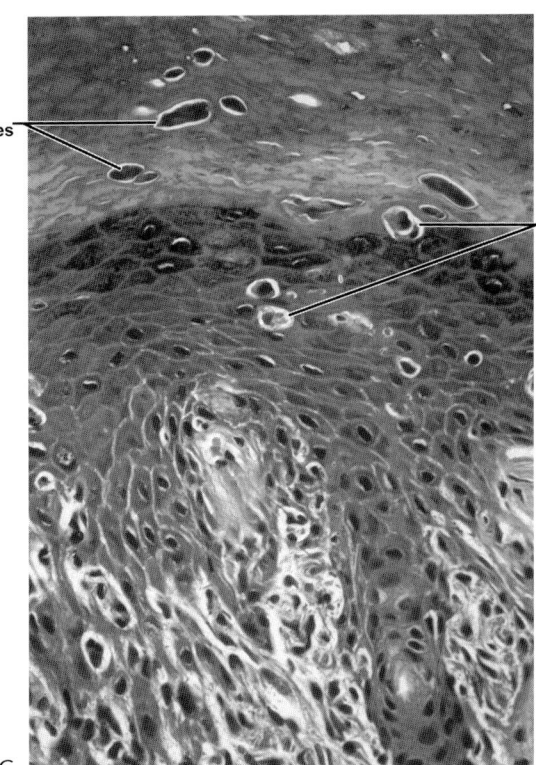

pyknotic
melanocytes

upward migration of
individual melanocytes

C

Figure 20-22. *Continued.* There are many individual melanocytes above the basal layer, with ascent into the cornified layer **(C)**.

Histopathologic Features

Nevus of Ota, nevus of Ito, and mongolian spots all have dendritic pigmented melanocytes sparsely scattered in both the superficial and deep dermis, aligned parallel to dermal collagen bundles along with a few melanophages (Fig. 20-23). Nevus fusco-caeruleus zygomaticus tends to have melanocytes mostly in the superficial dermis. Nevi of Ota and Ito have distinctive ultrastructural findings, namely, basement membranes complete with basal lamina and lamina lucida and extracellular sheaths that surround dermal melanocytes composed of filaments that vary from 2 to 4 nm in diameter.[68]

Clinicopathologic Correlation

The dusky, bluish color in these conditions is accounted for by the Tyndall effect, just as it is in blue nevi. The lesions are normal in consistency, reflecting the absence of sclerosis. Although mongolian spots fade over time, biopsy specimens of the sacral skin of adults who had these lesions show persistence of some dermal melanocytes.

Differential Diagnosis

These entities share with blue nevi the presence of dendritic, bipolar, pigmented melanocytes but are clinically distinctive. Blue nevi generally contain more numerous melanocytes, which are in most cases accompanied by sclerosis of the dermis. In contrast, the dermal collagen pattern is undisturbed in nevi of Ota and Ito, nevus fusco-caeruleus zygomaticus, and mongolian spots.

Pathophysiology

Nevi of Ota and Ito and mongolian spots are thought to derive from melanocytes whose migration from the neural crest to the dermoepidermal junction was incomplete. White infants, who do not tend to develop mongolian spots, nonetheless have incompletely melanized melanocytes in the dermis of the lumbosacral area, which do not produce a clinically evident lesion.

BLUE NEVI

Blue nevi are benign, acquired, or sometimes congenital melanocytic neoplasms that are entirely intradermal, or nearly so, from their outset. Pigmented, bipolar dendritic melanocytes are present in nearly all blue nevi, although they may be rare in some. Blue nevi have been described not only in the skin but also on mucosal surfaces and in the prostate gland. Blue nevi are usually classified as "common" when composed of dendritic melanocytes and "cellular" when spindled or ovoid ones are also present.[69]

Clinical Features

Although some blue nevi can be congenital lesions, most become clinically evident in the second decade of life or later. Blue nevi are twice as common in females as in males and have a predilection for darkly pigmented persons. Usually, common blue nevi are smooth surfaced, dome-shaped papules (less than 0.5 cm in diameter) that show symmetry and sharp peripheral circumscription. Their color may be dark brown, black, or blue-black. They tend to occur on the scalp, face, hands, and feet.

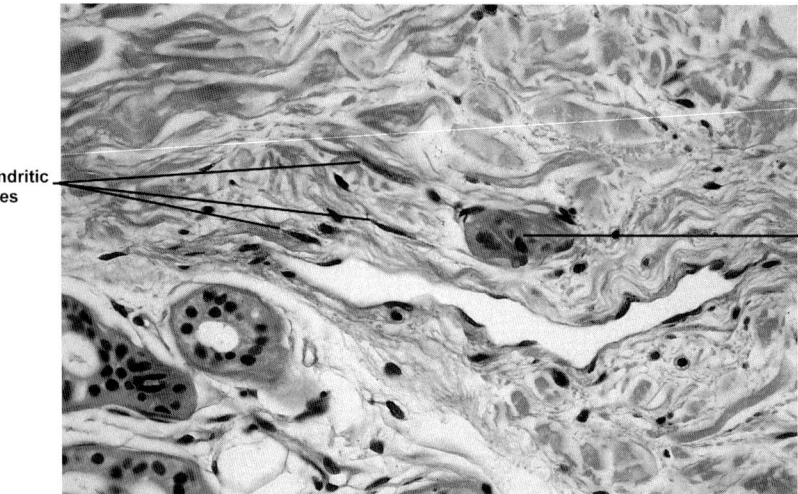

bipolar dendritic
melanocytes

oval and spindle
shaped melanocytes
with abundant
melanin in cytoplasm

Figure 20-23. Nevus of Ota. This nevus, as well as nevus of Ito and mongolian spots, are composed of scattered dendritic melanocytes in the reticular dermis. Their presence can be subtle histologically.

Cellular blue nevi occur as larger nodules or plaques, usually 1 to 2 cm in diameter. While they can be situated in many locations, the buttock is a common site.

There are exotically rare blue nevi that present as large plaques either at birth or later.[70] These plaque-type blue nevi can involve deep soft tissues including muscle. The lesions appear to be biologically benign.

Histopathologic Features

The traditional classification of blue nevi into common and cellular types oversimplifies the range of appearances of these lesions. The components that vary in proportion in all blue nevi include bipolar, dendritic, pigmented melanocytes; melanophages; and sclerosis. Unlike ordinary acquired and "dysplastic" nevi and Spitz nevi, maturation is not evident in blue nevi (perhaps the dendritic cells of a blue nevus can be said to already represent a mature phenotype). Components that are present only in some blue nevi include ovoid or spindled melanocytes and multinucleated melanocytes.

"Common" blue nevus is the term given to one composed largely of heavily pigmented, bipolar, dendritic melanocytes and melanophages. The dendritic processes of melanocytes are finer than those of melanophages and can be branched. Dendritic melanocytes are often arranged in parallel to reticular dermal collagen bundles, except around adnexal structures, where they are often vertically oriented. Sclerosis may be present and sometimes is even marked. The lesions are usually wedge shaped with their apex in the midreticular dermis, and, like congenital nevi, there is a tendency for periappendageal involvement. Mitoses are nearly always absent. The epidermis is generally uninvolved but, in exceptional lesions, increased numbers of single melanocytes or junctional nests of dendritic melanocytes are present (Fig. 20-24).

"Cellular" blue nevus has ovoid melanocytes arranged in oblong nests or fascicles in addition to the components of common blue nevi.[69] They, too, are largely centered in the reticular dermis, or in the deep dermis and subcutis, and can be densest around appendages. A range of appearances includes lesions with dendritic pigmented melanocytes and ovoid melanocytes in fascicles in different areas, lesions in which ovoid melanocytes in nests and fascicles are present nearly to the exclusion of dendritic ones, and lesions in which ovoid melanocytes are in nests in portions of the lesion and arranged between thickened collagen bundles in other areas. The ovoid melanocytes of blue nevi have monomorphous nuclei, scant chromatin along their nuclear membranes, and small nucleoli that are amphophilic in well-stained hematoxylin and eosin-stained sections (Fig. 20-25).

In addition to these stereotypic types, there are blue nevi composed of scattered dendritic melanocytes, dendritic melanocytes in small tangles, spindled melanocytes between thickened collagen bundles, spindled and dendritic melanocytes with sclerosis, and composite lesions with areas of any of the characteristics noted above.

The term *deep penetrating nevus* applies to a deep wedge-shaped type of nevus composed of fascicles of ovoid melanocytes that have abundant pale cytoplasm accompanied by melanophages. The apex of the wedge is usually in the superficial subcutis. A few junctional nests can be present. Because these are so inconspicuous as to imply that such nevi do not evolve from a junctional to a compound stage, they may well be a form of blue nevus.[70] They are a frequent component in combined nevi and are discussed in detail in that section.

A rare variant is Masson's blue neuronevus in which sinuous, elongated fascicles of spindled melanocytes simulate peripheral nerves. Peripheral to these neuroid structures are areas of sclerosis with bipolar, dendritic melanocytes and melanophages and nodules of ovoid melanocytes.

All of the variants of cellular blue nevus can have a rounded base that protrudes into the subcutaneous fat. Scattered multinucleated melanocytes with a peripherally arranged ring of nuclei are a frequent and helpful finding. Mitotic figures are rare and generally average less than two per 10 high power fields ($\times$ 400 magnification).[71] Foci of degeneration can occur in large lesions and resolve with stellate areas of acellular sclerosis, a process termed *encystification*.

Plaque-type blue nevi can feature both bipolar dendritic and

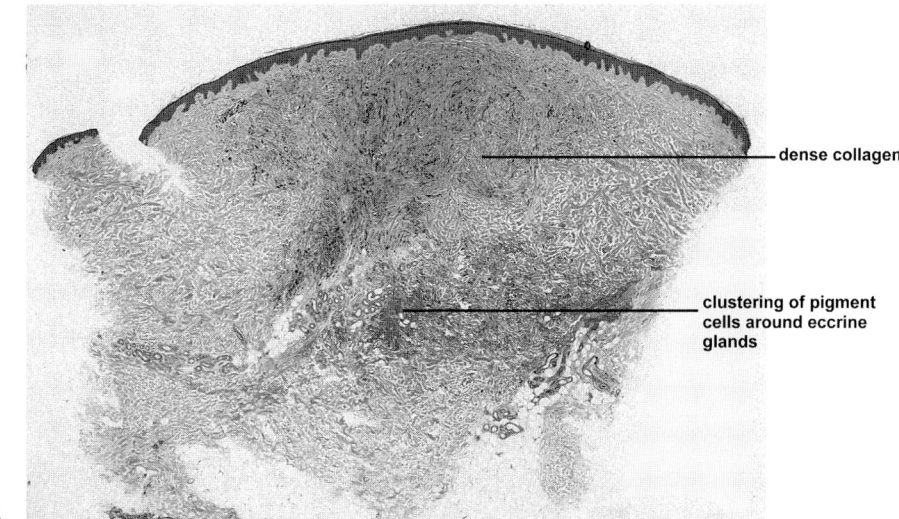

dense collagen

clustering of pigment
cells around eccrine
glands

A

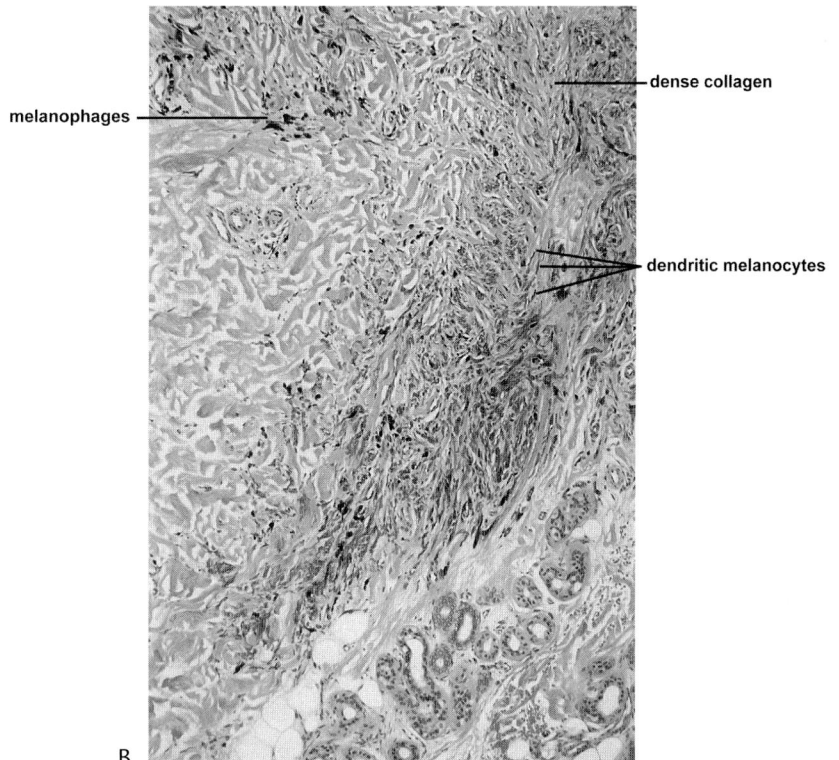

melanophages

dense collagen

dendritic melanocytes

B

Figure 20-24. Common blue nevus. The picture
of a dark blue-black or brown papular blue nevus
most often corresponds to a wedge-shaped zone
in which there are dendritic melanocytes,
melanophages, and sclerosis (**A**). The apex of the
wedge is deeply pigmented. In contrast to ordinary nevi, whether congenital or acquired,
melanin in blue nevi is frequently more abundant
in the deep portion of the lesion than in its superficial areas (**B**). *Continued.*

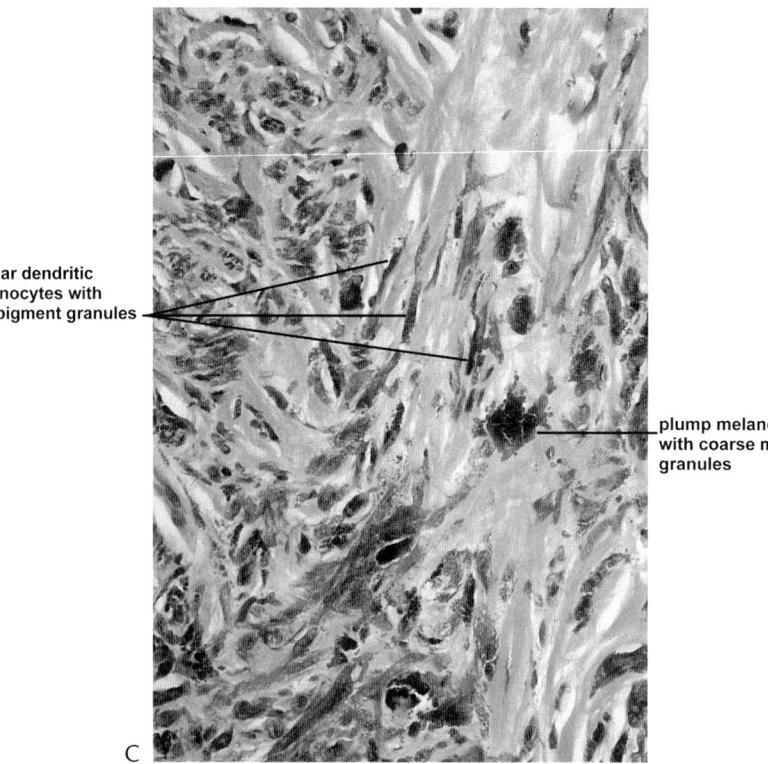

bipolar dendritic melanocytes with fine pigment granules

plump melanophages with coarse melanin granules

C

Figure 20-24. *Continued.* The dendritic melanocytes are the cells with delicate processes and smaller granules of melanin; those with blunt processes and coarser granules are melanophages. The collagen bundles in this area are thickened (**C**).

ovoid melanocytes, sometimes in conjunction with elongated rete ridges, basilar hyperpigmentation, and increased numbers of single basilar melanocytes.[72]

The melanocytes of all forms of blue nevi react with antisera to S-100 protein and with HMB-45. HMB-45 recognizes a glycoprotein found in melanosomes, and most blue nevi are composed of cells that actively synthesized melanin.

Differential Diagnosis

Common blue nevus histopathologically resembles mongolian spot, nevus of Ito, and nevus of Ota because all have bipolar dendritic melanocytes. The three latter conditions lack the sclerosis often seen in common blue nevi and have only sparsely distributed dermal melanocytes. Rarely, common blue nevi consist only of scattered dendritic melanocytes with melanophages and can only be distinguished from the other conditions on clinical grounds.

Blue nevi of several types are often mistaken for dermatofibromas because both lesions contain spindled cells, fibrosis, and pigment. The spindled cells of blue nevi often have an S-shaped nucleus. In contrast, the nuclei of spindled cells in a dermatofibroma are stellate or triangular. The dermal pigment in blue nevi is melanin and in dermatofibroma, hemosiderin. The epidermis above blue nevi is most often normal or, at most, slightly hyperplastic, while above dermatofibromas the epider-

mis is markedly hyperplastic and has broad, flat-based rete ridges and basilar hyperpigmentation.

The deposition of exogenous pigments can simulate a blue nevus. Tattoos have pigment that is deposited in macrophages or lies freely within the dermis and has a darker, more opaque appearance than does melanin. While macrophages can have elongated processes, these are not as fine as those of dendritic melanocytes. In traumatic tattoos there can be refractile material, and the fibrosis that results from traumatic implantation of foreign material has horizontally oriented fibroblasts and vertically oriented blood vessels, as does that of an ordinary dermal scar. Monsel's solution (ferrous subsulfate) is sometimes used to staunch bleeding following biopsies. Its use can result in a proliferation of spindled cells that contain pigment that is coarser and more refractile than melanin and can be stained for iron. Small granules of formalin pigment can be deposited on tissue sections when unbuffered formalin is used as fixative. Formalin pigment is anisotropic on examination with polarized light.

Blue nevi can resemble neurotized melanocytic nevi because both can have spindled melanocytes, mucin, and mast cells. Neurotized nevi often contain lipocytes, which are not a feature of blue nevi, and do not have melanophages, which are present in virtually all blue nevi. While the cells of blue nevi react with HMB-45, those of neurotized nevi do not.

Cellular blue nevus and its variants must be distinguished

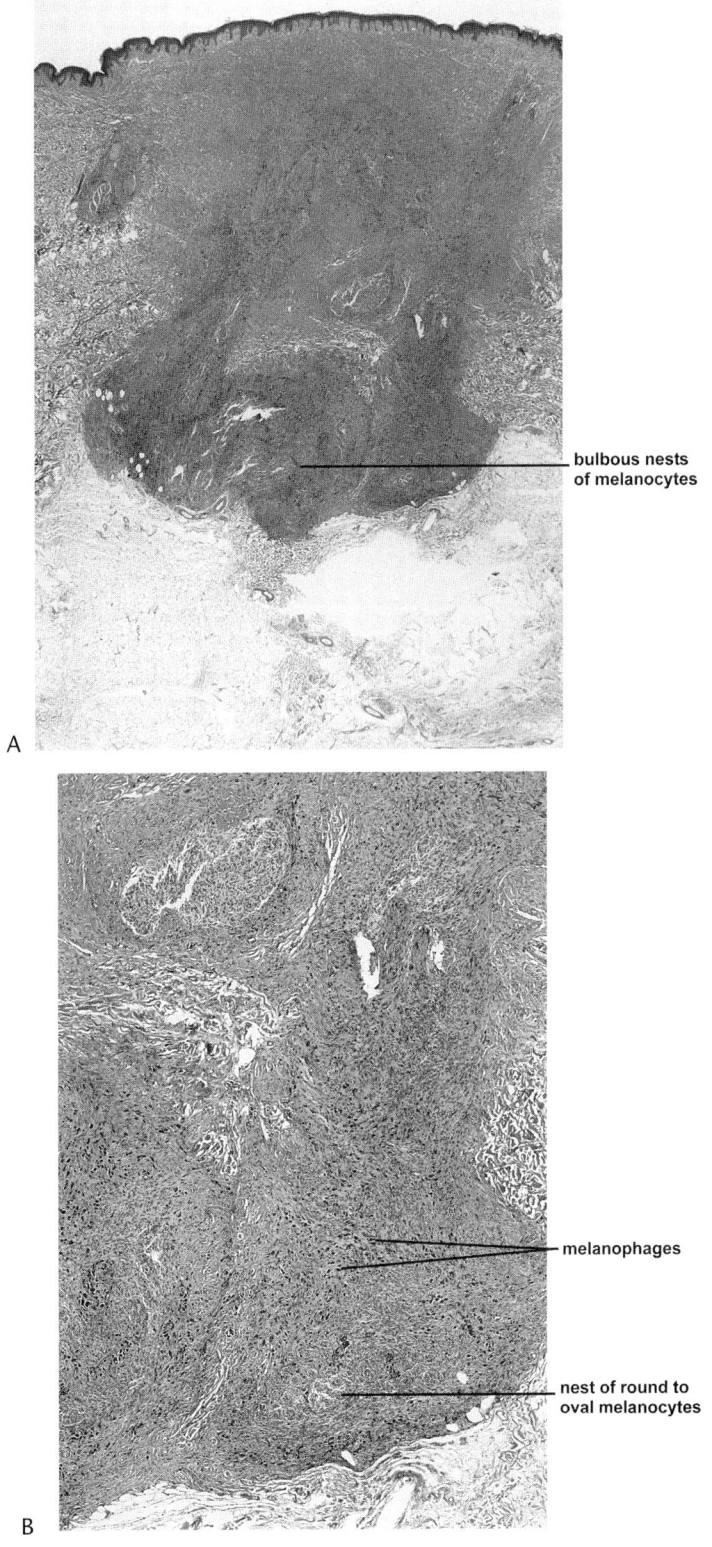

bulbous nests
of melanocytes

A

melanophages

nest of round to
oval melanocytes

B

Figure 20-25. Cellular blue nevus. The name cellular blue nevus can be applied to several patterns of blue nevus in which melanocytes are arranged compactly. Most often, it is used for lesions in which there are compact aggregations of spindled or ovoid melanocytes. A typical configuration, seen here, has dumbbell-shaped protrusions of cells extending into the subcutis. These protrusions may correspond to the sites of extinct hair follicles, reflecting the propensity of blue nevi to have cells distributed along the paths of adnexal structures **(A)**. The bulbous portions of the dumbbells have small but compact nests of melanocytes and are surrounded in this instance by less cellular, fibrotic areas containing dendritic melanocytes and melanophages **(B)**. *Continued.*

681

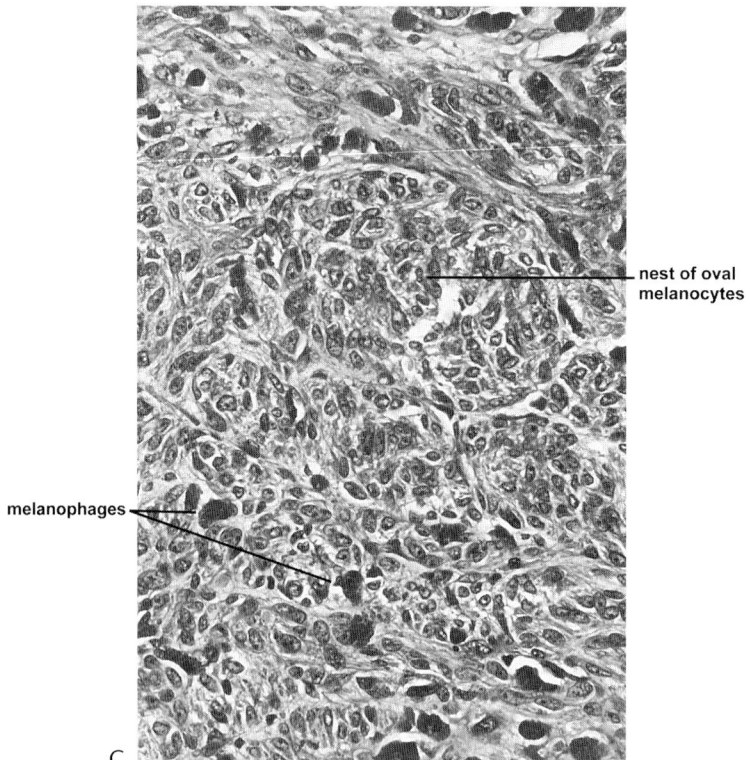

nest of oval melanocytes

melanophages

C

Figure 20-25. *Continued.* Spindled melanocytes in compact aggregations accompanied by melano-phages (**C**). Because both cellular blue nevi and melanoma can have large melanocytes compactly arranged, analysis of the overall pattern at scanning magnification is critical for telling them apart.

from malignant melanoma with spindled cells. The rounded protuberant lower border of cellular blue nevus, the scarcity of mitoses, and the absence of marked nuclear pleomorphism are useful features. Rarely, cellular blue nevi can have small foci of necrosis. Necrosis is also often seen in a melanoma arising in a pre-existent blue nevus. A lymphocytic infiltrate is not a usual feature of cellular blue nevus and its variants and raises the possibility of a malignant melanoma. Immunoperoxidase staining with HMB-45 has no utility in the differential diagnosis of spindle cell malignant melanoma versus blue nevus, as nearly all blue nevi will stain with this reagent but many melanomas will not.

Lastly, some cutaneous metastases of melanoma resemble blue nevi by virtue of having superficial wedge-shaped infiltrates that are roughly symmetric and many stromal melanophages.

Pathophysiology

Blue nevi are thought to derive from neural crest cells that migrate to the skin in the first trimester but do not reach the dermoepidermal junction. "Pools" of these melanocytes can be found in fetal skin, but involute during the second half of gestation. Blue nevi are thought to arise from incompletely involuted pools of these dermally arrested melanocytes.

COMBINED NEVI

A combined nevus is a benign melanocytic neoplasm composed of more than one cell type. Combinations of "ordinary" and blue or Spitz nevus, and Spitz nevus and blue nevus cells, are among the most frequent.

Clinical Features

Often combined nevi are clinically worrisome lesions because the degree of pigmentation or elevation of the surface of the skin imparted by the two (or sometimes three) populations of nevus cells differs from one part of the nevus to another. Often, areas of blue nevus appear as dark brown spots within a lighter lesion.

Histopathologic Features

In combined nevi, the different cell types usually occupy topographically distinct areas. Often areas of blue nevus will be present in the center or deep portion of an ordinary compound nevus.[73] In some combinations of ordinary and Spitz nevus there will be an intimate mixture of cell types.

In combined nevi in which a Spitz nevus-like component is situated superficially, the epidermis reacts with the same features it shows in uncomplicated Spitz nevus (i.e., irregular hyperplasia, compact hyperkeratosis with a thickened granular layer, and Kamino bodies). One component in a combined nevus, usually the Spitz nevus, can evoke a halo reaction. Lymphocytes permeate the lesion, ascend to the dermoepidermal junction, and are seen in direct apposition to melanocytes with karyorrhectic nuclei.

One newly described, benign melanocytic neoplasm considered by some to be a type of combined nevus has been termed *deep penetrating nevus*.[70] Deep penetrating nevi have a number of features in common with both Spitz and cellular blue nevi. Like Spitz nevi, they often have an inverted wedge shape and are likewise composed of large melanocytes with moderate nuclear pleomorphism. The epidermis overlying them does not show the typical reactive changes seen in Spitz nevi. Like cellular blue nevi, there are ovoid melanocytes and melanophages distributed throughout both the superficial and deep portions of the neoplasm. Unlike cellular blue nevi, junctional nests can be present. Because only one cell type is present, but the neoplasm

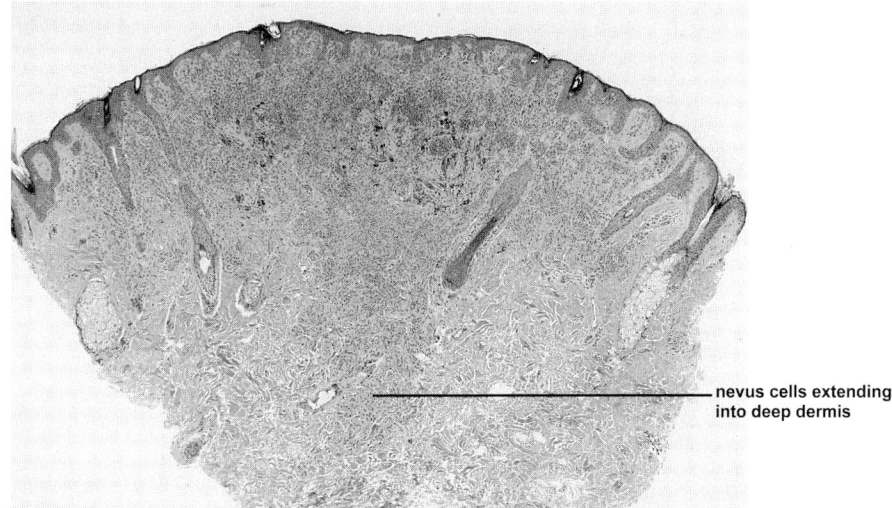

nevus cells extending into deep dermis

A

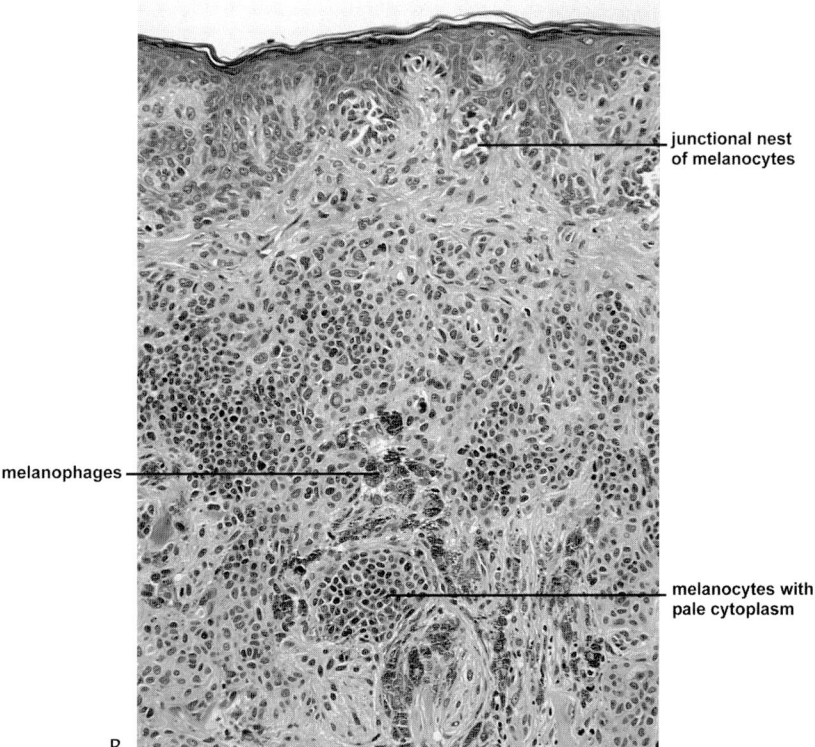

junctional nest of melanocytes

melanophages

melanocytes with pale cytoplasm

B

Figure 20-26. Combined nevus with a deep penetrating component. The overall contour of the lesion is that of a superficial congenital nevus **(A)**. Clusters of melanophages and nests of melanocytes with a pale appearance reflect the deep penetrating component **(B)**. *Continued.*

Figure 20-26. *Continued.* In a deep penetrating nevus, these elements constitute the entire lesion, which is wedge shaped and extends into the deep dermis or subcutis, hence its name. In this field, there are both ordinary and pagetoid melanocytes. The term pagetoid is used in this case to indicate that these cells have cytologic features similar to those of Paget's disease, i.e., abundant pale cytoplasm **(C)**.

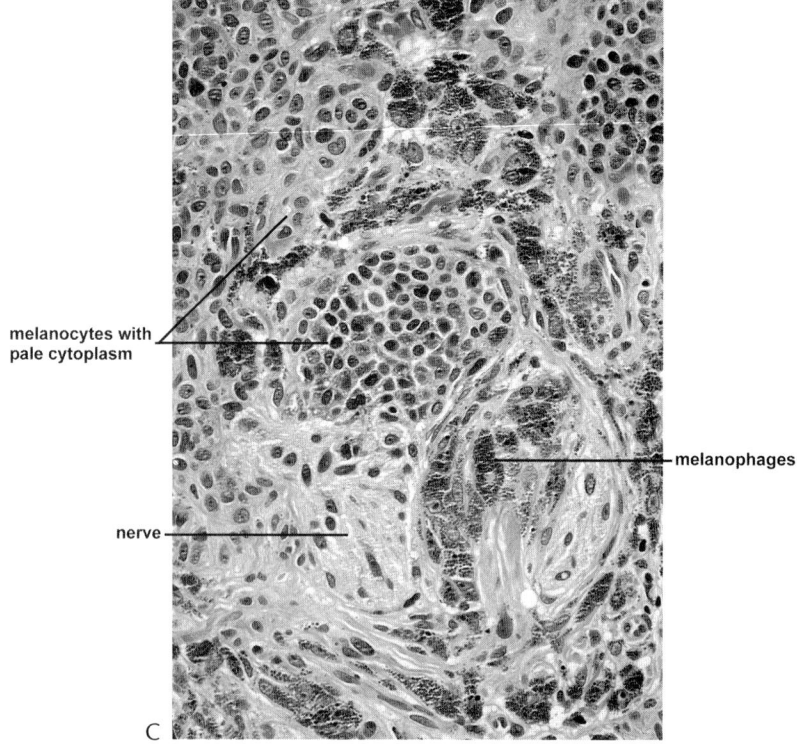

melanocytes with pale cytoplasm

melanophages

nerve

C

has features of both cellular blue nevus and Spitz nevus, deep penetrating nevus has also been termed *monomorphous combined nevus*[74] (Fig. 20-26).

In nearly all instances, balloon cell nevi are combined nevi. The balloon cell nevus is a compound or intradermal melanocytic nevus in which there are unusual nevus cells that have exceedingly abundant, pale-staining, clear or slightly reticulated cytoplasm (Fig. 20-27). These cells have a normal-sized, centrally situated nucleus. Transitional forms may be seen within a single nest of cells from ordinary nevus cells to typical balloon cells. Occasional balloon cells can be found in an otherwise ordinary melanocytic nevus. There can be but a few nests of balloon cells, or balloon cells or ordinary nevus cells can predominate. The peculiar appearance of balloon cells is due to an abnormality in the formation of their melanosomes.

Clinicopathologic Correlation

The marked focal pigmentation in combined nevi that have a blue nevus component is usually due to numerous melanophages. Despite the combination of different types of nevus cells, most combined nevi are sharply circumscribed and symmetric. Some combined nevi that have a component of the "dysplastic" nevus type may be poorly circumscribed and asymmetric. When accompanied by the variability of pigmentation seen in almost all combined nevi, the resemblance to malignant melanoma may be marked.

Differential Diagnosis

Combined nevi have, by definition, a biphasic pattern (i.e., an appearance that sharply varies from one part of a lesion to the other). All melanocytic neoplasms with biphasic patterns are worthy of close examination, as malignant melanomas that arise in nevi can also have a similar appearance. Features common to combined nevi but absent in malignant melanoma arising in preexistent nevi include sharp lateral circumscription, symmetry of each separate component of the nevus, and scarcity of mitoses. A lymphocytic host response is infrequent in combined nevi, but can be seen in combinations that include Spitz nevus, which can evoke a halo reaction. If the classic features of Spitz nevus are not all present in a lesion suspected to be a combined Spitz nevus, complete excision is warranted. Likewise, lesions suspected of being deep penetrating nevi and that show marked nuclear pleomorphism or more than rare mitoses should be completely removed.

RECURRENT (PERSISTENT) NEVI

Recurrent nevi are benign melanocytic neoplasms that regrow after their seeming removal.[75] The term *persistent nevus* is more accurate, as these nevi were never truly eradicated. Although nevi may recur after incomplete removal by any technique, superficial shave biopsy and electrocautery most often result in persistence.

Clinical Features

The most frequent clinical presentation of recurrent or persistent nevus is the appearance of a small, brown macule in the center of a scar several weeks to months after a procedure. In contrast, recurrent or persistent malignant melanoma is usually evident as a pigmented papule or nodule at the edge of a scar, sometimes years later.

Histopathologic Features

Recurrent or persistent nevi can simulate malignant melanoma, either in situ or invasive, because they can contain areas in which solitary melanocytes are more frequent than nested ones, and scattered melanocytes may be present above the dermoepidermal junction.[76,77] These changes are well circumscribed laterally and present above an area in which the dermis has been replaced by scar. The intraepidermal melanocytes generally do not have markedly atypical nuclei and often have a retracted cytoplasm and abundant pigment. Nests of melanocytes with similar nuclear features may be present in the most superficial, dermal portion of the scar. As a persistent nevus ages, the proportion of dermal cells becomes larger. Beneath the scar, or to the side of it (if the biopsy specimen includes these areas) are the remains of the original, incompletely removed nevus (Fig. 20-28). Spindled melanocytes that resemble fibroblasts but are identifiable using immunoperoxidase staining with S-100 protein antisera are present in the fibrotic zone between the junctional and dermal portions of the proliferation.[78] These cells may be melanocytes migrating in an upward direction from the unremoved portion of the nevus.

Clinically, recurrent blue nevi seldom occur, and their histopathologic features have not been described.

Persistent or recurrent Spitz nevi can show several different histologic patterns. In lesions removed by the shave biopsy technique, there can be pagetoid spread of single melanocytes as occurs in persistent nevi of other types. There can be nodular aggregates of spindled or epithelioid melanocytes, sometimes with a high mitotic rate. The epidermal changes seen overlying

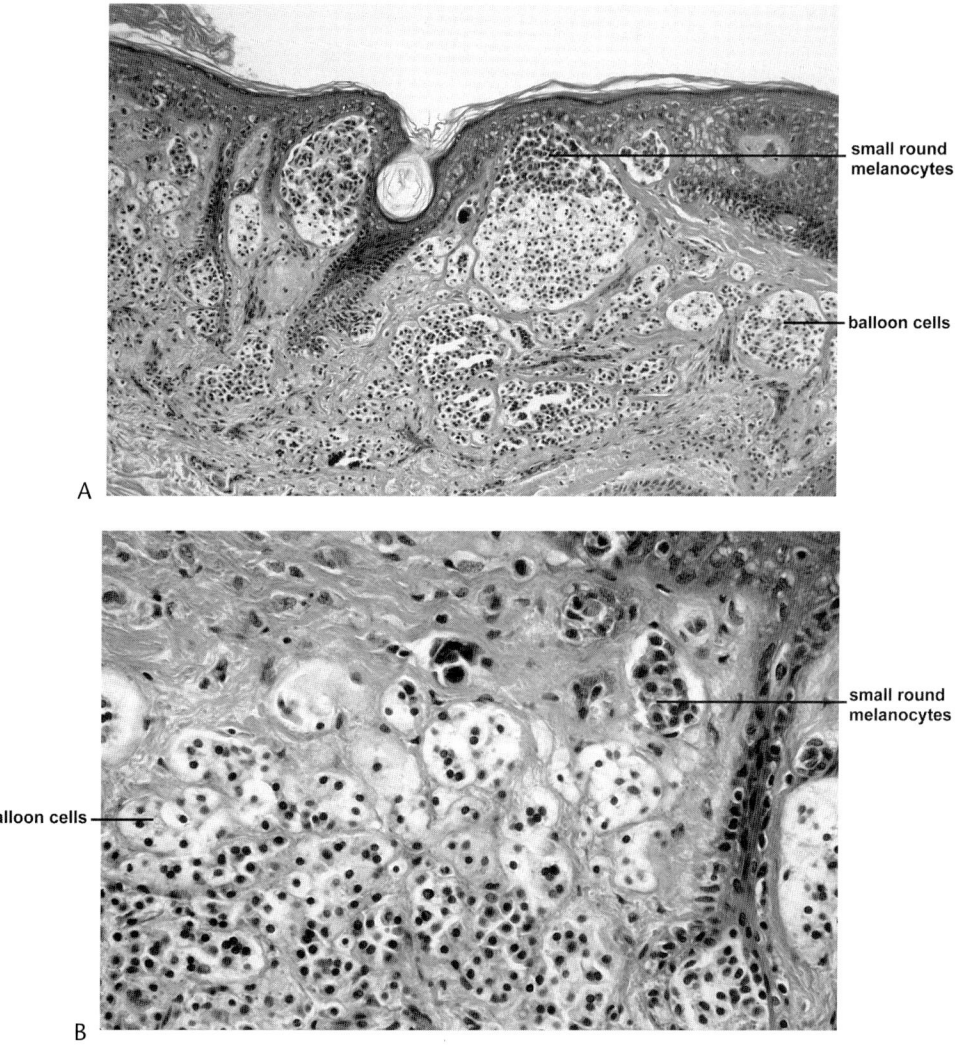

Figure 20-27. Combined nevus with balloon cells is usually termed balloon cell nevus, but is properly a combined nevus because there are two different types of melanocytes in virtually every example. In this one, ordinary (small round) melanocytes and balloon cells are present at the junction, whereas balloon cells predominate in the dermis **(A)**. Balloon cells have copious pale finely vacuolated cytoplasm, usually with small nuclei. Their cytoplasm is more abundant and less pigmented than that of pagetoid cells (contrast with those shown in Fig. 20-26C) **(B)**.

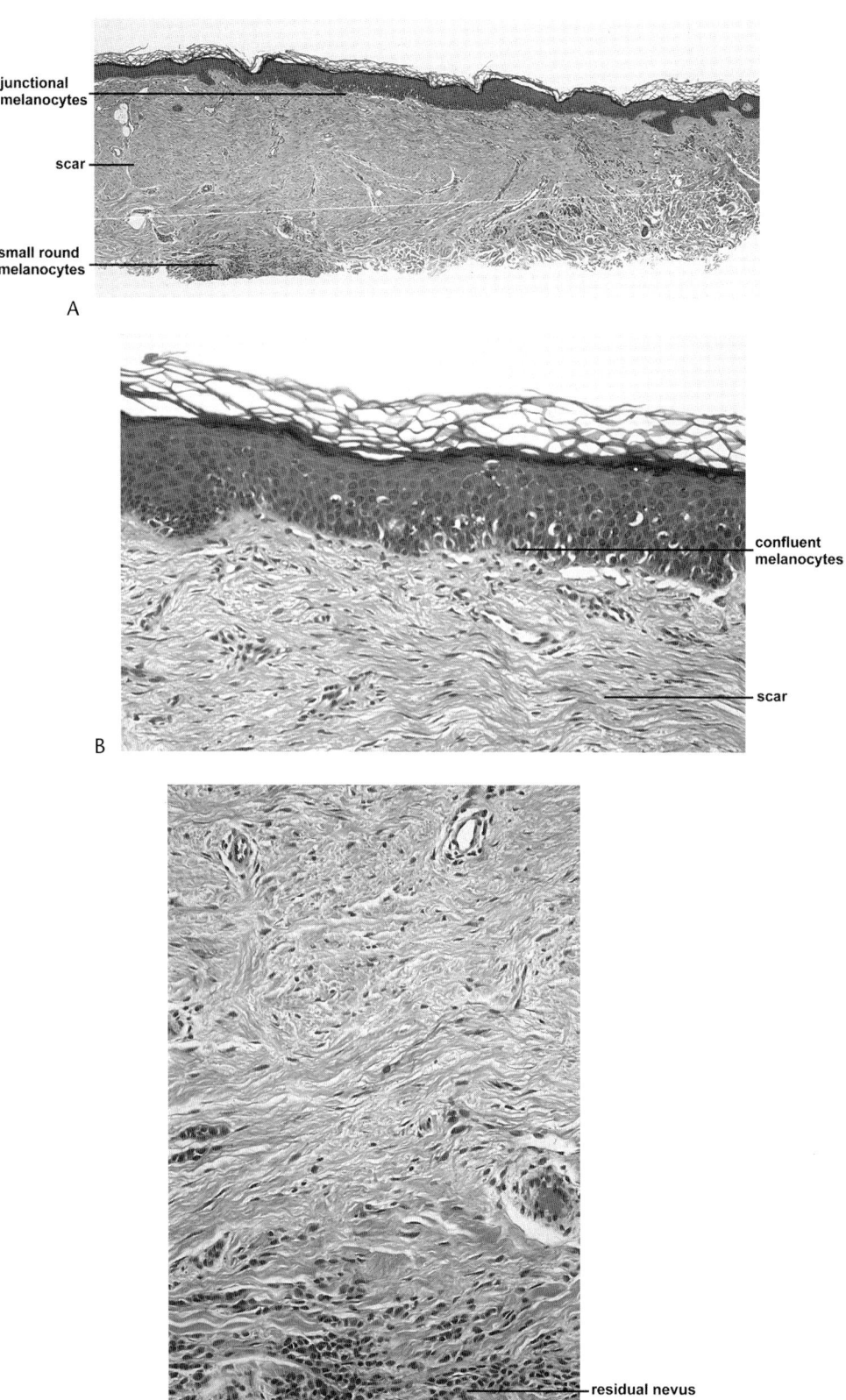

junctional
melanocytes

scar

small round
melanocytes

A

confluent
melanocytes

scar

B

residual nevus

C

Figure 20-28. Persistent compound melanocytic nevus. A scar separates the small round cells of the pre-existent nevus *(bottom)* from the persistent junctional proliferation. Note that the junctional proliferation is confined to a central zone overlying the scar **(A)**. The intraepidermal melanocytes in persistent nevi are usually single, pigmented, and situated near the junction. Florid pagetoid spread is exceptional **(B)**. Beneath the scar lies the residuum of a superficial congenital nevus **(C)**.

Spitz nevus may also be seen in recurrent examples. Some persistent Spitz nevi are only sparsely cellular and have desmoplastic stroma.[79]

Clinicopathologic Correlation

The intraepidermal portion of persistent nevi likely derives from melanocytes in hair follicles or sweat ducts beneath the portion removed by the biopsy. This would explain why persistent melanocytic nevi impart pigment to the center of the scar rather than to its edges.

Differential Diagnosis

Persistent or recurrent melanocytic nevi must be differentiated from malignant melanoma that is either in situ or superficially invasive. This similarity gave rise to the term *pseudomelanoma*.[76] Key to distinguishing these two conditions is an adequate biopsy specimen that extends beyond the intraepidermal portion of the lesion or, better yet, beyond the scar. Persistent melanocytic nevi seldom spread beyond the lateral confines of the dermal scar from the previous biopsy. Persistent malignant melanoma often extends beyond the scar, and more often still the center of the recurrent lesion is at the edge of the scar. In persistent, melanocytic nevi there are often dendritic, heavily pigmented melanocytes within the epidermis, and they are usually mostly in the lower half of the epidermis. In persistent malignant melanoma any cytologic type of intraepidermal melanocyte can be found. One particular pitfall occurs when the history of a prior biopsy is not obtained from the patient or from the clinician. If a scar is histologically subtle, as can be the result of trauma or incomplete ablation with liquid nitrogen or carbon dioxide laser treatment, the resultant lesion can easily be mistaken for malignant melanoma. Suspicion that a scar is present can be confirmed by the absence of fibers on an elastic tissue stain and by the diminished anisotropism of collagen bundles on examination with polarized light.

MELANOMA

Melanoma is a neoplasm of melanocytes that has the potential to metastasize or is in an evolutionary pathway in which the acquisition of that potential is likely. The word *malignant* is often used before melanoma, but as there is no benign melanoma in current medical terminology, *malignant melanoma* is redundant. Melanoma in situ refers to the stage at which the neoplasm is situated within the epidermis and/or epithelium of hair follicles or sweat ducts.

Clinical Features

A wide range of clinical appearances can be seen in melanoma. In situ lesions begin as macules with pigmentation that varies from pink to dark brown. If the cells of a melanoma enter the dermis early in the evolution of a lesion, a papule or nodule can form with or without a perceptible flat component. Variation in pigmentation is a hallmark of melanoma. Shades of brown and black are often seen; thick lesions have foci of red, white, or blue on occasion. Large nodules can be ulcerated.

Clark et al[80] described several histogenetic types of melanoma based largely on the pattern of their intraepithelial portions. This classification has been challenged by Ackerman and David[81] on the grounds that these types have a similar prognosis when matched for sex, thickness, and site and that many of the characteristics of each type are, in fact, secondary to the site of the neoplasm or caused by secondary changes such as solar elastosis. We review the "histogenetic" classification of melanoma because it is so entrenched in the literature and to a large extent correlates with the epidemiology of the disease. Whether this classification has any relevance to the management of individual patients is debatable. The following descriptions present the way that those who divide melanomas into histogenetic types view the subject and, taken together, provide an overview of the clinical presentations of melanoma.

Superficial spreading melanoma is said to occur anywhere on the cutaneous surface, but most often is on the trunk or extremities proximal to the wrists or ankles. A portion, or all, of the lesion is flat and usually is irregular in outline, poorly circumscribed, and variegated in pigmentation. Clinical criteria to distinguish most small superficial spreading melanomas from so-called dysplastic or Clark nevi do not exist. Superficial spreading melanoma is by far the most common subtype, estimated to comprise 67% of cases.

Nodular melanoma lacks a flat component clinically. The most frequent site is the trunk. The papule (or nodule) may have an intact or ulcerated surface, and its color can vary from pink, gray, or brown to black. Nodular melanoma, when diagnosed with strict histopathologic criteria (the absence of an intraepidermal component lateral to the dermal nodule), is relatively rare, comprising 10% of cases.[80] Superficial spreading and nodular melanoma can be viewed as a single disease from an epidemiologic perspective. Both are rare in nonwhite populations and occur mainly in middle-aged or older persons.

Lentigo maligna melanoma is said to evolve slowly as a tan to brown patch on sun-damaged skin, most often of the head or neck. Evolution of the flat component (lentigo maligna) to a large size over many years before papules or nodules (which can indicate involvement of the dermis) occur is frequent. On occasion amelanotic examples of lentigo maligna or lentigo maligna melanoma can present as scaly, erythematous patches simulating a dermatitis or Bowen's disease.[82] Lentigo maligna melanoma almost always occurs in whites, is directly related to chronic sun exposure, and is thus most common in the elderly. Its incidence varies with latitude, comprising 9% of the cases in the data of Clark et al.[80]

Acral lentiginous malignant melanoma is said to occur on the palms, soles, and nail beds and is similar to lesions on mucous membranes (mucosal lentiginous melanoma). Lesions are often dark brown and may spread indolently before papules or nodules arise. Subungual malignant melanoma presents as a pigmented streak in the nail or can involve the entire nail bed with spread of pigment over the proximal nail fold, known as Hutchinson's sign. Acral and mucosal lentiginous melanoma is uncommon (4% of melanomas), but has a similar incidence in all races.

While the schema outlined above depends to some extent on the site of the neoplasm, there is an imperfect correspondence between the location of a melanoma and its histogenetic type. Both superficial spreading and nodular melanomas, as defined by Clark, can occur on the face or hands; it is unclear if the epidemiologic features of nodular melanomas of the acra are different from those of acral lentiginous melanoma.

One can argue that the differences between these forms of melanoma are an artificial construct and that they are secondary to the area of skin involved. It is certainly true that it can be difficult to classify a melanoma accurately if a clinical photograph is masked so that the observer cannot see which part of the body is involved. Such tendencies as extension into follicular infundibula, which is conventionally associated with lentigo maligna, may simply be due to the presence of many follicles on facial skin. On the other hand, the finding that acral melanomas are roughly equal in incidence among the races and that lentigo maligna is found in light-skinned patients who have had a great deal of sun exposure suggests that there are important biologic, if not prognostic, differences.

Regression can occur in any form of melanoma.[83] Regression is an immunologically mediated destruction of a portion or all of the neoplasm. It is evident clinically as a flat, gray or white focus that may occupy any or all of the neoplasm's surface.

Because the dermatopathologist is often consulted for advice regarding biopsy, excision, and surgery for melanoma, some basic principles are worth stressing. A small partial biopsy showing a benign histopathologic picture does not necessarily vitiate a strong clinical suspicion of melanoma. Pigmented patches can be composed in part of solar lentigo and in part harbor melanoma in situ, and biopsy specimens of larger heterogeneous neoplasms can sample only the benign melanocytic nevus within which a melanoma began. In most cases, simple complete excision with minimal margins (perhaps 2 mm or so) results in a specimen whose histopathologic examination is uncompromised. Definitive excision with margins thought appropriate for melanoma should, in general, not be performed as a

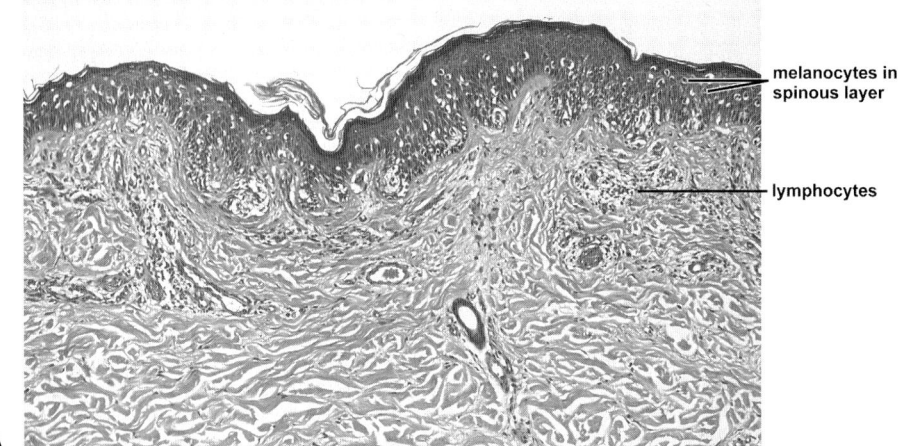

melanocytes in spinous layer

lymphocytes

A

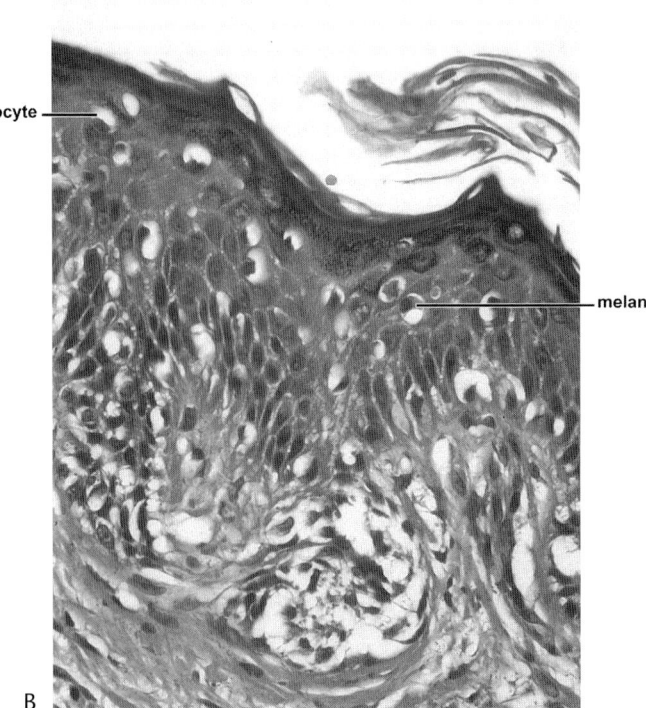

melanocyte

melanocyte

B

Figure 20-29. The features of early evolving melanoma in situ can be inferred from those at the periphery of more established lesions. In this example of melanoma in situ, there are both nested and single melanocytes in the center of the lesion, with prominent pagetoid spread of single cells **(A).** Many of the melanocytes are present in the granular and cornified layers, a more definative sign of upward spread than their presence in the midspinous zone. Individual melanocytes sometimes appear to be in the spinous layer when a section is tangential **(B).** *Continued.*

single procedure. All too often the clinical recognition of pigmented lesions is impaired, and pathologic examination reveals a simulant of melanoma such as an unusual seborrheic keratosis.

Histopathologic Features

A number of histologic features are common to melanoma in most locations and correspond to its evolution. For practical purposes, nearly all melanomas originate in the epidermis or in mucosal epithelium. There are extraordinarily rare instances in which melanoma begins in the dermis of a congenital or blue nevus, and these are exceptions to the pathway of evolution described below.

The earliest lesions of most melanomas in situ, small macules clinically, appear microscopically as proliferations of solitary melanocytes at or slightly above the dermoepidermal junction,

spaced at irregular intervals (Fig. 20-29). The nuclei of melanocytes in these early neoplasms may or may not be cytologically atypical, but are almost always larger than those of the non-neoplastic basilar melanocytes. As lesions of melanoma in situ evolve, melanocytes can aggregate to form nests and spread to the upper spinous, granular, and cornified layers. Often, single neoplastic melanocytes will be visible beyond the last nest on either side of the lesion, and some of these cells may be situated above the basal layer. Melanoma in situ typically involves follicular infundibula and acrotrychia in a given lesion with melanocytes distributed in the same pattern as they are within the interadnexal epidermis.

The most common form of melanoma in situ evolves to feature pagetoid upward migration of melanocytes into the upper spinous, granular, and cornified layers and is termed *superficial spreading melanoma in situ* by some. The melanocytes in this

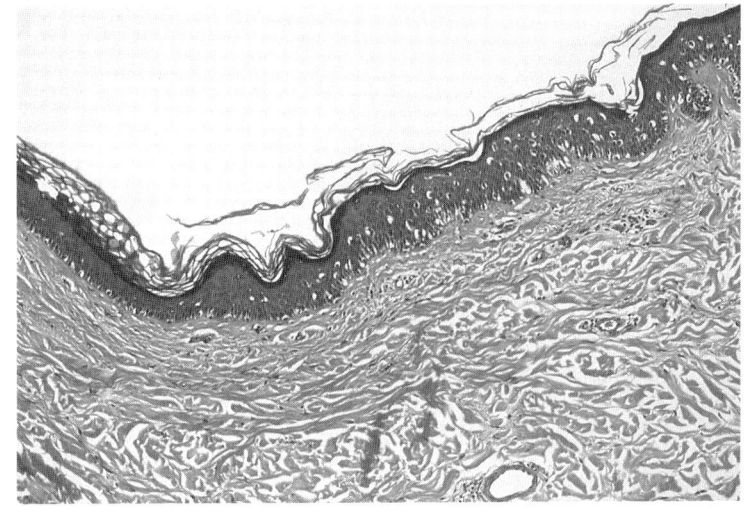

C

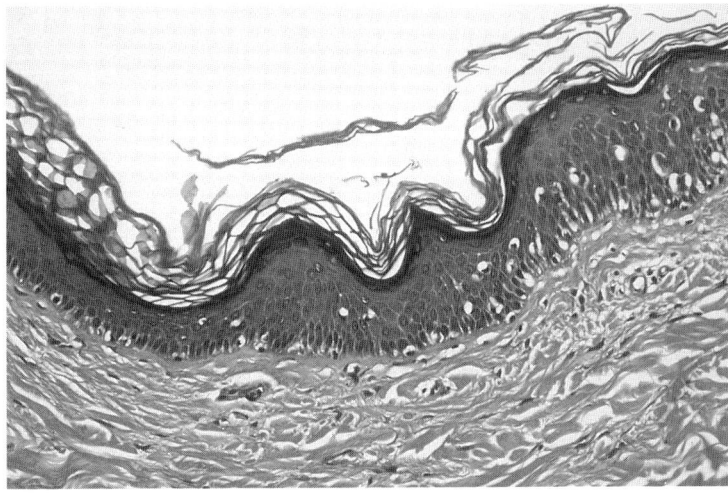

D

Figure 20-29. *Continued.* At the edge of the lesion, there are only single cells and no nests are present **(C).** Some of these are suprabasilar in location, but toward the edge of the lesion, most are in the basal zone **(D).** Note that lymphocytes are nearly absent at the edge of this lesion. They are usually present in melanoma in situ that has evolved to the formation of junctional nests, but are scant in areas in which single cells alone are seen.

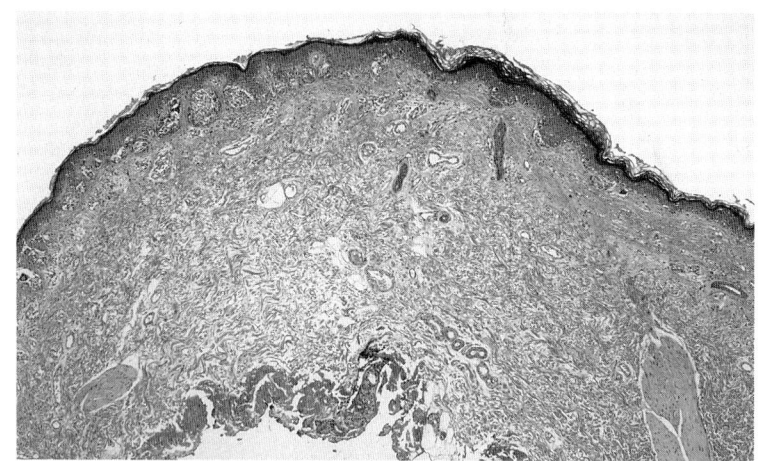

A

atypical melanocytes
above basal layer

nest of pleomorphic
spindle shaped
melanocytes

B

Figure 20-30. A nested pattern of melanoma in situ. At first glance one might mistake this lesion for a junctional nevus **(A)**. There are large nests of melanocytes situated above copious elastotic material **(B)**. *Continued.*

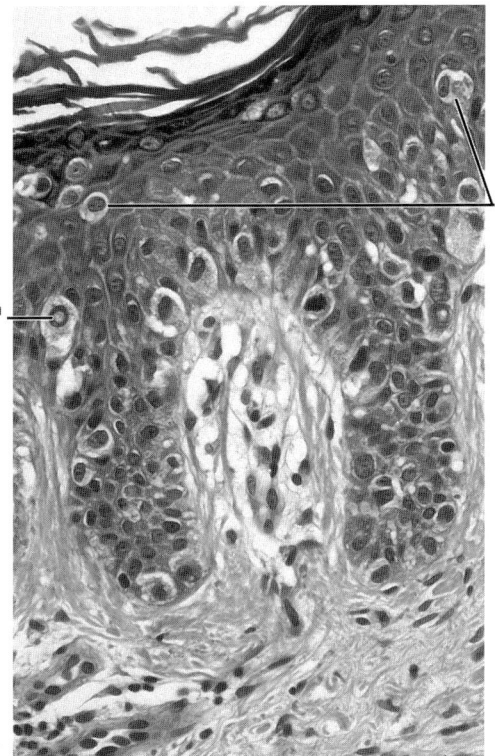

atypical melanocytes
above basal layer

nuclear pseudoinclusion
of cytoplasm in atypical
melanocyte

C

Figure 20-30. *Continued.* Note the uneven shapes and pigmentation of junctional nests. While these findings alone do not mandate a diagnosis of melanoma, they should cause the pathologist to strongly consider it. In another area of the same lesion, there is a pagetoid pattern **(C)**.

form of the disease have more abundant cytoplasm than in the other types, and the cytoplasm is frequently pale and finely vacuolated, with or without dusty-appearing melanin. This pattern of melanoma in situ is not limited to the trunk and nonacral extremities, but in fact can occur at any cutaneous site. Melanoma in situ has a broad range of histologic appearances, with a predominantly basilar distribution of cells in some examples and a mostly nested pattern in others.

Melanoma in situ most often occurs de novo but is found above a pre-existent melanocytic nevus in about one fifth of cases. All types of melanocytic nevi, with the exceptions of Spitz nevi and blue nevi, have been associated with melanoma in situ. Dysplastic or Clark nevus is the type most frequently found in association with melanoma in situ, followed by small, superficial congenital nevi.

As any of the patterns of melanoma in situ evolve, nests enlarge and become confluent with their neighbors, which can result in the formation of nests with odd shapes and discohesion between the epidermis and dermis (Fig. 20-30). The resultant junctional clefts are a valuable diagnostic feature as they rarely occur in benign nevi. Lymphocytic infiltrates often accumulate in the papillary dermis at the same time that nests form in melanoma in situ. The infiltrates are frequently beneath the nests and are distributed asymmetrically with respect to the rest of the neoplasm. The formation of both large nests and dense

lymphocytic infiltrates seems to occur just prior to invasion of the papillary dermis.

Neoplastic melanocytes first enter the papillary dermis as individual cells or as small nests, with or without a lymphocytic host response. These aggregates enlarge, and nodules of melanoma cells eventuate, bowing the papillary-reticular dermal interface downward. In early lesions the degree of cytologic atypia can be modest, but in most invasive lesions with large nodular aggregates melanocyte nuclei show the features of cytologic atypia: large nuclear size, irregular chromatin patterns, irregularly thickened nuclear membranes, and large nucleoli. Mitotic figures are not usually evident until intradermal nests are quite large, numerous, and deeply invasive. This limits their utility in the differential diagnosis of early lesions.

Regression of melanoma should be considered at this point as it can complicate lesions that otherwise appear to be in situ or either superficially or deeply invasive. It is manifest histologically as a zone within the epidermis (and sometimes papillary dermis) in which neoplastic melanocytes are diminished in number compared with the remainder of the lesion and accompanied by a band-like infiltrate of lymphocytes and melanophages, thickening of the papillary dermis, telangiectases, fibrosis, and loss of the rete ridge pattern in variable proportions.[83] Some regressed melanomas feature irregular epidermal hyperplasia and hyperkeratosis, which, in conjunction with band-like

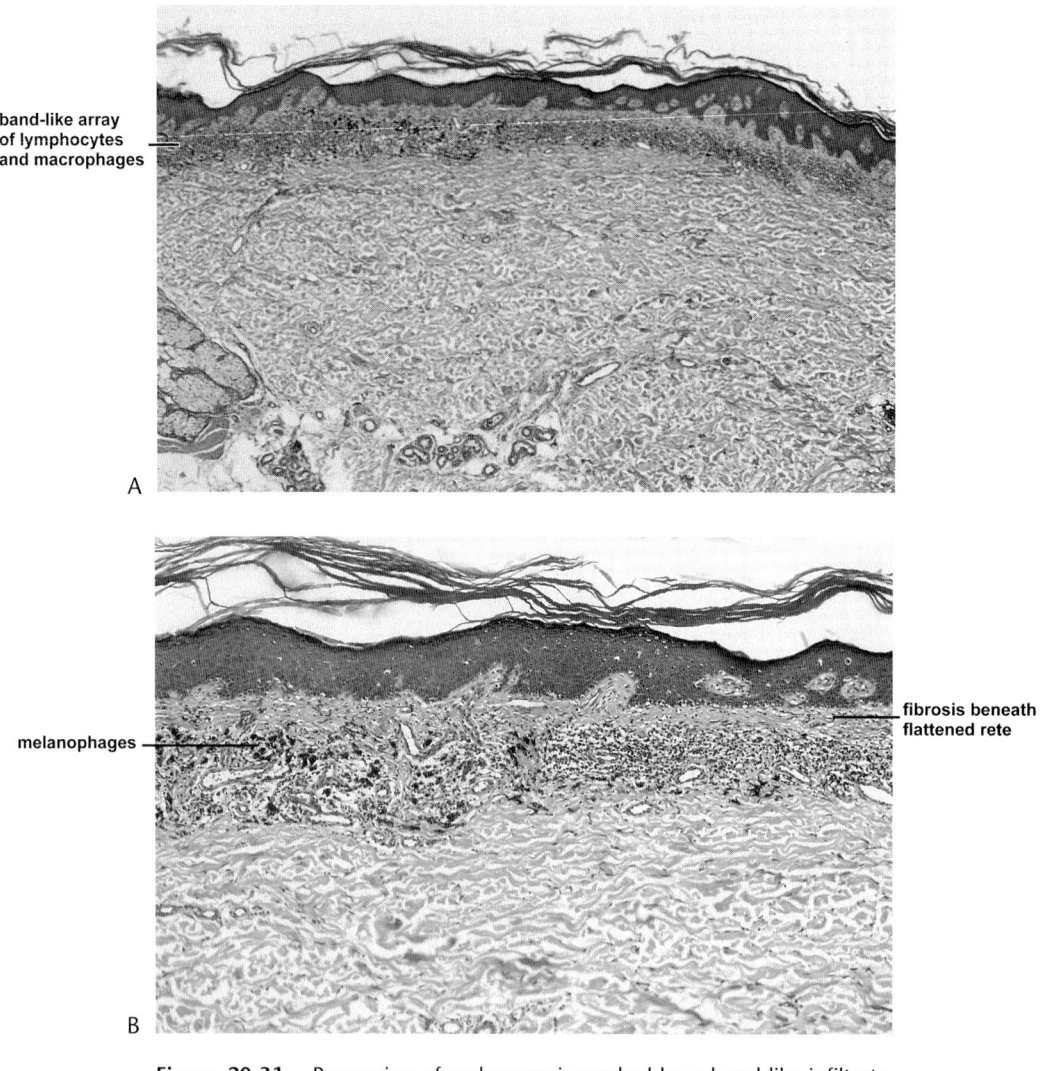

band-like array
of lymphocytes
and macrophages

A

melanophages

fibrosis beneath
flattened rete

B

Figure 20-31. Regression of melanoma is marked by a band-like infiltrate of lymphocytes and melanophages in a papillary dermis that is thickened and fibrotic, whether adjacent to a melanoma (either in situ or invasive) or by itself **(A)**. When these changes are seen alone, the diagnosis of regression of melanoma can be inferred if the infiltrate of melanophages is very dense (so-called melanosis) **(B)**.

infiltrates, can lead to a misdiagnosis of lichen planus–like keratosis. Regression is termed *partial* if melanoma cells obviously persist in these foci and *complete* if they do not (Fig. 20-31). A melanoma in situ or a superficially invasive lesion can regress in its entirety, leaving only these changes. Regression of a lesion in which nodular aggregations of melanocytes have accumulated in the dermis leads to a similarly nodular mass of melanophages beneath an epidermis devoid of neoplastic melanocytes, a finding sometimes called *tumoral melanosis.*

The dermal portion of melanoma has a range of histologic appearances. In most invasive melanomas, the dermal cells have an atypical nucleus and abundant cytoplasm and are arranged as single cells or nests. As the cells of an invasive malignant melanoma accumulate in the papillary dermis, nests often become compressed and may be less apparent as melanocytes take on a sheet-like or plaque-like growth pattern. The papillary-

reticular dermal interface is often a barrier to expanding melanomas and can become bowed downward before melanoma cells permeate the reticular dermis. Lymphocytes are often present beneath melanoma cells in the papillary dermis, but tend to become scant in cases in which the reticular dermis is involved.

Secondary changes include adnexal involvement, perineural invasion, lymphatic or vascular invasion, regression, and the presence of a melanocytic nevus. *Adnexal involvement* refers to extension of the neoplasm into hair follicles, sweat ducts, and then the adventitial dermis that surrounds them. The same distribution of melanocytes seen in the intraepidermal portions of these lesions occurs in these adnexal structures. Adnexal involvement of the perifollicular adventitial dermis can result in the positioning of melanoma cells deep in the dermis with only a small "tumor volume." Because the resultant thickness measurement may result in an exaggeratedly dire prognosis, one should use melanoma cells in other parts of the dermis to establish lesional thickness (see below).

Perineural invasion occurs in some thick melanomas, especially those in which the invasive component is spindled. It is important to note its occurrence, as perineural invasion beyond excision margins can result in loss of local surgical control of the neoplasm, especially in melanomas on the skin of the face, scalp, or ears. Perineural invasion with extension along cranial nerves can result in the spread of melanoma into the brain.

Invasion of lymphatic and blood vessels is similarly an attribute of deeply invasive lesions. The determination of whether lymphatic or vascular invasion is present should not be based solely on the presence of neoplastic cells in vessel lumens.

Signs that are specific for vascular or lymphatic invasion include the attachment of melanoma cells to vessel walls or fibrin strands between cells. Compact nests of melanoma cells can sometimes have small spindled cells around them, simulating the relationship between endothelial cells and intraluminal melanoma. Immunoperoxidase staining with antisera to endothelial determinants such as factor VIII, CD31, or CD34 or lectin staining with *Ulex europeus* agglutinin can clarify whether the peripheral spindled cells are indeed endothelial.

Remnants of a melanocytic nevus can be identified in some melanomas. Various authors have claimed that anywhere from 9% to 50% of melanomas arise in association with a pre-existent nevus.[80] These widely disparate figures doubtless reflect the difficulties in judging whether small melanocytes seen at the

Figure 20-32. Melanoma in situ on severely sun-damaged facial skin (also known as lentigo maligna). There is prominent involvement of follicular infundibular epithelium **(A)**. Melanocytes are present mostly in the basal layer of the epidermis and of the infundibulum **(B)**.

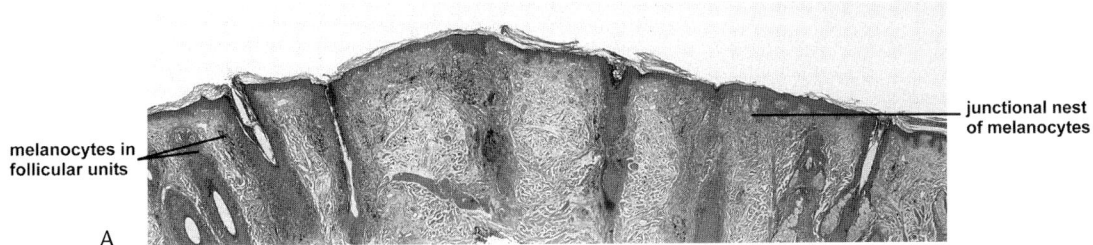

melanocytes in
follicular units

junctional nest
of melanocytes

A

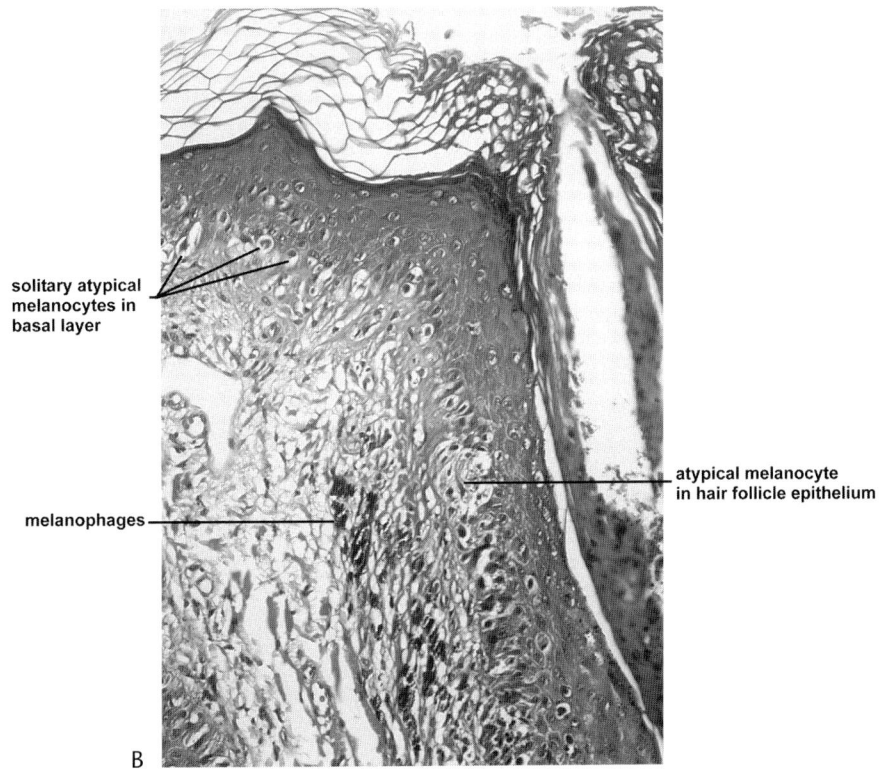

solitary atypical
melanocytes in
basal layer

atypical melanocyte
in hair follicle epithelium

melanophages

B

base of a melanoma are small melanoma cells or those of a pre-existent nevus. More recently, some groups have considered melanomas to arise in association with a nevus if evidence of "melanocytic dysplasia" was present at their periphery.[84] Until better criteria are developed to discriminate between small melanoma and nevus cells, the question of how many melanomas arise in nevi may not be solvable. If the small cells at the base of a melanoma lie above solar elastosis or newly formed vessels or are encased in fibrosis, they are more likely than not small melanoma cells; conversely, if they lie within elastosis or are clustered around adnexal structures they are more likely to represent a pre-existent nevus.

Because the histogenetic classification of melanoma is so entrenched in the literature, dermatopathologists should be familiar with it even if they do not choose to use it. The following is a brief summary of the main histologic features that those who believe in the usefulness of this classification apply to their evaluation of melanomas.

Lentigo maligna (better termed *melanoma in situ of sun-dam-aged skin of the head or neck*) is said to begin as a proliferation of single melanocytes in the basal layer of the epidermis, above a dermis in which there is usually abundant elastotic material. The melanocytes most often have hyperchromatic nuclei, scant cytoplasm, and angulated shapes. Melanocytic giant cells, with scalloped borders and nuclei distributed in a wreath-like configuration, are more commonly found in this setting than in truncal or acral melanomas. Neoplastic melanocytes frequently extend deeply into follicular infundibula and into acrosyringia. Melanin is usually more coarsely granular. The melanocytic nuclei tend to be hyperchromatic and angulated. Small, round nests of melanocytes and multinucleated melanocytes are more often found in this setting than in other forms of melanoma in situ. Patches of this form of melanoma in situ can be several centimeters across with no evident dermal involvement (Fig. 20-32). Only in more fully evolved foci just before invasion are nests, pagetoid upward migration, and lymphocytic infiltrates found. In some examples of lentigo maligna melanoma there are only a few invasive melanocytes in the papillary dermis, usually

Text continued on page 700

Figure 20-33. Invasive melanoma on severely sun-damaged facial skin (lentigo maligna melanoma). There is a nodular proliferation of atypical melanocytes flanked by a poorly circumscribed area in which melanocytes infiltrate the basilar epidermis above severe solar elastosis **(A)**. The atypical melanocytes in the basal layer have large hyperchromatic nuclei and scant cytoplasm **(B)**. *Continued.*

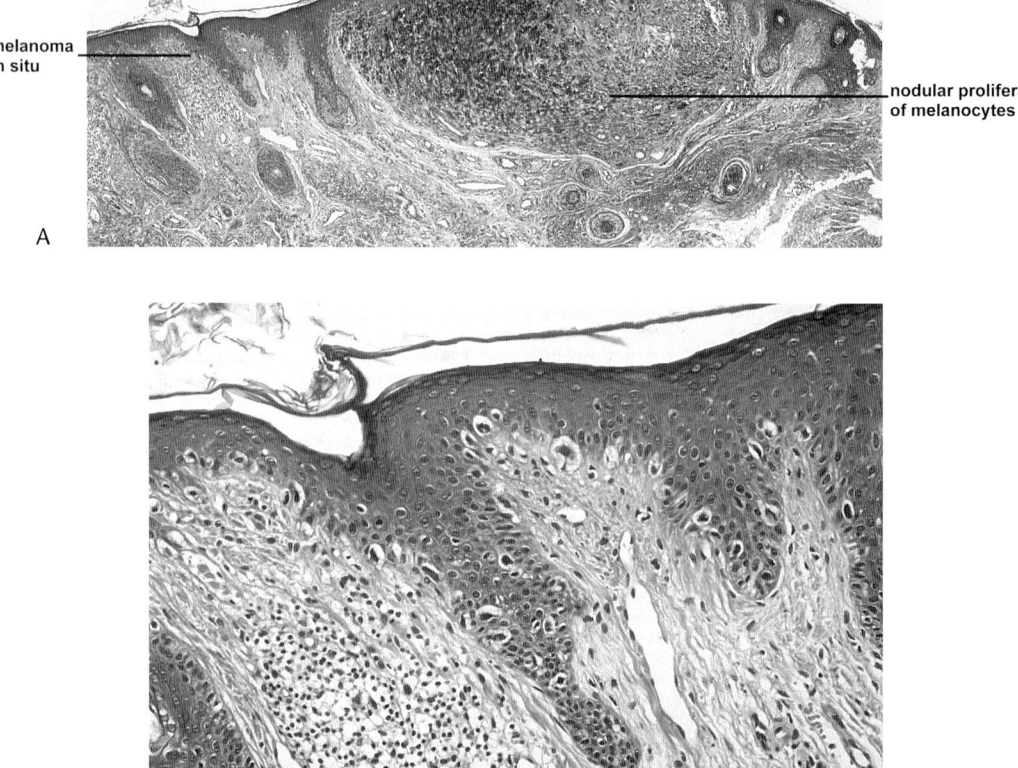

melanoma in situ

nodular proliferation of melanocytes

A

B

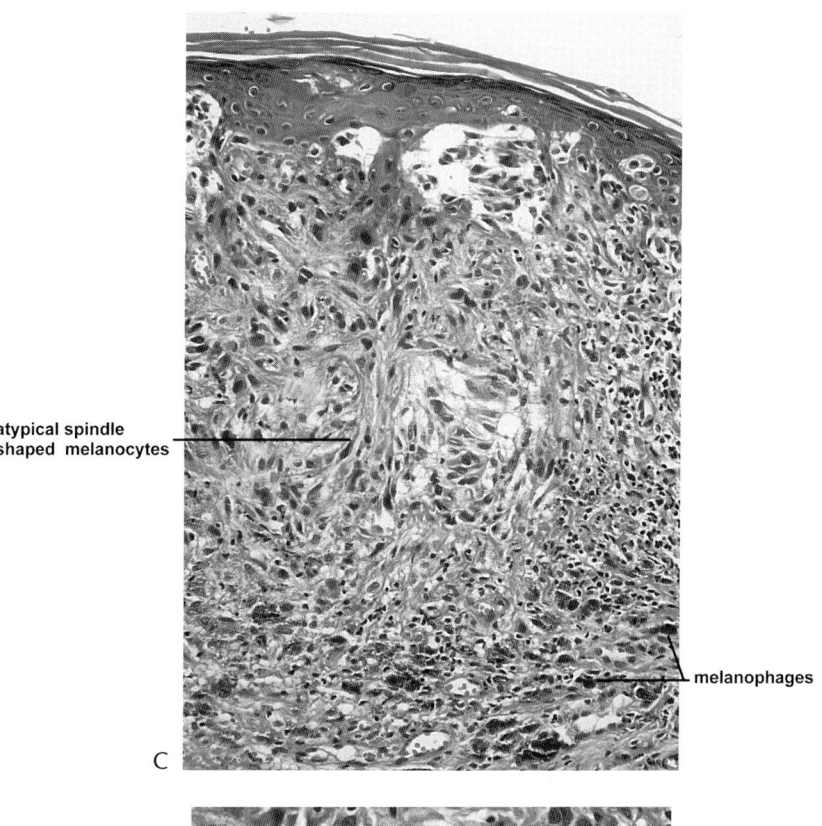

atypical spindle
shaped melanocytes

melanophages

C

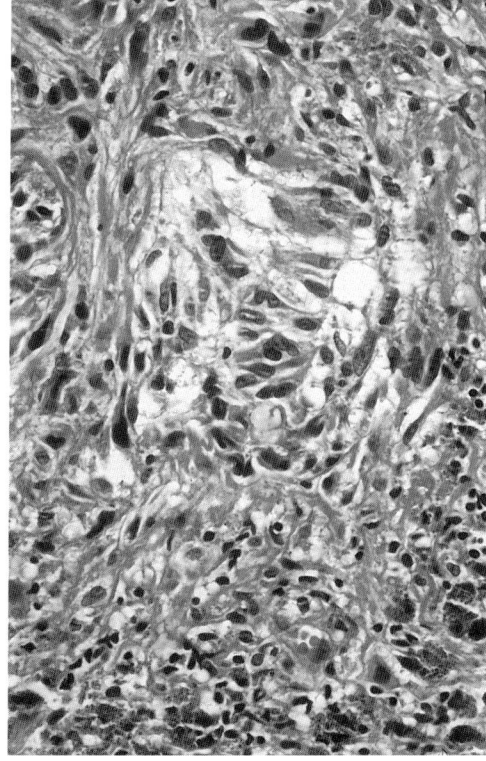

D

Figure 20-33. *Continued.* The nodule is composed of large spindled melanocytes with abundant pigment **(C)**, which is associated with many melanophages **(D)**.

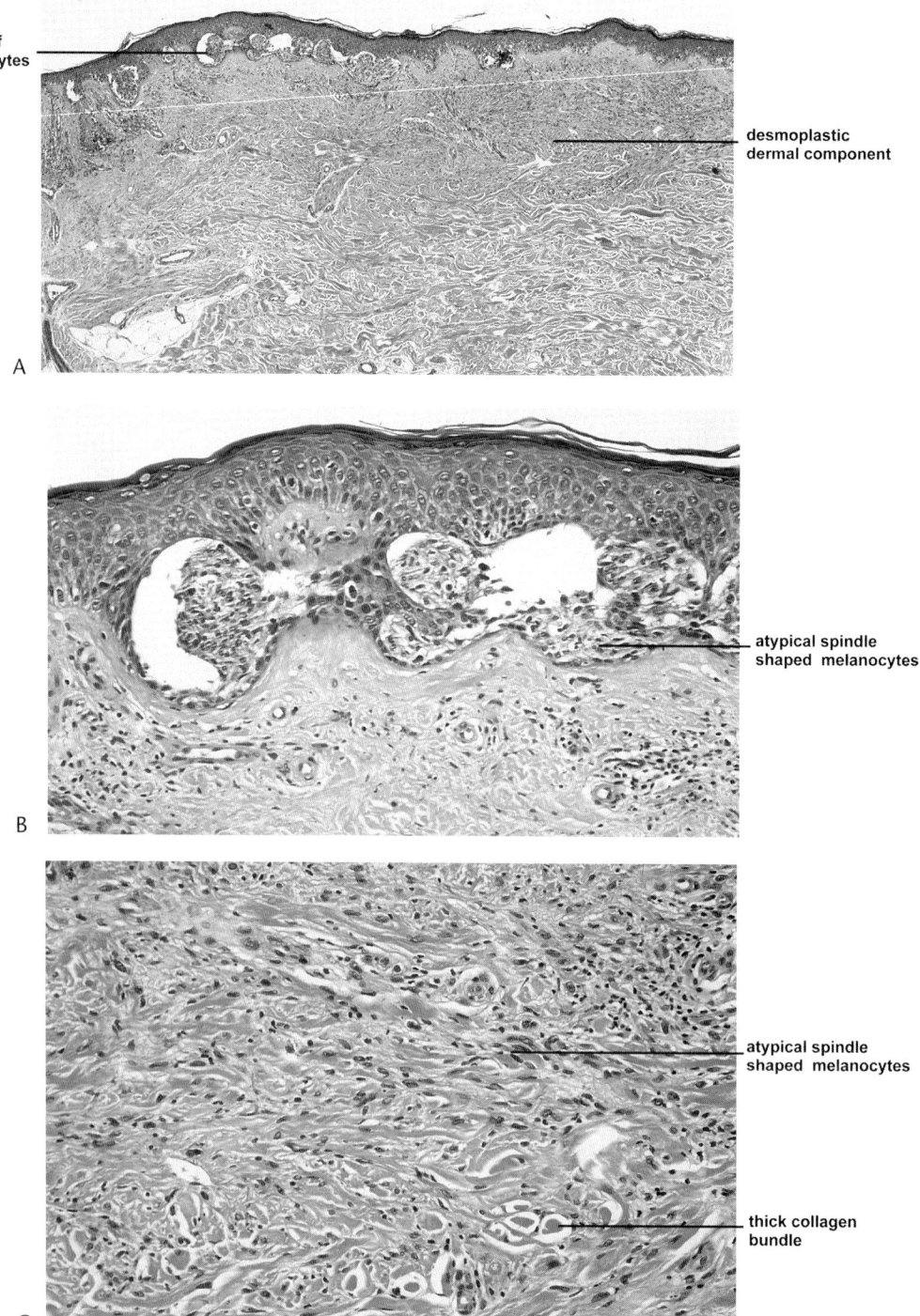

confluent nests of
atypical melanocytes

desmoplastic
dermal component

A

atypical spindle
shaped melanocytes

B

atypical spindle
shaped melanocytes

thick collagen
bundle

C

Figure 20-34. Desmoplastic melanoma. Many melanomas with a desmoplastic growth pattern in the dermis have only subtle signs of melanoma in
situ or have no appearant intraepidermal component (**A**). In this example,
the intraepidermal portion features lateral confluence of junctional nests
(**B**). Within the dermis are spindled melanocytes with pleomorphic nuclei,
which are situated between thickened collagen bundles (**C**). *Continued.*

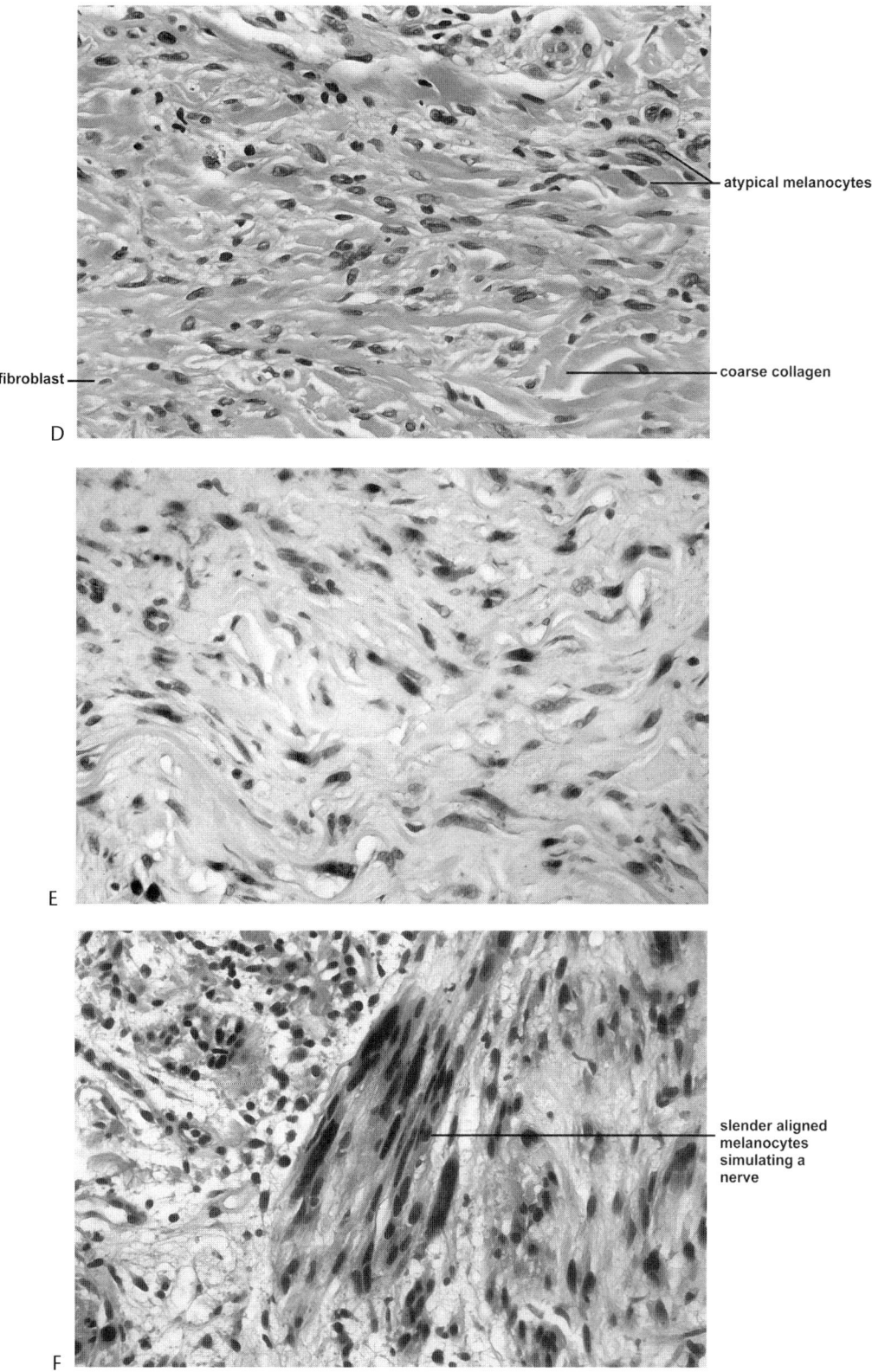

D

fibroblast ——

—— atypical melanocytes

—— coarse collagen

E

F

slender aligned
melanocytes
simulating a
nerve

Figure 20-34. *Continued.* The nuclei of melanocytes in this area are larger and hyperchromatic compared with those of dermal fibroblasts, but this is not always the case **(D)**. Desmoplastic areas can be amazingly subtle and sometimes require immunoperoxidase staining with S-100 protein for their delineation **(E)**. Areas in which the spindled cells simulate nerve fascicles can be present in desmoplastic melanomas **(F)**, as can foci of perineural invasion **(G)**.

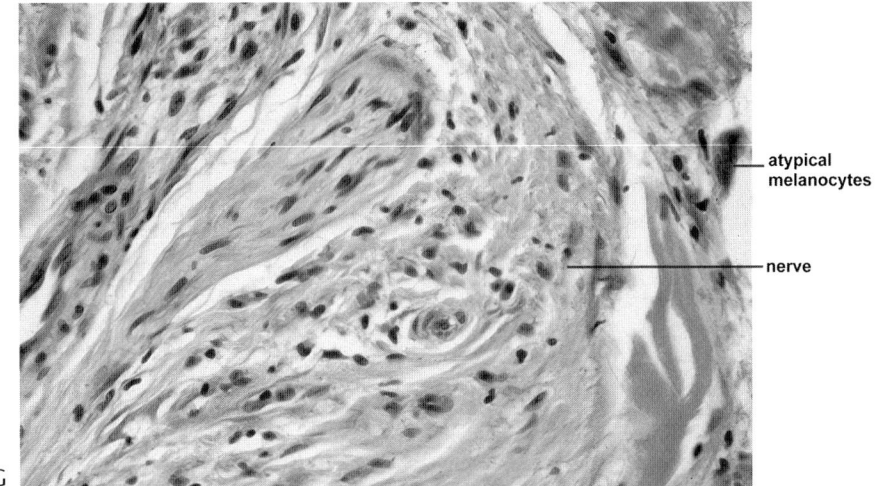

Figure 20-34. *Continued.*

Figure 20-35. Melanoma in situ on acral-volar skin. The center of this lesion has a nested pattern, while single melanocytes predominate at its edge **(A)**. The nests are laterally confluent, and lie above infiltrates of lymphocytes and melanophages **(B)**. *Continued.*

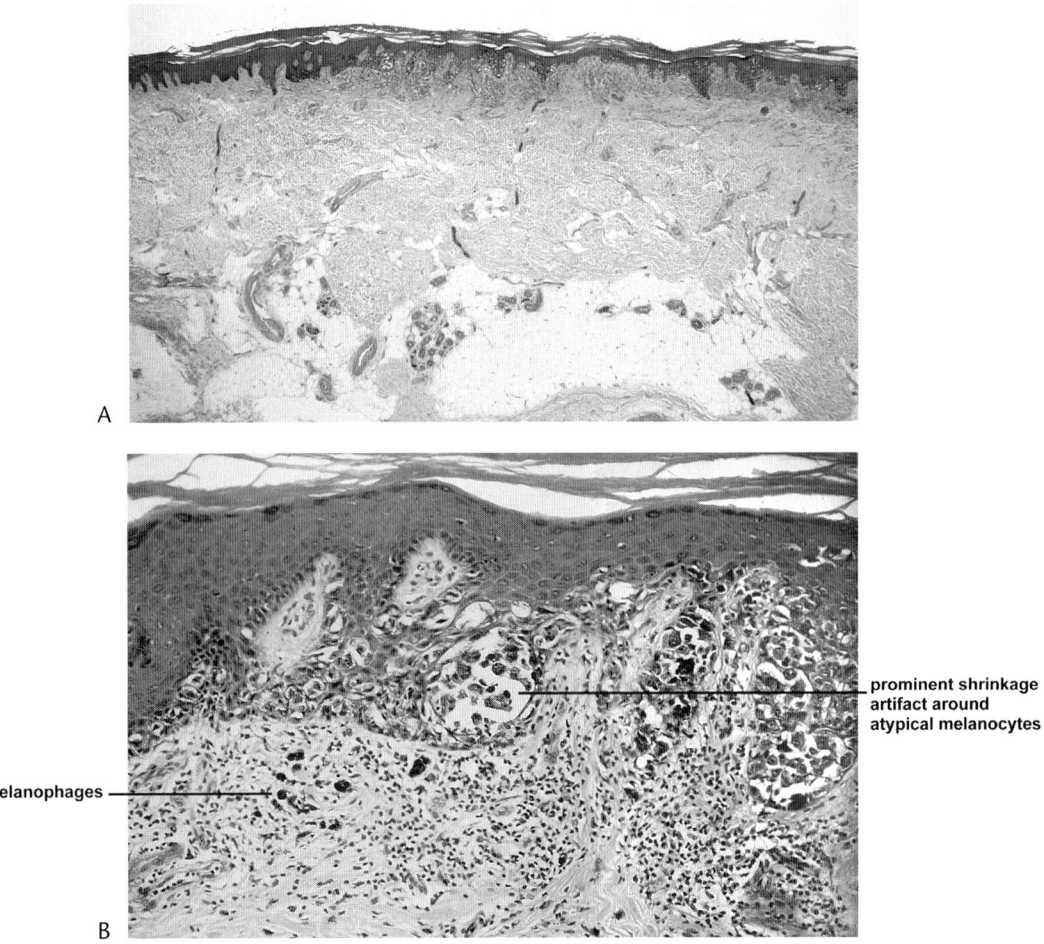

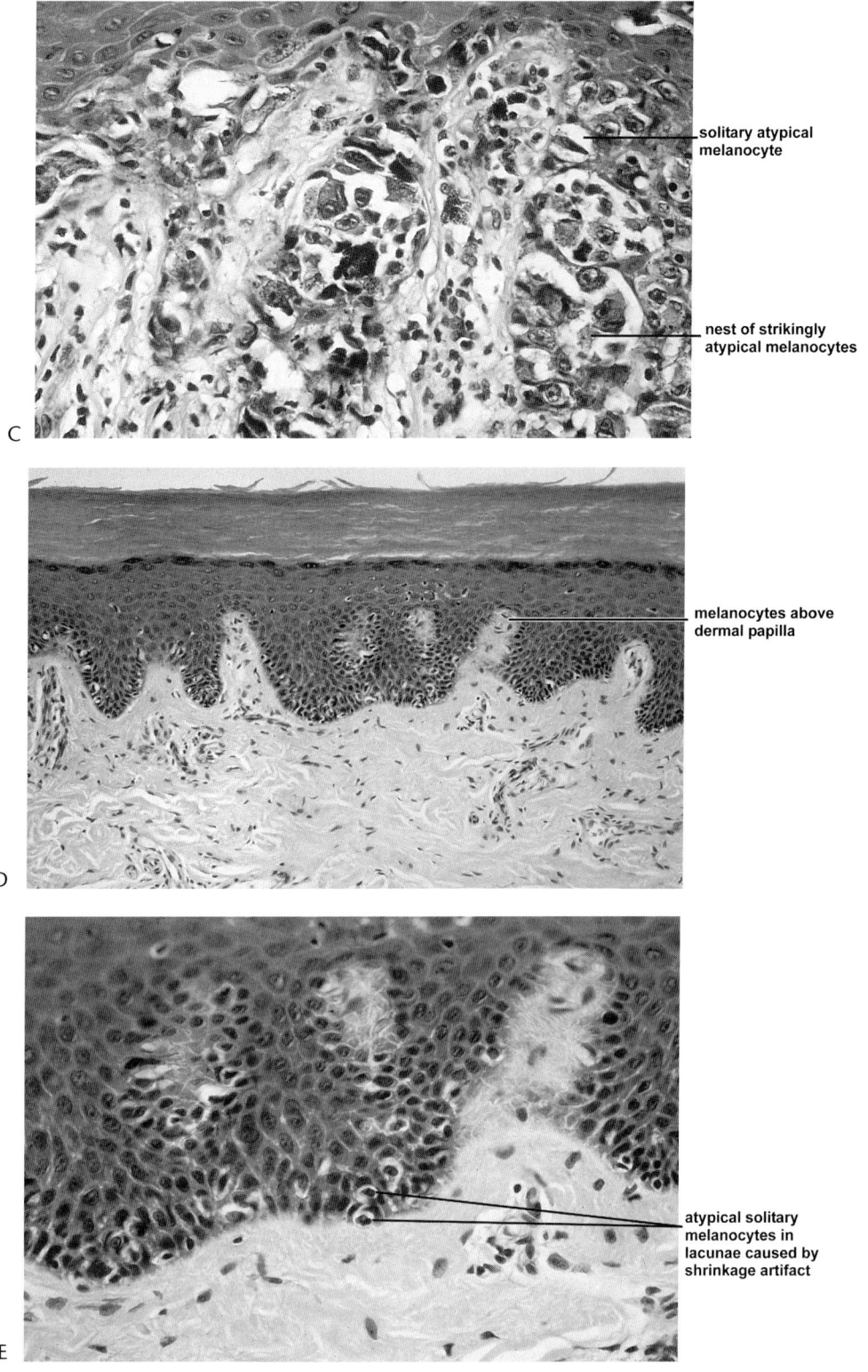

C — solitary atypical melanocyte

— nest of strikingly atypical melanocytes

D — melanocytes above dermal papilla

E — atypical solitary melanocytes in lacunae caused by shrinkage artifact

Figure 20-35. *Continued.* They are composed of strikingly atypical melanocytes with abundant pale cytoplasm **(C)**. At the periphery of the lesion, there are subtle changes that reflect the picture often seen in early melanoma in situ on acral skin. There are many solitary melanocytes in the basal layer, both at the bases of rete ridges and above dermal papillae **(D)**. These melanocytes are not markedly atypical. One must be careful in evaluating a broad and poorly circumscribed proliferation of single melanocytes on acral skin. Keep in mind that simple lentigines do occur on the acra but are small, well circumscribed, and have melanocytes mainly at the bases of rete **(E)**.

in areas of fibrosis. It can be difficult to identify melanocytes in these subepidermal foci of fibrosis without benefit of immuno-peroxidase staining with S-100 protein antisera because the melanocytes can be scattered singly, be difficult to distinguish from fibroblasts, dermal dendrocytes, or macrophages, or be obscured by lymphocytes and melanophages.[85] The invasive component in lentigo maligna melanoma may be indistinguishable from that seen in other types, or may be spindled (Fig. 20-33). Melanomas whose invasive components are spindled more frequently show neurotropism, simulate neural structures (neuronal differentiation) by growing in elongated, sinuous fascicles, or exhibit desmoplasia than other subtypes[86] (Fig. 20-34).

Acral lentiginous or mucosal lentiginous melanoma in situ also has, in its beginnings, a basilar pattern of growth in which single melanocytes predominate (Fig. 20-35). These melanocytes are likewise typically angulated in shape and feature hyperchromatic nuclei and scant cytoplasm. Occasionally, melanocytes with prominent branching dendrites are present; the finding of dendritic processes high in the spinous layer of the epidermis of acral skin or nail bed epithelium can alert the observer to the possibility of melanoma in situ. A similar basilar pattern, but without dendritic melanocytes, can also occur on the skin of the trunk, especially in elderly patients. As in other melanomas in which most neoplastic cells are in the basal layer, scatter of melanocytes in the upper spinous and cornified layers is generally seen in more advanced foci, which can also have nest formation, a lymphocytic infiltrate, and dermal invasion. Spindled dermal melanoma cells with or without neurotropism and desmoplasia are also seen in acral lentiginous melanoma. For those who use the histogenetic classification, the mere location of a neoplasm on an acral site is insufficient for a lesion to be typed as acral lentiginous because superficial spreading and nodular melanoma can also occur on acral skin.

Superficial spreading melanoma is defined as having an intraepidermal component that extends beyond the dermal one and does not show features of either lentigo maligna or acral lentiginous melanoma. Stereotypically there is extensive scattering of single cells or cell nests (pagetoid spread) within the epidermis and epithelial adnexa that extends laterally beyond the dermal component. The neoplastic cells typically have abundant cytoplasms with finely divided melanin and vesicular nuclei with prominent nucleoli. The cells of the invasive component are usually large and either round or polygonal (Fig. 20-36). A common misinterpretation of the histogenetic classification by those who would use it is to diagnose a superficial spreading melanoma in which a nodule is present as nodular melanoma.

Nodular melanoma appears as a large, protuberant nodule that often attenuates the overlying epidermis (Fig. 20-37). Usually there are only small foci of intraepidermal melanoma, but by definition these do not extend laterally much beyond the dermal neoplasm. Arbitrarily, three rete ridges was set as the limit for such extension.[80] The cytology of the dermal cells is indistinguishable from that of superficial spreading melanomas of similar depth. Rare nodules of malignant melanoma arise in the dermal portions of intradermal melanocytic nevi, without detectable intraepidermal involvement, although the majority of such reports may relate melanomas whose intraepidermal components have been removed by shave biopsy or inadvertent

trauma or combined nevi misinterpreted as melanoma.[87] To those who use the histogenetic schema, there is no distinct boundary that separates a superficial spreading melanoma with a dominant nodule from a nodular malignant melanoma with slight intraepidermal extension even in the view of those who propound the histogenetic classification of melanoma. The configuration of each lesion doubtless depends on the relative rates of proliferation of the intraepidermal and invasive components. Nodular melanomas are thought to have begun as an in situ melanoma, but the rapid evolution of the dermal component overtook and obscured the in situ portion.

While most melanomas can be classified into one of the histogenetic types described by Clark; a sizable number defy such classification and there is considerable inter- and intraobserver inconsistency in its application. The value of classifying malignant melanoma has been challenged, as has the concept that a classification should be based on its intraepithelial growth pattern. The proponents of preserving Clark's histogenetic classification hold that while superficial spreading and nodular malignant melanoma seem to represent a continuum in terms of their biologic behavior, acral lentiginous and lentigo maligna melanoma have distinct epidemiologic features. Acral lentiginous melanoma has similar rates of incidence in dark-skinned races that do not develop other forms of melanoma.[88] Lentigo maligna melanoma is epidemiologically related to sun exposure, and in at least some studies patients with this form have a more favorable prognosis even when compared with patients with melanomas of similar thickness.

Melanoma has a wide variety of appearances well beyond those delineated in the histogenetic classification, and several unusual types should be noted. The epidermis can proliferate, resulting in a verrucous profile and pseudocarcinomatous hyperplasia histologically.[89] Neoplasms can grow exophytically to form polyps both on the trunk and in mucosal or juxtamucosal sites. Melanoma cells can confluently replace the basal layer of the epidermis, resulting in the dyshesion of epidermis and dermis and the formation of blisters.[90]

Although melanomas confined to the papillary dermis generally evoke a lymphocytic infiltrate, invasion of the reticular dermis is often accompanied by an apparent loss of immunogenicity and the absence of such an infiltrate. In occasional malignant melanomas, dermal nodules are heavily infiltrated by lymphocytes, simulating a halo nevus. The infiltration of nodules of melanoma by these so-called tumor-infiltrating lymphocytes is thought by some to be a favorable prognostic sign.[91]

The cytologic features of primary melanoma are highly variable and include small round, large round, ovoid, spindled, and polygonal melanocytes. The evolution of nuclear atypia in a melanoma appears to be a stepwise progression, and it is common to see several cytologic appearances within the dermal portion of a malignant melanoma. The cytoplasms of melanoma cells vary from scant and amphophilic to abundant and can be brightly eosinophilic, clear, or finely vacuolated. Melanin can be absent or abundant. Balloon cells similar to those seen in benign melanocytic nevi can occur as small clusters or diffusely. Melanin can be detected in many melanomas in which it is not apparent in routinely stained sections either with the Fontana-Masson stain or with the Warthin-Starry stain, performed at pH 3.2.

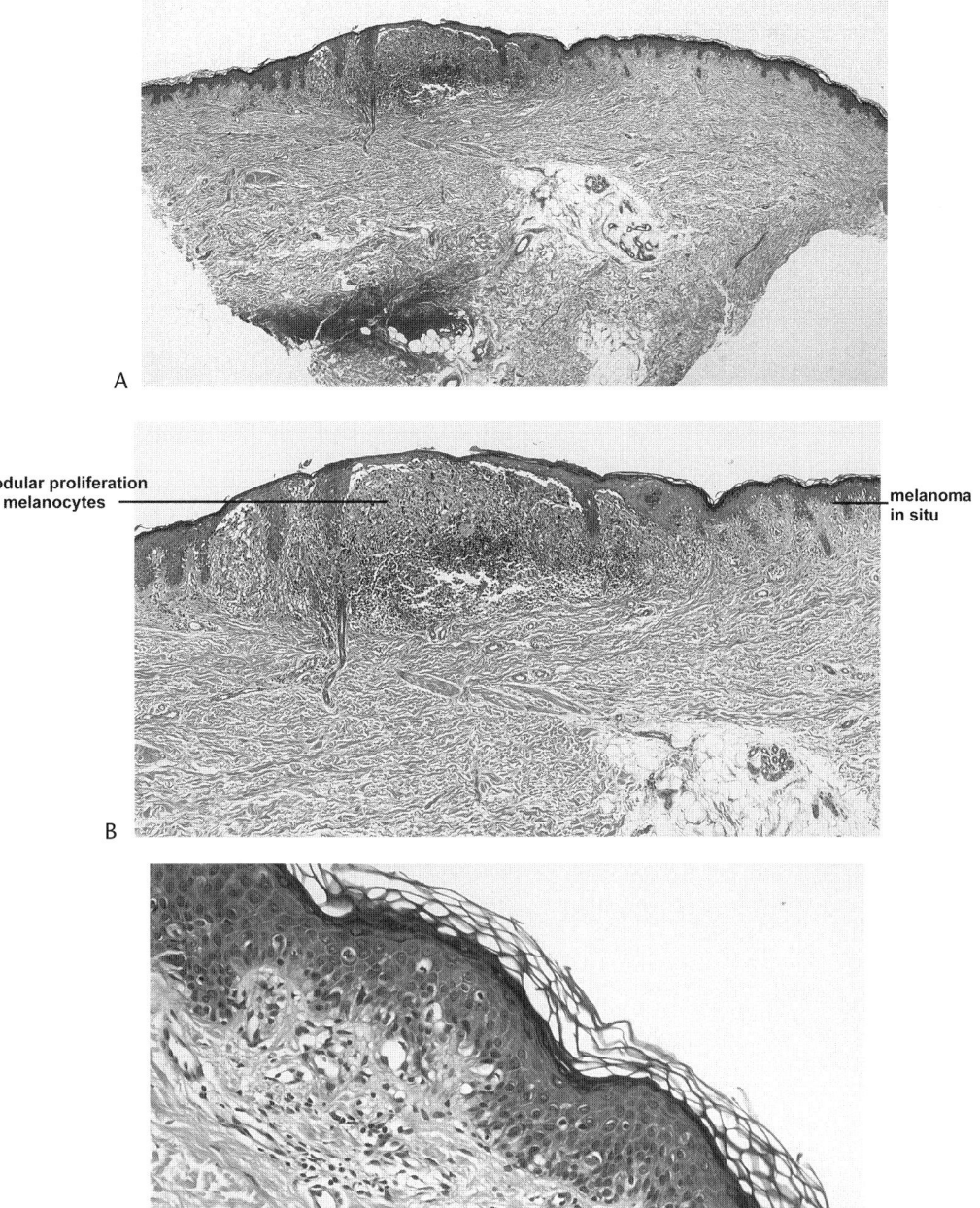

Figure 20-36. Melanoma with a superficial spreading growth pattern. It remains to be proven whether the histogenetic patterns outlined by Clark have prognostic value. At scanning magnification, there is a nodular proliferation of atypical melanocytes flanked by zones of melanoma in situ **(A)**. The epidermis is elevated above the nodular area **(B)**. Single melanocytes predominate at the periphery, some are above the basal layer, and there is poor lateral circumscription **(C)**. *Continued.*

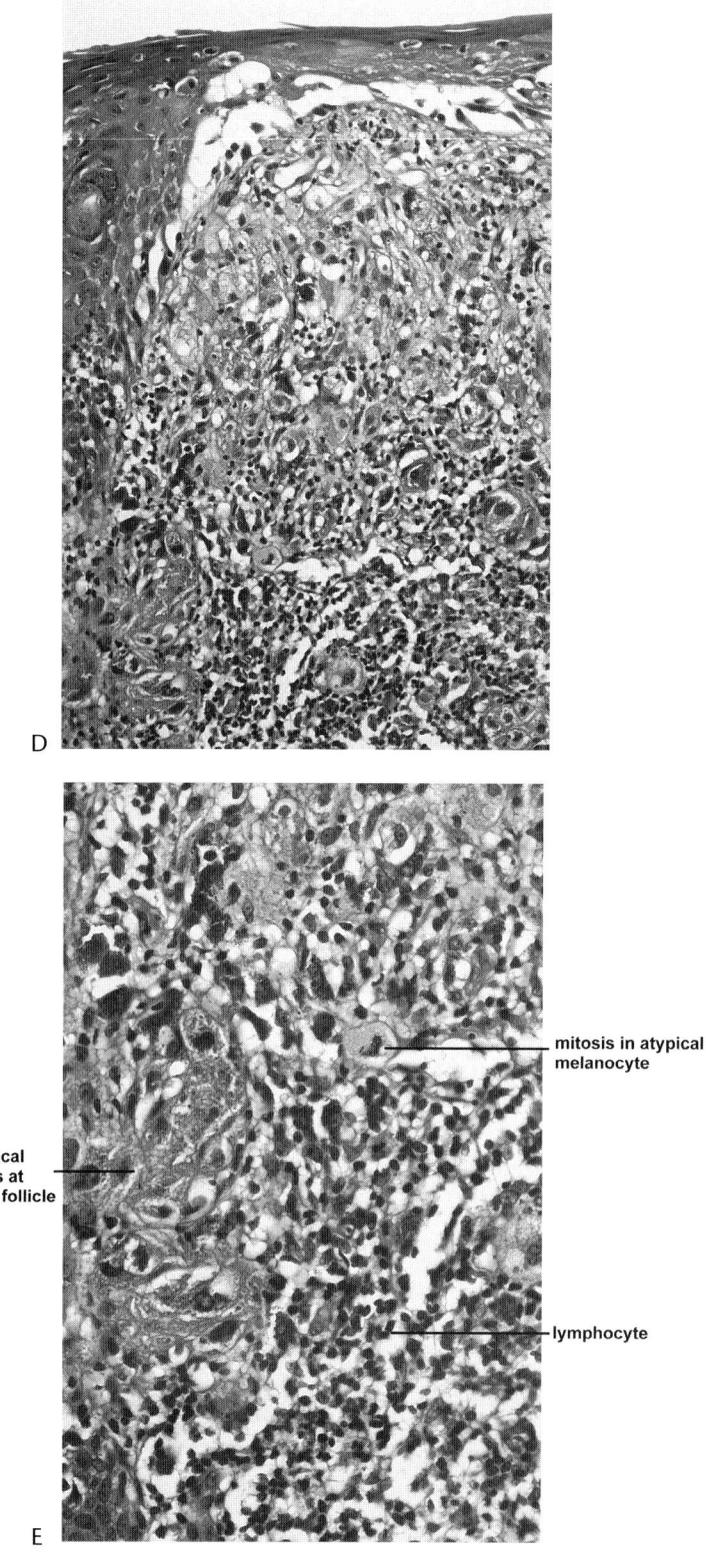

Figure 20-36. *Continued.* In the central area, maturation with descent is lacking **(D)**. Atypical nuclei and mitotic figures can be seen in this area **(E)**.

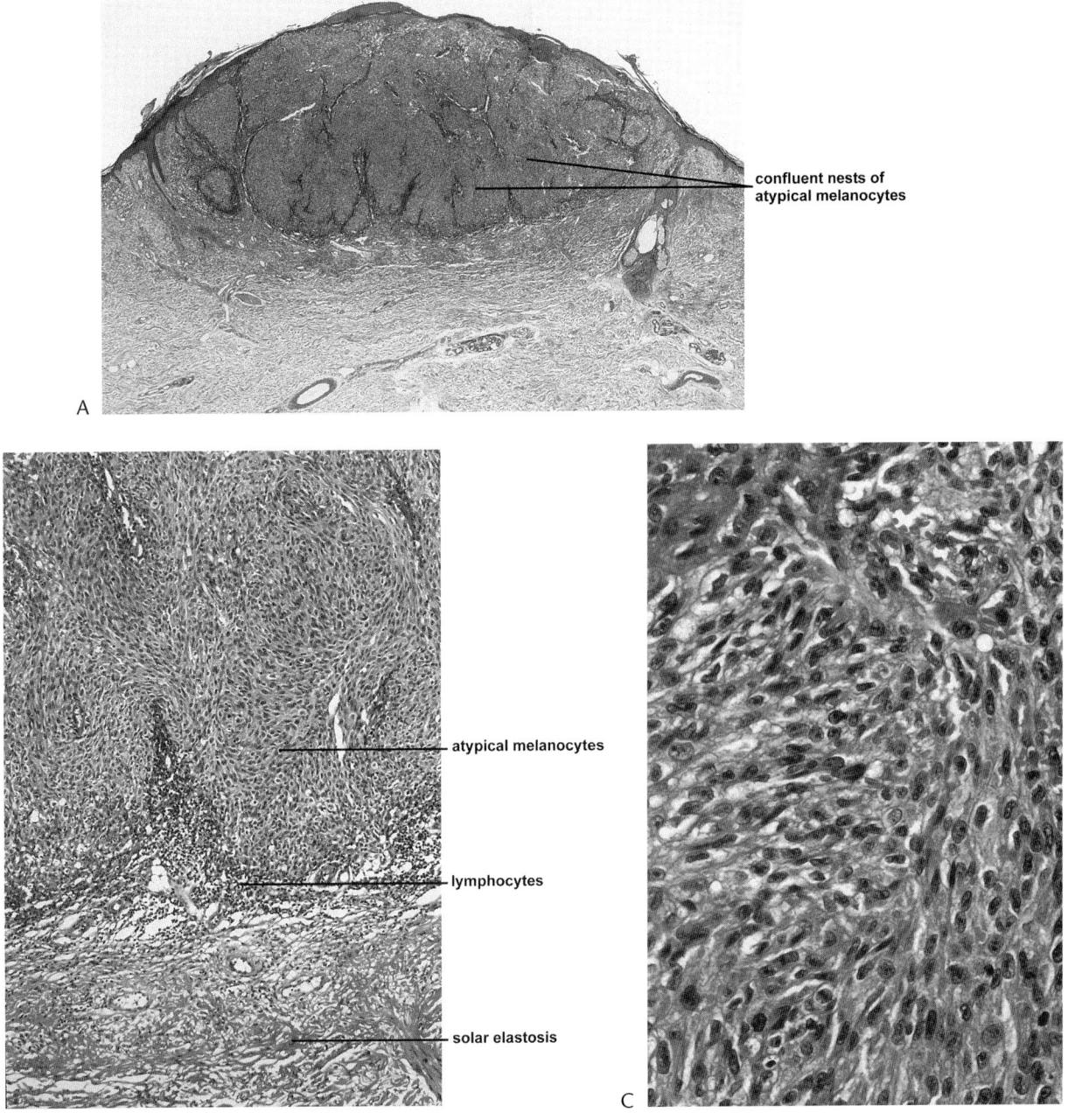

confluent nests of
atypical melanocytes

atypical melanocytes

lymphocytes

solar elastosis

A

B

C

Figure 20-37. Melanoma with a nodular growth pattern. There is no melanoma in situ in the adjacent epidermis. Presumably, the dermal proliferation eclipsed this earlier stage due to more rapid growth **(A)**. A sparse lymphocytic infiltrate is present at the blunt base of the lesion **(B)**. There is striking cytologic atypia of melanocytes even in the deep component **(C)**.

Stromal changes seen adjacent to dermal melanoma cells include desmoplasia and myxoid change. The latter can be so marked as to simulate such better-known myxoid neoplasms as liposarcoma and malignant schwannoma. Bony and cartilaginous foci, and even osteosarcomatous changes have been described, seemingly due to abnormal matrix production by aberrant melanocytes.[92]

Among the stromal changes seen in melanoma, desmoplasia is by far the most important. Desmoplastic melanoma occurs with no recognizable in situ component in almost one half of the reported cases. This may be due to abrasion removing the intraepidermal cells or to regression or to the neoplasm having a different evolutionary pathway than that of conventional melanoma. The dermal component of a desmoplastic melanoma appears as large spindled melanocytes intercalated between thickened collagen bundles. Usually the neoplasm involves both the superficial and deep dermis by the time that a lesion is sampled (Fig. 20-38). Elongated fascicles of spindled melanocytes are present in the more cellular areas; the least cellular ones can be difficult to distinguish from fibrosis, having slender spindled cells with bland nuclei. Nodular lymphocytic infiltrates are often present in the superficial subcutis if the process extends into the septa. Perineural invasion is so common in desmoplastic melanoma that it is sometimes termed *desmoplastic neurotropic melanoma.*

Various clinical features of primary melanoma are predictive of prognosis. Attributes that are important in this regard include the sex of the patient (women survive in greater numbers than do men, other attributes being equal) and site. Melanomas on the extremities (except for those on volar skin and nail beds) have the most favorable outcome, followed by lesions on the trunk. Particularly unfavorable locations include volar or subungual skin, scalp, ears, and mucous membranes or the skin adjacent to them. Perhaps the greater vascularity of these sites enables thinner lesions to generate metastases.

A number of histologic characteristics have also been investigated for their predictive value in prognostic models. Tumor thickness, as described by Breslow,[93] is of undisputed importance, although some patients with thin invasive tumors die of metastatic disease and others with thick lesions are long-term survivors. Thickness is measured with an ocular micrometer, although in very thick lesions a hand-held micrometer is preferable. The thickness measurement has been standardized as extending from the top of the granular layer of the epidermis to the deepest malignant melanocyte. There are many nuances of and exceptions to the standard application of this measurement, and it should be kept in mind that, as is the case with other prognostic factors, thickness measurements predict how a group of patients with melanoma will fare, not how an individual patient will do.[94]

Of lesser or disputed impact on prognosis are such features as mitotic rate, the presence, density, and distribution of the lymphocytic infiltrate, ulceration, ploidy, the presence of plasma cells, regression, and classification into "radial" or "vertical growth phase."

The mitotic rate of malignant melanoma is usually expressed in terms of mitoses/mm^2 and requires calibration of each individual microscope. One standard method is to scan the invasive portion of a melanoma for areas in which mitoses are frequent and then to count mitoses in contiguous nonoverlapping fields chosen in a random manner, beginning with a field in which mitoses are identified. This method is limited by the heterogeneity of mitotic activity within a neoplasm, the completion of cell division after biopsy, and other flaws. More objective measures of cellular proliferation, such as the percentage of cells in replicative phases of the cell cycle (assessed by immunoperoxidase staining for Ki-67) may eventually replace mitotic counts.

As noted above, a lymphocytic infiltrate is often present beneath early lesions of in situ and invasive melanoma, but is often absent beneath melanomas that invade deeply. Recent attention has been given to the role of tumor-infiltrating lymphocytes in the host response to neoplasia in general. In melanoma, tumor-infiltrating lymphocytes are those within rather than merely around or beneath nests of dermal melanoma cells. One study has shown a favorable prognostic influence of a dense infiltrate of tumor-infiltrating lymphocytes.[91] Plasma cells are usually seen only in infiltrates of thick tumors and are more common in ulcerated lesions. Their presence in melanomas whose surfaces are intact may be a reflection of exhaustion of T-cell–mediated immunity and seems to be an unfavorable prognostic influence in some studies.

Ulceration has long been known to be an adverse prognostic factor.[95] As with several other such markers, including the presence of plasma cells, its value as an independent variable is limited. Tumors generally do not ulcerate unless they are quite thick.

Ploidy, or relative DNA content of tumor cells, has a proven prognostic value in a number of neoplasms. Several studies have suggested that ploidy, as judged by flow or image analysis cytometry, may provide independent prognostic information.[96]

Regression has been viewed contradictorily as a marker of adverse and of favorable prognosis in several studies. Certainly metastatic disease has occurred in patients with completely regressed malignant melanomas and with in situ or partially regressed thin melanomas. Some of the conflicting data regarding the effect of regression on prognosis relate to the difficulty in recognizing partial regression and in quantifying regression in histopathologic cross sections. A more representative measurement of regression would be the area of skin involved, which would require clinical documentation and correlation with histopathologic features. At present it seems that small areas of partial regression do not substantially affect prognosis and that larger areas of regression in thin melanomas may be an unfavorable influence.[83,97]

Clark and co-workers[91] applied principles of tumor progression to classify malignant melanomas into radial and vertical growth phases. According to their definition, radial growth occurs in in situ lesions as well as in neoplasms in which the dermal cells do not form large (greater than 15 cells in diameter) aggregates or nests that exceed junctional ones of the same lesion in size (Fig. 20-39). Further characteristics of radial growth phase lesions include cytologic features that are similar to those in the intraepidermal portion of the neoplasm and dense lymphocytic infiltrates. A radial growth phase melanoma lacks the capacity to metastasize. Vertical growth phase lesions, in contrast, are capable of metastasis and have aggregates of dermal melanoma cells that are large and exceed junctional nests in size or in the atypia of their cells. Simply put, if the cells of a melanoma are capable of forming a mass in the dermis, they are capable of doing the same in a distant site, and if they are not, metastasis cannot occur.

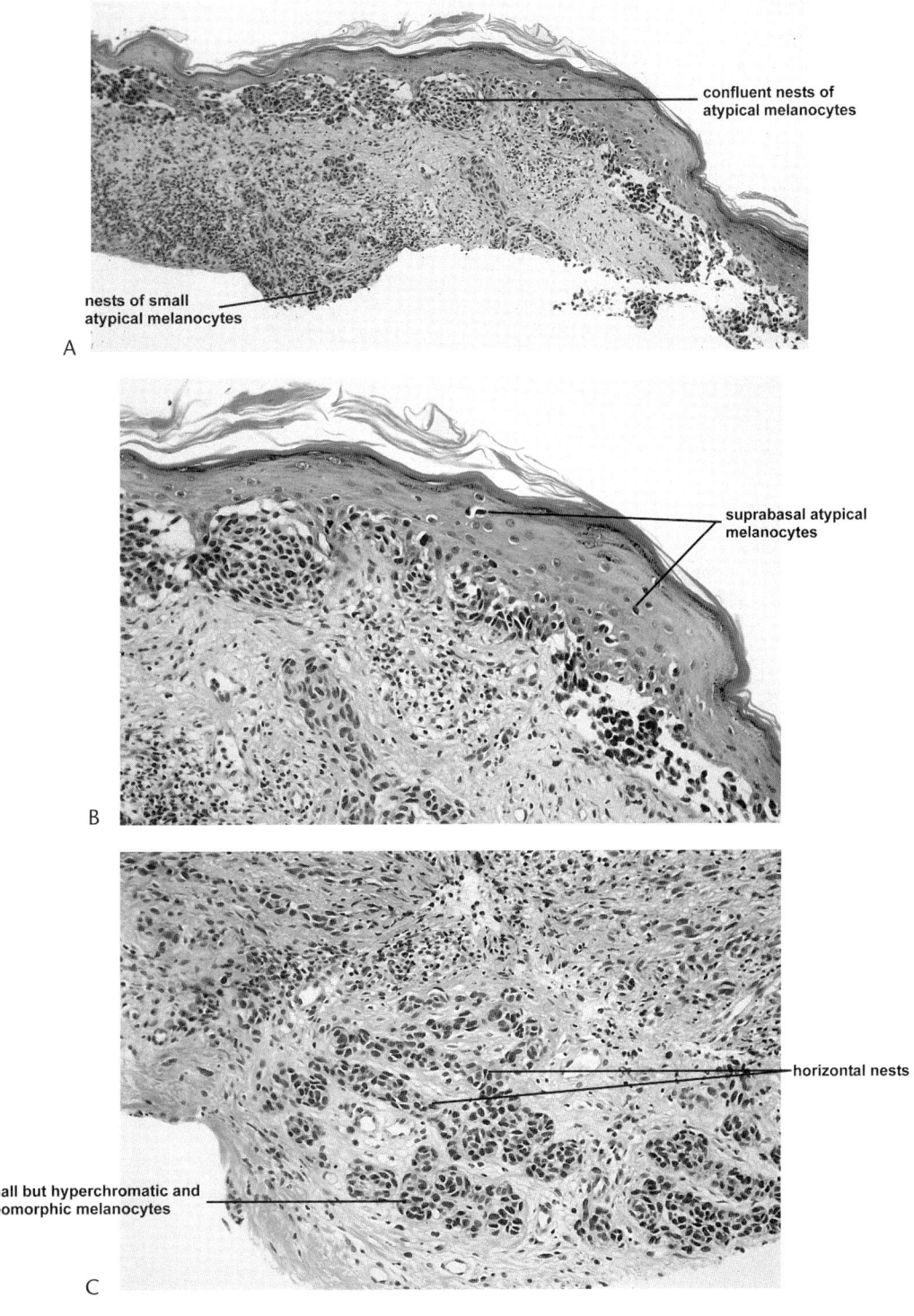

Figure 20-38. Melanoma with a dermal component of small, round cells—so-called nevoid melanoma. At first glance, one could easily mistake this lesion for a compound nevus **(A).** However, there are confluence of junctional nests and single melanocytes with hyperchromatic nuclei are present above the junction **(B).** The dermal component is compactly arranged, with many horizontally elongated aggregations **(C).** *Continued.*

Figure 20-38. *Continued.* The nuclei of these cells are hyperchromatic compared with those of a compound nevus **(D)**. Melanomas such as this one, in which small, round or nevoid cells represent the dermal component have also been termed minimal deviation melanoma. The evidence that their behavior is different from those of conventional melanomas is tenuous.

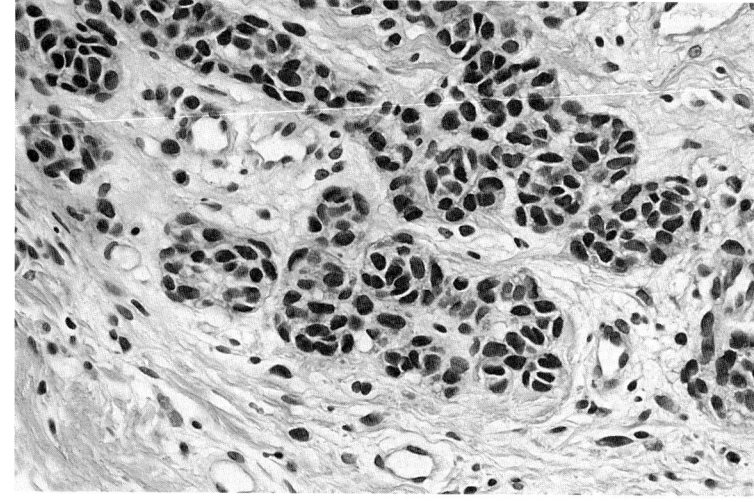

D

Figure 20-39. An invasive melanoma that would be classified as being in radial growth phase by the criteria of Clark and associates. At scanning magnification, there is a broad zone of melanoma in situ **(A)**. In one area, small clusters of atypical melanocytes are present in the papillary dermis **(B)**. *Continued.*

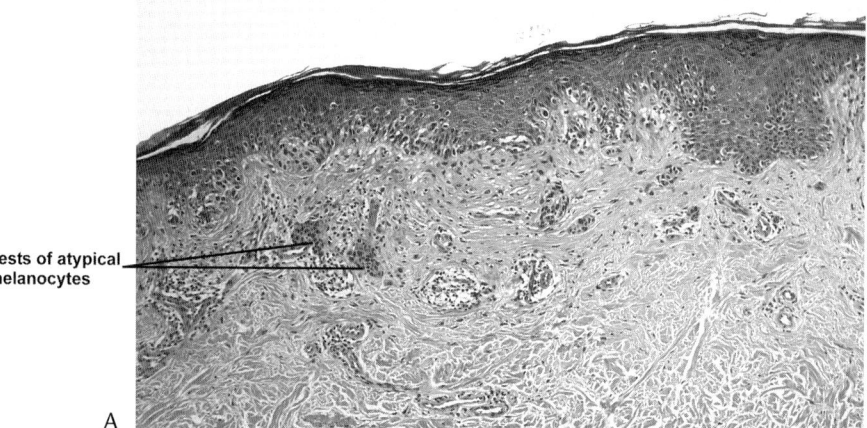

nests of atypical melanocytes

A

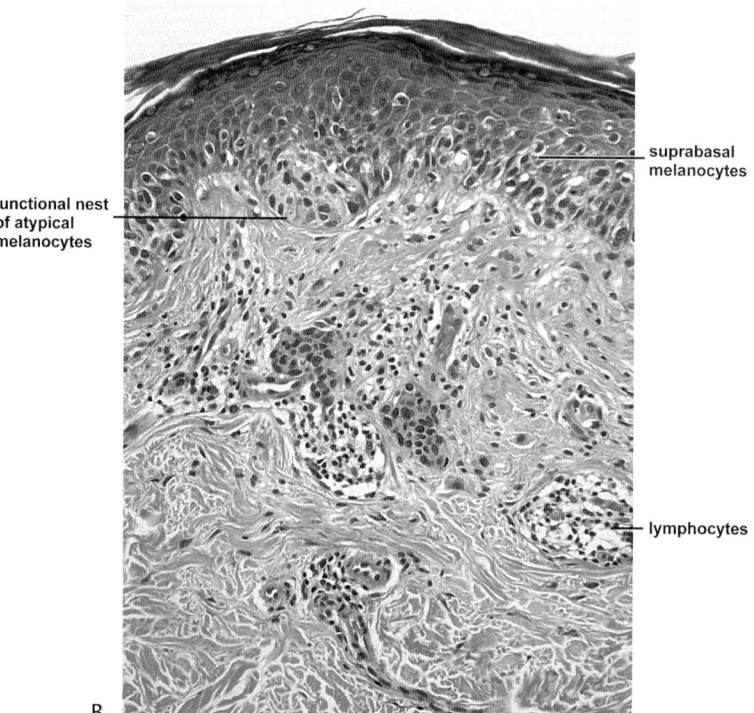

suprabasal melanocytes

junctional nest of atypical melanocytes

lymphocytes

B

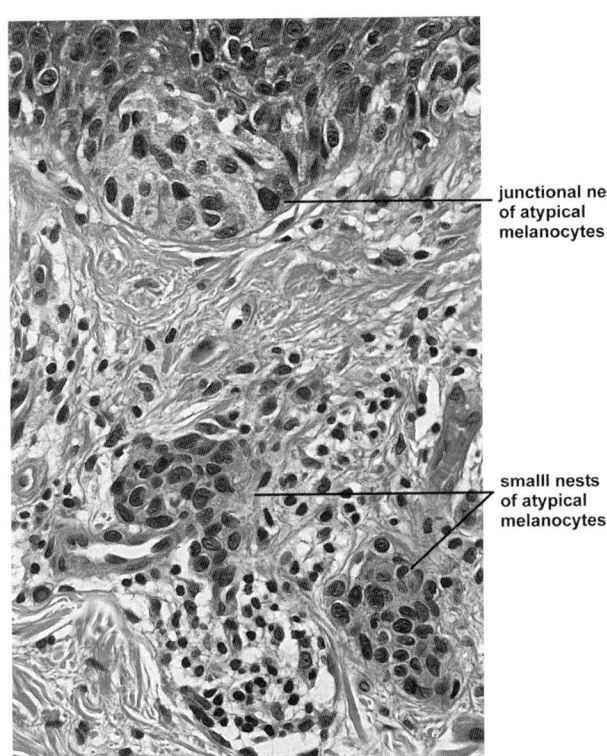

junctional nest
of atypical
melanocytes

smalll nests
of atypical
melanocytes

C

Figure 20-39. *Continued.* The size of these clusters does not exceed those at the junction **(C)**. Whether melanomas in which the invasive component meets the criteria of Clark and colleagues never metastasize is controversial.

Although conceptually appealing, there are reasons to be hesitant in accepting this schema entirely. Most malignant melanomas that are invasive, and yet would still be classified as being in radial growth phase, are thin, and metastases from these tumors would be expected to be rare in any event. Another explanation of the infrequency of metastases from "radial growth phase" melanomas is that metastatic potential is simply dependent on tumor volume and that the criteria that discriminate between radial and vertical growth simply distinguish between lesions with few and many dermal melanoma cells rather than reflect on the biology of intralesional tumor progression. A recent study of 167 cases demonstrated metastasis in three cases that reportedly fulfilled Clark's criteria for radial growth phase malignant melanoma.[98] As most of these were thin lesions using Breslow's thickness measurement, this finding calls into question whether pathologists can judge microscopically which thin melanomas will or will not metastasize.

At present, the intricacies of prognosis far exceed clinical utility. The simple strategy of complete removal of primary melanomas with a reasonable border of uninvolved skin, the removal of lymph nodes only if clinically involved, and the counseling of patients on their prognosis based on sex, site, and thickness has not yet been improved on. Adjuvant therapy for very thick melanomas may be beneficial, but quite coarse measurements of metastatic risk seem to suffice for making this decision.

Clinicopathologic Correlation

Each of the clinical features of malignant melanoma has a histologic correlate. The large size (compared with most acquired nevi) and asymmetry of many malignant melanomas are best appreciated in sections taken through the long axis of the lesion rather than by the "breadloaf" method of sectioning. The poor lateral circumscription evident clinically can be seen histologically as singly disposed neoplastic melanocytes that extend irregularly laterally beyond the last junctional nest or as junctional nests that are widely and irregularly spaced at the periphery of a tumor. The variability of color in many malignant melanomas reflects the amount of melanin within melanophages, melanocytes, and the epidermis, as well as inflammation (red or pink), and regression (white or blue-gray). Areas of invasion are frequently palpable as plaques, papules, or nodules. Desmoplastic melanomas are often firm or hard, and neurotropic ones can be painful.

Differential Diagnosis

The differential diagnosis of malignant melanoma in situ is covered in part in the sections on lentigo simplex and junctional nevi. Given that melanoma in situ regardless of histogenetic type begins as a proliferation of solitary melanocytes and only later eventuates in nests, it is exceptional for a lesion of melanoma in situ to be less than 3 mm in width and mostly nested. Larger in situ lesions, and the intraepidermal portions of invasive ones, can be mostly nested and can be mistaken for ordinary or Spitz nevi. Clues that such lesions are melanomas include the large size and irregular shapes of nests, variable spacing between them, lateral confluence of nests, and necrotic melanocytes.

Melanoma in situ must also be distinguished from other intraepidermal neoplasms that have a pagetoid pattern (i.e., the scatter of neoplastic cells, either singly or in small nests or both, within the epidermis). Mammary and extramammary Paget's disease differs from pagetoid malignant melanoma in that nests of cells often compress the basal layer of the epidermis rather than occupy a truly junctional position. Ductular spaces may be evident, and mucin (more often neutral mucin in mammary Paget's disease and acidic mucin in extramammary Paget's disease) can be detected with appropriate stains in the majority of cases. Pagetoid examples of Bowen's disease have dyskeratotic cells, multinucleated cells, and foci in which cells with atypical nuclei have visible intercellular bridges. Pagetoid spread can be present in Merkel cell carcinomas, which can rarely be mostly intraepidermal. As in Paget's disease, compression of basal cells is a valuable diagnostic clue, as are the cytologic features of this neuroendocrine carcinoma, namely, scant cytoplasm, homogeneous or smudged chromatin, and tiny nucleoli.[99] Pagetoid reticulosis, or Woringer-Kolopp disease, is an indolent, epidermotropic cutaneous T-cell lymphoma. It most often presents as a verrucous plaque on the hands or feet. Biopsy specimens show large, convoluted lymphocytes within the epidermis and sometimes within the dermis as well. Immunohistochemical studies have refined the differential diagnosis of pagetoid neoplasms. While most pagetoid malignant melanomas mark with antisera to S-100 protein, they do not express keratin filaments or leukocyte common antigen. On occasion, the cells of mammary Paget's disease can react with antisera to S-100 protein, but also contain keratin filaments and carcinoembryonic antigen.[100] Pagetoid Merkel cell carcinoma has a distinctive paranuclear dot-like pattern of deposition when stained with antisera to low-molecular-weight keratins and does not react with antisera to S-100 protein.

The differential diagnosis of invasive malignant melanoma versus benign melanocytic neoplasms is discussed in detail in the sections on Spitz nevus, blue nevus, halo nevus, and ordinary nevi.

Several pitfalls lie in the recognition of features within lesions in which the diagnosis of melanoma has already been made. The determination of whether small melanocytes at the base of a lesion of malignant melanoma are those of malignant melanoma or of a pre-existent nevus is often difficult. Features that favor cells of melanoma include horizontally oriented nests, cells with hyperchromatic nuclei, nuclei more than 10 μm in diameter, a lymphocytic infiltrate beneath the cells, and marked fibrosis around them. Mitotic figures or necrosis of melanocytes obviously favor small melanoma cells but are seldom present. Adnexocentric or vasocentric distribution and splaying of melanocytes between reticular dermal collagen bundles are hallmarks of the congenital type of melanocytic nevus and are infrequently mimicked by the small cells of a malignant melanoma. In many cases determining whether such cells are melanoma or pre-existent nevus does not matter, as the difference in the thickness measurements including and exempting these cells is prognostically trivial. In other cases the distinction can be between an in situ and a moderately thick lesion.

Another pitfall is in the identification of perineural invasion. Perineural invasion should be carefully looked for in a melanoma whose invasive portions are spindled. Normal or hypertrophic perineural cells can easily be mistaken for a perineurally invasive melanoma. Immunoperoxidase stains may be of help. Perineural melanoma cells stain with antiserum to S-100 protein, while perineural fibroblasts are S-100 protein negative but do express epithelial membrane antigen.[101]

Desmoplasia in malignant melanoma can be mistaken for the scar of a previous biopsy or vice versa. The collagen bundles of desmoplastic areas in malignant melanoma are generally thick and often randomly oriented, while the collagen of young scars is thin and the bundles are generally parallel to the epidermal surface. Fibroblast nuclei are monomorphous, thin, and tapered and arranged in parallel in recent scars, while the nuclei of desmoplastic malignant melanoma are pleomorphic and haphazardly arranged or grouped in fascicles. Immunoperoxidase staining for S-100 protein is of value, but care must be taken not to mistake dermal Langerhans cells for melanoma cells. Both mark with anti-S-100 antibodies, but Langerhans cells have dendritic processes. Desmoplastic Spitz nevus is usually well circumscribed and wedge shaped and has only solitary cells at its base. The aggregations of cells at any given depth within the dermis are of roughly the same size, unlike the case in desmoplastic melanoma.

Pathophysiology

Several studies suggest biological differences between the cells of so-called radial and vertical growth phase melanomas. Radial growth phase melanoma cells are said to lack the ability to produce tumors when injected into nude, athymic mice, fail to anchor in soft agar, and are purportedly composed of diploid rather than aneuploid cells. Whether these differences truly reflect biologic differences or are an artifact of the scant and, perhaps, heterogeneous population of dermal melanocytes in early invasive lesions awaits further study.

METASTATIC MELANOMA

Melanoma may spread from its site of origin by either the lymphatic or vascular route. Microsatellites are metastases to the dermis or fat immediately adjacent to a primary melanoma and, thus, are included in the excision of it. Satellite or "in transit" metastases are those seen clinically in the skin adjacent to a primary malignant melanoma. Melanoma can, of course, generate distant metastases either to lymph nodes or viscera.

Clinical Features

Most cutaneous metastases of melanoma present as papules or nodules, varying from a few millimeters to several centimeters in size. Unlike most primary melanomas, cutaneous metastases are generally well circumscribed, symmetric, and of uniform color, which can range from blue-white to brown to black. Ulceration can occur in large or long-standing cutaneous metastases.

Satellite metastases are most often seen with primary melanomas of the extremities or with melanomas in highly vascular areas such as the scalp or ears. On the extremities, satellites spread proximally.

There are several unusual forms of metastatic melanoma. In diffuse melanosis the patient's entire integument becomes pigmented, sometimes accompanied by melanuria.[102] Slate-gray macules can be produced by the spontaneous regression of metastatic melanoma, a condition termed *melanophagic dermatitis and panniculitis*.[103] In inflammatory melanoma there are erythematous plaques similar to those in inflammatory carcinoma of the breast or produced by other malignancies.[104]

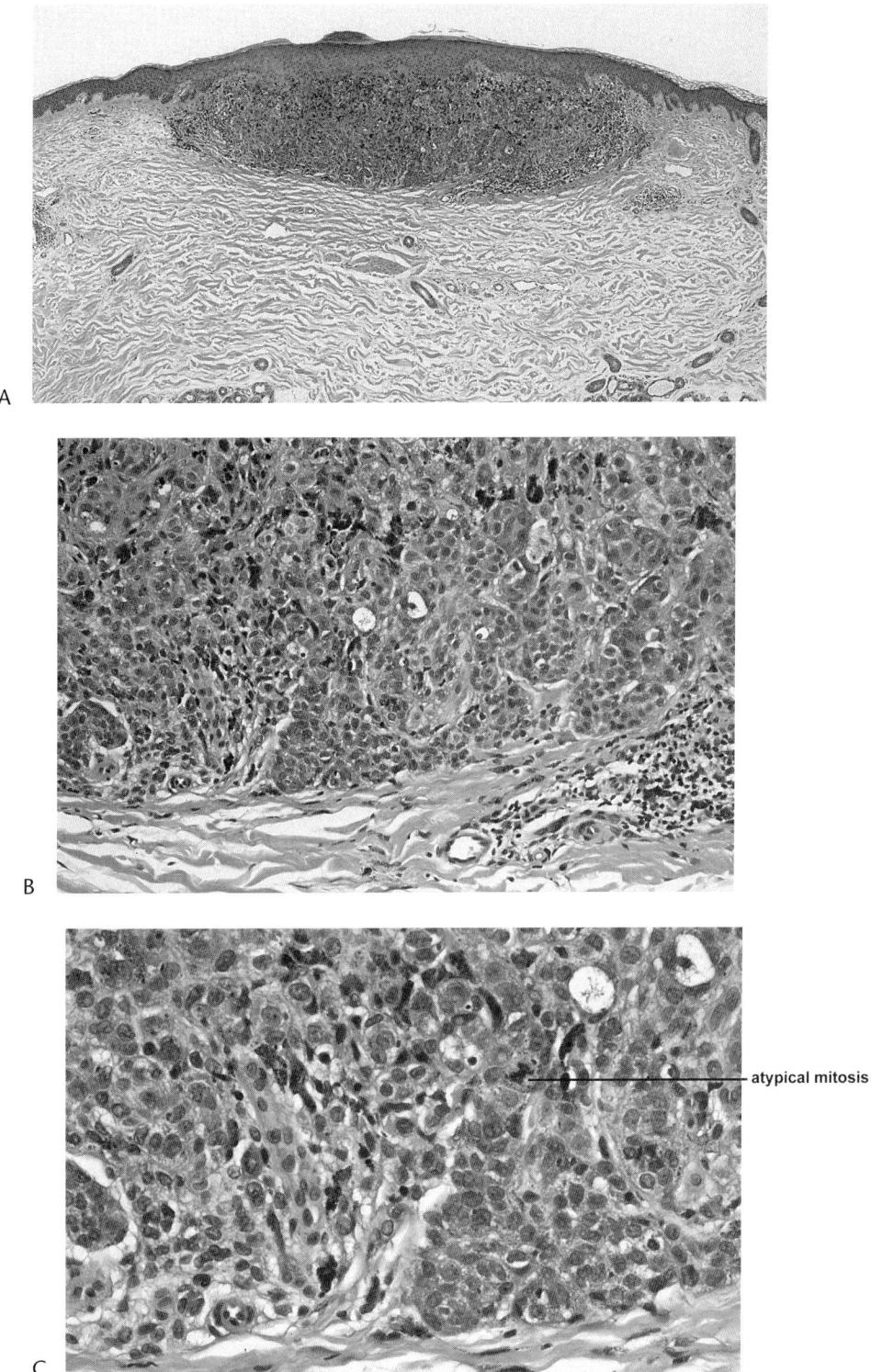

atypical mitosis

Figure 20-40. Metastatic melanoma. This relatively small lesion is composed of cells with striking cytologic atypia. Most primary melanomas do not contain such cells until they have evolved to become broader. The symmetric contour and sharp circumscription is characteristic of a metastasis **(A)**. The cells at the base of a metastatic melanoma in the skin are often smaller than those above, simulating maturation of a nevus **(B)**, but unlike the case in a nevus mitotic figures can be present.

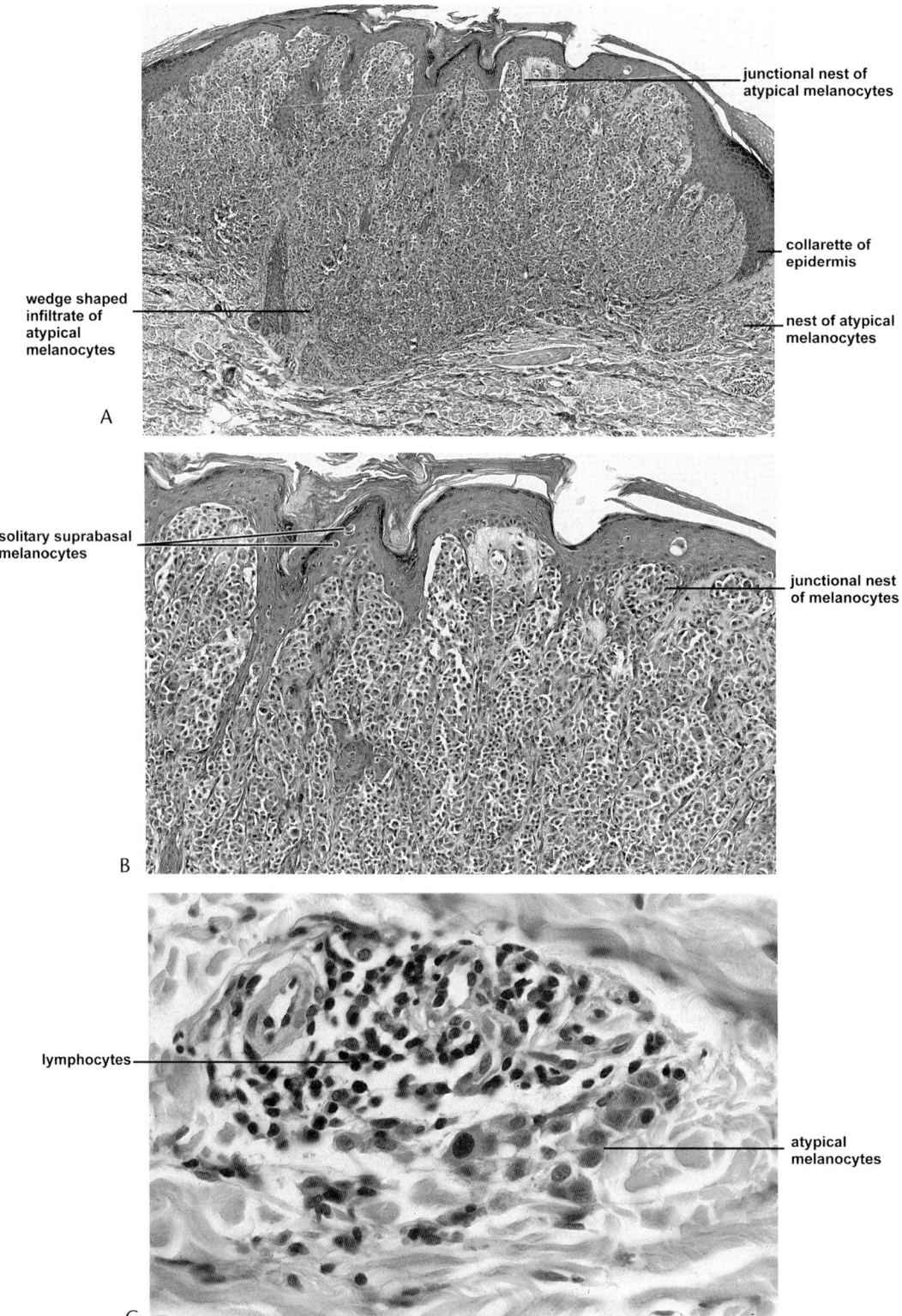

junctional nest of
atypical melanocytes

collarette of
epidermis

wedge shaped
infiltrate of
atypical
melanocytes

nest of atypical
melanocytes

A

solitary suprabasal
melanocytes

junctional nest
of melanocytes

B

lymphocytes

atypical
melanocytes

C

Figure 20-41. Epidermotropic metastatic melanoma. **(A)** At scanning magnification the dermal component extends laterally beyond the intradermal component of this papule. **(B)** Higher magnification reveals nests of atypical melanocytes at the dermo-epidermal junction and single melanocytes at higher levels in the epidermis. **(C)** Atypical melanocytes are present around vessels of the superficial plexus.

Histopathologic Features

Many cutaneous metastases of melanoma seem to grow in a spherical manner. They can lie entirely within the dermis or can abut the epidermis, which is often thinned. Many cutaneous metastases in close proximity to the epidermis are surrounded by epithelial collarettes as a result of their rapid growth (Fig. 20-40). Infiltration of the overlying epidermis is seen in epidermotropic metastatic melanoma.[105] In rare cases there are many metastases that histopathologically resemble primary malignant melanoma, with most of the metastatic cells colonizing the epidermis[106] (Fig. 20-41). Often, melanoma cells are evident in lymphatic spaces at the base of a cutaneous metastasis of malignant melanoma.

The cells of a single lesion of metastatic melanoma are generally of a single cytologic type (e.g., large, polygonal cells with pink cytoplasm or ovoid cells with abundant cytoplasm and dusty-appearing melanin) within a given metastasis. As a group, the nuclear atypia evident in metastatic melanoma exceeds that in primary malignant melanoma. There have been many reports of unusual cytologic findings in metastases of malignant melanoma, including signet ring cells, metastases composed of spindled cells, sometimes producing desmoplasia or simulating neoplasms of neural origin, numerous giant cells resulting in a picture resembling that of malignant fibrous histiocytoma, or concentrically arranged cells (tumor cell cannibalism) simulating keratin pearl formation.[107]

In patients with diffuse melanosis, the discoloration appears to be produced by melanin in macrophages and in endothelial cells and in some cases additionally by dissemination of melanoma cells.[102] In melanophagic dermatitis only melanophages persist in the dermis or subcutis as the residuum of a regressed metastasis.[103] Inflammatory melanoma features aggregations of melanoma cells enmeshed in fibrin within the lumens of small dermal vessels.[104]

Melanoma metastatic to lymph nodes can result in small deposits of cells in the subcapsular sinus, sometimes so subtle that their detection is only possible with immunohistochemical methods. The finding of so-called "occult tumor cells" in lymph nodes stained with antisera to S-100 protein is an unfavorable prognostic finding.[108] Nodules of melanoma cells in the lymph node cortex, complete nodal replacement, and extension of melanoma cells into the perinodal fat signify that melanoma cells are successfully proliferating within a lymph node.

Clinicopathologic Correlation

The symmetric, domed shape of metastatic melanoma is the result of the proliferation of a single cell or small group of cells, in contrast to most primary malignant melanomas in which lateral spread of neoplastic cells and variable rates of proliferation of different cells within a given lesion result in a less orderly appearance. The color of metastatic melanoma is dependent on the pigmentation of its cells and on the depth of the neoplasm beneath the surface of the skin.

The differential diagnosis of melanophagic dermatitis or panniculitis secondary to regression of metastatic malignant melanoma includes postinflammatory pigmentary alteration in which melanophages are present in the papillary dermis only. This is in contrast to the dense nodular aggregations of melanophages seen in melanophagic dermatitis.

The differential diagnosis of inflammatory melanoma includes those conditions in which disseminated neoplastic cells plug the lumens of cutaneous venules. Inflammatory carcinoma can derive from adenocarcinomas of the breast or pancreas, and the cells of malignant lymphoma can occlude vascular lumens in intravascular lymphomatosis. Immunoperoxidase staining can be used to resolve this differential diagnosis if melanin is not present in the intravascular cells.

Small subcapsular deposits of metastatic melanoma are usually found in elective lymph node dissections or in clinically uninvolved nodes in a therapeutic lymph node dissection. Larger deposits of melanoma cells that take up more than one fourth of a node's cross-sectional area and are palpable have a worse prognosis than microscopic metastases.[109]

Differential Diagnosis

The differential diagnosis of metastatic versus primary melanoma can be a difficult one as both can be symmetric, well-circumscribed nodules with epidermal infiltration. Features that favor metastatic over primary malignant melanoma include a "starburst" distribution of cells in which melanocytes seem to radiate from a central point, melanocytes within lymphatic spaces at the base of the nodule, and a few melanocytes within the epidermis above the center of the nodule. In epidermotropic metastatic melanoma, small nests of melanocytes can outnumber singly disposed cells in the suprabasilar epidermis. A dense lymphocytic infiltrate is rare in cutaneous metastases of malignant melanoma.

Rarely, epidermotropically metastatic melanoma can result in lesions in which melanocytes spread laterally to the dermal portion of the metastasis, further simulating primary melanoma.[106] The clinical presentation is obviously that of metastatic melanoma in most such cases. Melanoma cells in lymphatic spaces beneath a melanoma that is only superficially invasive is another clue to this form of epidermotropic metastatic melanoma.

The differential diagnosis of melanoma metastatic to lymph nodes or other organs is vast and lies more within the sphere of the surgical pathologist than it does the dermatopathologist. A familiarity with the many unusual guises of metastatic melanoma, such as the pseudopapillary, pseudoalveolar, and pseudoglandular patterns, metastases with myxoid stroma or metaplastic changes, branching vessels simulating hemangiopericytoma, or ribbon-like arrangements simulating neuroendocrine neoplasms can prevent many dilemmas.[107] While there is only a limited use for immunoperoxidase staining with HMB-45 in cutaneous melanocytic neoplasms, this antiserum is a relatively specific marker of melanocytic lineage in evaluating metastatic lesions. Antibodies to S-100 protein are also useful and are more sensitive, but less specific, marking a variety of carcinomas.[110] Hence, they should be used along with antikeratin antisera.

REFERENCES

1. Masson P: My conception of cellular nevi. Cancer 4:9–38, 1951
2. van der Esch EP, Rampen FHJ: Punch biopsy of melanoma. J Am Acad Dermatol 13:899–902, 1985
3. Lund HZ, Stobbe GD: The natural history of the pigmented nevus: factors of age and anatomic location. Am J Pathol 25:1117, 1949
4. Connelly J, Smith JL Jr: Malignant blue nevus. Cancer 67:2653–2657, 1991
5. Abernethy JL, Soyer HP, Kerl H, Jorizzo JL, White NL: Epidermotropic metastatic melanoma simulating melanoma in situ: a report of 10 examples from two patients. Am J Surg Pathol 18:1140–1149, 1994
6. Echevarria R, Ackerman LV: Spindle and epithelioid nevi in the adult. Clinicopathologic report of 26 cases. Cancer 20:175–189, 1967
7. Weedon D, Little JH: Spindle and epithelioid cell nevi in children and adults. A review of 211 cases of the Spitz nevus. Cancer 40:217–225, 1997
8. Bolognia JL: Reticulated black solar lentigo ("ink spot lentigo"). Arch Dermatol 128:934–940, 1992
9. Sison-Torre EO, Ackerman AB: Melanosis of the vulva: a clinical simulator of malignant melanoma. Am J Dermatopathol 7(suppl):51–60, 1985
10. Wolinsky S, Silvers DIV: The small lentiginous nevus. Am J Dermatopathol 7(suppl):5–11, 1985
11. Rhodes AR, Harrist TJ, Momtaz TK: The PUVA-induced pigmented macule: a lentiginous proliferation of large, sometimes cytologically atypical, melanocytes. J Am Acad Dermatol 9:47–58, 1983
12. Stern JB, Peck GL, Haupt HM et al: Malignant melanoma in xeroderma pigmentosum: search for a precursor lesion. J Am Acad Dermatol 28:591–594, 1995
13. Montagna W, Hu F, Carlisle K: A reinvestigation of solar lentigines. Arch Dermatol 116:1151–1154, 1980
14. Maize JC: Mucosal melanosis. Dermatol Clin 6:283–293, 1988
15. Maize JC, Foster G: Age-related changes in melanocytic nevi. Clin Exp Dermatol 4:49–58, 1979
16. Orkin M, Frichot BC III, Zelickson AS: Cerebriform intradermal nevus. A case of cutis verticis gyrata. Arch Dermatol 110:575, 1974
17. Guzzo C, Johnson B, Honig P: Cockarde nevus: a case report and review of the literature. Pediatr Dermatol 4:250–253, 1988
18. Haupt HM, Stern JB: Pagetoid melanocytosis: histologic features in benign and malignant lesions. Am J Surg Pathol 19:792–797, 1995
19. Clark WH, Reimer RR, Greene M et al: Origin of familial malignant melanomas from hereditable melanocytic lesions. "The B-K mole syndrome." Arch Dermatol 114:732–738, 1978
20. Clark WH, Elder DE, Guerry D et al: A study of tumor progression: the precursor lesions of superficial spreading and nodular melanoma. Hum Pathol 15:1147–1165, 1984
21. Elder DE, Goldman LI, Goldman SC et al: Dysplastic nevus syndrome: a phenotypic association of sporadic cutaneous melanoma. Cancer 46:1787–1794, 1980
22. Ackerman AB, Mihara I: Dysplasia, dysplastic melanocytes, dysplastic nevi, the dysplastic nevus syndrome, and the relation between dysplastic nevi and malignant melanomas. Hum Pathol 16:87–91, 1985
23. Ackerman AB: What naevus is dysplastic, a syndrome and the commonest precursor of malignant melanoma? A riddle and an answer. Histopathology 13:241–256, 1988
24. Piepkorn M, Meyer L, Goldgar D et al: The dysplastic nevus: a prevalent lesion that correlates poorly with clinical phenotype. J Am Acad Dermatol 20:407–415, 1989
25. Klein LJ, Barr RJ: Histologic atypia in clinically benign nevi; a prospective study. J Am Acad Dermatol 2:275–282, 1990
26. Kraemer KH, Greene MH, Tarone R et al: Dysplastic nevi and cutaneous melanoma risk. Lancet 2:1076–1077, 1983
27. Clark WH Jr, Ackerman AB: An exchange of views regarding the dysplastic nevus controversy. Semin Dermatol 8:229–250, 1989
28. Sagebiel RW, Bonda PW, Schneider JS et al: Age distribution and histologic patterns of dysplastic nevi. J Am Acad Dermatol 13:975–982, 1985
29. Ackerman AB, Magana-Garcia M: Naming acquired melanocytic nevi. Unna's, Miescher's, Spitz's, Clark's. Am J Dermatopathol 12:193–209, 1990
30. National Institutes of Health: Consensus Development Conference Statement on Diagnosis and Treatment of Early Melanoma, January 27–29, 1992. Am J Dermatopathol 15:34–43, 1992
31. Harley S, Walsh N: A new look at nevus-associated melanomas. Am J Dermatopathol 18:137–141, 1996
32. Christensen WN, Friedman KJ, Woodruff JD et al: Histologic characteristics of vulvar nevocellular nevi. J Cutan Pathol 14:87–91, 1987
33. Meyerson LB: A peculiar papulosquamous eruption involving pigmented nevi. Arch Dermatol 103:510–512, 1971
34. Gray MH, Smoller BR, McNutt NS, Hsu A: Immunohistochemical demonstration of factor XIIIa expression in neurofibromas. A practical means of differentiating these tumors from neurotized intradermal melanocytic nevi and schwannomas. Arch Dermatol 126:472–476, 1990
35. Pierard GE, Pierard-Franchimont C: The proliferative activity of cells of malignant melanomas. Am J Dermatopathol 6:317S–23S, 1984
36. Smolle J, Soyer H-P, Kerl H: Proliferative activity of cutaneous melanocytic tumors defined by Ki-67 monoclonal antibody. A quantitative immunohistochemical study. Am J Dermatopathol 11:301–307, 1989
37. Goovaerts G, Buyssens N: Nevus cell maturation or atrophy? Am J Dermatopathol 10:20–27, 1988
38. Wayte DM, Helwig EB: Halo nevi. Cancer 22:69–90, 1968
39. Pennys NS, Mayoral F, Barnhill R et al: Delineation of nevus cell nests in inflammatory infiltrates by immunohistochemical staining for the presence of S100 protein. J Cutan Pathol 12:28–32, 1985
40. Schmitt D, Ortonne JP, Haftek M et al: Halo nevus and halo melanoma. Immunocytochemical study of the inflammatory cell infiltrate. pp. 333–340. In Ackerman AB (ed): Pathology of Malignant Melanoma. New York: Masson Publications, 1981

41. Walton RG, Jacobs AH, Cox AJ: Pigmented lesions in newborn infants. Br J Dermatol 95:389–396, 1976

42. Pers M: Nevus pigmentosus giganticus. Ugeskr Laeger 125:613–619, 1963

43. Kopf AW, Bart RS, Hennessey P: Congenital melanocytic nevi and malignant melanomas. J Am Acad Dermatol 1:123–130, 1979

44. Stewart DM, Altman J, Mehregan AH: Speckled lentiginous nevus. Arch Dermatol 114:895–896, 1978

45. Stenn KS, Arons M, Hurwitz S: Patterns of congenital nevocellular nevi. A histologic study of thirty-eight cases. J Am Acad Dermatol 9:388–393, 1983

46. Clemmenson OJ, Kroon S: The histology of "congenital features" in early acquired melanocytic nevi. J Am Acad Dermatol 19:642–666, 1988

47. Mark GJ, Mihm MC, Liteplo MG et al: Congenital melanocytic nevi of the small and garment type: clinical, histologic and ultrastructural studies. Hum Pathol 4:394–418, 1973

48. Silvers DN, Helwig EB: Melanocytic nevi in neonates. J Am Acad Dermatol 4:166–175, 1981

49. Hendrikson MR, Ross JC: Neoplasms arising in congenital pigmented nevi. Am J Surg Pathol 5:109–135, 1981

50. Elder DE, Murphy GF: Atlas of Tumor Pathology (AFIP). Third Series. Fascicle 2. Melanocytic Tumors of the Skin. Bethesda, Armed Forces Institute of Pathology (AFIP), Washington, D.C. pp 95–96, 1991

51. National Institutes of Health. Consensus Development Conference Statement, October 24–26, 1984. Precursors of malignant melanoma. J Am Acad Dermatol 10:683–688, 1984

52. Stenzinger W, Suter L, Schumann J: DNA aneuploidy in congenital melanocytic nevi: suggestive evidence for premalignant changes. J Invest Dermatol 82:569–572, 1984

53. Ellis DL, Wheeland RG, Solomon H: Estrogen and progesterone receptors in congenital melanocytic nevi. J Am Acad Dermatol 12:235–244, 1985

54. Burket JM: Multiple benign juvenile melanoma. Arch Dermatol 115:229, 1979

55. Paniago-Pereira C, Maize J, Ackerman AB: Nevus of large spindle and/or epithelioid cells (Spitz's nevus). Arch Dermatol 114:1811–1823, 1978

56. Kamino H, Misheloff E, Ackerman AB et al: Eosinophilic globules in Spitz's nevi. New findings and a diagnostic sign. Am J Dermatopathol 1:319–324, 1979

57. Arbuckle S, Weedon D: Eosinophilic globules in the Spitz nevus. J Am Acad Dermatol 7:324–327, 1982

58. Sagebiel RW, Chinn EK, Egbert BM: Pigmented spindle cell nevus. Clinical and histologic review of 90 cases. Am J Surg Pathol 8:645–653, 1984

59. Spitz S: Melanomas of childhood. Am J Pathol 24:591–609, 1948

60. Barr RJ, King DF: The significance of pseudoinclusions within the nuclei of melanocytes of certain neoplasms. pp. 269–272. In Ackerman AB (ed): Pathology of Malignant Melanoma. New York: Masson Publications, 1981

61. Barr RJ, Morales RV, Graham JH: Desmoplastic nevus. A distinct histologic variant of mixed spindle cell and epithelioid cell nevus. Cancer 46:557–564, 1980

62. Merot Y, Frenk E: Spitz nevus (large spindle and/or epithelioid cell nevus). Age related involvement of the suprabasilar epidermis. Virchow's Arch A (Pathol Anat) 415:97–101, 1989

63. Okun MR: Melanoma resembling spindle and epithelioid cell nevus. Arch Dermatol 115:1416–1420, 1979

64. Howat AJ, Variend S: Lymphatic invasion in Spitz nevi. Am J Surg Pathol 9:125–128, 1985

65. Smith KJ, Skelton HG, Lupton GP et al: Spindle cell and epithelioid cell nevus with atypia and metastasis (malignant Spitz nevus). Am J Surg Pathol 13:931–939, 1989

66. LeBoit PE, Fletcher HV: A comparative study of Spitz nevus and nodular malignant melanoma using image analysis cytometry. J Invest Dermatol 88:753–757, 1987

67. Sun C-C, Lu Y-C, Lee EF et al: Nevus fusco-caeruleus zygomaticus. Br J Dermatol 117:545–553, 1987

68. Okawa Y, Yokota R, Ymauchi A: On the extracellular sheath of dermal melanocytes in nevus fuscoceruleus acromiodeltoideus (Ito) and mongolian spot. An ultrastructural study. J Invest Dermatol 73:224–230, 1979

69. Rodriguez HA, Ackerman LV: Cellular blue nevus. Clinicopathologic study of 45 cases. Cancer 21:393–405, 1968

70. Seab JA, Graham JH, Helwig EB: Deep penetrating nevus. Am J Surg Pathol 13:39–44, 1989

71. Temple-Camp CRE, Saxe N, King H: Benign and malignant cellular blue nevus. A clinicopathologic study of 30 cases. Am J Dermatopathol 10:289–296, 1988

72. Ishibashi A, Kimura K, Kukita A: Plaque-type blue nevus combined with lentigo (nevus spilus). J Cutan Pathol 17:241–245, 1990

73. Fletcher V, Sagebiel RW: The combined nevus. p. 273. In Ackerman AB (ed): Pathology of Malignant Melanoma. New York, Masson Publishing 1981

74. Cooper PH: Deep penetrating (plexiform spindle cell) nevus: a frequent participant in combined nevus. J Cutan Pathol 19:172–180, 1992

75. Schoenfeld RJ, Pinkus H: The recurrence of nevi after incomplete removal. Arch Dermatol 78:30–35, 1958

76. Kornberg R, Ackerman AB: Pseudomelanoma: recurrent melanocytic nevus following partial surgical removal. Arch Dermatol 111:1588–1590, 1975

77. Park HK, Leonard DD, Arrington III JH et al: Recurrent melanocytic nevi: clinical and histologic review of 175 cases. J Am Acad Dermatol 17:285–292, 1987

78. Estrada JA, Pierard-Franchimont C, Pierard G: Histogenesis of recurrent nevus. Am J Dermatopathol 12:370–372, 1990

79. Stern JB: Recurrent Spitz's nevi. Am J Dermatopathol 7 (suppl):49–50, 1985

80. Clark WH Jr, Elder DE, Van Horn M: The biologic forms of malignant melanoma. Hum Pathol 17:443–450, 1986

81. Ackerman AB, David KM: A unifying concept of malignant melanoma: Biologic aspects. Hum Pathol 17:438–440, 1986

82. Tschen JA, Fordice DB, Reddick M, Stehlin J: Amelanotic melanoma presenting as inflammatory plaques. J Am Acad Dermatol 27:464–465, 1992

83. Cooper PH, Wanebo JH, Hagar RW: Regression in thin malignant melanoma. Microscopic diagnosis and prognostic importance. Arch Dermatol 121:1127–1131, 1985

84. Rhodes AR, Harrist TJ, Day CL et al: Dysplastic melanocytic nevi in histologic association with 234 primary cutaneous melanomas. J Am Acad Dermatol 9:563–574, 1983

85. Penneys NS: Microinvasive lentigo maligna melanoma. J Am Acad Dermatol 17:675–680, 1987

86. Reed RJ, Leonard DD: Neurotropic melanoma (a variant of desmoplastic melanoma). Am J Surg Pathol 3:301–311, 1979

87. Benisch B, Peison B, Kannerstein M, Spivack J: Arch Dermatol 116:696–698, 1980

88. Arrington JH II, Reed RJ, Ichinose H et al: Plantar lentiginous melanoma: a distinctive variant of cutaneous malignant melanoma. Am J Surg Pathol 1:131–143, 1977

89. Kamino H, Tam St, Alvarez L: Malignant melanoma with pseudocarcinomatous hyperplasia–an entity that can simulate squamous cell carcinoma. A light-microscopic and immunohistochemical study. Am J Dermatopathol 12:446–451, 1990

90. Pierard GE: Melanome malin bulleux. Dermatologica 170:48–50, 1985

91. Clark WH Jr, Elder DE, Guerry DG et al: A model predicting survival in stage I melanoma based upon tumor progression. JNCI 81:1893–1904, 1989

92. Chung EB, Enzinger FM: Malignant melanoma of soft parts: reassessment of clear cell sarcoma. Am J Surg Pathol 7:405–413, 1983

93. Breslow A: Thickness, cross-sectional area and depth of invasion in the prognosis of cutaneous melanoma. Ann Surg 172:902–908, 1970

94. Green MS, Ackerman AB: Thickness is not an accurate gauge of prognosis of primary cutaneous melanoma. Am J Dermatopathol 15:461–473, 1993

95. Balch CM: The prognostic significance of ulceration of cutaneous melanoma. Cancer 45:3012–3017, 1980

96. Kheir SM, Bines SD, Vonroenn JH et al: Prognostic significance of DNA aneuploidy in stage I cutaneous melanoma. Ann Surg 207:455–461, 1988

97. Ronan SG, Eng Am, Briele HA et al: Thin malignant melanomas with regression and metastases. Arch Dermatol 1326–1330, 1987

98. Barnhill RL, Fine JA, Roush GC et al: Predicting five-year outcome for patients with cutaneous melanoma in a population-based study. Cancer 78:427–432, 1996

99. LeBoit PE, Crutcher W, Shapiro P: Pagetoid intraepidermal spread in cutaneous (neuroendocrine) carcinoma. Am J Surg Pathol 16:584–592, 1992

100. Guarner J, Cohen C, DeRose PB: Histogenesis of extramammary and mammary Paget cells: an immunohistochemical study. Am J Dermatopathol 11:313–318, 1989

101. Erlandson RA: The enigmatic perineural cell and its participation in tumors and tumorlike entities. Ultrastruct Pathol 15:335–351, 1991

102. Steiner A, Rappersberger K, Groh V et al: Diffuse melanosis in metastatic malignant melanoma. J Am Acad Dermatol 24:625–628, 1991

103. Pierard GE: Melanophagic dermatitis and panniculitis. A condition revealing an occult metastatic malignant melanoma. Am J Dermatopathol 10:133–136, 1988

104. Haupt HM, Hood AF, Cohen MH: Inflammatory melanoma. J Am Acad Dermatol 10:52–55, 1984

105. Kornberg R, Harris M, Ackerman AB: Epidermotropically metastatic malignant melanoma. Arch Dermatol 114:67–69, 1978

106. Heenan PJ, Clay CD: Epidermotropically metastatic malignant melanoma simulating multiple primary melanomas. Am J Dermatopathol 13:396–402, 1991

107. Nahkleh RE, Wick MR, Rocamora A et al: Morphologic diversity in malignant melanoma. Am J Clin Pathol 93:731–740, 1990

108. Cochran AJ, Wen DR, Morton DL: Occult tumor cells in the lymph nodes of patients with pathological stage I malignant melanoma. An immunohistochemical study. Am J Surg Pathol 12:612–618, 1988

109. Cochran AJ, Lana AMA, Wen DR: Histomorphometry in the assessment of prognosis in stage II melanoma. Am J Surg Pathol 13:600–604, 1989

110. Gown AM, Vogel AM, Hoak D et al: Monoclonal antibodies specific for melanocytic tumors distinguish subpopulations of melanocytes. Am J Pathol 123:195–203, 1986

21

CUTANEOUS LYMPHOPROLIFERATIVE DISEASES, LYMPHOMAS, AND LEUKEMIA

GENERAL CONSIDERATIONS

In the last two decades there has been a quantum leap in our understanding of the immune system and the cells that comprise it. From theories about humoral and cellular immunity, we have progressed to the routine application of immunohistochemical and molecular biologic tests on clinical specimens.

It is difficult to understand cutaneous lymphomas and leukemias in depth without understanding lymph node and bone marrow histology and histopathology. There are several excellent summaries of this information.[1]

Definitions

A *lymphoproliferative disease* is one in which lymphocytes replicate in the absence of a known stimulus or persist in doing so after removal of the stimulus. Most lymphoproliferative diseases are malignant in the sense that they can result in death if unchecked, but many progress slowly. Unequivocally benign, cutaneous lymphocytic neoplasms have not been described. *Lymphoma* is thus a synonym for *malignant lymphoma*. Lymphomas are sometimes referred to as "low grade" or "high grade," depending on the degree of atypicality of their cells. Most low-grade lymphomas in lymph nodes have a less aggressive course than high-grade neoplasms, but the latter are sometimes curable by chemotherapy as their proliferative rate is higher and agents that attack replicating cells are effective. In the skin, the critical determination for many lymphomas is not histologic grade but whether the neoplasm is primary in the skin or secondary to systemic disease. *Primary cutaneous lymphomas* are often curable with local modalities, such as excision or radiation therapy. Many conditions formerly regarded as "pseudomalignancies," such as lymphomatoid papulosis (LYP), are now widely considered to be low-grade lymphomas, as are some cutaneous lymphomas with small clusters of neoplastic cells in a background of reactive lymphocytes. Immunopheno-typic and genotypic studies have been critical in the reassessment of such cases.

Leukemias are malignant neoplasms of the hematopoietic cells, which form the bone marrow. These neoplasms usually spread to the peripheral blood, but can infiltrate the skin or viscera late in their course. Blood-borne cells in number occur in some lymphomas and are regarded therein as indicating leukemic phase.

Clonality is the resemblance of neoplastic cells to one another, implying a common precursor. A neoplasm is said to be *monoclonal* when all of its cells resemble each other. In *clonal evolution*, additional mutations occur that affect subsets of cells differently. *Oligoclonal* infiltrates are those in which clones are present, but comprise only a minority of cells. *Polyclonal* infiltrates characterize a normal immune response due to the recruitment of lymphocytes of many different antigenic specificities. Current technologies cannot distinguish the thousands of individual clones that comprise polyclonal infiltrates. Analysis of clonality in clinical practice is currently limited to lymphoid infiltrates, but several laboratories are currently developing methods to evaluate clonality in solid tumors.

Epidermotropism refers to the property of lymphocytes to migrate into the epidermis (or hair follicle epithelium). Broadly used, it can refer to the infiltration of the epidermis by lymphocytes as seen in inflammatory skin diseases such as allergic contact dermatitis. Most authors use *epidermotropism* to refer to lymphocytic infiltration of the epidermis accompanied by disproportionately slight spongiosis, as in mycosis fungoides (MF). Epidermotropism can vary in degree, from slight epidermotropism in some early patch stage lesions of MF to striking epidermotropism in some cases of pagetoid reticulosis (PR).

Atypical lymphocytes have nuclear enlargement, hyperchromasia, or changes in nuclear shape beyond that seen in lymphocytes during an immune response. Some authors naively refer to large follicular center cells and immunoblasts as *atypical lymphocytes.*

Patterns of Cutaneous Lymphoid Infiltration

Two major patterns of cutaneous lymphoid infiltration occur in both benign and malignant disease. In the so-called T-cell pattern, lymphocytes amass around vessels and infiltrate into the adventitial dermis, epidermis, and, sometimes, hair follicle epithelium. In the so-called B-cell pattern, nodular lymphocytic infiltrates are present in the reticular dermis, but spare the adventitial dermis and epidermis. The "non-T-, non-B-cell pattern" has features of both. The predictive value of these patterns in determining the immunophenotype of a lymphoma is limited. While biopsy specimens of MF, the most common cutaneous T-cell lymphoma (CTCL), and Sezary syndrome have a typical T-cell pattern, those of other peripheral T-cell lymphomas often have a B-cell pattern of infiltration.[2] Rare B-cell lymphomas may infiltrate the papillary dermis and epidermis.

Several other patterns may be discerned on sections from some lymphomas at scanning magnification. Infiltrates surrounding pilosebaceous units that simulate folliculitis and perifolliculitis, or clustering of cells around eccrine coils, are evident in some patients with MF.[3] Chronic lymphocytic leukemia can resemble perivascular dermatitis without epidermal involvement. Angiocentric lymphoma can simulate vasculitis, T-cell lymphomas with a granulomatous reaction can be mistaken for sarcoidosis or other granulomatous dermatitides, and subcutaneous lymphoma can resemble panniculitis.

Immunophenotypic Aspects

Both the diagnosis and classification of cutaneous lymphoid infiltrates is increasingly becoming dependent on immunophenotypic and genotypic studies. The demonstration of clonality is essential for diagnosis in some cases, especially when the question is whether it is a low-grade lymphoma. The determination of whether an infiltrate is that of B- or T-cell lymphoma is important for determining the type of lymphoma, which can give the clinician a sense of the natural history that the patient's disease might follow. Many immunohistochemical reagents have now evolved from laboratory tools that could only be used in frozen sections to commercially available antibodies that can be used to stain paraffin-embedded sections in community hospital or independent laboratories. Most lymphocyte antigens have been assigned "cluster designations" (CD numbers) for ease of communication. Some of the most important ones are listed in Table 21-1.

CUTANEOUS LYMPHOID HYPERPLASIA

Cutaneous lymphoid hyperplasia (CLH) is a condition in which nodules or plaques occur as a result of dense, reactive lymphocytic infiltrates. Usually, the infiltrates in CLH include B cells and T cells, and the infiltrates partially or wholly recapitulate the relationship between germinal centers, mantle zones, and paracortex seen in lymph nodes.[4] Less commonly, nodular infiltrates of T cells are present.[5] Other terms for CLH include *pseudolymphoma, lymphadenosis benigna cutis*, and *lymphocytoma cutis*. It should be kept in mind that many cases considered to be CLH in the past were not adequately studied by modern techniques and might today be reclassified as low-grade B-cell lymphomas.

Table 21-1. Commonly Used Immunohistochemical Reagents Applied to Lymphoid Infiltrates

CD No.	Normal Cells Stained	Diagnostic Use
CD1	Langerhans cells, cortical thymocytes	Langerhans cell histiocytosis
CD3	T cells	T- versus B-cell lymphoma
CD4	T-helper cells	Classic mycosis fungoides versus CD8+ lymphoma
CD5	T cells, B-cell subset	Abnormal expression by B cells in chronic lymphocytic leukemia
CD7	T cells	Loss of antigen in mycosis fungoides, but not in inflammatory infiltrates (controversial); presence or absence determines prognosis in CD8+ lymphoma
CD10	B cells	Expressed by nodal follicular center lymphoma, but not by primary cutaneous follicular lymphoma
CD15	Macrophages, monocytes	Expressed by the cells of Hodgkin disease, but not by those of lymphomatoid papulosis
CD20	B cells	Lineage specific marker; B- versus T-cell lymphoma
CD30	Large paracortical cells, activated lymphocytes	Rare cells in reactive infiltrates, Hodgkin cells, lymphomatoid papulosis (esp. type A cells), cells of anaplastic large cell lymphoma
CD33	Myeloid cells	Leukemic infiltrates
CD45	Leukocytes	"Leukocyte common antigen," lymphoid or leukemic infiltrate versus other lineages
CD45RO	T cells	T-cell lineage marker, but not as specific as CD3
CD79a	B cells	Lineage-specific marker, similar to CD20
BCL-2	Cells resistant to apoptosis	Mantle zone lymphocytes, T cells, cells of nodal follicle center lymphoma
Kappa	B cells, plasma cells	Clonal restriction; only plasma cells, plasmacytoid lymphocytes, and some immunoblasts stainable in paraffin sections in most laboratories
Lambda	B cells, plasma cells	Clonal restriction; only plasma cells, plasmacytoid lymphocytes, and some immunoblasts stainable in paraffin sections in most laboratories
Ulex europeus agglutinin	Erythroid precursors	Normoblasts in extramedullary hematopoiesis

Clinical Features

The lesions of CLH are usually firm, red to purple nodules or plaques of up to several centimeters in size. Lesions may be single or multiple. Patients with multiple lesions of CLH most often have only a few lesions affecting a circumscribed area (most often the skin of the head or neck), but rare patients have generalized lesions.[6]

The majority of cases of CLH are idiopathic. Known causes include hypersensitivity reactions to tattoos, gold earrings, insect bites, infections, folliculitis, trauma, or infection with the spirochete *Borrelia burgdorferi*.[7–9] CLH is a late complication of borreliosis, and it occurs in patients with borreliosis more frequently in Europe than in North America, where it appears to be a reaction to *B. burgdorferi afzelius*, a local strain of the spirochete. A distinctive presentation of borrelia-induced CLH is bilateral ear lobe lesions.

Histopathologic Features

CLH may have either a nodular or a diffuse pattern. Generally the infiltrate is denser in the superficial dermis than in the deep dermis or subcutis, resulting in a "top heavy" pattern of infiltration at scanning magnification (Fig. 21-1). The histologic lesions produced by the infiltrates of CLH range from those with conspicuous lymphoid follicles to those without any apparent follicular differentiation. In the follicular pattern of CLH, distinct germinal centers, identical in composition to secondary follicles in reactive lymph nodes, are present. Primary follicles are collections of small round lymphocytes that have not been exposed to antigen. Secondary follicles are formed by antigen-stimulated lymphocytes. The follicles are composed of small cleaved and large lymphocytes (*centrocytes* and *centroblasts* in the terminology of the Kiel classification) and tingible body macrophages, which have in their cytoplasm nuclear debris from karyorrhectic

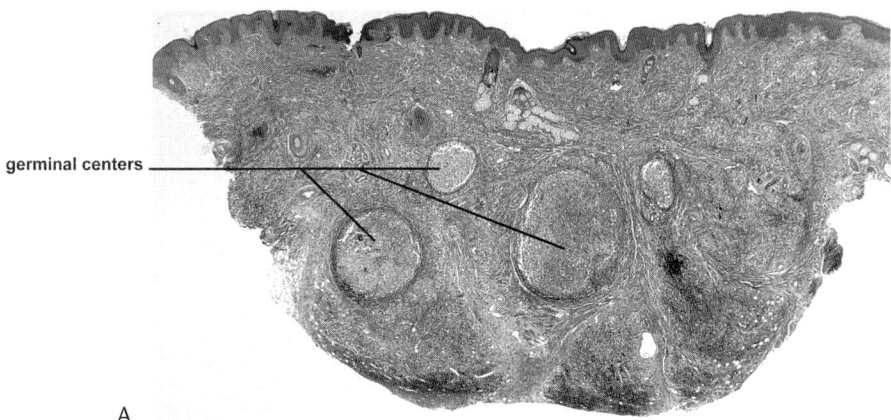

germinal centers

A

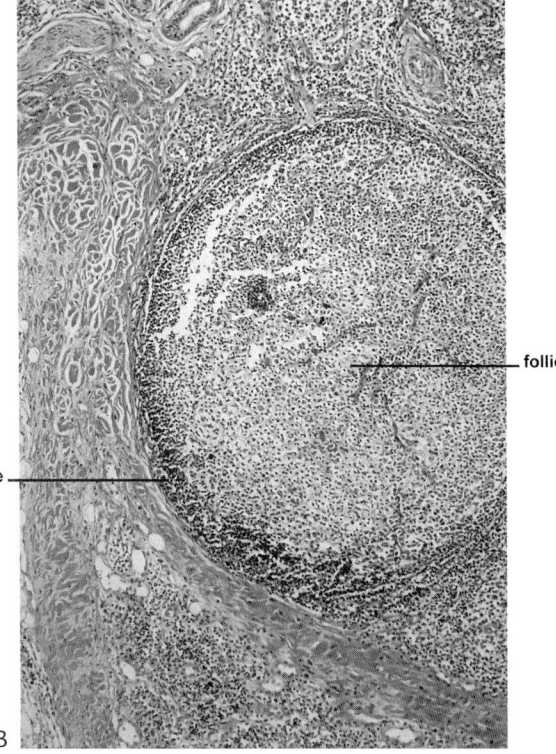

follicle center cells

mantle zone

B

Figure 21-1. Cutaneous lymphoid hyperplasia, follicular pattern. There are distinct, rounded lymphoid follicles (germinal centers) in the superficial and mid-dermis (**A**). Most reactive follicles are surrounded by a collar of B cells with small round nuclei, termed the mantle zone (**B**). *Continued.*

Figure 21-1. *Continued.* The follicles consist of follicular center cells (centrocytes, or small cleaved cells, and centroblasts, or large noncleaved cells), tingible body macrophages (histiocytes that have ingested the debris from apoptotic lymphocytes) and in this example, polykaryons (multinucleated T cells) (C).

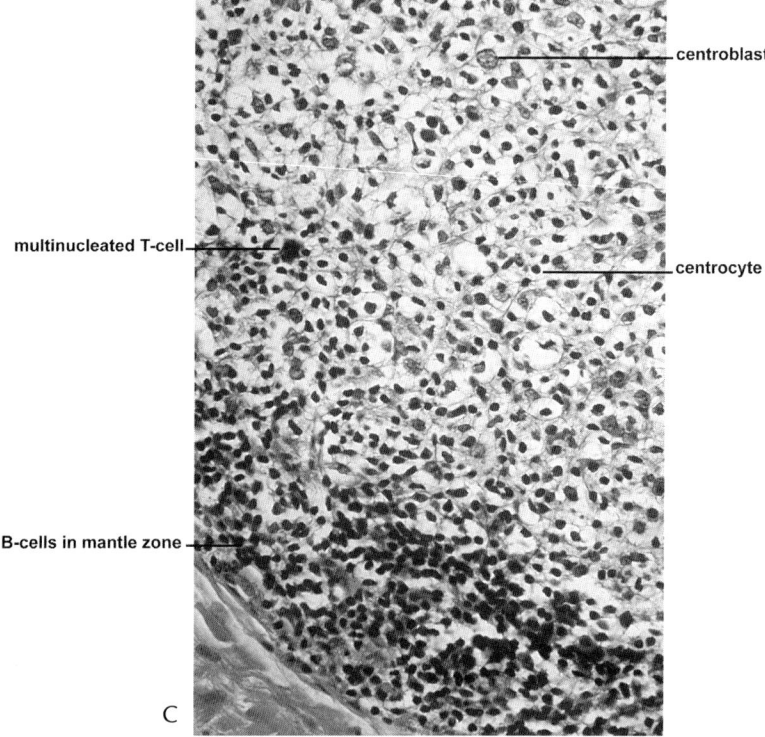

lymphocytes. Mitotic figures are commonly found in reactive follicles. The follicles in CLH are surrounded, as they are in lymph nodes, by a ring of small round lymphocytes, termed the *mantle zone*. Between the mantles of adjacent follicles lie a mixture of cells that can include small, convoluted lymphocytes, immunoblasts, macrophages, and, sometimes, giant cells, eosinophils, plasma cells, and so-called plasmacytoid monocytes.[10] Venules in interfollicular areas often have swollen endothelial cells. Rarely, large atypical cells that resemble Hodgkin cells and express the Reed-Sternberg cell–associated antigen Ki-1 (CD30) are found in interfollicular areas.[11]

In the nonfollicular form of CLH, there are nodular or diffuse dermal infiltrates of follicular center cells, often admixed with eosinophils, macrophages, and plasma cells (Fig. 21-2). Sometimes these cells are grouped in irregularly shaped clusters, their pale staining distinguishing them from their neighbors.

The immunophenotypic structure of CLH has been well characterized. Both follicular center cells and mantle zone cells are polyclonal B cells. A scattering of T cells (mostly helper cells) are seen within the germinal centers themselves. Currently, staining for cell membrane-bound immunoglobulin is usually performed on frozen, freeze-dried, or plastic-embedded tissue, although some groups claim success with routinely processed tissues using microwave antigen retrieval methods. Cytoplasmic immunoglobulin, as seen in plasma cells, plasmacytoid lymphocytes, and some immunoblasts, can readily be demonstrated using formalin-fixed, paraffin-embedded tissue, as can κ or λ messenger RNA. When frozen sections of CLH are stained with antisera to κ or λ light chains, cells bearing each can be identified in both follicles and interfollicular areas. The ratio of κ:λ positive cells is usually 2:1 in reactive B-cell infiltrates, but the range seen in CLH is from 5:1 to 1:1.

When specimens of nonfollicular CLH are stained with antisera that demonstrate B cells, mantle zone cells, or follicular dendritic cells (immune cells that reside in germinal centers and have a role in presenting antigen to B lymphocytes), a rudimentary follicular pattern often becomes apparent.

Clinicopathologic Correlation

The nodules of CLH generally spare the epidermis and papillary dermis. This pattern corresponds to their smooth-surfaced appearance clinically. Dense lymphoid infiltrates impart a red-purple color to the skin. Nodules of CLH and cutaneous lymphoma can be indistinguishable in their clinical appearances, except for the occurrence of ulceration in lymphoma.

Differential Diagnosis

The follicular pattern of CLH can be more easily recognized than the nonfollicular pattern. The major entity in the differential diagnosis of follicular CLH is follicular lymphoma. In follicular lymphoma the deep dermis and subcutis may be more extensively involved, and follicles are often closely packed together. The follicles of follicular lymphoma are composed of either a monomorphous population of small cleaved cells (centrocytes) or small cleaved and large lymphocytes (centrocytes and centroblasts) in contrast to the mixture of cell types seen in follicular CLH. Mitoses are rare in follicular lymphoma of the small cleaved cell type, more common in mixed small cleaved and large cell lymphoma, and frequent in the follicular pattern of CLH and in follicular large cell lymphoma. Mitotic figures cannot, therefore, be used to discriminate between benign and malignant follicles without reference to the cellular composition of the follicles. Mantle zones are more apt to be incomplete or absent in follicular lymphoma than in follicular CLH. The intervening areas between follicles in follicular lymphoma sometimes do not have the heterogeneous cell types seen in follicular CLH or can be infiltrated by small cleaved cells. In cases that defy diagnosis by routine microscopy, immunoperoxidase staining reveals light chain restriction in follicular lymphoma and a mixture of κ and λ light chain-bearing cells in follicular CLH. In some cases of follicular lymphoma, the interstitial polyclonal immunoglobulins that are normally detected in follicles are absent, resulting in so-called immunoglobulin-negative follicular lymphoma. Southern blot studies using probes to the immunoglobulin heavy and light chain genes can further confirm the presence or absence of clonality. Occasionally, CLH can appear polyclonal in immunophenotypic studies, but a clonal expansion can result in genotypic studies.[12] Some such infiltrates have eventuated in cutaneous lymphoma.

Other conditions may be mistaken for CLH because they have conspicuous germinal centers. Angiolymphoid hyperplasia with eosinophilia has congeries of muscular vessels with protuberant endothelial cells, infiltrates containing numerous eosinophils, and prominent lymphoid follicles. In some cases of morphea, dermatofibroma, and necrobiosis lipoidica, germinal centers may distract from other, more specific findings. Necrobiotic xanthogranuloma with paraproteinemia has massive degeneration of collagen, xanthomatous infiltrates, and lymphoid germinal centers. Rarely, malignant lymphomas will have reactive germinal centers at the periphery of the malignant infiltrate.

Nonfollicular CLH typically has an admixture of cell types that are not found in many B-cell lymphomas, including eosinophils, plasma cells, and histiocytic giant cells. Even in paraffin-embedded material, immunoperoxidase staining can demonstrate small foci of germinal center cells in many cases of nonfollicular CLH. Cytologic features are sometimes helpful, as CLH can have large cells (centroblasts and immunoblasts) but lacks cells with striking cytologic atypia.

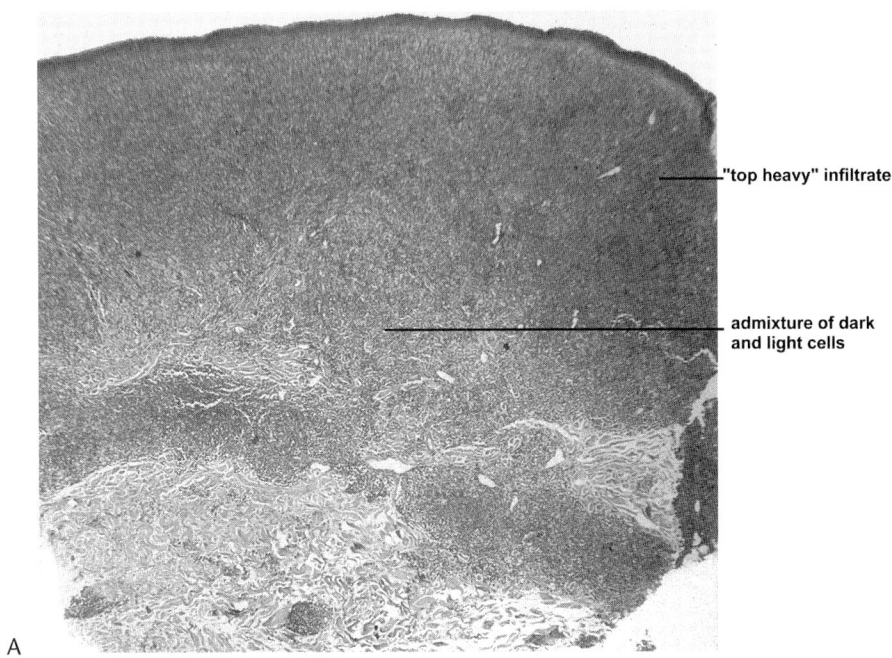

"top heavy" infiltrate

admixture of dark and light cells

A

Figure 21-2. Cutaneous lymphoid hyperplasia, nonfollicular pattern. There is a top-heavy, wedge-shaped infiltrate in the dermis, composed of a mixture of cell types, which can be seen at scanning magnification by a mixture of darkly and lightly staining cells **(A)**. Although well-demarcated follicles are not present, there are follicular center cells (centrocytes and centroblasts, also known as small cleaved and large noncleaved cells) mixed with small lymphocytes and plasma cells in this field **(B)**. Note the venule with swollen endothelial cells at upper left.

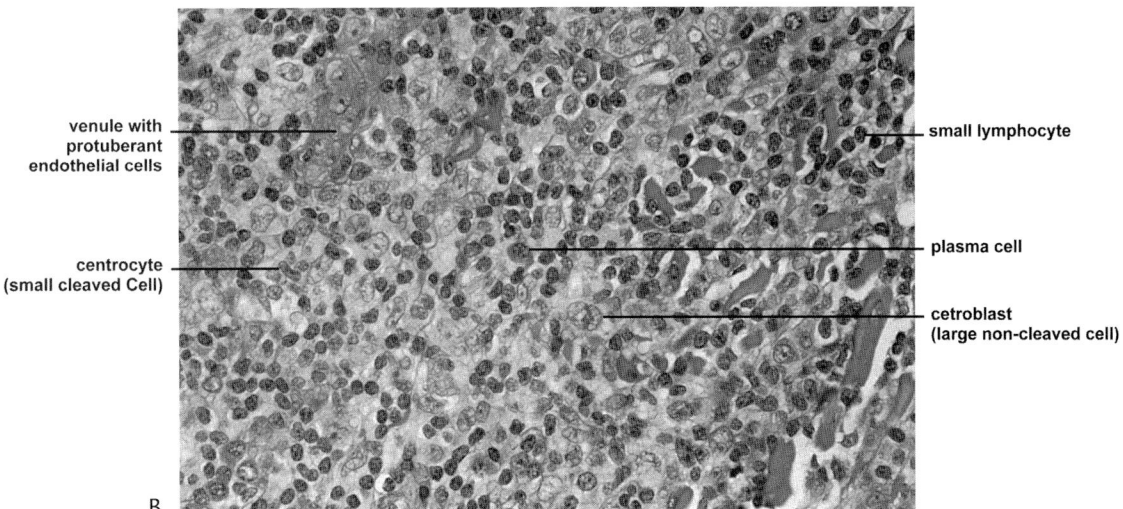

venule with protuberant endothelial cells

centrocyte (small cleaved Cell)

small lymphocyte

plasma cell

cetroblast (large non-cleaved cell)

B

THE "GENERIC" CUTANEOUS LYMPHOMAS

The malignant lymphomas are a group of diseases in which lymphocytes proliferate with partial to complete loss of their normal control mechanisms. We have grouped cutaneous lymphomas other than Hodgkin disease into four categories: nonepidermotropic cutaneous lymphomas of either B- or T-cell origin, which are considered herein and below; MF and its variants and other epidermotropic T-cell lymphomas (see below); remitting and relapsing T-cell proliferations (see below); lymphomas whose infiltrates are centered around blood vessels (see below); and Hodgkin disease (see below). This schema reflects the pattern of infiltration in cutaneous lymphomas, or the "compartment" affected by them, rather than their immunophenotype or grade.

Early classifications of malignant lymphoma were based solely on histopathologic features. More recent classifications, such as those developed by the Working Group and the modified Kiel classification of T-cell lymphoma[13] correlate morphology with prognosis. The prognoses implied by the older classifications often do not apply to patients with primary cutaneous lymphoma. As a rule, patients with primary extranodal lymphoma have a more favorable prognosis than do patients with the same histopathologic type of lymphoma based in lymph node. The more recent revised European-American lymphoma (REAL) classification is based on cohesive clinicopathologic entities and is more useful to dermatopathologists and dermatologists than are past attempts[14] (Table 21-2).

A group of dermatopathologists and clinicians interested in cutaneous lymphoma has preferred a classification of primary cutaneous lymphoma. The resultant European Organization for Research and Treatment of Cancer classification presupposes that a workup for disseminated disease is negative and that the patient has remained free of disease for 6 months[15] (Table 21-3).

Table 21-2. List of Lymphoid Neoplasms Recognized by the International Lymphoma Study Group

B-cell neoplasms
  Precursor B-cell neoplasm: precursor B-lymphoblastic leukemia/lymphoma
  Peripheral B-cell neoplasms
    B-cell chronic lymphocytic leukemia/prolymphocytic leukemia/small lymphocytic lymphoma
    Lymphoplasmacytoid lymphoma/immunocytoma
    Mantle cell lymphoma
    Follicle center lymphoma, follicular
    Provisional cytologic grades: 1 (small cell), 2 (mixed small and large cell), 3 (large cell)
    Marginal zone B-cell lymphoma
    Extranodal (MALT-type with or without monocytoid B cells)
    Provisional entity: splenic marginal zone lymphoma (with or without villous lymphocytes)
    Hairy cell leukemia
    Plasmacytoma/plasma cell myeloma
    Diffuse large B-cell lymphoma[a]
    Subtype: primary mediastinal (thymic) B-cell lymphoma
    Burkitt lymphoma
    Provisional entity: high-grade B-cell lymphoma, Burkitt-like[a]
T-Cell and Putative NK-Cell Neoplasms
  Precursor T-cell neoplasm: precursor T-lymphoblastic lymphoma/leukemia
  Peripheral T-cell and natural killer cell neoplasms
    T-cell chronic lymphocytic leukemia/prolymphocytic leukemia
    Large granular lymphocyte leukemia
    T-cell type
    NK-cell type
    Mycosis fungoides/Sezary syndrome
    Peripheral T-cell lymphomas, unspecified[a]
    Provisional cytologic categories: medium-sized cell, mixed medium and large cell, large cell, lymphoepithelioid cell
    Provisional subtype: Hepatosplenic T-cell lymphoma
    Provisional subtype: Subcutaneous panniculitic T-cell lymphoma
    Angioimmunoblastic T-cell lymphoma
    Angiocentric lymphoma
    Intestinal T-cell lymphoma (with or without enteropathy)
    Adult T-cell lymphoma/leukemia
    Anaplastic large cell lymphoma, CD30, T- and null-cell types
    Provisional entity: anaplastic large-cell lymphoma, Hodgkin-like
Hodgkin disease
  Lymphocyte predominance
  Nodular sclerosis
  Mixed cellularity
  Lymphocyte depletion
  Provisional entity: lymphocyte-rich classic Hodgkin disease

[a] These categories are thought likely to include more than one disease entity.

Table 21-3. European Organization for Research and Treatment of Cancer Classification for Primary Cutaneous Lymphomas

Primary CTCL	Primary CBCL
Indolent	Indolent
MF	Follicle center cell lymphoma
MF + follicular mucinosis	
Pagetoid reticulosis	Immunocytoma and marginal zone B-cell lymphoma
Large cell CTCL, CD30+	
Anaplastic	
Immunoblastic	
Pleomorphic	Intermediate
Lymphomatoid papulosis	Large B-cell lymphoma of the leg
Aggressive	
Sezary syndrome	
Large cell CTCL, CD30−	
Immunoblastic	
Pleomorphic	
Provisional	Provisional
Granulomatous slack skin	Intravascular CBCL
CTCL, pleomorphic small/medium-sized	Plasmacytoma
Subcutaneous panniculitis-like T-cell lymphoma	

CTCL, cutaneous T-cell lymphoma; CBCL, cutaneous B-cell lymphoma; MF, mycosis fungoides.

Clinical Features

Cutaneous lymphomas other than Hodgkin disease and MF usually present with red to purplish papules, nodules, or tumors. Ulceration, eschars, hemorrhage, and scaling may also occur. The lesions are often restricted to a single area of skin, such as the head and neck, trunk, or an extremity. Some lymphomas present as subcutaneous masses. Annular plaques with central clearing and mamillated plaques are among the unusual manifestations of cutaneous lymphoma. Most types of cutaneous lymphoma other than MF and its variants cannot be distinguished from each other clinically.

Primary cutaneous lymphomas have highly variable clinical courses. Low-grade lymphomas involving a single area of skin often grow indolently and local therapy such as excision, radiation, or intralesional injection can result in complete remission, if not a cure. The 5-year survival rate for patients with localized cutaneous lymphoma (stage IE using the TNM classification) can approach 100%. Most medium- and high-grade cutaneous lymphomas that are not accompanied by systemic disease have a more favorable prognosis than do their node-based counterparts. Secondary spread of malignant lymphoma to the skin is a sign of advanced disease and portends a poor prognosis, especially if the lymphoma is of high grade histologically and viscera are involved by it.

Histopathologic Features

The infiltrates of most cutaneous lymphomas, whether primary or secondary, and of B- or T-cell origin, present with either the so-called B-cell or non-B-, non-T-cell histologic patterns (Fig. 21-3). The B-cell pattern is more common and features dense

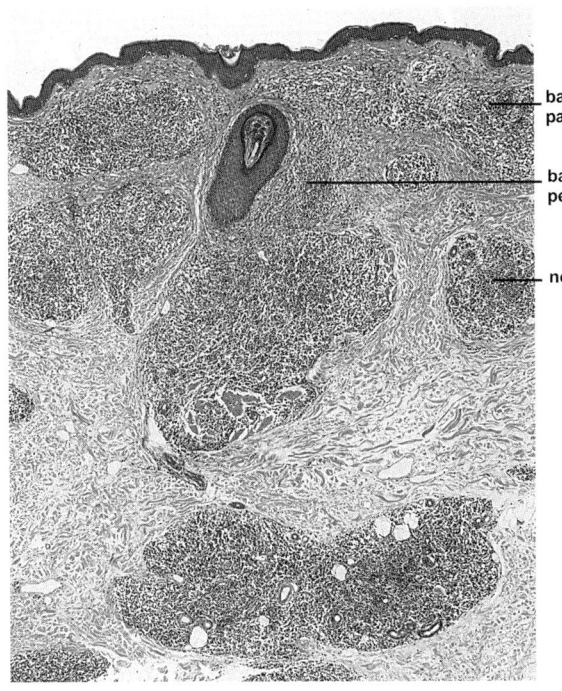

bandlike infiltrate in papillary dermis

bandlike infiltrate in perifollicular adventitial dermis

nodules of lymphocytes

A

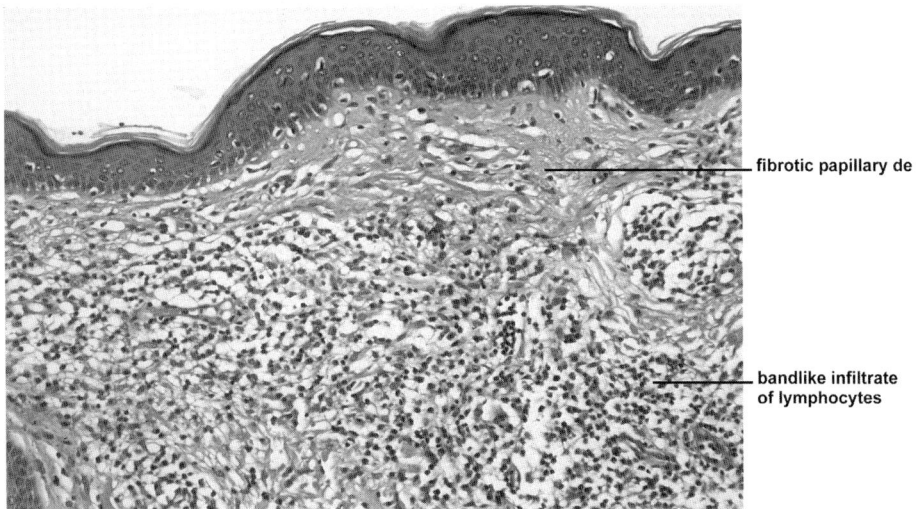

fibrotic papillary de

bandlike infiltrate of lymphocytes

B

Figure 21-3. The pattern at scanning magnification does not always predict the immunophenotype of a cutaneous lymphoma. In this example, the pattern is non-B-cell, non-T-cell because there are multiple nodules throughout the dermis (**A**), while the papillary dermis is involved by a band-like infiltrate (**B**).

nodular or diffuse infiltrates that efface adnexal structures but spare the papillary dermis. Large plaques or tumors of cutaneous lymphoma may contain "bottom-heavy" infiltrates whose centers of gravity appear to lie in the deep reticular dermis or subcutaneous fat. Smaller papules and nodules tend to have "top heavy" infiltrates, similar at scanning magnification to those of CLH or other simulants of malignant lymphoma; however, large lesions of cutaneous lymphoplasmacytic lymphoma and secondary deposits of many other types of lymphoma can have top-heavy patterns. An assessment of whether a lesion contains top- or bottom-heavy infiltrates is best made on an incisional biopsy specimen. The pattern of infiltration should be considered in the context with the clinical setting (e.g., the top-heavy histologic pattern seen on biopsy of a small papule may not be representative of the changes in large nodules in the same patient). Ulceration may be evident in the large nodules of a high-grade cutaneous lymphoma, but this finding is often superfluous as a diagnostic clue.

Monomorphous populations of cells are evident in most types of cutaneous lymphoma because lymphomatous cells usually proliferate more rapidly than reactive cells accumulate. In most B-cell lymphomas, reactive T cells are scattered throughout the infiltrate, and in some other types of lymphoma, such as lymphoplasmacytic lymphoma, Lennert lymphoma, and some other T-cell lymphomas, reactive cells of various types in addition to T cells (e.g., eosinophils, plasma cells, or macrophages) are typically present. While it has heretofore been assumed that non-neoplastic T cells represent a valiant "host response" battling the neoplasm, recent evidence suggests that in so-called T-cell-rich B-cell lymphoma these cells may be the source of cytokines that actually further proliferation of the neoplastic cells.

The cytologic features of the malignant cells in cutaneous lymphomas are the same as their node-based counterparts or, in the case of many B-cell lymphomas, similar to the cells seen in mucosal lymphomas.[16] The cytologic and immunophenotypic features of many types of B-cell lymphoma correspond to stages of B-cell differentiation. In intermediate- and high-grade lymphomas, there are cytologically atypical lymphocytes that differ in appearance from those seen in reactive nodes.

The following are descriptions of several variants of cutaneous lymphoma and their differential diagnoses. The term listed first is that of the REAL classification.

Clinical and Pathologic Features of Specific Types of Cutaneous Lymphoma Resulting in Nodular or Diffuse Dermal Infiltrates

Small Lymphocytic Lymphoma (Tissue Infiltrates of B-Cell Chronic Lymphocytic Leukemia)

Small lymphocytic lymphoma is a low-grade lymphoma, characterized histologically by a proliferation of B cells morphologically identical to those of lymphocytic leukemia. It presents with cutaneous nodules or tumors or diffuse infiltrates that can cause a leonine facies.[2] The cells of small lymphocytic lymphoma have scant cytoplasm and small, round to oval nuclei with small, dark blocks of chromatin and a small nucleolus. In instances of massive cutaneous infiltration, there are so-called proliferation centers, nodular areas seen in lymph nodes involved by small lymphocytic lymphoma wherein slightly larger

cells, termed *prolymphocytes* and *paraimmunoblasts,* impart a more pallid appearance to the infiltrate. Proliferation centers are far more common in lymph node infiltrates of small lymphocytic lymphoma.

The principal entities to be distinguished from small lymphocytic lymphoma are those that produce either perivascular or perivascular and interstitial lymphocytic infiltrates without much epidermal change (e.g., polymorphous light eruption, tumid lesions of lupus erythematosus, erythema annulare centrifugum, and early inflammatory lesions of morphea in which sclerosis has not supervened). Small lymphocytic lymphoma tends to produce monomorphous infiltrates, as opposed to the polymorphous infiltrates seen in many other reactive conditions in which small lymphocytes abound. Cytologic features are valuable diagnostic indicators, as small lymphocytic lymphomas have round nuclei, while most reactive infiltrates are composed of T cells with slightly convoluted nuclei. Immunohistochemical staining can be of help in difficult cases, as the cells of small lymphocytic lymphoma often aberrantly co-express the T-cell-associated antigens CD43 and CD5, as well as the B-cell determinant CD20. These antigens are preserved in formalin-fixed, paraffin-embedded tissue.

Extranodal Marginal Zone Lymphoma (Lymphoplasmacytoid Lymphoma, Immunocytoma)

This condition is a low-grade lymphoma whose cells have the features of plasmacytoid lymphocytes (i.e., their appearance is between small lymphocytes and plasma cells and they have cytoplasmic rather than cell surface immunoglobulin). Many believe that this neoplasm and cases reported as "cutaneous immunocytoma" are within a spectrum of marginal zone lymphoma. *Splenic marginal zone* refers to a ring of pale-staining cells peripheral to the mantle zone in lymphoid follicles in that organ. The small lymphocytes have indented nuclei and slightly more cytoplasm than do centrocytes of lymph node follicles. These lymphomas further resemble those arising in mucosal-associated lymphoid tissue (MALT).[16]

Immunocytoma/marginal zone lymphoma usually has an unremarkable clinical appearance and frequently presents as a solitary lesion. In Europe, where cutaneous immunocytoma is more common than in North America, nodules arising within patches of acrodermatitis chronica atrophicans (an atrophying dermatitis occurring late in the course of infection with the spirochete *B. burgdorferi afzelius*) have been reported.[2] While the prognosis of patients with primary cutaneous involvement is favorable, some develop immunoblastic lymphoma or leukemia. IgM κ immunoglobulin is present in the cytoplasm of plasmacytoid lymphoma cells in most cases, but rarely IgG κ is produced.[17] In some cases, the cells secrete IgM, resulting in Waldenstrom macroglobulinemia.

Immunocytoma/marginal zone lymphoma can be difficult to diagnose histologically because it shares many features with CLH.[18] Its infiltrates are seldom bottom heavy, but consist instead of small nodules of cells that sometimes surround hair follicles but spare their epithelium (Fig. 21-4). It is only occasionally monomorphous and often displays an admixture of eosinophils and macrophages. Even the neoplastic cells can have a range of differentiation, sometimes resembling small lymphocytes, plasmacytoid lymphocytes, immunoblasts, or plasma cells.

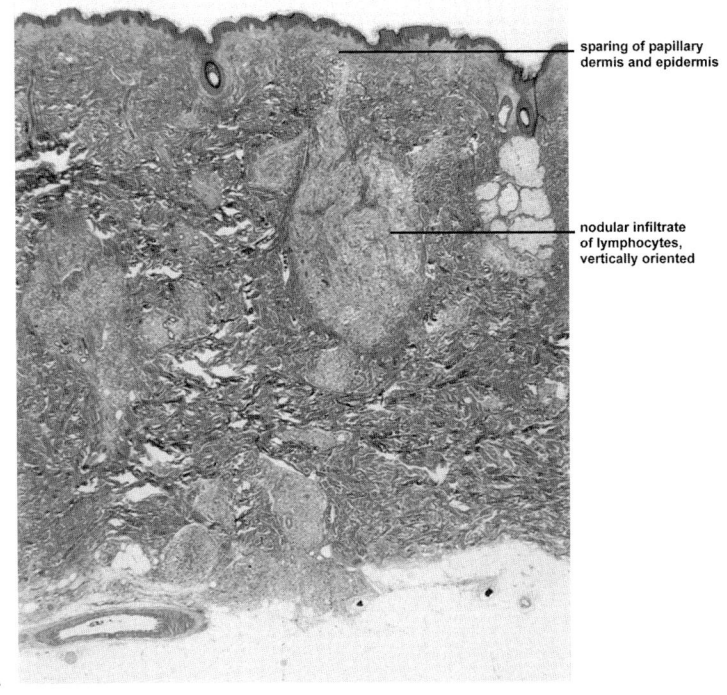

sparing of papillary dermis and epidermis

nodular infiltrate of lymphocytes, vertically oriented

A

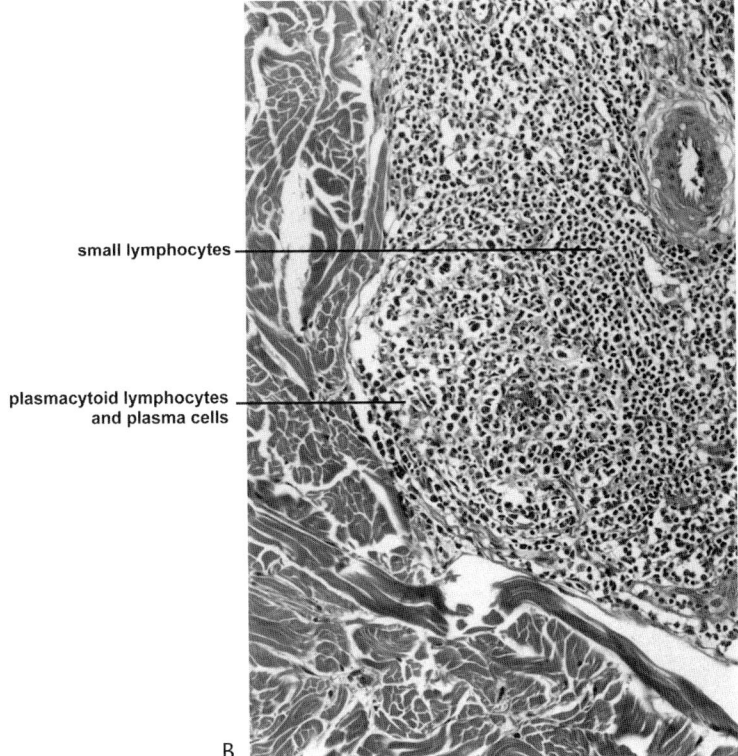

small lymphocytes

plasmacytoid lymphocytes and plasma cells

B

Figure 21-4. Marginal zone lymphoma, also known as lymphoplasmacellular lymphoma or immunocytoma. This condition is low-grade form of B-cell lymphoma that was often misdiagnosed as cutaneous lymphoid hyperplasia in the past because of its admixture of cell types. At scanning magnification, there are several nodules of pale staining cells in the dermis, with some aggregations that are vertically oriented with respect to the skin surface **(A)**. The aggregations are composed of small lymphocytes in their centers, with plasma cells and plasmacytoid lymphocytes (cells with features intermediate between small lymphocytes and plasma cells) at the periphery **(B)**. *Continued.*

Figure 21-4. *Continued.* The plasma cells and plasmacytoid lymphocytes both have eccentric rims of cytoplasm and compose the clonal population in this form of lymphoma (**C**).

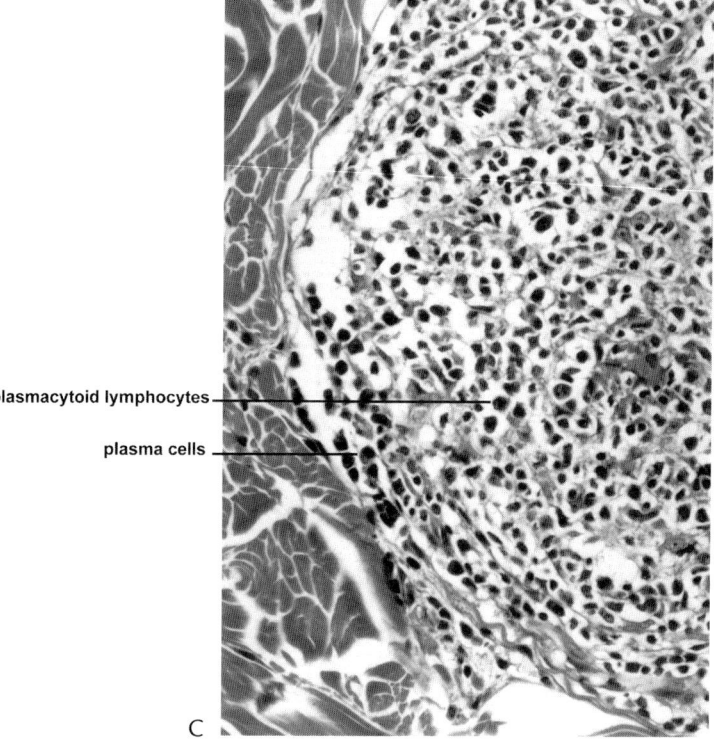

plasmacytoid lymphocytes

plasma cells

C

The differential diagnosis of immunocytoma includes inflammatory diseases in which plasma cells occur and multiple myeloma (MM). Rarely, plasmacytoid lymphocytes are present in secondary syphilis, leishmaniasis, erythema chronicum migrans, the inflammatory stage of morphea, reactions to ruptured cysts, and other inflammatory diseases. An unusual cytologic feature unique to plasmacytoid lymphoma is the occurrence of cells with eccentric cytoplasm and convoluted or indented nuclei.[19] Because cytoplasmic (as opposed to cell surface) immunoglobulin is preserved in routinely processed tissue, staining with anti-light-chain reagents can demonstrate clonality in immunocytoma.

Follicular Center Lymphoma

Primary cutaneous follicular lymphomas have only been recognized recently.[20] Indeed, many authors prior to the mid-1980s doubted the existence of such lesions. They were initially considered to be proliferations of B cells of the type also found in follicles (e.g., small cleaved cells [centrocytes in the Kiel classification] or large cleaved or noncleaved cells [centroblasts]). Based on the behavior of lymphomas that arise in lymph nodes, the Working Formulation categorized nodular small cleaved cell and small cleaved and large cell lymphomas as low-grade neoplasms and their diffuse counterparts as well as the nodular and diffuse forms of large cell lymphoma as intermediate-grade neoplasms.[13] Cutaneous lymphoma resembling follicular center lymphoma in lymph nodes behaves more indolently than does its node-based counterpart. Recently, immunophenotypic and genotypic evidence has shown that the cells of many so-called primary cutaneous follicular lymphomas resemble those of mucosal lymphomas (MALTomas) more than they do true follicular center lymphomas in lymph nodes.[16] It seems likely that cutaneous lymphomas with a follicular pattern are a heterogeneous group, including true follicular center lymphomas, MALToma-like neoplasms with colonized follicles, and mantle zone lymphomas with compressed residual follicles. The discussion that follows ignores the distinction between these lesions, as indolent behavior is the rule. Distinguishing between these entities, which seem to share a follicular pattern, is not yet practical with routinely processed tissues and can be problematic even with fresh material in some cases. We use the term *cutaneous follicular lymphoma* to refer to malignant infiltrates that show a follicular pattern regardless of the exact subtype.

Cutaneous follicular lymphomas present clinically as plaques, nodules, and tumors. Ulceration is rare. The course of patients with follicular large cell (centroblastic) lymphoma is so indolent that some have advocated the use of the term *large cell lymphocytoma* rather than *lymphoma.*[22]

The skin is involved in just under 4% of cases of systemic follicular lymphoma. Cutaneous infiltrates can be of a higher histologic grade than the nodal infiltrates from which they arose, which diminishes survival from 100% to 60% at 5 years.[23]

The histopathologic features of follicular center lymphomas depend on its cellular composition. The infiltrates are often bottom heavy, a finding whose evaluation depends on the willingness of the clinician to perform an incisional biopsy including the deep subcutis. In some cases that probably are true follicular center lymphomas (Fig. 21-5), the neoplastic follicles are of similar sizes throughout the infiltrate, mantles of smaller lymphocytes are attenuated or absent, and tingible body macrophages are rare.[20] In cases where the cells are small, mitoses are scant; in examples with intermediate or larger cells, they are more numerous. The cells that compose the neoplastic follicles

Figure 21-5. Cutaneous B-cell lymphoma, follicular type. This particular example is primary in the skin, but secondary spread to the skin by a nodal follicular B-cell lymphoma might look identical histologically. At low power, there are distinct follicles of varying sizes that are only partly surrounded by mantles of small lymphocytes **(A)**. The absence of a mantle zone around portions of the follicle is evident at higher magnification **(B)**. *Continued.*

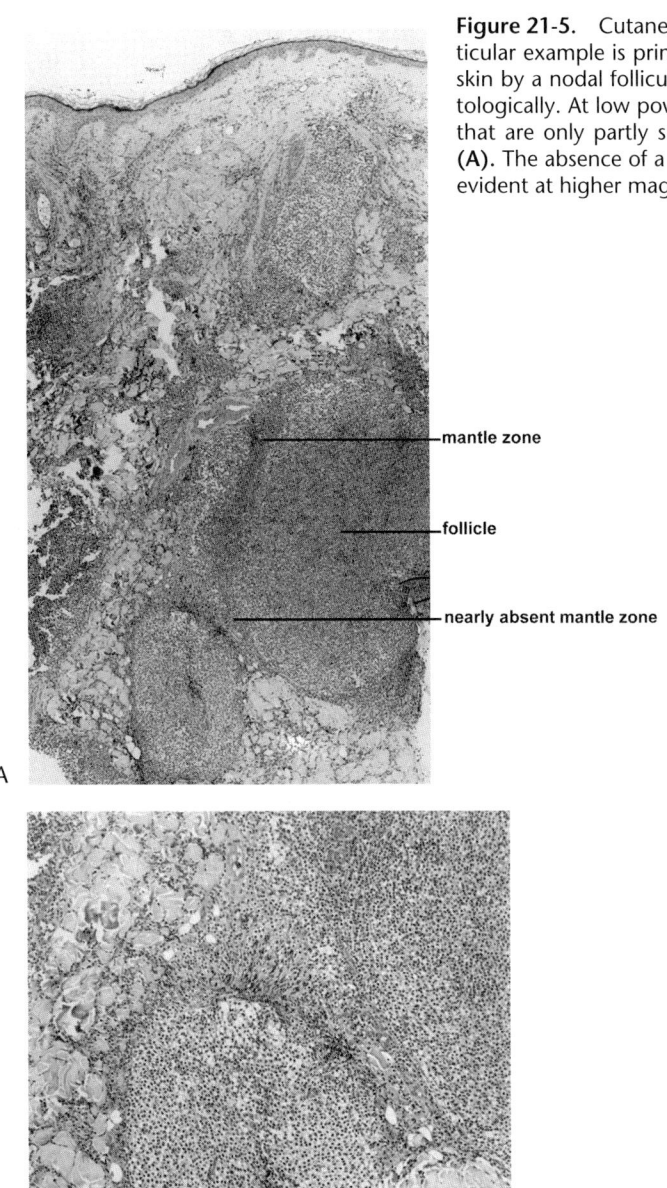

Figure 21-5. *Continued.* The monomorphous composition of the neoplastic follicle is evident at high magnification. The constituent cells in this case have small, slightly irregular nuclei. Unlike the case in a reactive follicle in a lymph node, there is no admixture of centroblasts (noncleaved cells), mitotic figures are rare, and so are tingible body macrophages (macrophages that have ingested cellular debris from lymphocytes that undergo apoptosis in a reactive follicle) **(C).**

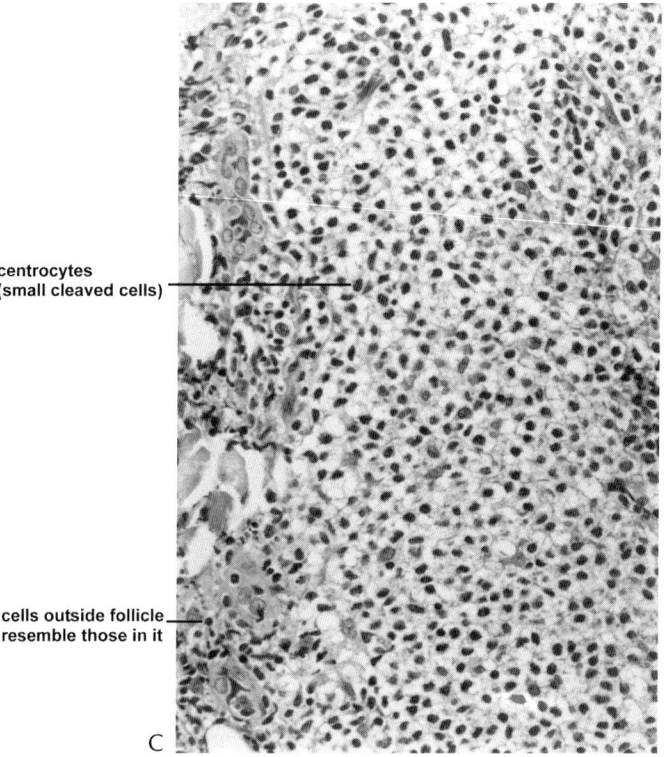

centrocytes (small cleaved cells)

cells outside follicle resemble those in it

C

vary from centrocytes and centroblasts, to cells resembling centrocytes but with slightly more abundant cytoplasm (so-called centrocytoid cells), to cells with slightly irregular, somewhat larger nuclei and stippled chromatin resembling those seen in mantle zone lymphoma.

The most important simulant of cutaneous follicular lymphoma is the follicular pattern of CLH. Key features that occur in CLH but not in follicular lymphoma include greater variability in the size of follicles, preservation of mantle zones, presence of tingible body macrophages and appropriate numbers of mitotic figures in follicules, and the presence of eosinophils, plasma cells, or multinucleated macrophages in interfollicular zones. Immunophenotyping can help as the cells of neoplastic follicles express either κ or λ light chain exclusively, in contradistinction to the mixture of light chain types present on the surfaces of cells in reactive follicles. In "immunoglobulin-negative" follicular lymphoma neither light chain can be detected; however, these lymphomas can still be diagnosed by the absence of interstitial polyclonal immunoglobulin, which is present in reactive follicles.[24] If immunophenotypic studies are equivocal, genotypic studies can often be performed using the same frozen tissue specimen to detect clonal rearrangement of the immunoglobulin heavy or light chain genes, or both.

The majority of follicular lymphomas in lymph nodes have a t(14;18) translocation, which brings an oncogene situated on chromosome 14, *bcl*-2, in apposition to the heavy chain joining gene (J_H) on chromosome 14. This results in increased production of the protein bcl-2. *Bcl*-2 confers resistance to apoptosis, and B cells with high levels of *bcl*-2 are particularly long lived. *Bcl*-2 can be detected immunohistochemically in the cells of many nodal follicular lymphomas and in their cells in cutaneous

deposits. This translocation is rare in primary cutaneous follicular lymphoma, and the CD10-,*bcl*-2-phenotype of its cells is opposite that found in node-based follicular lymphoma.[21]

Diffuse Large B-Cell Lymphoma (Centroblastic Lymphoma and B-Cell Immunoblastic Lymphoma)

Nodal B-cell lymphomas in which large cells predominate are high-grade neoplasms. Many authors have separated lymphomas of large non-cleaved B cells (centroblastic lymphoma) from immunoblastic lymphomas. Immunoblasts were first described as B cells that had large, vesicular nuclei with prominent central nucleoli and distinct nuclear membranes and a rim of amphophilic cytoplasm, which can contain immunoglobulin. B immunoblasts are thought to be precursors of plasma cells. T cells with similar cytologic features are known as *T immunoblasts*. T immunoblasts are antigen-stimulated cells that do not evolve into plasma cells. Immunoblastic lymphomas can be of either B- or T-cell derivation, and both are categorized as high-grade neoplasms by the Working Formulation and in the modified Kiel classification of T-cell lymphomas.[13,14] Because of a lack of reproducibility even among expert hematopathologists, the REAL classification does not attempt to separate large noncleaved (centroblastic) lymphoma from immunoblastic lymphoma.[15] This differential would rest on an assessment of the size and position of nucleoli, which are larger and more centrally placed in immunoblasts than in centroblasts. In many cases there is a mixture of centroblast-like and immunoblast-like cells.

The histopathologic appearance of large cell lymphoma of the B-cell type is most often as a dense, diffuse infiltrate that in-

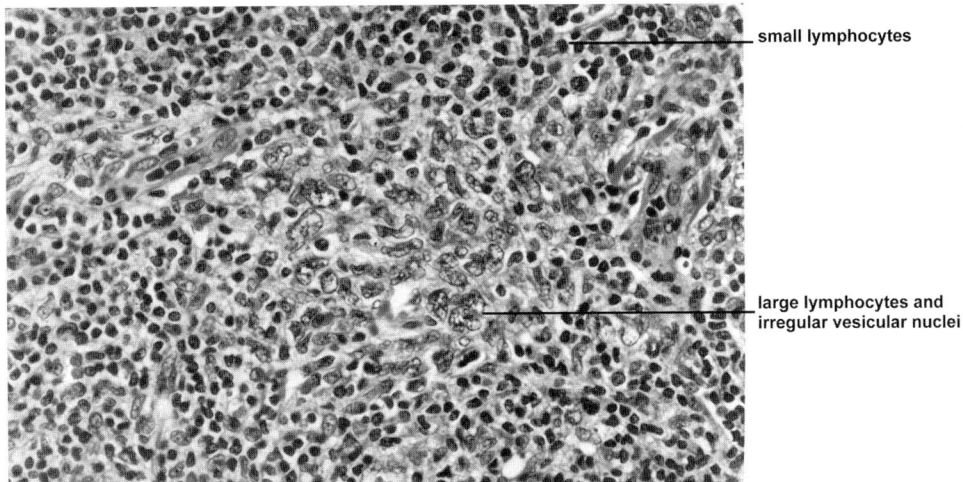

small lymphocytes

large lymphocytes and irregular vesicular nuclei

Figure 21-6.   A high-grade B-cell lymphoma. There is a cluster of neoplastic cells with scant cytoplasm and pleomorphic vesicular nuclei, surrounded by small lymphocytes. The cytologic irregularity of these cells exceeds that seen in nearly all reactive follicles.

volves the dermis and subcutis (Fig. 21-6). In rare cases the infiltrates efface the papillary dermis and infiltrate the epidermis or induce pseudocarcinomatous epidermal hyperplasia. The chromatin pattern of the cells of large cell lymphoma can be even more coarse than that of reactive immunoblasts. Mitotic figures are numerous.

Despite the classification of diffuse large cell lymphoma as an intermediate-grade lymphoma and of immunoblastic lymphoma as high grade by the Working Formulation, large B-cell lymphoma of the skin, when primary in the skin and confined to one area, carries a favorable prognosis, with the possible exception of patients who present with tumors of the lower legs.[25] Large cell lymphoma affecting the skin of the back has been referred to as "reticulohistiocytoma of the dorsum (of Crosti)" in the European literature.[26] The infiltrates of this condition are clonally restricted and histologically indistinguishable from those of other cutaneous large B-cell lymphomas.

The differential diagnosis of large B-cell lymphoma includes nonlymphoid malignancies because of the large size of the cells. Its cells are usually disposed in sheets rather than in nests, as would be seen in malignant melanoma or poorly differentiated squamous cell carcinoma. Immunophenotyping is not usually necessary for a diagnosis of lymphoma (as opposed to melanoma or carcinoma), unless fixation is poor or only a small sample is available. Some immunoblastic lymphomas do not react with antisera to leukocyte common antigen (CD45RB), a potential pitfall if the differential diagnosis being investigated is lymphoma versus carcinoma or melanoma. As large cell lymphomas can be of either T- or B-cell derivation, immunohistochemical studies are needed to differentiate these neoplasms, although the answer may not be of great clinical relevance. Most will express either the T-cell antigen CD3 or react with the B-cell marker L26 (CD20). In some cases, immunophenotyping with currently available panels will not demonstrate lineage, and either frozen section immunohistochemistry or gene rearrangement studies can be done to classify the lesion. Only a mi-

nority of B-cell immunoblastic lymphomas will contain enough cytoplasmic immunoglobulin to stain with anti-light-chain reagents after being fixed in formalin and embedded in paraffin.

Lymphoblastic Lymphoma

Lymphoblastic lymphoma was originally considered a neoplasm of lymphocytes whose appearance resembled those of "pre-B-cells" (i.e., B lymphocytes that contain intracytoplasmic IgM heavy chains but no light chains). Recently, the concept of lymphoblastic lymphoma has been expanded to include T-cell proliferations of similarly primitive cells. Whether of T- or B-cell derivation, lymphoblastic lymphomas are considered high-grade neoplasms in the Working Formulation.[13]

B-cell lymphoblastic lymphoma presents in children as red to plum colored, smooth-surfaced nodules often involving the skin of the head and neck. The prognosis is poor for children with disseminated disease, but for those in whom cutaneous lesions are the only manifestation (stage IE) the prognosis is excellent following treatment.[27] T-cell lymphoblastic lymphoma, which comprises 70% of cases, most often presents in male children, adolescents, or young adults as a mediastinal mass accompanied by infiltration of the bone marrow and circulating lymphoblasts.

Regardless of immunophenotype, the cutaneous infiltrates of lymphoblastic lymphoma are diffuse far more often than they are nodular, and neither the T- nor the B-cell form is epidermotropic. The cells of lymphoblastic lymphoma may be difficult for the uninitiated to recognize. They have scant cytoplasm and slightly to moderately convoluted nuclei with finely dispersed chromatin. Some T-cell lymphoblastic lymphomas have an admixture of eosinophils.

Lymphoblastic lymphoma can be maddeningly difficult to distinguish from small, noncleaved cell (also known as *undifferentiated*) lymphoma, which can be of the Burkitt or so-called non-Burkitt type. Both lymphoblastic and small noncleaved cell lymphomas are high-grade neoplasms. Distinguishing these two forms of lymphoma can be important, as the management of patients with them can differ. The cytoplasms of cells of small non-cleaved lymphoma stain more intensely than do those of lymphoblastic lymphoma with methyl-green pyronine and contain vacuoles that can be discerned on touch imprints of cut sections of skin biopsy specimens. The nuclei of cells of small non-cleaved lymphoma have slightly more coarse chromatin patterns. Immunophenotypic studies can be useful, as lymphoblastic lymphomas can express either T- or B-cell phenotypes, and small noncleaved cell lymphomas are B-cell neoplasms exclusively. The enzyme terminal deoxynucleotidyl transferase can be detected by immunohistochemistry in the cells of lymphoblastic lymphoma, but not in those of other types of lymphoma.

Peripheral T-Cell Lymphoma (Nonepidermotropic T-Cell Lymphoma; Small, Medium, and Large Cell; Lennert Lymphoma; Subcutaneous Panniculitic T-Cell Lymphoma)

The correlation of clinical, histologic, and immunophenotypic data has made it possible to recognize a variety of T-cell lymphomas that are unrelated to MF and Sezary syndrome. The term *nonepidermotropic* is imperfect, as limited epidermal infiltration occurs in some examples. The most extensive consideration of these neoplasms is the Kiel classification, the revised version of which recognizes a number of types whose reproducible diagnosis is difficult.[14] Some of these types are recognized as provisional categories within the REAL classification.[15]

Lennert or lymphoepithelioid lymphoma is a low-grade T-cell neoplasm in which epithelioid macrophages proliferate in reaction to the neoplasm. Systemic involvement can include cervical lymphadenopathy, hepatosplenomegaly, bone marrow infiltration, and fever. The skin is involved in less than 10% of cases.[28] There are no features that distinguish the cutaneous lesions from those of other lymphomas clinically. Dense nodular and diffuse infiltrates of lymphocytes with convoluted, elongated, or twisted-appearing nuclei, with clusters of epithelioid macrophages and rare plasma cells, typify Lennert lymphoma. Large atypical lymphocytes are often directly apposed to the clusters of macrophages. In addition to nodular or diffuse dermal infiltrates, there can be band-like infiltrates in the papillary dermis, and lymphocytes may occasionally infiltrate the epidermis.[29] Lennert lymphoma can resemble granulomatous MF histologically, but the patches seen in the latter clinically are never found. The clusters of epithelioid macrophages that typify Lennert lymphoma are evenly dispersed throughout the infiltrate, while those of granulomatous MF are randomly distributed. Immunophenotyping is not useful for differentiating these conditions, as both are T-helper cell neoplasms. The clusters of macrophages are smaller than those found in sarcoidosis or other sarcoidal granulomatous dermatitides.

Angioimmunoblastic lymphadenopathy (AILD) is a condition characterized by fever, lymphadenopathy, and dysproteinemia. Infiltrates in lymph nodes are polymorphous and feature immunoblasts, plasma cells, small lymphocytes, and a background in which there are increased numbers of small blood vessels with extravascular accumulations of periodic acid-Schiff diastase-positive material. Overt T-cell lymphomas evolve in many patients with this condition. Large atypical lymphocytes with clear cytoplasm are found next to small vessels in AILD-like T-cell lymphoma. It is conceivable that many cases of AILD without these atypical cells have minor clonal populations and are already low-grade lymphomas. Roughly 40% of patients develop cutaneous macules and papules, with one observer claiming that the histopathology was that of lymphocytic vasculitis and another showing atypical lymphocytes in the infiltrates.

Pleomorphic T-cell lymphoma was first described in Japanese patients infected with HTLV-1, but it is now known that it can occur in noninfected patients also.[30] The disease is defined by its cytologic features: irregular nuclear size and shape, small nucleoli, and hyperchromasia. In the modified Kiel classification the small cell (3 to 7 μm) variant of pleomorphic T-cell lymphoma is a low-grade lymphoma and the medium (7 to 11 μm) and large (over 11 μm) cell variants are high-grade lymphomas.[14] The REAL classification recognizes the difficulty that many pathologists have in classifying these lesions and consolidates them in a group termed *peripheral T-cell lymphoma, unspecified.*[15]

The clinical lesions of pleomorphic T-cell lymphoma do not have a distinctive appearance. Patches, as seen in MF, are not present. The infiltrates of pleomorphic T-cell lymphoma have a T-cell pattern histologically, and infiltration of the epidermis and hair follicle epithelium is usually found (Fig. 21-7). Multi-lobated T-cell lymphoma is a type of large cell, pleomorphic, T-cell lymphoma with a propensity to involve the skin and bones of elderly patients.[31,32]

Subcutaneous panniculitic or lipotropic T-cell lymphoma presents with subcutaneous masses, usually on the extremities. Many patients with this condition have a hemophagocytic syndrome, which in one series was fatal in the majority of patients.[33] There may be considerable overlap with angiocentric lymphoma, as infiltration of vessel walls often accompanies subcutaneous infiltrates (see angiocentric lymphoma, below). Histopathologic features include dense subcutaneous infiltrates with a mixed septal and lobular pattern, composed largely of cells with cytologic features similar to those of the medium or large cell type of pleomorphic T-cell lymphoma (Fig. 21-8); rarely, anaplastic large cells are prominent. Foci of karyorrhexis and fat necrosis are prominent, the later resulting in granulomatous areas in some specimens. Phagocytosis of erythrocytes by non-neoplastic macrophages is present in the subcutaneous infiltrates, but is more prominent in bone marrow biopsies from these patients. The neoplastic cells mark as mature helper T cells in most cases, but can show loss of the CD5 and CD7 antigens or a natural killer cell phenotype (CD16+, CD56+) and evidence of Epstein-Barr viral infection by immunohistochemistry or in situ hybridization. Genotypic findings have been mixed, with some cases demonstrating clonal rearrangements of the T-cell receptor β-chain gene and others having germline configurations.

One unusual case[2] of subcutaneous T-cell lymphoma was composed of cells that produced interferon-γ, expressed the δ T-cell receptor, expressed neither CD4 nor CD8, but instead had a natural killer cell phenotype. Subcutaneous T-cell lymphomas resemble panniculitis at scanning magnification, and, in the cases in which small pleomorphic T cells predominate, their infiltrates may not be obviously malignant even on closer scrutiny. Karyorrhexis can also be a feature of subcutaneous lupus erythematosus. Careful attention to cytologic detail and a search for morphologic and laboratory evidence of erythrophagocytosis can be of help with these difficult cases.

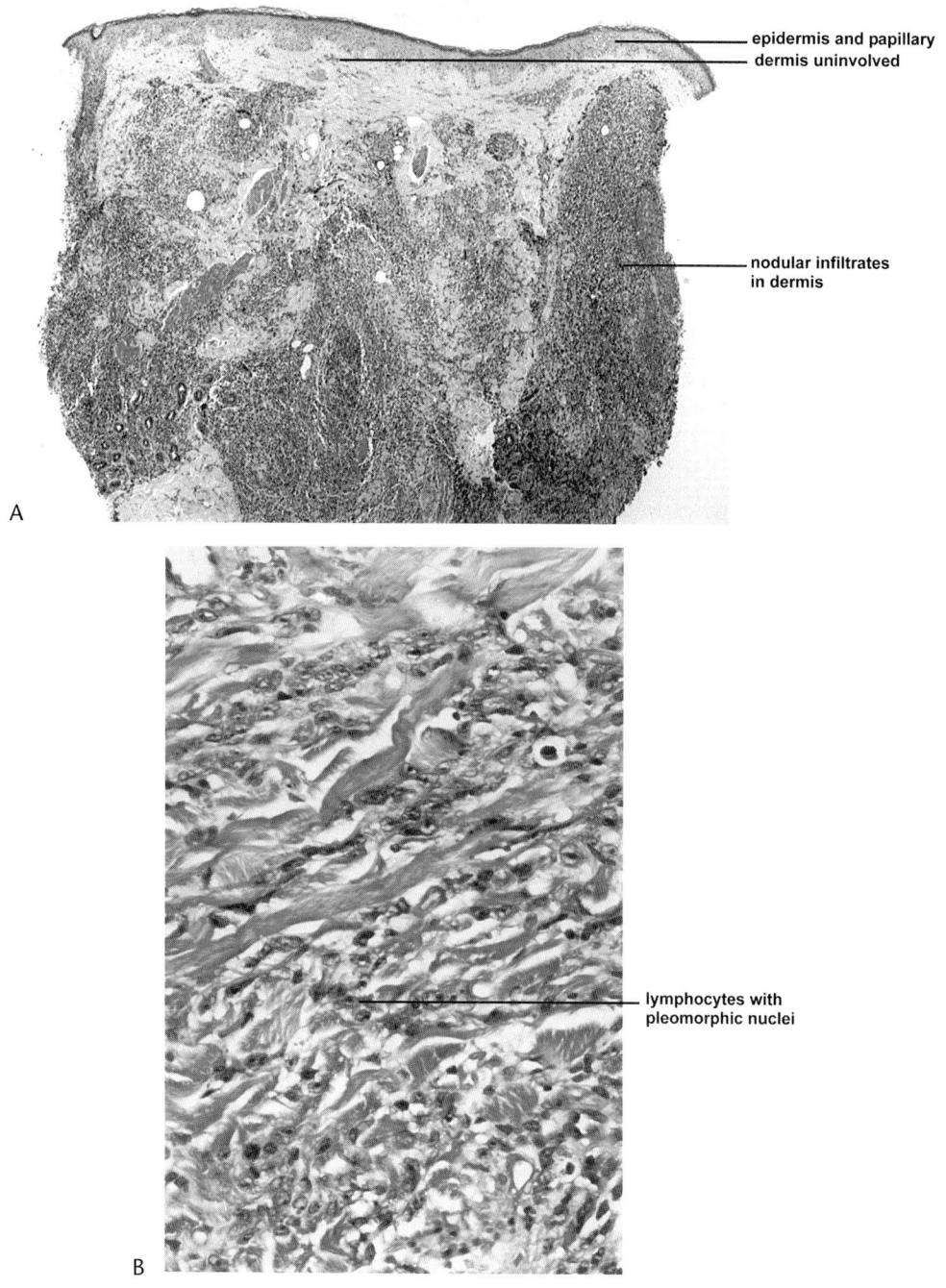

Figure 21-7. Pleomorphic T-cell lymphoma. There are confluent nodular infiltrates of cells with hyperchromatic nuclei and scant cytoplasm, hence the dark appearance of the infiltrates at scanning magnification **(A)**. The cells of pleomorphic T-cell lymphoma have irregularly shaped nuclei but are not cerebriform as the cells of mycosis fungoides are **(B)**.

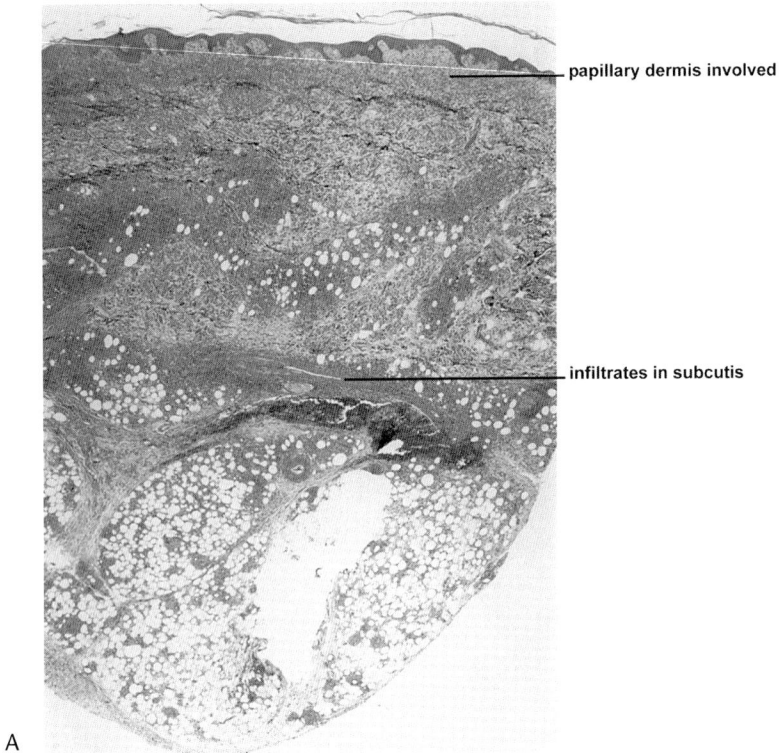

papillary dermis involved

infiltrates in subcutis

A

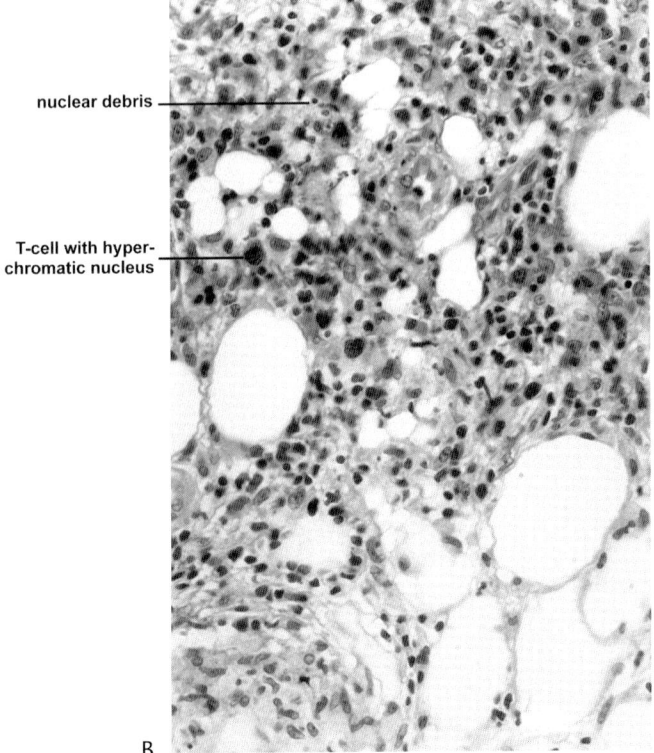

nuclear debris

T-cell with hyper-chromatic nucleus

B

Figure 21-8. Subcutaneous T-cell lymphoma. This form of T-cell lymphoma is associated with the hemophagocytic syndrome and has a poor prognosis. It is important not to confuse it with a lobular panniculitis, such as lupus profundus. There are patchy infiltrates of neoplastic cells throughout the superficial and deep dermis and subcutis **(A)**. The cytologic features of this lymphoma overlap with those of pleomorphic T-cell lymphoma. Note the abundant nuclear debris **(B)**. Phagocytosis of nuclear dust by macrophages has given rise to the term cytophagic panniculitis, which is a misnomer.

MULTIPLE MYELOMA AND CUTANEOUS PLASMACYTOMAS

Multiple myeloma (MM) is a malignant neoplasm of plasma cells, which may be either well or poorly differentiated. Criteria for the diagnosis of MM include a combination of clinical, laboratory, and histologic findings, including infiltration of the marrow by plasma cells, a biopsy-proven plasmacytoma, a paraprotein in plasma or urine, osteolytic bone lesions, or circulating plasma cells.

Cutaneous plasmacytomas are masses of plasma cells that have arisen in the skin rather than having reached it by direct extension from an osseous focus of myeloma. Cutaneous plasmacytomas may precede disseminated disease or MM by many years.

Clinical Features

Cutaneous lesions of MM or plasmacytoma are usually circumscribed, violaceous papules or nodules. More diffusely infiltrative lesions are occasionally seen.[34]

Patients with MM may also have a variety of nonspecific cutaneous lesions, including amyloid or cryoglobulin deposition, pyoderma gangrenosum, leukocytoclastic vasculitis, Sweet syndrome, erythema elevatum diutinum, and plane xanthomas. Conditions often accompanied by monoclonal gammopathies, such as scleromyxedema, necrobiotic xanthogranuloma with paraproteinemia, POEMS (polyneuropathy, organomegaly, endocrinopathy, M protein, and skin lesions) syndrome, or scleredema may develop into full-blown MM.

Figure 21-9. Plasmacytoma. There is a nodular infiltrate of plasma cells in the dermis (**A**). Unlike immunocytoma (lymphoplasmacellular lymphoma, marginal zone lymphoma), the infiltrate is entirely composed of plasma cells, without plasmacytoid lymphocytes or small lymphocytes. Some of the plasma cells have atypical nuclei (**B**).

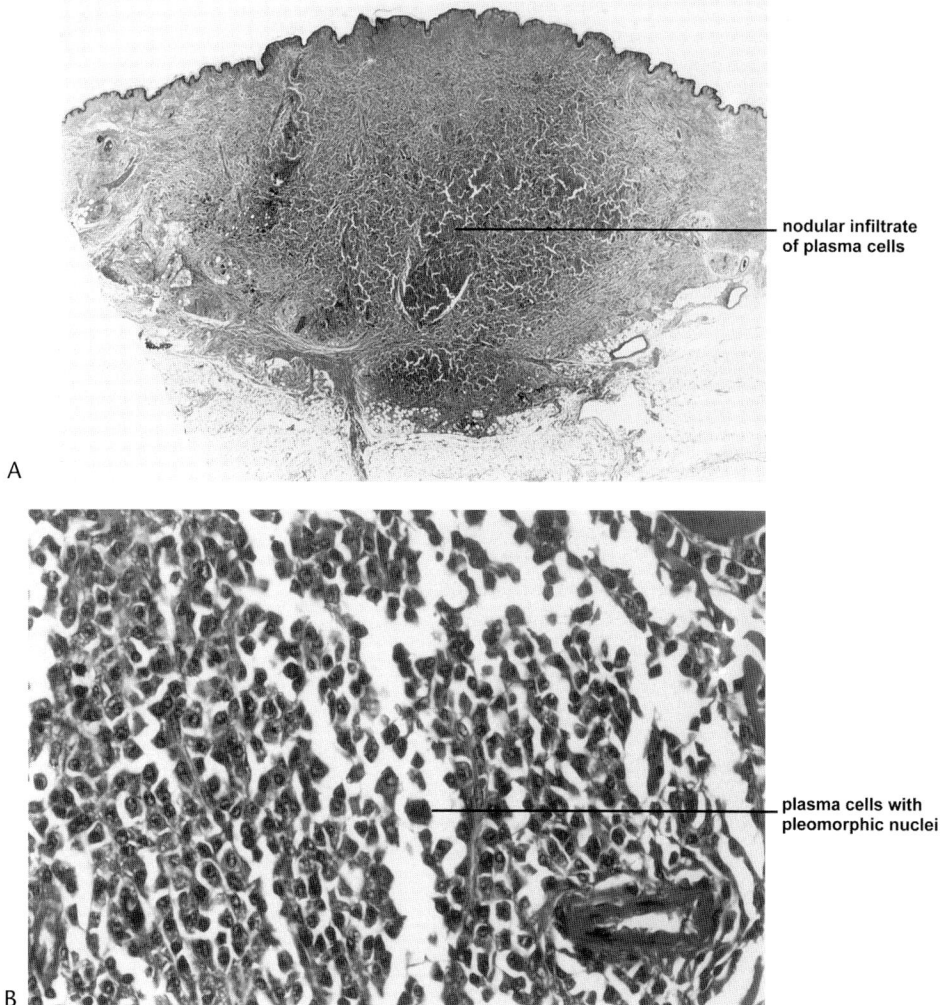

A — nodular infiltrate of plasma cells

B — plasma cells with pleomorphic nuclei

Histopathologic Features

Biopsies from cutaneous lesions of MM and plasmacytomas show monomorphous infiltrates of plasma cells either as densely cellular nodules (Fig. 21-9) or as an arrangement of single cells or cords of cells distributed between collagen bundles.[35] In the nodular pattern, clusters of macrophages are sometimes present. Nodular lesions may be composed of well-differentiated plasma cells. They may also have multinucleated cells, cells with large atypical nuclei, or mitotic figures. So-called plasma cell bodies, which are round, anucleated, eosinophilic-staining clumps of plasma cell cytoplasm, can be present. Intranuclear inclusions of immunoglobulin, known as Dutcher bodies, which can be mistaken for eosinophilic nucleoli, are rare in MM. In lesions of MM that show the infiltrative patterns, it can be difficult to recognize the neoplastic cells; they can have angulated shapes, vacuolated cytoplasms, and nuclei that lack the "clock-face" clumping of chromatin typical of mature plasma cells.

Differential Diagnosis

A variety of cutaneous conditions that include infiltrates composed predominantly of mature plasma cells can simulate MM or plasmacytomas. Some specimens of CLH contain many plasma cells, and, rarely, plasma cells are the predominant cell type. In these specimens, clusters of immunoblasts, small cleaved and large lymphocytes, and even fully formed germinal centers may provide clues to the correct diagnosis. A variety of inflammatory reactions on the scalp or near mucous membranes also feature conspicuous plasma cells. This phenomenon is known as *orificial plasmacytosis*.[36] Another condition, systemic plasmacytosis, has been described in Japanese patients, who have developed cutaneous plaques, lymphadenopathy, and polyclonal hypergammaglobulinemia.[37] The cutaneous infiltrates in these cases were perivascular or dermal nodules of cytologically normal-appearing plasma cells.

These stimulants of MM and plasmacytoma are composed of polyclonal plasma cells. Cytoplasmic, as opposed to cell membrane-bound, immunoglobulin is often well preserved in formalin-fixed, paraffin-embedded tissue and can be detected in most plasma cell infiltrates, so that the diagnosis of MM can usually be confirmed or excluded using routinely processed tissue.

Staining with antisera to κ and λ light chains is also useful in identifying cases of MM or plasmacytoma when plasma cells are distorted by fixation or are poorly differentiated. Distorted plasma cells can resemble the cells of melanoma, carcinoma, or other neoplasms. The demonstration of cytoplasmic immunoglobulin is especially useful in such cases because some antigens found on B lymphocytes are lost as the cells differentiate into plasma cells.

Two closely related lymphomas, immunoblastic lymphoma and marginal zone lymphoma, can be mistaken for MM and cutaneous plasmacytoma. In immunoblastic lymphoma, the nuclei of the neoplastic cells are larger and more vesicular than those of plasma cells, and, while chromatin is marginated around the nuclear membrane, it does not have the "clock-face" pattern seen in plasma cells. Immunoblastic lymphoma cells have less cytoplasm than do plasma cells, and their nuclei are not eccentrically positioned. Marginal zone lymphoma (immunocytoma) has a far better prognosis than MM. While the cells of marginal zone lymphoma may have eccentrically placed nuclei and fan-shaped cytoplasm, the nuclei have a more dispersed chromatin pattern, and a perinuclear clear zone (hof) is not as pronounced. A range of differentiation may be present in some cases of marginal zone lymphoma, with some cells having scant cytoplasm and others resembling well-differentiated plasma cells. In contrast, in a single lesion of MM or cutaneous plasmacytoma, the neoplastic cells are usually monomorphous.

MYCOSIS FUNGOIDES

MF is a T-cell lymphoma that invades the epidermis and papillary dermis and subsequently acquires the ability to grow into the reticular dermis, lymph nodes, and viscera. Such terms as *parapsoriasis en plaques, poikiloderma vasculare atrophicans, prereticulotic poikiloderma, chronic superficial dermatitis, large plaque parapsoriasis,* and *parapsoriasis variegata* predate the recognition of the histologic criteria for patch stage MF. While some still regard them as valid diagnostic categories for an early, preneoplastic stage of MF, we believe that most patients described as having these conditions actually had MF.

Clinical Features

MF is most commonly detected in patients who are in late middle age or elderly. However, the disease has been reported in all age groups, including children.

The earliest lesions of MF are pink to red, slightly scaly patches, often on the trunk or proximal extremities. The buttocks and breasts are often involved by MF, perhaps because they are "double-clothed" sites. The infiltrates of MF in its early stages are sensitive to ultraviolet light, and these sites may be refuges for patch stage infiltrates of the neoplasm.

Patients with patch stage MF usually have at least a few lesions larger than an adult palm (approximately 10 cm). In many patients, the lesions remain stable or may slowly involute as new lesions emerge. In some patients, patches become poikilodermatous, with an atrophic, wrinkled appearance, telangiectases, and mottled pigmentation. This appearance has been called *poikiloderma vasculare atrophicans,* a term that may be confusing in that it is also used to refer to atrophic lesions in dermatomyositis and other conditions. Some patches of MF have a reticulated appearance, referred to as *parapsoriasis variegata.*

It is currently unknown what proportion of patients with patches of MF will develop plaques. Plaques of MF can be pink, red, or brown and are slightly raised, often sharply circumscribed, and annular.

Once patients with MF develop plaques they usually will also develop nodules and tumors of MF if not treated. These lesions can be clinically indistinguishable from the nodules and tumors of other cutaneous lymphomas. They tend to be pink, red, red-brown, or plum colored, firm, and sometimes ulcerated. MF in such patients can be best diagnosed by the presence of residual patches, which do not occur in other forms of lymphoma. Patients with the sudden onset of tumors of cutaneous lymphoma that had cells with scant cytoplasm and irregular nuclei were formerly regarded as *mycosis fungoides d'emblee*; such patients most likely had pleomorphic T-cell lymphoma (see above) and not MF.

Some patients with limited cutaneous disease become diffusely erythrodermic, either transiently or persistently. These cases illustrate the overlap between MF and the closely related Sezary syndrome and engendered the term *cutaneous T-cell lymphoma* as a unifying concept.[38] Initially, CTCL referred to neoplasms in which epidermotropism and a composition of helper T cells were important features. The utility of that term is limited by the heterogeneity of the lesions that further study has revealed also to be T-cell neoplasms but nonepidermotropic and not necessarily helper cell in nature, such as the angiocentric, subcutaneous, pleomorphic, and anaplastic large cell lymphomas.

Lymphadenopathy may be present both in patients with erythrodermic MF and in those with extensive cutaneous involvement. Hepatosplenomegaly is only evident in patients with advanced disease.

It is difficult to evaluate the natural history of MF from the studies performed to date. Early studies focused on patients with late patch, plaque, and tumor stage disease.[39] The evolution of criteria for early patch stage lesions has resulted in an increased rate of diagnosis, which has been sometimes interpreted as indicative of increased incidence.[40] What the prognosis is for such patients presenting with early patch stage disease requires further studies. The median survival for patients with patch or plaque stage disease is greater than a decade, but those with tumors, histologically evident lymph node or visceral involvement, or erythroderma usually live less than 5 years.

Histopathologic Features

Sparse lymphocytic infiltrates are present around vessels of the superficial plexus and are scattered within the papillary dermis in early macules or patches of MF (Fig. 21-10). A few to many lymphocytes with small irregular nuclei, accompanied by slight spongiosis, may also be present within the epidermis.[41] One characteristic intraepidermal arrangement of the cells of patch stage MF is a linear array of lymphocytes on the epidermal side of the dermoepidermal junction, with little vacuolar change and only rare necrotic keratinocytes, in contrast to an interface dermatitis.[42] In another pattern, small, well-circumscribed clusters of lymphocytes are present within the epidermis (Fig. 21-11). The epidermis in patches of MF is often slightly hyperplastic, with evenly elongated rete that have rounded bases. Eosinophils and plasma cells are generally absent in early patch stage MF, and easily discernible cytologic atypia of lymphocytes is the exception rather than the rule.[41] Even in sparsely infiltrated patches of MF, the collagen bundles of the papillary dermis are often coarse and are either haphazardly arranged or are parallel to the surface of the epidermis.

Fully developed patches of MF often show band-like papillary dermal infiltrates and psoriasiform hyperplasia of the epidermis. There rete ridges are usually only moderately elongated, relatively narrow, and have rounded bases. Foci with scant spongiosis containing numerous lymphocytes can also be present in the epidermis. Papillary dermal fibrosis is similar in nature to that seen in early patch stage disease but is often more marked. Nuclei of lymphocytes in fully developed patches may be demonstrably larger, more convoluted, and stain darker than their reactive counterparts in the underlying papillary dermis. Eosinophils and plasma cells may also be found in fully developed patches.

In poikilodermatous MF there are fibrosis and thickening of the papillary dermis, loss of the normal rete ridge pattern, and deposition of melanophages (Fig. 21-12). Specific features of MF can be entirely absent in biopsies from poikilodermatous areas. Lymphocytes with large, hyperchromatic nuclei, either in clusters or a linear basilar distribution along the dermoepider-

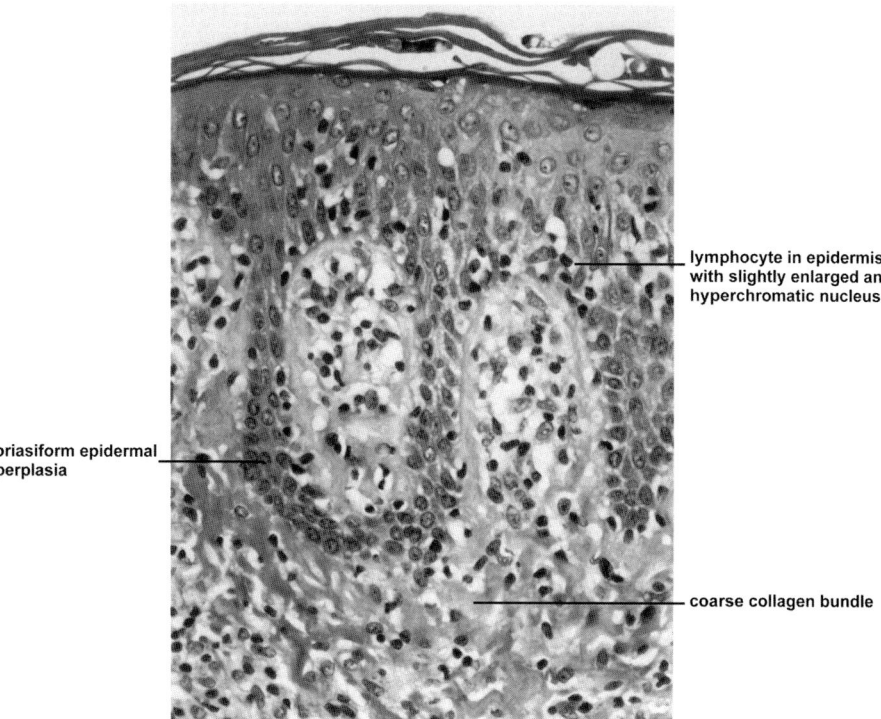

psoriasiform epidermal hyperplasia

lymphocyte in epidermis with slightly enlarged and hyperchromatic nucleus

coarse collagen bundle

Figure 21-10. Mycosis fungoides, patch stage. Slender elongated rete ridges that overly a papillary dermis in which collagen bundles are thickened and separated by clefts is a typical finding. Note lymphocytes in the epidermis with slightly larger and darker nuclei than those of their dermal counterparts. There is spongiosis, but it is slight considering the number of lymphocytes within the epidermis in this field.

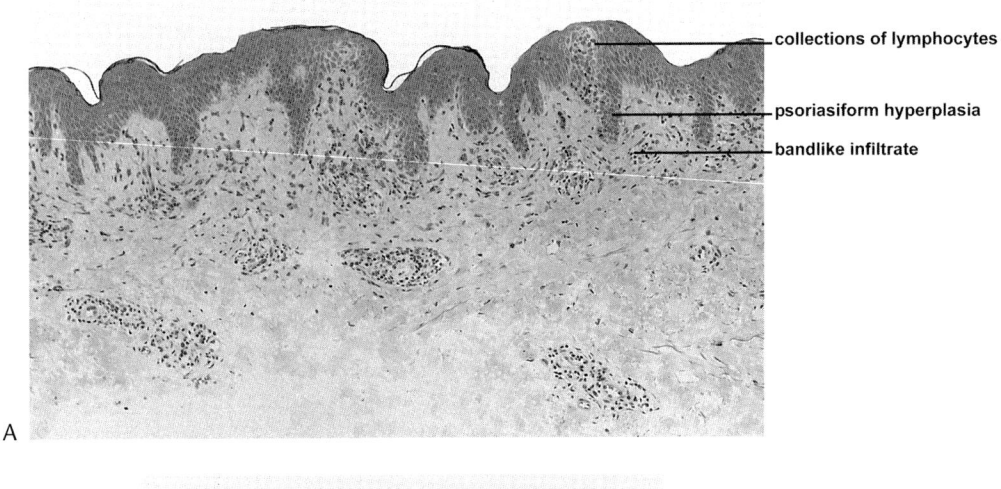

collections of lymphocytes

psoriasiform hyperplasia

bandlike infiltrate

A

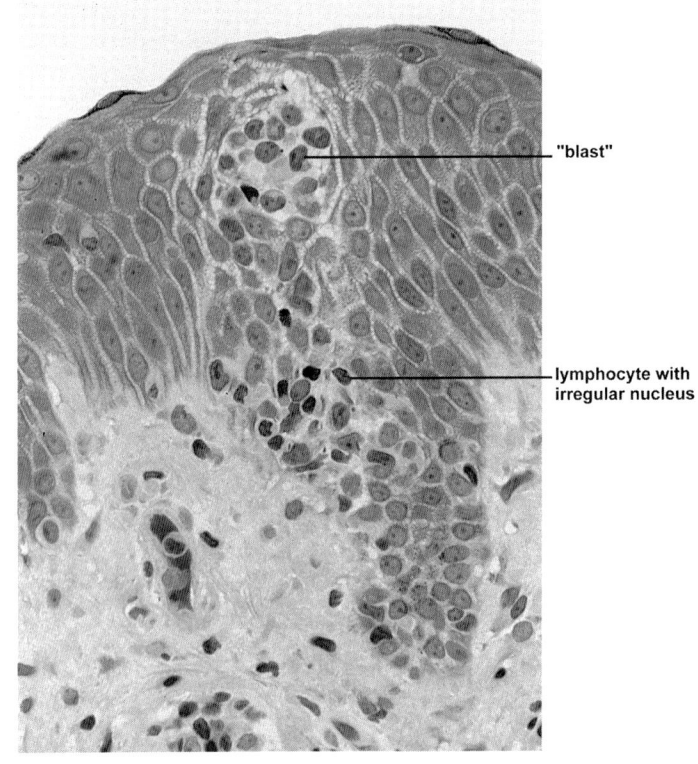

"blast"

lymphocyte with
irregular nucleus

B

Figure 21-11. Mycosis fungoides, patch stage. In this pattern, lymphocytes are present in tightly packed aggregations in the epidermis. There is psoriasiform epidermal hyperplasia, and a patchy band-like infiltrate is present in the papillary dermis **(A)**. The collection of cells within the epidermis includes several blasts, which are lymphocytes with large round nuclei and dispersed chromatin **(B)**.

mal junction, may enable a specific diagnosis of MF. Poikilodermatous MF can be thought of as MF altered by regression, the result of reactive T cells eliminating the neoplastic T cells of MF and altering the dermis and epidermis. The histologic changes in poikilodermatous MF resemble those seen in other forms of lymphocyte-mediated regression, such as regressed malignant melanoma, the findings in the papillary dermis between the nests of superficial basal cell carcinoma, in the centers of lesions of actinic porokeratosis, and in atrophic lichen planus.

In plaques of MF, the reticular dermis harbors infiltrates that may be perivascular or nodular, and the band-like papillary dermal infiltrates are denser than they are in patch stage MF (Fig. 21-13). Cytologically atypical lymphocytes, with large hyperchromatic and hyperconvoluted nuclei, are the rule in plaque stage disease. Dense infiltrates often outline the vertically oriented vessels of the intercommunicating vascular plexus. Follicular mucinosis, the abnormal production of mucin (mostly hyaluronic acid) by hair follicle epithelium, is an unusual occurrence in plaques of MF. In specimens of MF with follicular

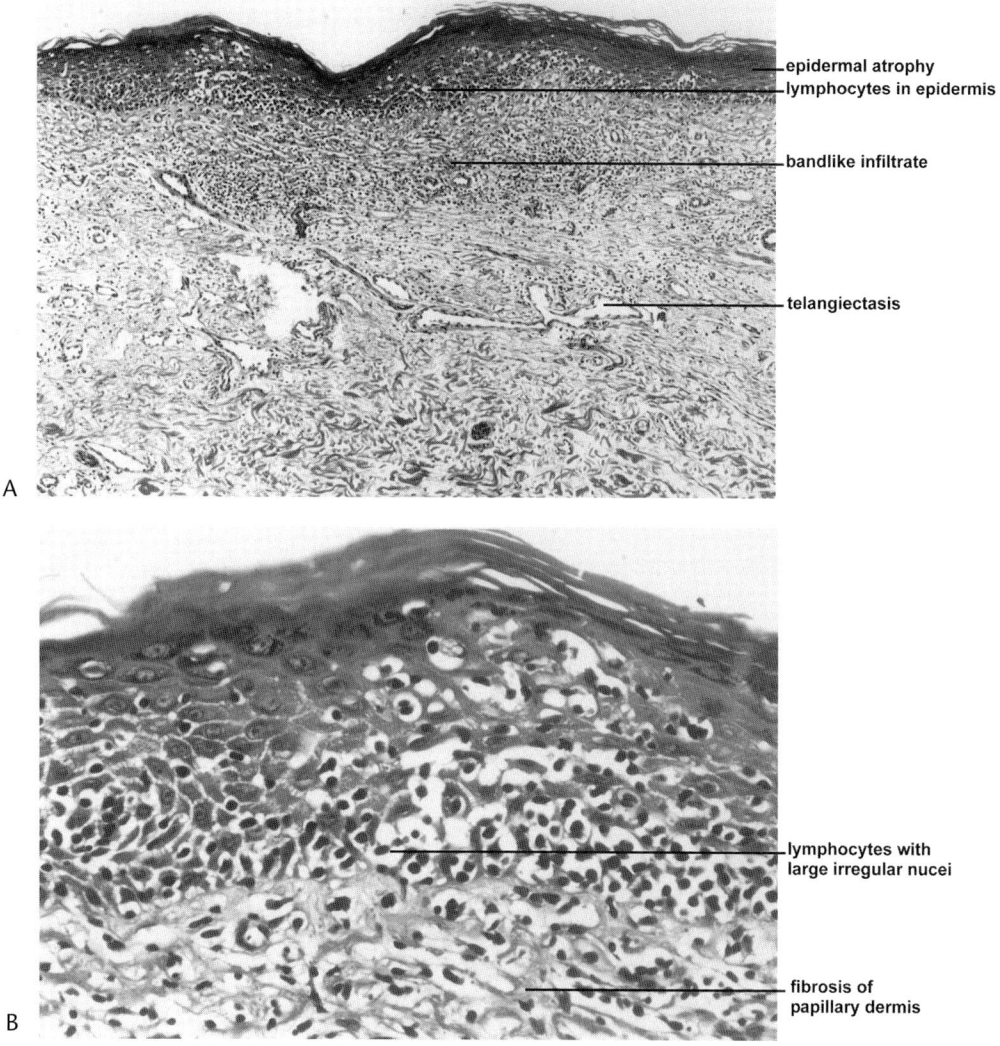

epidermal atrophy
lymphocytes in epidermis

bandlike infiltrate

telangiectasis

A

lymphocytes with
large irregular nucei

fibrosis of
papillary dermis

B

Figure 21-12. Mycosis fungoides, atrophic patch stage. The rete ridge pattern is effaced, and the epidermis riddled with innumerable lymphocytes which have slightly enlarged and hyperchromatic nuclei. There are prominent telangiectases in the papillary dermis **(A)**. The papillary dermis contains coarse collagen bundles **(B)**.

mucinosis the outer root sheath of the follicle is expanded, and interstices between keratinocytes are widened by accumulations of mucin. Follicular keratinocytes are attenuated and their intercellular bridges stretched. In MF with follicular mucinosis there are usually diagnosable findings of MF other than in the follicular epithelium itself.

In nodules and tumors of MF the neoplastic cells densely infiltrate the reticular dermis, often losing their affinity for the papillary dermis and the epidermis. The epidermis in such cases may even be thinned. The dermal infiltrates contain lymphocytes with nuclei that are larger and considerably more atypical than those in patches and most plaques of MF. There is often a range of cells from small ones with convoluted nuclei to large convoluted forms, to "blasts" with rounded nuclei, coarse chromatin, and large nucleoli. Eosinophils and plasma cells are found in the dermal infiltrates of most nodules or tumors of MF.[3]

One approach to the histopathologic evaluation of tumors of

MF is to evaluate the infiltrates using the modified Kiel classification.[14] Three forms of large cell lymphoma can be discerned in tumors of MF. T-cell lymphoma of the medium or large pleomorphic type (medium to large cells with folded or lobulated nuclei); T-cell lymphoma, immunoblastic type (monomorphous large cells with vesicular nuclei and prominent central nucleoli); and T large cell lymphoma of the anaplastic type (large cells with abundant cytoplasm and large irregularly shaped nuclei, sometimes with several large nucleoli). Despite the frequent presence of CD30 (Ki-1) in the cells of large cell anaplastic lymphoma developing in MF, the prognosis is less favorable than that of CD30+ lymphoma. However, the survival of patients with tumors of MF and histopathologic features of transformation is not necessarily worse than of those with tumors composed of small convoluted lymphocytes.[42]

MF has a large repertoire of various clinical and histologic guises, and the stereotypical evolution of lesions noted above does little justice to the variety of appearances that the der-

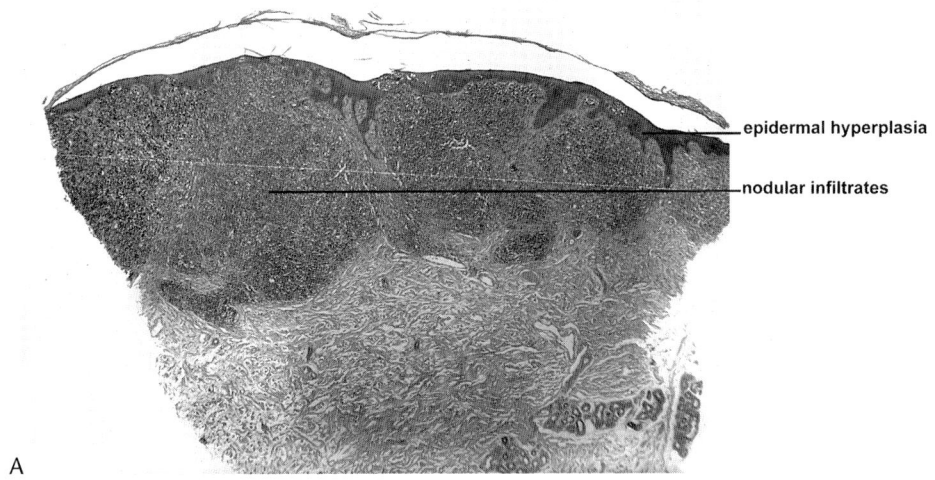

epidermal hyperplasia

nodular infiltrates

A

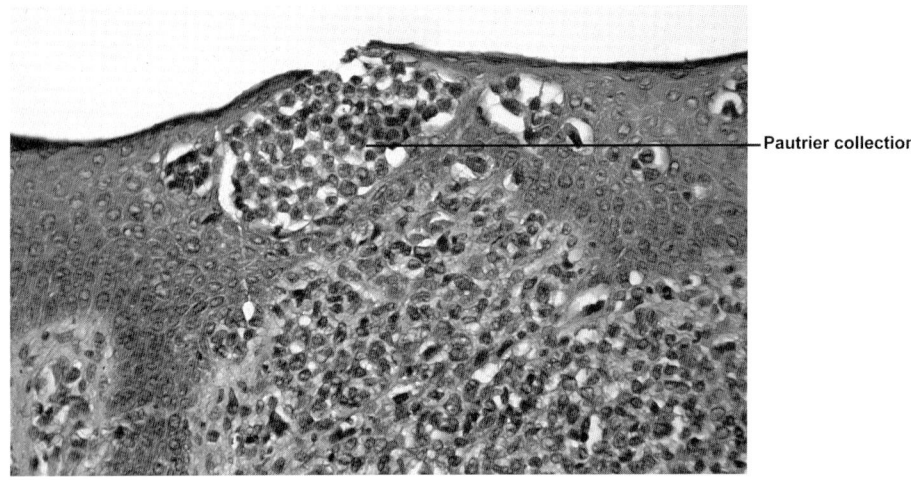

Pautrier collection

B

Figure 21-13. Mycosis fungoides, plaque stage. Lymphocytic infiltrates now form large nodules in the superficial dermis, with focal epidermal hyperplasia **(A)**. There are large collections of cerebriform lymphocytes in the epidermis. Note that the cells that comprise this Pautrier microabscess or collection are monomorphous and tightly packed **(B)**.

matopathologist can encounter. One notable variant is granulomatous MF, in which aggregates of macrophages and giant cells comprise a portion of the dermal infiltrate. One patient with this variant survived for an extraordinarily long time despite widespread tumors, but other studies have not shown any benefit to having this variant.[43,44] Closely related to granulomatous MF is granulomatous slack skin in which pendulous bags of skin are found in flexural areas.[44]

Occasionally, patients with otherwise typical MF have presented with large, verrucous plaques that histologically showed pseudocarcinomatous hyperplasia. Vasculitis with atypical lymphocytes, acanthosis nigricans–like lesions, bullous lesions, follicular papules, and other unusual morphologies have all been reported.[45]

There are a number of adjunctive techniques that were developed in the hope of improving diagnostic accuracy in early MF. Immunophenotyping of fresh-frozen sections, the evaluation of nuclear infoldings using 1 μm plastic sections or electron microscopy, and the measurement of nuclear DNA content by image analysis cytometry have all had proponents and opponents.

Of these, immunophenotyping is the most commonly used. The vast majority of patches and plaques of MF are neoplasms of lymphocytes with a mature helper T-cell phenotype. Early studies held out hope that a high helper/suppressor ratio in the infiltrating cells might be specific for MF, but it is apparent that rare cases of MF are suppressor cell neoplasms, that some lesions of MF are infiltrated by reactive suppressor T cells, and that some inflammatory skin diseases, in their early stages, are composed nearly entirely of helper T cells. The simultaneous expression of both helper and suppressor markers by the same T cells, while rare, may indicate a neoplastic infiltrate. Claims have been made that the cells of MF aberrantly fail to express CD7, an antigen found on mature helper T cells; however, other workers have not found the absence of CD7 to be a reliable marker for MF.[46] Plaques and tumors of MF, which are easier to diagnose with certainty by routine methods, often have lymphocytes with abnormal immunophenotypes, lacking T-cell antigens such as CD2, CD3, and CD5.

A new technique, clonal analysis, may become an important adjunct to the diagnosis of MF in difficult cases. Studies of the configuration of the T-cell receptor genes has shown that densely infiltrated patches, plaques, and tumors of MF are produced by single clones of neoplastic T cells.[47] Because early patches of MF are sparsely infiltrated, it has been difficult to use the Southern blot method to assay these lesions for clonality. The polymerase chain reaction (PCR) may make it possible to detect clonal populations in early patch stage lesions and comprehensively answer the question of whether the very earliest lesions of MF are clonal (neoplastic) or nonclonal (inflammatory) in nature. Because minor clones can be amplified by PCR, quantification of clonal populations will likely be key for reliably using this technique as an ancillary test.[48] Antisera are available against only a few of the variable regions of the T-cell receptor β-chain. Biopsy specimens from patch stage lesions of MF stained with these antisera by the immunoperoxidase technique have shown a preponderance of Vβ usage in some cases, supporting the clonal nature of patch stage MF.

Clinicopathologic Correlation

The clinical and histologic faces of MF correlate with a wide range of pathologic situations. The pink color of macules and patches derives largely from vascular dilation. The surfaces of patches and plaques are scaly but usually not weeping. Histologically, lamellar or compact hyperkeratosis and, occasionally, parakeratosis can be seen, but not much serum is present in the cornified layer. The dusky color of plaques and tumors derives from dermal infiltration by lymphocytes. Plaques with follicular mucinosis may have the same peau d'orange appearance as those of alopecia mucinosa. Patches of poikilodermatous MF have epidermal atrophy, papillary dermal fibrosis, melanophages, and telangiectases. The verrucous hyperkeratotic form of MF has pseudocarcinomatous hyperplasia and hyperkeratosis, which can sometimes result in biopsies being misinterpreted as keratoacanthoma or squamous cell carcinoma. Papules of MF may be folliculocentric microscopically, with

the hair follicle epithelium rather than epidermis serving as the target of lymphocytic infiltration.[49] In MF with vasculitis, the clinical lesions may be hemorrhagic. In bullous MF, lymphocytes so confluently replace the basilar epidermis that dermoepidermal separation occurs.[50] The extreme laxity of flexural skin in granulomatous slack skin is due to elastolysis by the numerous giant cells that pepper the dermal infiltrates of that condition.[44]

Differential Diagnosis

The main simulants of patch stage MF are the spongiotic dermatitides and conditions with lichenoid infiltrates. Chronic allergic contact and nummular dermatitis both can have superficial perivascular and interstitial infiltrates of small lymphocytes in the papillary dermis, as well as a few lymphocytes in the epidermis, as can be seen in patch stage MF. Additionally, fibrosis of the papillary dermis and compact or lamellar hyperkeratosis are present in both of these disorders. Specimens of patch or plaque stage MF often have a lichenoid pattern of papillary dermal infiltration accompanied by slight psoriasiform epidermal hyperplasia, which is not seen in these spongiotic simulants. A so-called psoriasiform, lichenoid, or spongiotic psoriasiform lichenoid pattern in which lymphocytes predominate favors MF over any of the primary spongiotic dermatitides.[51] Slight spongiosis usually occurs in MF in areas infiltrated by lymphocytes, but in spongiotic dermititis the spongiosis is diffuse and occurs in noninfiltrated areas as well. In MF, the number of lymphocytes infiltrating the epidermis in a given high power field is greater than that seen in the spongiotic dermatitides. Spongiotic vesiculation is seldom seen in MF, but, if it is, one should require lymphocytes with unequivocal nuclear atypia to make a diagnosis (Fig. 21-14).

In spongiotic dermatitis, intraepidermal aggregates of mononuclear cells are sometimes present, which superficially mimic the Pautrier microabsesses seen in MF.[52] These collec-

Figure 21-14. Spongiotic vesiculation in mycosis fungoides. In this example, the striking nuclear atypia makes the diagnosis clear. Spongiosis and indeed spongiotic vesiculation can occur in mycosis fungoides; but the diagnosis should not be made in the latter context in the absence of cells with striking cytologic atypia.

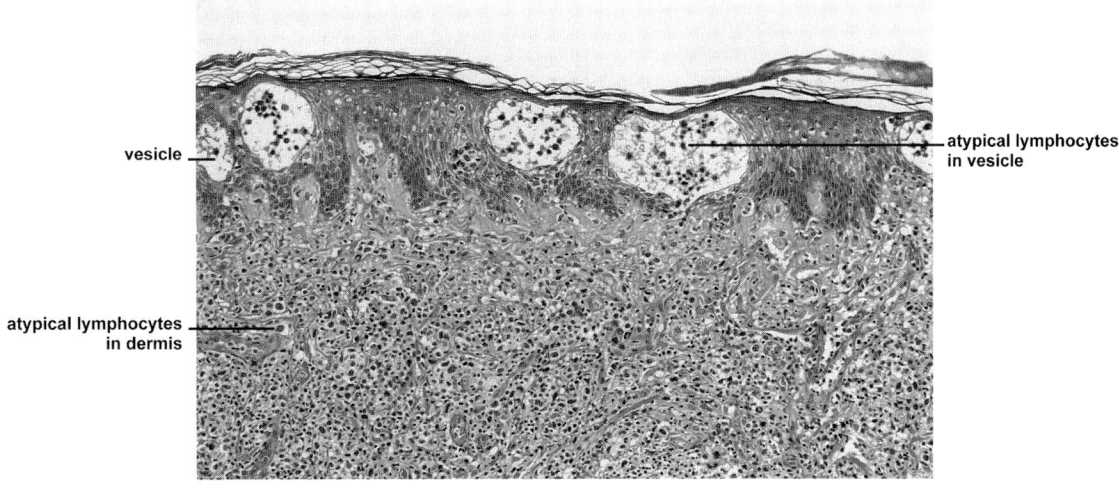

tions are surrounded by plasma, which can extrude laterally, creating a vase-shaped pattern as the aggregates reach the cornified layer. They are more loosely packed than true Pautrier microabsesses and contain an admixture of cells, including Langerhans or indeterminate cells, macrophages, lymphocytes, and degenerating keratinocytes. In contrast, true Pautrier microabscesses are compact and are composed mainly of lymphocytes, although a Langerhans cell may be at the center of the collection.

The lichenoid interface dermatitides may also simulate patch stage MF. Lichenoid drug eruptions generally damage the basilar epidermis, as evidenced by vacuolization and the presence of necrotic keratinocytes. As a result, the rete ridges become pointed, a change that is only rarely present in MF. On occasion, infiltration of the epidermis by lymphocytes may occur with only scant spongiosis. Lichenoid purpura and lichen aureus, two of the persistent pigmented purpuric dermatitides, can produce lesions with a psoriasiform lichenoid pattern and numerous lymphocytes in a nonspongiotic epidermis. The presence of siderophages, especially deep to the band-like infiltrate, is a key diagnostic finding. Edema of the papillary dermis, the finding of many extravasated erythrocytes within the papillary dermis and epidermis, the presence of eosinophils, and an absence of lymphocytes with cytologically atypical nuclei are all features favoring pigmented purpuric dermatitis over MF. Confounding this situation is the presence of clonal T-cell populations in some cases of lichenoid purpura.[53] Some lichenoid simulants of MF presenting as solitary lesions defy specific classification, but can be separated histologically from MF.[54]

MF can occasionally simulate vasculitis, folliculitis, panniculitis, and granulomatous dermatitis and should enter into the differential diagnosis of inflammatory skin disease that show these histologic patterns.[3] One comforting thought is that a delay in the diagnosis of this often indolent condition is outweighed by the harm that can be done by treating patients with inflammatory skin diseases for lymphoma.

Pathophysiology

Lymphocytes that circulate between lymph nodes and the epidermis, so-called cutaneous T cells, seem to be the most likely cell of origin of MF. Staining with antisera to Ki-67, which marks cells that are actively cycling, reveals that in patch stage disease most cellular replication is within the epidermis.[55] There is no firm evidence that environmental exposure causes MF. Small portions of the DNA of HTLV-1 provirus have been identified in the cells of patients with MF who lack antibodies to HTLV-1.[56]

PAGETOID RETICULOSIS

PR (Woringer-Kolopp disease) is an indolent form of T-cell lymphoma in which lesions are usually present on acral skin and show striking infiltration of epidermis histologically. The Ketron-Goodman variant has more widespread cutaneous lesions, but demonstrates marked epidermotropism.

Clinical Features

The lesions of PR are most often verrucous, scaling plaques that can have an annular or polycyclic configuration. Long-standing lesions may be fungating or crusted. The lesions of the Ketron-Goodman variant resemble those of conventional MF, being scaly patches or plaques. Persistence of disease is the rule for both variants. The existence of the Ketron-Goodman variant has been called into question as some cases develop a clinical course indistinguishable from that of MF. PR responds well to radiation therapy, surgical removal of lesions, and other localized treatments.

Histopathologic Features

The name *pagetoid reticulosis* derives from the propensity of the neoplastic lymphocytes to infiltrate the epidermis, some-

Figure 21-15. Pagetoid reticulosis or Woringer-Kolopp disease. This condition is marked in many specimens by striking pagetoid epidermotropism on the part of the neoplastic cells, seen here within the epidermis, while only small lymphocytes remain in the papillary dermis.

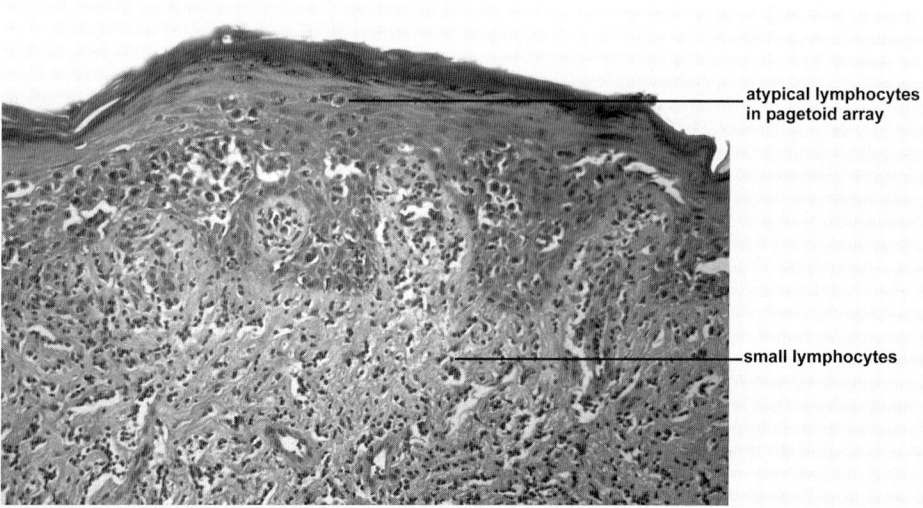

atypical lymphocytes in pagetoid array

small lymphocytes

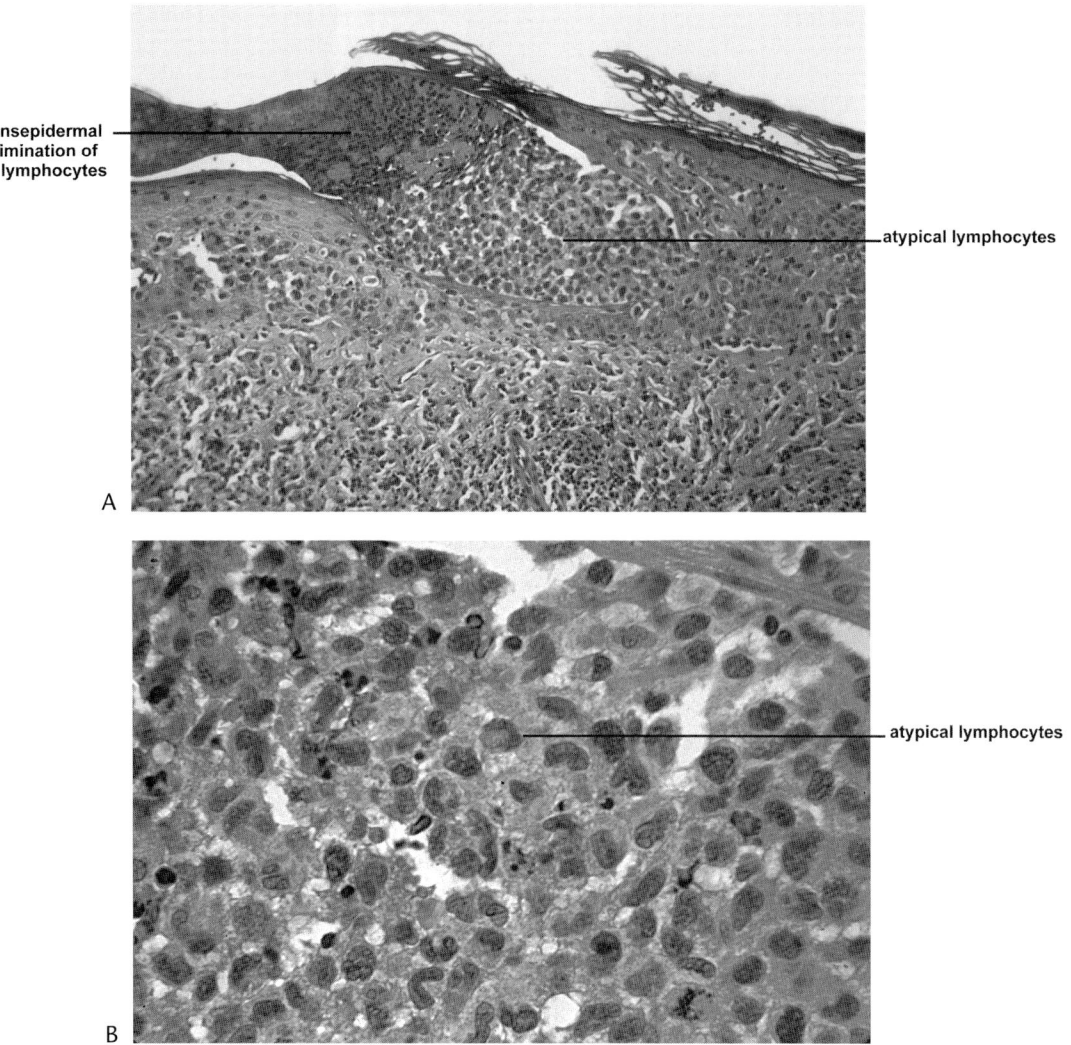

Figure 21-16. Disseminated pagetoid reticulosis (Ketron-Goodman disease) differs immunophenotypically from the localized (Woringer-Kolopp disease) form but also shows striking epidermotropism. A large intraepidermal mass of lymphocytes is expelled through the epidermis **(A)**. Some of the lymphocytes have bizarre shapes **(B)**.

times with little dermal involvement (Fig. 21-15). The clear halos around these cells impart an appearance that reminded early observers of Paget disease. The neoplastic cells in PR usually have intermediate-sized, convoluted nuclei and scant cytoplasm. The epidermis generally is hyperplastic, often strikingly so, and hyperkeratotic. The dermal infiltrates of PR may sometimes be composed of only small lymphocytes, presumably reactive cells. Eosinophils and plasma cells, which can be seen in late patches, plaques, and tumors of MF, are not present in PR.[57] Some cases with the classic clinical appearance of PR may not have striking epidermotropism. Marked epidermotropism is present by definition in the Ketron-Goodman variant and distinguished the condition from ordinary MF (Fig. 21-16).

From 1939, when Woringer and Kolopp first described PR,[58] to the early 1980s, controversy has existed regarding the cell of origin. The melanocyte, Merkel cell, and histiocyte have all had

their champions. Immunophenotypic studies have clearly shown that PR is a T-cell neoplasm. Analysis of one case using a probe to the T-cell antigen receptor indicated clonality.[59] The immunophenotype of PR appears to be heterogeneous. Most cases mark as CD4+ helper T-cell neoplasms, while some are CD8+ proliferations of suppressor cells.[60] Unlike the cells of MF, Sezary syndrome, and adult T-cell leukemia/lymphoma, those of localized PR do not express leukocyte common antigen (CD45) or the related T-cell-restricted epitope of leukocyte common antigen (CD45RO) recognized by the antibody UCHL1.[61] CD45 may interact with a protein kinase involved in cellular proliferation, which may explain the indolent clinical behavior of PR. The cells of the Ketron-Goodman variant express CD45, and in some cases there is a primitive T-cell phenotype in which the $\gamma\delta$, but not the $\alpha\beta$ form of the T-cell receptor is expressed.[62] This is in contrast to MF, in which the $\alpha\beta$ T-cell receptor is expressed.

Clinicopathologic Correlation

Marked verrucous hyperplasia and hyperkeratosis correspond to the clinical appearance of warty lesions.

Differential Diagnosis

The Woringer-Kolopp form of PR has some features in common with MF, such as lymphocytes within the epidermis accompanied by only slight spongiosis, lymphocytes with atypical nuclei, and epidermal hyperplasia. With the exception of rare patients with disseminated MF who have lesions of the verucous/hyperkeratotic type, the degree of epidermal hyperplasia, papillomatosis, and hyperkeratosis is more marked in Woringer-Kolopp disease. In many cases nearly all of the atypical lymphocytes are intraepidermal, while in lesions of conventional MF, wherein comparably atypical lymphocytes are present, the cells are located in the papillary dermis as well. Eosinophils and plasma cells, which can be present in all but early patches of MF, are seldom seen in Woringer-Kolopp disease. The absence of CD45-related antigens in Woringer-Kolopp disease is also in contrast to MF. This can be most easily assessed by staining for leukocyte common antigen (CD45RB) or the T-cell-associated antigen UCHL-1 (CD45RO) in formalin-fixed, paraffin-embedded sections. A cytotoxic-suppressor (CD8+) phenotype is often present in Woringer-Kolopp disease but not in MF.

Distinguishing between the Ketron-Goodman form of PR and MF is more problematic. Indeed, some authors hold that the two are indistinguishable. Regardless, the degree of pagetoid epidermotropism is greater than is generally seen in conventional MF. Vasculitis has been reported in some cases, manifested by fibrin in the walls of dermal venules, surrounded and infiltrated by lymphocytes with large and hyperchromatic nuclei.[63] Immunophenotyping of some cases of this type has revealed a natural killer cell phenotype. As is the case with some natural killer cells, the neoplastic lymphocytes have cytoplasmic granules in Wright-Giemsa-stained touch imprints and express CD56 but bear neither helper (CD4) nor suppressor (CD8) subset markers. Cases of this type appear to overlap features in a subset of those with angiocentric lymphoma (see below).

SEZARY SYNDROME

Sezary syndrome is a form of T-cell lymphoma characterized by erythroderma and the presence of neoplastic cells in the peripheral blood. Because its cells share many features with those of MF (epidermotropism, nuclear hyperconvolution, and helper T-cell phenotype), some consider Sezary syndrome and MF to be two forms of a single entity, CTCL.[38] Others contend that the concept of CTCL has outlived its usefulness because the spectrum of CTCL now includes so many other entities, such as adult T-cell leukemia/lymphoma, angiocentric lymphoma, pleomorphic T-cell lymphoma, and anaplastic large cell lymphoma.

Clinical Features

Strictly defined Sezary syndrome is a rare entity, perhaps 20 times less common than MF. Some patients with MF complicated by transient erythroderma and other patients with idiopathic erythrodermas have doubtless been misdiagnosed as having Sezary syndrome. The age at onset is similar to that of MF, with a peak in the seventh decade.[64] Rare cases occur in children and young adults.

In addition to erythroderma, the salient clinical signs of Sezary syndrome include lymphadenopathy, hepatomegaly, alopecia, and palmoplantar keratoderma. Patients with advanced disease may have leonine facies.

Survival with Sezary syndrome has been estimated at 2.5 to 5 years. During the course of the disease, plaques and tumors indistinguishable from those of MF may arise. Death is often from a breakdown of the immune system and resultant sepsis.

Histopathologic Features

The histologic findings in the erythrodermic skin of patients with Sezary syndrome often resemble those seen in patch stage MF, including band-like lymphocytic infiltrates with disproportionately little spongiosis and papillary dermal edema. Eosinophils and plasma cells can be present. Distinctly large, hyperchromatic, and hyperconvoluted nuclei are evident in the lymphocytes of many cases.[65] Pautrier microabscesses as seen in MF can also be seen in biopsy specimens from Sezary syndrome patients. The plaques and tumors that arise in advanced cases of Sezary syndrome are indistinguishable histologically from those of MF.

Some patients with clinical and hematologic evidence of Sezary syndrome have findings, even on repeated biopsies, that suggest spongiotic dermatitis rather than epidermotropic T-cell lymphoma.[66] Whether the erythroderma in these patients was caused by a cutaneous hypersensitivity reaction to the circulating cells of a lymphoma or whether the lymphocytic infiltrates accompanying the spongiosis are themselves part of the lymphoma awaits further study.

The peripheral blood of patients with Sezary syndrome contains an increased number of lymphocytes with hyperconvoluted nuclei, or Sezary cells. Sezary cells were at first thought to be unique to MF and Sezary syndrome; however, they have since been detected in the blood of patients with inflammatory skin diseases such as lichen planus and lupus erythematosus. Several methods have been proposed to measure the degree of hyperconvolution, including the nuclear contour index, which compares the perimeter of the nuclear membrane, as measured on an electron micrograph, to nuclear radius. Thin plastic-embedded sections stained to mask monocytes have to be used to more reliably identify the percentage of Sezary cells.[67]

The number of circulating Sezary cells considered diagnostic of the syndrome is controversial. Counts of more than $100/mm^2$ and 30% of circulating lymphocytes have been advocated. The failure of most observers to reproducibly count Sezary cells and the absence of a diagnostic "gold standard" have made it inadvisable to diagnose Sezary syndrome on the basis of blood smears alone unless large Sezary cells are present.

Immunophenotypic studies have also shown limited utility. While an increased helper suppressor ratio among peripheral blood lymphocytes is characteristic of Sezary syndrome, it is not specific for it. The circulating cells in most cases have mature T-helper-cell phenotypes. As is the case with infiltrates of MF, many cases feature diminished expression of CD7 in both tissue and blood. The percentage of CD7- T cells in either skin or blood that indicates Sezary syndrome needs to be refined by studying appropriate control populations of patients with erythrodermas of diverse causes.

Clonal rearrangements of the T-cell receptor β gene have been detected in most cases of Sezary syndrome.[68] A limited number of samples from patients with erythrodermic inflammatory skin diseases that could be confused clinically with Sezary syndrome have been analyzed and have not yet shown clonal populations.

As this time, the diagnosis of Sezary syndrome can be considered certain given the presence of erythroderma, increased numbers of hyperconvoluted lymphocytes in the peripheral blood, and either a skin biopsy showing features that are diagnostic of T-cell lymphoma or clonal rearrangement of the T-cell receptor β-chain gene.

Clinicopathologic Correlation

Biopsies from erythrodermic skin show a degree of infiltration equivalent to that of patch stage MF. Biopsies of palmar or plantar skin may show marked hyperkeratosis and epidermal hyperplasia as well as lymphocytic infiltration. While onychodystrophy can be seen in some patients, biopsies of the nail unit are not performed.

Differential Diagnosis

The cutaneous infiltrates seen in patients with Sezary syndrome so closely resemble those of MF that many consider the two conditions to be variants of CTCL. Two studies have compared the cutaneous histopathology of Sezary syndrome with that of MF.[65,69] Both found that Pautrier microabscesses were more common in Sezary syndrome. Papillary dermal edema may also be more common in Sezary syndrome than in MF, perhaps because biopsies are performed sooner in patients with erythroderma than they are in those with localized patches in whom topical treatments are often tried before a lesion is biopsied. Sentis and co-workers[65] noted monotonous infiltrates of large mononuclear cells with cerebriform nuclei in 7 of 11 cases of Sezary syndrome but in none of four cases of erythrodermic MF. Eosinophils and plasma cells appeared in fewer cases of Sezary syndrome than of MF.

Patients with erythroderma with underlying inflammatory skin diseases such as psoriasis, pityriasis rubra pilaris, or allergic contact dermatitis pose a more difficult diagnostic challenge. Some patients have had an apparent erythrodermic "chronic dermatitis," but have been shown to have band-like infiltrates of lymphocytes in the papillary dermis. T-cell receptor gene rearrangement studies on skin biopsies or peripheral blood mononuclear cell preparations may prove useful in such cases.

Hyperconvoluted nuclei are not unique to Sezary syndrome. Even more striking nuclei, with clover leaf shapes and pedunculated nuclear lobes, are often present in the blood of patients with adult T-cell leukemia/lymphoma (ATLL) due to HTLV-1 infection. Circulating Sezary cells are present in erythrodermic follicular mucinosis, a rare condition involving widespread cutaneous lesions of alopecia mucinosa and peripheral blood eosinophilia. A patient with B-cell lymphoma developed circulating hyperconvoluted cells indistinguishable from those that infiltrated the lymph nodes.[70] Another patient was described as having non-neoplastic Sezary cells as evidenced by the absence

of a clonal band in T-cell gene rearrangement studies. This patient did, in fact, have Sezary syndrome, but with circulating clonal lymphocytes that were not hyperconvoluted.[71]

ADULT T-CELL LEUKEMIA/LYMPHOMA

ATLL is a high-grade T-cell lymphoma induced by infection with the retrovirus HTLV-1. ATLL largely affects adults in areas endemic for HTLV-1 infection, including the southern islands of Japan, other areas in southeastern Asia, and the Caribbean. Infection has also been noted to affect African-Americans in the southeastern United States. The virus is transmissible through exchange of bodily fluids. Serologic testing reveals that cases of subclinical infection with HTLV-1 vastly outnumber those of overt ATLL.

Clinical Features

ATLL usually has an abrupt onset and an aggressive clinical course. *H*ypercalcemia, *o*steolytic bone lesions, *T*-cell leukemia, and *s*kin lesions (HOTS) are found in many cases, as well as lymphadenopathy. ATLL can be complicated by opportunistic infections. Most patients live less than 3 years following the onset of their disease.[72]

The cutaneous lesions of ATLL appear abruptly as papules, nodules, and tumors. Patches, which are the initial lesions of MF, are not generally a feature of ATLL. Unusual findings include purpuric plaques, subcutaneous tumors, and pompholyx-like vesicles on acral skin.[73]

Histopathologic Features

Papules are the earliest lesions of ATLL to have been depicted histologically. They are comprised of dense, superficial, dermal infiltrates, mostly of lymphocytes with small- or intermediate-sized convoluted nuclei (Fig. 21-17). Band-like infiltrates are present in the papillary dermis, often accompanied by slight to moderate epidermal hyperplasia and infiltration of the epidermis by lymphocytes singly or in clusters, as seen in MF.

Nodules and tumors of ATLL may contain lymphocytes with large, vesicular nuclei and clumped chromatin, resembling the cells of anaplastic large cell lymphoma. Infiltration of the walls of large vessels at the dermal-subcutaneous junction is sometimes seen in nodules or tumors.[74]

The peripheral blood in most patients with ATLL contains lymphocytes with distinctive multilobated nuclei. Eosinophilia appears to be more frequent than in other forms of cutaneous lymphoma.[75]

Immunostaining of the lymphocytes of ATLL mark them as T helper cells, expressing CD3 and CD4. Paradoxically, they may exert suppressor activity in vitro. Southern blot analysis of the T-cell receptor gene reveals clonality in the vast majority of cases. The circulating cells of ATLL often express CD25, the interleukin-2 receptor, in higher percentages than do the cells of Sezary syndrome.[76]

Clinicopathologic Correlation

As in other lymphomas and lymphoproliferative disorders, densely infiltrated lesions of ATLL are purplish, usually smooth-surfaced masses. Detailed histologic descriptions of

Figure 21-17. Adult T-cell leukemia and lymphoma. In this papule, atypical lymphocytes plug the lumen of a superficial lymphatic vessel. Even though the lymphocytes of this condition have a distinctive cloverleaf-shaped nucleus in peripheral blood smears, it is nearly impossible to distinguish them cytologically from those of mycosis fungoides.

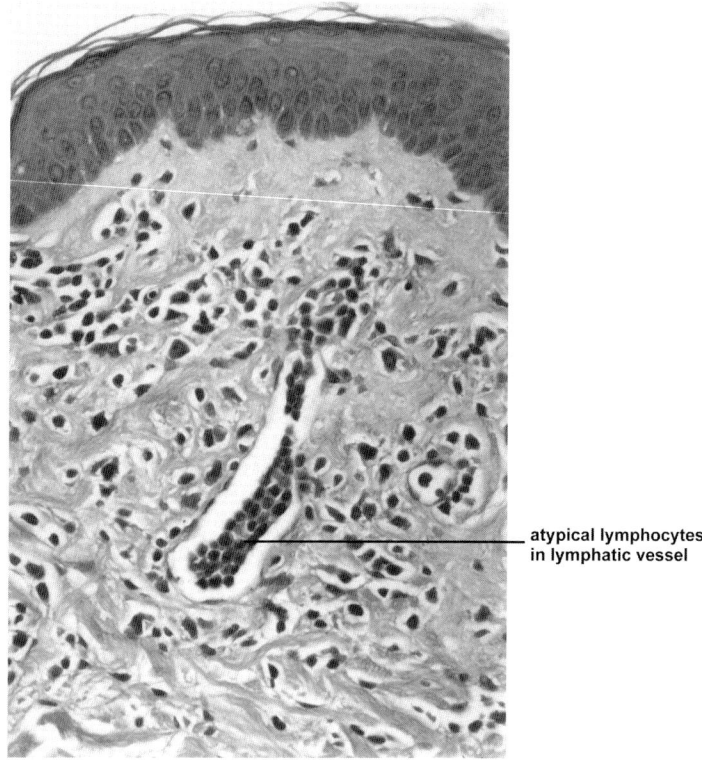

atypical lymphocytes in lymphatic vessel

some of the more unusual clinical presentations, such as the pompholyx-like vesicles, have not been recorded. Osteolytic bone lesions and hypercalcemia are due to osteoclastic overactivity rather than invasion of bone by lymphocytes.

Differential Diagnosis

ATLL is most easily confused with MF Sezary syndrome. It is important to distinguish ATLL from other entities, as it has a far worse clinical course and is transmissible by transfusion or sexual contact. The insidious rather than abrupt onset of skin lesions and the presence of patches rather than papules as the initial lesions are clinical features that favor MF over ATLL. Histologic features alone do not enable differentiation between plaques or tumors of MF and ATLL. The changes seen in patches of MF have not been reported in ATLL, in which the earliest lesions are papules.

Because some cases of ATLL present with erythroderma, a distinction between ATLL and Sezary syndrome based only on clinical grounds may be difficult. Immunophenotypic studies may be helpful. The cutaneous infiltrates of ATLL mark as immunologically naive T cells, and those of MF or Sezary syndrome have a pattern of antigen expression similar to that of memory T cells. A positive serologic test for HTLV-1 antibodies does not always indicate ATLL in an erythrodermic patient, as the prevalence of such antibodies in endemic populations is high, and occasional patients with MF or Sezary syndrome have such antibodies. Peripheral blood smears may be useful, as the clover-leaf-like lobated nuclei of ATLL are not seen in the lymphocytes of Sezary syndrome. The "reference test" for ATLL is the demonstration of clonal integration of the HTLV-1 genome

into the malignant cells of ATLL.[77] Clonal integration is so-called because the retrovirus inserts itself into a T lymphocyte early in the neoplastic process, and all of the progeny of that lymphocyte carry the virus in the exact same point in their genome. Testing for clonal integration can be performed on either lesional skin or blood from ATLL patients, using the Southern blot method. Patients with the smoldering form of ATLL, in which cutaneous lesions precede leukemic involvement, may not have circulating retrovirus-infected cells, and, thus, a skin biopsy specimen from such patients is the preferred substrate.

Pathophysiology

Interleukin-2 may drive the proliferation of T cells in ATLL. The cells of ATLL have high levels of expression of the receptor for interleukin-2 (Tac or CD25), and antibodies against the receptor have been successfully used to block interleukin-2 binding, resulting in remission of the disease.

LYMPHOMATOID PAPULOSIS

LYP consists of cutaneous papules and nodules that simulate lymphoma histologically, but spontaneously involute.

Clinical Features

The spectrum of patients affected with LYP ranges from infants to the elderly, but it most commonly occurs in adults. It affects men nearly twice as frequently as women.[78] Most patients with LYP have crops of papules and nodules on the trunk and proximal extremities, with the palms, soles, face, and scalp exceptionally involved. Many lesions begin as red papules, become ulcerated, and resolve with scars, sometimes with pigmentary changes. Vesicular or pustular lesions and large plaques are sometimes seen. Individual lesions can take from 3 weeks to several months to resolve.[79]

While most patients with LYP have a condition limited to the skin that resolves in 10 to 20 years, a small minority develop malignant lymphoma, usually MF or Hodgkin disease, before the onset of LYP, concomitantly with it, or after LYP. Other lymphomas have been sporadically associated with LYP, but many reports have used what is now archaic terminology and have not included immunohistochemical data. Some studies have shown an association of lymphoma with LYP in up to 20% of cases, but such cases are far more likely to be referred to an academic center and be included in published series. In one study, none of 22 patients with uncomplicated LYP developed lymphoma over several years.[80]

Histopathologic Features

Two main histopathologic patterns can be discerned in fully formed lesions of lymphomatoid papulosis, termed types A and B by Willemze.[78] Type A lesions are typically dense and wedge shaped and have polymorphous infiltrates of neutrophils, eosinophils, small lymphocytes, and large lymphocytes with vesicular nuclei, large central nucleoli, and abundant cytoplasm (Fig. 21-18). The atypical cells are occasionally multinucleated or bizarre in shape. Mitotic figures are frequent. The epidermis is only sparsely infiltrated, can have slight spongiosis, and sometimes ulcerated.

Both early and waning type A lesions have few atypical cells and superficial and deep perivascular lymphocytic infiltrates with interstitial eosinophils, neutrophils, and spongiosis. Other findings in type A lesions include vasculitis and dermal mucin deposition.[81]

Type B lesions have band-like or nodular rather than wedge-shaped configurations (Fig. 21-19). The pattern of infiltration is more monotonous, predominated by lymphocytes with large cerebriform nuclei. Eosinophils and neutrophils are rare. Infiltration of the lower portion of the epidermis is more extensive than it is in type A lesions, although necrotic keratinocytes are rare and vacuolar change at the dermoepidermal junction is slight.

A third histopathologic form, the type C lesion, is rare. It is composed of sheets of lymphocytes that resemble those of anaplastic T-cell lymphoma.

While some patients with LYP consistently produce type A lesions and others type B or C ones, infiltrates with mixed features are sometimes encountered, and some patients have lesions of each type concurrently.

The nature of the large, atypical cells in LYP, once debated, has been resolved by immunohistochemical studies. The atypical cells with vesicular nuclei seen in type A lesions usually mark as T lymphocytes with some of the defects in antigen expression usually seen in high-grade T-cell lymphomas (e.g., lack of expression of CD2 or CD3). The cells also are similar to the Reed-Sternberg cells of most types of Hodgkin disease in that they express activation antigens such as Ki-1 (CD30). Rather than being postmitotic, as was once thought, they are rapidly cycling as evidenced by nuclear staining with the proliferation marker Ki-67.[82] The small lymphocytes in type A lesions have an activated but not aberrant phenotype, suggesting that they represent a host response to the large atypical cells. The large cerebriform cells in type B lesions are less likely to be CD30 positive, but also can have aberrant T-cell phenotypes.

Studies of clonality in LYP support the idea that the disease is lymphoproliferative rather than inflammatory in nature.[83] While some lesions have no detectable clonal populations, others may have a T-cell clone or, occasionally, several clones.[84] In some patients different clonal populations are evident in each

Figure 21-18. Lymphomatoid papulosis, type A lesion. There are many cell types present, including both large and small lymphocytes, neutrophils, and eosinophils in a background of edema. The characteristic type A cell described by Willemze has a large vesicular nucleus and prominent eosinophilic nucleolus, resembling a Hodgkin cell.

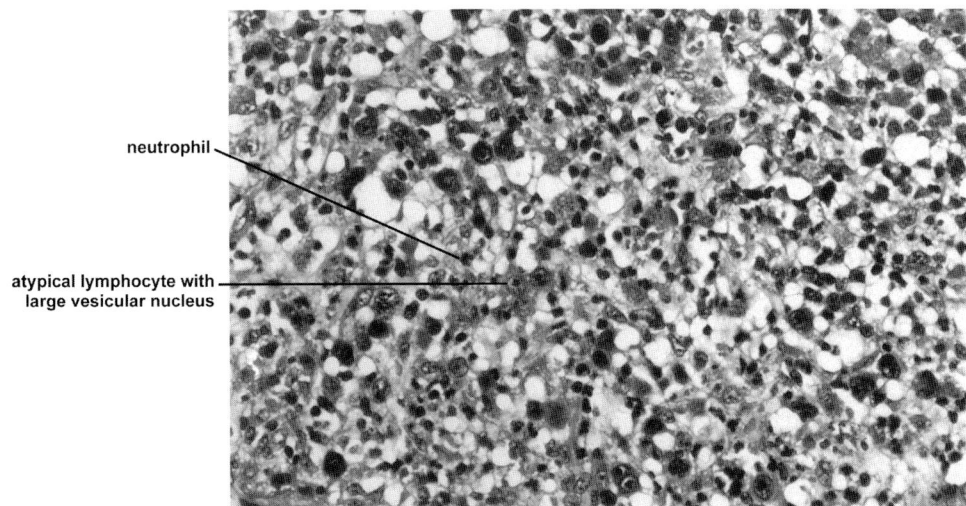

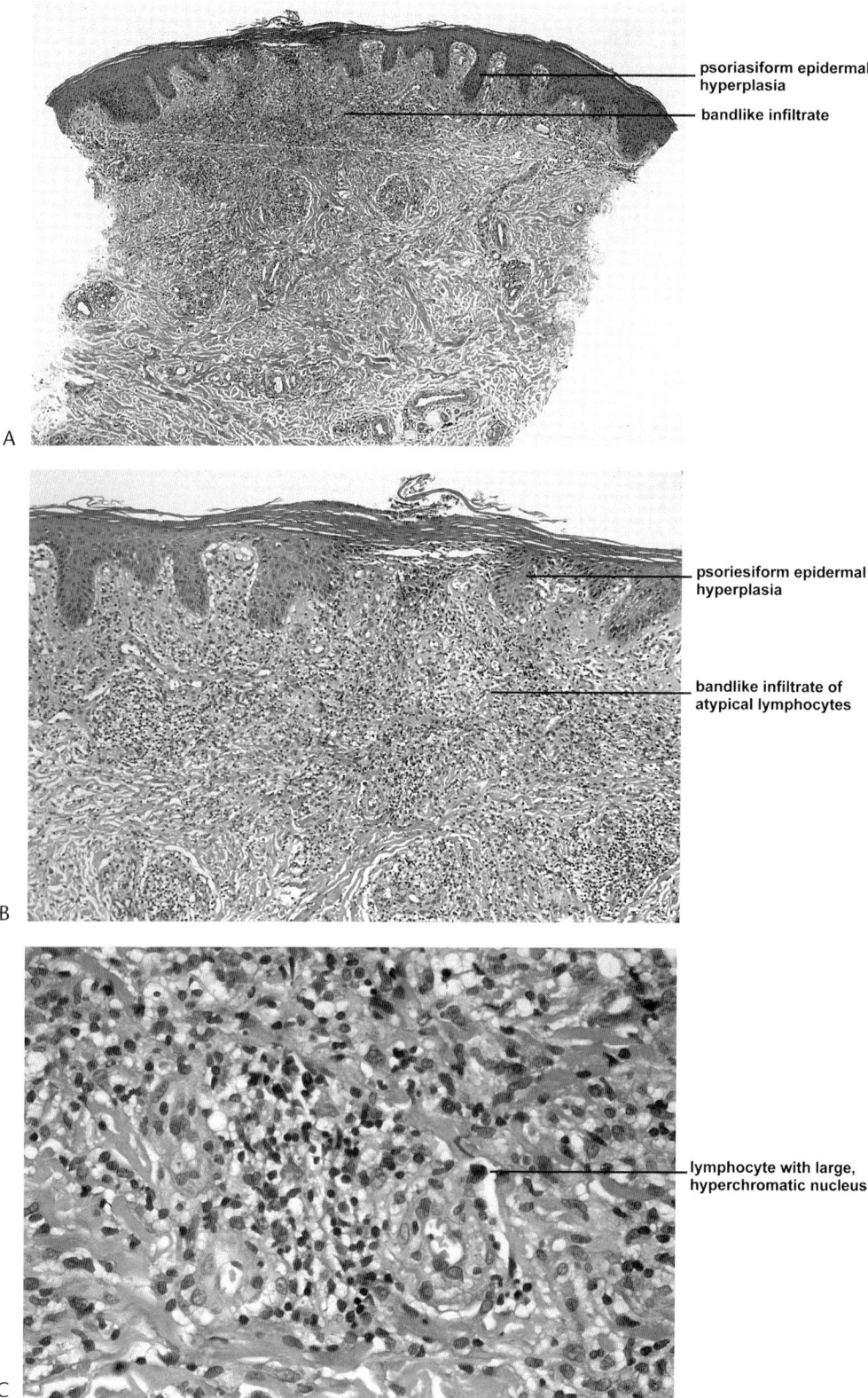

psoriasiform epidermal
hyperplasia

bandlike infiltrate

A

psoriesiform epidermal
hyperplasia

bandlike infiltrate of
atypical lymphocytes

B

lymphocyte with large,
hyperchromatic nucleus

C

Figure 21-19.   Lymphomatoid papulosis, type B lesion. There is a psoriasiform, lichenoid pattern similar to that seen in many lesions of mycosis fungoides **(A).** The papillary dermis is thickened and fibrotic **(B).** Unlike the
vesicular nuclei present in the cells of type A lesions, those of type B lesions
have hyperconvoluted and hyperchromatic nuclei **(C).** *Continued.*

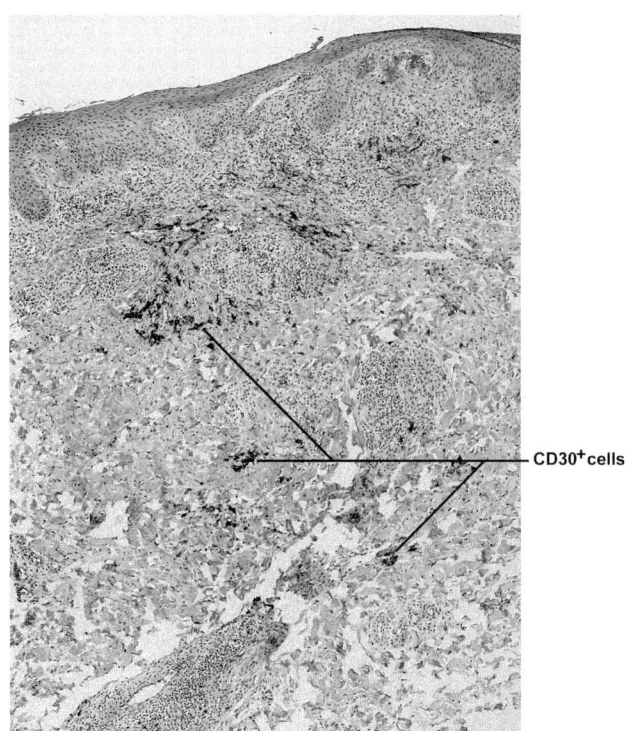

CD30⁺cells

Figure 21-19.   *Continued.* A CD30 immunoperoxidase stain highlights clusters of neoplastic cells **(D)**. The CD30+ cells do not form sheets in most cases of lymphomatoid papulosis, unlike the case in anaplastic large cell lymphoma but are instead arranged singly or in discrete clusters **(E)**.

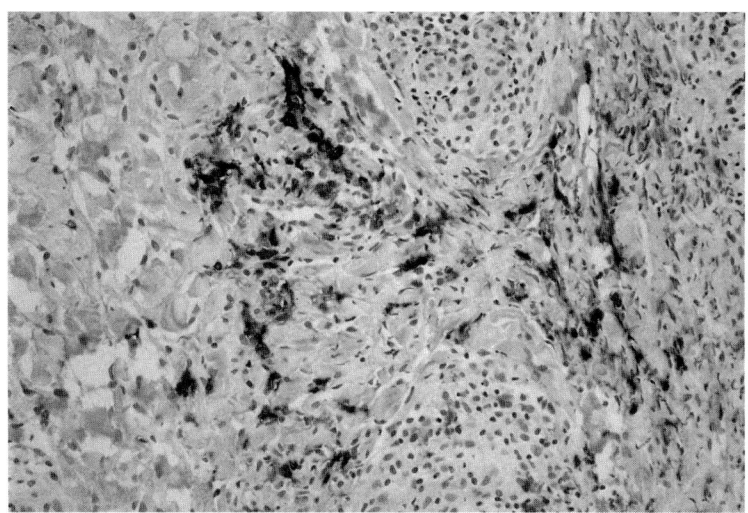

E

lesion. These findings differ from those seen in most lymphomas, in which the same clone is evident in each lesion, and suggest that emerging clones may be held in check by the host's immune response.

Clinicopathologic Correlation

While the earliest lesions of LYP are small, smooth-surfaced papules, later lesions include papulovesicles, papulopustules, and ulcerated papules or nodules. Papulovesicles often have edema of the papillary dermis and spongiosis. In papulopustules the neutrophils that are scattered in type A lesions coalesce beneath or within the epidermis. In ulcerating papules or nodules, small vessel vasculitis is frequently present and may contribute to ulceration.

Some authors have suggested that type B lesions persist longer than type A lesions, sometimes requiring months to involute. The larger numbers of small lymphocytes in type A lesions (presumably present as a host response to the neoplasm) is consistent with the hypothesis that involution is mediated by these cells.

While the atypical cells of type A lesions resemble those of Hodgkin disease and the cells of type B lesions resemble those of MF, the type of LYP lesion imperfectly predicts the type of lymphoma that a given patient is most likely to develop, should one ensue.

Differential Diagnosis

LYP was at one time thought to be a variant of pityriasis lichenoides, with which it shares many features. Both conditions have crops of papules on the trunk and extremities that tend to ulcerate or crust and sometimes heal with scars. Both have superficial and deep infiltrates that sometimes obscure the dermoepidermal junction. Both conditions have been associated with clonal populations of T lymphocytes, although studies using T-cell receptor β-chain gene probes and fresh tissue and ones using γ-chain probes and PCR do not agree.

A number of distinctions mark LYP and pityriasis lichenoides as separate entities. LYP is associated with another form of lymphoma in up to 10% of cases, while only a few patients with pityriasis lichenoides have developed lymphoma, and conceivably those patients had LYP rather than Mucha-Habermann disease. Pityriasis lichenoides tends to occur in younger patients than does LYP, and, on average, there are more lesions at any one time and they tend to be smaller. While only 6% of patients with pityriasis lichenoides had their disease for over a decade in one study, fully 50% of patients with LYP did.[85] Histologic evidence also points to the two diseases being distinct entities. In LYP, especially in type A lesions, the infiltrates often contain neutrophils and eosinophils. While neutrophils inhabit ulcerated or crusted examples of pityriasis lichenoides, eosinophils are almost never present. Vacuolar change and necrotic keratinocytes are evident at the dermoepidermal junction in pityriasis lichenoides and can be prominent even when only a few lymphocytes are present. In contrast, even in type B lesions of LYP with moderate infiltration of the lower portion of the epidermis, vacuolar change is minimal, and dyskeratotic cells are few.

The presence of lymphocytes with markedly atypical nuclei favors LYP over pityriasis lichenoides. The diagnosis of LYP can be missed because early and late lesions can be devoid of atypical lymphocytes.[81] The "small cell" variant of LYP has dense infiltrates of cells only slightly larger than most reactive lymphocytes accompanied by neutrophils and eosinophils. It seems that biopsies of early or late lesions or the small cell variant account for some of the reported cases in which pityriasis lichenoides was said to progress to LYP.

Reactions to arthropod assaults may resemble LYP clinically, and wedge-shaped, mixed cellular infiltrates can be found in both conditions. Features favoring the diagnosis of an arthropod assault over LYP include focal epidermal necrosis around the puncture site, lymphocytic vasculitis (i.e., lymphocytes around venules with fibrin in their walls or lumens) limited to superficial vessels, and many immunoblasts in the infiltrate.

Immunophenotypic studies help to differentiate LYP from these two conditions. While not all biopsies of LYP show CD30 expression by the atypical lymphoid cells, CD30+ cells are rare in either pityriasis lichenoides or in reactions to arthropod assaults,[86] although these data need to be re-evaluated using antigen retrieval methods, which are more sensitive.

Hodgkin disease involving the skin may be difficult to discriminate from LYP. The clinical situation may help, as some cases of cutaneous Hodgkin disease are the result of direct extension from massively involved lymph nodes. Cutaneous papules and nodules can complicate Hodgkin disease, and the diagnosis in such cases is between Hodgkin disease and lymphomatoid papulosis following Hodgkin disease. Reed-Sternberg cell variants such as the popcorn-like cells seen in the mixed cellularity type of Hodgkin disease and lacunar cells are not seen in LYP and favor Hodgkin disease. Immunophenotypic studies are of little help, as both Reed-Sternberg cells and the atypical cells of LYP can express the Ki-1 (CD30) and Leu-M1 (CD15) antigens, as well as some T-cell antigens. Cutaneous involvement of the rare lymphocyte-predominant, nodular variant of Hodgkin disease can be distinguished from LYP, as its atypical cells have a B-cell phenotype. Gene rearrangement studies need to be interpreted with care, as the infiltrates of Hodgkin disease can engender an oligoclonal pattern on analysis of the T-cell receptor γ gene. Some cases of LYP with a type A appearance can lack T-cell receptor rearrangements, as those of Hodgkin disease most often do.

Pathophysiology

LYP has been posited as the "missing link" between MF and Hodgkin disease.[87] The cells of MF have a mature helper T-cell phenotype in most cases, as do those of lymphomatoid papulosis. Those of Hodgkin disease can on occasion also have a helper T-cell phenotype, and, like the cells of LYP, express the CD30 antigen. In patients who have both Hodgkin disease and LYP, or Hodgkin disease and CD30+ lymphoma, the atypical cells can be immunophenotypically or even genotypically identical.[88,89] Although a viral pathogenesis of LYP has appealed to many observers, studies to date have not revealed a role for either HTLV-1 or Epstein-Barr virus. The cells of LYP lack the t(2,5) translocation present in systemic CD30+ anaplastic large cell lymphoma.

CUTANEOUS CD30+ (KI-1) LYMPHOMA

Cutaneous CD30+ or Ki-1+ lymphoma is characterized by persistent cutaneous nodules composed of lymphocytes with large, anaplastic nuclei. The cells usually express markers of T-cell lineage and, by definition, the CD30 (Ki-1) antigen. Cases in which large nodules of mononuclear cells with anaplastic nuclei arise in the skin and sometimes spontaneously regress, as they do in LYP, have been termed *regressing atypical histiocytosis* (RAH). Most authors regard RAH as a subset of the condition now known as *CD30+ lymphoma*. While a more precise name would be *CD30+* anaplastic large cell lymphoma, that term is unwieldy. It is worth remembering that pleomorphic T-cell lymphomas, and cells in tumors of MF can be CD30+ and that CD30+ lymphoma does not simply equal a lymphoma with CD30+ cells.

The CD30 or Ki-1 antigen is a marker of activation and can be induced on both T and B cells by a variety of antigens and is not specific for any lineage. Because the atypical cells of LYP, RAH, and cutaneous CD30+ lymphoma all share aberrant T-cell phenotypes, clonal rearrangement of the T-cell receptor α and β genes (in most cases), and CD30 expression, a strong case can be made that the three conditions comprise a disease spectrum in which patients with LYP usually have a relapsing and remitting course with only rare systemic dissemination, those with RAH have a similar tendency to remit and relapse but an intermediate rate of systemic dissemination, and those with cutaneous CD30+ lymphoma have persistent disease, either primary in the skin or metastatic to it.

Clinical Features

Lesions of CD30+ lymphoma tend to be large nodules, tumors, or subcutaneous masses that often ulcerate and crust. Most are located on the extremities. Fewer lesions are present than in LYP, and often only one cutaneous lesion is present at a time. The ages of onset have spanned the first seven decades of life. Many cases of systemic CD30+ lymphoma are in children, while primary cutaneous disease is more common in adults. The patients with RAH or primary cutaneous disease are not usually ill, in contrast with those having nodal involvement at presentation.[90] The courses of patients with RAH favor the proposition that RAH and CD30+ lymphoma are two expressions of the same neoplasm. The two patients who were described in the initial report of RAH died with systemic lymphoma.[91,92] Some patients with cutaneous CD30+ lymphoma involving lymph nodes have spontaneous regression and relapse of the cutaneous lesions, but persistence of nodal disease. CD30+ anaplastic large cell lymphoma appears to be the most common cutaneous lymphoma in patients with human immunodeficiency virus (HIV) disease.[93] Patients with CD30+ lymphoma complicating HIV disease have a dismal prognosis.

Histopathologic Features

Both RAH and cutaneous CD30+ lymphoma have massive dermal and sometimes subcutaneous infiltrates of lymphocytes that have abundant, faintly basophilic cytoplasm; large, irregularly shaped vesicular nuclei with coarsely clumped chromatin along nuclear membranes; and large, irregularly shaped nucleoli (Fig. 21-20). Wreath-shaped multinucleated cells are often present, as are embryo-shaped nuclei. In the initial report,[91] erythrophagocytosis was cited as a diagnostic sign, but this has been downplayed in subsequent reports and is much more common in subcutaneous T-cell lymphoma. Rare cases of CD30+ lymphoma have spindled neoplastic cells that simulate a sarcoma.[94] Lesions of RAH that ulcerate prior to regression often have pseudocarcinomatous hyperplasia, foci of granulation tissue, and an admixture of neutrophils.

The large cells of CD30+ lymphoma can be stained using the immunoperoxidase method in frozen tissue or with the clone Ber-H2 in paraffin-embedded sections. Intense staining of the Golgi region in addition to cell membranes indicates a specific reaction. Using antigen retrieval techniques, CD30+ cells are present in small numbers in a variety of reactive infiltrates and in large numbers in some inflammatory lesions in some HIV-infected patients. Their mere presence does not indicate a malignancy.

Immunophenotypic and genotypic studies have indicated a T-cell lineage in the majority of cases of CD30+ lymphoma. Even though the neoplastic cells have abundant cytoplasm, and on rare occasion exhibit erythrophagocytosis, suggesting a histiocytic origin to early observers, antigens such as Mac-387 and CD68 found on macrophages are not present. An interesting observation in some cases has been the presence of CD1, an antigen found on immature T cells and on Langerhans cells.[95]

Clinicopathologic Correlation

The regression of lesions in RAH is reflected histologically by necrosis and ulceration. Pseudocarcinomatous hyperplasia and formation of granulation tissue occur in slowly regressing lesions and impart a verrucous or vegetating appearance. Nodules of CD30+ lymphoma, which show no tendency toward involution, often have smooth surfaces.

Differential Diagnosis

While LYP is closely related to RAH and CD30+ lymphoma, its course unless complicated by another lymphoproliferative disease is benign, and hence it is valuable to distinguish these conditions. Lesions of LYP are far smaller than those of either RAH or CD30+ lymphoma, and subcutaneous masses are not present. Histologically, LYP often has an admixture of inflammatory cells, and, in many cases, atypical cells are in the minority. In CD30+ lymphoma, the atypical cells usually comprise a large majority of the infiltrate and often form sheets. Cells with multiple nuclei arranged in wreaths at the periphery of each cell are more often found in CD30+ lymphoma than in LYP.

Cutaneous lesions of Hodgkin disease may be difficult to distinguish from those of RAH and CD30+ lymphoma. Hodgkin disease most often involves the skin by direct extension from involved lymph nodes; however, patients with Hodgkin disease and either RAH or CD30+ lymphoma may present with concurrent cutaneous and nodal disease. Reed-Sternberg cells are nearly always found in infiltrates of Hodgkin disease but are not present in CD30+ lymphoma. If there are enlarged lymph nodes, biopsy of them is often helpful, as nodes involved by CD30+ lymphoma often have a sinusoidal pattern of infiltration distinct from the interfollicular or diffuse patterns seen in Hodgkin disease.

A note of caution is warranted with regard to the use of staining for CD30 without regard to other findings. CD30 can be expressed by embryonal carcinoma and those of the breast, stomach, lung, bladder, and endometrium.[96] Thus, the diagnosis of metastatic carcinoma should be considered before concluding that a cutaneous infiltrate of large anaplastic cells that express CD30 is RAH or lymphoma. Cutaneous B-cell lymphomas of the immunoblastic, Burkitt, and large, noncleaved types can also express CD30, making it imperative that a panel of lymphoid and nonlymphoid markers be used in cases when histopathologic features are equivocal.

Pathophysiology

Segments of the HTLV-1 genome, or in some cases the entire genome, have been found in the cells of cutaneous Ki-1 lymphoma in patients from areas in which the virus is not endemic.[97] The Epstein-Barr virus is present in the cells of CD30+ lymphoma in immunosuppressed patients, but not in those of immunocompetent ones.[98] As in situ hybridization studies show the viral genome in most of the cells of such infiltrates, it seems likely that there is clonal integration of viral DNA in the neoplastic cells. HIV may have a role in the upregulation of CD30+ in these lymphomas in immunosuppressed patients.

Progression from LYP to CD30+ lymphoma has occurred in some patients and is marked clinically by the advent of larger, persistent lesions. The failure of these lesions to involute may

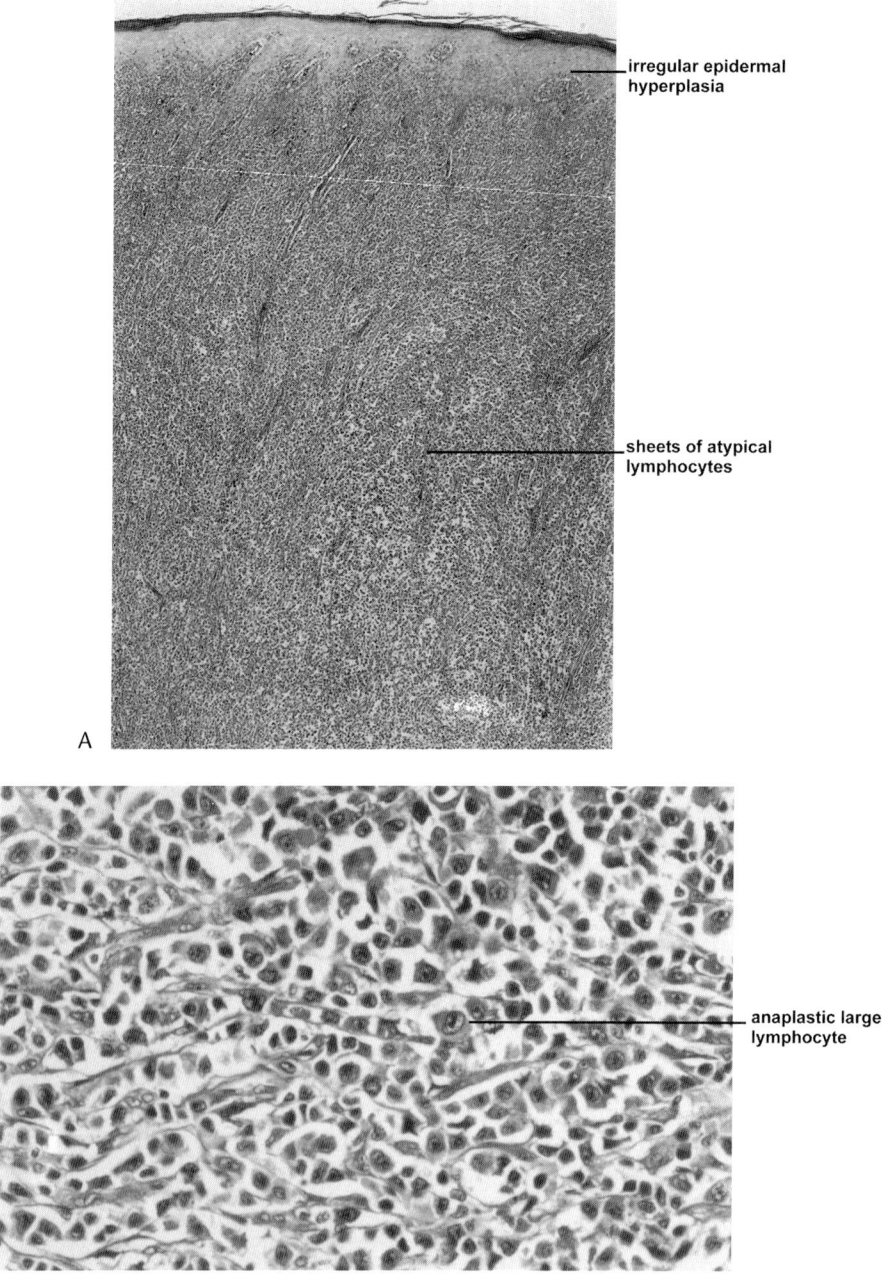

irregular epidermal
hyperplasia

sheets of atypical
lymphocytes

anaplastic large
lymphocyte

A

B

Figure 21-20. Anaplastic large cell lymphoma, CD 30+. The dermis is effaced by sheets of large lymphocytes. Irregular epidermal hyperplasia is frequently seen above the infiltrate **(A)**. The cells of anaplastic large cell lymphoma usually have abundant cytoplasm and large pleomorphic nuclei with large nucleoli **(B)**.

reflect loss of the receptor for transforming growth factor-β, which has an inhibitory effect on the cells of LYP.[99]

ANGIOCENTRIC LYMPHOMA

In angiocentric lymphoma, neoplastic cells infiltrate blood vessel walls, although other structures are often involved. Systemic disease is nearly always evident. The terms *lymphomatoid granulomatosis* and *angiocentric immunoproliferative lesion* have been used by those authors who believe that there is a spectrum of diseases with similar histopathologic patterns, ranging from reactive infiltrates to frank lymphoma. The findings of clonal rearrangement of the T-cell receptor γ–gene and clonal integration of the Epstein-Barr virus genome in many Asian cases favors the use of the term *angiocentric lymphoma*,[100] as it seems that in at least one important subset of the disease it is a lymphoma ab initio. Angiocentricity seems to be a pattern expressed by several different lymphomas. Some are conventional T-cell neoplasms; others, especially pulmonary examples, are T-cell-rich B-cell neoplasms; and yet others are proliferations of natural killer–like cells.

Clinical Features

Cutaneous lesions of angiocentric lymphoma are often subcutaneous or dermal nodules, but a range of appearances from macules and papules to ulcerated tumors has been described.[101] Pulmonary disease is frequent and can be presaged by, occur simultaneously with, or follow cutaneous lesions. The central nervous system is involved in one third of patients. Infiltration of peripheral nerves simulating tuberculoid leprosy has been reported. Curiously, the lymph nodes, spleen, and bone marrow, organs involved in many conventional lymphomas, are spared by the disease. The prognosis of angiocentric lymphoma is dire, with 94% of patients in one series dying within 3 years of presentation.[100]

Histopathologic Features

Lesions of angiocentric lymphoma contain perivascular lymphocytic infiltrates with variable proportions of atypical cells.[102] In some cases, the lymphocytes show scant cytologic atypia, and the diagnosis is only suggested by systemic findings. In other cases, lymphocytes with medium-sized nuclei with rounded or irregularly shaped borders can be seen. They often have deep clefts, but are usually not cerebriform.[100] In most cases, medium-sized and small vessels usually have lymphocytes within their walls, although this finding can be subtle (Fig. 21-21). Concentric, onion skin-like fibrosis around venules, fibrin deposits in vessel walls or lumens, expansion of the intima of arteries or arterioles by lymphomatous infiltration, and the formation of vascular tufts reminiscent of glomeruli are evi-

dence of damage to blood vessels.[100] Infiltration into the epidermis occurs on occasion. Some cases in which there is a prominent pagetoid pattern may have been reported as the disseminated (Ketron-Goodman) form of PR.[63] In other cases, instead of epidermotropism there is an interface reaction with necrotic keratinocytes. In many cases with a natural killer cell phenotype, there are prominent subcutaneous infiltrates, and some of these patients have been reported as having subcutaneous T-cell lymphoma. Coagulation necrosis of neoplastic cells, or of the dermis, epidermis, or subcutis, may be evident when vascular lumens are compromised.

Immunophenotypic studies have revealed aberrant T-cell phenotypes in many cases of angiocentric lymphoma, with loss of the CD3, CD5, and CD7 antigens.[73] Especially in Asian patients, the cells can have a natural killer-like phenotype, failing to express most T-cell markers but staining in frozen sections for CD16 and CD56. Touch imprints of these infiltrates show large granular lymphocytes when stained by the Wright-Giemsa method.[103] Although the cells do not have CD3 on their surfaces, and frozen sections will be negative when stained for that antigen, paraffin section immunohistochemistry will be positive for cytoplasmic CD3. Occasional cases have a B-cell phenotype and exhibit rearrangement of immunoglobulin genes. Despite the appellation of *lymphomatoid granulomatosis* initially given to this disease, granulomatous inflammation is not usually present, and immunophenotypic studies on cutaneous lesions have not revealed significant numbers of macrophages.

Clinicopathologic Correlation

Biopsy specimens taken from macules and papules of angiocentric lymphoma viewed at scanning magnification reveal su-

Figure 21-21. Angiocentric lymphoma. Infiltrates of atypical lymphocytes within the walls of cutaneous vessels, as seen here, are present in several types of lymphomas with differing phenotypes—classic lymphomatoid granulomatosis, which appears to be a B-cell lymphoma with reactive T-cell infiltrates; some T-cell lymphomas; and lymphomas with a natural killer cell phenotype. Lymphomatous vasculitis can sometimes complicate mycosis fungoides. Given the findings seen here, one should only make the diagnosis of lymphomatous vasculitis and perform immunoperoxidase staining to delineate which of these angiocentric lymphomas is the culprit.

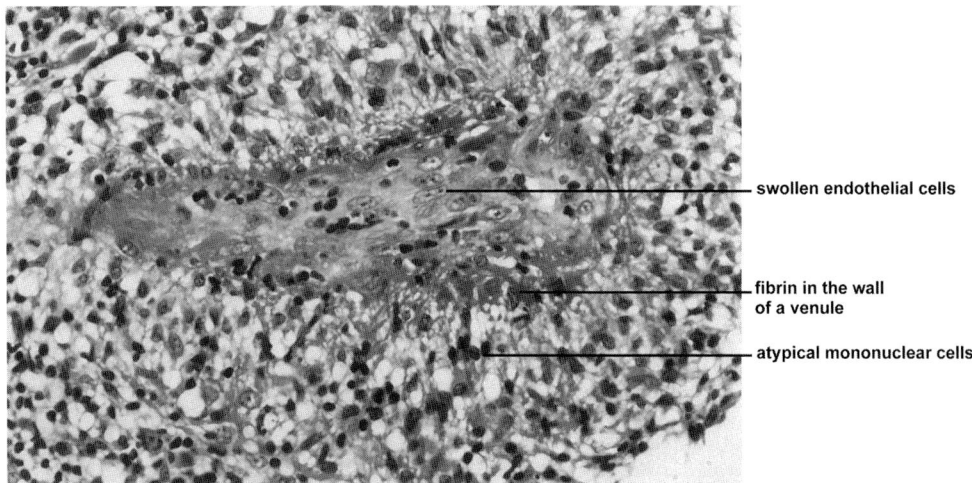

swollen endothelial cells

fibrin in the wall of a venule

atypical mononuclear cells

perficial and deep perivascular lymphocytic infiltrates. Large nodules, plaques, and tumors often have diffuse infiltration of the dermis or subcutis or both in addition to perivascular infiltrates. Intact lesions are often smooth surfaced, owing to sparing of the papillary dermis and epidermis in the majority of cases. Ulcerated lesions have occluded vessels that have caused infarction of the neoplastic infiltrate and of the skin.

Differential Diagnosis

Cases of angiocentric lymphoma with sparse infiltrates and only a few atypical cells can be mistaken for conditions that show superficial and deep perivascular dermatitis such as erythema annulare centrifugum (which it may also simulate clinically), tumid lupus erythematosus, Jessner lymphocytic infiltrate, erythema chronicum migrans, and polymorphous light eruption. If fibrin is present in vessel walls, resulting in a true lymphocytic vasculitis, perniosis and pityriasis lichenoides also need to be considered. Careful examination of the infiltrate for cells with larger nuclei that are prominently indurated is the best way to discriminate between angiocentric lymphoma and its simulants, but requires caution and experience.

LYP has several features in common with angiocentric lymphoma, including lymphocytes with large atypical nuclei, infiltration of vessel walls, and, sometimes, fibrin deposition. LYP displays more prominently wedge-shaped infiltrates than does angiocentric lymphoma, and papillary dermal and epidermal involvement is far more frequent. The neoplastic cells of LYP express CD30 more often than those of angiocentric lymphoma.

Vasculitis may be seen in rare cases of epidermotropic CTCL or MF.[3,45] These cases tend to have a suppressor/cytotoxic cell phenotype in contrast to the helper cell phenotype evident in the vast majority of cases of MF and Sezary syndrome. The epidermotropism of angiocentric lymphoma tends to be more spotty than that seen in MF with vasculitis.

Angiocentric lymphoma is often confused with angiotropic lymphoma or, as it has been traditionally known, malignant angioendotheliomatosis. In this condition, which is best termed *intravascular lymphomatosis*, the lesions are bruise-like patches and the lymphomatous infiltrates are confined almost entirely to vessel lumens. The large majority of cases of intravascular lymphomatosis are B-cell neoplasms.

Pathophysiology

Infection with Epstein-Barr virus may play an important role in angiocentric lymphoma. Not only is the viral genome present in most cases, but it is clonally integrated into the DNA of host lymphocytes, much in the same manner as HTLV-1 is integrated into the genome of lymphocytes of ATLL. In situ hybridization for EBER-1 or immunoperoxidase staining for Epstein-Barr virus latent membrane protein-1 can be used to establish this connection in routinely processed specimens.

INTRAVASCULAR LYMPHOMA

Intravascular lymphoma is the most straightforward of the many terms used for this rare condition, in which the cells of malignant lymphoma show a peculiar tendency to accumulate in the lumens of small blood vessels in several organs, including the skin. Other terms for intravascular lymphoma include *malignant angioendotheliomatosis, angioendotheliomatosis proliferans systemisata, intravascular lymphomatosis*, and *intravascular endothelioma*.

Clinical Features

Intravascular lymphoma most often affects the skin and brain. Systemic signs include fever and an elevated sedimentation rate. Neurologic abnormalities include dementia and disturbances of vision, speech, and sensation. Cutaneous lesions produced by intravascular lymphoma are often hemorrhagic plaques, with or without telangiectasia, scale, or ulceration, most frequently affecting the skin of the trunk or extremities.

Histopathologic Features

Small vessels throughout the dermis and subcutis are distended by cells that accumulate in their lumens but usually neither infiltrate their walls nor extend beyond them (Fig. 21-22). The neoplastic cells in most cases have been large, with scant cytoplasm, irregular nuclear membranes, hyperchromatic nuclei, and prominent nucleoli. They are frequently enmeshed in fibrin. In some cases the lumens of vessels show infolding, resulting in papillary structures lined by prominent endothelial cells, and a glomeruloid configuration.[104]

Intravascular lymphoma is most often a neoplasm of B cells, but there are rare cases that have a T-cell phenotype.[105]

Clinicopathologic Correlation

The lesions of intravascular lymphoma appear as hemorrhagic plaques because the occlusion of small vessels results in extravasation of erythrocytes, as it does in the noninflammatory thrombotic disorders such as the lupus anticoagulant syndrome and purpura fulminans. Intravascular lymphoma results in smooth-surfaced lesions in most cases, as the epidermis is spared by the neoplastic cells. Infarction of the dermis and epidermis leads to ulceration in large plaques.

Differential Diagnosis and Pitfalls

Other conditions that result in the accumulation of neoplastic cells in the lumens of blood vessels can be distinguished from intravascular lymphoma. *Inflammatory carcinoma* and *inflammatory melanoma* are the names given to those neoplasms whose metastatic cells lodge in the lumens of dermal venules instead of exiting them. In the absence of melanin to identify the cells of inflammatory melanoma, immunoperoxidase staining is the best method to resolve this differential diagnosis. The cells of intravascular lymphoma express leukocyte common antigen (CD45), while those of carcinoma and melanoma do not, but contain keratin filaments and S-100 protein, respectively.

Reactive angioendotheliomatosis is a condition in which cutaneous endothelial cells proliferate and form glomeruloid structures.[104] As the clinical lesions are bruise-like, just as those of intravascular lymphoma are, and the histopathologic changes of intravascular lymphoma can include endothelial proliferation, the two conditions were confused for many years.[106] Reactive angioendotheliomatosis has been linked to endocarditis, allergy, and lumenal occlusion by fibrin or cryoglobulin.[104] In optimally cut and stained sections it is apparent that the prolif-

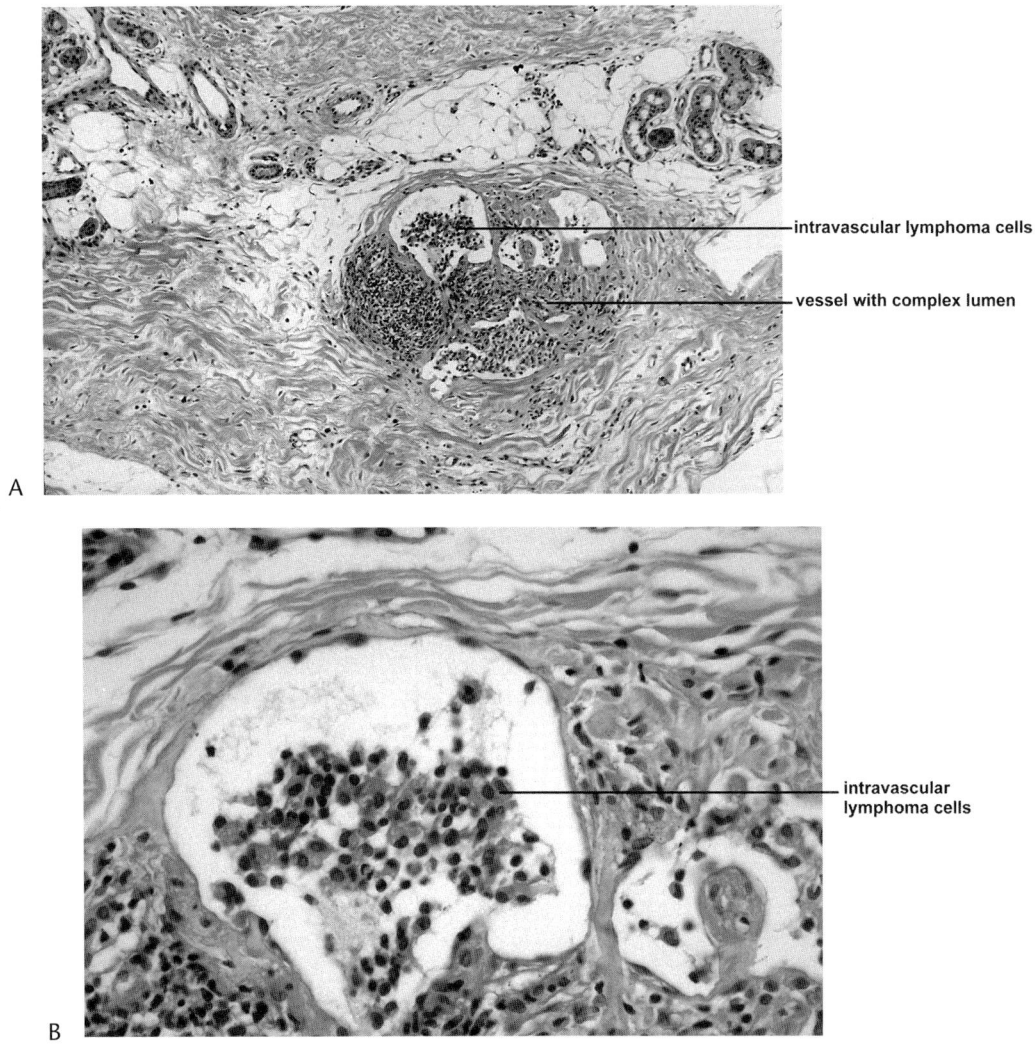

Figure 21-22. Intravascular lymphoma, also known as malignant angioen-dotheliomatosis or angiotropic lymphoma. Lymphocytes with atypical nuclei are present in the lumen of a complex vascular structure **(A)**. Thrombosis of the partially occluded lumen may be responsible at least in part for the presence of several vascular channels. The atypical lymphocytes, usually B cells, form a mass in the center of the lumen, but several appear attached to its wall **(B)**.

erating cells in reactive angioendotheliomatosis line vascular spaces, and, while they may bulge into them, they do not appear actually to lie within them, in contrast to intravascular lymphoma. Immunoperoxidase staining shows that these cells express vascular endothelial determinants such as factor VIII–related antigen and blood group substances, but do not contain leukocyte common antigen.

Pathophysiology

It seems likely that an inability to exit the walls of small vessels on the part of the intravascular lymphoma cells results in their distinctive intraluminal accumulation. This defect does not appear to be lineage specific. Although the vast majority of cases have been proliferations of B cells, a few cases of intravascular T-cell lymphoma have now been described. The interplay be-

tween circulating cells and endothelial cells is highly specific and dependent on cell surface molecules. One analysis demonstrated that the Hermes-3 homing receptor, which plays a role in the binding of lymphocytes to high endothelial venules in lymph nodes, is present on the surfaces of the cells of intravascular lymphoma.[107] The inability of the neoplastic cells to exit from vessels may explain the sparing of parenchymal tissues by this peculiar condition.

HODGKIN DISEASE

Hodgkin disease is a form of lymphoma characterized by a contiguous pattern of spread from one lymphoid organ to another and by the presence of highly atypical cells of unknown lineage termed *Reed-Sternberg* cells in its infiltrates. Four histologic types are recognized in the Rye classification: lymphocyte-pre-

Figure 21-23.   Hodgkin disease involving the skin. The patient had known systemic Hodgkin disease. There are geographic zones of necrosis surrounded by a mixed infiltrate that includes many Hodgkin cells **(A)**. Although the large pale nuclei simulate a palisaded granulomatous infiltrate, even at an intermediate magnification, there is striking nuclear atypia **(B)**. *Continued.*

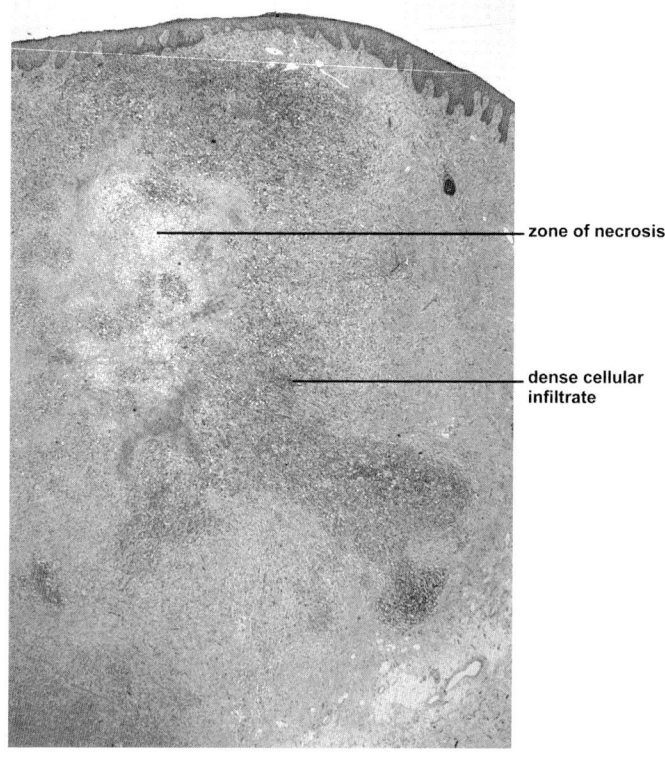

zone of necrosis

dense cellular
infiltrate

A

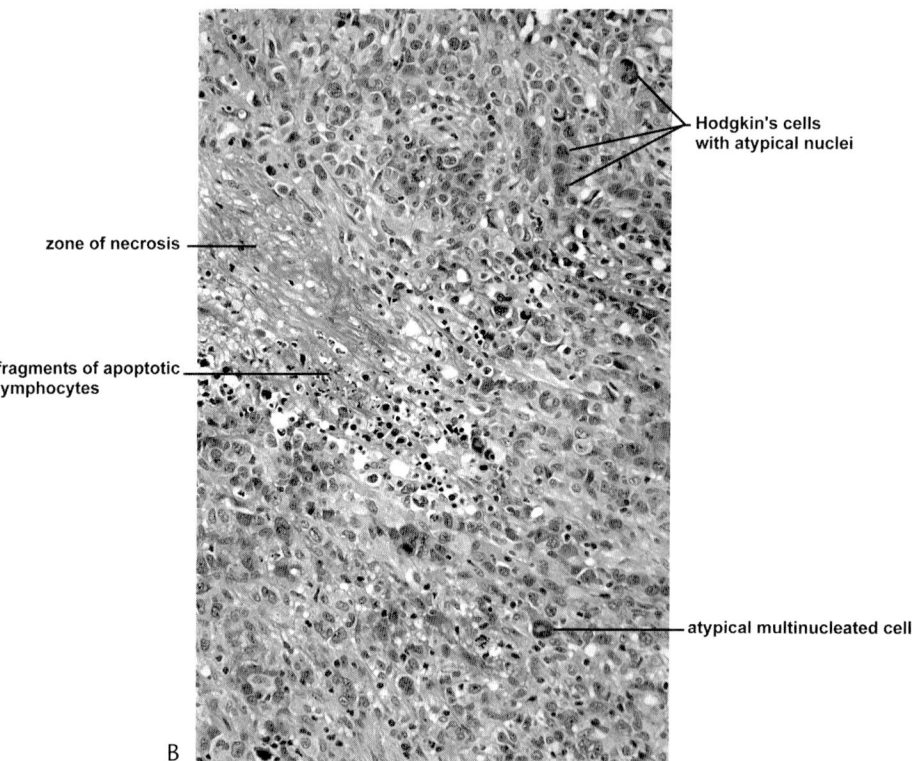

Hodgkin's cells
with atypical nuclei

zone of necrosis

fragments of apoptotic
lymphocytes

atypical multinucleated cell

B

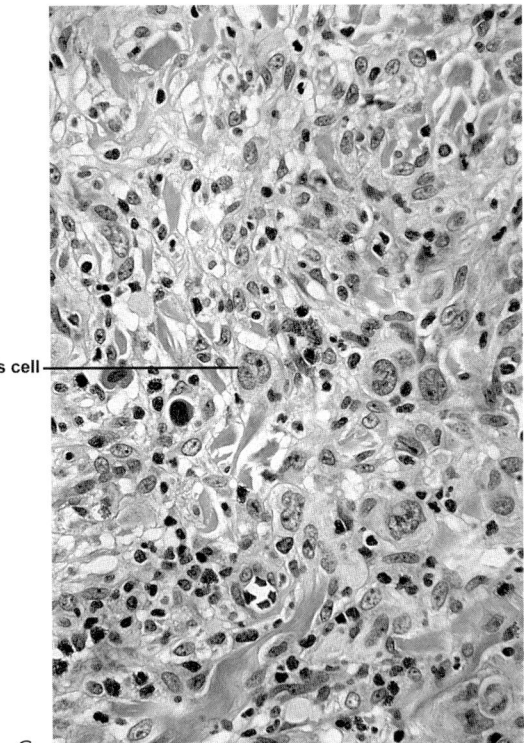

binucleate Hodgkin's cell

C

Figure 21-23. *Continued.* The Hodgkin cells in this example have multilobated, vesicular nuclei and large eosinophilic nucleoli. One is binucleate *(arrow)*. Their nature could be proven by immunohistochemistry. Like the cells of lymphomatoid papulosis, they express CD30, but unlike them, they also express CD15 **(C)**.

dominant, nodular sclerosing, mixed cellularity, and lymphocyte-depleted Hodgkin disease.

Clinical Features

Hodgkin disease can present with lymphadenopathy, hepatosplenomegaly, abdominal or thoracic masses, or systemic symptoms. Secondary cutaneous lesions are uncommon, with a prevalence in two recent series of 0.5% and 3.4%.[108,109] In most cases of secondary cutaneous Hodgkin disease, the skin distal to involved lymph nodes develops papules, nodules, plaques, or subcutaneous nodules. In rare cases, the skin is involved by direct extension from involved lymph nodes, an event that seems to have been more frequent prior to the advent of effective therapy. Also uncommon are scattered papules or nodules unrelated to involved lymph nodes, which are thought to be the result of hematogenous spread. Cutaneous involvement by Hodgkin disease usually accompanies other signs of disseminated disease and is a poor prognostic sign, except in those cases in which cutaneous lesions are evident at the time systemic disease first manifests.

While there are many older reports of primary cutaneous Hodgkin disease in the literature, most of these appear to be of cases of LYP or of CD30+ lymphoma. Recently developed histologic and immunohistochemical criteria have enabled the identification of what seems to be authentic primary cutaneous Hodgkin disease. These patients present with papules or nodules, some of which spontaneously involute. Several patients with this disorder have gone on to develop mixed cellularity Hodgkin disease of lymph nodes, while in others the condition has remained confined to the skin.[110]

Histopathologic Features

The Reed-Sternberg cell is a distinctive finding seen in all types of Hodgkin disease. Reed-Sternberg cells are large (up to 50 μm in diameter) and binucleate. The nuclei are vesicular with chromatin condensed along their membranes, which are often irregular. The size of the nucleoli is an important criterion; true Reed-Sternberg cells have brightly eosinophilic nucleoli that measure over one third of the diameter of the nucleus. Immunoblasts in conditions that may be mistaken for Hodgkin disease, such as infectious mononucleosis, often have nucleoli that do not meet this test. The term *Hodgkin cell* is used for cells that have the other features of Reed-Sternberg cells but are not binucleate (Fig. 21-23). There are three variants of Hodgkin cells that can be found in cutaneous infiltrates. Lymphocytic-histiocytic cells, seen in lymphocyte-predominant Hodgkin disease, have large, multilobated vesicular nuclei with minute nucleoli and moderate amounts of pale cytoplasm. The lacunar cell of the nodular sclerosing form of Hodgkin disease is so named because it has clear cytoplasm that often appears retracted from a sharply defined peripheral margin and multilobated, distinct nuclei in formalin-fixed samples. In the reticular type of lymphocyte-depleted Hodgkin disease, Hodgkin cells can appear "sarcomatoid" (i.e., spindled and pleomorphic). Extreme variation in the appearance of nuclei typifies the pleomorphic variant of lymphocyte-depleted Hodgkin disease.

Cutaneous lesions of each subtype of Hodgkin disease show the same histologic findings as nodal infiltrates, except that occasionally the skin will harbor an infiltrate whose prognosis is worse than that suggested by the patient's lymph nodes or viscera. Lymphocyte-predominant Hodgkin disease is only rarely seen in the skin; but, when it is seen, it has sheets of small, convoluted lymphocytes and scattered Reed-Sternberg cells.

In the nodular sclerosing variant of Hodgkin disease, affected nodes have bands of polarizable collagen traversing them. While this feature is not evident in cutaneous infiltrates, the lacunar variant of the Reed-Sternberg cell, which has a space around it formed by retraction due to formalin fixation, can be seen.

Lymphocyte-depleted Hodgkin disease present in the skin as relatively monomorphous infiltrates of Reed-Sternberg or Hodgkin cells. Necrosis is often present.

Immunophenotypic studies have not succeeded in conclusively identifying the cell of origin of Hodgkin disease, but a consistent immunophenotype has been established. Reed-Sternberg cells in all types of Hodgkin disease express CD30 (for a discussion of this antigen, see the sections on LYP and on CD30+ lymphoma, above).[111] Leu-M1 recognizes another activation antigen, CD15, present on Reed-Sternberg cells in all types of Hodgkin disease except on the nodular lymphocyte-predominant type, wherein only a minority of cases have Reed-Sternberg cells that are positive for Leu-M1.[112] Reed-Sternberg cells have been stained for T- and B-cell antigens with spotty results. Gene rearrangement studies have shown clonal rearrangements of T-cell receptor or immunoglobulin genes in a minority of cases, and the rearranged bands are often faint, suggesting that they could derive from oligoclonal populations of reactive cells.

Clinicopathologic Correlation

Ulcerated lesions of Hodgkin disease often have large areas of necrosis histologically. Rare bullous lesions of Hodgkin disease[113] may be due to lymphatic obstruction.

Differential Diagnosis

The principal differential diagnosis of Hodgkin disease is the spectrum of fellow CD30+ conditions ranging from LYP to anaplastic large cell lymphoma. LYP may precede, occur simultaneously with, or follow Hodgkin disease. Occasional patients have had both LYP and CD30+ lymphoma, as well as Hodgkin disease. The differential diagnosis of these conditions with Hodgkin disease is discussed in detail above. Because primary cutaneous Hodgkin disease can be overdiagnosed if its features are not rigorously defined, it is worth mentioning that Reed-Sternberg cells in its infiltrates mark for CD15 and CD30, but not for the leukocyte common antigen CD45RA.

The tumor stage of MF can be confused histopathologically with Hodgkin disease, especially since the two diseases can occur in the same patient.[114] Tumor stage MF often has cells with large vesicular nuclei and eosinophilic nucleoli, resembling variants of Reed-Sternberg cells. The distinction between tumor stage MF and disseminated cutaneous Hodgkin disease is important, as treatments of the two conditions differ. Features that favor Hodgkin disease include a background of small lymphocytes that are not especially convoluted, the presence of several unequivocal Reed-Sternberg cells or Hodgkin cells, or the presence of distinctive Reed-Sternberg

variants such as lymphocytic-histocytic or lacunar cells. Features that favor the tumor stage of MF include the presence of convoluted lymphocytes intermediate in size between those of the smallest and largest cells of the infiltrate and involvement of the epidermis or hair follicle epithelium. Immunophenotypic studies may also be helpful. A predominance of CD8+ (suppressor/cytotoxic) T cells was evident in two cases of Hodgkin disease involving the skin. While the large cells of MF sometimes express CD30 or CD15, in Hodgkin disease their expression is the rule. The same features apply in distinguishing systemic spread of MF from Hodgkin disease arising in the setting of MF.

Pathophysiology

The non-neoplastic counterpart of the Reed-Sternberg cell may be a dendritic cell found in the paracortex of the lymph node that expresses CD30 and has a high rate of proliferation. The role of the Epstein-Barr virus in transforming these cells is suggested by the presence of the viral genome in Reed-Sternberg cells. Perhaps Epstein-Barr-infected lymphocytes undergo clonal proliferation, express activation markers, and induce a polyclonal host response.[115] This theory would explain the association of Hodgkin disease with different forms of lymphoma, the detection of B- and T-cell antigens on the cells of some cases, and the finding of occasional T-cell or immunoglobulin gene rearrangements. Epstein-Barr virus can be found in Hodgkin cells but is more common in immunosuppressed patients and those in the third world.

LEUKEMIA CUTIS

The leukemias are malignant neoplasms of hematopoietic or lymphoid cells that replace the bone marrow, circulate in the peripheral blood in large numbers, or both. The leukemias can be broadly grouped into myelogenous and lymphocytic forms. Myelogenous leukemia comprises a spectrum of differentiation toward myelocytes, monocytes, and megakaryocytes. Acute leukemias cause replacement of the marrow by primitive-appearing cells (blasts); in chronic leukemias a range of differentiation can occur, and more of the marrow is spared.

Clinical Features

The wide range of clinical lesions caused by cutaneous leukemic infiltrates includes papules, macules, plaques, nodules, ecchymotic or purpuric lesions, and ulcers. Unusual manifestations include gingival hypertrophy most commonly seen with acute myelogenous leukemia or acute myelomonocytic leukemia. Erythroderma and bullous lesions, which may be unusual reactions to insect bites, are restricted to patients with chronic lymphocytic leukemia or monocytic leukemia.[116] Nodules or tumors of myeloblasts are termed *granulocytic sarcoma* or *chloroma*. Rarely, chloromas may precede the appearance of blasts in the peripheral blood or marrow. The occurrence of a leukemic skin infiltrate prior to its appearance in the blood is known as *aleukemic leukemia cutis*. A variety of inflammatory skin diseases may occur in conjunction with leukemia, including leukocytoclastic vasculitis, pyoderma gangrenosum, perniosis, urticaria, exfoliative erythroderma, erythema nodosum, hyperpigmentation, and erythema multiforme.

Histopathologic Features

Several patterns characterize leukemic infiltrates of the skin. The most distinctive pattern is a diffuse dermal infiltrate in which the leukemic cells are seen in linear array between reticular dermal collagen bundles (Fig. 21-24). Compact, nodular infiltrates can also be found. Band-like infiltrates that affect the superficial dermis are occasionally present, as are sparse perivascular infiltrates. Each of the specific types of leukemia has a propensity to one or more of these patterns.

Acute myelogenous leukemia usually presents with dense, diffuse infiltration by cells in a linear array between collagen bundles or in a nodular pattern. Infiltration of the epidermis is rare, but in the majority of cases cells extend into the subcutis. Myeloblasts may be difficult to recognize in tissue sections. They have scant cytoplasm, large vesicular nuclei, and prominent nucleoli. Cells with either folded nuclei or strikingly atypical nuclei may occur, but in many biopsies the infiltrates are monomorphous and cytologically bland.

Chronic myelogenous leukemia also has a diffuse or nodular pattern, but is less likely to involve the epidermis than is acute myelogenous leukemia. The infiltrates contain both band-like and mature neutrophils as well as blasts and eosinophilic myelocytes, which are cells with a single nucleus and granular cytoplasm indistinguishable from that of mature eosinophils.

Acute myelomonocytic and monocytic leukemia may be difficult to distinguish from acute myelogenous leukemia on the basis of histomorphology alone. Some cases of acute monocytic leukemia have pale, reniform nuclei.

Both acute and chronic lymphocytic leukemia most often show dense, diffuse, pan-dermal infiltrates. Unusual patterns include nodular infiltrates and, in chronic lymphocytic leukemia, either band-like or sparse perivascular infiltrates. The latter may simulate a superficial and deep perivascular dermatitis. The

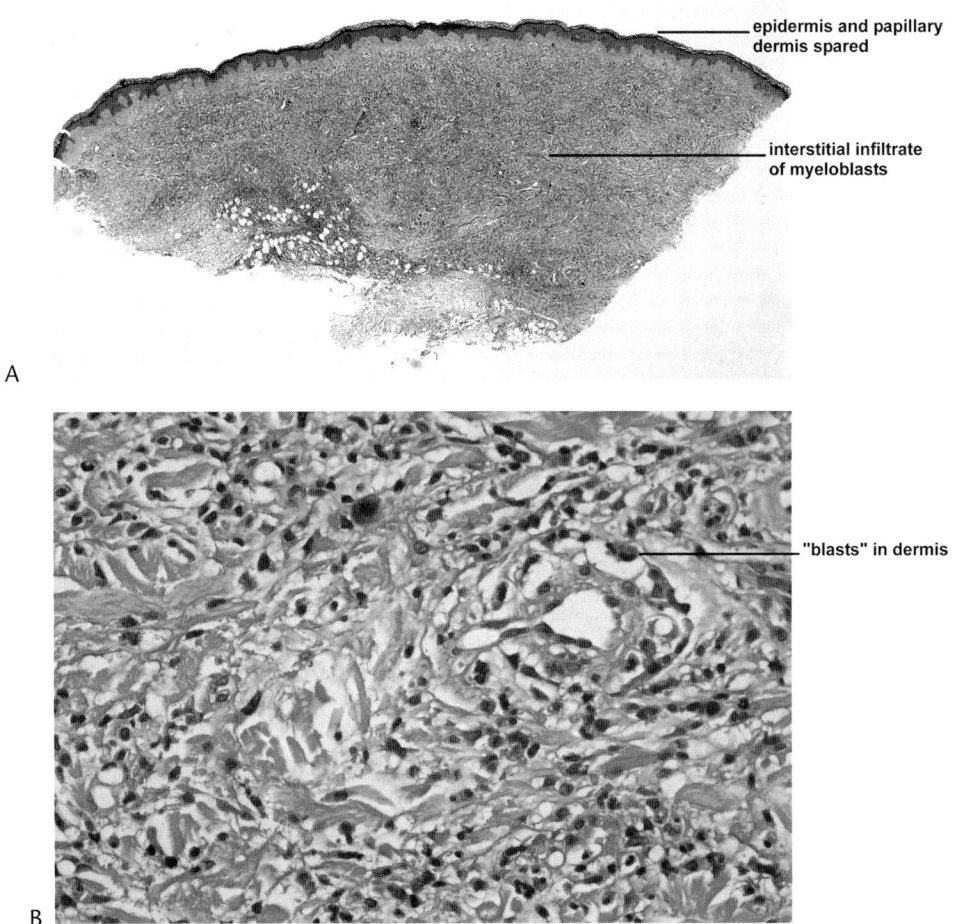

epidermis and papillary
dermis spared

interstitial infiltrate
of myeloblasts

A

"blasts" in dermis

B

Figure 21-24. Myeloblastic leukemia cutis. Hematogenously borne infiltrates, including those of leukemia and some metastatic melanomas and carcinomas, have a prominently interstitial or reticular pattern in which cells are aligned alongside collagen bundles in the reticular dermis **(A)**. The myeloblasts have enlarged nuclei with smudgy chromatin **(B)**. Either enzyme histochemical or immunohistochemical studies would need to be done to prove their identity.

cells of acute lymphocytic leukemia appear in tissue sections as having scant, basophilic cytoplasm and large, round, hyperchromatic nuclei. Those of chronic lymphocytic leukemia are roughly the size of normal lymphocytes. In cells of B-cell chronic lymphocytic leukemia, the cytoplasm is extremely scant, and peripheral clumping of chromatin within round or ovoid nuclei occurs. Some cells that resemble prolymphocytes with prominent nucleoli are generally present. In the T-cell type of chronic lymphocytic leukemia, nuclear convolutions are more apparent. Infiltration of the epidermis may also occur in T-cell chronic lymphocytic leukemia, resembling the histologic picture seen in Sezary syndrome or MF.[117]

Hairy cell leukemia is so named because of the hair-like cytoplasmic projections that its cells have in peripheral blood. In the rare reports of cutaneous infiltration, small- to medium-sized hyperchromatic nuclei were present with scant, nondescript cytoplasm.[118] The characteristic hairs cannot be seen in tissue sections. The infiltrates of hairy cell leukemia in the spleen, lymph nodes, and bone marrow have a distinctive pattern with clear cytoplasm and evenly separated monomorphous nuclei. This pattern has not yet been seen in the skin.

Clinicopathologic Correlation

The reddish to purple lesions of leukemia cutis appear to be the result of dermal infiltration. Submucosal infiltration results in the gingival hypertrophy common in acute monocytic leukemia. The greenish color of chloroma is due to the presence of myeloperoxidase. The bullous lesions thought to be unusual reactions to arthropod assaults in patients with chronic lymphocytic leukemia show dense, superficial and deep infiltrates as well as papillary dermal edema and spongiosis. Eosinophils may be present in the blister cavity as well as in the dermal infiltrates.[119]

Differential Diagnosis

The diffuse, interstitial, and nodular patterns of leukemic infiltration are shared by malignant lymphoma. It can be exceedingly difficult to tell if an infiltrate of monomorphous cells with atypical, discohesive nuclei are those of leukemia or lymphoma. The diffuse pattern seen in some cases of follicular center lymphoma with intermediate-sized nuclei closely resembles acute myelogenous leukemia. The presence of bands and mature neutrophils or eosinophilic myelocytes favors chronic myelocytic leukemia, while pale-staining, reniform nuclei favor monocytic leukemia. In general, an Indian-file arrangement of cells between collagen bundles favors leukemia over lymphoma.

Myelogenous leukemic infiltrates can be differentiated from lymphocytic leukemia by both histochemical and immunophenotypic studies. The peroxidase reaction can be used to identify myeloid cells in unfixed or frozen sections and may be applied to touch imprints from skin biopsies. The chloroacetate esterase or Leder stain marks myeloid cells (and mast cells) but not lymphocytes. Unfortunately, many myelogenous leukemic infiltrates, especially outside the bone marrow, fail to mark with this method. Immunoperoxidase staining using Mac-387 is a relatively sensitive and specific way to detect cells of myeloid lineage. Lysozyme, MY-9, and elastase antisera are also specific but less sensitive markers of myeloid cells. Because no one stain

of antibody has 100% sensitivity for detecting myelocytes, a panel of at least three antisera may yield the best results.[120] CD34, also known as the *human progenitor cell antigen*, is expressed by blasts in several types of leukemia, but not by the cells of most types of malignant lymphoma. It can be detected in paraffin-embedded sections.[121]

The Indian-file arrangement of cells in leukemia cutis can also be seen in some examples of metastatic adenocarcinoma, especially ductal carcinoma of the breast. The cells of metastatic adenocarcinoma are more frequently contiguous than those seen in leukemic infiltrates, and at least a few nests are generally present. Glandular lumens, staining of intracytoplasmic mucin, or staining with antikeratin by the immunoperoxidase method can characterize metastatic adenocarcinoma.

When chronic lymphocytic leukemia presents with superficial and deep perivascular infiltrates, its differential diagnosis includes erythema annulare centrifugum, reticular erythematous mucinosis, polymorphous light eruption, Jessner lymphocytic infiltrate, tumid lupus erythematosus, and erythema chronicum migrans of Lyme disease. In some cases of chronic lymphocytic leukemia the infiltrate extends into the subcutis with focal necrosis of adipocytes, a feature not seen in the other conditions. Optimally fixed thin sections may demonstrate the characteristic nuclear features of small lymphocytes in B-cell chronic lymphocytic leukemia, as opposed to the diffuse hyperchromasia and irregular shape seen in reactive infiltrates of T cells. Immunoperoxidase staining may help to make the diagnosis, as the cells of B-cell chronic lymphocytic leukemia coexpress the B-cell marker L26 and the T-cell marker Leu-22 (CD43).[122] The sparse perivascular infiltrates of hairy cell leukemia can be distinguished by histochemical staining for tartrate-resistant acid phosphatase. This stain does not work well in formalin-fixed, paraffin-embedded tissue. In routinely processed specimens the cells of hairy cell leukemia mark with B-cell lineage specific antibodies such as L26.[123]

DERMAL ERYTHROPOIESIS AND HEMATOPOIESIS

Dermal erythropoiesis refers to the presence of red blood cell precursors in the dermis and is usually seen in newborns as a reaction to stress. Precipitating events include congenital infections (rubella, Coxsackie virus, cytomegalovirus) or hematologic disease (hemolysis due to ABO or Rh incompatibility, twin transfusion syndrome, hereditary spherocytosis). The term *dermal hematopoiesis* is used when either myelocytic or megakaryocytic cell lines are also present.

Dermal hematopoiesis occurs mainly in adults with acute myelofibrosis due to megakaryocytic leukemia, but cases due to chronic myelogenous leukemia have also been reported. Many authors have used the term *extramedullary hematopoiesis* to refer to either dermal erythropoiesis or dermal hematopoiesis.

Clinical Features

The macules and papules of either dermal erythropoiesis or dermal hematopoiesis are most often reddish-blue, and nodules can be present in dermal hematopoiesis in adults. There is a propensity for the head and neck area in dermal erythropoiesis in neonates and for the trunk in dermal hematopoiesis in adults.

Histopathologic Features

Dermal erythropoiesis has a perivascular and interstitial pattern (Fig. 21-25). The infiltrate consists of erythroblasts, which have scant cytoplasm and round nuclei, and nucleated erythrocytes. These cells are key to recognizing this condition, as they have homogeneously eosinophilic cytoplasm and small, round,

darkly staining nuclei. In some cases in neonates, small numbers of myeloid precursors may also be present, but megakaryocytes are not usually seen.[124]

In dermal hematopoiesis secondary to myelofibrosis, all these cell lines are often evident. Megakaryocytes have voluminous cytoplasm and multilobulated nuclei. Infiltrates with numbers of atypical megakaryocytes have been described, but

Figure 21-25. Extramedullary hematopoiesis. As in the case of leukemia cutis, a reticular pattern is often present **(A)**. Two cell lines are seen in this field—normoblasts (erythrocyte precursors) with round hyperchromatic nuclei, and myeloblasts (neutrophilic precursors) with somewhat larger nuclei **(B)**.

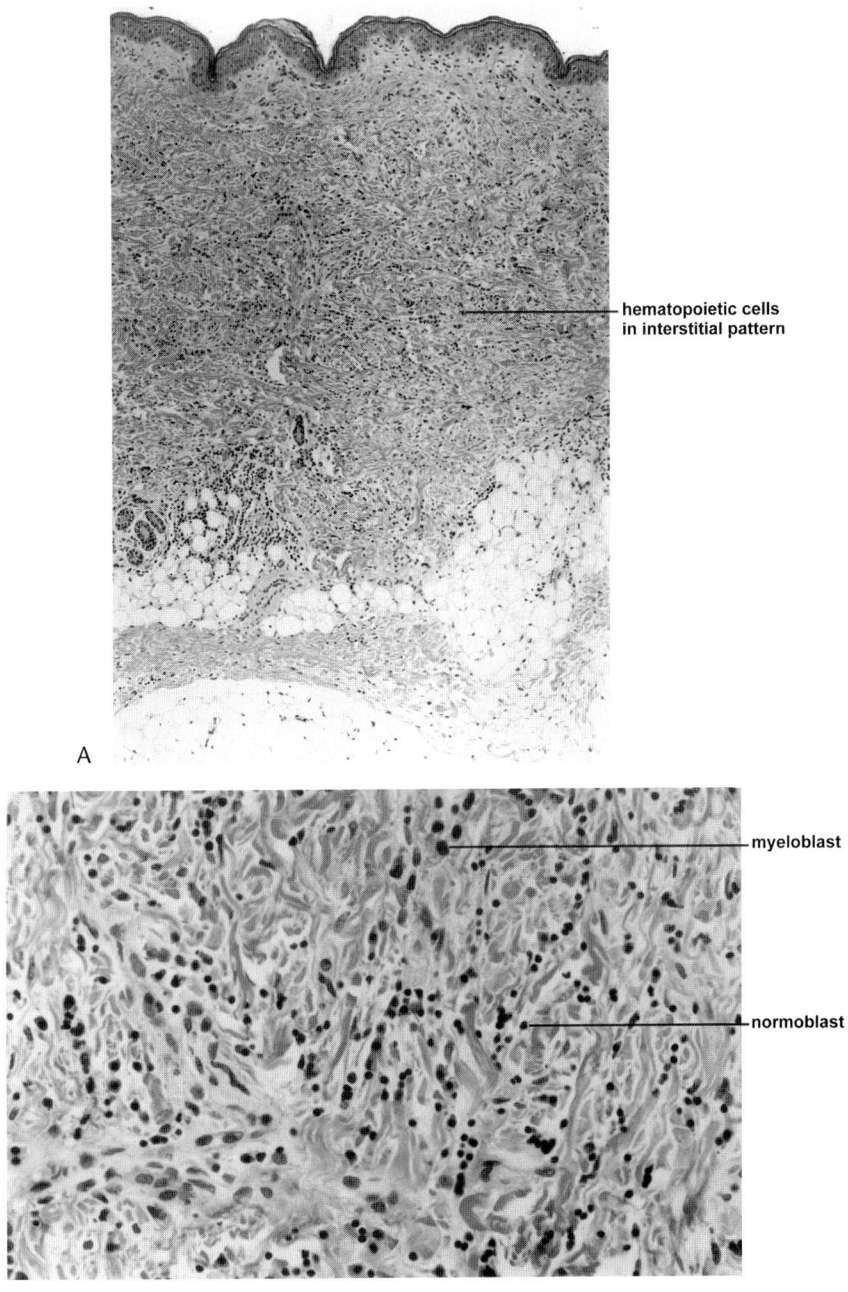

these may actually be specific infiltrates of megakaryocytic leukemia.[125]

Clinicopathologic Correlation

The term *blueberry muffin baby* has been coined to note the appearance of the red-blue macules in dermal erythropoiesis in neonates. In adults, splenectomy may accelerate the spread of marrow elements to the skin. Several cases of dermal hematopoiesis have occurred in postsplenectomy surgical scars.

Differential Diagnosis

The perivascular and interstitial patterns of dermal hematopoiesis and dermal erythropoiesis resemble those of leukemia cutis, especially when cords of cells lie between collagen bundles. Nucleated red blood cells are not present in leukemic infiltrates and can be discerned in well-prepared tissue sections. Staining with *Ulex europeus* lectin using the peroxidase method can identify erythroid precursors. Megakaryocytes are also distinctive histologically and mark with antisera to platelet glycoprotein IIB/IIIA.

REFERENCES

1. Warnke RA, Weiss LM, Chan JKC et al: Tumors of the Lymph Nodes and Spleen. Vol 14, 3rd ed. Washington, DC: Armed Forces Institute of Pathology. 1995
2. Burg G, Braun-Falcoll O: Cutaneous Lymphomas, Pseudolymphomas, and Related Disorders. New York: Springer-Verlag, 1983
3. Shapiro PE, Pinto FJ: The histologic spectrum of mycosis fungoides/Sezary's syndrome (cutaneous T-cell lymphoma). A review of 222 biopsies, including newly described patterns and the earliest pathologic changes. Am J Surg Pathol 18:6645–6667, 1994
4. Smolle J, Torne R, Soyer HP et al: Immunohistochemical classification of cutaneous pseudolymphomas: delineation of distinct patterns. J Cutan Pathol 17:149–159, 1990
5. van der Putte SC, Toonstra J, Felten PC: Solitary nonepidermotropic T cell pseudolymphoma of the skin. J Am Acad Dermatol 14:444–453, 1986
6. Torne R, Roura M, Umbert P: Generalized cutaneous B-cell pseudolymphoma. Report of a case studied by immunohistochemistry. Am J Dermatopathol 11:544–548, 1989
7. Blumental G, Okun MR, Ponitch JA: Pseudolymphomatous reaction to tattoos. Report of three cases. J Am Acad Dermatol 6:485–488, 1982
8. Hovmark A, Asbrink E, Olsson I: The spirochetal etiology of lymphadenosis benigna cutis sotaria. Acta Derm Venereol (Stockh) 66:479–484, 1986
9. Iwatsuki K, Yamada M, Takigawa M et al: Benign lymphoplasia of the earlobes induced by gold earrings: immunohistologic study on the cellular infiltrates. J Am Acad Dermatol 16:83–88, 1987
10. Eckert F, Schmid U: Identification of plasmacytoid T cells in lymphoid hyperplasia of the skin. Arch Dermaol 125:1518–1524, 1989
11. Ecker F, Schmid U, Kaudewitz P et al: Follicular lymphoid hyperplasia of the skin with high content of Ki-1 positive lymphocytes. Am J Dermatopathol 11:345–352, 1989
12. Wood GS, Ngan BY, Tun R et al: Clonal rearrangements of immunoglobulin genes and progress to B cell lymphoma in cutaneous lymphoid hyperplasia. Am J Pathol 135:9–13, 1989
13. Lennert K, Feller AC: Histopathology of Non-Hodgkin's Lymphomas. 2nd Ed. New York: Springer-Verlag, 1992
14. Harris NL, Jaffe ES, Stein H et al: A revised European-American classification of lymphoid neoplasms. A proposal from the international lymphoma study group. Blood 84:1361–1392, 1994
15. Willemze R, Kerl H, Sterry W et al: EORTC classification for primary cutaneous lymphomas. Blood 90:354–371, 1997
16. LeBoit PE, McNutt NS, Reed JA et al: Primary cutaneous immunocytoma: a B-cell lymphoma that can easily be mistaken for cutaneous lymphoid hyper plasia. Am J Surg Pathol 18:969–978, 1994
17. Bailey EM, Ferry JA, Harris NL et al: Marginal zone lymphoma (low-grade B-cell lymphoma of mucosa-associated lymphoid tissue type) of skin and subcutaneous tissue. Am J Surg Pathol 8:1011–1023, 1996
18. van der Putte SC: Immunocytoma of the skin simulating lymphadenosis benigna cutis. Arch Dermatol 277:36–43, 1982
19. van der Putte SC, De KE, Go DM et al: Primary cutaneous lymphoplasmacytoid lymphoma (immunocytoma). Am J Dermatopathol 6:15–24, 1984
20. Garcia CF, Weiss LM, Warnke RA et al: Cutaneous follicular lymphoma. Am J Surg Pathol 10:454–463, 1986
21. Giannotti B, Santucci M: Skin-associated lymphoid tissue (SALT)-related B-cell lymphoma (primary cutaneous B-cell lymphoma). A concept and a clinicopathologic entity [editorial]. Arch Dermatol 129:353–355, 1993
22. English JS, Smith NP Spaull J et al: Large cell lymphocytoma—a clinicopathological study. Clin Exp Dermatol 14:181–185, 1989
23. Dabski K, Banks PM, Winkelmann RK: Clinicopathologic spectrum of cutaneous manifestations of systemic follicular lymphoma. A study of 11 patients. Cancer 64:1480–1485, 1989
24. Ngan B, Warnke A, Cleary ML: Variability of immunoglobulin expression in follicular lymphoma. An immunohistologic and molecular genetic study. Am J Pathol 135:1139–1144, 1989
25. Willemze R, Meijer CJ, Sentis JH et al: Primary cutaneous large cell lymphomas of follicular center cell origin. A clinical follow-up study of nineteen patients. J Am Acad Dermatol 16:518–526, 1987
26. Pimpinelli N, Santucci M, Bosi A et al: Primary cutaneous follicular centre-cell lymphoma—a lymphoproliferative disease with favorable prognosis. Clin Exp Dermatol 14:12–19, 1989
27. Sander CA, Medeiros LJ, Abruzzo LV et al: Lymphoblastic lymphoma presenting at cutaneous sites. A clinicopathologic analysis of six cases. J Am Acad Dermatol 25:1023–1031, 1991
28. Roundtree JM, Burgdorf W, Harkey MR: Cutaneous involvement in Lennert's lymphoma. Arch Dermatol 116:1291–1294, 1982

29. Kiesewetter F, Haneke E, Lennert K et al: Cutaneous lymphoepithelioid lymphoma (Lennert's lymphoma). Combined immunohistological, ultrastructural, and DNA-flow cytometric analysis. Am J Dermatopathol 11:549–554, 1989

30. Sterry W, Wiebel A, Mielke V: HTLV-1-negative pleomorphic T-cell lymphoma of the skin: the clinicopathological correlations and natural history of 15 patients. Br J Dermatol 126:456–462, 1992

31. van der Putte SC, Toonstra J, De WR et al: Cutaneous T-cell lymphoma, multibated type. Histopathology 6:35–54, 1982

32. Goldman BD, Bari M, Candor GR et al: Cutaneous multilobated T-cell lymphoma with aggressive course. J Am Acad Dermatol 25:345–349, 1991

33. Gonzalez CL, Medeiros LJ, Braziel RM et al: T-cell lymphoma involving subcutaneous tissue. A clinicopathologic entity commonly associated with hemophagocytic syndrome. Am J Surg Pathol 15:17–27, 1991

34. Kois JM, Sexton FM, Lookingbill DP: Cutaneous manifestations of multiple myeloma. Arch Dermatol 127:69–74, 1991

35. Patterson JW, Parsons JM, White RM: Cutaneous involvement of multiple myeloma and extramedullary plasmacytoma. J Am Acad Dermatol 19:879–890, 1988

36. White JJ, Olsen KD, Banks PM: Plasma cell orificial mucositis. Report of a case and review of the literature. Arch Dermatol 122:1321–1324, 1986

37. Watanbe S, Ohara K, Kukita A, Mori S: Systemic plasmacytosis. A syndrome of peculiar multiple skin eruptions, generalized lymphadenopathy, and polyclonal hypergammaglobulinemia. Arch Dermatol 122:1314–1320, 1986

38. Edelson RL: Cutaneous T-cell lymphoma. Mycosis fungoides, Sezary's syndrome and other variants. J Am Acad Dermatol 2:89–106, 1980

39. Epstein EH, Devin DL, Croft JD et al: Mycosis fungoides. Survival, prognostic findings, response to treatment, and autopsy findings. Medicine 51:61–72, 1972

40. Weinstock MA, Horm JW: Mycosis fungoides in the United States. Increasing incidence and descriptive epidemiology. JAMA 260:26–42, 1988

41. Sanchez J, Ackerman AB: The patch stage of mycosis fungoides: criteria for histologic diagnosis. Am J Dermatopathol 1:5–26, 1979

42. Cerroni L, Rieger E, Hodl S et al: Clinicopathologic and immunologic features associated with transformation of mycosis fungoides to large-cell lymphoma. Am J Surg Pathol 16:543–552, 1992

43. Ackerman AB, Flaxman BA: Granulomatous mycosis fungoides. Br J Dermatol 82:397–401, 1970

44. LeBoit PE, Zackheim HS, White CRJ: Granulomatous variants of cutaneous T-cell lymphoma. The histopathology of granulomatous mycosis fungoides and granulomatous slack skin. Am J Surg Pathol 12:83–95, 1988

45. LeBoit PE: Variants of mycosis fungoides and related cutaneous T-cell lymphomas. Semin Diagn Pathol 8:73–81, 1991

46. Ralfkiaer E: Immunohistological markers for the diagnosis of cutaneous lymphomas. Semin Diagn Pathol 8:62–73, 1991

47. Weiss LM, Hu E, Wood GS et al: Clonal rearrangements of T-cell receptor genes in mycosis fungoides and dermatopathic lymphadenopathy. N Engl J Med 313:539–544, 1985

48. Chan WC, Greiner TC: Diagnosis of lymphomas by the polymerase chain reaction. Am J Clin Pathol 102:273–274, 1994

49. Kim SY: Follicular mycosis fungoides [letter]. Am J Dermatopathol 7:300–301, 1985

50. Kartsonis J, Brettschneider F, Weissmann A, Rosen L: Mycosis fungoides bullosa. Am J Dermatopathol 12:76–80, 1990

51. Ackerman AB, Guo Y, Vitale PA: A spongiotic lichenoid, psoriasiform lichenoid, or spongiotic psoriasiform lichenoid pattern in which lymphocytes predominate overwhelmingly is a clue to mycosis fungoides. pp. 241–244. In Clues to Diagnosis in Dermatopathology. Vol, 2, 1st Ed. Chicago: American Society of Clinical Pathology, 1992

52. LeBoit PE, Epstein BA: A vase-like shape characterizes the epidermal-mononuclear cell collections seen in spongiotic dermatitis. Am J Dermatopathol 12:612–616, 1990

53. Toro JR, Sander CA, LeBoit PE: Persistent pigmented purpuric dermatitis and mycosis fungoides. Simulant, precursor or both? Am J Dermatopathol 19:108–118, 1997

54. Rijilaarsdam JU, Scheffer E, Meijer CJ et al: Cutaneous pseudo-T-cell lymphomas. A clinicopathologic study of 20 patients. Cancer 69:717–724, 1992

55. Nickoloff BJ, Griffiths CE: Intraepidermal but not dermal T lymphocytes are positive for a cell-cycle-associated antigen (Ki-67) in mycosis fungoides. Am J Pathol 136:261–266, 1990

56. Hall WW, Liu CR, Schneewind O et al: Deleted HTLV-1 provirus in blood and cutaneous lesions of patients with mycosis fungoides [see comments]. Science 253:317–320, 1991

57. Mandojana RM, Helwig EG: Localized epidermotropic reticulosis (Woringer-Kolopp disease). J Am Acad Dermatol 8:813–829, 1983

58. Woringer F, Kolopp P: Lesion erythemato-squameuse polycyclique de l'avant bras evoulant depuis 6 ans chez un garconnet de 13 ans. Histologiquiement infiltrat intraepidermiquie d-apparance tumorale. Ann Dermatol Venereol 10:9245–9958, 1939

59. Wood GS, Weiss LM, Hu CH et al: T-cell antigen deficiencies and clonal rearrangements of T-cell receptor genes in pagetoid reticulosis (Woringer-Kolopp disease). N Engl J Med 318:164–167, 1988

60. Deneau DG, Wood GS, Beckstead J et al: Woringer-Kolopp disease (pagetoid reticulosis). Four cases with histopathologic, ultrastructural, and immunohistologic observations. Arch Dermatol 120:1045–1051, 1984

61. Sterry W, Hauschild A: Loss of leucocyte common antigen (CD45) on atypical lymphocytes in the localized but not disseminated type of Pagetoid reticulosis. Br J Dermatol 125:238–242, 1991

62. Berti E, Cerri A, Cavicchin S et al: Primary cutaneous gamma/delta T-cell lymphoma presenting as disseminated pagetoid reticulosis. J Invest Dermatol 96:718–723, 1991

63. Fujiwara Y, Abe Y, Kuyama M et al: CD8+ cutaneous T-cell lymphoma with pagetoid epidermotropism and angiocentric and angiodestructive infiltration. Arch Dermatol 126:801–804, 1990

64. Wieselthier JS, Koh HK: Sezary syndrome: Diagnosis, prognosis, and critical review of treatment options [see comments]. J Am Acad Dermatol 22:381–401, 1990

65. Sentis HJ, Willemze R, Scheffer E: Histopathologic studies in Sezary syndrome and erythrodermic mycosis fungoides: a comparison with benign forms of erythroderma. J Am Acad Dermatol 15:1217–1226, 1986

66. Buechner SA, Winkelmann RK: Sezary syndrome. A clinico-pathologic study of 39 cases. Arch Dermatol 119:979–986, 1983
67. Fletcher V, Zackheim HS, Beckstead JH: Circulating Sezary cells. A new preparatory method for their identification and enumeration. Arch Pathol Lab Med 108:954–958, 1984
68. Weiss LM, Wood GS, Hu E, Abel EA, Hoppe RT, Skylar J: Detection of clonal T-cell receptor gene rearrangements in the peripheral blood of patients with mycosis fungoides/Sezary syndrome. J Invest Dermatol 92:601–604, 1989
69. Imai S, Burg G, Braun FO: Mycosis fungoides and Sezary's syndrome show distinct histomorphological features. Dermatologica 173:131–135, 1986
70. O'Brian DS, Lawlor E, Sarsfield P et al: Circulating cerebriform lymphoid cells (Sezary-type cells) in a B-cell malignant lymphoma. Cancer 61:1587–1593, 1988
71. Bendelac A, O'Connor NT, Daniel MT et al: Nonneoplastic circulating Sezary-like cells in cutaneous T-cell lymphoma. Ultrastructural immunologic, and T-cell receptor gene-rearrangement studies. Cancer 60:980–986, 1987
72. Bunn PJ, Schechter GP, Jaffe E et al: Clinical course of retrovirus-associated adult T-cell lymphoma in the United States. N Engl J Med 309:257–264, 1983
73. Chan HL, Su IJ, Juo TT et al: Cutaneous manifestations of adult T cell leukemia/lymphoma. Report of three different forms. J Am Acad Dermatol 13:213–219, 1985
74. Manabe T, Hirokawa M, Sugihara K et al: Angiocentric and angiodestructive infiltration of adult T-cell leukemia/lymphoma (ATLL) in the skin. Report of two cases. Am J Dermatopathol 8:813–829, 1983
75. Murata K, Yamada Y, Kamihira S et al: Frequency of eosinophilia in adult T-cell leukemia/lymphoma. Cancer 69:966–971, 1992
76. Waldman TA, Greene WC, Sarin PS et al: Functional and phenotypic comparison of human T cell leukemia/lymphoma virus positive adult T cell leukemia with human T cell leukemia/lymphoma virus negative Sezary leukemia, and their distinction using anti-Tac. Monoclonal antibody identifying the human receptor for T cell growth factor. J Clin Invest 73:1711–1718, 1984
77. Gessain A, Noulonguet I, Flageul B et al: Cutaneous type of adult T cell leukemia/lymphoma in a French West Indian woman. Clonal rearrangement of T-cell receptor beta and gamma genes and monclonal integration of HTLV-1 proviral DNA in the skin infiltrate. J Am Acad Dermatol 23:994–1000, 1990
78. Willemze R: Lymphomatoid papulosis. Dermatol Clin 3:735–747, 1985
79. Sanchez NP, Pittelkow MR, Muller SA et al: The clinicopathologic spectrum of lymphomatoid papulosis: study of 31 cases. J Am Acad Dermatol 8:81–94, 1983.
80. Thomasen K, Wantzin GL: Lymphomatoid papulosis. A follow-up study of 30 patients. J Am Acad Dermatol 17:632–636, 1987
81. Weinman VF, Ackerman AB: Lymphomatoid papulosis. A critical review and new findings. Am J Dermatopathol 3:129–163, 1981
82. Ralfkiaer E, Stein H, Wantzin GL: Lymphomatoid papulosis.

Characterization of skin infiltrates by monoclonal antibodies. Am J Clin Pathol 84:587–593, 1985
83. Whittaker S, Smith N, Jones RR et al: Analysis of beta, gamma, and delta T-cell receptor genes in lymphomatoid papulosis: cellular basis of two distinct histologic subsets. Invest Dermatol 96:786–791, 1991
84. Weiss LM, Wood GS, Trela M et al: Clonal T-cell populations in lymphomatoid papulosis. Evidence of a lymphoproliferative origin for a clinically benign disease. N Engl J Med 315:475–479, 1986
85. Willemze R, Scheffer E: Clinical and histologic differentiation between lymphomatoid papulosis and pityriasis lichenoides. J Am Acad Dermatol 13:418–428, 1985
86. Smoller BR, Stewart M, Warnke R: A case of Woringer-Kolopp disease with Ki-1 (CD30)+ cytotoxic/suppressor cells. Arch Dermatol 128:526–529, 1992
87. Kadin M, Nasu K, Sako D et al: Lymphomatoid papulosis. A cutaneous proliferation of activated helper T cells expressing Hodgkin's disease-associated antigens. Am J Pathol 119:315–325, 1985
88. Davis TH, Morton CC, Miller CR et al: Hodgkin's disease, lymphomatoid papulosis, and cutaneous T-cell lymphoma derived from a common T-cell clone. N Engl J Med 326:1115–1122, 1992
89. Kaudewitz P, Stein H, Plewig G et al: Hodgkin's disease followed by lymphomatoid papulosis. Immunophenotypic evidence for a close relationship between lymphomatoid papulosis and Hodgkin's disease. J Am Acad Dermaol 22:999–1006, 1990
90. Pileri S, Falini B, Delsol G et al: Lymphohistiocytic T-cell lymphoma (anaplastic large cell lymphoma CD30+/Ki-1+ with a high content of reactive histiocytes). Histopathology 16:383–391, 1990
91. Flynn KJ, Dehner LP, Gajl PK et al: Regressing atypical histiocytosis: a cutaneous proliferation of atypical neoplastic histiocytes with unexpectedly indolent biologic behavior. Cancer 49:959–970, 1982
92. Headington JT, Roth MS, Schnitzer B: Regressing atypical histiocytosis: a review and critical appraisal. Semin Diagn Pathol 4:28–37, 1987
93. Kerschman RL, Berger TG, Weiss LM et al: Cutaneous lymphoma in human immunodeficiency viral disease. Predominance of T-cell lineage with two clinicopathological presentations. Arch Dermatol 131:1281–1288, 1995
94. Chan JK, Buchanan R, Fetcher CD: Sarcomatoid variant of anaplastic large-cell Ki-1 lymphoma [see comments]. Am J Surg Pathol 14:983–988, 1990
95. Jaworsky C, Cirillo HV, Petrozzi JW et al: Regressing atypical histiocytosis. Aberrant prothymocyte differentiation, T-cell receptor gene rearrangements, and nodal involvement. Arch Dermatol 126:1609–1616, 1990
96. Palesen G: The diagnostic significance of the CD30 (Ki-1) antigen [see comments]. Histopathology 16:409–413, 1990
97. Anagnostopoulos I, Humel M, Kaudewitz P et al: Detection of HTLV-1 proviral sequences in CD30-positive large cell cutaneous T-cell lymphomas. Am J Pathol 137:1317–1322, 1990
98. Kerschmann RL, Berger TG, Weiss LM et al: Cutaneous pre-

sentations of lymphoma in human immunodeficiency virus disease. Predominance of T-cell lineage. Arch Dermatol 131:1281–1288, 1995

99. Kadin ME, Cavaille CM, Gertz R et al: Loss of receptors for transforming growth factor beta in human T-cell malignancies. Proc Natl Acad Sci USA 91:6002–6006, 1994

100. Chan JK, Ng CS, Ngan KC et al: Angiocentric T-cell lymphoma of the skin. An aggressive lymphoma distinct from mycosis fungoides. Am J Surg Pathol 12:861–876, 1988

101. James WD, Odom RB, Katzenstein AL: Cutaneous manifestations of lymphomatoid granulomatosis. Report of 44 cases and a review of the literature. Arch Dermatol 117:196–202, 1981

102. Jambrosic J, From L, Assaad DA et al: Lymphomatoid granulomatosis. J Am Acad Dermatol 17:621–631, 1987

103. Wong KF, Chan JK, Ng CS et al: CD56 (NkH1)-positive hematolymphoid malignancies: in aggressive neoplasm featuring frequent cutaneous/mucosal involvement, cytoplasmic azurophilic granules, and angiocentricity. Hum Pathol 23:798–804, 1992

104. Bhwan J: Angioendotheliomatosis proliferans systemisata: an angiotropic neoplasm of lymphoid origin. Semin Diagn Pathol 4:18–27, 1987

105. Sepp N, Schuler G, Romani N et al: "Intravascular lymphomatosis" (angioendotheliomatosis): evidence for a T-cell origin in two cases. Hum Pathol 21:1051–1058, 1990

106. Wick MR, Mills SE, Scheithauer BW et al: Reassessment of malignant "angioendotheliomatosis." Evidence in favor of its reclassification as "intravascular lymphomatosis." Am J Surg Pathol 10:112–123, 1986

107. Ferry JA, Harris NL, Picker LJ et al: Intravascular lymphomatosis (malignant angioendotheliomatosis). A B-cell neoplasm expressing surface homing receptors. Mod Pathol 1:444–452, 1988

108. Smith JJ, Butler JJ: Skin involvement in Hodgkin's disease. Cancer 45:354–361, 1980

109. White RM, Patterson JW: Cutaneous involvement in Hodgkin's disease. Cancer 55:1135–1145, 1985

110. Sioutos N, Kerl H, Murphy SB: Primary cutaneous Hodgkin's disease. Unique clinical, morphologic, and immunophenotypic findings. Am J Dermatopathol 16:2–8, 1994

111. Moretti S, Pimpinelli N, Di LS et al: In situ immunologic characterization of cutaneous involvement in Hodgkin's disease. Cancer 63:661–666, 1989

112. Timens W, Visser L, Poppema S: Nodular lymphocyte pre-

dominance type of Hodgkin's disease is a germinal center lymphoma. Lab Invest 54:457–461, 1986

113. Hanno R, Bean SF: Hodgkin's disease with specific bullous lesions. Am J Dermatopathol 2:363–366, 1980

114. Simrell CR, Boccia RV, Long DL et al: Coexisting Hodgkin's disease and mycosis fungoides. Immunohistochemical proof of its existence. Arch Pathol Lab Med 110:1029–1034, 1986

115. Harris NL: Epstein-Barr virus in lymphoma. Protagonist or passenger? [editorial; comment]. Am J Clin Pathol 98:278–281, 1992

116. Su SP, Buechner SA, Li CY: Clinicopathologic correlations in leukemia cutis. J Am Acad Dermatol 11:121–128, 1984

117. Cote J, Trudel M, Gratton D: T cell chronic lymphocytic leukemia with bullous manifestations. J Am Acad Dermatol 8:874–878, 1983

118. Arai E, Ikeda S, Itoh S, Katayama I: Specific skin lesions as the presenting symptom of hairy cell leukemia. Am J Clin Pathol 90:459–464, 1988

119. Cerroni L, Zenatolik P, Hofler G et al: Specific cutaneous infiltrates of B-cell chronic lymphocytic leukemia. A clinicopathologic and prognostic study of 42 patients. Am J Surg Pathol 20:1000–1010, 1996

120. Davey FR, Olson S, Kurec AS et al: The immunophenotyping of extramedullary myeloid cell tumors in paraffin-embedded tissue sections. Am J Surg Pathol 12:699–707, 1988

121. Hanson CA, Ross CW, Schnitzer B: Anti-CD34 immunoperoxidase staining in paraffin sections of acute leukemia: comparison with flow cytometric immunophenotyping. Hum Pathol 23:26–32, 1992

122. Picker LJ, Michie SA, Rott LS et al: A unique phenotype of skin-associated lymphocytes in humans. Preferential expression of the HECA-452 epitope by benign and malignant T cells at cutaneous sites. Am J Pathol 136:1053–1068, 1990

123. Stroup R, Sheibani K: Antigenic phenotypes of hairy cell leukemia and monocytoid B-cell lymphoma: an immunohistochemical evaluation of 66 cases. Hum Pathol 23:172–177, 1992

124. Bowden JB, Hebert AA, Rapini RP: Dermal hematopoiesis in neonates: report of five cases. J Am Acad Dermatol 20:1104–1110, 1989

125. Schofield JK, Shun JL, Cerio R et al: Cutaneous extramedullary hematopoiesis with a preponderance of atypical megakaryocytes in myelofibrosis. J Am Acad Dermatol 22:334–337, 1990

22

PROLIFERATIVE DISORDERS OF MONONUCLEAR PHAGOCYTES AND LANGERHANS CELLS

Concepts of "histiocytic" diseases have undergone a great deal of revision in the past several years, and even the word *histiocyte* has been criticized as anachronistic and unmeaningful.[1] While it is true that a histiocyte is more properly designated as a *mononuclear phagocyte* or a *macrophage*, it would be unreasonable to expect that the former term will disappear from diagnostic use. Indeed, a meaningful body of data exists on the clinicopathologic features of "histiocytic" proliferations in the skin and other sites.[2–7] Moreover, current research continues to address the relationship between cutaneous histiocytes and dendritic cells, both of which demonstrate similar enzyme-histochemical, immunologic, functional, and, perhaps, neoplastic potentialities.[8] It is possible that these elements of the phagocytic system represent points in a spectrum of cellular differentiation, as influenced by variable environmental factors and soluble products derived from other hematologic cell types.

FUNCTIONAL AND PHENOTYPIC ASPECTS IN THE SKIN AND OTHER ANATOMIC SITES

Cells of the mononuclear phagocyte system (MPS) are found normally in many topographic sites, including the skin, lymph nodes, bone marrow, spleen, liver, and lungs. These cells derive from monoblasts of the bone marrow and circulating monocytes, the latter of which emigrate to become transitory or fixed residents of the above-cited organs.

Functionally, MPS cells (hereafter called *histiocytes*) are responsible for the phagocytosis of foreign microorganisms, indigenous cellular debris, immune complexes, and human cells to which antibodies or complement proteins have been attached or that have become altered antigenically. Ingested intracellular material is digested by histiocytic lysosomal enzymes of the acid hydrolase class. Because they express class I and II major histocompatibility (HLA-A, -B, -C, -DR, -DP, and -DQ) antigens and produce interleukin-1 (lymphocyte-activating factor), histiocytes are capable of "presenting" processed antigens to T lymphocytes, allowing the latter cells to recognize and respond to them.[9] This process is a crucial step in the "afferent" arm of the immune response. In turn, T cells often elaborate soluble cytokines after activation, which may "recruit" or further stimulate histiocyte activity. Lastly, histiocytes often exhibit direct cellular cytotoxicity with respect to other cell types or microorganisms through their production of exportable neutral proteases, interferon, and prostaglandins.

Normally, there are few resident histiocytes in the skin, at least as visualized by conventional microscopy; these are disposed around dermal blood vessels. Dermal "dendrocytes," which are characterized by their formation of dentritic cellular processes and synthesis of clotting factor XIIIa, represent other cutaneous denizens in the MPS family.[8] They are dispersed throughout the corium, are similarly inconspicuous on routine histologic examination of normal skin, and are thought to function principally in antigen presentation.

Langerhans cells (LCs; named after their discoverer, Dr Paul Langerhans) are also dendritic in nature. They are localized to several epithelia, including that of the epidermis and cutaneous appendages, and serve a role in the afferent limb of immune responses that is remarkably similar to that of histiocytes. LCs share with histiocytes several cellular determinants, such as complement receptors, immunoglobulin Fc receptors, and class I and II histocompatibility molecules.

Nevertheless, there also are several pertinent functional and phenotypic differences between LCs and histiocytes. The former do not display direct cytotoxicity or appreciable phagocytic activity and have only a limited intracellular complement of hydrolytic enzymes. Moreover, they show an exclusively intimate

763

association with epithelial cells and possess at least two antigenic markers that are lacking in MPS histiocytes. These are represented by S-100 protein (an intracellular mediator of calcium flux) and the CD1 (prethymocyte) antigen. Normal LCs also contain characteristic intracytoplasmic organelles (Birbeck granules) on an ultrastructural level, whereas MPS histiocytes do not. These inclusions are derived by invagination and detachment of the cellular plasmalemma; consequently, they have a zipper-like configuration, often with bulbous ends. The function of Birbeck granules has not been discerned to date, but it is conceivable that they are a by-product of antigenic attachment to the LC surface and subsequent internalization.

Because of the aforementioned overlaps in cellular characteristics between LCs and MPS histiocytes, the historical convention was to label all proliferations involving such elements as "histiocytoses." "Histiocytosis-X" is the outmoded term for what is now called *Langerhans cell disease* (LCD); similarly, "non-X histiocytosis" was used in the past to denote a proliferation of MPS cells.

PROLIFERATIONS OF MONONUCLEAR PHAGOCYTIC CELLS

Eruptive and Tuberous (Hyperlipoproteinemic) Xanthomas

Lipoprotein Metabolism

Plasma lipoproteins represent a heterogeneous population of complex macromolecules, containing variable amounts of lipid and protein. The former of these two components is present as either cholesterol or triglyceride. The latter, apoprotein, may function as an enzyme cofactor or as a ligand for tissue receptors that are involved in lipoprotein metabolism. The balance of contributions to the circulating lipoproteinaceous milieu from ingested fat and hepatic synthesis ultimately determines the peripheral and tissue levels of these moieties.

Triglyceride-rich chylomicrons that are synthesized in the gut from dietary cholesterol and fatty acids are coated with various apoproteins (apo-B48, -AI, -AII, and -AIV) before lymphatic secretion. Within the venous circulation, chylomicrons accept the transfer of apo-CII, apo-CIII, and apo-E from high-density lipoproteins (HDL). In capillary endothelia, the chylomicrons are transformed into cholesterol-rich "remnants" by progressive hydrolysis with lipoprotein lipase. Activation of the latter enzyme requires the presence of apo-CII. Deficiency of this cofactor severely impairs the clearance of triglycerides, creating an excess in the plasma and an enhanced risk of pancreatitis. In normal circumstances, apo-E chyloremnants are catabolized in the liver after recognition of apo-E ligands via hepatocellular receptors. They are degraded by lysosomal enzymes into cholesterol esters, which are used in the synthesis of bile acids, steroid hormones, cell membranes, and endogenous lipoproteins. Thus, defects in the synthesis or function of apo-E impair hepatic clearance of circulating triglyceride by reducing their uptake by the liver. Exogenous estrogenic compounds and other steroids may diminish the activity of lipoprotein lipase, again favoring secondary elevations of plasma triglycerides.[10,11]

Endogenous lipoprotein is produced in the liver as triglyceride-rich, very-low-density lipoprotein (VLDL), requiring functional apoproteins (apo-B100, apo-CI, apo-CII, apo-CIII, and apo-E) for assembly and secretion. VLDL synthesis may be modulated by exogenous (e.g., dietary) factors,[10,11] resulting in *secondary hyperlipoproteinemic states*. Hepatic VLDL serves as a source of metabolic energy for muscle cells and adipocytes via generation of fatty acids. Again, this is accomplished by endothelial lipoprotein lipase with apo-CII as an activating cofactor. VLDL is degraded into triglyceride-rich remnants and cholesterol-rich, intermediate-density lipoprotein (IDL). Hepatocytes remove apo-E from the latter molecules, and triglyceride lipase hydrolyzes IDL into low-density lipoproteins (LDL), which accounts for most circulating cholesterol under normal conditions. Tissue uptake of LDL requires the recognition of receptors for these lipoproteins by apo-E. Hence, abnormally low levels of apo-E or mutant forms of it impair the metabolism of LDL cholesterol peripherally. *Dysbetalipoproteinemia* is caused by combined defects of lipoprotein metabolism, especially aberrant apo-EII synthesis (with low receptor affinity) with coexisting overproduction of VLDL or abnormal, low-affinity LDL receptors.[12]

Clinical Features

Hyperlipoproteinemic xanthomas (HLX) of the *eruptive, tuberous*, and *intertriginous types* are a manifestation of disturbed lipid metabolism, with elevated levels (usually by a factor of three or more above normal) of serum triglycerides or cholesterol, or both. As such, these lesions are encountered in patients who have familial (genetically determined) or acquired (secondary) hyperlipoproteinemic states. Six electrophoretic patterns of pathologic lipoprotein distribution have been defined,[13] as follows: type I hyperlipidemia (HL) features an excess in plasma chylomicrons; type IIa HL shows elevated β-lipoprotein LDL; type IIb HL is characterized by elevations in LDL and pre-β VLDL lipoproteins; type III HL patients have augmented IDL levels with "broad β" electrophysical migration properties; type IV disease shows high levels of pre-β VLDL; and type V HL is recognized by excessive values of chylomicrons and VLDL in the plasma. These nosologic designations are supplemented by others that are predicated on the topographic distribution of HLX or on predisposing conditions for them (Table 22-1).

The subcategorization of xanthomas into distinctive clinical groups has prognostic importance as well as diagnostic utility (Table 22-1). In addition to the dyslipoproteinemias, two rare autosomal recessive normolipidemic states, cerebrotendinous xanthomatosis and β-sitosterolemia, are linked to cutaneous lesions containing lipidized histiocytes. Deep xanthomas, xanthelasmas (special forms of xanthomas affecting the periorbital skin), and hematologic, neurologic, or endocrinologic abnormalities constitute the other clinical aberrations seen in the latter genetic conditions.

Eruptive xanthomas may serve as cutaneous indicators of various other diseases that produce biochemical abnormalities in the synthesis or utilization of chylomicrons and VLDL. The former of these lipids may accumulate because of deranged lipoprotein lipase activity or apo-CII deficiency or as a result of competitive displacement by VLDL that are constitutively overproduced by the liver. Diabetes mellitus, biliary obstruction, hypothyroidism, renal disease, pancreatitis, ethanol abuse, and the

Table 22-1. Primary and Secondary Lipid Disorders Associated with Cutaneous Xanthomas

Xanthelasma
    Familial hypercholesterolemia
    Secondary hypercholesterolemia[a]
    Normolipidemia
    β-Sitosterolemia
    Cerebrotendinous xanthomatosis
Eruptive xanthoma
    Hyperlipoproteinemia, types I and V
        Familial hypertriglyceridemia
        Familial combined hyperlipoproteinemia
        Lipoprotein lipase deficiency
        Lipoprotein lipase inhibitor
        Apoprotein (apo)-CII deficiency
        Abnormal Apo-CIII
        Apo-EIV phenotype
    Hyperlipoproteinemia, type IV
        Familial hypertriglyceridemia
        Familial combined hyperlipidemia
        Abnormal apo-CIII
Tuberous and tendinous xanthomas
    Hyperlipoproteinemia, type II
        Familial hypercholesterolemia
        Familial combined hyperlipoproteinemia
    Hyperlipoproteinemia, type III (broad β disease)
    β-Sitosterolemia
    Cerebrotendinous xanthomatosis
Intertriginous xanthoma
    Hyperlipoproteinemia, type II
Palmar xanthoma
    Hyperlipoproteinemia, type III
        Familial dysbetalipoproteinemia
        Hepatic lipase deficiency

[a] Exacerbated by exogenous factors and disease states.
(Modified from Schaefer and Levy,[99] with permission.)

use of exogenous estrogen[14] or retinoids[15,16] produce these metabolic defects secondarily, whereas familial HL of types III through V is the principal cause of primary eruptive xanthomatosis. Clinically, both constitutional and secondary eruptive xanthomas are associated with the appearance of multiple, discrete, clustered red to yellow papules, usually measuring less than 5 mm in diameter. They show a predilection for extensor surfaces of the extremities and the buttocks and are less often located in flexural or acral skin, or mucocutaneous sites.

The finding of HLX in the skin of the elbows, knees, or buttocks, together with others in the palmar creases and tendons, is pathognomonic for type III HL (broad β disease). By contrast, type II HL features the presence of intertriginous HLX; these manifest themselves as yellowish cerebriform plaques on the hands, flexural surfaces of the extremities, and axillary skin, and they appear in childhood. As noted above, the xanthomas in both of these dyslipoproteinemias are associated with premature atherosclerosis and are therefore important clinical indicators of this systemic disease.

In light of the widespread availability of laboratory tests to measure and fractionate plasma lipids, biopsies of suspected xanthomas are usually not performed. However, in selected cir-

cumstances, such as those wherein the lesions may have an atypical clinical appearance, the dermatopathologist may be presented with such a specimen for microscopic interpretation.

Histopathologic Features

Eruptive and tuberous xanthomas differ only in size and the relative bulk of lesional cells comprising them. Both are constituted by dermal sheets of lipidized histiocytes with "foamy" cytoplasm and bland, compact, single, peripherally placed nuclei (Figs. 22-1 and 22-2). Neutrophils and mature lymphocytes are commonly dispersed throughout the xanthoma cell population, but eosinophils are rarely observed. A grenz zone is inconstantly present beneath the overlying epidermis, which is often atrophic, and the surrounding corium may demonstrate variable degrees of fibrosis. Multinucleated giant cells are reproducibly absent in these lesions. Xanthomas in deeper tissues, such as fascia, have similar histologic attributes, but regularly exhibit more striking fibrosis. Ocular xanthelasmas have been said to lack appreciable numbers of inflammatory cells, but this has not been our experience (Fig. 22-3).

Differential Diagnosis

On microscopic grounds alone, it is usually not possible to distinguish eruptive and tuberous xanthomas from the lesions of xanthoma disseminatum or the "histiocytic" variant of juvenile xanthogranuloma (see below). Clinical information should be sought to accomplish this task; among the disorders just cited, only eruptive and tuberous xanthomas are accompanied by abnormalities in serum lipids.

Xanthoma Disseminatum

Clinical Features

Xanthoma disseminatum (XD) was fully recognized as a distinctive clinicopathologic entity in 1938,[17] although it had been described initially by von Graefe 70 years earlier. It is currently categorized as a systemic proliferation of histiocytes that manifests itself with diabetes insipidus, cutaneous xanthomas, and xanthomatous lesions of the mucous membranes. XD has a propensity to affect adolescents (50% of whom are prepubescent) and young adults, but has been reported in patients of all ages.[18]

Macroscopically, one observes multiple red-brown coalescing plaques or nodules, showing a tendency to involve flexural and intertriginous skin. These vary markedly in size, but may attain dimensions of several centimeters. Among extracutaneous sites, the epiglottis, larynx, tracheobronchial tree, conjunctivae, lips, tongue, buccal surfaces, gingivae, soft and hard palates, uvula, tonsils, and pharynx all are involved in up to 40% of cases. Respiratory obstruction with dyspnea is possible when the disease is localized inopportunely in the airway or when such lesions are inordinately large. XD is seen rarely in the cornea, hepatobiliary tree, stomach, skeletal muscle, and hypothalamus or pituitary gland.[18,19] Some reported examples of the disorder have been linked with osseous lesions,[20–22] but their separation from LC proliferations was less than satisfactory in these accounts.[19] The concurrence of XD and Walden-

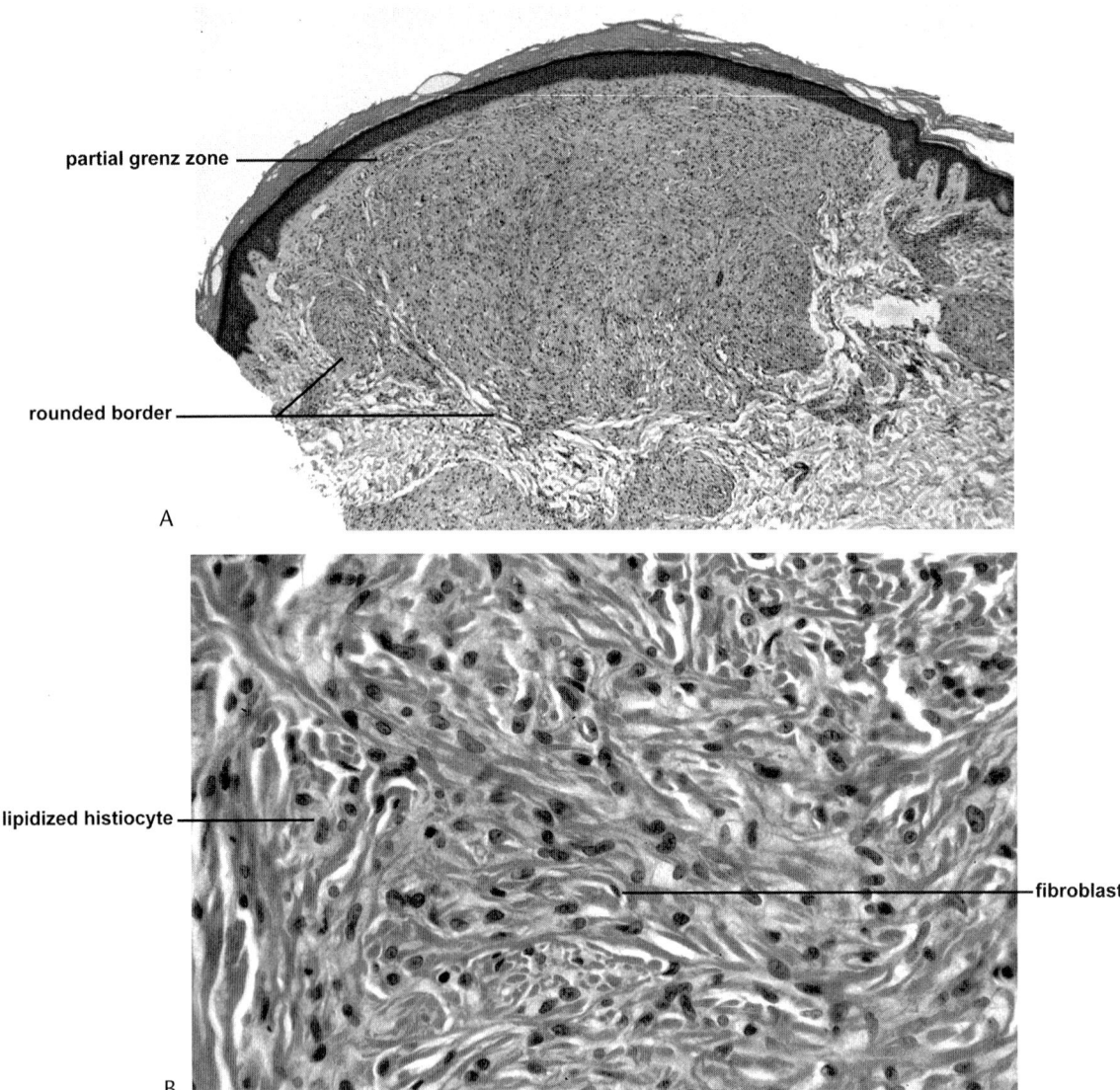

partial grenz zone

rounded border

A

lipidized histiocyte

fibroblast

B

Figure 22-1. (**A**) Punch biopsy specimen of a tuberous xanthoma. There is an irregular nodule of lipidized histiocytes and fibroblasts occupying most of the papillary and some of the reticular dermis. Many of these lesions would display a grenz zone, which is poorly defined in this example. (H&E, × 40.) (**B**) Higher power view of the lipidized histiocytes and fibroblasts. As the lesion ages, more collagen develops. (H&E, × 150.)

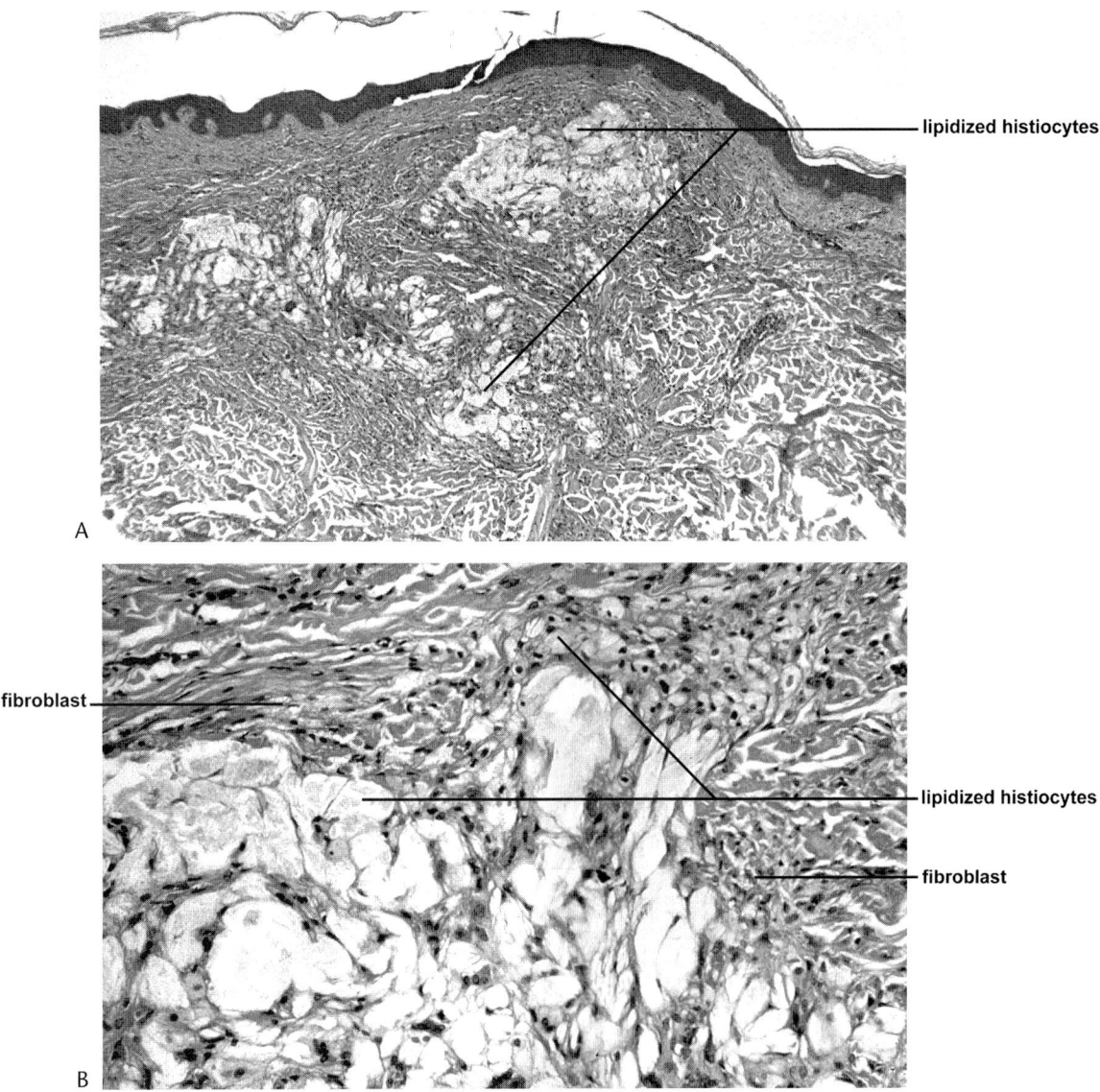

Figure 22-2. Eruptive xanthoma. (**A**) Irregular nodules of lipidized histiocytes in the papillary and reticular dermis. An inflammatory infiltrate and a grenz zone are present. (H&E, × 40.) (**B**) Higher power view showing the lipidized histiocytes. Collagenization is less than in a tuberous xanthoma. (H&E, × 150.)

Figure 22-3. Orbital xanthelasma showing lipidized histiocytes in clusters around appendages and blood vessels. The lipidized histiocytes are superficially placed and usually fail to form large sheets. (H&E, × 100.)

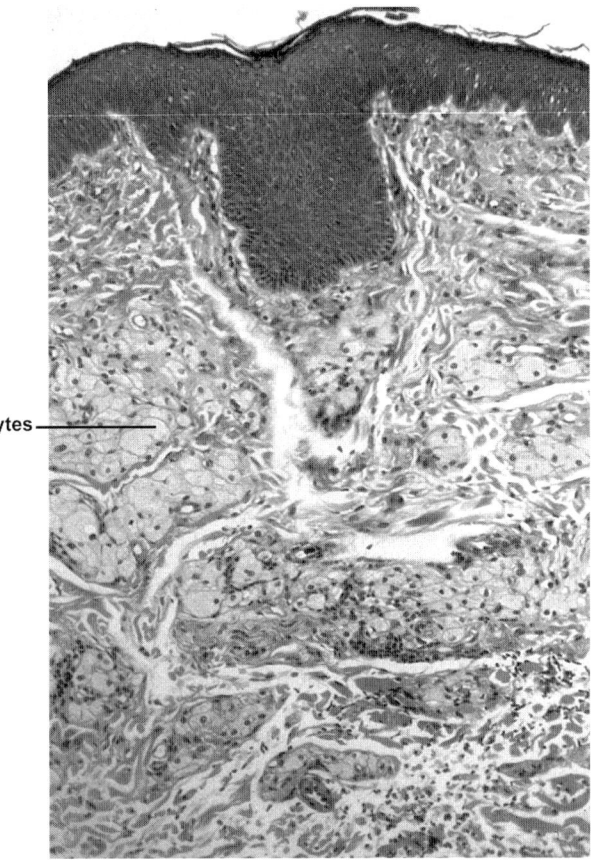

lipidized histiocytes——————

ström's macroglobulinemia also has been documented.[23] Patients with XD characteristically have a normal serum lipid profile biochemically.

Histopathologic Features

XD demonstrates numerous lipidized histiocytes in sheets and clusters in the dermis or, more rarely, in the corium and subcutis, that usually are separated from the overlying epidermis by a grenz zone (Fig. 22-4). Slight atrophy may be noted in the surface epidermis. Dermal appendages are surrounded by lesional elements. The closely apposed proliferating cells contain finely vacuolated cytoplasm and are separated only by an inconspicuous fibrovascular stroma. Their nuclei are amitotic, bland, and, for the most part, single. However, scattered multinucleated elements are often present within the infiltrates, having the appearance of Touton-like or foreign body-type cells. Early examples of "classic" XD show variable numbers of mature lymphocytes, neutrophils, and nonvacuolated histiocytes that are admixed with the lipidized cells. Eosinophils are extremely sparse or altogether absent in this disorder. Older lesions may demonstrate dermal fibrosis and tend to have more multinucleated cells.

Results of Special Pathologic Studies

There are no distinctive ultrastructural characteristics of XD cells that demonstrate the array of degradative lysosomal inclu-

sions that one would expect of phagocytic histiocytes. Immunohistologically, they express hematopoietic antigens in the CD11b, CD11c, CD14, CD45, and CD68 groups.[19] Vimentin and HLA-A, -B, -C, and -DR antigens also are apparent in XD cells, but CD1 and CD43 determinants, as well as S-100 protein, are lacking.

Differential Diagnosis

Depending on the biologic stage of XD at which a biopsy is performed, this disorder can be confused with other xanthomas of the eruptive, papular, or tuberous types or with "burned-out" lesions of LCD and juvenile xanthogranuloma (JXG). Eruptive and tuberous xanthomas do not contain multinucleated cells. Moreover, they occur in patients with HL, in contrast to individuals with XD. *Papular xanthomatosis* (which is distinguished from XD by some observers, but occurs in a similar clinical setting) does manifest Touton-like giant cells, but lacks the neutrophils and lymphocytes that may be seen in XD. Moreover, the former of these two disorders features discrete yellow papules that do not coalesce, representing a macroscopic dissimilarity from XD.

Advanced LCD and JXG are not easy to separate from XD on purely histologic grounds. It is true that eosinophils are a common constituent of LC lesions in their classic forms; however, they commonly disappear in time and are replaced by lipidized cells and multinucleated histiocytes. The latter may represent histiocytes that are recruited to the area and thus serve to obfuscate the original identity of the lesion. Clinical information is often necessary to distinguish between LCD, JXG, and XD, if it can be obtained. When this is not possible, immunohistologic analyses may be beneficial. The observation of significant numbers of lesional cells that conjointly express S-100 protein, HLA-DR, CD43, and CD76 would favor the diagnosis of LCD. CD45 is absent in the lipidized histiocytes of JXG, whereas it is present in lesional cells of XD.

Verruciform Xanthoma

Clinical Features

Verruciform xanthoma (VX) is typically a solitary exophytic lesion of the skin or squamous mucosal surfaces, first described in the oral cavity in 1971.[24] Other common sites for VX include the mucocutaneous genital region (particularly the perineum and vulvar labia in women),[25–29] the digits,[30] and the skin of the legs.[31] It principally affects adults, but shows no predilection for a particular age group in this context. Both men and women may develop VX. This lesion has been reported in association with linear epidermal nevus,[25,32] epidermolysis bullosa dystrophica,[33] and inflammatory verrucous nevus.[34] Such concurrences suggest that VX may represent a secondary cutaneous reaction pattern in likeness to cornoid lamellae in porokeratosis.[35]

Histopathologic Features

Aside from verrucoid changes in the overlying epidermis, the histologic appearance of VX is virtually identical to that of eruptive or tuberous xanthoma. The surface of the skin is exuberantly hyperplastic in VX, as the name suggests. Epidermal acanthosis and papillomatosis are prominent, and a sparse lichenoid band of subepidermal lymphocytes is often observed as well (Fig. 22-5). Xanthoma cells are packed between the epidermal rete.

Figure 22-4. Xanthoma disseminatum also consists of sheets and clusters of lipidized histiocytes. (**A**) Slight atrophy of the surface epidermis, lacking a grenz zone. (H&E, × 40). (**B**) Constituent elements of the xanthoma are present. Multinucleate lipidized histiocytes of the Touton type are present. Touton giant cells are not seen in either tuberous xanthoma or eruptive xanthomas. The histologic appearance shown here overlaps with that of the juvenile xanthogranuloma. (H&E, × 150).

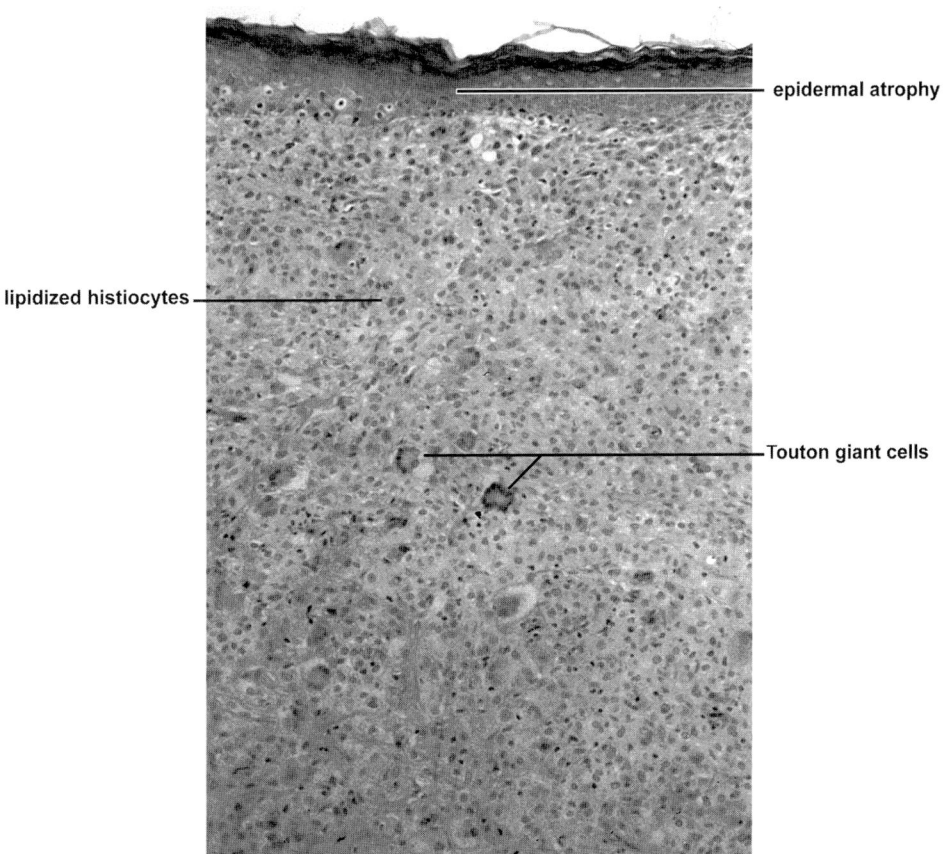

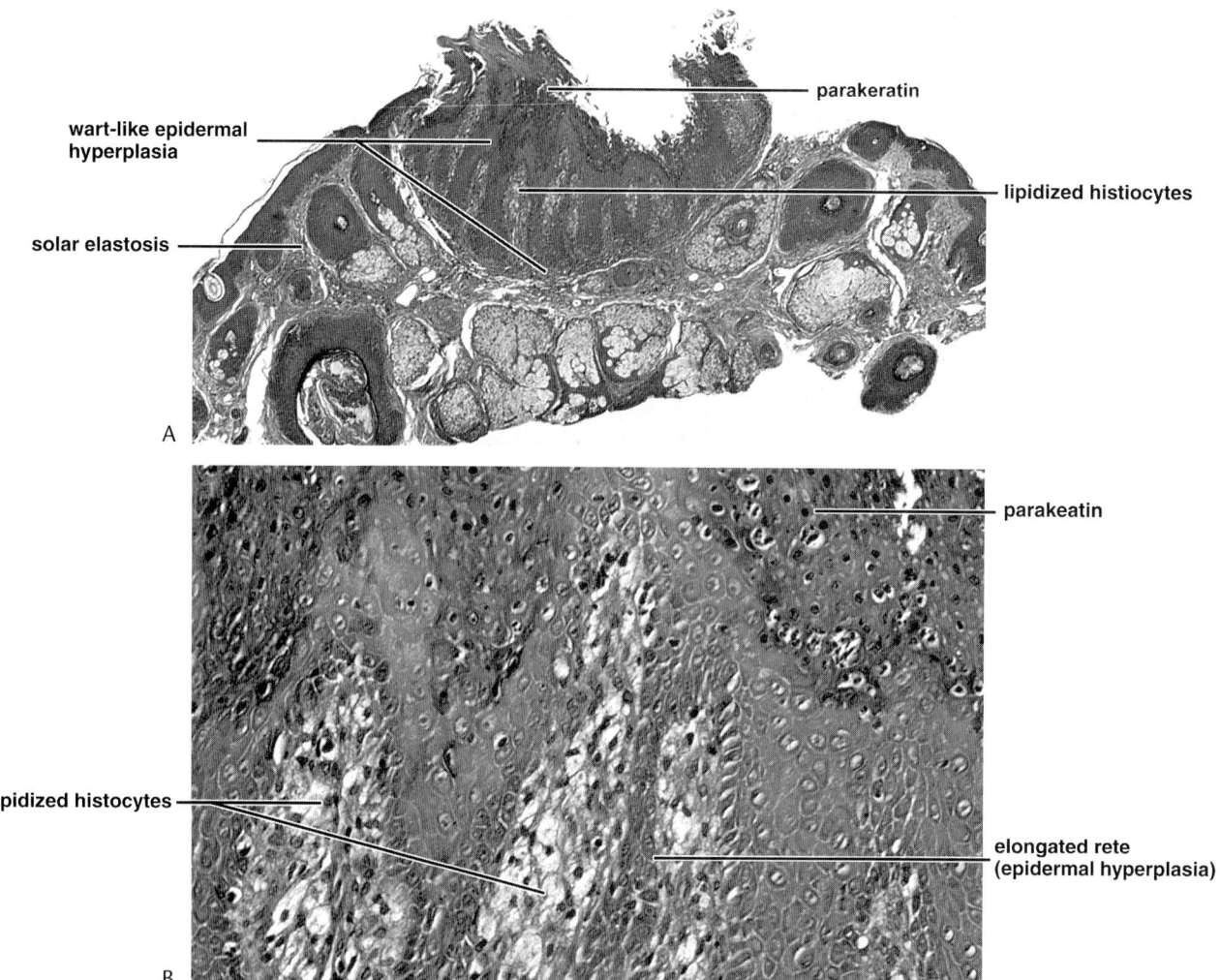

Figure 22-5. Verruciform xanthoma is an unusual type of xanthoma. (**A**) Verruciform xanthoma of sun-damaged skin. The lesion has a wart-like surface and a rounded base. Elastosis of the dermis is prominent. (H&E, × 40). (**B**) Lipidized histiocytes between the elongate epidermal rete. Parakeratosis is present in the stratum corneum. A slight mononuclear infiltrate is also present. (H&E, × 100).

Differential Diagnosis

Aside from other forms of xanthoma, as mentioned above, there are two major differential diagnostic considerations in cases of VX. These are granular cell tumor and metastatic renal cell carcinoma.

In the former, pseudoepitheliomatous epidermal hyperplasia is also a striking feature, and subjacent groups of granular cells may bear a passing resemblance to the lipidized histiocytes of VX. However, on closer inspection, the proliferating cells of granular cell tumor are not foamy but instead show dense aggregates of lysosomal granules. Moreover, the neoplastic elements tend to be arranged in distinct nests and cords in granular cell tumor, whereas lesional cells of VX assume a medullary or sheet-like configuration. Immunohistologic studies are useful in this particular differential diagnostic setting; the majority of granular cell tumors exhibit positivity for S-100 protein, while VX is negative.

Neoplastic cells in metastatic renal cell carcinoma likewise lack the multivacuolated appearance of histiocytes in VX and instead show the presence of uniform cytoplasmic lucency. Carcinomas of the kidney display a rich stromal vasculature; as a consequence, hemorrhagic "pools" of erythrocytes are common in such tumors. These cellular aggregates are not observed in VX. Lastly, renal cell carcinomas are usually intensely reactive with periodic acid-Schiff (PAS) and keratin, whereas lipidized cells of VX are negative.

Dysproteinemic Plane Xanthoma

Clinical Features

Also known as *atypical xanthoma disseminatum* and *generalized xanthelasma*, dysproteinemic plane xanthoma (DPX) is a relatively uncommon disorder that is associated with multiple myeloma and paraproteinemia.[18] Most patients with this condition are men between 40 and 60 years of age,[36] although children may rarely be affected. The typical clinical presentation of DPX is that of a generalized eruption of discrete yellow-brown papules and plaques. These can be seen at any cutaneous site, but favor the eyelids, lateral neck, and upper torso; they also have a peculiar tendency for secondary deposition in scars. Involvement of the ocular skin is universal and may precede the onset of more systemic disease by many years. Unlike patients with eruptive and tuberous xanthomas, the great majority of those with DPX show normal biochemical lipid profiles in serum.[37,38] Although myeloma is the usual underlying disease process,[18,37,38] anecdotal cases have been linked with renal cell carcinoma[39] and cutaneous T-cell lymphoma.[40]

Histopathologic Features and Differential Diagnosis

The histopathologic features of DPX are not diagnostic of this entity because of significant similarities to the microscopic attributes of HLX. Lipidized histiocytes in DPX may fill the superficial dermis, or they may be localized to perivascular areas in the corium. One typically does not see lymphocytes, neutrophils, or eosinophils in these lesions, and multinucleated cells of the Touton or foreign-body types are also totally lacking in almost all cases. Correlation of histologic observations with clinical information is essential for the proper recognition of DPX.

Necrobiotic Xanthogranuloma with Dysproteinemia

Clinical Features

Necrobiotic xanthogranuloma (NXG) was first described by Kossard and Winkelmann[41] in 1980 as another distinctive cutaneous indicator of paraproteinemic states. In this regard, it is similar to DPX. Prior to its seminal description, NXG had been represented variably in the literature as an atypical variant of multicentric reticulohistiocytosis[42] or necrobiosis lipoidica.[43,44] However, its distinction from the latter two conditions is now generally accepted.

Patients with NXG are typically adults between 30 and 60 years of age (average age, 55 years), with no predilection for either gender. However, this disease has been seen in individuals as young as 17 years of age and also in very elderly patients. Monoclonal paraproteins are found in the serum in approximately 80% of cases, usually being isotypes of IgG; some may have the properties of cryoglobulins or serve as the substrate for visceral amyloidosis. Surprisingly, only 10% to 15% of NXG cases are associated with underlying myeloma or lymphoproliferative states.[45,46]

Cutaneous lesions in this disease are indurated, sometimes ulcerated, xanthomatous papulonodules or plaques. They are violaceous to red-orange and multiple and range in size from 0.5 to 25 cm. The central aspects of older lesions may demonstrate atrophy or clearing. Involvement of the periorbital skin is characteristic of NXG,[41,45,46] and secondary ocular inflammation may result in glaucoma, iritis, scleritis, uveitis, and ptosis. Extracutaneous abnormalities may include sensory polyneuropathy,

myositis, and arthritis, and some fatal cases have demonstrated evidence of visceral involvement by NXG.[45]

Histopathologic Features

Well-developed NXG has a characteristic microscopic appearance. It is typified by replacement of the reticular dermis, or subcutis, or both, by lipidized histiocytes that are arranged in a granuloma-like configuration. As such, they tend to aggregate peripherally around foci of necrobiosis and extracellular cholesterolosis, which often become hyalinized as the lesions progress (Fig. 22-6). Touton-type and foreign-body multinucleated giant cells are abundant. Moreover, the nuclei within such elements are often hyperchromatic and tend to become polarized within the cytoplasm. The overall contours of the giant cells are irregular. Rarely, transepithelial elimination of xanthomatized histiocytes or amorphous debris may be observed through the ostia of hair follicles.[46]

Early lesions of NXG can be more difficult to recognize with certainty, especially if a relatively superficial biopsy is performed. In these instances, dermal necrobiotic arrays of histiocytes may bear a striking resemblance to those of granuloma annulare or necrobiosis lipoidica. As in the second of these disorders, the central portions of granuloma-like cell clusters in NXG are found to contain lipid with the oil red O or Sudan IV methods.

At least 50% of fully evolved cases show prominent lymphoid aggregates. These are usually centered on the junction between the dermis and subcutis and may be so notable that a diagnosis of lymphocytoma cutis is considered. In addition, perivascular or periappendigeal aggregates of plasma cells are often seen; occasionally, these may "dissect" through dermal collagen in a manner similar to that observed in cutaneous myeloma.[45,46]

Subcuticular deposits of NXG are virtually pathognomonic of the disorder. They contain a mixture of Touton giant cells, lipidized histiocytes, cholesterol clefts, and macrophages and are lobular in distribution. Subjacent granulomatous inflammation in fasciae or muscles is evident in 10% of NXG cases.[45] Less frequently, it may surround large blood vessels in the soft tissues, eventuating in luminal thrombosis.[47] However, true intramural vasculitis is not seen.

Although the above-cited microscopic findings appear to be distinctive when they are well represented in any given biopsy specimen, Mehregan and Winkelmann[48] have recommended that three lesions in separate locations should be sampled before a definitive diagnosis of NXG is rendered. Such an approach is understandable in view of the adverse prognosis attending this condition.

Differential Diagnosis

Because of the clinical similarities between DPX and NXG, the differential diagnosis between them rests in the procurement of a biopsy specimen. As stated previously, the xanthomatous infiltrate of DPX is much more superficial than that of NXG, and it lacks multinucleated giant cells. Necrobiosis lipoidica and granuloma annulare may be simulated by NXG in superficial locations, but the characteristic atypical giant cells of NXG and associated extracellular cholesterolosis should suffice to sepa-

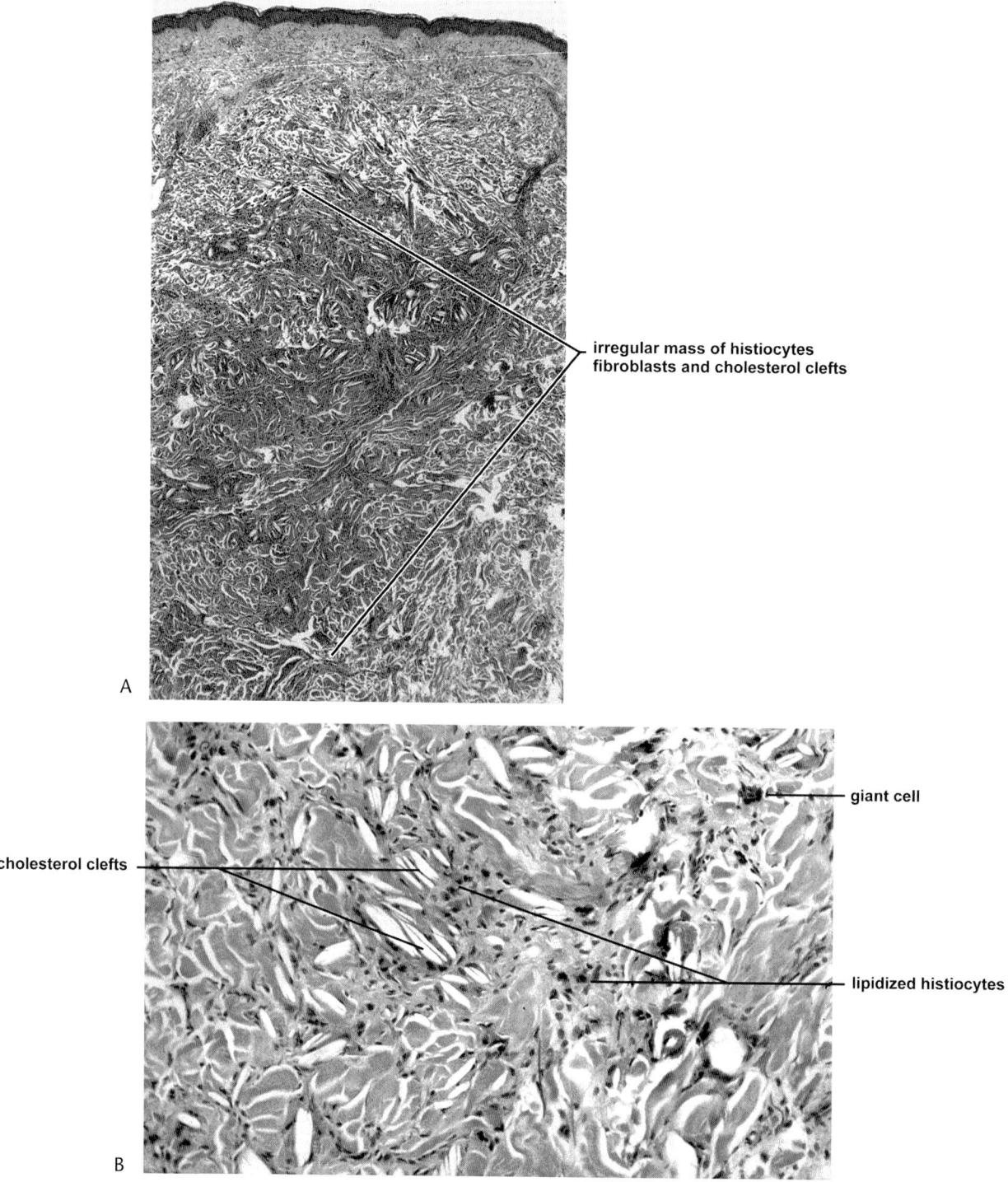

Figure 22-6. Necrobiotic xanthogranuloma has a distinctive appearance. (**A**) The lesion is centered in the reticular dermis. (H&E, × 40). (**B**) The lesion is characterized by lipidized histiocytes with occasional giant cells. As a characteristic feature, numerous cholesterol clefts are also present. Other forms of xanthoma do not display the cholesterol clefts.

rate these diseases. Moreover, granulomatoid cellular arrays in granuloma annulare contain stromal mucin, unlike those of necrobiosis lipoidica and NXG. Finally, the clinical presentations of DPX, necrobiosis lipoidica, granuloma annulare, and NXG are sufficiently dissimilar so that historical data are reliable in distinguishing between them.

Juvenile Xanthogranuloma

Clinical Features

As its name suggests, JXG is a proliferation that is seen predominantly in childhood and adolescence (average age, 4.5 years), and many cases occur in children under the age of 1 year[49] but may occur in adults. There is no preference for JXG to affect either males or females.

Classically, this disorder has been described as one featuring multiple, firm, yellow-brown to red-violet papulonodules, which typically show a short clinical evolution (3.5 months) before coming to medical attention. They most often arise in the skin of the head, neck, and upper trunk, as well as other sites.[50]

JXG tends to undergo spontaneous "self-regression" with time, a phenomenon that has not been studied well histologically until recently.[50] Experience has shown that this process is not, in fact, one of regression. Instead, it appears that JXG *mature* with time to acquire the microscopic characteristics of nodular histiocytoma or dermatofibroma. Hence, one can justifiably consider these lesions to represent a spectrum of "fibrohistiocytic" proliferations. The recurrence of JXG after excision has been reported, but this seems to be a rare event.

Histopathologic Features

Three subtypes or stages of JXG have been established: "classic," "transitional," and "xanthomatous" lesions. Classic JXG is a dermal lesion that may involve the superficial subcutis as well. It is composed of a mixed infiltrate of compact or lipidized mononuclear histiocytes and Touton- or foreign body-type multinucleated giant cells, with scant numbers of lymphocytes and eosinophils being dispersed throughout (Fig. 22-7). Although some authors have suggested that lipid-containing histiocytes and Touton cells are absent in "early" classic JXG, experience has shown that the latter elements can indeed be found in nearly every case if an excisional biopsy specimen is examined.[50] Giant cells in JXG lack nuclear atypicality. Their nuclei are nonpolarized within the cytoplasm; instead, they assume a distinctive wreath-like configuration. The peripheral borders of the infiltrate are distinct. Hyperplastic change may be seen in the epidermis along with an increased melanin. Spindle cells should not be present in abundance in classic JXG.

By contrast, transitional JXG exhibits a notable proportion of bland, fibroblast-like spindle cells, and there are more foreign body-type giant cells than Touton cells in the lesional infiltrate. Lipidized histiocytes and admixed lymphocytes complete the microscopic picture of this proliferation.

Finally, xanthomatous JXG is remarkably similar to XD or popular xanthomatosis histologically. One sees a predominance of lipid-laden histiocytes, scant numbers of multinucleated giant cells, and a few dispersed lymphocytes in this variant of JXG (Fig. 22-8). However, it is more expansile and shows greater circumscription than XD or popular xanthomatosis.

Neither the age of the lesion in any given case nor its macroscopic size correlates with any one histologic subtype, as just described. However, biopsies done after a "JXG" has been present for more than 6 or 7 months are likely to show a histologic pattern more like that of "nodular histiocytoma" (see below).

Differential Diagnosis

The primary reason for subdividing JXG nosologically is to remind oneself of the differential diagnostic considerations that each histologic subtype invokes. Classic JXG may be confused with NXG, but the former lesion lacks necrobiosis, cholesterolosis, and nuclear atypia. Transitional JXG is said to "mimic" nodular histiocytoma, but the distinction between these two lesions may be more fancy than fact. Xanthomatous JXG is potentially simulated by late-stage LCD, HLX, XD, and papular xanthomatosis. In general, JXG is better delimited microscopically than the other lesions; moreover, it does not have an epidermal component as seen in LCD and usually contains scattered lymphocytes, unlike HLX variants.

Immunohistology may be necessary to make the distinction between these proliferations in selected instances. JXG lacks S-100 protein, whereas LC lesions express this determinant. Lipidized cells in XD, HLX, and papular xanthomatosis are positive for CD45 antigens, in contrast to LCD.

Subcutaneous Xanthogranuloma

Clinical Features

Several examples of a rare disorder with xanthogranulomatous microscopic features, termed *subcutaneous xanthogranuloma* (SXG), have been reported.[51,52] This condition appears to primarily affect men between 50 and 70 years of age and takes the form of multiple, deep, firm, blue-red nodules on the upper torso, proximal extremities, or face. Some cases have shown extracutaneous involvement of the larynx or conjunctiva as well. There is no apparent association with underlying systemic diseases, and patients are normolipemic.[48,52]

Histopathologic Features and Differential Diagnosis

Reported microscopic observations in cases of SXG are very similar to those of JXG, featuring circumscription on scanning microscopy, lipidized histiocytes, and multinucleated giant cells. Nevertheless, the former of these two lesions shows more internal fibrosis, central necrosis, and an acute inflammatory component. Perivascular lymphoid aggregates also may be evident, and stromal vascular thrombosis is sometimes seen. A minority of SXG contain admixed eosinophils. The differential diagnosis of these lesions is substantively that of JXG, and their immunohistologic attributes are identical. Whether SXG represents yet another variant of JXG in adults remains to be proven.

Nodular Histiocytoma (of Woringer)

Clinical Features

Nodular histiocytoma has also been termed *subepidermal fibrosis* or *sclerosing hemangioma* in the older literature. It is a relatively common proliferation that is seen in adults of all ages and

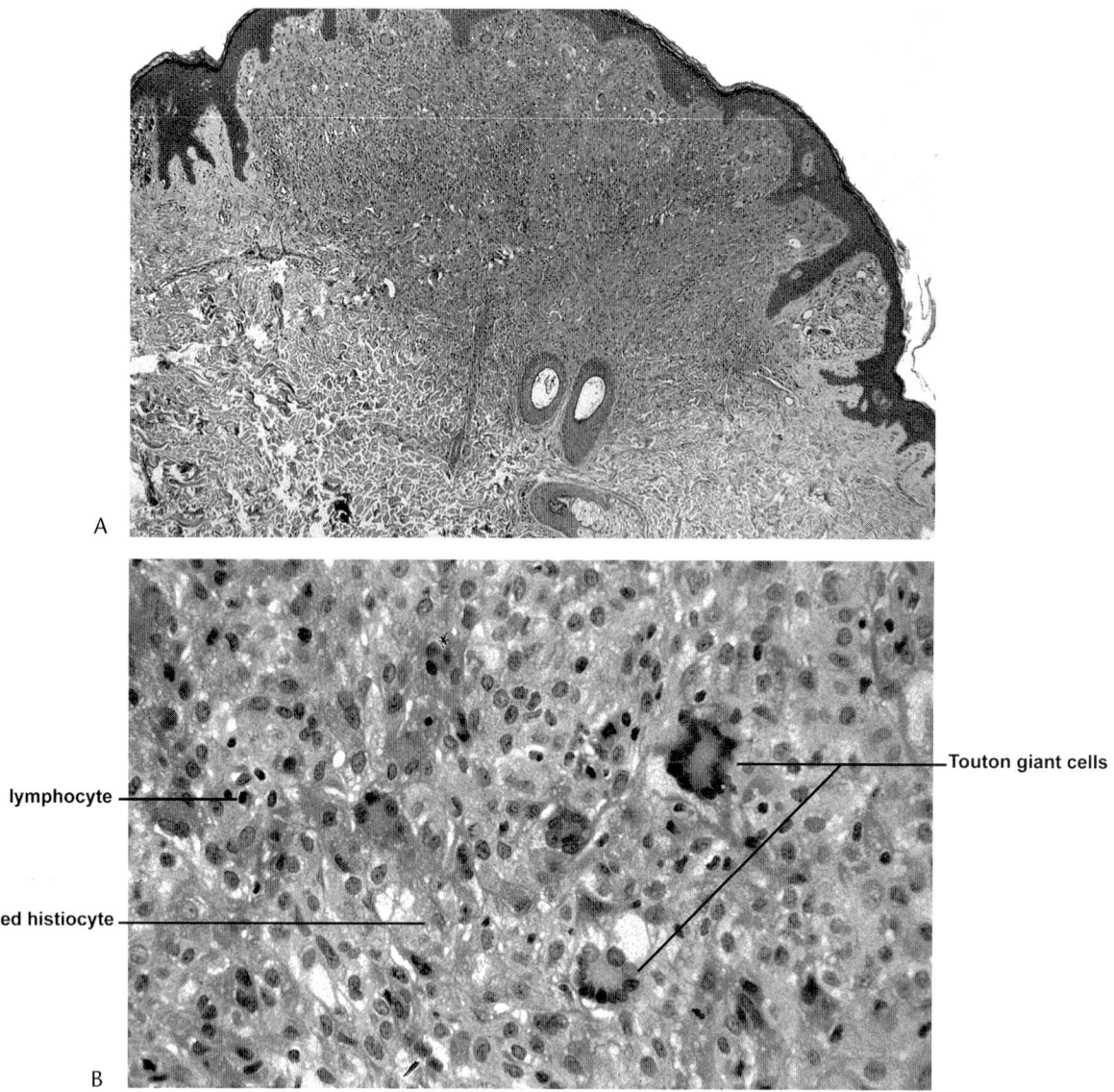

Figure 22-7. The histologic features of the juvenile xanthogranuloma overlap with some of the other xanthogranulomas. (**A**) A distinct nodule in a papule formation is present beneath the epidermis. (H&E, × 40). (**B**) Constituent elements are lipidized histiocytes, lymphocytes, and Touton giant cells. The proportion of giant cells to smaller lipidized histiocytes can vary greatly. Older lesions display increasing numbers of spindle fibroblast-like cells.

both sexes, usually on the lower extremities. The lesions are solitary, firm, and tan-pink and usually are less than 1 cm in greatest dimension.

Histopathologic Findings and Differential Diagnosis

Nodular histiocytomas are composed of storiform arrays of bland spindle cells, some of which are lipidized, and they are typically confined to the dermis. Lipidized histiocytes also are scattered randomly throughout the proliferating cell population, with a small number of chronic inflammatory cells. Multinucle-

ated giant cells may be present infrequently. The overlying epidermis is usually hyperplastic.

The distinction between transitional JXG, nodular histiocytoma, and dermatofibroma is, in our opinion, an arbitrary one. Based on careful comparative studies,[50] these lesions are part of a single histologic spectrum. Past dogma held that nodular histiocytoma was probably an idiosyncratic tissue response to trauma or arthropod bites, whereas JXG and dermatofibroma have been classified as histiocytic proliferations of a presumably neoplastic nature.[49] Immunohistologic studies have shown factor XIIIa reactivity in nodular histiocytomas.[53]

Isolated Cutaneous Reticulohistiocytoma

Clinical Features

Isolated cutaneous reticulohistiocytoma (ICR) is a disease of adults in which solitary or multiple lesions are observed in the skin of the head and neck. These are red-brown papulonodules that on occasion may demonstrate central ulceration. There is no gender predilection, and patients are usually older than 30 years of age at presentation.[50,51] ICR does not show an association with underlying systemic conditions[42]; specifically, there is no evidence of arthritis or another rheumatologic disease. The lesions may persist for several months and tend to be self-resolving.

Histopathologic Features

ICR has distinctive microscopic characteristics. It is typified by aggregates of large, rounded or polygonal histiocytes in the dermis and superficial subcutis. The infiltrates are circumscribed on low-power microscopy, and they often abut and elevate the overlying epidermis (Fig. 22-9). Atrophy of rete ridges may accompany this observation.

Constituent histiocytes contain brightly eosinophilic, homogeneous cytoplasm that often exhibits a granular or "ground-glass" appearance. Multinucleated elements, with up to 10 nuclei having bland vesicular chromatic and small nucleoli, are abundant in the proliferating cell population, and these are mixed with other histiocytes showing single eccentric nuclear profiles. Florid lesions of ICR manifest a generous admixture of lymphocytes, with lesser numbers of eosinophils and neutrophils. With time it loses its inflammatory character and gains a fibroblastic component that is intimately intertwined with the multinucleated cells. In the latter stage, giant cells commonly acquire artifactual "halos" around them because of retraction.

The granular nature of the multinucleated elements is apparently a result of the intracellular accumulation of phospholipids, in likeness to cutaneous granular cell tumors. Accordingly, the PAS stain with diastase is positive in ICR.

Differential Diagnosis

There are three principal differential diagnostic considerations in cases of ICR. These are the classic variant of JXG, granular cell tumor of the skin, and cutaneous lesions of sinus histiocytosis with massive lymphadenopathy (SHML).

JXG differs from ICR in showing classic Touton-type giant cells rather than eosinophilic multinucleated cells with "glassy" features. Moreover, there are typically more lipidized histiocytes in JXG than in ICR; the converse applies to the amount of inflammation seen in these two lesions. Granular cell tumor does not have multinucleated cells, lacks inflammation, and has a more infiltrative appearance. SHML bears a marked microscopic likeness to ICR in many respects, but almost invariably demonstrates the pathognomonic finding of lymphemperipolesis, as discussed subsequently. This feature allows for adequate distinction between the latter two proliferations. In cases where additional objectification for a diagnosis of SHML is desired,

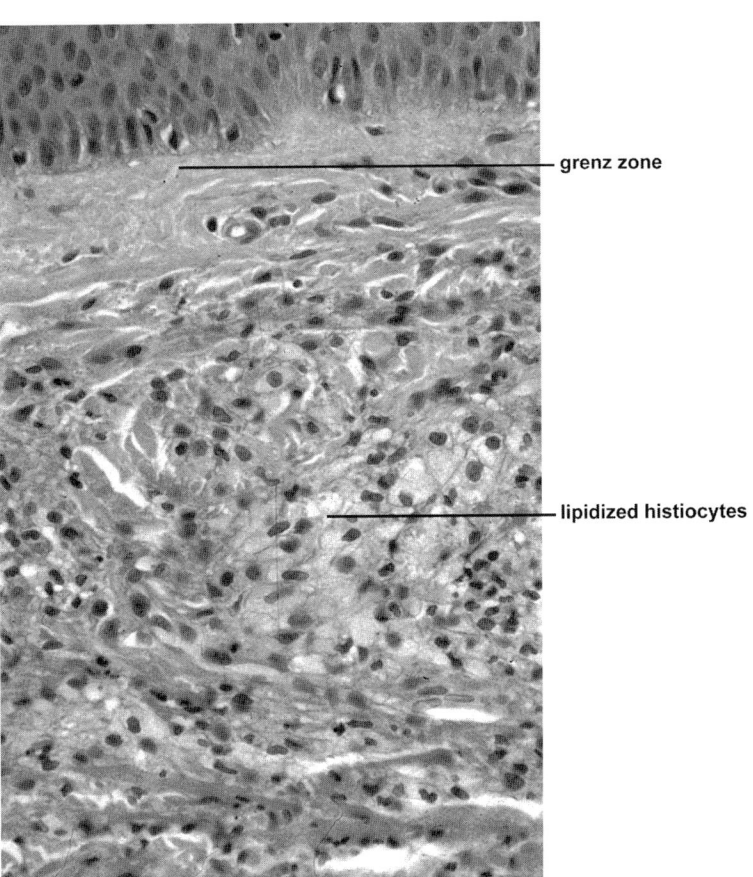

grenz zone

lipidized histiocytes

Figure 22-8. Xanthomatous juvenile xanthogranuloma. A remarkable similarity to xanthoma disseminatum is apparent because of the predominance of lipid-laden histiocytes. (H&E, × 100).

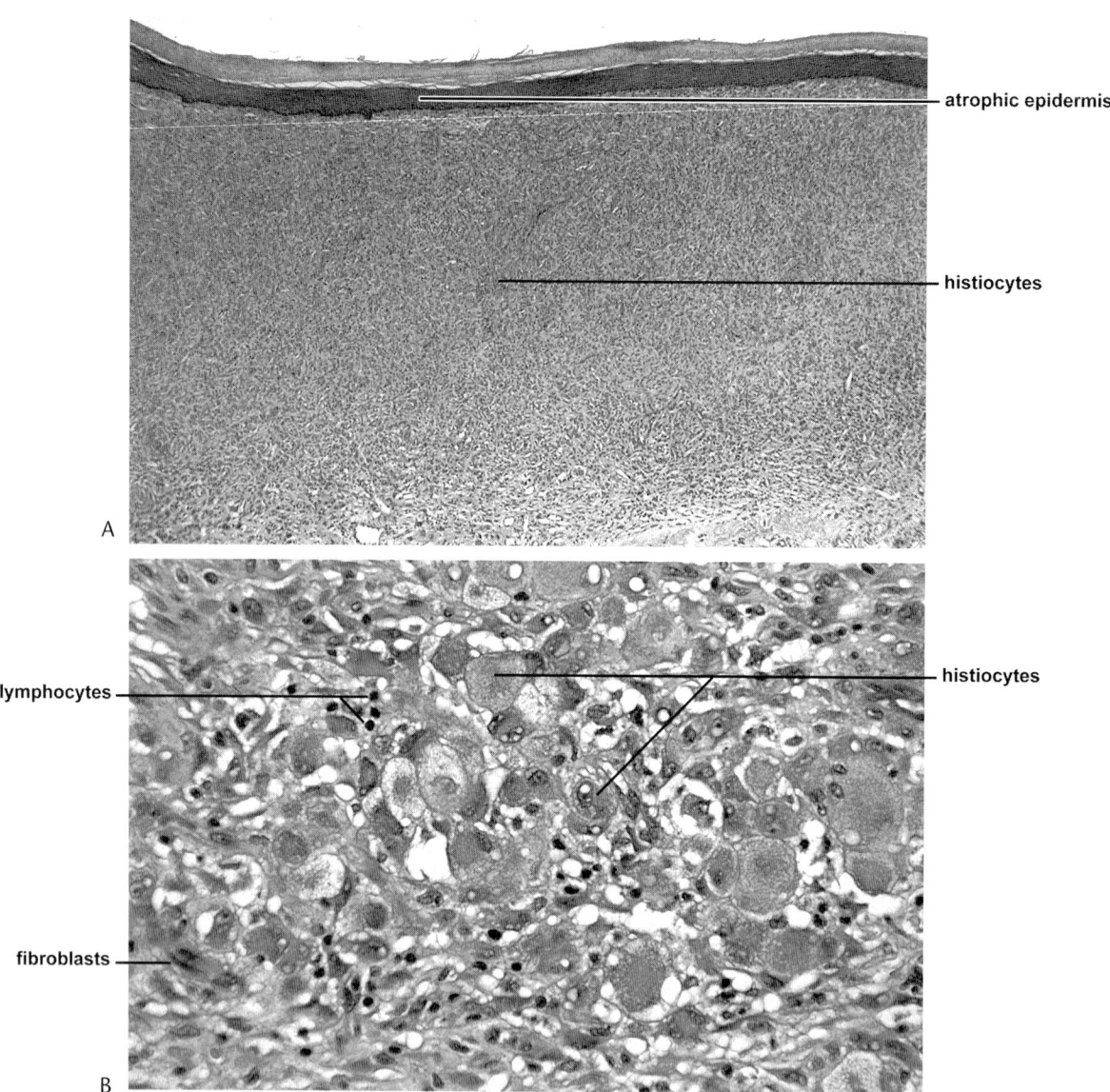

Figure 22-9. Cutaneous reticulohistiocytoma (regardless of whether isolated or multiple). (**A**) Atrophic epidermis overlies the sheets of histiocytes. (H&E, × 40). (**B**) Eosinophilic, homogeneous histiocytes are present, as well as small numbers of lymphocytes. With time, the lymphocytes disappear and an increased number of fibroblasts become intertwined with the histiocytic element. (H&E, × 150).

immunohistologic stains for S-100 protein are useful (see below).

Multicentric Reticulohistiocytosis

Clinical Features

Multicentric reticulohistiocytosis is the generalized counterpart of ICR, in which several histologically similar lesions are seen in the skin and the synovium of various joints. The latter result in symmetric, destructive, mutilating arthritis that typically affects the small interphalangeal joints. More uncommonly, the joints of the girdle bones, the large bones of the extremities, or the spine are involved.

Skin lesions in multicentric reticulohistiocytosis are dome-shaped, red-brown or flesh-colored papulonodules, sometimes attaining a size of several centimeters in greatest dimension. They tend to cluster over joints of the hands, but also may affect the face, scalp, pinnae of the ears, and torso. One-half of patients also exhibit mucosal lesions of the lips, mouth, and nose. Ulceration of the lesions is only exceptionally observed.[54,55]

With time, both the cutaneous and arthritic elements of this condition resolve spontaneously, but often this does not occur before irretrievable joint damage has been incurred. The resulting clinical rheumatologic appearance may be confused with that of end-stage rheumatoid or psoriatic arthritis.[54] Very rarely, cellular infiltrates in the viscera have been reported in necropsied cases of multicentric reticulohistiocytosis, which superficially resemble those seen in the skin.[55]

Histopathologic Findings and Differential Diagnosis

The microscopic features and differential diagnoses of multicentric reticulohistiocytosis are identical to those of ICR with regard to findings in skin biopsies. There are no major morphologic differences between the cutaneous and periarticular foci of disease except that a greater degree of fibrosis is observed in synovial lesions with the passage of time. Some authors have implied that less inflammation accompanies the multinucleated cells in the multicentric variant of reticulohistiocytosis.[54] Accordingly, each patient in whom a diagnosis of ICR is considered must be subjected to a thorough rheumatologic examination.

Generalized Eruptive Histiocytoma

Clinical Features

Generalized eruptive histiocytoma is a rare cutaneous proliferation of the MPS that is seen in adults of all ages. It is characterized by hundreds of rapidly evolving, small, discrete, red-brown or violaceous papules, which usually assume a symmetric distribution over the lower torso and proximal limbs and do not have a tendency to coalesce. The mucous membranes are only uncommonly involved.

Although the disorder is self-limited and does not affect the visceral organs, it may take over a decade for total resolution.[56–58] Atrophic, slightly pigmented macules result from regression in eruptive histiocytoma. Patients have normal serum lipid profiles. A single case has been reported in which eruptive histiocytosis was observed in an individual with normolipemic xanthelasmas.[58]

Histopathologic Features

Microscopic findings in eruptive histiocytosis include the presence of a dense, monomorphic, interstitial infiltrate of polygonal mononuclear histiocytes that is confined to the dermis, together with a small number of background lymphocytes and a limited amount of stromal mucin. Eosinophils are not seen in this disorder; lipidized histiocytes and giant cells also are absent. The proliferating histiocytes have homogeneous eosinophilic cytoplasm, oval eccentric nuclei, dispersed chromatin, and distinct but small nucleoli. There is no nuclear atypia, and mitoses are infrequently seen.

Immunohistologically, the constituent cells in eruptive histiocytosis demonstrate reactivity for CD11b, CD11c, CD45, and CD68 antigens. They lack CD1 determinants and S-100 protein.

Differential Diagnosis

Primary considerations in the differential diagnosis center on LCD, disseminated granuloma annulare, and "early" lesions of classic JXG. The absence of eosinophils and S-100 positivity in eruptive histiocytosis militates against a diagnosis of LC proliferations, as does the lack of any intraepidermal infiltrate. In dif-

ficult cases, immunophenotyping of constituent histiocytes provides a definitive means of separating these two conditions from one another. Early JXG can be recognized by a thorough search for lipidized histiocytes and Touton giant cells. These elements are nearly invariably present in xanthogranulomas but are not present in eruptive histiocytosis. Generalized granuloma annulare, when seen in its cellular phase, is admittedly very similar to eruptive histiocytosis microscopically. Nonetheless, one never observes necrobiosis in the latter disorder. If biopsies are done on lesions that have been present for several weeks, central collagenous degeneration should be apparent in granuloma annulare but not in eruptive histiocytosis.

Benign Cephalic Histiocytosis

Clinical Features

Benign cephalic histiocytosis (BCH) was first described by Gianotti et al[59] in 1971. It represents a self-healing cutaneous proliferation of histiocytes that shows a predilection for the skin of the face, eyelids, and forehead. Both sexes are affected equally, but the disease appears to be limited below the age of 5 years. BCH pursues a chronic and relapsing course in two-thirds of cases, although a significant proportion of individual lesions regress spontaneously within 1 to 2 years.[60]

Multiple skin-colored to yellow-brown papules or macules smaller than 1 cm are observed in this disorder. The torso and proximal limbs are uncommonly involved. Patients are uniformly normolipemic and do not have lesions of the mucous membranes, palms, soles, or viscera, in contrast to individuals with other MPS proliferations or LCD.[60]

Histopathologic Features

BCH is characterized by a monomorphic infiltrate of mononuclear cells in the superficial and reticular dermis, associated with admixed lymphocytes and a small number of eosinophils. The epidermis and adnexal structures are typically spared. Proliferating cells in this disorder show mild nuclear pleomorphism and evenly dispersed nuclear chromatin.[60] They do not exhibit the folded, notched, or coffee bean-shaped nuclear profiles of LC. Cytoplasm is scanty and amphophilic. Multinucleated giant cells are observed occasionally, but are most often present in clinically regressing lesions. Lipidized histiocytes are uniformly absent.

Results of Special Studies

Because of the patient population that is affected by BCH and the presence of eosinophils in this process, its distinction from LCD may be difficult. This is particularly true in those rare instances of BCH that do involve the epidermis. Immunohistologic studies and electron microscopy may be employed in difficult cases to resolve such uncertainty.

Differential Diagnosis

BCH does not show Birbeck granules in proliferating cells by ultrastructural analysis, but rather demonstrates intracellular organelles that are more typical of cells in the MPS. Cytoplasmic vesicles, short profiles of rough endoplasmic reticulum, and phagolysosomes are observed in this disorder on electron microscopy.[61] This point is particularly important, because some examples of BCH share S-100 protein immunoreactivity with LCD.[5,60]

Reactivity with antibodies in the CD11b, CD11c, CD45, and CD68 groups is also typical of BCH.[5,60] By contrast, CD1 antigens are absent, unlike the expected findings in LCD.

Aside from LC proliferations, as mentioned, several other conditions may be considered in the histologic differential diagnosis of BCH. These include JXG, eruptive xanthomatosis, reticulohistiocytosis, and mast cell disease.

We have repeatedly stated in this discussion that JXG and eruptive xanthomatosis uniformly feature the presence of at least some lipidized histiocytes, if these cells are sought carefully. By contrast, BCH lacks such elements. Moreover, well-formed Touton-type giant cells are typical of JXG, but not of BCH.

Sinus Histiocytosis with Massive Lymphadenopathy

Clinical Features

SHML (Rosai-Dorfman disease) is a peculiar proliferation of the MPS that was first described as a lymph nodal disorder in 1969.[62] Although it was initially thought to be more common in children than in adults, this opinion has been modified over the succeeding decades (mean age at onset, 20 years).[63,64] Early data that showed an apparent predilection for black patients have not held true.[64] Men are very slightly more often affected by SHML than are women.

In addition to causing striking enlargement of lymph nodes, the disease is often associated with clinical evidence of immune dysfunction. Autoimmune arthritides, glomerulonephritis, insulin-dependent (juvenile-onset) diabetes mellitus, and erythrocyte autoantibodies are overrepresented in the population of patients with SHML.[64]

This disorder is self-limited or persistent but stable in most cases (90%), but it may take many years for clinical abnormalities to resolve themselves. Lesions in the skin do not appear to affect survival adversely; however, SHML of the kidney, lungs, or liver is linked to an increased likelihood of progressive disease and potential fatality.[64]

Lesions of the skin are seen in up to 15% of cases, and skin involvement is the most common extralymph nodal manifestation of SHML.[63,64] Indeed, some patients may *present* with cutaneous disease. There is no predilection for any particular skin site. Many individuals with SHML of the skin also will develop extranodal disease in the soft tissue, paranasal sinuses, nasal cavity, or other locations.[64]

Cutaneous lesions range in size and description from small red-brown macules to large red-yellow plaques up to 15 cm in diameter. They are commonly scaly and may resemble lesions of cutaneous T-cell lymphomas microscopically.[63]

Histopathologic Features

Well-developed dermal or subcuticular lesions of SHML are extremely distinctive on low-power microscopy in that they resemble nodal involvement. A fibrous pseudocapsule often envelops the infiltrate, which is circumscribed and composed of large, pale, bland mononuclear cells with homogeneous, sometimes "glassy" eosinophilic cytoplasm arranged in sheets or clusters[63,64] (Fig. 22-10). Their nuclei are oval or reniform with vesicular chromatin; nucleoli are variably present. Mitotic activity is usually scanty, and there is no cellular pleomorphism or necrosis. The most diagnostically salient finding in SHML is the presence of "*lymphemperipolesis*," where intact small lymphocytes are observed within the cytoplasm of the large histiocytic cells (Fig. 22-11). Rarely, erythrocytes may be phagocytosed as well.[64]

The aggregates of histiocytes are separated from one another by dense groupings of mature lymphocytes, yielding the above-cited similarity to nodal tissue in cutaneous SHML. A minor admixture of plasma cells and neutrophils is not uncommon. The overlying epidermis is intact and usually unremarkable in appearance, although some cases may exhibit acanthosis and elongation of the rete ridges. Dermal blood vessels within the infiltrate and around it may show ectasia or proliferation.

Results of Special Studies and Differential Diagnosis

Immunohistochemically, the large histiocytes display uniform reactivity for antigens in the CD45 (leukocyte common antigen), CD14, CD15, and CD68 groups. In addition, they show variable positivity for CD11b, CD30, CD43, CD45RO, and CD74 determinants.[65] Knowledge of this phenotype is important, because some of the specified reactants (particularly CD30) may lead to a misdiagnosis of *malignant lymphoma* if considered in isolation. Virtually all examples of this disorder exhibit S-100 protein reactivity in large constituent histiocytes, a finding that is essentially diagnostic of SHML. The alternative interpretation of LCD (which is also S-100 protein positive) may be dismissed by the size and cytologic characteristics of the proliferating histiocytes in SHML. Also, electron microscopy fails to disclose cytoplasmic Birbeck granules in SHML. *Malignant melanoma* is also reactive for S-100 protein, but it lacks CD45 antigens and would not be expected to show lymphemperipolesis.

"Malignant Histiocytosis" and Related Disorders

Clinical Features and Controversies

A sizable body of dermatopathologic literature exists on the disease entity that is variably known as *histiocytic medullary reticulosis*, *true histiocytic lymphoma*, or *malignant histiocytosis* (MH).[66–70] It was originally described in 1939 by Scott and Robb-Smith[71] and has been the subject of controversy ever since. In its classic form, MH is a progressive, systemic disorder that can affect patients of any age. It presents with fever, weight loss, peripheral cytopenias, organomegaly, and lymphadenopathy and may be accompanied by striking laboratory abnormalities of the coagulation system. Cutaneous lesions have been documented in approximately 15% of reported cases and are usually described as red to violaceous, variably ulcerative papulonodules.[72] These can appear in virtually any skin field and are characteristically multiple. Unlike monocytic

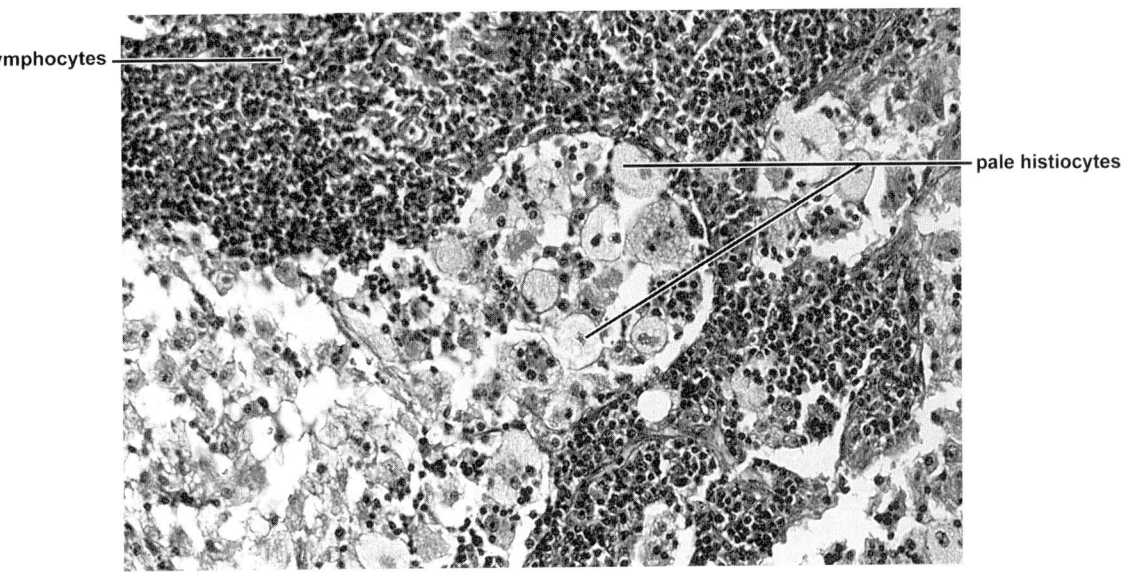

Figure 22-10. Sinus histiocytosis with massive lymphadenopathy. Circumscribed infiltrate of large, pale, bland mononuclear cells with eosinophilic cytoplasm surrounded by adjacent sheets of lymphocytes. (H&E, × 120).

Figure 22-11. Sinus histiocytosis with massive lymphadenopathy. Lymphemperipolesis. Intact small lymphocytes and other cells are observed in the cytoplasm of the large histiocytic cells. (H&E, × 200).

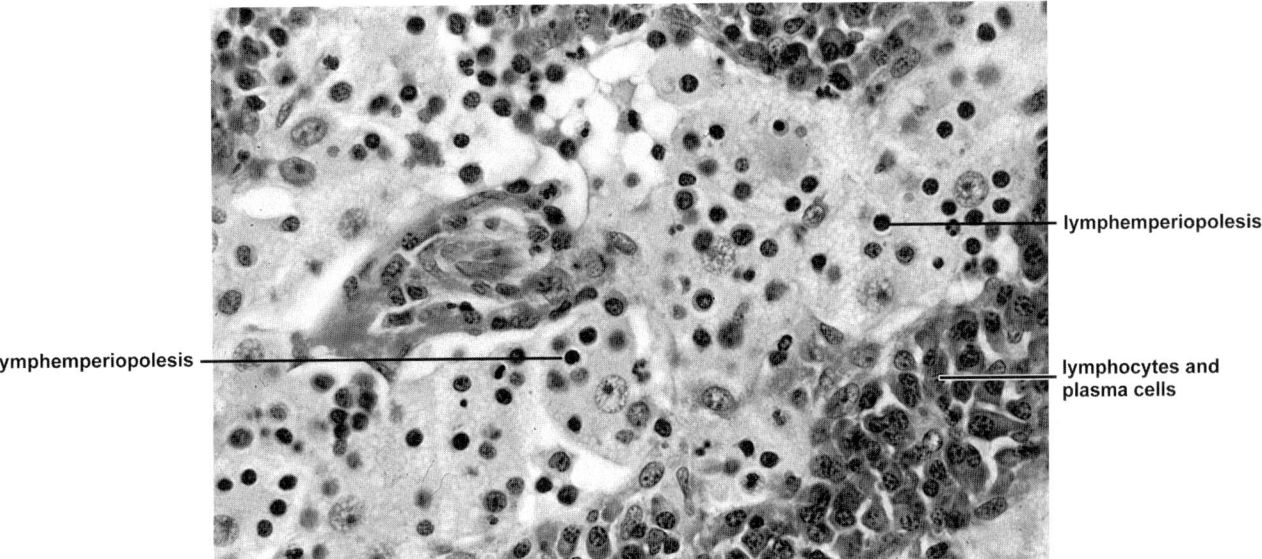

leukemia, which also may involve the skin, MH is not associated with gingival lesions or circulating tumor cells in the peripheral blood; these differences represent helpful clinical points of distinction between the two disorders. With proper therapy, patients with MH may attain remission from the disease; however, untreated individuals universally succumb within 24 months of diagnosis.

A peculiar variant of MH is that reported by Flynn et al[73] in 1982 as *regressing atypical histiocytosis* (RAH).[73] The latter disorder tends to affect adolescents or young adult patients (under 40 years of age). They develop large, deep, nodular lesions of the skin that progress through an ulcerated phase to self-healing, only to be replaced by new tumors at adjacent or distant cutaneous sites. This cycle may be perpetuated over several years (up to 10). Nevertheless, RAH will involve the viscera with time, and sufficient follow-up invariably demonstrates its malignant behavioral properties.

Using immunophenotyping studies and gene rearrangement analyses, several authors have proven conclusively that many published cases of subcutaneous "MH" and "RAH" were, in fact, not histiocytic in nature.[74–76] Instead, many lesions with the clinical and conventional histologic features of MH/cytophagic panniculitis/RAH have exhibited a T-cell phenotype in their malignant cellular elements, sometimes with the additional expression of the Ki-1 antigen, an activation-related determinant in the CD30 group.[74] Associated tissue macrophages in these cases were thought to be non-neoplastic and could have been "recruited" by cytokines released by the tumor cells.[77] The entity described by Winkelmann and Bowie[78] as "cytophagic panniculitis" is probably smoldering T-cell lymphoma that involves the subcutaneous tissue and features numerous recruited phagocytic macrophages.[77,79]

All cases cannot necessarily be dismissed as T-cell lymphomas. A small number of cutaneous lesions in this category—with unequivocally malignant cytologic and clinical characteristics—did *not* demonstrate T-cell differentiation upon specialized laboratory analysis. Instead, their immunologic and genotypic properties were those of monocytes/macrophages.[80] Hence, it would appear that the *clinical* entities of "MH" and "RAH" are, in fact, mixtures of two lineage-unrelated processes (T cell and histiocytic), neither of which is distinguishable from the other by conventional histologic evaluation.

Histopathologic Features

MH has a microscopic appearance like that of other malignant hematolymphoid disease in the skin. In its early stages, one sees an intact epidermis, with dermal perivascular and periappendigeal dyscohesive aggregates of large, pleomorphic, cytologically atypical cells (Fig. 22-12). The neoplastic cells have high nucleocytoplasmic ratios, irregular nuclear membranes, coarse chromatin, and prominent nucleoli and may be seen in mitosis (Fig. 22-13). Multinucleated forms also may be appreciable, particularly with wreath-like arrays of the nuclei. The adjacent dermis sometimes contains a moderate number of small mature lymphocytes, with or without bland macrophages. In some instances, the macrophages demonstrate striking cytophagocytosis, with engulfed erythrocytes or leukocytes in their cytoplasm.[72]

More advanced lesions of MH commonly show variable epidermal ulceration, effacement of the dermis, and involvement of the subcutis; adnexae may be engulfed or destroyed by the malignant cellular infiltrate.[68,72] When present, cytophagic macrophages tend to be disposed at the advancing periphery of the lesion. The RAH subtype of MH attains this histologic configuration more slowly, allowing the overlying epidermis to develop reactive hyperplasia.[73] Hence, this variant usually exhibits striking acanthosis and elongation of the rete ridges over the atypical cellular infiltrate (Fig. 22-12).

Some histologic features tend to militate *against* the diagnosis of true histiocytic malignancy and *for* an interpretation of T-cell lymphoma. These include marked tissue eosinophilia, as mentioned above; large areas of coagulative necrosis in the dermis or subcutis (usually caused by the angiocentricity of tumor cells in these compartments); and a spectrum of nuclear atypia in both large *and* small lymphoid cells in the proliferation.[66] Conversely, the absence of these findings does *not* imply that the histiocytic lineage of the lesion has been assured.

Results of Specialized Studies

True histiocytic lesions fail to express antigens in the CD2, CD3, CD4, CD5, CD7, CD8, CD19, and CD20 groups upon flow cytometric or frozen tissue immunophenotyping.[80,81] Moreover, they lack surface light chain immunoglobulins, and, if present, cytoplasmic immunoglobulins are polytypic in nature. Instead, immunoreactivity is observed with antibodies in the CD11b, CD11c, CD13, CD14, CD32, CD64, or CD68 groups, with CD64 markers being the most specific of the group.[81] Genotypic data in histiocytic proliferations fail to show rearrangements of B-cell or T-cell genes and demonstrate only a "germ-line" (nonrearranged) configuration of cellular DNA.[81,82]

Differential Diagnosis

Aside from pleomorphic T-cell lymphomas of the skin (and lymphomatoid papulosis, which is pathologically similar to the latter disorders), as just considered, there are few *cutaneous* lesions that can be confused microscopically with MH. These principally include poorly differentiated carcinoma of squamous or sweat glandular types and malignant melanoma. Such tumors characteristically show much more intercellular cohesion and are not usually associated with accompanying infiltrates of cytophagic macrophages. Moreover, they are solitary growths and do not exhibit the tendency for self-resolution that may be observed in MH. When diagnostic uncertainty exists, immunohistochemical studies for leukocyte common antigen, keratin, S-100 protein, and the HMB-45 antigen are valuable in this context.[83]

PROLIFERATIONS OF LANGERHANS CELLS ("HISTIOCYTOSIS-X")

In 1953, Lichtenstein[84] verified under the designation of *histiocytosis-X* three diseases that were originally described by Hand,[85] Schüller,[86] Christian,[87] Letterer,[88] and Siwe.[89] They featured cellular proliferations with cytologic attributes that he believed were identical to one another and that were thought to be those of a peculiar type of histiocyte. Accordingly, Lichten-

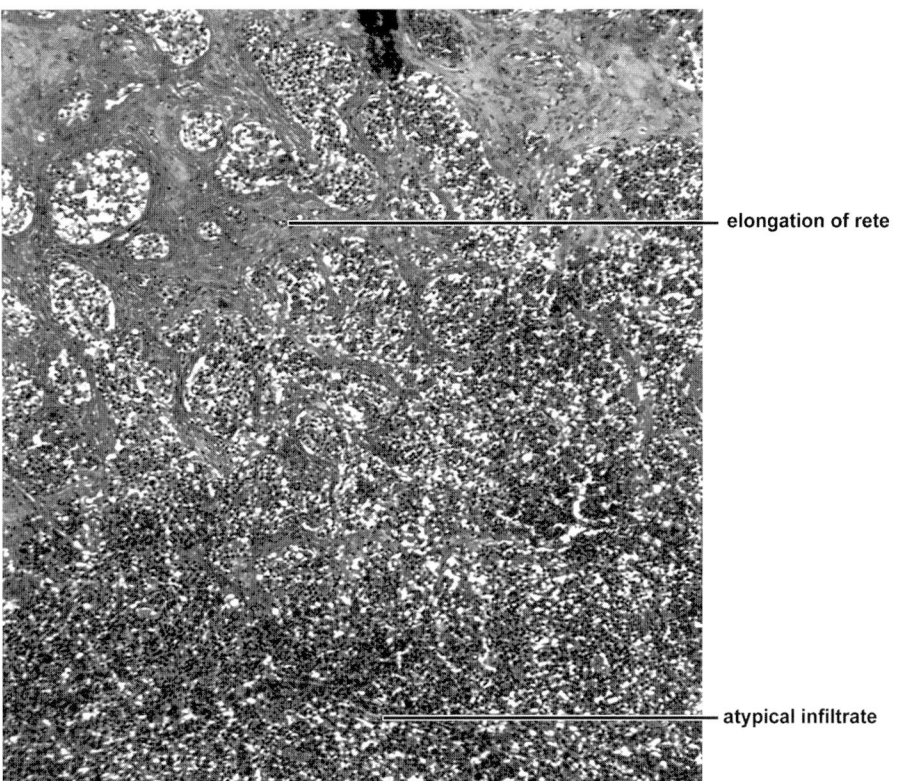

Figure 22-12. Malignant histiocytosis from a child with the regressing atypical histiocytosis variant. Prominent elongation of epidermal rete and exocytosis of the atypical histiocytes are present. The infiltrate extended into the deep dermis. (H&E, × 80).

elongation of rete

atypical infiltrate

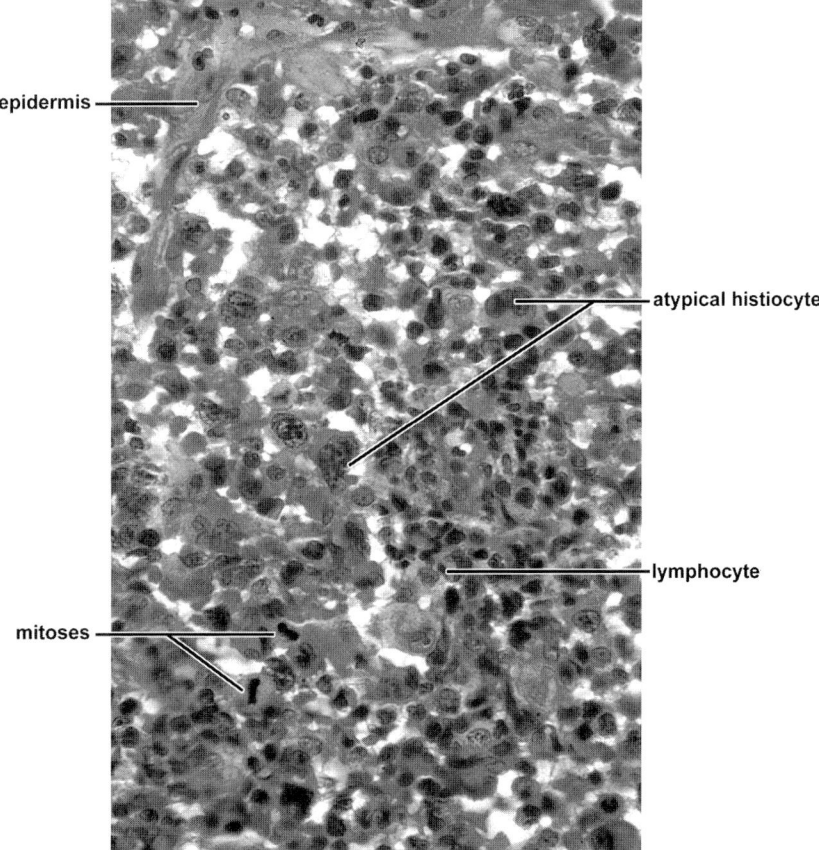

Figure 22-13. Malignant histiocytosis. The neoplastic cells have high nuclear cytoplasmic ratios, irregular nuclear membranes, coarse chromatin, and prominent nucleoli. The atypical cells are S-100 negative. (H&E, × 200).

epidermis

atypical histiocytes

lymphocyte

mitoses

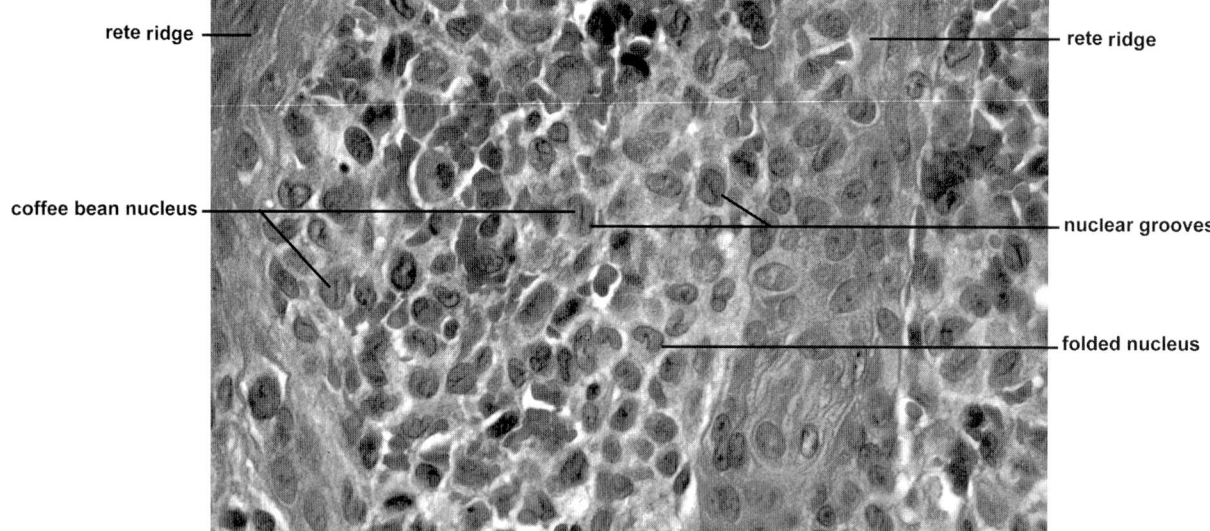

rete ridge

coffee bean nucleus

rete ridge

nuclear grooves

folded nucleus

Figure 22-14. All forms of Langerhans cell disease have large polygonal dyscohesive histiocyte-like cells having characteristic nuclear features. These include lobulated, notched, grooved, or folded nuclear contours often like those of a coffee bean. (H&E, × 250).

stein created the unifying term *histiocytosis-X*. Subsequent evaluations have shown that the proliferating cells in this condition possess the morphologic, ultrastructural, and immunohistologic properties of LCs, as seen in the normal skin. Thus, the preferred nomenclature for histiocytosis-X is currently *Langerhans cell disease*.

The three classic forms of LCD include *eosinophilic granuloma, Hand-Schüller-Christian syndrome*, and *Letterer-Siwe disease*.[90] They differ only in the scope of systemic involvement in any given case, such that eosinophilic granuloma is typically localized to one tissue site (e.g., the skin, bones, or lungs), whereas the other two subtypes of LCD affect several organs. Hand-Schüller-Christian syndrome features lesions of the hypothalamus, skull, and orbits, with or without extracranial disease, and is associated with a clinical triad of diabetes insipidus, exophthalmos, and lytic defects in the calvarium. Letterer-Siwe disease is more disseminated and, by definition, exhibits involvement of multiple visceral organs (liver, spleen, lungs, bones, bone marrow, thymus, lymph nodes, meninges, and internal mucosae) as well as the skin. Associated clinical findings include peripheral eosinophilia, anemia, thrombocytopenia, fever, weight loss, and general malaise. Eosinophilic granuloma and Hand-Schüller-Christian syndrome are most often observed in school-aged children or young adults, whereas classic Letterer-Siwe disease is typically seen in very young children. Males tend to be more often affected by LCD than females. There are also reports in the literature on all forms of LCD in middle-aged or even elderly adults as well.

Several authors have attempted to discern histologic nuances (see below) that might be used to predict the clinical evolution of LCD.[90,91] For the most part, these have not been productive. It would appear that the best predictors of potentially aggressive behavior in such cases are the age of the patient, the scope of organ involvement, and the rapidity with which the disease progresses.[92,93] Also, one is not always justified in making a diagnosis of LCD simply because aggregates of LCs are identified in biopsy specimens. Neumann and Frizzera[94] have shown that the

latter elements may represent a reactive cellular component that can be juxtaposed to deposits of non-Hodgkin's lymphomas or Hodgkin's disease in lymph nodes and other tissue sites.

Clinical Features

The skin is commonly involved in Hand-Schüller-Christian syndrome and Letterer-Siwe-disease, but it is typically free of abnormalities in patients with eosinophilic granuloma of the bones or lungs. Conversely, cutaneous or mucosal lesions may represent the only manifestation of this disorder; indeed, "*congenital self-healing reticulohistiocytosis*" is a limited variant of LCD that affects only the skin in infants.[95,96] Several cases of isolated cutaneous LCD in adults have been observed.

Involvement of the skin and mucosal surfaces may assume several clinical appearances.[90] These include a diffuse, scaly, papular erythematous eruption simulating seborrheic dermatitis; noduloulcerative lesions; multiple yellow-brown papules like those of the xanthomatoses; a vesiculopustular eruption occurring in "crops"; generalized "bronzing" of the skin; and numerous petechial or purpuric lesions. Purpuric lesions may well reflect bone marrow involvement by the disease with resulting thrombocytopenia rather than direct infiltration of the skin. However, *all* lesions of LCD do have the potential to appear hemorrhagic at their peripheries. The scalp, temples, ears, perioral area, and intertriginous skin fields of the extremities and torso are the preferred sites of involvement by LCD. Oral lesions may simulate simple ulcers or gingivitis.

Histopathologic Features

Similar to its clinical manifestations, the histopathologic appearances of LCD are varied. All have a unifying attribute, the preponderance of large, polygonal, dyscohesive histiocyte-like cells having characteristic nuclear features. These include lobulated, notched, grooved, or folded nuclear contours, often like those of a "coffee bean" (Fig. 22-14); evenly distributed chromatin; variable mitotic activity (without pathologic forms); and usually indistinct nucleoli. The cytoplasm of these cells is amphophilic and moderate in amount, without discernible inclusions or vacuolation.

The proliferating LCs invariably are seen within the epidermis in "early" lesions of LCD, and they are dispersed or aggregated in small clusters at all levels of the surface epithelium (Fig. 22-15). Cutaneous adnexae may be similarly affected. In the corium, the cells may be grouped into broad sheets, confined to perivascular and periappendageal areas, or disposed as a subepidermal "band." Subcuticular involvement is apparent only in clinically nodular lesions. Foci of regional necrosis are distinctly uncommon, although apoptotic changes in individual LCs are frequently observed.

The tissue background of typical LCD is edema, both in the epidermis and the dermis. Ulceration and extravasation of erythrocytes also may be evident. Accompanying inflammatory cells are mixed, including eosinophils, lymphocytes, and a small number of neutrophils. Although some inexperienced observers will not make a diagnosis of LCD if eosinophils are absent or scarce, these cells are by no means mandatory for such an interpretation.

As individual lesions "mature," they show a marked lessening or absence of epidermal involvement by infiltrates of LCs. The surface epithelium may appear regenerative and acanthotic at this stage. Typical dermal aggregates give way to a mixed population of LCs, lymphocytes, and macrophages, and xanthomatized "foamy" histiocytes make their appearance in late-stage LCD (Fig. 22-16). The dermis also may be fibrotic (although this is relatively rare), and pigment incontinence in its superficial aspect is a common finding.

Multinucleated giant cells of the Touton or foreign body types are sometimes apparent, and these may lead to histologic confusion of "mature" LCD with xanthogranulomatous lesions. However, giant cells in LCD tend to be randomly distributed throughout the infiltrate, whereas xanthogranulomas demonstrate more evenly dispersed multinucleated elements.

The existence of a cytologically "malignant" form of LCD has been addressed. Ben-Ezra et al[97] reported the largest series on this variant to date and defined it by the presence of prominent nucleoli, increased nucleocytoplasmic ratios, and nuclear pleomorphism in otherwise typical LCs associated with unusual patterns of tissue involvement (such as the invasion of intestines, pancreas, renal parenchyma, or muscle). Mitotic activity alone does not appear to correlate quantitatively with aggressive behavior, but the presence of pathologic division figures (e.g., multipolar forms) *is* seemingly restricted to "atypical" LCD.

The main problem accompanying the classification of any given case of this disorder as "malignant" is that clinical behavior does not follow suit in a predictable fashion. In the aforementioned series reported by Ben-Ezra and colleagues,[97] seven patients had cytologically atypical LCD and aggressive evolution of the disease, but two manifested "malignant" proliferations that were unattended by adverse clinical progression. Nevertheless, it would seem advisable to make special note of any atypical cytologic features in reports on LCD, with suggestions that the attending physicians should be alert for possibly aggressive behavior.

Results of Special Studies and Differential Diagnosis

LCs have a distinctive ultrastructural appearance and immunophenotype. Birbeck granules, which are peculiar and distinctive invaginations of the cellular surface membrane (Fig. 22-17), are confined to LCD and therefore serve as pathognomonic markers of it.[91] However, the diagnosis should not be withheld simply because these inclusions are absent, because they are manifested in only 50% to 60% of patients. Immunohistology is a more universally effective means of identifying LCD in that the proliferating cells show a unique antigenic constituency. They are nonreactive for lysozyme and CD45 antigens, but exhibit conjoint positivity for S-100 protein, CD1, CD74, and class II histocompatibility (HLA-DR) antigens.[98] This profile is unlike that of cells in the MPS, including those that characterize all other diseases considered in this chapter.

Figure 22-15. The early lesion of Langerhans cell disease displays clusters of the atypical cells in the papillary dermis and extending through the epidermis. (H&E, × 80).

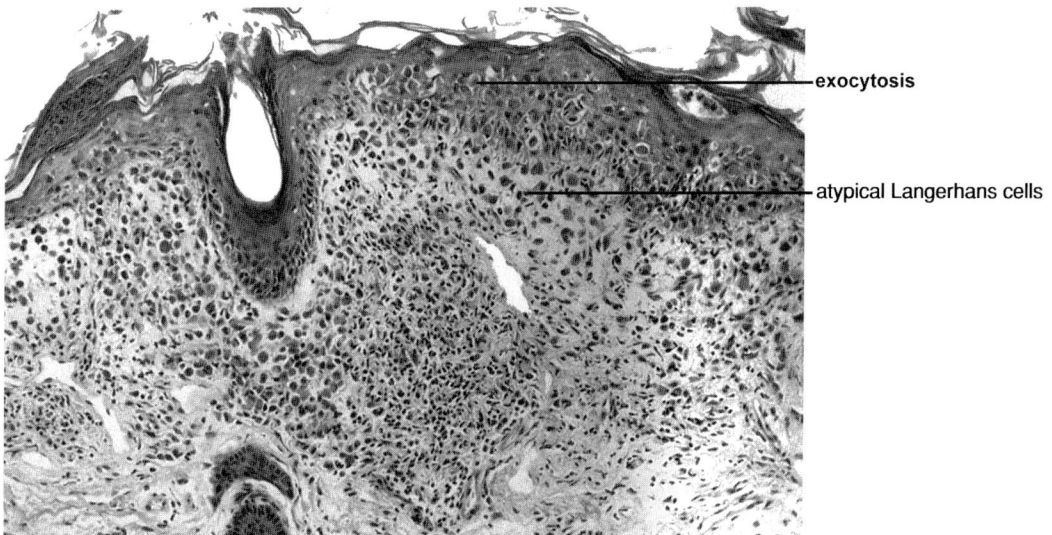

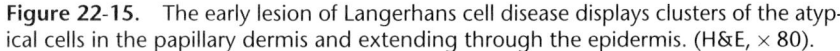
exocytosis

atypical Langerhans cells

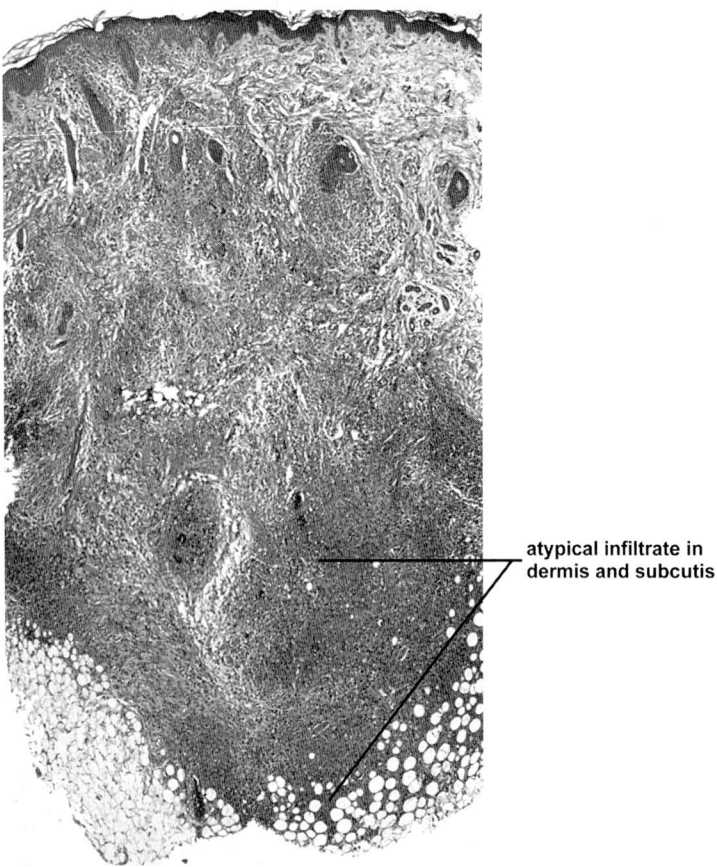

Figure 22-16. A later, nodular lesion of Langerhans cell disease. The infiltrate is based in the deep dermis and subcutis. (H&E, × 40).

atypical infiltrate in
dermis and subcutis

Figure 22-17. Electron micrograph showing the Birbeck granule, a distinctive and peculiar invagination of the cellular surface membrane. Only about 50% to 60% of cases show such granules. Immunohistochemistry is a much more practical method of identifying Langerhans cell disease.

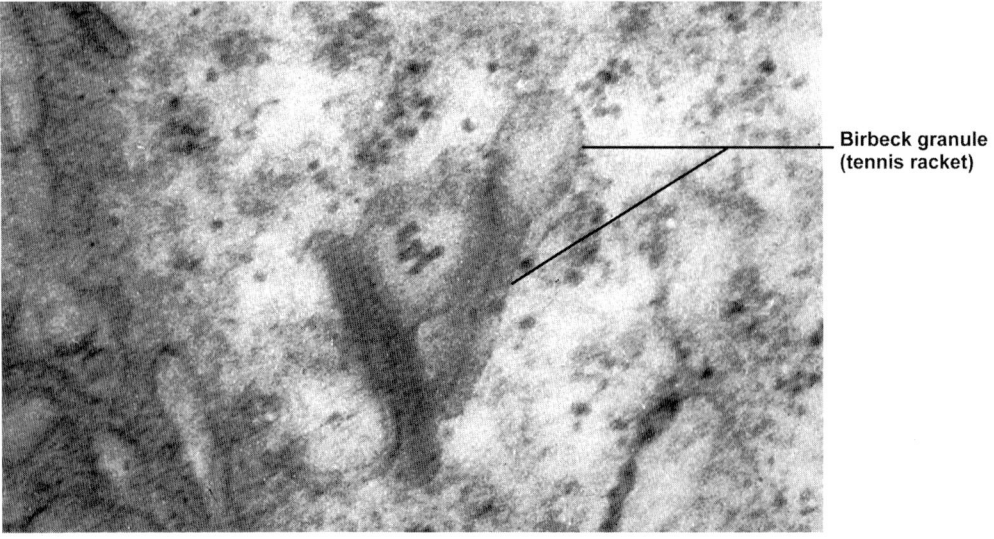

Birbeck granule
(tennis racket)

REFERENCES

1. Headington JT: The histiocyte: in memoriam. Arch Dermatol 122:532–533, 1986
2. Basset F, Escaig J, LeCrom M: A cytoplasmic membranous complex in histiocytosis X. Cancer 48:287–305, 1972
3. Favara BE, McCarthy RE, Mierau GW: Histiocytosis X. Hum Pathol 14:663–676, 1983
4. Gianotti F, Caputo R: Histiocytic syndromes: a review. J Am Acad Dermatol 13:383–404, 1985
5. Murphy GF, Messadi D, Fonferko E et al: Phenotypic transformation of macrophage to Langerhans' cells in the skin. Am J Pathol 123:401–406, 1986
6. Roper SS, Spraker MK: Cutaneous histiocytosis syndromes. Pediatr Dermatol 3:19–30, 1985
7. Winkelmann RK: Cutaneous syndromes of non-X histiocytosis: a review of the macrophage-histiocyte diseases of the skin. Arch Dermatol 117:667–672, 1981
8. Headington JT, Cerio R: Dendritic cells and the dermis. Am J Dermatopathol 12:217–220, 1990
9. Lasser A: The mononuclear phagocytic system: a review. Hum Pathol 14:108–126, 1983
10. Parker F: Xanthomas and hyperlipidemias. J Am Acad Dermatol 13:1–30, 1985
11. Cruz PD, East C, Bergstresser PR: Dermal, subcutaneous, and tendon xanthomas: diagnostic markers for specific lipoprotein disorders. J Am Acad Dermatol 19:95–111, 1988
12. Fortmann SP, Maron DJ: Disorders of lipid metabolism. Sci Am 9:1–21, 1991
13. Frederickson DS, Lees RS: A system for phenotyping hyperlipoproteinemia. Circulation 31:321–327, 1965
14. Fleischmajer R: Familial hyperlipidemias. Arch Dermatol 110:43–49, 1974
15. Dicken CH, Connolly SM: Eruptive xanthomas associated with isotretinoin (13-cis-retinoic acid). Arch Dermatol 116:951–952, 1980
16. Marsden J: Hyperlipidemia due to isotretinoin and etretinate: possible mechanisms and consequences. Br J Dermatol 114:401–407, 1986
17. Montgomery H, Osterberg AE: Xanthomatosis: correlation of clinical, histopathologic, and chemical studies of cutaneous xanthoma. Arch Dermatol 337:373–402, 1938
18. Altman J, Winkelmann RK: Xanthoma disseminatum. Arch Dermatol 86:582–596, 1962
19. Varotti C, Bettoli V, Berti E et al: Xanthoma disseminatum: a case with extensive mucous membrane involvement. J Am Acad Dermatol 25:433–436, 1991
20. Blodstein SH, Cladwell D, Carter DM: Bone lesions in xanthoma disseminatum. Arch Dermatol 121:1313–1317, 1985
21. Mishkel MA, Cockshott WP, Nazir DJ et al: Xanthoma disseminatum. Arch Dermatol 113:1094–1100, 1977
22. Pinol J, Mascaro JM, Romeguera C et al: Xanthoma disseminatum avec lesions osseuses. Bull Soc Fr Dermatol Syphilgr 76:555, 1969
23. Goodenberger ME, Piette WW, MacFarlane DE et al: Xanthoma disseminatum and Waldenstrom's macroglobulinemia. J Am Acad Dermatol 23:1015–1018, 1990
24. Shafer WG: Verruciform xanthoma. Oral Surg 31:784–789, 1971
25. Barr RJ, Plank CJ: Verruciform xanthoma of the skin. J Cutan Pathol 7:422–428, 1980
26. Harrington AC, Fitzpatrick JE, Werness BA et al: Verruciform xanthoma of the scrotum. J Assoc Military Dermatol 114:22–24, 1988
27. Kimura S: Verruciform xanthoma of the scrotum. Arch Dermatol 120:1378–1379, 1984
28. Kraemer BB, Schmidt WA, Foucar E et al: Verruciform xanthoma of the penis. Arch Dermatol 117:516–518, 1981
29. Santa Cruz DJ, Martin SA: Verruciform xanthoma of the vulva. Am J Clin Pathol 71:224–225, 1979
30. Mountcastle EA, Lupton GP: Verruciform xanthoma of the digits. J Am Acad Dermatol 20:313–317, 1989
31. Chyu J, Medenica M, Witney DH: Verruciform xanthoma of the lower extremity. J Am Acad Dermatol 17:695–698, 1987
32. Palestine RF, Winkelmann RK: Verruciform xanthoma in an epithelial nevus. Arch Dermatol 118:686–691, 1982
33. Cooper TW, Santa Cruz DJ, Bauer EA: Verruciform xanthoma: occurrence in eroded skin in a patient with recessive dystrophic epidermolysis bullosa. J Am Acad Dermatol 8:463–467, 1983
34. Grosshans E, Laplanche G: Verruciform xanthoma or transformation of inflammatory epidermal nevus. J Cutan Pathol 8:382–384, 1981
35. Wade TR, Ackerman AB: Cornoid lamellation: a histologic reaction pattern. Am J Dermatopathol 2:5–15, 1980
36. Lynch PJ, Winkelmann RK: Generalized plane xanthoma and systemic disease. Arch Dermatol 93:639–646, 1966
37. Marien KJC, Smeenk G: Plane xanthomata associated with multiple myeloma and hyperlipoproteinemia. Br J Dermatol 93:407–415, 1975
38. Feiwel M: Xanthomatosis in cryoglobulinemia and other paraproteinemias with report of a case. Br J Dermatol 80:719–729, 1968
39. Hu CH, Winkelmann RK: Unusual normolipidemic cutaneous xanthomatosis. Acta Derm Venereol (Stockh) 57:421–429, 1977
40. Winkelmann RK, Welborn WR: Xanthome und maligne reticulosen. Hautarzt 20:550–555, 1969
41. Kossard S, Winkelmann RK: Necrobiotic xanthogranuloma with paraproteinemia. J Am Acad Dermatol 3:257–270, 1980
42. Winkelmann RK: Cutaneous syndromes of non-X histiocytosis. A review of the macrophage-histiocyte diseases of the skin. Arch Dermatol 117:667–672, 1981
43. Gibson LE, Reizner GT, Winkelmann RK: Necrobiosis lipoidica diabeticorum with cholesterol clefts in the differential diagnosis of necrobiotic xanthogranuloma. J Cutan Pathol 15:18–21, 1988
44. Finan MC, Winkelmann RK: Necrobiotic xanthogranuloma with paraproteinemia. A review of 22 cases. Medicine 65:376–388, 1986
45. Finan MC, Winkelmann RK: Necrobiotic xanthogranuloma with paraproteinemia: a review of 22 cases. Medicine 65:376–388, 1986

46. Dupre A, Viraben DA: Necrobiotic xanthogranuloma: a case without paraproteinemia but with transepithelial elimination. J Cutan Pathol 15:116–119, 1988
47. Finan MC, Winkelmann RK: Histopathology of necrobiotic xanthogranuloma with paraproteinemia. J Cutan Pathol 14:92–99, 1987
48. Mehregan DA, Winkelmann RK: Necrobiotic xanthogranuloma. Arch Dermatol 128:94–100, 1992
49. Nomland R: Nevoxanthoendothelioma. J Invest Dermatol 22:207–217, 1959
50. Marrogi AJ, Dehner LP, Coffin CM et al: Benign cutaneous histiocytic tumors in childhood and adolescence, excluding Langerhans' cell proliferations. Am J Dermatopathol 14:8–18, 1992
51. Fleischmajer R, Schaefer EJ, Gal AE et al: Normolipemic subcutaneous xanthomatosis. Am J Med 75:1065–1070, 1983
52. Winkelmann RK, Fergus-Oliver G: Subcutaneous xanthogranulomatosis: an inflammatory non-X-histiocytic syndrome (subcutaneous xanthomatosis). J Am Acad Dermatol 21:924–929, 1989
53. Cerio R, Spaull J, Fergus-Oliver G et al: A study of factor XIIIa and MAC-387 immunolabelling in normal and pathological skin. Am J Dermatopathol 12:221–233, 1990
54. Barrow MV, Holubar K: Multicentric reticulohistiocytosis: a review of 33 patients. Medicine (Baltimore) 48:287–305, 1969
55. Lesher JL, Allen BS: Multicentric reticulohistiocytosis. J Am Acad Dermatol 11:713–723, 1984
56. Winkelmann RK, Muller SA: Generalized eruptive histiocytoma. Arch Dermatol 88:154–163, 1963
57. Caputo R, Alessi E, Allegra F: Generalized eruptive histiocytoma. Arch Dermatol 117:216–221, 1981
58. Unbert PJ, Winkelmann RK: Eruptive histiocytoma. J Am Acad Dermatol 20:958–963, 1989
59. Gianotti F, Caputo R, Ermacora E: Singuliere "histiocytose infantile acellules avec particules vermiformes intracytoplasmiques." Bull Soc Fr Dermatol Syphilgr 78:232–233, 1971
60. Gianotti F, Caputo R, Ermacora E et al: Benign cephalic histiocytosis. Arch Dermatol 122:1038–1043, 1986
61. Caputo R, Gianotti F: Cytoplasmic markers: ultrastructural features in histiocytic proliferations in skin. G Ital Dermatol Venereol 115:107–120, 1980
62. Rosai J, Dorfman R: Sinus histiocytosis with massive lymphadenopathy. Arch Pathol 87:63–70, 1969
63. Thawerani H, Sanchez RL, Rosai J et al: The cutaneous manifestations of sinus histiocytosis with massive lymphadenopathy. Arch Dermatol 114:191–197, 1978
64. Foucar E, Rosai J, Dorfman R: Sinus histiocytosis with massive lymphadenopathy (Rosai-Dorfman disease): review of the entity. Semin Diagn Pathol 7:19–73, 1990
65. Eisen RN, Buckley PJ, Rosai J: Immunophenotypic characterization of sinus histiocytosis with massive lymphadenopathy (Rosai-Dorfman disease). Semin Diagn Pathol 7:74–82, 1990
66. Jaffe ES: Malignant histiocytosis and true histiocytic lymphomas. pp. 381–411. In Jaffe ES (ed): Surgical Pathology of the Lymph Nodes and Related Organs. WB Saunders, Philadelphia, 1985

67. Risdall RJ, Sibley RK, McKenna RW et al: Malignant histiocytosis: a light and electron microscopic and histochemical study. Am J Surg Pathol 4:439–450, 1980
68. Ducatman BS, Wick MR, Morgan TW et al: Malignant histiocytosis. Hum Pathol 15:319–329, 1984
69. van der Valk P, Meijer CJLM, Willemze R et al: Histiocytic sarcoma (true histiocytic lymphoma): a clinicopathologic study of 20 cases. Histopathology 8:105–123, 1984
70. Mirchandani I, Shah I, Palutke M et al: True histiocytic lymphoma: a report of four cases. Cancer 52:1911–1918, 1983
71. Scott RB, Robb-Smith AHT: Histiocytic medullary reticulosis. Lancet 2:194–198, 1939
72. Wick MR, Sanchez NP, Crotty CP, Winkelmann RK: Cutaneous malignant histiocytosis. J Am Acad Dermatol 8:50–62, 1983
73. Flynn KJ, Dehner LP, Gajl-Peczalska KJ et al: Regressing atypical histiocytosis. Cancer 49:959–970, 1982
74. Agnarsson B, Kadin ME: Ki-1-positive large cell lymphoma: a morphologic and immunologic study of 19 cases. Am J Surg Pathol 12:264–274, 1988
75. Chan JC, Ng CS, Ngan KC et al: Angiocentric T-cell lymphoma of the skin. Am J Surg Pathol 12:861–876, 1988
76. Headington JT, Roth MS, Ginsburg D et al: T-cell receptor gene rearrangement in regressing atypical histiocytosis. Arch Dermatol 123:1183–1187, 1987
77. Gonzalez CL, Medeiros LJ, Braziel RM et al: T-cell lymphoma involving subcutaneous tissue: a clinicopathologic entity commonly associated with hemophagocytic syndrome. Am J Surg Pathol 15:17–22, 1991
78. Winkelmann RK, Bowie EJW: Hemorrhagic diathesis associated with benign histiocytic cytophagic panniculitis and systemic histiocytosis. Arch Intern Med 140:1460–1466, 1980
79. Aronson IK, West DP, Variakojis D et al: Panniculitis associated with cutaneous T-cell lymphoma and cytophagic histiocytosis. Br J Dermatol 112:87–96, 1985
80. Norton AJ, Isaacson PG: Immunohistology of lymphoid tissue and lymphomas. pp. 277–302. In Filipe IM, Lake BD (eds): Histochemistry in Pathology. Churchill-Livingstone, New York, 1990
81. Hanson CA, Jaszcz W, Kersey JH et al: True histiocytic lymphoma: histopathologic, immunophenotypic, and genotypic analysis. Br J Haematol 73:187–198, 1989
82. Weiss LM, Trela MJ, Clearly ML et al: Frequent immunoglobulin and T-cell receptor gene rearrangements in "histiocytic" neoplasms. Am J Pathol 121:369–373 1985
83. Wick MR, Kaye VN: The role of diagnostic immunohistochemistry in dermatology. Semin Dermatol 5:346–358, 1986
84. Lichtenstein L: Histiocytosis X. Arch Pathol 56:84–102, 1953
85. Hand A Jr: Polyuria and tuberculosis. Arch Pediatr 10:673–675, 1893
86. Schüller A: Über eigenartige Schädeldefekte im Jugendalter. Fortschr Geb Roentgenstr 23:12–18, 1915
87. Christian HA: Defects in membranous bones, exophthalmos, and diabetes insipidus: an unusual syndrome of dyspituitarism, a clinical study. pp. 1390–1401. In Contributions to Medical and Biological Research. Paul B. Hoeber, New York, 1919

88. Letterer E: Aleukämische Retikulose. [Ein Beitrag zu den proliferativen Erkrankungen des Retikuloendothelialapparates.] Frankfurt Z Pathol 30:377–394, 1924

89. Siwe SA: Die Reticuloendotheliose–ein neues Krankheitsbild unter den Hepatosplenomegalien. Z Kinderheilkd 55:212–247, 1933

90. Newton WA Jr, Hamoudi AB: Histiocytosis: a histologic classification with clinical correlation. Perspect Pediatr Pathol 1:251–283, 1973

91. Risdall RJ, Dehner LP, Duray P et al: Histiocytosis X (Langerhans' cell histiocytosis). Arch Pathol Lab Med 107:59–63, 1983

92. Lahey ME: Prognostic factors in histiocytosis X. Am J Pediatr Hematol Oncol 3:57–60, 1981

93. Nezelof C, Frileux-Herbet F, Cronier-Sachot J: Disseminated histiocytosis X: analysis of prognostic factors based on a retrospective study of 50 cases. Cancer 44:1824–1838, 1979

94. Newmann MP, Frizzera G: The coexistence of Langerhans' cell granulomatosis and malignant lymphoma may take different forms. Hum Pathol 17:1060–1065, 1986

95. Hashimoto K, Takahashi S, Lee RG et al: Congenital self-healing reticulohistiocytosis. J Am Acad Dermatol 11:447–454, 1984

96. Dehner LP: Morphologic findings in the histiocytic syndromes. Semin Oncol 18:8–17, 1991

97. Ben-Ezra J, Bailey A, Azumi N et al: Malignant histiocytosis X: a distinct clinicopathologic entity. Cancer 68: 1050–1060, 1991

98. Azumi N, Sheibani K, Swartz WG et al: Antigenic phenotype of Langerhans' cell histiocytosis. Hum Pathol 19: 1376–1382, 1988

99. Schaefer EJ, Levy RI: Pathogenesis and management of lipoprotein disorders. N Engl J Med 312:1300–1310, 1985

INDEX

Note: Page numbers followed by *t* and *f* indicate tables and figures, respectively.

Fibroadenoma(s) (*continued*)
  histopathology of, 601–603
  recurrent, 601
Fibroblasts, dermal, 25
Fibroepithelioma, 456–457, 458*f*
  of Pinkus, 537, 539*f*
    differential diagnosis of, 442
Fibrofolliculoma, associated syndrome with, 496,
    566
  clinical features of, 496
  cystic, 540
  diagnosis of, 568
  histology of, 496, 497*f*
Fibroma(s), calcifying aponeurotic, clinical
      features of, 573
    histopathology of, 575
  perifollicular, 502, 573
    syndrome associated with, 566
  peripheral ossifying, 429
  sclerotic, 625
  subepidermal, 592
  tendon sheath. *See* Giant cell tumors of tendon
      sheaths.
  trichoblastic, 486–489, 488*f*, 569
  unguioblastic. *See* Onychomatricoma.
Fibromatosis, desmoid-type (aggressive), clinical
      features of, 573–574
    histopathology of, 574, 575*f*
  histopathology of, 574–575, 575*f*
  hyaline, clinical features of, 573
    histopathology of, 575
  palmar-plantar, clinical features of, 574
    histopathology of, 575, 576*f*
Fibronectin, 22
Fibrosing dermatitis, clinicopathologic
    correlation in, 69
Fibrosis, subepidermal, 773. *See also* Nodular
    histiocytoma (of Woringer).
Fibrous hamartoma of infancy, clinical features
    of, 575
  differential diagnosis of, 589
  histopathology of, 575, 576*f*
Fibrous histiocytoma, 592
  aneurysmal, 593, 595*f*
  angiomatoid malignant, clinical features of,
      603
    differential diagnosis of, 604
    histopathology of, 603–604, 604*f*
  atypical, 593–594
  benign, recurring, clinical features of, 594
      histopathology of, 594
    with potential for local recurrence, 594, 601
  malignant, clinical features of, 619–620
    differential diagnosis of, 621, 622*t*
    electron microscopy of, 622*t*
    giant cell, 620, 621*f*
    histopathology of, 620–621, 621*f*
    immunohistochemistry of, 622*t*
    inflammatory, 620
    monomorphic-histiocytic, 620
    myxoid, 620–621, 621*f*
    occupational exposures and, 572
    spindle cell/pleomorphic, 620, 621*f*
  plexiform, clinical features of, 603
    histopathology of, 603
    metastases of, 603
    recurrence of, 603
Fibrous papule, clinical features of, 572
  histopathology of, 572–573, 574*f*
  of nose, 395, 396*f*
Fibrous tumor of digits. *See* Myofibromatosis,
    acquired digital.
Fibroxanthoma, atypical, clinical features of,
    618–619

Fibroxanthoma (*continued*)
    course of, 619–620
    differential diagnosis of, 619
    electron microscopy of, 622*t*
    histopathology of, 619, 620*f*
    immunohistochemistry of, 622*t*
  clinical features of, 571
  differential diagnosis of, 608–609
Filaggrin, 6, 108, 122–123, 363
FITC. *See* Fluorescein isothiocyanate.
Fixation, of biopsy specimens, 34*t*, 36–39
    general considerations for, 36, 49
    specimen size and, 37–38, 38*f*, 49
    temperature and, 37
    tissue : fixative solution ratio and, 37–38
    of frozen sections, 35
Fixative(s), 34*t*. *See also specific fixative.*
  antibacterial effects of, 36
  aqueous, 36
  coagulating, 36
  nonaqueous, 36
  noncoagulating, 36
  pH of, 38
Flame figures, 85
Flat wart(s). *See* Verruca plana.
Flegel's disease, differential diagnosis of, 380
Floaters, 40
Floret cells, 589, 591*f*
Florid papillomatosis, of nipple ducts. *See* Nipple
    adenoma.
Fluorescein isothiocyanate, 47
Fluoroderma, 235
Focal acantholytic dyskeratosis, conditions
    associated with, 68
Focal acral hyperkeratosis, 403
  differential diagnosis of, 380
Focal dermal hypoplasia, 385
  clinical features of, 396
  definition of, 395
  differential diagnosis of, 397
  histopathology of, 397, 397*f*
Focal mucinosis, 422*f*, 422–423
Fogo selvagem. *See* Pemphigus foliaceus.
Follicular atrophoderma, 401
Follicular cyst. *See* cyst(s), follicular.
Follicular degeneration syndrome, 315
Follicular hamartomas, 566
Follicular mucinosis, associated with cutaneous
      T-cell lymphoma, 300
  clinical features of, 300
  differential diagnosis of, 300
  histopathology of, 300, 301*f*
  inflammatory reaction patterns in, 54
Follicular myomas, 502*f*, 502–503
Follicular papilla, 7, 10*f*, 13*f*, 14
Follicular poromas, 497
Follicular unit, 303*f*–304*f*, 305
Folliculitis, 291–300. *See also*
      Infundibulofolliculitis; Scalp, dissecting
      cellulitis of.
  acneiform, 296–300
    definition of, 296–297
    pathophysiology of, 296–297
  bacterial (staphylococcal), clinical features of,
      291
    differential diagnosis of, 296, 297*t*
    histopathology of, 291, 293*f*
  classification of, 292*f*
  cutaneous lymphoid hyperplasia caused by,
      717
  eosinophilic, inflammatory reaction patterns
      in, 54

Folliculitis (*continued*)
  eosinophilic pustular, clinical features of, 296
    differential diagnosis of, 296, 297*t*
    histopathology of, 296, 296*f*
  epilating, 318
  fungal, clinical features of, 291–294
    differential diagnosis of, 296, 297*t*
    histopathology of, 293*f*–294*f*, 295
  herpetic, clinical features of, 295
    differential diagnosis of, 296, 297*t*
    histopathology of, 295, 295*f*
  perforating, 291
  pityrosporon, 294, 294*f*
  pustule formation in, 66
Folliculitis decalvans, clinical features of, 318
  histopathology of, 319–320, 320*f*
  microscopic findings in, 320*t*
Folliculosebaceous cystic hamartoma, 484, 547
Folliculo-sebaceous unit(s), 2*f*, 7, 13*f*, 14
  divisions of, 7, 8*f*
  fetal, 29
  terminal, 7, 8*f*
  vellus, 7, 8*f*
Folliculo-sebaceous-apocrine unit(s), 1, 7–14
  components of, 7, 17*f*
  distribution of, 7
Fonsecaea compactum, 229
Fonsecaea pedrosoi, 229
Fontana-Masson technique, 43
Fordyce spots, 15
Foreign body granulomas, clinical features of,
    225
  differential diagnosis of, 225
  histopathology of, 224*f*, 225
Foreign body reactions, 221
Formalin, advantages and disadvantages of, 36,
    49
  chemistry of, 36
  exposure limit for, 36
Formvar, 50
Fox-Fordyce disease, clinical features of, 295
  differential diagnosis of, 296, 297*t*
  histopathology of, 295–296
  inflammatory reaction patterns in, 54
Freckle(s). *See* Ephelis.
Friction blisters, 263, 287
Frozen sections, artifacts in, 34–35, 35*f*
  fixation of, 35
  labeling of, 35–36
  microtomy technique for, 35–36
  preparation of, 34–36
  stained, 35
  unstained, 35
Fungal infection(s), 221
  deep, 228–229
    clinical features of, 228
    differential diagnosis of, 228–229
    histopathology of, 228
  localized, 229–231
  systemic, 231–234
Fungi, histochemical identification of, 46*t*

Ganglion cell choristoma, 583
Ganglioneuroma(s), 583–585
  clinical features of, 583
  histopathology of, 584
  solitary, 583
Gardner syndrome 540–541, 567
  cutaneous mesenchymal neoplasia with, 571,
    589
  dystrophic calcification in, 427

Photodermatitis *(continued)*
definition of, 108
histopathology of, 109
pathophysiology of, 110
Photoirritation dermatitis. *See* Phototoxic
dermatitis.
Phototoxic contact dermatitis, cause of, 94
clinical features of, 94
Phototoxic dermatitis, cause of, 94, 148
clinical features of, 94, 153
clinicopathologic correlation in, 94
differential diagnosis of, 94
histopathology of, 94, 95f, 153–154, 154f
pathophysiology of, 94
postinflammatory pigmentary alteration with,
71
Phytanic acid storage disease. *See* Refsum
syndrome.
Picker's nodule, clinical features of, 179
histopathology of, 181
Piebaldism, 346
differential diagnosis of, 359
Pigmentation, abnormalities of. *See also*
Hyperpigmentation; Hypopigmentation.
differential diagnosis of, 69
postinflammatory, 71–72, 72f, 357–358
disorders of, 345–362
Pigmented purpuric dermatosis, clinical features
of, 72
differential diagnosis of, 72
histopathology of, 72, 73f
Pigmented purpuric eruptions, clinical features
of, 211
differential diagnosis of, 211
histopathology of, 211, 211f–212f
Pigmented purpuric lichenoid dermatosis of
Gougerot and Blum, 72, 125, 127, 211, 211f
Pigments, stains for, 43
Pilar sheath acanthoma. *See* Acanthoma(s), pilar
sheath.
Pilar tumor. *See* Cyst(s), proliferative tricholemmal.
Piloleiomyomas. *See* Follicular myomas.
Pilomatricoma(s), 497–499
associated syndromes with, 497, 566
clinical features of, 497
cystic, 540
diagnosis of, 568
diagnosis of, 569
differential diagnosis of, 499
dystrophic calcification in, 427
histology of, 499, 500f–501f
ossification with, 429
shadow cells of, 499, 500f–501f
treatment of, 497
Pinta, 359
Pityriasis alba, 357
clinical features of, 155
histopathology of, 155–156, 156f
Pityriasis capitis, 159
Pityriasis lichenoides, 100
acute, clinical features of, 98
clinicopathologic correlation in, 100
differential diagnosis of, 98–100, 131
histopathology of, 98f–99f, 98–100
chronic, clinical features of, 98
clinicopathologic correlation in, 100
differential diagnosis of, 100, 227
histopathology of, 98–100
course of, 98
differential diagnosis of, 746
histopathology of, 89
pathophysiology of, 100

Pityriasis lichenoides chronica. *See* Pityriasis
lichenoides, chronic.
Pityriasis lichenoides et varioliformis acuta. *See*
Pityriasis lichenoides, acute.
Pityriasis lichenoides subacuta, 100
Pityriasis rosea, clinical features of, 159
differential diagnosis of, 100
epidermal hyperplasia in, 186–187, 187f
healing stage of, hyperpigmentation due to,
357
herald patch, 100, 159
parakeratosis in, 58
histopathology of, 159–160, 160f
mother patch. *See* Pityriasis rosea, herald
patch.
papules in, Christmas tree distribution of, 159
Pityriasis rubra pilaris, acquired, 177
clinical features of, 177
clinicopathologic correlations in, 178
differential diagnosis of, 167
distribution of lesions in, 177
familial, 177
histopathology of, 178, 179f
juvenile types of, 177
parakeratosis in, 58
pathophysiology of, 178
prognosis for, 177
types of, 177
Pityrosporum orbiculare. See Malassezia furfur.
Pityrosporum ovale. See Malassezia furfur.
Plantar wart(s). *See* Verruca plantaris.
Plasma cell bodies, 732
Plasmacytomas, cutaneous, clinical features of,
731
definition of, 731
differential diagnosis of, 732
histopathology of, 731f, 732
Plasmacytosis, orificial, differential diagnosis of,
732
systemic, differential diagnosis of, 732
Plastic sections, of tissue specimens, 40
Platysma muscle, 28
PLC (pityriasis lichenoides chronica). *See*
Pityriasis lichenoides, chronic.
Plectin, disease associated with, 268t
in basement membrane, 267, 268f
Pleomorphic fibroma, 593
PLEVA (pityriasis lichenoides et varioliformis
acuta). *See* Pityriasis lichenoides, acute.
PLP solution, 36
PNCS. *See* Primary neuroendocrine carcinoma of
skin.
POEMS syndrome, 387, 581
multiple myeloma and, 731
Poikiloderma, 387
chemotherapy-related, 139
clinical features of, 139
clinicopathologic correlations in, 139
definition of, 139
hereditary sclerosing, 59
histopathology of, 139
of Civatte, 403
clinical features of, 139
of dyskeratosis congenita, 371–372, 373f
pathophysiology of, 140
radiotherapy-related, 139
variants of, 139
Poikiloderma congenitale, differential diagnosis
of, 59
of Rothmund and Thomson, clinical features
of, 139
histopathology of, 139, 139f

Poikiloderma vasculare atrophicans. *See* Mycosis
fungoides.
Poikilodermatomyositis, clinical features of, 139
Poikilodermatous conditions, 139–140
Poliosis, 483
Polyarteritis nodosa, 198
musculocutaneous, cutaneous lesion in, 199
differential diagnosis of, 206
histopathology of, 206, 207f
systemic, cutaneous lesion in, 199
Polyclonal infiltrate(s), definition of, 715
Polymorphous light eruption, 269
clinical features of, 76
differential diagnosis of, 76, 78, 94, 122, 135,
167t, 750
histopathology of, 76
inflammatory reaction patterns in, 54
plaque form, clinical features of, 76
histopathology of, 76, 77f
spongiosis in, 167, 167t
Polymorphous sweat gland carcinoma, 534
Polyneuropathy, organomegaly, endocrinopathy,
monoclonal gammopathy, and skin lesions.
See POEMS syndrome.
Porocarcinoma, clinical features of, 534
diagnosis of, 569–570
epidermotropic, diagnosis of, 570
histology of, 534, 538f
Porokeratosis, 364t, 375–378
actinic, differential diagnosis of, 139
disseminated superficial, 143, 376–378
clinical features of, 376
clinicopathologic correlations in, 68, 378
definition of, 375
discrete palmar-plantar, clinical features of,
377
disseminated, clinical features of, 377
disseminated superficial actinic, 143, 376–378
histopathology of, 377f, 377–378
linear, clinical features of, 377
of Mibelli, 143
clinical features of, 376
punctate plantar, clinical features of, 377
types of, 376–377
Poroma, 513, 519f
clear cell, differential diagnosis of, 497
clinical features of, 518
cystic, 540
definition of, 518
dermal, 518, 521f
diagnosis of, 568
diagnosis of, 568–570
eccrine, 518
differential diagnosis of, 451
epidermal, 518
follicular, 497
histology of, 518, 520f–522f
immunohistochemistry of, 518
intraepidermal, 518, 520f–521f
diagnosis of, 568
juxtaepidermal, 518, 520f
Poromatosis, syndrome associated with, 566
Porphyria(s), definition of, 277–280
differential diagnosis of, 80
histopathology of, 281–282
inheritance of, 281t
Porphyria cutanea tarda, 268t, 387
clinical features of, 269, 280
definition of, 280
differential diagnosis of, 282
histopathology of, 65, 281f, 281–282, 282f
in HIV-infected (AIDS) patients, 280
sclerodermoid, 386
subepidermal vesicles in, 64, 65f

ISBN 0-443-08717-2

90038